Register Now for Online Access to Your Book!

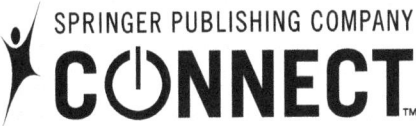

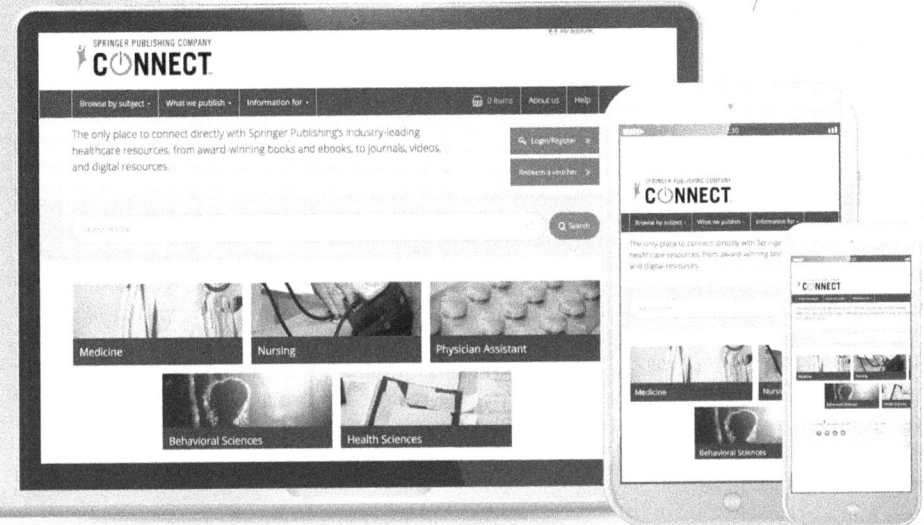

Your print purchase of *Canadian Family Practice Guidelines* **includes online access to the contents of your book**—increasing accessibility, portability, and searchability!

Access today at:

https://connect.springerpub.com/content/reference-book/978-0-8261-9498-5
or scan the QR code at the right with your smartphone
and enter the access code below.

DKXARVYW

Scan here for quick access.

If you are experiencing problems accessing the digital component of this product, please contact our customer service department at cs@springerpub.com

The online access with your print purchase is available at the publisher's discretion and may be removed at any time without notice.

Publisher's Note: New and used products purchased from third-party sellers are not guaranteed for quality, authenticity, or access to any included digital components.

SPRINGER PUBLISHING COMPANY
View all our products at springerpub.com

Jill C. Cash, MSN, APN, FNP-BC, a family nurse practitioner for over 26 years, currently practices at Vanderbilt University Medical Center for the Vanderbilt Medical Group at Westhaven Family Practice in Franklin, Tennessee. She is a faculty member for the School of Nursing at Vanderbilt University. She has been a clinical preceptor for nurse practitioner students for a variety of programs over the past several years. Her previous experience includes high-risk obstetrics as a clinical nurse specialist in maternal–fetal medicine, as well as practicing as a nurse practitioner in women's health, family practice, and rheumatology. In 2017, Ms. Cash was awarded the 2017 American Association of Nurse Practitioners State Award for Excellence in Illinois. Ms. Cash has authored several chapters in a variety of nursing and nurse practitioner textbooks. She is the coeditor of *Family Practice Guidelines* (first, second, third, and fourth editions) and *Adult-Gerontology Practice Guidelines* (first and second editions). Ms. Cash is an active member of the American Association of Nurse Practitioners and Sigma Theta Tau International Honor Society.

Cheryl A. Glass, MSN, APRN, WHNP, RN-BC, a women's health nurse practitioner for over 22 years, currently practices as a clinical research specialist for KEPRO in TennCare's Medical Solutions Unit in Nashville, Tennessee. She is also adjunct faculty at Vanderbilt University School of Nursing. Previously, Ms. Glass was a clinical trainer and trainer manager for Healthways. Her previous nurse practitioner practice was as clinical research coordinator on pharmaceutical clinical trials at Nashville Clinical Research. She also worked in a Collaborative Clinical OB Practice with the director and assistant directors of maternal–fetal medicine at Vanderbilt University Medical Center Department of Obstetrics-Gynecology. Ms. Glass is the coeditor of *Family Practice Guidelines* (first, second, third, and fourth editions) and *Adult-Gerontology Practice Guidelines* (first and second editions). She has published five refereed journal articles. In 1999, Ms. Glass was named Nurse of the Year by the Tennessee chapter of the Association of Women's Health, Obstetric and Neonatal Nurses. Ms. Glass is an active member of the American Association of Nurse Practitioners and Nurse Practitioners in Women's Health.

Debbie Fraser, MN, CNEON(C), RNC-NIC, is director of the Nurse Practitioner Program at Athabasca University. In addition, Ms. Fraser is executive director and chief nurse planner, at the Academy of Neonatal Nursing, and as adjunct faculty, she is responsible for teaching and supervising medical students and residents from Pediatrics, Obstetrics, and Anesthesia, in the Department of Pediatrics at the University of Manitoba. Ms. Fraser serves as editor-in-chief for the *Neonatal Network* journal. She has received many awards, including the Canadian Nurses Association Order of Merit for Nursing Education (2014); the St. Boniface General Hospital Nursing Excellence Award for Education and Research (2010); the University of Manitoba Graduate Nursing Students Association Excellence in Teaching Award; and the *AJN* BOTY award for *Neonatal Infections: A Comprehensive Guide to Assessment, Management and Nursing Care* (2004). She has authored other texts, including *Neonatal Infections: A Clinical Guide,* second edition, (2016). She also is widely published in peer-reviewed journals and is a regular chapter contributor to many undergraduate textbooks, including Lowdermilk and Perry (Eds.), *Maternity & Women's Health Care,* 11th edition; Hockenberry, Wilson, and Winkelstein (Eds.), *Wong's Essentials of Pediatric Nursing*; and Kozier and Erb (Eds.), *Fundamentals of Nursing: The Nature of Nursing Practice in Canada.* She is a professional affiliate of the Manitoba Nursing Research Institute.

Lynn Corcoran, PhD, RN, is assistant professor, faculty of Health Disciplines, at Athabasca University. Dr. Corcoran has more than 25 years of experience in the areas of nursing practice, education, and research. She earned a PhD in the Graduate Division of Education Research, Werklund School of Education at the University of Calgary. Her research and scholarly interests include a variety of topics in the areas of women's health and public health.

Margaret Edwards, PhD, RN, is dean of the Faculty of Health Disciplines at Athabasca University, where she has been instrumental in establishing what are regarded as Canada's leading online nursing programs, playing a key role in developing and delivering exemplary online education offering rich learning experiences to build the capacity of nurses. Extensive long-term committee involvement with CARNA (College and Association of Registered Nurses of Alberta) includes leading the review of Nursing Practice Standards and developing entry-to-practice competencies and serving for 10 years as the CARNA representative for Netcare developing the provincial electronic health record. Her ongoing research and scholarly activity focuses on nursing informatics and strengthening online learning. Dr. Edwards is the author and/or coauthor of four books and their later editions and translations published by Springer Publishing Company, in addition to numerous peer-reviewed publications.

Canadian Family Practice Guidelines

Jill C. Cash, MSN, APN, FNP-BC
Cheryl A. Glass, MSN, APRN, WHNP, RN-BC
Debbie Fraser, MN, CNEON(C), RNC-NIC
Lynn Corcoran, PhD, RN
Margaret Edwards, PhD, RN

Editors

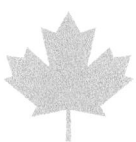

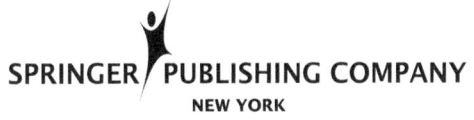

Copyright © 2020 Springer Publishing Company, LLC

All rights reserved.

No part of this publication may be reproduced, stored in a retrieval system, or transmitted in any form or by any means, electronic, mechanical, photocopying, recording, or otherwise, without the prior permission of Springer Publishing Company, LLC, or authorization through payment of the appropriate fees to the Copyright Clearance Center, Inc., 222 Rosewood Drive, Danvers, MA 01923, 978-750-8400, fax 978-646-8600, info@copyright.com or on the Web at www.copyright.com.

Springer Publishing Company, LLC
11 West 42nd Street
New York, NY 10036
www.springerpub.com
http://connect.springerpub.com

Acquisitions Editor: Adrianne Brigido
Compositor: diacriTech

ISBN: 9780826194961
e-book ISBN: 9780826194978
DOI: 10.1891/9780826194978

19 20 21 22 / 5 4 3 2 1

Digital Client Teaching Guides are available at http://connect.springerpub.com/content/reference-book/978-0-8261-9498-5

The author and the publisher of this Work have made every effort to use sources believed to be reliable to provide information that is accurate and compatible with the standards generally accepted at the time of publication. Because medical science is continually advancing, our knowledge base continues to expand. We recommend that the reader always consult current research and specific institutional policies before performing any clinical procedure The author and publisher shall not be liable for any special, consequential, or exemplary damages resulting, in whole or in part, from the readers' use of, or reliance on, the information contained in this book. The publisher has no responsibility for the persistence or accuracy of URLs for external or third-party Internet websites referred to in this publication and does not guarantee that any content on such websites is, or will remain, accurate or appropriate.

Library of Congress Cataloging-in-Publication Data is on file with the Library of Congress.

Library of Congress Control Number: 2019908766

Contact us to receive discount rates on bulk purchases.
We can also customize our books to meet your needs.
For more information please contact: sales@springerpub.com

Publisher's Note: New and used products purchased from third-party sellers are not guaranteed for quality, authenticity, or access to any included digital components.

Printed in the United States of America.

Contents

Contributors xi
Reviewers xiii
Foreword xv
Acknowledgments xvi

PART I. GUIDELINES

1. Health Maintenance Guidelines

Culture, Cultural Safety, and Cultural Diversity 3
Health Maintenance Across the Life Span 4
Interprofessional Collaborative Practice 22

2. Public Health Guidelines

Homelessness 29
Obesity 31
Postbariatric Surgery Long-Term Follow-Up 34
Substance Use Disorders 41
Violence: Children 49
Violence: Intimate Partner (IPV) 52
Violence: Older Adults 56

3. Pain Management Guidelines

Pain 59
Acute Pain 59
Chronic Pain 61
Lower Back Pain 65

4. Dermatology Guidelines

Acne Rosacea 69
Acne Vulgaris 70
Animal Bites, Mammalian 72
Benign Skin Lesions 73
Candidiasis 74
Contact Dermatitis 76
Eczema or Atopic Dermatitis 77
Erythema Multiforme 79
Folliculitis 80
Hand, Foot, and Mouth Syndrome 81
Herpes Simplex Virus Type 1 82
Herpes Zoster or Shingles 83
Impetigo 84
Insect Bites and Stings 85
Lice (Pediculosis) 86
Lichen Planus 88
Pityriasis Rosea 89
Precancerous or Cancerous Skin Lesions 90
Psoriasis 91
Scabies 93
Seborrhoeic Dermatitis 95
Tinea Corporis (Ringworm) 96
Tinea Versicolour 97
Warts 98
Wound Care 99
Wounds of the Skin 103
Xerosis (Winter Itch) 105

5. Eye Guidelines

Amblyopia 107
Blepharitis 108
Cataracts 109
Chalazion 110
Conjunctivitis 110
Corneal Abrasion 112
Dacryocystitis 113
Dry Eyes 114
Excessive Tears 116
Eye Pain 116
Glaucoma, Acute Angle-Closure 118
Hordeolum (Stye) 119
Strabismus 120
Subconjunctival Haemorrhage 121
Uveitis 122

6. Ear Guidelines

Acute Otitis Media 125
Cerumen Impaction (Earwax) 126
Hearing Loss 127
Otitis Externa 129
Otitis Media With Effusion 131
Tinnitus 132

7. Nasal Guidelines

Allergic Rhinitis   135
Epistaxis   137
Nonallergic Rhinitis   138
Acute Sinusitis/Rhinosinusitis   139

8. Throat and Mouth Guidelines

Avulsed Tooth   143
Dental Abscess   144
Epiglottitis   145
Oral Cancer   146
Pharyngitis   147
Stomatitis, Minor Recurrent Aphthous
    Stomatitis   149
Thrush   150

9. Respiratory Guidelines

Asthma   153
Bronchiolitis: Child   158
Bronchitis, Acute   160
Chronic Obstructive Pulmonary
    Disease (COPD)   162
Common Cold/Upper Respiratory Infection   166
Cough   168
Croup, Viral   170
Obstructive Sleep Apnoea (OSA)   172
Pneumonia (Bacterial)   175
Pneumonia (Viral)   177
Respiratory Syncytial Virus (RSV) Bronchiolitis   179
Shortness of Breath (SOB)   181
Tuberculosis (TB)   183

10. Cardiovascular Guidelines

Acute Myocardial Infarction   189
Arrhythmias   191
Atherosclerosis and Hyperlipidaemia   194
Atrial Fibrillation (AF)   197
Chest Pain   200
Chronic Venous Insufficiency (CVI) and Varicose Veins   205
Deep Vein Thrombosis (DVT)   207
Heart Failure (HF)   209
Hypertension (HTN)   213
Lymphoedema   217
Murmurs   218
Palpitations   221
Peripheral Arterial Disease (PAD)   222
Superficial Thrombophlebitis   225
Syncope   227

11. Gastrointestinal Guidelines

Abdominal Pain   231
Appendicitis   235
Celiac Disease   238
Cholecystitis   241
Colic   243
Colorectal Cancer Screening   245
Constipation   246
Crohn's Disease   250
Cyclosporiasis   256
Diarrhoea   258
Diverticulosis and Diverticulitis   260
Elevated Liver Enzymes   262
Gastroenteritis, Bacterial and Viral   264
Gastro-esophageal Reflux Disease   268
Giardiasis   271
Haemorrhoids   273
Hepatitis A   275
Hepatitis B   278
Hepatitis C   282
Hernias, Abdominal   286
Hernias, Pelvic   288
Hirschsprung's Disease or Congenital Aganglionic
    Megacolon   291
Hookworm   292
Irritable Bowel Syndrome (IBS)   294
Jaundice   298
Malabsorption   301
Nausea and Vomiting   303
Peptic Ulcer Disease (PUD)   306
Pinworm   309
Roundworm   311
Ulcerative Colitis   312

12. Genitourinary Guidelines

Benign Prostatic Hypertrophy   317
Chronic Kidney Disease (CKD) in Adults   319
Epididymitis   323
Erectile Dysfunction (ED)   325
Haematuria   329
Hydrocele   331
Interstitial Cystitis (IC)   333
Premature Ejaculation (PE)   335
Prostatitis   336
Proteinuria   339
Pyelonephritis   341
Renal Calculi or Kidney Stones (Nephrolithiasis)   344
Testicular Torsion   347
Undescended Testes or Cryptorchidism   348
Urinary Incontinence (UI)   350
Urinary Tract Infection (Acute Cystitis)   354
Varicocele   358

13. Obstetrics Guidelines

Preconception Counselling: Identifying Clients
    at Risk   361
Routine Prenatal Care   363
Anaemia, Iron Deficiency   365
Gestational Diabetes Mellitus   366
Preeclampsia   369
Preterm Labour   371
Pyelonephritis in Pregnancy   372
Vaginal Bleeding: First Trimester   374
Vaginal Bleeding: Second and Third Trimesters   376
Breast Engorgement   378
Endometritis   379
Secondary Postpartum Haemorrhage   381
Mastitis   382
Postpartum Care: Six Weeks Postpartum
    Examination   383
Postpartum Depression   384
Wound Infection   387

14. Gynecologic Guidelines

Amenorrhoea 389
Atrophic Vaginitis 391
Bacterial Vaginosis (or Gardnerella) 392
Bartholin's Cyst or Abscess 394
Breast Pain (Mastalgia) 395
Cervicitis 397
Contraception 398
Dysmenorrhoea 402
Dyspareunia 404
Emergency Contraception (EC) 406
Endometriosis 408
Female Sexual Dysfunction 409
Infertility 412
Menopause 415
Pap Smear Screening Guidelines and Interpretation 418
Pelvic Inflammatory Disease (PID) 420
Premenstrual Syndrome (PMS) and Premenstrual Dysphoric Disorder (PMDD) 423
Vulvovaginal Candidiasis 425

15. Sexually Transmitted Infections Guidelines

General Approach to Sexually Transmitted Infections 429
Chlamydia 430
Gonorrhoea 431
Herpes Simplex Virus Type 2 433
Human Papillomavirus 434
Syphilis 436
Trichomoniasis 438

16. Infectious Disease Guidelines

Cat Scratch Disease (CSD) 441
Cytomegalovirus (CMV) 443
Encephalitis 446
H1N1 Influenza A 449
Influenza (Flu) 451
Kawasaki Disease (KD) 454
Lyme Disease 457
Meningitis 459
Mononucleosis (Epstein–Barr) 463
Mumps 465
Parvovirus B19 (Fifth Disease, Erythema Infectiosum) 467
Rheumatic Fever 469
Rocky Mountain Spotted Fever (RMSF) 472
Roseola (Exanthem Subitum) 474
Rubella (German Measles) 475
Rubeola (Red Measles) 477
Scarlet Fever (Scarlatina) 480
Toxoplasmosis 482
Varicella (Chickenpox and Shingles) 485
West Nile Virus (WNV) 488
Zika Virus Infection 490

17. Systemic Disorders Guidelines

Chronic Fatigue Syndrome (Systemic Exertion Intolerance Syndrome) 495
Fevers of Unknown Origin 497
Human Immunodeficiency Virus (HIV) 499
Idiopathic (Autoimmune) Thrombocytopaenic Purpura 504
Iron-Deficiency Anaemia (Microcytic, Hypochromic) 506
Lymphadenopathy 509
Pernicious Anaemia (Megaloblastic Anaemia) 512

18. Musculoskeletal Guidelines

Neck and Upper Back Disorders 515
Plantar Fasciitis 517
Sciatica 519
Sprains: Ankle and Knee 520

19. Neurologic Guidelines

Alzheimer's Disease 523
Bell's Palsy 525
Carpal Tunnel Syndrome (CTS) 527
Dementia 528
Guillain–Barré Syndrome (GBS) 531
Headache 534
Migraine Headache 538
Mild Traumatic Brain Injury (Concussion) 542
Multiple Sclerosis (MS) 546
Myasthenia Gravis (MG) 550
Parkinson's Disease (PD) 552
Restless Legs Syndrome (RLS) 554
Seizures 556
Seizure, Febrile (Child) 561
Transient Ischaemic Attack (TIA) 563
Vertigo 565

20. Endocrine Guidelines

Addison's Disease 571
Cushing's Syndrome 573
Diabetes Mellitus 575
Galactorrhoea 584
Gynaecomastia 585
Hirsutism 586
Hypogonadism 588
Metabolic Syndrome/Insulin Resistance Syndrome 589
Polycystic Ovarian Syndrome (PCOS) 592
Thyroid Disease: Hyperthyroidism 595
Thyroid Disease: Hypothyroidism 598
Thyrotoxicosis/Thyroid Storm 602

21. Rheumatological Guidelines

Ankylosing Spondylitis (AS) 605
Fibromyalgia (FM) 607
Gout 609
Osteoarthritis (OA) 610
Osteoporosis/Kyphosis/Fracture 612
Polymyalgia Rheumatica (PMR) 615
Pseudogout 616
Psoriatic Arthritis (PsA) 618
Raynaud's Phenomenon (RP) 619
Rheumatoid Arthritis (RA) 622
Systemic Lupus Erythematosus (SLE) 625
Temporal Arteritis/Giant Cell Arteritis (GCA) 628
Vitamin D Deficiency 630

22. Psychiatric Guidelines

Generalized Anxiety Disorder (GAD)　633
Attention Deficit Disorder (ADD)/Attention Deficit
　　Hyperactivity Disorder (ADHD)　635
Bipolar Disorder　637
Depression　641
Failure to Thrive　645
Grief　647
Sleep Disorders　649
Suicide　652

23. Assessment Guide for Sport Participation

Appendix A. Normal Laboratory Values　661
Appendix B. Diet Recommendations　667
Appendix C. Tanner's Sexual Maturity Stages　677

Index　679

PART II: CLIENT TEACHING GUIDELINES

**Client Teaching Guides are available as downloadable PDF forms at
http://connect.springerpub.com/content/reference-book/978-0-8261-9498-5**

Abdominal Pain: Adults
Abdominal Pain: Children
Acne Rosacea
Acne Vulgaris
Acute Otitis Media
Addison's Disease
ADHD: Coping Strategies for Teens and Adults
ADHD: Tips for Caregivers of a Child with ADHD
Adolescent Nutrition
Allergic Rhinitis
Amenorrhea
Ankle Exercises
Aphthous Stomatitis
Atherosclerosis and Hyperlipidemia
Asthma
Asthma: Action Plan and Peak Flow Monitoring
Asthma: How to Use a Metered-Dose Inhaler
Atrial Fibrillation
Atrophic Vaginitis
Back Stretches
Bacterial Vaginosis
Bell's Palsy
Bipolar Disorder
Bronchiolitis: Child
Bronchitis, Acute
Bronchitis, Chronic
Cerumen Impaction (Earwax)
Cervicitis
Chickenpox (Varicella)
Childhood Nutrition
Chlamydia
Chronic Obstructive Pulmonary Disease
Chronic Venous Insufficiency
Colic: Ways to Soothe a Fussy Baby
Common Cold
Conjunctivitis
Constipation Relief
Contraception: How to Take Birth Control Pills
Cough
Crohn's Disease
Croup, Viral
Cushing's Syndrome
Deep Vein Thrombosis

Dementia
Dermatitis
Diabetes
Diarrhoea
Dysmenorrhoea
Dyspareunia
Eczema
Emergency Contraception: Levonogestrel
Emergency Contraception: Ulipristal Acetate
Emphysema
Epididymitis
Erythema Multiforme
Exercise
Eye Medication Administration
Febrile Seizures: Child
Fibrocystic Breast Changes and Breast Pain
Fibromyalgia
Folliculitis
Gastro-oesophageal Reflux Disease
Gonorrhoea
Gout
Grief
Head Injury: Mild Concussion
Haemorrhoids
Herpes Simplex Virus
Herpes Zoster or Shingles
Human Papillomavirus (HPV)
Infant Nutrition
Influenza
Insect Bites and Stings
Irritable Bowel Syndrome
Jaundice and Hepatitis
Kidney Disease, Chronic
Knee Exercises
Lactose Intolerance and Malabsorption
Lice (Pediculosis)
Lichen Planus
Lyme Disease and Removal of a Tick
Lymphoedema
Menopause
Migraine Headache
Mononucleosis
Myasthenia Gravis

Nicotine Dependence
Nosebleeds
Oral Thrush in Children
Osteoarthritis
Osteoporosis
Otitis Externa
Otitis Media with Effusion
Parkinson's Disease Management
Pelvic Inflammatory Disease
Peripheral Arterial Disease
Pernicious Anaemia
Pharyngitis
Pityriasis Rosea
Pneumonia, Bacterial: Adult
Pneumonia, Bacterial: Child
Pneumonia, Viral: Adult
Pneumonia, Viral: Child
Polymyalgia Rheumatica
Premenstrual Syndrome
Problematic Substance Use
Prostatic Hypertrophy/Benign
Prostatitis
Pseudogout
Psoriasis
Respiratory Syncytial Virus
Rice Therapy and Exercise Therapy
Ringworm (Tinea)
Rocky Mountain Spotted Fever and Removal of a Tick

Roundworms and Pinworms
Scabies
Seborrhoeic Dermatitis
Shortness of Breath
Sinusitis
Skin Care Assessment
Sleep Apnoea
Sleep Disorders/Insomnia
Superficial Thrombophlebitis
Syphilis
Systemic Lupus Erythematosus
Testicular Self-Examination
Tinea Versicolour
Tinnitus
Toxoplasmosis
Transient Ischaemic Attack
Trichomoniasis
Trigeminal Neuralgia
Ulcer Management
Urinary Incontinence: Women
Urinary Tract Infection (Acute Cystitis)
Varicose Veins
Warts
Wound Care: Lower-Extremity Ulcers
Wound Care: Pressure Ulcers
Wound Care: Wounds
Xeriosis (Winter Itch)
Zika Virus Infection

Contributors

Julie Adkins, DNP, APRN, FNP-BC, FAANP
Certified Family Nurse Practitioner
Adkins Family Practice, LLC
West Frankfort, Illinois

Rhonda Arthur, DNP, CNM, WHNP-BC, CNE
Associate Professor
Frontier Nursing University
Hyden, Kentucky

Luisa Barton, NP-PHC, BScN, MN, DNP
Assistant Professor
Faculty of Health Disciplines, Nurse Practitioner Program
Athabasca University
Athabasca, Alberta, Canada

Julia Blake, BScN, MN, DNP, PHC-NP
School of Health Science
Seneca College
Toronto, Ontario, Canada

Krista A. Bradley, BN, MSc, MD, FCFPC
Family Physician
Kamloops, British Columbia, Canada

Amy C. Bruggemann, MSN, APRN-BC, CWS
Director of Clinical Operations
Specialized Wound Management
Chesterfield, Missouri

Kate Burkholder, BN, MN, NP
Family/All Ages Nurse Practitioner
Sessional Instructor, Athabasca University
Athabasca, Alberta, Canada

Beverly R. Byram, MSN, FNP
Clinical Instructor
Vanderbilt University School of Nursing
Director, Ryan White Part D
Comprehensive Care Center
Nashville, Tennessee

Jill C. Cash, MSN, APN, FNP-BC
Vanderbilt Medical Group Westhaven Family Practice
Franklin, Tennessee; and
Vanderbilt University Medical Center
Nashville, Tennessee

Donna Clare, MN, NP
Academic Coordinator, Family/All Ages Nurse
    Practitioner
Athabasca University
Athabasca, Alberta, Canada

Moya Cook, APN, CNP
Morthland College Health Services
West Frankfort, Illinois

William Diehl-Jones, BSc, MSc, PhD, BScN
Associate Professor
Sessional Instructor, Athabasca University
Athabasca, Alberta, Canada

Susan Drummond, RN, MSN, C-EFM
Associate in Obstetrics
Department of Obstetrics and Gynecology
Vanderbilt University Medical Center
Nashville, Tennessee

Elsie Duff, NP, BScN, MEd, PhD
Nurse Practitioner Instructor
Sessional Instructor, Athabasca University
Athabasca, Alberta, Canada

Valda Duke, MN, NP
Nurse Educator
Centre for Nursing Studies
Memorial University
St. John's, Newfoundland, Canada

Wanda Emberley-Burke, RN, MEd, PCNP
Nurse Educator
Centre for Nursing Studies
Memorial University
St. John's, Newfoundland, Canada

Cindy Fehr, BSN, MEd, MScN, RN(NP)
Nurse Practitioner, Southern Health Sante-Sud
CEO, Nurse Practitioner Association of Manitoba
Winnipeg, Manitoba, Canada

Cheryl A. Glass, MSN, WHNP, RN-BC
Clinical Research Specialist
KEPRO Peer Review
Medical Solutions Unit
Nashville, Tennessee

Debbie Gunter, APRN, FNP-BC, ACHPN
Nurse Practitioner
Emory University
Atlanta, Georgia

Mellisa A. Hall, DNP, APN-BC, FNP-BC, ACHPN
University of Southern Indiana
Evansville, Indiana

Kristen Heise, NP-PHC, BScN, BScHK
Primary Health Care Nurse Practitioner
Planned Parenthood
Toronto, Ontario, Canada

Paul Jeffrey, DNP, NP-Adult
Professor, Nursing
Humber College Institute of Technology & Advanced Learning
Toronto, Ontario, Canada

Julie Johnson, MN(NP), RN, CPHIMS-CA
Sessional Instructor
Sessional Instructor, Athabasca University
Athabasca, Alberta, Canada

Daris Klemmer, RN, BN-with distinction, MN-Family All Ages, GNC (c)
Nurse Practitioner Clinical Lead, Alberta Health Services
Sessional Instructor, Athabasca University
Athabasca, Alberta, Canada

Kimberley Lamarche, RN, NP, DNP
Associate Professor/Nurse Practitioner
Athabasca University
Athabasca, Alberta, Canada

Audra C. Malone, DNP, FNP-BC
Assistant Professor
Frontier Nursing University
Hyden, Kentucky

Lynn Miller, DNP, NP, FRE
Nurse Practitioner
Policy, Practice and Legislative Services, College of Registered Nurses of Nova Scotia
Gulf Shore, Nova Scotia, Canada
Sessional Instructor, Athabasca University

Kristie A. D. Morydz, MN, NP
Nurse Practitioner
Cancer Care Manitoba
Sessional Instructor, Athabasca University
Winnipeg, Manitoba, Canada

Robertson Nash, PhD, ACNP, BC
Director, PATHways Clinic
Nurse Practitioner Medicine/Infectious Diseases
Comprehensive Care Clinic
Vanderbilt University Medical Center
Nashville, Tennessee

Laura A. Petty, MSN, GNP-BC
Gerontological Nurse Practitioner
Lebanon, Tennessee

Darlene Pierce, DNP, MN, BN, RN, NP
Program Director Nurse Practitioner Program
University of Manitoba
Winnipeg, Manitoba, Canada
Sessional Instructor, Athabasca University

Roger Pilon, PhD, NP-PHC
Assistant Professor
Laurentian University
Sudbury, Ontario, Canada

Bunny Pounds, DNP, FNP, BC
Frontier Nursing University
Hyden, Kentucky

Kelly Power-Kean, RN, BN, MHS, NP
Professional Associate
Centre for Nursing Studies
Memorial University
St. John's, Newfoundland, Canada

Susan Prendergast, MN, NP, PhD(C)
Dalhousie University
University of Alberta
Edmonton, Alberta, Canada

Margaret Ellen Rauliuk, BScN, MN, RN, NP
Academic Coordinator and Family Nurse Practitioner
Faculty of Health Disciplines
Athabasca University
Athabasca, Alberta, Canada

Monakshi Sawhney, NP (Adult), PhD
Assistant Professor
School of Nursing
Queen's University
Kingston, Ontario, Canada

Angelito Tacderas, APN
Marion, Illinois

Shelley Ann Walkerley, NP-PHC, PhD
Assistant Professor of Nursing
Faculty of Health, School of Nursing
York University
Toronto, Ontario, Canada

Nancy Pesta Walsh, DNP, CNP
Frontier Nursing University
Hyden, Kentucky

Kimberly D. Waltrip, PhD(c), APRN- BC
Instructor of Nursing
Southeast Missouri State University
Cape Girardeau, Missouri

Jocelyn T. Whittier, BSC, BScN, MN, PNP, FNP
Nurse Practitioner (Family Practice and Pediatrics)
Sessional Instructor, Athabasca University
Athabasca, Alberta, Canada

Alyson Wolz, DNP, APN, PMHCNS, BC
Harrisburg Medical Center
Harrisburg, Illinois

Erin Ziegler, PhD, NP-PHC
Nurse Practitioner
Associate Member of the Yeates School of Graduate Studies
Ryerson University
Toronto, Ontario, Canada

Reviewers

Luisa Barton, NP-PHC, BScN, MN, DNP
Assistant Professor
Faculty of Health Disciplines, Nurse Practitioner Program
Athabasca University
Athabasca, Alberta, Canada

Kate Burkholder, BN, MN, NP
Family/All Ages Nurse Practitioner
Sessional Instructor, Athabasca University
Athabasca, Alberta, Canada

Donna Clare, MN, NP
Academic Coordinator, Family/All Ages Nurse Practitioner
Athabasca University
Athabasca, Alberta, Canada

Elsie Duff, NP, BScN, MEd, PhD
Nurse Practitioner Instructor
Sessional Instructor, Athabasca University
Athabasca, Alberta, Canada

Sandi Engi, RN, MN, NP
Nurse Practitioner
Edmonton, Alberta, Canada

Paul Jeffrey, DNP, NP-Adult
Professor, Nursing
Humber College Institute of Technology & Advanced Learning
Toronto, Ontario, Canada

Julie Johnson, MN(NP), RN, CPHIMS-CA
Sessional Instructor
Athabasca University
Athabasca, Alberta, Canada

Lynn Miller, DNP, NP, FRE
Nurse Practitioner
Sessional Instreuctor, Athabasca University
Consultant
Policy, Practice and Legislative Services, College of Registered Nurses of Nova Scotia
Gulf Shore, Nova Scotia, Canada

Kristie A. D. Morydz, MN, NP
Nurse Practitioner
Cancer Care Manitoba
Winnipeg, Manitoba, Canada
Sessional Instructor, Athabasca University

Bonnie Myslik, RN, MN, NP
Nurse Practitioner
Adjunct Professor
University of Waterloo
Windsor, Ontario, Canada

Kristy Naulls, RN, MN, NP
Nurse Practitioner
Belleville Nurse Practitioner-Led Clinic
Belleville, Ontario, Canada

Kelly Power-Kean, RN, BN, MHS, NP
Professional Associate
Centre for Nursing Studies
Memorial University
St. John's, Newfoundland, Canada

Margaret Ellen Rauliuk, BScN, MN, RN, NP
Academic Coordinator and Family Nurse Practitioner
Faculty of Health Disciplines
Athabasca University
Athabasca, Alberta, Canada

Paul Sawchuk, MD, MBA, CCFP, FCFP
President
The College of Family Physicians Canada
Winnipeg, Manitoba, Canada

Vicky Stooke, RN, MN, NP
Nurse Practitioner
Calgary Foothills Primary Care Network
Calgary, Alberta, Canada

Nancy Watts, RN, MN
Clinical Nurse Specialist
Mount Sinai Hospital
Toronto, Ontario, Canada

Jocelyn T. Whittier, BSC, BScN, MN, PNP, FNP
Nurse Practitioner (Family Practice and Pediatrics)
Sessional Instructor, Athabasca University
Athabasca, Alberta, Canada

Erin Ziegler, PhD, NP-PHC
Nurse Practitioner, Associate Member of the Yeates School of Graduate Studies
Ryerson University
Toronto, Ontario, Canada

Foreword

We know from Barbara Starfield's groundbreaking research that primary care is the foundation of a high-functioning health-care system, but there are many challenges involved for those who strive to provide high-quality primary care.

First, the potential scope of primary care is daunting. Generalist primary care providers see patients from all stages of life—children and adults, high-performance athletes, and the frail elderly. A good primary care system serves everybody, whether they are looking for immunizations, fertility control, chronic disease monitoring, or mental health counseling.

Scope of practice is not the only challenge. Patients do not present with clear diagnoses. They usually present with symptoms of undifferentiated clinical problems. They do not come in to the office complaining of asthma. They complain of cough or dyspnoea. To take it from symptoms to diagnosis and management is the value of the skilled primary care provider. As we work to limit our patients' exposure to potentially harmful tests or treatments, and avoid unnecessary referrals to specialists, primary care providers need to lean on their judgment and clinical skills.

The challenge can be further complicated by potential confounding factors. Is the presentation just a variation of normal physiology? Or an early presentation of pathology that has not yet fully manifested? Are there emotional, psychological, or social factors that are influencing the presentation? Some patients may overemphasize their symptoms while others underreport how the condition is impacting their lives.

Between the variations of normal, the transient illnesses, the differences in how and when a problem presents, the impact of psychosocial overlay, issues in primary care frequently move from the complicated, where answers exist but are difficult to determine, to the complex, where there is no clear solution.

How do primary care providers manage all of these challenges?

One of the greatest advantages of the primary care provider is their relationship with their patients. They are familiar with their past history. They know how the most recent presentation compares to previous presentations. They know their patient social context and life situation.

A second advantage of the primary care provider is the judicious use of time. Watchful waiting is often a legitimate clinical tool as illnesses resolve or evolve. Primary care providers are in a position to provide easy access to follow up if issues are not resolving.

Relationship with patients over time is not only a great clinical strength, it is also excellent motivation. Continuity of relationship is valuable to not only patients but also to providers. The experience of serving patients in relatively straightforward ways, such as renewing medications or even filling out forms, can be very rewarding if we focus on the significant benefit to the patients. Other interactions can be much more demanding and intense. Primary care providers sometimes need to share bad news with patients or listen to patients tell them about traumatic events. Even when the primary care provider is not able to resolve the issues, it is at these times when primary care providers may have their greatest value. To connect with patients during difficult times, to be a witness to their experience, to let them know that whatever happens, they will have at least one ally, you, their primary care provider. More powerful than we know.

This fourth edition of *Family Practice Guidelines* by Cash and Glass has been updated and adapted to the Canadian context to help you navigate the challenges of providing high-quality primary care. It includes new evidence-based guidelines on a variety of topics including rheumatology, population health, sports medicine, and psychiatric disorders. It contains the definitions, incidence, pathogenesis, signs, symptoms, diagnostic tests, and care plans for more than 200 diagnoses. It also offers numerous printable Client Teaching Guides. It will serve as a valuable companion on your journey to becoming an excellent clinician.

Paul Sawchuk, MD, MBA, CCFP, FCFP

Reference

Starfield, B. (2005, September). Contribution of primary care to health systems and health. *Milbank Quarterly, 83*(3), 457–502.

Acknowledgment

Our thanks to Nicole Askin, MLIS, for assistance with research and copy editing.

Guidelines

1. Health Maintenance Guidelines
2. Public Health Guidelines
3. Pain Management Guidelines
4. Dermatology Guidelines
5. Eye Guidelines
6. Ear Guidelines
7. Nasal Guidelines
8. Throat and Mouth Guidelines
9. Respiratory Guidelines
10. Cardiovascular Guidelines
11. Gastrointestinal Guidelines
12. Genitourinary Guidelines
13. Obstetrics Guidelines
14. Gynecologic Guidelines
15. Sexually Transmitted Infections Guidelines
16. Infectious Disease Guidelines
17. Systemic Disorders Guidelines
18. Musculoskeletal Guidelines
19. Neurologic Guidelines
20. Endocrine Guidelines
21. Rheumatological Guidelines
22. Psychiatric Guidelines
23. Assessment Guide for Sport Participation

1 Health Maintenance Guidelines

Culture, Cultural Safety, and Cultural Diversity

Margaret Ellen Rauliuk

Culture, cultural safety, and diversity are important considerations when providing health care to Canadians across the lifespan. In a country whose population comprises Indigenous populations as well as generations of immigrants and refugees from across the globe, an understanding of cultural diversity is essential.

Culture is complex. Culture is influenced by values, beliefs, habits, common practices, community, and societal norms, as well as family loyalties and responsibilities. Culture influences how we think and how we make decisions as individuals, communities, and populations. What each of us experiences as culture is, in part, acquired over time from close personal relations with family, friends, and members of society.

Canada is culturally diverse. Cultural diversity exists when people of many cultures coexist within an environmental area (e.g., family, neighbourhood, township, city, or country). Health-care providers who are able to respect varying cultural ways of knowing and empower the person receiving care bring a cultural safety lens to their practice. This involves the ability to meet people where they are and recognize that power imbalances exist between most health-care providers and the people seeking or receiving care. It is important to remember that significant differences may exist in the way health care is perceived and practiced because of differing values and beliefs about health and illness inherent among people of varying cultural backgrounds.

Factors Contributing to Cultural Diversity
- Urbanization of Canada's Indigenous people (e.g., First Nations, Métis, and Inuit).
- Multiethnic economic immigration and increasing refugee populations.
- Cultural variations in gender roles and gender identities.
- Changes in family structures recognizing single parents, different/same sex marriage, and multigenerational parenting.
- Diverse religious and spiritual beliefs.
- Differing values for the individual compared to the collective.
- Increasing representation of health-care providers from a variety of cultural backgrounds.
- Legislation and regulations.

Cultural competence is the responsibility of all health-care providers. Each visit with a client is an opportunity to gain more knowledge about a client's health beliefs and practices. Inadequate awareness of the client's health beliefs and practices influenced by culture may lead to mistrust. This may result in barriers including inappropriate delivery of care, increased cost, noncompliance, seeking care elsewhere, or not seeking care at all. For vulnerable populations, lack of access to a culturally competent health-care provider can contribute to social exclusion that can in turn contribute to unfavourable health outcomes.

Thoughtful Consideration
Providing care without being sensitive to the cultural needs of a client may suggest that the health-care provider's values and beliefs are superior to those of the client and may lead to disparity of care. The limited involvement of the client in their care may result in noncompliance, placing the client at greater risk of health-related complications. The delay in provision of health care can result in life-threatening complications.

Numerous cultural resources are available throughout the literature and online. Many Canadian universities now require an undergraduate level course in Indigenous studies as part of a commitment to the calls to action arising from Canada's Truth and Reconciliation Commission. Preference as to which educational/assessment tools are most appropriate for use with clients and families can be decided by the health-care provider.

The following are suggestions for promoting cultural sensitivity in the clinical setting:

A. Provide a cultural diversity self-assessment/practice opportunity:
  1. Consult online self-assessment tools such as the *Cultural Competence Self-Assessment Checklist for Primary Care Practitioners*, which can be found on the National Center for Cultural Competence website, at nccc.georgetown.edu/assessments/.
  2. If applicable, review this excerpt from Peggy McIntosh's classic paper, *White Privilege: Unpacking the Invisible Knapsack,* at www.racialequitytools.org/resourcefiles/mcintosh.pdf.
  3. Learn about the Truth and Reconciliation Commission of Canada: nctr.ca/reports.php.
B. Identify the needs of the population:
  1. Seek out information to help you understand the community and the health status of its members. Most regional health authorities in Canada conduct a community needs assessment every five years. Documents detailing the findings of these needs assessments may be accessed on the health region website in the jurisdiction of the health-care provider. The community health assessment will often report at the neighbourhood cluster level and may include information such as general

health, death rates, chronic disease, mental health and substance use, injury, sexually transmitted infections, health behaviours, and health determinants.
2. Evaluate resources, attitudes, and barriers inside the community and practice location:
   a. Access to resources.
   b. Range of assistance options:
      i. Transportation.
      ii. Communication: Consider accessing the services of an interpreter:
         1) Identify bilingual and multilingual staff.
         2) Consider use of family members or personal acquaintances as interpreters (adults only) when formal interpreter services are not available.
         3) Provide multilingual written materials.
      iii. Education (meaningful/multilingual). Consider general and health literacy level when providing education or educational materials.
C. Employers will often provide some cultural safety training for new employees. Those in leadership roles should ensure staff receive education regarding cultural safety and diversity:
   1. Assessments should consider the client's health values and beliefs:
      a. Consider cultural variations in family member roles, gender roles, and interpersonal dynamics.
      b. Consider delaying questions or discussion about potentially sensitive topics (e.g., relationships and sexuality) until you are more familiar with the individual or family and their culture, and a relationship of trust is established. Avoid cultural generalizations; do not make assumptions.
      c. Consider the LEARN model for cross-cultural discussions as described by the Canadian Paediatric Society:
         i. **Listen**: Bring your curiosity to the encounter, draw out the individual's understanding of the health issue that has brought him or her to clinic.
         ii. **Explain**: Share your understanding of what is going on from a medical perspective recognizing that cultural beliefs can influence how illness may be perceived.
         iii. **Acknowledge**: There may be disparities between your understanding and how the issue might be perceived by the individual or family. Respectful discussion can help to identify differing beliefs and their potential impact on the therapeutic plan.
         iv. **Recommend**: A planned course of care to the individual or family.
         v. **Negotiate**: With the individual or family to reach agreement on a plan of care that recognizes cultural beliefs or practices relating to health and healing.
   2. Communication should be meaningful. The following suggestions apply to all clinical encounters:
      a. A client-centred approach allows flexibility in communication.
      b. Maintain eye contact when culturally appropriate during conversations.
      c. Use plain language.
      d. Observe facial expressions and body language.
      e. Use short sentences to explain lengthy information.
      f. Avoid medical jargon.
      g. Use repetition for emphasis.
      h. Ask questions to confirm understanding or have the individual explain the key messages.
D. Schedule longer appointments if needed.
E. Health-care providers should clarify the limitations of a health-care provider's role.
F. Clearly identify alternatives offered by health-care provider.

Bibliography

Andrews, M. M., & Boyle, J. S. (2015). *Transcultural concepts in nursing care* (7th ed.). Philadelphia, PA: Lippincott Williams & Wilkins.

Douglas, M. K., Rosenkoetter, M., Pacquiao, D. F., Callister, L. C., Hattar-Pollara, M., Lauderdale, J., . . . Purnell, L. (2014). Guidelines for implementing culturally competent nursing care. *Journal of Transcultural Nursing: Official Journal of the Transcultural Nursing Society/Transcultural Nursing Society, 25*(2), 109–121. doi:10.1177/1043659614520998

Guerra, O., & Kurtz, D. (2017). Building collaboration: A scoping review of cultural competency and safety education and training for healthcare students and professionals in Canada. *Teaching & Learning in Medicine, 29*(2), 129–142. doi:10.1080/10401334.2016.1234960

Huber, D. L. (2013). *Leadership and nursing care management* (5th ed.). St. Louis, MO: Saunders.

Ladha, T., Zubairi, M., Hunter, A., Audcent, T., Johnstone, J., & Global Child and Youth Health Section Executive. (2018, February 16). *Cross-cultural communication: Tools for working with families and children* [Practice Point]. Retrieved from https://www.cps.ca/en/documents/position/cross-cultural-communication

McIntosh, P. (1988). *White privilege: Unpacking the invisible knapsack*. Retrieved from www.racialequitytools.org/resourcefiles/mcintosh.pdf

Mikkonen, J., & Raphael, D. (2010). *Social determinants of health: The Canadian facts*. Toronto, ON, Canada: York University School of Health Policy and Management. Retrieved from http://thecanadianfacts.org/the_canadian_facts.pdf

Muronda, V. (2016). The culturally diverse nursing student: A review of the literature. *Journal of Transcultural Nursing, 4*, 400–412. doi:10.1177/1043659615595867

National Centre for Truth & Reconciliation. (n.d.). *University of manitoba. Truth & reconciliation commission. Reports*. Retrieved from http://nctr.ca/reports.php

Purnell, L. D., & Paulanka, B. J. (2013). *Transcultural health care: A culturally competent approach* (4th ed.). Philadelphia, PA: F.A. Davis.

Spector, R. E. (2012). *Cultural diversity in health and illness* (8th ed.). Upper Saddle River, NJ: Prentice-Hall.

Vollman, A., Anderson, E., & McFarlane, J. (Eds.). (2012). *Canadian community as partner: Theory and multidisciplinary practice* (3rd ed.). Philadelphia, PA: Lippincott, Williams, & Wilkins.

Health Maintenance Across the Lifespan

Margaret Ellen Rauliuk

Health maintenance involves identifying individuals who are at risk of health problems and encouraging behaviours that reduce these risks. An important aspect of health maintenance is education, including teaching individuals about their risk factors for disease and ways to modify their behaviours to reduce their risks of comorbidities. In approaching this work, it is essential for the practitioner to consider the impact of health determinants. The experience of health is complex as many factors influence health including income and social status, social support networks, education, employment and working conditions, physical environment, personal health practices and coping skills, healthy child development, and access to primary health-care services. These factors must be considered when working with individuals, families, and communities (Hamilton & Bhatti, 1996).

Paediatric Well-Child Examination

The Rourke Baby Record (Exhibit 1.1) is designed for use with newborns and young children up to 5 years old. When complications arise, a detailed Subjective, Objective, Assessment, and Plan (SOAP) note is required for documentation in the medical chart. Growth charts for children are available on the *Rourke Baby Record* website: www.rourkebabyrecord.ca/growth_charts.

Anticipatory Guidance by Age

The anticipatory guidance tool (Exhibit 1.2) provides a quick reference for the practitioner from the child's initial visit at one month throughout the well-child visits until age 15 years. It lists topics that the practitioner should discuss with the caregiver. This information should be supplemented with booklets, teaching guides, and brochures for the caregiver.

Nutrition

Proper nutrition is an essential part of maintaining health and preventing diseases. Essential to this is experiencing food security, a social determinant of health that relates to being able to afford and have access to healthy foods. The Dieticians of Canada reported that one out of every eight households in Canada experience food insecurity; there is a direct link between food insecurity and poverty. Currently, there is work underway to support the development of a national food policy for Canada.

Well-balanced diets should be promoted for all clients, with an emphasis on the prevention of obesity. Diet modification may be an important part of disease or disorder management. The Government of Canada provides a variety of interactive educational tools on nutrition the Canada's Food Guide website: www.canada.ca/en/health-canada/services/canada-food-guides.html. It is recommended that clients use these tools for family education on healthy diet and lifestyle. Diet information is found in Tables 1.1 to 1.3.

Teaching parents the correct serving sizes for children will help guide their children's eating habits for life. Serving sizes for children, teens, and adults are delineated in Canada's Food Guide. Use the food guide to teach and reinforce proper nutrition. Some helpful websites about nutrition are as follows:

A. Canada's Food Guide: www.canada.ca/en/health-canada/services/canada-food-guides.html Food Guide Basics, How much food you need every day: www.canada.ca/en/health-canada/services/food-nutrition/canada-food-guide/food-guide-basics/much-food-you-need-every-day.html.
B. On the Canada's Food Guide, main page is a link to the Eat Well Plate, which will allow people to build a healthy meal using the food guide.

Encouraging healthy eating and physical activity is part of a well-child visit and adult or older adult periodic health examination. Each office visit is an opportunity to evaluate the client's weight and to encourage healthy lifestyles. As the pain assessment becomes the "fifth vital sign" in the hospital setting, the body mass index (BMI) becomes the fifth vital sign in the outpatient setting. Height and weight are used to calculate BMI. The mathematical calculation is $BMI = kg/m^2$; many easy-to-use BMI calculators can be found online.

C. The Dietitians of Canada website includes a BMI tool:
Children and teens: www.dietitians.ca/Your-Health/Assess-Yourself/Assess-Your-BMI/BMI-Children.aspx.
Adults: www.dietitians.ca/Learn/BMI-Adult.aspx.

D. Malnutrition and vitamin and mineral deficiency are commonly seen in older adults. Vitamins B6, B12, D, E, folic acid, zinc, calcium, and iron are often deficient in the elderly diet, along with protein and calorie deficiencies.

Identification of factor(s) contributing to an elderly client's malnutrition assists you, the client, and the client's family in resolving them. For links to ministers responsible for all issues related to seniors in your province/territory refer to the Federal/Provincial/Territorial Ministers Responsible for Seniors Forum: www.canada.ca/en/employment-social-development/corporate/seniors/forum.html.

Exercise

Physical exercise is a vital component of health maintenance. Exercise provides cardiovascular fitness and weight control, prevents osteoporosis through weight-bearing exercise, decreases lipids and can help lower high blood pressure. Exercise is important for flexibility, strength, and coordination. Exercise can also be used for both weight control and reduction. Approximately 3,500 calories must be burned to lose 0.45 kg of fat. Therefore, along with exercise, caloric intake must remain the same or decrease to result in weight loss.

Planning an Exercise Program

Most Canadians start exercise plans without consulting health-care professional. The 2018PAR-Q+ questionnaire (Exhibit 1.3) will indicate if assessment by a health professional is indicated prior to embarking on an exercise program. Providers may need to evaluate the client using screening tests before prescribing an exercise program. Consider the client's age and all comorbidities for any investigations. Examples of investigations might include the following:

A. Bloodwork: Complete blood count (CBC) or Haemoglobin A1C.
B. Exercise stress test.
C. EKG.
D. X-ray.
E. Urinalysis.

Persons with a heart murmur or other abnormal physical findings should defer exercise until the full nature of the disorder is evaluated. The best measure of an exercise work capacity is the determination of oxygen consumption at maximal activity, which is measured with an exercise stress test. Hypertension, elevated resting blood pressures, and chronic obstructive pulmonary disease are other factors that require attention before participation in exercise. Persons with hypertensionshould undergo a thorough evaluation, have antihypertensive agent(s) prescribed, and be monitored periodically during their prescribed graded exercise program. Refer to the PARmed-X for the list of absolute and relative contradictions as well as when special exercise prescriptions might be required.

Measurement of the heart rate during exercise is an easy and inexpensive method to evaluate cardiovascular fitness. Target heart rates vary by physical condition and a person's age. The following formula is used to evaluate target heart/aerobic activity level:

$[220 - (\text{Age of individual})] \times 0.65 = $ Maximum heart rate range.

Maximum heart rate $\times\ 0.65 = $ Minimum aerobic effect.
Maximum heart rate $\times\ 0.85 = $ Maximum aerobic effect.

EXHIBIT 1.1 Rourke Baby Record

©2017 Drs. L Rourke, D Leduc and J Rourke
Revised January 24, 2017
www.rourkebabyrecord.ca

  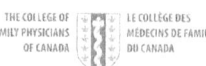 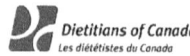

See RBR parent web portal for corresponding parent resources

Rourke Baby Record: Evidence-Based Infant/Child Health Maintenance

GUIDE I: 0–1 mo (National)

NAME: _____ Birth Day (d/m/yy): _____ M [ ] F [ ]
Gestational Age: _____ Birth Length: _____ cm Birth Weight: _____ g
Head Circumference: _____ cm Discharge Weight: _____ g

Pregnancy/Birth remarks/Apgar	Risk factors/Family history

DATE OF VISIT ___/___/20___	DATE OF VISIT ___/___/20___	DATE OF VISIT ___/___/20___
within 1 week	2 weeks (optional)	1 month

GROWTH[1] use WHO growth charts. Correct age until 24–36 months if < 37 weeks gestation

Length	Weight	HC (avg 35 cm)	Length	Weight (regains BW 1–3 weeks)	Head Circ.	Length	Weight	Head Circ.

PARENT/CAREGIVER CONCERNS

NUTRITION[1] For each ○ item discussed, indicate "✓" for no concerns, or "X" if concerns

○ Breastfeeding (exclusive)[1]
  ○ Vitamin D 400 IU/day[1]
○ Formula Feeding (iron-fortified)/preparation[1]
  [150 mL(5 oz) /kg/day[1]]
○ Stool pattern and urine output
	○ Breastfeeding (exclusive)[1]
	  ○ Vitamin D 400 IU/day[1]
	○ Formula Feeding (iron-fortified)/preparation[1]
	  [150 mL(5 oz) /kg/day[1]]
	○ Stool pattern and urine output
		○ Breastfeeding (exclusive)[1]
		  ○ Vitamin D 400 IU/day[1]
		○ Formula Feeding (iron-fortified)/preparation[1]
		  [450–750 mL(15–25 oz) /day[1]]
		○ Stool pattern and urine output

EDUCATION AND ADVICE Repeat discussion of items is based on perceived risk or need

Injury Prevention[1] ○ **Motorized vehicles/Car seat**[1] ○ Carbon monoxide/*Smoke detectors*[1] ○ **Firearm safety**[1] ○ *Hot water <49°C/Bath safety*[1] ○ **Choking/Safe toys**[1] ○ Pacifier use[1] ○ **Safe sleep** (*position, room sharing, avoid bed sharing, crib safety*)[1] ○ *Falls (stairs, change table)*[1]	Behaviour and Family Issues[2] ○ Crying[2] ○ Healthy sleep habits[2] ○ Night waking[2] ○ Soothability/Responsiveness ○ Parenting/Bonding[2] ○ Family conflict/Stress ○ Siblings ○ Parental fatigue/Postpartum depression[2] ○ High risk infants/Assess home visit need[2] ○ Inquire re difficulty making ends meet or feeding your family[2]	Environmental Health[1] ○ **Second hand smoke**[1] ○ Sun exposure[1] Other Issues[1] ○ **No OTC cough/Cold medicine**[1] ○ Inquiry on complementary/Alternative medicine[1] ○ Temperature control and overdressing ○ Fever advice/Thermometers[1] ○ **Supervised tummy time while awake**[1]

DEVELOPMENT[2] (Inquiry and observation of milestones)
Tasks are set after the time of normal milestone acquisition. Absence of any item suggests consideration for further assessment of development. NB–Correct age if < 37 weeks gestation

○ Sucks well on nipple	○ Sucks well on nipple ○ No parent/caregiver concerns	○ Focuses gaze ○ Startles to loud noise ○ Calms when comforted ○ Sucks well on nipple ○ No parent/caregiver concerns

PHYSICAL EXAMINATION[2] An appropriate age-specific physical examination is recommended at each visit. Evidence-based screening for specific conditions is highlighted.

○ Fontanelles[2] ○ Skin (jaundice[2], bruising[2]) ○ **Eyes (red reflex)**[2] ○ Ears (TMs) Hearing inquiry/screening[2] ○ Tongue mobility[2] ○ Neck/Torticollis[2] ○ Heart/Lungs ○ Abdomen/Femoral pulses ○ Umbilicus ○ **Hips (Barlow/Ortolani)**[2] ○ Testicles/Genitalia ○ Male urinary stream/Foreskin care ○ Patency of anus ○ Muscle tone[2]	○ Fontanelles[2] ○ Skin (jaundice[2], bruising[2]) ○ **Eyes (red reflex)**[2] ○ Ears (TMs) Hearing inquiry/screening[2] ○ Tongue mobility[2] ○ Neck/Torticollis[2] ○ Heart/Lungs ○ Abdomen/Femoral pulses ○ Umbilicus ○ **Hips (Barlow/Ortolani)**[2] ○ Testicles/Genitalia ○ Male urinary stream/Foreskin care ○ Muscle tone[2]	○ Skin (jaundice[2], bruising[2]) ○ Fontanelles[2] ○ **Eyes (red reflex)**[2] ○ **Corneal light reflex**[2] ○ Hearing inquiry/Screening[2] ○ Tongue mobility[2] ○ Heart/Abdomen ○ Neck/Torticollis[2] ○ **Hips (Barlow/Ortolani)**[2] ○ Muscle tone[2]

PROBLEMS AND PLANS/CURRENT & NEW REFERRALS[4] E.g. medical specialist, dietitian, speech, audiology, PT, OT, eyes, dental, social-determinants resources

INVESTIGATIONS/SCREENING[2] AND IMMUNIZATION[3] Discuss immunization pain reduction strategies[3] Record Vaccines on Guide V

○ **Newborn screening as per province** ○ Hemoglobinopathy screen (if at risk)[2] ○ **Universal newborn hearing screening (UNHS)**[2] ○ If HBsAg-positive parent/sibling Hep B vaccine #1[3]		○ If HBsAg-positive parent/sibling Hep B vaccine #2[3]

SIGNATURE

Strength of recommendation is based on literature review using the classification: **Good (bold type)**; *Fair (italic type)*; Inconclusive evidence/Consensus (plain type). See literature review table at www.rourkebabyrecord.ca
[1]Resources 1: Growth, Nutrition, Injury Prevention, Environment, Other [2]Resources 2: Family, Behaviour, Development, P/E, Investigations [3]Resources 3: Immunization [4]Resources 4: ECD Resources System and Table

Disclaimer: Given the constantly evolving nature of evidence and changing recommendations, the Rourke Baby Record is meant to be used as a guide only.
Financial support has been provided by the Government of Ontario. For fair use authorization, see www.rourkebabyrecord.ca

EXHIBIT 1.1 Rourke Baby Record (*continued*)

©2017 Drs. L Rourke, D Leduc and J Rourke
Revised January 24, 2017
www.rourkebabyrecord.ca

 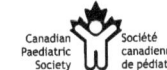 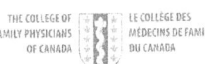 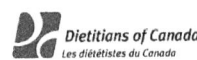

See RBR parent web portal for corresponding parent resources

Rourke Baby Record: Evidence-Based Infant/Child Health Maintenance   **GUIDE II: 2–6 mos** (National)

NAME: _____   Birth Day (d/m/yy): _____ M [ ] F [ ]

Gestational Age: _____ Birth Length: _____ cm Birth Wt: _____ g Birth Head Circ: _____ cm

Past problems/Risk factors:	Family history:

DATE OF VISIT ___/___/20___	DATE OF VISIT ___/___/20___	DATE OF VISIT ___/___/20___
2 months	4 months	6 months

GROWTH[1] use WHO growth charts. Correct age until 24–36 months if < 37 weeks gestation

Length	Weight	Head circ.	Length	Weight	Head Circ.	Length	Weight (x2 BW)	Head Circ.

PARENT/CAREGIVER CONCERNS

NUTRITION[1]
For each ○ item discussed, indicate "✓" for no concerns, or "X" if concerns

2 months	4 months	6 months

○ Breastfeeding (exclusive)[1]
  ○ Vitamin D 400 IU/day[1]
○ Formula Feeding (iron-fortified)/preparation[1] [600–900 mL(20–30 oz) /day[1]]
	○ Breastfeeding (exclusive)[1]
	  ○ Vitamin D 400 IU/day[1]
	○ Formula Feeding (iron-fortified)/preparation[1] [750–1080 mL(25–36 oz) /day[1]]
	○ Discuss future introduction of solids[1]
		○ Breastfeeding[1] – introduction of solids[1]
		  ○ Vitamin D 400 IU/day[1]
		○ Formula Feeding – iron-fortified/preparation[1] [750–1080 mL(25–36 oz) /day[1]]
		○ Iron containing foods[1] (iron fortified infant cereals, meat, tofu, legumes, poultry, fish, whole eggs)
		○ Fruits, vegetables and milk products (yogurt, cheese) to follow
		○ No honey[1] ○ Choking/Safe food[1]
		○ Avoid juices/sweetened liquids[1] ○ No bottles in bed

EDUCATION AND ADVICE Repeat discussion of items is based on perceived risk or need

Injury Prevention[1] ○ Poisons[1]; PCC#[1] ○ Firearm safety[1] ○ Hot water <49°C/Bath safety[1] ○ Choking/Safe toys[1] ○ Pacifier use[1] ○ Electric plugs/Cords ○ Motorized vehicles/Car seat[1] ○ Carbon monoxide/Smoke detctors[1] ○ Safe sleep (position, room sharing, avoid bed sharing, crib safety)[1] ○ Falls (stairs, change table, unstable furniture/TV, no walkers)[1]	**Behaviour and Family Issues[2]** ○ Crying[2] ○ Healthy sleep habits[2] ○ Night waking[2] ○ Soothability/Responsiveness ○ Parenting/Bonding[2] ○ Family conflict/Stress ○ Siblings ○ Child care[2]/Return to work ○ Encourage reading[2] ○ Parental fatigue/Postpartum depression[2] ○ High risk infants/Assess home visit need[2] ○ Inquire re difficulty making ends meet or feeding your family[2] ○ Family healthy active living/Sedentary behaviour/Screen time[2]	**Environmental Health[1]** ○ Second hand smoke[1] ○ Pesticide exposure[1] ○ Sun exposure/sunscreens/insect repellent[1] **Other Issues[1]** ○ OTC/Complementary/Alternative medicine[1] ○ No OTC cough/Cold medicine[1] ○ Temperature control and overdressing ○ Fever advice/Thermometers[1] ○ Teething/Dental cleaning/Fluoride[1] ○ Supervised tummy time while awake[1]

DEVELOPMENT[2] (Inquiry and observation of milestones)
Tasks are set *after* the time of normal milestone acquisition. Absence of any item suggests consideration for further assessment of development. NB–Correct for age if < 37 weeks gestation

○ Follows movement with eyes ○ Coos – throaty, gurgling sounds ○ Lifts head up while lying on tummy ○ Can be comforted & calmed by touching/rocking ○ Sequences 2 or more sucks before swallowing/breathing ○ Smiles responsively ○ No parent/caregiver concerns	○ Follows a moving toy or person with eyes ○ Responds to people with excitement (leg movement/panting/vocalizing) ○ Holds head steady when supported at the chest or waist in a sitting position ○ Holds an object briefly when placed in hand ○ Laughs/smiles responsively ○ No parent/caregiver concerns	○ Turns head toward sounds ○ Makes sounds while you talk to him/her ○ Vocalizes pleasure and displeasure ○ Rolls from back to side ○ Sits with support (e.g., pillows) ○ Reaches/grasps objects ○ No parent/caregiver concerns

PHYSICAL EXAMINATION[2]
An appropriate age-specific physical examination is recommended at each visit. Evidence-based screening for specific conditions is highlighted.

○ Fontanelles[2] ○ Eyes (red reflex)[2] ○ Corneal light reflex[2] ○ Hearing inquiry/screening[2] ○ Heart/Abdomen ○ Neck/Torticollis[2] ○ Muscle tone[2] ○ Hips (Barlow/Ortolani)[2] ○ Skin (jaundice[2], bruising[2])	○ Anterior fontanelle[2] ○ Eyes (red reflex)[2] ○ Corneal light reflex[2] ○ Hearing inquiry/screening[2] ○ Neck/Torticollis[2] ○ Hips (limited hip abd'n)[2] ○ Muscle tone[2] ○ Bruising[2]	○ Anterior fontanelle[2] ○ Eyes (red reflex)[2] ○ Hearing inquiry/screening[2] ○ Bruising[2] ○ Corneal light reflex/Cover-uncover test & inquiry[2] ○ Hips (limited hip abd'n)[2] ○ Muscle tone[2] ○ Teeth[2]

PROBLEMS AND PLANS/CURRENT & NEW REFERRALS[4]
E.g. medical specialist, dietitian, speech, audiology, PT, OT, eyes, dental, social-determinants resources

INVESTIGATIONS/SCREENING[2] AND IMMUNIZATION[3]
Discuss immunization pain reduction strategies[3]   Record Vaccines on Guide V

		○ Hemoglobin (If at risk)[2] ○ Inquire about risk factors for TB[2] ○ If HBsAg-positive parent/sibling Hep B vaccine #3[3]

SIGNATURE

Strength of recommendation is based on literature review using the classification: **Good (bold type)**; *Fair (italic type)*; Inconclusive evidence/Consensus (plain type). See literature review table at www.rourkebabyrecord.ca
[1]Resources 1: Growth, Nutrition, Injury Prevention, Environment, Other   [2]Resources 2: Family, Behaviour, Development, P/E, Investigations   [3]Resources 3: Immunization   [4]Resources 4: ECD Resources System and Table

Disclaimer: Given the constantly evolving nature of evidence and changing recommendations, the Rourke Baby Record is meant to be used as a guide only.
Financial support has been provided by the Government of Ontario.   For fair use authorization, see www.rourkebabyrecord.ca

EXHIBIT 1.1 Rourke Baby Record (continued)

©2017 Drs. L Rourke, D Leduc and J Rourke
Revised January 24, 2017
www.rourkebabyrecord.ca

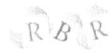 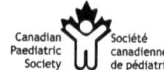 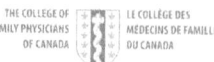 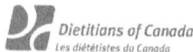

See RBR parent web portal for corresponding parent resources

Rourke Baby Record: Evidence-Based Infant/Child Health Maintenance   **GUIDE III: 9–15 mos** (National)

NAME: _____ Birth Day (d/m/yy): _____ M [ ] F [ ]

Gestational Age: _____ Birth Length: _____ cm   Birth Wt: _____ g   Birth Head Circ: _____ cm

Past problems/Risk factors:	Family history:

DATE OF VISIT ___/___/20___	DATE OF VISIT ___/___/20___	DATE OF VISIT ___/___/20___
9 months (optional)	12–13 months	15 months (optional)

GROWTH[1] use WHO growth charts. Correct age until 24–36 months if < 37 weeks gestation

Length	Weight	Head Circ.	Length	Weight (x3 BW)	HC (avg 47 cm)	Length	Weight	Head Circ.

PARENT/CAREGIVER CONCERNS

NUTRITION[1]
For each ○ item discussed, indicate "✓" for no concerns, or "X" if concerns

9 months:
- ○ Breastfeeding[1]/Vitamin D 400 IU/day[1]
- ○ Formula Feeding – iron-fortified/preparation[1] [720–960 mLs (24–32 oz)/day[1]]
- ○ Iron containing foods[1], fruits, vegetables
- ○ Cow's milk products (e.g., yogurt, cheese, homogenized milk)
- ○ Encourage change from bottle to cup
- ○ Eats a variety of textures
- ○ Avoid juices/sweetened liquids[1]
- ○ Independent/self-feeding[1]
- ○ No honey[1]
- ○ No bottles in bed
- ○ Choking/Safe foods[1]

12–13 months:
- ○ Breastfeeding[1]/Vitamin D 400 IU/day[1]
- ○ Homogenized milk [500–750 mLs (16–24 oz)/day[1]]
- ○ Appetite reduced
- ○ Choking/safe foods[1]
- ○ Avoid juices/sweetened liquids[1]
- ○ Promote open cup instead of bottle
- ○ Inquire re: vegetarian diets[1]
- ○ Eats family foods with a variety of textures.
- ○ Independent/self-feeding[1]

15 months:
- ○ Breastfeeding[1]/Vitamin D 400 IU/day[1]
- ○ Homogenized milk [500–750 mLs (16–24 oz)/day[1]]
- ○ Choking/safe foods[1]
- ○ Avoid juices/sweetened liquids[1]
- ○ Promote open cup instead of bottle
- ○ Inquire re: vegetarian diets[1]
- ○ Independent/self-feeding[1]

EDUCATION AND ADVICE
Repeat discussion of items is based on perceived risk or need

Injury Prevention[1]
- ○ Poisons[1]; PCC#[1]
- ○ Hot water <49°C/bath safety[1]
- ○ Carbon monoxide/Smoke detectors[1]
- ○ Motorized vehicles/Car seat[1]
- ○ Firearm safety[1]
- ○ Pacifier use[1]

Childproofing, including:
- ○ Falls (stairs, change table, unstable furniture/TV, no walkers)[1]
- ○ Electric plugs/Cords
- ○ Choking/safe toys[1]

Behaviour and Family Issues[2]
- ○ Crying[2]
- ○ Night waking[2]
- ○ Siblings
- ○ Parenting[2]
- ○ Child care[2]/Return to work
- ○ Parental fatigue/Depression[1]
- ○ High risk children/assess home visit need[2]
- ○ Family healthy active living/sedentary behaviour/screen time[2]
- ○ Inquire re difficulty making ends meet or feeding your family[2]
- ○ Healthy sleep habits[2]
- ○ Soothability/Responsiveness
- ○ Encourage reading[2]
- ○ Family conflict/Stress

Environmental Health[1]
- ○ Second hand smoke[1]
- ○ Sun exposure/Sunscreens/insect repellent[1]
- ○ Pesticide exposure[1]

Other Issues[1]
- ○ Teething/Dental cleaning/Fluoride/Dentist[1]
- ○ Complementary/Alternative medicine[1]
- ○ No OTC cough/Cold medicine[1]
- ○ Footwear[1]
- ○ Fever advice/Thermometers[1]

DEVELOPMENT[2] (Inquiry and observation of milestones)
Tasks are set *after* the time of normal milestone acquisition. Absence of any item suggests consideration for further assessment of development. NB–Correct for age if < 37 weeks gestation

9 months:
- ○ Looks for an object seen hidden
- ○ Cries or shouts for attention
- ○ Babbles a series of different sounds (e.g., baba, duhduh)
- ○ Responds differently to different people
- ○ Makes sounds/gestures to get attention or help
- ○ Stands with support when helped into standing position
- ○ Opposes thumb and fingers when grasps objects and finger foods
- ○ Plays social games with you (e.g., nose touching, peek-a-boo)
- ○ Sits without support
- ○ No parent/caregiver concerns

12–13 months:
- ○ Responds to own name
- ○ Understands simple requests, (e.g., Where is the ball?)
- ○ Makes at least 1 consonant/vowel combination
- ○ Says 3 or more words (do not have to be clear)
- ○ Crawls or 'bum' shuffles
- ○ Pulls to stand/walks holding on
- ○ Has pincer grasp to pick up and eat finger foods
- ○ Shows distress when separated from parent/caregiver
- ○ Follows your gaze to jointly reference an object
- ○ No parent/caregiver concerns

15 months:
- ○ Says 5 or more words (words do not have to be clear)
- ○ Walks sideways holding onto furniture
- ○ Shows fear of strange people/places
- ○ Crawls up a few stairs/steps
- ○ Tries to squat to pick up toys from the floor
- ○ No parent/caregiver concerns

PHYSICAL EXAMINATION[2]
An appropriate age-specific physical examination is recommended at each visit. Evidence-based screening for specific conditions is highlighted.

9 months:
- ○ Anterior fontanelle[2]
- ○ Corneal light reflex/Cover-uncover test & inquiry[2]
- ○ Hearing inquiry/screening[2]
- ○ Hips (limited hip abd'n)[2]
- ○ Eyes (red reflex)[2]
- ○ Teeth[2]

12–13 months:
- ○ Anterior fontanelle[2]
- ○ Corneal light reflex/Cover-uncover test & inquiry[2]
- ○ Hearing inquiry/screening[2]
- ○ Tonsil size/Sleep-disordered breathing[2]
- ○ Eyes (red reflex)[2]
- ○ Teeth[2]

15 months:
- ○ Anterior fontanelle[2]
- ○ Corneal light reflex/Cover-uncover test & inquiry[2]
- ○ Hearing inquiry/screening[2]
- ○ Tonsil size/Sleep-disordered breathing[2]
- ○ Hips (limited hip abd'n)[2]
- ○ Eyes (red reflex)[2]
- ○ Teeth[2]

PROBLEMS AND PLANS/CURRENT & NEW REFERRALS[4]
E.g. medical specialist, dietitian, speech, audiology, PT, OT, eyes, dental, social-determinants resources

INVESTIGATIONS/SCREENING[2] AND IMMUNIZATION[3]
Discuss immunization pain reduction strategies[3] Record Vaccines on Guide V

- ○ If HBsAg positive mother check HBV antibodies and HBsAg[3] (at 9 or 12 months)
- ○ Hemoglobin (If at risk)[2]
- ○ Blood lead if at risk[1]

SIGNATURE

Strength of recommendation is based on literature review using the classification: **Good (bold type)**; *Fair (italic type)*; Inconclusive evidence/Consensus (plain type). See literature review table at www.rourkebabyrecord.ca
[1]Resources 1: Growth, Nutrition, Injury Prevention, Environment, Other [2]Resources 2: Family, Behaviour, Development, P/E, Investigations [3]Resources 3: Immunization [4]Resources 4: ECD Resources System and Table

Disclaimer: Given the constantly evolving nature of evidence and changing recommendations, the Rourke Baby Record is meant to be used as a guide only.
Financial support has been provided by the Government of Ontario.   For fair use authorization, see www.rourkebabyrecord.ca

EXHIBIT 1.1 Rourke Baby Record (continued)

©2017 Drs. L Rourke, D Leduc and J Rourke
Revised January 24, 2017
www.rourkebabyrecord.ca

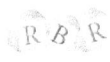  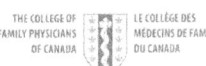 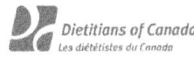

See RBR parent web portal for corresponding parent resources

Rourke Baby Record: Evidence-Based Infant/Child Health Maintenance GUIDE IV: 18 mo–5 yr (National)

NAME: _____ Birth Day (d/m/yy): _____ M[ ] F[ ]

Gestational Age: _____ Birth Length: _____ cm Birth Wt: _____ g Birth Head Circ: _____ cm

Past problems/Risk factors:	Family history:

DATE OF VISIT ___/___/20___	DATE OF VISIT ___/___/20___	DATE OF VISIT ___/___/20___
18 months	2-3 years	4-5 years

GROWTH[1] use WHO growth charts. Correct age until 24–36 months if < 37 weeks gestation

Length	Weight	Head Circ. (HC)	Height	Weight	HC if prior abN	BMI	Height	Weight	BMI

PARENT/CAREGIVER CONCERNS

NUTRITION[1] For each ○ item discussed, indicate "✓" for no concerns, or "X" if concerns

○ Breastfeeding[1]/Vitamin D 400 IU/day[1] ○ Homogenized milk [500–750 mLs(16–24 oz) /day[1]] ○ Avoid juices/sweetened liquids[1] ○ No bottles ○ Inquire re: vegetarian diets[1] ○ Independent/self-feeding[1]	○ Breastfeeding[1]/Vitamin D 400 IU/day[1] ○ Canada's Food Guide[1] ○ Avoid juices/sweetened liquids[1] ○ Inquire re: vegetarian diets[1] ○ Gradual transition to lower fat diet[1] ○ Skim, 1% or 2% milk [~ 500 mLs(16 oz) /day[1]]	○ Skim, 1% or 2% milk [~ 500 mLs(16 oz) /day[1]] ○ Avoid juices/sweetened liquids[1] ○ Inquire re: vegetarian diets[1] ○ Canada's Food Guide[1]

EDUCATION AND ADVICE Repeat discussion of items is based on perceived risk or need

Injury Prevention[1] ○ Motorized vehicles/Car seat (child/booster)[1] ○ Bath safety[1] ○ Choking/Safe toys[1] ○ Wean from pacifier[1] ○ Falls (stairs, change table, unstable furniture/TV)[1] ○ Poisons[1]; PCC#[1] Behaviour[2] ○ Parent/child interaction ○ Healthy sleep habits[2] ○ Discipline/Parenting skills programs[2] Family[2] ○ High-risk children[2] ○ Encourage reading[2] ○ Parental fatigue/Stress/Depression[2] ○ Socializing/Peer play opportunities ○ Family healthy active living/Sedentary behaviour/Screen time[2] ○ Inquire re difficulty making ends meet or feeding your family[2] Environment Health[1] ○ Second-hand smoke[1] ○ Pesticide exposure[1] ○ Sun exposure/Sunscreens/ISnsect repellent[1] Other[1] ○ Dental care/Dentist[1] ○ Toilet learning[2]	Injury Prevention[1] ○ Bike helmets[1] ○ Firearm safety[1] ○ Matches ○ Poisons[1]; PCC#[1] ○ Carbon monoxide/smoke detectors[1] ○ Water safety[1] ○ Falls (stairs, unstable furniture/TV, trampolines)[1] ○ Motorized vehicles/Car seat (child/booster)[1] ○ No pacifiers[1] Behaviour[2] ○ Parent/Child interaction ○ Discipline/Parenting skills programs[2] ○ High-risk children[2] ○ Parental fatigue/Depression[2] ○ Family conflict/Stress ○ Siblings Family[2] ○ Healthy sleep habits[2] ○ Assess child care/Preschool needs/school readiness[2] ○ Socializing opportunities ○ Encourage reading[2] ○ Family healthy active living/sedentary behaviour/Screen time[2] ○ Inquire re difficulty making ends meet or feeding your family[2] Environment Health[1] ○ Second-hand smoke[1] ○ Sun exposure/Sunscreens/insect repellent[1] ○ Pesticide exposure[1] Other[1] ○ Dental cleaning/Fluoride/Dentist[1] ○ Complementary/Alternative medicine[1] ○ Toilet learning[2] ○ No OTC cough/Cold medicine[1]	

DEVELOPMENT[2] (Inquiry and observation of milestones)
Tasks are set after the time of normal milestone acquisition. Absence of any item suggests consideration for further assessment of development. NB–Correct for age if < 37 weeks gestation

	2 years[2]	3 years	4 years	5 years
Social/Emotional[2] ○ Interested in other children ○ Usually easy to soothe ○ Child's behaviour is usually manageable ○ Comes for comfort when distressed Communication Skills[2] ○ Points to several different body parts ○ Tries to get your attention to show you something ○ Turns/Responds when name is called ○ Points to what he/she wants ○ Looks for toy when asked or pointed in direction ○ Imitates speech sounds and gestures ○ Says 15 or more words (words do not have to be clear) ○ Produces 4 consonants, (e.g., B D G H N W) Motor Skills ○ Feeds self with spoon with little spilling ○ Walks alone Adaptive Skills ○ Removes hat/Socks without help ○ No parent/caregiver concerns	○ Combines 2 or more words ○ Understands 1 and 2 step directions ○ Walks backward 2 steps without support ○ Tries to run ○ Puts objects into small container ○ Uses toys for pretend play (e.g., give doll a drink) ○ Continues to develop new skills ○ No parent/caregiver concerns	○ Understands 2 and 3 step directions (e.g., "Pick up your hat and shoes and put them in the closet.") ○ Uses sentences with 5 or more words ○ Walks up stairs using handrail ○ Twists lids off jars or turns knobs ○ Shares some of the time ○ Plays make-believe games with actions and words (e.g., pretending to cook a meal, fix a car) ○ Turns pages one at a time ○ Listens to music or stories for 5–10 minutes ○ No parent/caregiver concerns	○ Understands 3-part directions ○ Asks and answers lots of questions (e.g., "What are you doing?") ○ Walks up/down stairs alternating feet ○ Undoes buttons and zippers ○ Tries to comfort someone who is upset ○ No parent/caregiver concerns	○ Counts out loud or on fingers to answer "How many are there?" ○ Speaks clearly in adult-like sentences most of the time ○ Throws and catches a ball ○ Hops on 1 foot several times ○ Dresses and undresses with little help ○ Cooperates with adult requests most of the time ○ Retells the sequence of a story ○ Separates easily from parent/Caregiver ○ No parent/caregiver concerns

PHYSICAL EXAMINATION[2] An appropriate age-specific physical examination is recommended at each visit. Evidence-based screening for specific conditions is highlighted.

○ Anterior fontanelle closed[2] ○ Eyes (red reflex)[2] ○ Corneal light reflex/Cover-uncover test & inquiry[2] ○ Hearing inquiry ○ Teeth[2] ○ Tonsil size/Sleep-disordered breathing[2]	○ Blood pressure if at risk[2] ○ Teeth[2] ○ Eyes (red reflex)/Visual acuity[2] ○ Hearing inquiry ○ Corneal light reflex/Cover-uncover test & inquiry[2] ○ Tonsil size/Sleep-disordered breathing[2]	○ Blood pressure if at risk[2] ○ Teeth[2] ○ Eyes (red reflex)/Visual acuity[2] ○ Hearing inquiry ○ Corneal light reflex/Cover-uncover test & inquiry[2] ○ Tonsil size/Sleep-disordered breathing[2]

PROBLEMS AND PLANS/CURRENT & NEW REFERRALS[4] E.g. medical specialist, dietitian, speech, audiology, PT, OT, eyes, dental, social-determinants resources

INVESTIGATIONS/SCREENING[2] AND IMMUNIZATION[3] Discuss immunization pain reduction strategies[3] Record Vaccines on Guide V

○ Hemoglobin (If at risk)[2] ○ Blood lead if at risk[1]		

SIGNATURE

Strength of recommendation is based on literature review using the classification: **Good (bold type)**; *Fair (italic type)*; Inconclusive evidence/Consensus (plain type). See literature review table at www.rourkebabyrecord.ca
[1]Resources 1: Growth, Nutrition, Injury Prevention, Environment, Other   [2]Resources 2: Family, Behaviour, Development, P/E, Investigations   [3]Resources 3: Immunization   [4]Resources 4: ECD Resources System and Table

Disclaimer: Given the constantly evolving nature of evidence and changing recommendations, the Rourke Baby Record is meant to be used as a guide only.
Financial support has been provided by the Government of Ontario.   For fair use authorization, see www.rourkebabyrecord.ca

EXHIBIT 1.1 Rourke Baby Record (*continued*)

©2017 Drs. L Rourke, D Leduc and J Rourke
Revised January 24, 2017
www.rourkebabyrecord.ca

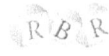 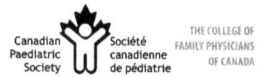 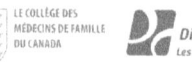 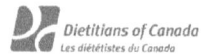

See RBR parent web portal for corresponding parent resources

For additional information, refer to the National Advisory Committee on Immunization website.

Provincial guidelines vary and are available at the Public Health Agency of Canada (PHAC).

Rourke Baby Record: Evidence-Based Infant/Child Health Maintenance **GUIDE V: Immunization**
Canadian Immunization Guide as per NACI Recommendations (as of October 2016) **(National)**

NAME: _____ Birth Day (d/m/yy): _____ M [ ] F [ ]

Vaccine	NACI recommendations	Date given	Injection site	Lot number	Expiry date	Initials	Comments
Rotavirus[3] 2 or 3 doses # doses varies with manufacturer	dose #1 (6 weeks–14 weeks/6 days)						
	dose #2						
	± dose #3 (by 8 months/0 days)						
DTaP/IPV/[3] 4 doses (2, 4, 6, 18 months) Hib[3]	dose #1 (2 months)						
	dose #2 (4 months)						
	dose #3 (6 months)						
	dose #4 (18 months)						
Pneu-C-13[3] 3 or 4 doses (2, 4, ±6, 12–15 months)	dose #1 (2 months)						
	dose #2 (4 months)						
	±dose #3 (6 months)						
	dose #4 (12–15 months)						
Men-Conjugate[3] MCV-C: 1 dose at 12 months MCV-C or MCV-4:1 dose at 12 years or during adolescence If at increased risk: - MCV-C: 3 doses at 2, 4 & 12 months - MCV-4: at 2 years or older - 4CMenB: at 2 months or older	MCV-C: 2 doses at 2 and 4 months only if at increased risk ± dose #1 (2 months) ± dose #2 (4 months)						
	MCV-C: 1 dose at 12 months						
	MCV-C or MCV-4: 1 dose at 12 years or during adolescence						
Hepatitis B[3] 3 doses in infancy OR 2–3 doses preteen/teen Can be combined with Hep A vaccine	dose #1						
	dose #2						
	± dose #3						
MMR or MMRV[3] 2 doses (12 months, 18 months OR 4 years)	dose #1 (12 months)						
	dose #2 (18 months OR 4 years)						
Varicella[3] 2 doses (12 months–12 years – MMRV or univalent) OR 2 doses (>13 years–univalent)	dose #1						
	dose #2						
DTaP/IPV[3]	1 dose (4–6 years)						
dTap[3]	1 dose (14–16 years)						
Influenza[3] 1 dose annually (6–59 months and high risk > 5 years) First yr only for < 9 years – give 2 doses 1 month apart							
HPV Starting at 9 years of age, as per provincial/territorial guidelines	dose #1						
	dose #2						
	±dose #3						
Other							

Disclaimer: Given the constantly evolving nature of evidence and changing recommendations, the Rourke Baby Record is meant to be used as a guide only.
[3]Resources 3: Immunization
Financial support has been provided by the Government of Ontario. For fair use authorization, see www.rourkebabyrecord.ca

EXHIBIT 1.1 Rourke Baby Record (*continued*)

©2017 Drs. L Rourke, D Leduc and J Rourke
Revised January 24, 2017
www.rourkebabyrecord.ca

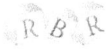

Rourke Baby Record: **RESOURCES 1:**

Growth, Nutrition, Injury Prevention, Environmental Health, Other (National)

See RBR parent web portal for corresponding parent resources

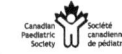

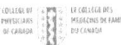

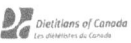

GROWTH

- **Important:** Corrected age should be used at least until 24 to 36 months of age for premature infants born at <37 weeks gestation.
- *Measuring growth:* The growth of all term infants, both breastfed and non-breastfed, and preschoolers should be evaluated using Canadian growth charts from the 2006 World Health Organization Child Growth Standards (birth to 5 years) with measurement of recumbent length (birth to 2–3 years) or standing height (≥ 2 years), weight, head circumference (birth to 2 years) and calculation of BMI (2–5 years). WHO Growth Charts Adapted for Canada (DC) Growth Monitoring (CTFPHC) Optimal growth monitoring (CPS)

NUTRITION: Nutrition for healthy term infants (NHTI): 0–6 months 6–24 months NutriSTEP® Overview NHTI 0–6 months (CPS) Nutrition Guidelines 0-6 years (OSNPPH) Dietitians of Canada

- **Breastfeeding: Exclusive breastfeeding** is recommended for the first six months of life for healthy term infants. Introduction of solids should be led by the infant's signs of readiness – a few weeks before to just after 6 months. Breast milk is the optimal food for infants, and breastfeeding (with complementary foods) may continue for up to two years and beyond unless contraindicated. Breastfeeding reduces gastrointestinal and respiratory infections and helps to protect against SIDS. Maternal support (both antepartum and postpartum) increases breastfeeding and prolongs its duration. Early and frequent mother-infant contact, rooming in, and banning handouts of free infant formula increase breastfeeding rates.
  - Baby-Friendly Initiative (Breastfeeding Committee for Canada)
  - Ankyloglossia and breastfeeding (CPS)
  - Maternal medications when breastfeeding: Drugs and Lactation Database (TOXNET)
  - Weaning: Weaning from the breast (CPS)
- **Vitamin D supplementation** of 400 IU/day (800 IU/day in high-risk infants) is recommended for infants/children for as long as they are breastfed. Breastfeeding mothers should continue to take Vitamin D supplements for the duration of breastfeeding. Vitamin D supplementation (CPS)
- *Infant formula:* Discourage the use of homemade infant formulas.
  - Formula composition and use Alberta Health Services Compendium and Summary Sheet
  - Formula preparation and handling: Powdered formula preparation and handling (HC)
- Milk consumption range is consensus only & is provided as an approximate guide.
- Soy-based formula is not recommended for routine use in term infants as an equivalent alternative to cow's milk formula, or for cow milk protein allergy, and is contraindicated for preterm infants. Soy-based formulas (CPS)
- **Avoid all sweetened fruit drinks, sport-drinks, energy drinks and soft-drinks**; restrict fruit juice consumption to a maximum of 1/2 cup (125 mL) per day.
- Colic: Dietary interventions for colic (CPS)
- **Introduction to solids:** A few weeks before to just after 6 months, start iron containing foods to avoid iron deficiency. A variety of soft texture foods, ranging from purees to finger foods, can be introduced.
- **Allergenic foods:** Delaying the introduction of priority food allergens is not currently recommended to prevent food allergies, including for infants at risk of atopy. Dietary exposures & allergy prevention (CPS)
- **Avoid honey until 1 year of age** to prevent botulism.
- *Dietary fat content:* Restriction of dietary fat during the first 2 years is not recommended since it may compromise the intake of energy and essential fatty acids, required for growth and development. After 2 years, a gradual transition begins from a high fat milk diet to a lower fat milk diet, as per Canada's Food Guide.
- Promote family meals with independent/self-feeding while offering a variety of healthy foods. NHTI: 6–24 months
- Vegetarian diets: Vegetarian diets in children and adolescents (CPS)
- Fish consumption: 2 servings/week of low mercury fish: Fish consumption and mercury (HC)

ENVIRONMENTAL HEALTH

- **Second-hand smoke exposure:** There is no safe level of exposure. Advise caregivers to stop smoking and/or reduce second-hand smoke exposure, which contributes to childhood respiratory illnesses, SIDS and neuro-behavioural disorders. Offer smoking cessation resources.
- Sun exposure/sunscreens/insect repellents: Minimize sun exposure. Wear protective clothing, hats, properly applied sunscreen with SPF ≥ 30 for those > 6 months of age. No DEET in < 6 months; 6–24 months 10% DEET apply max once daily; 2–12 years 10% DEET apply max TID. Preventing mosquito and tick bites (CPS)
- *Pesticides:* Avoid pesticide exposure. Encourage pesticide-free foods. Pesticide Exposure in Children (AAP)
- *Lead:* There is no safe level of lead exposure in children. Evidence suggests that low blood lead levels can have adverse health effects on a child's cognitive function. Prevention of Childhood Lead Toxicity (AAP), Lead and Children (CFP)
  Blood Lead Screening is recommended for children who:
  - in the last 6 months lived in a house or apartment built before 1978;
  - live in a home with recent or ongoing renovations or peeling or chipped paint;
  - have a sibling, housemate, or playmate with a prior history of lead poisoning;
  - live near point sources of lead contamination;
  - have household members with lead-related occupations or hobbies;
  - are refugees aged 6 months–6 years, within 3 months of arrival and again in 3–6 months.
- Websites about environmental issues:
  - Canadian Partnership for Children's Health and Environment (CPCHE)
  - AAP Council on Environmental Health

INJURY PREVENTION: In Canada, unintentional injuries are the leading cause of death in children and youth. Most of these preventable injuries are caused by motor vehicle collisions, drowning, choking, burns, poisoning, and falls. Unexplained injuries (e.g. fractures, bruising, burns) or injuries that do not fit the rationale provided or developmental stage raise concern for child maltreatment.

- **Transportation in motorized vehicles including cars, ATVs, snowmobiles, etc.:** Child passenger safety (AAP) Preventing ATV injuries (CPS) Snowmobile safety (CPS)
  - Children < 13 years should sit in the rear seat. Keep children away from all airbags.
  - Install and follow size recommendations as per specific car seat model and keep child in each stage as long as possible.
  - Use rear-facing infant/child seat that is manufacturer approved for use until at least age 2 years.
  - Use forward-facing child seat after 2 years for as long as manufacturer specifications will allow.
  - After this, use booster seat for children 18-36 kg (40-80 lbs) and up to 145 cm (4'9").
  - Use lap and shoulder belt in the rear middle seat for children over 8 years who are at least 36 kg (80 lb) and 145 cm (4' 9") and *fit vehicle restraint system.*
- **Bicycle:** wear **bike helmets** and advocate for helmet legislation for all ages. Replace if heavy impact or damage. Bicycle helmet legislation (CPS)
- <u>Drowning:</u> Prevention of drowning (AAP)
  - *Bath safety:* Never leave a young child alone in the bath. Do not use infant bath rings or bath seats.
  - *Water safety:* Recommend adult supervision, training for adults, 4-sided pool fencing, lifejackets, swimming lessons, and boating safety to decrease the risk of drowning.
- <u>Choking:</u> Avoid hard, small and round, smooth and sticky solid foods until age 3 years. Encourage child to remain seated while eating and drinking. Use safe toys, follow minimum age recommendations, and remove loose parts and broken toys. Preventing choking and suffocation in children (CPS)
- *Burns:* Install smoke detectors in the home on every level. Keep hot water at a temperature < 49°C.
- **Poisons:** Keep medicines and cleaners locked up and out of child's reach. Have Poison Control Centre number handy. Use of ipecac is contraindicated in children.
- *Falls:* Assess home for hazards – never leave baby alone on change table or other high surface; use window guards and stair gates. Baby walkers are banned in Canada and should never be used. Ensure stability of furniture and TV. Advise against trampoline use at home. Trampoline use (CPS)
- **Safe sleeping environment:** Joint statement on safe sleep (CPS/CFSIDS/CICH/HC/PHAC)
  - **Sleep position, bed sharing and SIDS:** Healthy infants should be positioned on their backs for sleep. Counsel parents on the dangers of other contributory causes of SIDS such as bed sharing, overheating, maternal smoking or second-hand smoke.
  - **Positional plagiocephaly:** While supine for sleep, the orientation of the infant's head should be varied to prevent positional plagiocephaly. Sleep positioners should not be used. After umbilical cord stump has detached, infants should have supervised tummy time while awake.
  - **Crib safety/Room sharing:** Infants should sleep in a crib, cradle or bassinette, without soft objects, loose bedding and similar items that meet current 2016 Health Canada regulations in parents' room for the first 6 months of life. Room sharing is protective against SIDS.
  - Swaddling: Proper swaddling of the infant for the first 2 months of life may promote longer sleep periods but could be associated with adverse events (hyperthermia, SIDS, or development of hip dysplasia) if misapplied. A swaddled infant must always be placed supine with free movement of hips and legs, and the head uncovered. Swaddling (AAP)
  - *Pacifier use* may decrease risk of SIDS and should not be discouraged in the 1st year of life after breastfeeding is well established, but should be restricted in children with chronic/recurrent otitis media. Pacifier recommendations (CPS)
- **Firearm safety:** Advise on removal of firearms from home or safe storage to decrease risk of unintentional firearm injury, suicide, or homicide. Youth and firearms in Canada (CPS)

OTHER

- Advise parents against using **OTC cough/cold medications:** Restricting Cough and Cold Medicines in Children (PCH)
- *Complementary and alternative medicine (CAM):* Questions should be routinely asked about the use of complementary and alternative medicine, therapy, or products, especially for children with chronic conditions. Natural Health Products (CPS); Homeopathy (CPS); Chiropractic care (CPS)
- Fever advice/thermometers: Fever ≥ 38°C in an infant < 3 months needs urgent evaluation. Ibuprofen and acetaminophen are both effective antipyretics. Acetaminophen remains the first choice for antipyresis under 6 months of age; thereafter ibuprofen or acetaminophen may be used. Alternating acetaminophen with ibuprofen for fever control is not recommended in primary care settings as this may encourage fever phobia, and the potential risks of medication error outweigh measurable clinical benefit. Temperature measurement (CPS)
- Footwear: Shoes are for protection, not correction. Walking barefoot develops good toe gripping and muscular strength. Footwear for children (CPS)
- **Oral Health** - Smiles for Life
  - **Dental Cleaning:** As excessive swallowing of toothpaste by young children may result in dental fluorosis, children under 3 years of age should have their teeth and gums brushed twice daily by an adult using either water (if low risk for tooth decay) or a rice grain sized portion of fluoridated toothpaste (if at caries risk). Children 3–6 years of age should be assisted during brushing and only use a small amount (e.g., pea-sized portion) of fluoridated toothpaste twice daily. Caregiver should brush child's teeth until they develop the manual dexterity to do this alone, and should continue to intermittently supervise brushing after children assume independence. Begin flossing daily when teeth touch.
  - Caries risk factors include: child has caries or enamel defects, hygiene or diet is concerning, parent has caries, premature or LBW infant, or no water fluoridation.
  - **To prevent early childhood caries:** avoid juices/sweetened liquids and constant sipping of milk or natural juices in both bottle and cup.
  - Fluoride varnish should be used for those at caries risk. Consider dietary fluoride supplements only for high risk children who do not have access to systemic community water fluoridation. Caries-risk assessment (AAPDA), Fluoride and your child (CDA)
  - Consider the first dentist visit by 6 months after eruption of 1st tooth or at age 1 year.

Disclaimer: Given the constantly evolving nature of evidence and changing recommendations, the Rourke Baby Record is meant to be used as a guide only.
Financial support has been provided by the Government of Ontario. For fair use authorization, see www.rourkebabyrecord.ca.

EXHIBIT 1.1 Rourke Baby Record (continued)

©2017 Drs. L Rourke, D Leduc and J Rourke
Revised January 24, 2017
www.rourkebabyrecord.ca

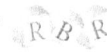
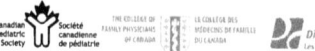

Rourke Baby Record: RESOURCES 2: Family, Behaviour, Development, Physical exam, Investigations/Screening
See RBR parent web portal for corresponding parent resources (National)

BEHAVIOUR
<u>Crying</u>: Excessive crying may be caused by behavioural or physical factors or be the upper limit of the normal spectrum. Caregiver frustration with infant crying can lead to child maltreatment/inflicted injury (head injury, fractures, bruising). The Period of Purple Crying. See Prevention of child maltreatment.
<u>Assess healthy sleep habits</u>: Normal sleep (quality and quantity for age) is associated with normal development and leads to better health outcomes. Sleeping Behaviour (EECD).
Recommended sleep duration per 24 hrs: 12-14 hrs (infants 4–12 months); 11-14 hrs (1–2 yrs); 10-13 hrs (3–5 yrs); 9-12 hrs (6–12 yrs); 8-10 hrs (13–18 yrs). Turn off computer/TV screens 60 minutes before bedtime. No computer/TV screens in bedroom. Recommended amount of sleep (AASM)
<u>Night waking</u>: occurs in 20% of infants and toddlers who do not require night feeding. Counselling around positive bedtime routines (including training the child to fall asleep alone), removing nighttime positive reinforcers, keeping morning awakening time consistent, and rewarding good sleep behaviour has been shown to reduce the prevalence of night waking, especially when this counselling begins in the first 3 weeks of life. Behaviour modification & sleep (MJA)   Sleep problems & night wakings (Sleep)

PARENTING/DISCIPLINE
Inform parents that warm, responsive, flexible & consistent discipline techniques are associated with positive child outcomes. Over reactive, inconsistent, cold & coercive techniques are associated with negative child outcomes. Use of any physical punishment including spanking should be discouraged in all ages. Effective discipline for children (CPS)
Refer parents of children at risk of, or showing signs of, behavioural or conduct problems to structured parenting programs which have been shown to increase positive parenting, improve child compliance, and reduce general behaviour problems. Access community resources to determine the most appropriate and available research-structured programs. Parenting skills (EECD)
e.g., The Incredible Years®, Right from the Start, COPE program, Triple P®, Strongest Families

HIGH RISK INFANTS/CHILDREN/PARENTS/CAREGIVERS/FAMILIES
- **Maternal depression:** Physicians should have a high awareness of maternal depression, which is a risk factor for the socio-emotional and cognitive development of children. Although less studied, paternal factors may compound the maternal-infant issues. Maternal depression and child development (CPS)
- **Fetal alcohol spectrum disorder (FASD).** Fetal alcohol syndrome (CPS)
- **Adoption/Foster care:** Children newly adopted or entering foster care are a high risk population with special needs for health supervision. Foster Care (CPS); Transracial Adoption (CPS)
- **Immigrants/refugees:** Caring for kids new to Canada (CPS); CCIRH-Clinical Guidelines
- **Aboriginal children:** Social determinants of health in Aboriginal children in Canada (PCH)
- **Social determinants of health (SDH):** Inquiry about impact of poverty: "Do you have difficulty in making ends meet? Do you have trouble feeding your family?" Child Poverty Tool (OCFP)
Social determinants of health (CFPC)   Infrastructure to address SDH (PCH)
- **Prevention of child maltreatment:**
  - Risk factors for child maltreatment:
    - Parent (low socio-economic status, maternal age <19 years, single parent family, non-biological parents, abused as child, substance abuse, lack of social support, unplanned pregnancy or negative parental attitude towards pregnancy).
    - Family (spousal violence, poor marital relations, poor child-parent relationship, unhappy family life).
    - Child (behaviour problems, disability).
  - Discuss with parents of preschoolers teaching names of genitalia, appropriate and inappropriate touch, and normal sexual behaviour for age.
  - Exposure to personal violence and other forms of violence has significant impact on physical and emotional well-being of children.
  - **Assess home visit need:** There is good evidence for home visiting by nurses during the perinatal period through infancy for first-time mothers of low socioeconomic status, single parents or teenaged parents to prevent physical abuse and/or neglect.
Child maltreatment interventions (USPSTF)   Bruising in suspected maltreatment cases (CPS)
Abusive head trauma (CPS)   INSPIRE: 7 strategies for ending violence against children (WHO)

NONPARENTAL CHILD CARE
Inquire about current child care arrangements. High quality child care is associated with improved paediatric outcomes in all children.
Factors enhancing quality child care include: practitioner general education and specific training; group size and child/staff ratio; licensing and registration/accreditation; infection control and injury prevention; and emergency procedures.
- Health implications of children in child care centres (CPS): Part A and Part B
- Guide to child-care in Canada (CPS): Well Beings

LITERACY
Encourage parents to read to their children within the first few months of life and to limit TV, video and computer games to provide more opportunities for reading.
- Read, speak, sing: promoting literacy (CPS)
- Literacy Promotion (AAP)
- Reading aloud to children: the evidence (Arch Dis Child)

FAMILY HEALTHY ACTIVE LIVING/SEDENTARY BEHAVIOUR/SCREEN TIME
Encourage increased physical activity, with parents as role models, through interactive floor-based play for infants and a variety of activities for young children, and decreased sedentary pastimes.
- **Media use** – Counsel on appropriate screen time: <2 years avoid; 2–4 years <1 h/day. Less is better. Educational and prosocial programming is better.
- Healthy active living (CPS)   CSEP guidelines

DEVELOPMENT
Maneuvers are based on evidence-based literature on milestone acquisition. Evidence-based milestone ages (PCH). They are not a developmental screen, but rather an aid to developmental surveillance. They are set after the time of normal milestone acquisition. Thus, absence of any one or more items is considered a high-risk marker and indicates consideration for further developmental assessment, as does parental or caregiver concern about development at any stage.
- Best Start website contains resources for maternal, newborn, and early child development
- Improving the Odds: Healthy Child Development (OCFP) toolkit for primary healthcare providers
- Centre of Excellence for Early Childhood Development Encyclopedia on Early Childhood Development
- Getting it right at 18 months (CPS)   Measuring in support of early childhood development (CPS)

TOILET LEARNING
The process of toilet learning has changed significantly over the years and within different cultures. In Western culture, a child-centred approach is recommended, where the timing and methodology of toilet learning is individualized as much as possible.
Toilet learning (CPS)   Toilet-training strategy (PCH): Part A   Part B

AUTISM SPECTRUM DISORDER
Specific screening for ASD at 18–24 months should be performed on all children with any of the following: failed items on the social/emotional/communication skills inquiry, sibling with autism, or developmental concern by parent, caregiver, or physician.
Use the revised M-CHAT-R™ and if abnormal, use the follow-up M-CHAT-R/F™ to reduce the false positive rate and avoid unnecessary referrals and parental concern. Electronic M-CHAT-R™ is available.

PHYSICAL EXAMINATION
- *Jaundice:* Bilirubin testing (total and conjugated) if persists beyond 2 wks of age.
  Neonatal Hyperbilirubinemia Guidelines (CPS)   Newborn screening for biliary atresia (AAP).
- *Bruising:* Unexplained bruising warrants evaluation re child maltreatment or medical illness.
- *Check blood pressure if at risk* – High blood pressure in children (NIH Working Group)
- *Fontanelles:* The posterior fontanelle is usually closed by 2 months and the anterior by 18 months.
- *Vision inquiry/screening:* Vision screening (CPS)
  - Check Red Reflex for serious ocular diseases such as retinoblastoma and cataracts.
  - **Corneal light reflex/cover-uncover test & inquiry for strabismus:** With the child focusing on a light source, the light reflex on the cornea should be symmetrical. Each eye is then covered in turn, for 2–3 seconds, and then quickly uncovered. The test is abnormal if the uncovered eye "wanders" OR if the covered eye moves when uncovered.
  - Check visual acuity at age 3–5 years.
- *Hearing inquiry/screening:* Any parental concerns about hearing acuity or language delay should prompt a rapid referral for hearing assessment. Formal audiology testing should be performed in all high-risk infants, including those with normal UNHS. Older children should be screened if clinically indicated.
- Inspect tongue mobility for ankyloglossia. Ankyloglossia and breastfeeding (CPS)
- Check neck for torticollis.
- *Tonsil size/sleep-disordered breathing:* Screen for sleep problems. Behavioural sleep problems and snoring in the presence of sleep-disordered breathing warrants assessment re obstructive sleep apnea (OSA). OSA (AAP)
- *Muscle tone:* Physical assessment for spasticity, rigidity, and hypotonia should be performed.
- *Hips:* There is insufficient evidence to recommend routine diagnostic imaging for screening for developmental dysplasia of the hips, but examination of the hips should be included until at least one year, or until the child can walk. Screening for developmental hip dysplasia (USPSTF)   DDH (CTFPHC)
- *Dental:* Examine for problems including dental caries, oral soft tissue infections or pathology; and for normal teeth eruption sequence.

FIRST TEETH	When teeth "come in"	When teeth "fall out"
Upper		
Central incisors	7-12 mos	6-8 yrs
Lateral incisors	9-13 mos	7-8 yrs
Canines	16-22 mos	10-12 yrs
First molars	13-19 mos	9-11 yrs
Second molars	25-33 mos	10-12 yrs
Lower		
Second molars	20-31 mos	10-12 yrs
First molars	12-18 mos	9-11 yrs
Canines	16-23 mos	9-12 yrs
Lateral incisors	7-16 mos	7-8 yrs
Central incisors	6-10 mos	6-8 yrs

INVESTIGATIONS/SCREENING
Anemia screening: All infants/children from high-risk groups for iron deficiency anemia require screening between 6 and 18 months of age. E.g. Lower SES; Asian; First Nations children; low-birth-weight and premature infants; infants/children fed whole cow's milk before 9 months of age or at quantities > 750 mls/day, or if iron containing foods are not provided.
Hemoglobinopathy screening: Screen all neonates from high-risk groups: Asian, African & Mediteranean.
Universal newborn hearing screening (UNHS) effectively identifies infants with congenital hearing loss and allows for early intervention & improved outcomes. Universal newborn hearing screening (CPS)
Tuberculosis – TB skin testing: for up-to-date information, see Tuberculosis (Gov't Canada)
Canadian TB Standards: 7th Edition 2013

Disclaimer: Given the constantly evolving nature of evidence and changing recommendations, the Rourke Baby Record is meant to be used as a guide only. Financial support has been provided by the Government of Ontario. For fair use authorization, see www.rourkebabyrecord.ca

EXHIBIT 1.1 Rourke Baby Record (*continued*)

©2017 Drs. L Rourke, D Leduc and J Rourke
Revised January 24, 2017
www.rourkebabyrecord.ca

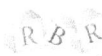

Rourke Baby Record: RESOURCES 3: Immunization
See RBR parent web portal for corresponding parent resources

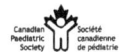 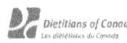

(National)

ROUTINE IMMUNIZATION
- See the Canadian Immunization Guide for recommended immunization schedules for infants, children, youth, and pregnant women, from the National Advisory Committee on Immunization (NACI)
- **Provincial/territorial immunization schedules** may differ based on funding differences. Provincial/territorial immunization schedules are available at the Public Health Agency of Canada.
- **Immunization pain reduction strategies:** During vaccination, pain reduction strategies with good evidence include breastfeeding or use of sweet-tasting solutions, use of the least painful vaccine brand, and consideration of topical anaesthetics.
Reducing vaccine pain (CMAJ)
- Acetaminophen or ibuprofen should not be given prior to, but after vaccination as required. Prophylactic Antipyretic Administration (PLOS ONE)
- Information for physicians on vaccine safety:
  - Canada's vaccine safety program (CPS)
  - Autism spectrum disorder: No causal relationship with vaccines (CPS)
- Information for parents on vaccinations can be accessed through:
  - ImmunizeCA
  - Caring for Kids website (CPS) including Your Child's Best Shot
  - A Parent's Guide to Vaccination (PHAC)
  - Working with vaccine-hesitant parents (CPS)

VACCINE NOTES
(Adapted websites of NACI and the Canadian Immunization Guide October 2016)

- **Diphtheria, Tetanus, acellular Pertussis, inactivated Polio virus vaccine and Haemophilus influenzae B (DTaP-IPV-Hib):** DTaP-IPV-Hib vaccine may be used for all doses in the vaccination series in children < 2 years of age, and for completion of the series in children < 5 years old who have received ≥ 1 dose of DPT (whole cell) vaccine (e.g., recent immigrants).
- **Diphtheria, Tetanus, acellular Pertussis, inactivated Polio virus vaccine, Haemophilus influenzae B and Hepatitis B (Hep B) (DTaP-IPV-Hib-Hep B)** is used for 3 of the 4 initial doses in some jurisdictions with routine infant Hep B vaccination programs.
- **Diphtheria, Tetanus, acellular Pertussis, inactivated Polio virus vaccine (DTaP-IPV)** may be used up to age 7 years and for completion of the series in incompletely immunized children 5-7 years old (healthy children ≥5 years of age do not require Hib vaccine).
- **Tetanus, Diphtheria, Pertussis, Polio (Tdap-IPV) Vaccine,** a quadrivalent vaccine containing less pertussis and diphtheria antigen than the preparations given to younger children and less likely to cause local reactions, is used for the preschool booster at 4-6 years of age in some jurisdictions and should be used in all individuals > 7 years of age receiving or completing their primary series.
- **Diphtheria, Tetanus, acellular Pertussis vaccine – (dTap):** is used for booster doses in people ≥ 7 years of age. All adults should receive at least one dose of pertussis containing vaccine (excluding the adolescent booster). Immunization with dTap should be offered to pregnant women (≥ 26 weeks of gestation) who have not received an adult dose of pertussis vaccine, to provide immediate protection to infants less than 6 months of age. In an outbreak situation it may be offered regardless of immunization history.
- **Haemophilus influenzae type b conjugate vaccine (Hib):** Hib is usually given as a combined vaccine (DTaP-IPV-Hib above). If required and not given in combination, Hib is available as Haemophilus b capsular polysaccharide – PRP conjugated to tetanus toxoid (Act-HIBTM or HiberixTM). The number of doses required depends on the age at vaccination and underlying health status.
- **Rotavirus vaccine:** Universal rotavirus vaccine is recommended by NACI and CPS. Two oral vaccines are currently authorized for use in Canada: Rotarix (2 doses) and RotaTeq (3 doses). Dose #1 is given between 6 weeks and 14 weeks/6 days with a minimum interval of 4 weeks between doses. Maximum age for the last dose is 8 months/0 days.
Recommendations for the use of rotavirus vaccines in infants (CPS)
- **Measles, Mumps and Rubella vaccine (MMR) and MMR-varicella (MMRV):** The first dose is given at 12-15 months and a second dose should be given with the 18 month or preschool dose of DTaP-IPV (±Hib) (depending on the provincial/territorial policy), or at any intervening age that is practical but at least 4 weeks after the first if MMR, or 3 months after the first if MMRV. If MMRV is not used, MMR and varicella vaccines should be administered concurrently, at different sites, or separated by at least 4 weeks.
- **Varicella vaccine:** Children aged 12 months to 12 years who have not had varicella should receive 2 doses of varicella vaccine (univalent varicella or MMRV). Unvaccinated individuals ≥ 13 years who have not had varicella should receive two doses at least 28 days apart (univalent varicella only). Consult NACI guidelines for recommended options for catch-up varicella vaccination. Varicella and MMR vaccines should be administered concurrently, at different sites if the MMRV [combined MMR/varicella] vaccine is not available, or separated by at least 4 weeks. Preventing varicella (CPS)
- **Hepatitis B vaccine (Hep B):**
  - Hepatitis B vaccine can be routinely given to infants or preadolescents, depending on the provincial/territorial policy. The first dose can be given at 1 month, or at 2 months of age to fit more conveniently with other routine infant immunization visits. The second dose should be administered at least 1 month after the first dose, and the third at least 2 months after the second dose, but again may fit more conveniently into the 4- and 6-month immunization visits. Alternatively, Hep B can be administered as DTaP-IPV-Hib-HepB vaccine in infants, with the first dose at 2 months of age. A two-dose schedule for adolescents is an option.
  - For high-risk children, 3 or 4 doses of higher dose of monovalent hepatitis B vaccine is recommended (immunocompromising conditions, chronic renal failure, dialysis).
  - For infants born to a mother with acute or chronic hepatitis B (HBsAg-positive), the first dose of Hep B vaccine should be given at birth (with Hepatitis B immune globulin, below) and repeat doses of vaccine at 1 and 6 months of age. Premature infants of birthweight less than 2,000 grams, born to HB- infected mothers, require four doses of HB vaccine at 0, 1, 2 and 6 months. The last dose should not be given before 6 months of age. Infants of HBsAg-positive mothers also require Hepatitis B immune globulin at birth and follow-up immune status at 9–12 months for HBV antibodies and HBsAg.
  - Infants with HBsAg-positive fathers, siblings or other household contacts require Hepatitis B vaccine at birth, and at 1 month, and 6 months of age.
  - Hepatitis B vaccine should also be given to all infants from high-risk groups, such as:
    - infants where at least one parent has emigrated from a country where Hepatitis B is endemic;
    - infants of mothers positive for Hepatitis C virus;
    - infants of substance-abusing mothers.
  - Children in other high risk groups, if not vaccinated in infancy, should be vaccinated as soon as the risk factor is recognized. See Hepatitis B chapter in the Canadian Immunization Guide for a list of high risk groups.

- **Hepatitis A or A/B combined (HAHB - when Hepatitis B vaccine has not been previously given):**
  - Children 6 months and older in high-risk groups should receive 2 doses of the hepatitis A vaccine given 6-36 months apart (depending on product used). HAHB is the preferred vaccine for individuals with indications for immunization against both hepatitis A and hepatitis B, who are ≥ 12 months unless medical condition indicates high dose Hep B vaccine required.
  - These vaccines should also be considered when traveling to countries where Hepatitis A or B are endemic.
  - Possible HAHB schedules include 12 months to 18 years: 2 doses at months 0 and 6-12; OR 3 doses at months 0, 1, and 6 depending on age and product used.

- **Pneumococcal vaccine: conjugate (Pneu-C-13) and polysaccharide (Pneu-P-23):** Recommended schedule, number of doses and product depend on the age of the child, risk for pneumococcal disease, and when vaccination is begun. Consult NACI guidelines. Routine infant immunization: administer three doses of Pneu-C-13 vaccine at minimum 8-week intervals beginning at 2 months of age, followed by a fourth dose at 12 to 15 months of age. For healthy infants, a three-dose schedule may be used, with doses at 2 months, 4 months, and 12 months of age. Children 2 years and above who are at highest risk of invasive pneumococcal disease should receive Pneu-P-23. Consult NACI guidelines for eligibility and dosing schedule.

- **Meningococcal vaccine:**
  - Canadian children should be immunized with a MCV-C at 12 months of age, or earlier depending on provincial/territorial vaccine programs; suggested one dose at 12 months of age.
  - MCV-4 (A, C, Y, W) should be given to children two months of age and older who are at increased risk for meningococcal disease or who have been in close contact with a case of invasive meningococcal A,C,Y or W disease. MCV-4-CRM (MenveoTM) should be used for those less than 2 years old; any MCV-4 may be used for older children.
  - A routine booster dose with MCV-4 or MCV-C is recommended at approximately 12 years of age. High risk children require boosters at 5 year intervals.
  - MCV-4 should be given to children two months of age and older travelling to areas where meningococcal vaccine is recommended. MCV-4 CRM is recommended for immunization of children 2 months to less than 2 years of age. Any MCV-4 may be used for older children.
  - Multi-component meningococcal serogroup B (4CMenB) vaccine should be considered for active immunization of children ≥ 2 months of age who are at high risk of meningococcal disease or who have been in close contact with a case of invasive meningococcal B disease or travelling to an area where risk of transmission of meningococcus B is high. Two to 3 doses are required at 4 or 8 wk intervals depending on age.
  - Routine prophylactic administration of acetaminophen after immunization and/or separating 4CMenB vaccination from routine vaccination schedule may be considered for preventing fever in infants and children up to 3 years of age.

- **Influenza vaccine:** Recommended for all children between 6 and 59 months of age, and for older high-risk children.
  - Previously unvaccinated children up to 9 years of age require 2 doses with an interval of at least 4 weeks. The second dose is not required if the child has received one or more doses of influenza vaccine during the previous immunization season. A quadrivalent vaccine should be used if available.
  - For children between 6 and 23 months, the quadrivalent inactivated influenza vaccine (QIV) should be used, and if not available, either unadjuvanted or adjuvanted trivalent inactivated vaccine (TIV).
  - Children 2-18 years of age should be given QIV, or quadrivalent live attenuated influenza vaccine (LAIV) if not contraindicated. Egg allergy is not a contraindication to vaccination with QIV, TIV, or LAIV.
  - Immunization with TIV or QIV in the second or third trimester to provide protection for the pregnant woman and infant <6 months of age.

- **Respiratory syncytial virus (RSV) vaccine:** Palivizumab (Synagis) prophylaxis during RSV season for children with chronic lung disease, congenital heart disease or born preterm.
Preventing hospitalizations for respiratory syncytial virus infection (CPS)

Disclaimer: Given the constantly evolving nature of evidence and changing recommendations, the Rourke Baby Record is meant to be used as a guide only.
Financial support has been provided by the Government of Ontario. For fair use authorization, see www.rourkebabyrecord.ca

EXHIBIT 1.1 Rourke Baby Record (*continued*)

©2017 Drs. L Rourke, D Leduc and J Rourke
Revised January 24, 2017
www.rourkebabyrecord.ca

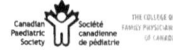 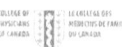 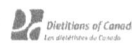

Rourke Baby Record: RESOURCES 4: (National)
Early Child Development and Parenting Resource System and Local Resources/Referrals Table

See RBR parent web portal for corresponding parent resources

Early Child Development and Parenting Resource System

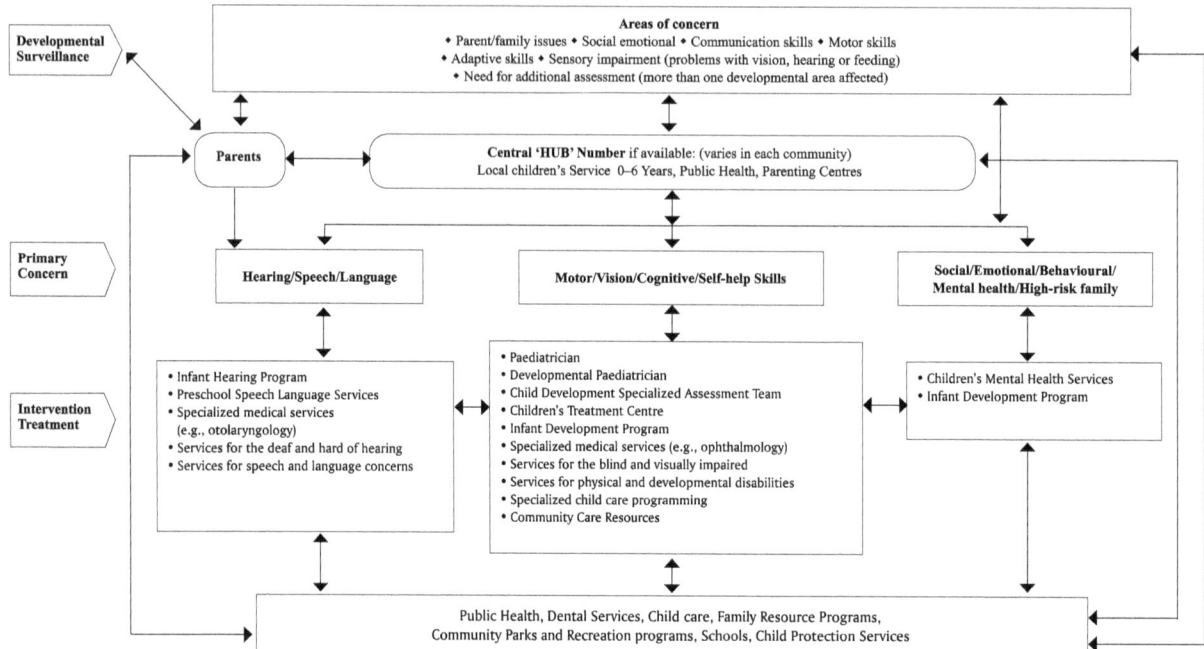

Local Resources and Referrals

Service	Contact person	Phone number	Website	Other

Disclaimer: Given the constantly evolving nature of evidence and changing recommendations, the Rourke Baby Record is meant to be used as a guide only. Financial support has been provided by the Government of Ontario. For fair use authorization, see www.rourkebabyrecord.ca

Source: The Rourke Baby Record, 2017 edition. www.rourkebabyrecord.ca. Accessed June 2019

EXHIBIT 1.2   Anticipatory Guidance

Immunizations: Refer to the *Canadian Immunization Guide* for recommended immunizations: www.canada.ca/en/public-health/services/canadian-immunization-guide.html.
For information related to immunization schedules in the provinces and territories, refer to the following: www.canada.ca/en/public-health/services/provincial-territorial-immunization-information.html.

Initial Visit: Two Weeks to One Month
A. *Safety*:
 1. Review sleeping position.
 2. Avoid placing newborn on top of tables, counters, bed. Discuss risk of fall.
 3. Avoid toys, pillows in crib.
 4. Discuss car seat safety. Use rear-facing car seat.

B. *Nutrition*:
 1. Breastfeeding with vitamin D supplementation or bottle-feeding.
 2. Feeding patterns/frequency.
 3. Regurgitation.
 4. Avoid propping bottles.

C. *Development*:
 1. Handling fussy periods.
 2. Soothing techniques: Music, reading.
 3. Reaction to pain.

D. *Health-Care Management*:
 1. Use of thermometer.
 2. Fever.
 3. Vomiting.
 4. Diarrhoea.
 5. Skin: Sun safety and insect protection.

E. *Family Dynamics*:
 1. The new role of parenting.
 2. Exhaustion. Screen for postpartum depression.
 3. Sleeping patterns of the newborn and parents.
 4. Sibling reactions, anticipated jealousy.

Two Months
A. *Safety*:
 1. Review sleeping habits.
 2. Use rails on cribs.
 3. Do not leave baby unattended (e.g., on bed, changing table).
 4. Discuss car seat safety.

B. *Nutrition*:
 1. Breastfeeding/formula intake.

C. *Development*:
 1. Head control.
 2. Eyes follow moving object to midline.

D. *Health-Care Management*:
 1. Use of thermometer.
 2. Fever.
 3. Vomiting.
 4. Diarrhoea.
 5. Skin: Sun and insect protection.

E. *Family Dynamics*:
 1. Child care.
 2. Relaxation and personal time for the parents.
 3. Sleeping patterns of infant and parents.
 4. Sibling rivalry/relationships.
 5. Screen for postpartum depression.

Four Months
A. *Safety*:
 1. Car seat safety.
 2. Choking, suffocation.
 3. Ways to assist in an emergency.
 4. Water safety: Do not leave baby unattended around water (e.g., tub, sink, bucket, pool).
 5. Use of safety gates.
 6. Poison control: Provide poison control number for parent.
 7. Covering electrical outlets.

B. *Nutrition*:
 1. Begin solids (infant cereal).
 2. Breastfeeding/formula intake.

C. *Development*:
 1. Sits with support.
 2. Follows moving object past midline.
 3. Social smile, squeals.
 4. Lifts head up.
 5. Rolls over supine to prone.

D. *Health-Care Management*:
 1. Patterns of sleep.
 2. Digestive changes.

E. *Family Dynamics*:
 1. Parents' time away.
 2. Child care.
 3. Sibling rivalry.
 4. Screen for postpartum depression.

Six Months
A. *Safety*:
 1. Review of four-month information.
 2. Car seat safety.
 3. Reinforce home safety.
 4. Security of chemicals, toxins, detergents.
 5. Use of cabinet and door locks, or gates for stairs.
 6. High-chair safety.
 7. Poison control phone number.

B. *Nutrition*:
 1. Breastfeeding/formula intake.
 2. Cereals/fruits/vegetable introduction.
 3. May introduce water.

C. *Development*:
 1. No head lag.
 2. Turns to rattle noise.
 3. Reaches toward object.
 4. Sits without support.
 5. Transfers object from hand to hand.
 6. Rolls over prone to supine.
 7. Shows stranger anxiety.

(continued)

EXHIBIT 1.2   **Anticipatory Guidance** (*continued*)

D. *Health-Care Management*:
  1. Dental care.
  2. Footwear.
E. *Family Dynamics*:
  1. Parents' time away.
  2. Child care.
  3. Sibling rivalry.
  4. Screen for postpartum depression.

Nine Months
A. *Safety*:
  1. Childproofing the home.
  2. Use of gates, locks, cabinet locks.
  3. Poison control phone number.
B. *Nutrition*:
  1. Breastfeeding/formula intake.
  2. Solid foods and choking hazards.
  3. Healthy snacks.
  4. Avoid sweetened drinks, encourage water only, restrict fruit juice.
C. *Development*:
  1. Takes two cubes, pincer grasp.
  2. Verbalizes "mama."
  3. Crawls, cruises.
  4. Weight-bearing legs.
  5. Imitates sound.
  6. Setting limits with "no."
D. *Health-Care Management*:
  1. Elimination patterns.
  2. Sleeping habits.
  3. Dental care.
  4. Screen for anaemia, if increased risk is identified.
E. *Family Dynamics*:
  1. Sibling interactions.
  2. Child care.

12 Months
A. *Safety*:
  1. Accident prevention (e.g., poison control, windows, outlets, and water).
  2. Poison control phone number.
B. *Nutrition*:
  1. Introduction to cow's milk.
  2. Use of cup.
  3. Solid food intake.
C. *Development*:
  1. Read books with caregiver.
  2. Playtime.
  3. Praising behaviour.
  4. Stranger and separation anxiety.
  5. Encourage speech.
  6. Walking.
D. *Health-Care Management*:
  1. Exercise.
  2. Elimination patterns.
  3. Sleeping habits.
  4. Dental care.
E. *Family Dynamics*:
  1. Sibling relationships.
  2. Child care.

15 Months
A. *Safety*:
  1. Accident prevention review.
  2. Water safety.
  3. Choking hazards.
  4. Plastic bags.
  5. Electrical safety.
B. *Nutrition*:
  1. Feeding patterns and habits.
  2. Dental care.
C. *Development*:
  1. Socialization-skills changing.
  2. Goes up steps in childlike manner.
  3. Bedtime routines.
  4. Looking at/reading books.
  5. Establishing hand preference.
D. *Health-Care Management*:
  1. Treating small injuries at home (e.g., abrasions and falls).
  2. Exercising/activities.
  3. Elimination patterns.
  4. Sleeping habits.
E. *Family Dynamics*:
  1. Child care.
  2. Parent relaxation/time alone.
  3. Extended family.

18 Months
A. *Safety*:
  1. Review 12-month information.
  2. Window safety.
  3. Falls.
B. *Nutrition*:
  1. Feeding patterns and habits.
  2. Dental care.
C. *Development*:
  1. Pretend play.
  2. Temper tantrums.
  3. Reinforce self-care.
  4. Self-comforting behaviour.
  5. Peer interactions/sharing skills.
  6. Kick, throw a ball.
D. *Health-Care Management*:
  1. Exercise/activity.
  2. Sleeping habits.
  3. Elimination patterns.
E. *Family Dynamics*:
  1. Child care.
  2. Parent relaxation/time alone.
  3. Extended family.

(*continued*)

EXHIBIT 1.2 Anticipatory Guidance (*continued*)

24 Months
A. *Safety*:
1. Review 18-month information.
2. Crib-to-bed transition.
3. Car seat and helmet safety.
4. Water safety.
5. Storage of hazardous household supplies.
6. Poison control.
7. Street safety.
8. Playground (e.g., slides, swings, and bikes).
9. Firearm safety.
10. Climbing.
11. Lighters and matches.
12. Motorized toys.
13. Electronic media (e.g., screen time and hearing protection).

B. *Nutrition*:
1. Fun foods to eat.
2. Feeding habits/daily intake.
3. Dental care.

C. *Development*:
1. Peer interaction.
2. Toileting habits.
3. Common routines for eating.
4. Bedtime routines.
5. Story time.
6. Praising good behaviour.
7. Two-word sentences, knowledge of approximately 250 words.

D. *Health-Care Management*:
1. Lead screening.
2. Skin care.
3. Elimination and voiding habits.

E. *Family Dynamics*:
1. Day care/child care.
2. Extended family interactions.
3. Sibling rivalry.

Three to Four Years
A. *Safety*:
1. Review 24-month information.

B. *Nutrition*:
1. Daily dietary intake.
2. Healthy snacks.

C. *Development*:
1. Pretend play.
2. Fears.
3. Fantasy.
4. Sleeping habits (night terrors).
5. Setting realistic limits.
6. Praising good behaviour.
7. Reading.
8. Music.
9. Child care.

D. *Health-Care Management*:
1. Dental.
2. Vision.
3. Hearing.
4. Speech evaluation.
5. Lead screen.

E. *Family Dynamics*:
1. Sibling rivalry.
2. Child care.
3. Parent time alone/relaxation.

Five to Six Years
A. *Safety*:
1. Review relevant topics as discussed at previous visits.
2. Safety with strangers.
3. Trampoline safety.

B. *Nutrition*:
1. Healthy eating habits.
2. Healthy snacks.

C. *Development*:
1. School readiness.
2. Sexual curiosity.
3. Peer interactions.
4. Good health habits (e.g., dental, diet, exercise, and sleep).
5. Praise good behaviour.
6. Adult role models.
7. Fears.
8. Lying.

D. *Health-Care Management*:
1. Dental.
2. Vision.
3. Hearing.

E. *Family Dynamics*:
1. Family traditions.
2. Changes in the family household (e.g., pets, moving, and divorce).
3. Sibling rivalry.
4. Extended family interactions.

10 Years
A. *Safety*:
1. Review relevant topics as discussed at previous visits.
2. Car and bike safety.
3. Pedestrian safety.

B. *Nutrition*:
1. Daily intake.
2. Healthy snacks.
3. Healthy nutrition for athletes.

(*continued*)

EXHIBIT 1.2 **Anticipatory Guidance** (*continued*)

C. *Development*:
1. School adjustments.
2. Social interactions.
3. Communications skills.
4. Health habits. Review relevant topics as previously discussed at five to six years visit.
5. Menstrual issues (female).

D. *Health-Care Management*:
1. Vision.
2. Hearing.
3. Scoliosis.

E. *Family Dynamics*:
1. Sibling rivalry.
2. Extended family.
3. Parenting.
4. Family responsibilities/chores.
5. Family rituals.
6. Changes in family household (e.g., pets, moving, and divorce).

15 Years

A. *Safety*:
1. Stranger awareness.
2. Car and bike safety.
3. Cyber awareness.
4. Review relevant topics as previously discussed at 10 years visit.

B. *Nutrition*:
1. Diet, healthy habits.

C. *Development*:
1. Relationships with peers.
2. Body image.
3. Sexuality.
4. Self-esteem.
5. Peer pressure.
6. Decision-making.

7. Role models.
8. School adjustments.
9. Extracurricular activities (e.g., sports, hobbies, and exercise).
10. Drug, alcohol, tobacco use.
11. Suicide.

D. *Health-Care Management*:
1. CPR.
2. Emergency numbers.
3. Skin care.
4. Vision.
5. Hearing.
6. Scoliosis.

E. *Family Dynamics*:
1. Change in family household (e.g., pets, moving, and divorce).
2. Family responsibilities/chores.
3. Identifying role models.
4. Family events.
5. Earning an allowance.

Sources: American Academy of Family Physicians, American Academy of Pediatrics, American College of Sports Medicine, American Medical Society for Sports Medicine. (2010). *Preparticipation physical evaluation* (4th ed.). Elk Grove Village, IL: American Academy of Pediatrics. Copyright © 2010 American Academy of Pediatrics. Canadian Paediatric Society & College of Family Physicians of Canada. (2016). *Greig health record*. Retrieved from https://www.cps.ca/en/tools-outils/greig-health-record; Rourke, L., Leduc, D., & Rourke, J. (2017, January). *Rourke baby record: Evidence-based infant/child health maintenance*. Retrieved from http://www.rourkebabyrecord.ca/pdf/RBR%202017%20National%20English%20-%20Black%2017 0926.pdf.

TABLE 1.1 Nutrition for Kids: Guidelines for a Healthy Diet

	Daily Guidelines for Ages 2–3 Years	Daily Guidelines for Ages 4–8 Years		Daily Guidelines for Ages 9–13 Years		Daily Guidelines for Ages 14–18 Years	
	Girls and Boys	Girls	Boys	Girls	Boys	Girls	Boys
Calories dependent on growth and activity level	1,000–1,400	1,200–1,800	1,200–2,000	1,400–2,200	1,600–2,600	1,800–2,400	2,000–3,200
Protein	2–4 oz.	3–5 oz.	3–5.5 oz.	4–6 oz.	5–6.5 oz.	5–6.5 oz.	5.5–7 oz.
Fruits	1–1.5 cups	1–1.5 cups	1–2 cups	1.5–2 cups	1.5–2 cups	1.5–2 cups	2–2.5 cups
Vegetables	1–1.5 cups	1.5–2.5 cups	1.5–2.5 cups	1.5–3 cups	2–3.5 cups	2.5–3 cups	2.5–4 cups
Grains	3–5 oz.	4–6 oz.	4–6 oz.	5–7 oz.	5–9 oz.	6–8 oz.	6–10 oz.
Dairy	2–2.5 cups	2.5–3 cups	2.5–3 cups	2.5–3 cups	3 cups	3 cups	3 cups

Notes: **Protein:** Choose seafood, lean meat and poultry, eggs, beans, peas, soy products, and unsalted nuts and seeds.
Fruits: Encourage your child to eat a variety of fresh, canned, frozen, or dried fruits.
Vegetables: Serve a variety of fresh, canned, or frozen vegetables—especially dark-green, red, and orange vegetables; beans; and peas.
Grains: Choose whole grains, such as whole-wheat bread, oatmeal, popcorn, quinoa, or brown or wild rice.
Dairy: Encourage your child to eat and drink fat-free or low-fat dairy products, such as milk, yogurt, cheese, or fortified soy beverages.
Source: Reprinted with permission from the Mayo Foundation for Medical Education and Research. (2017, June). *Nutrition for kids: Guidelines for a healthy diet.* Retrieved from http://www.mayoclinic.com/health/nutrition-for-kids/NU00606. All rights reserved.

TABLE 1.2 Recommended Number of Food Servings per Day

	Children			Teens		Adults			
	2–3 Years	4–8 Years	9–13 Years	14–18 Years		19–50 Years		51+ Years	
	Girls and Boys		Boys	Female	Male	Female	Male	Female	Male
Vegetables and fruits	4	5	6	7	8	7–8	8–10	7	7
Grain products	3	4	6	6	7	6–7	8	6	7
Milk and alternatives	2	2	3–4	3–4	2	2	3	3	3
Meat and alternatives	1	1	1–2	2	3	2	3	2	3

Source: © All rights reserved. Eating Well with Canada's Food Guide. Health Canada, 2007. Adapted and reproduced with permission from the Minister of Health, 2019.

TABLE 1.3   Food Sources for Common Vitamin and Mineral Deficiencies

Common Nutritional Deficiencies	Food Sources
Calcium	Dairy sources of calcium include yogurt and cheese.
	Nondairy sources of calcium are vegetables, including kale, broccoli, and Chinese cabbage.
	Calcium is also found in fortified sources, including breakfast cereals, fruit juices, and tofu.
Folate	Found naturally in vegetables (especially dark-green leafy vegetables), fruits, fruit juices, nuts, beans, peas, dairy products, poultry and meat, eggs, seafood, and grains.
	In January 1998, the U.S. Food and Drug Administration began requiring manufacturers to add folic acid to enriched breads, cereals, flours, cornmeal, pasta, rice, and other grain products.
Iron	Haeme iron is found in animal foods that originally contained haemoglobin, including red meat, fish, and poultry.
	Nonhaeme iron is found in plant foods, including lentils and beans.
	Iron is also found in fortified ready-to-eat cereals.
Magnesium	Widely distributed in plant and animal foods, including green leafy vegetables, legumes, nuts (almonds, peanuts, and cashews), seeds, and whole grains.
	Magnesium is also found in fortified breakfast cereals.
Vitamin A	Concentrations of preformed vitamin A are highest in liver, fish oils, leafy green vegetables, orange and yellow vegetables, tomato products, fruits, and some vegetable oils.
	Vitamin A is also found in fortified breakfast cereals.
Vitamin B6	Richest sources include fish; beef, liver, and other organ meats; potatoes and other starchy vegetables such as chickpeas; and fruit (except for citrus).
	Vitamin B6 is also found in fortified breakfast cereals.
Vitamin B12	Found naturally in animal products, including fish, meat, poultry, eggs, and milk and milk products.
	Generally not present in plant foods.
	Vitamin B12 is found in fortified breakfast cereals.
Vitamin D	Very few foods in nature contain vitamin D; it is found primarily in fortified foods.
	Almost all of the U.S. milk supply is voluntarily fortified with vitamin D.
	Both the United States and Canada mandate the fortification of infant formula with vitamin D.
Vitamin E	Found in nuts and seeds (sunflower seeds, almonds, hazelnuts, and peanuts), green leafy vegetables, and vegetable oils.
	Vitamin E is found in fortified breakfast cereals.
Zinc	Red meat and poultry provide the majority of zinc in American diets; however, oysters contain more zinc per serving than any other food. Other food sources include beans, nuts, seafood (crab and lobster), and dairy products.
	Zinc is also found in fortified breakfast cereals.

Source: National Institutes of Health, Office of Dietary Supplements. (2015). *Food sources for common vitamin and mineral deficiencies*. Retrieved from https://ods.od.nih.gov/factsheets/Mvms-HealthProfessional/.

Client Education Before Exercise

All exercise program prescriptions should include frequency, duration, intensity. Persons should be educated on the signs and symptoms of heat exhaustion and should be advised when to seek first aid. Visit the Canadian Society of Exercise Physiology (2019) website for the most up-to-date recommendations for early years, children and youth, adults, and older adults at https://csepguidelines.ca/.

Women engaged in regular physical exercise before pregnancy may safely continue exercise throughout pregnancy. The target heart rate for a pregnant woman during exercise should not exceed 140 beats per minute. Activities should also be limited to low-impact aerobics and activities that do not require agility, because a woman's center of balance changes throughout pregnancy, leaving the woman at risk of falling and injury.

Swimming is ideal for upper and lower body conditioning, with low impact on joints. Swimming is not well suited for women at risk of osteoporosis, because it is not a weight-bearing exercise. Examples of weight-bearing exercise to help prevent osteoporosis include dancing, impact aerobics, and resistance training.

For exercise to benefit individuals, it must be continued lifelong. The health-care provider should evaluate individual lifestyle and preferences in designing an exercise program. One exercise program can become boring over a period and probably will not be continued. Cross-training with a variety of sports and activities will decrease boredom, decrease the risk of overuse injuries, increase participation, and provide positive reinforcement help to keep physical activity fun as an integral part of a healthy lifestyle.

Health-care professionals who will be monitoring and prescribing exercise plans for large numbers of individuals are encouraged to seek special training and certification.

Adult and Older Adult Periodic Health Examination

Adult Risk Assessment

The Adult Risk Assessment Form (Exhibit 1.4) should be used for all adults and older adults as part of an initial assessment with new clients. It is used to evaluate risk for particular diseases. The practitioner should interview the client, assessing for the risk factors listed on the Adult Risk Assessment Form. The family history of first-degree relatives (parents, siblings, and children) should also be discussed, as many diseases are related to genetic factors. Keep a copy of the Adult Risk Assessment Form in the front of the client's chart, or the information might be gathered in personal and family history component of the client's electronic medical record. The information should be updated at periodic health examinations or as needed. When complete, this tool may guide the practitioner in determining periodic health screening. Many electronic medical record or electronic charting systems will have a preventative screening function or window that tracks when periodic screening is due.

Adult Preventive Health Care

The Preventive Care Checklist Forms take an evidence-informed approach to the periodic health examination. The traditional annual physical examination is not supported by evidence and has the potential for more harm than good. Planning periodic visits that take more of a health promotion/disease prevention approach and includes screening based on age, gender, and risk factors is in keeping with best practice. This "less is more" approach is endorsed by Choosing Wisely Canada, an organization committed to decreasing unnecessary tests and treatments where there are recommendation specifically for family medicine and nurse practitioner practice: choosingwiselycanada.org/.

Screening guidelines for each of these can be found in the associated chapters in this book and are informed by national clinical practice guidelines and the Canadian Task Force on Preventive Health Care.

The Canadian College of Family Physicians offers excellent resources including adult female and male periodic health examination forms that are updated regularly, and are informed by best current evidence for health maintenance (e.g., immunization, laboratory work, physical examination, and health promotion). The most current version of the preventive health care forms can be found at https://www.cfpc.ca/projectassets/templates/resource.aspx?id=1184&langType=4105. Additional evidence informed screening guidelines can be found on the Canadian Task Force for Preventive Health Care website at https://canadiantaskforce.ca/ or through their app.

Immunizations The Public Health Agency of Canada (PHAC) is the primary source for the current immunization and catch-up schedules, in addition to provincial ministries of health. The *Canadian Immunization Guide* is available online at www.canada.ca/en/public-health/services/canadian-immunization-guide.html.

This guide has 54 chapters. Chapters are updated as new evidence becomes available. It is organized into five sections:
- Key immunization information.
- Vaccine safety.
- Vaccination of specific populations.
- Active vaccines.
- Passive immunization.

Immunizations for Travel The PHAC recommends certain vaccines to protect travelers from illnesses present in other parts of the world and to protect others on return to Canada. The government of Canada's travel vaccination information can be found at travel.gc.ca/travelling/health-safety/vaccines, an interactive website to individualize the needs of travelers to their specific destination. Vaccinations required are dependent on several factors.

A. Travel destination.
B. Travel season.
C. Age.
D. Pregnancy or breastfeeding.
E. Traveling with infants or children.
F. Immunocompetent secondary to diabetes or HIV.

Medication Use in Older Adults It is important to conduct a comprehensive medication review when completing periodic health examinations with older adults. Visit the Canadian Deprescribing Network for tools to reduce medication use in older adults: www.deprescribingnetwork.ca/algorithms.

Bibliography

American Academy of Family Physicians, American Academy of Pediatrics, American College of Sports Medicine, American Medical Society for Sports Medicine. (2010). *Preparticipation physical evaluation* (4th ed.). Elk Grove Village, IL: American Academy of Pediatrics.

Birtwhistle, R., Bell, N., Thombs, B., Grad, R., & Dickinson, J. (2017). Periodic preventative health visits: A more appropriate approach to delivering preventative services. *Canadian Family Physician, 63*(11), 824–826. Retrieved from http://www.cfp.ca

Canadian Paediatric Society & College of Family Physicians of Canada. (2016). *Greig health record*. Retrieved from https://www.cps.ca/en/tools-outils/greig-health-record

Canadian Society for Exercise Physiology. (2017). *Canadian 24-hour movement guidelines: An integration of physical activity, sedentary behavior, and sleep*. Retrieved from http://csepguidelines.ca/

Canadian Deprescribing Network. (2019). *Deprescribing algorithms*. Retrieved from www.deprescribingnetwork.ca/algorithms

Dietitians of Canada. (2016). *Prevalence, severity and impact of household food insecurity: A serious public health issue*. [Background Paper]. Retrieved from https://www.dietitians.ca/Dietitians-Views/Food-Security/Household-Food-Insecurity.aspx

Dubey, V., Mathew, R., Iglar, K., & Duerksen, A. (2015). Preventive Care Checklist Forms. Retrieved from https://www.cfpc.ca/ProjectAssets/Templates/Resource.aspx?id=1184&langType=4105

Government of Canada. (2018a, December). *Canadian immunization guide*. Retrieved from https://www.canada.ca/en/public-health/services/canadian-immunization-guide.html

Government of Canada. (2018b, December). *Health, food & nutrition. Healthy eating. Canada's food guides. Food guide basics. How much food you need every day*. Retrieved from http://www.hc-sc.gc.ca/fn-an/food-guide-aliment/basics-base/quantit-eng.php

Greig, A., Constantin, E., LeBlanc, C., Riverin, B., Tak-Sam, P., Cummings, C., . . . Canadian Paediatric Society Community Paediatrics Committee. (2016). An update to the greig health record: Executive summary. *Paediatric Child Health, 21*(5), 265–268. Retrieved from https://www.cps.ca/en/documents/position/greig-executive-summary

Hamilton, N., & Bhatti, T. (1996). *Population health promotion: An integrated model of population health and health promotion*. Ottawa, ON, Canada: Government of Canada. Retrieved from https://www.canada.ca/en/public-health/services/health-promotion/population-health/population-health-promotion-integrated-model-population-health-health-promotion.html

Health Canada. (2007). *Eating well with Canada's food guide*. Retrieved from www.hc-sc.gc.ca/fn-an/food-guide-aliment/order-commander/eating_well_bien_manger-eng.php

Mayo Foundation for Medical Education and Research. (2016, January). *Nutrition for kids: Guidelines for a healthy diet*. Retrieved from http://www.mayoclinic.com/health/nutrition-for-kids/NU00606

Miller, N., Reicks, M., Redden, J. P., Mann, T., Mykerezi, E., & Vickers, Z. (2015). Increasing portion sizes of fruits and vegetables in an elementary school lunch program can increase fruit and vegetable consumption. *Appetite, 91*, 426–430. doi:10.1016/j.appet.2015.04.081

Mirabelli, M. H., Devine, M. J., Singh, J., & Mendoza, M. (2015). The preparticipation sports evaluation. *American Family Physician, 92*(5), 371–376. Retrieved from https://www.aafp.org/journals/afp.html

National Heart Lung and Blood Institute. (n.d.). *Obesity education initiative: BMI calculator*. Retrieved from http://www.nhlbi.nih.gov/health/educational/lose_wt/BMI/bmicalc.htm

Ritchie, C. (2015, October 22). Geriatric nutrition: Nutritional issues in older adults. *UpToDate*. Retrieved from http://www.uptodate.com/contents/geriatric-nutrition-nutritional-issues-in-older-adults

Rourke, L., Leduc, D., & Rourke, J. (2017). *Rourke baby record: Evidence-based infant/child health maintenance*. Retrieved from http://www.rourkebabyrecord.ca/downloads

Sanders, B., Blackburn, T. A., & Boucher, B. (2013). Preparticipation screening: The sports physical therapy perspective. *International Journal of Sports Physical Therapy, 8*(2), 180–193. Retrieved from https://spts.org/member-benefits-detail/enjoy-member-benefits/journals/ijspt

Sharma, S., Merghani, A., & Gati, S. (2015). Cardiac screening of young athletes prior to participation in sports: Difficulties in detecting the fatally flawed among the abulously fit. *JAMA Internal Medicine, 175*(1), 125–127. doi:10.1001/jamainternmed.2014.6023

Warburton, D., Jamnik, V., Bredin, S., McKenzie, D., Stone, J., Shephard, R., . . . Gledhill, N. (2011). Evidence-based risk assessment and recommendations for physical activity clearance: An introduction. *Applied Physiology Nutrition and Metabolism, 36*, S1–S2. doi:10.1139/H11-060

Interprofessional Collaborative Practice

Margaret Ellen Rauliuk

Most primary care providers' work as part of a larger, integrated team that embrace the five foundations for integrated care: patient-centred care; access; informational continuity; management continuity; and relational continuity with the overall goal of "better health, better care, and better value for Canadians" (Canadian Nurses Association, Canadian Medical Association & Health Action Lobby, 2013). Interprofessional primary care teams can include RNs, nurse practitioners, family physicians, respiratory therapists, physiotherapists, dietitians, dentists, optometrists, and others. Interprofessional competencies required to achieve effective interprofessional collaboration include role clarification, interprofessional conflict resolution, collaborative leadership, and attention to team functioning. For more information, review the National Interprofessional Competency Framework (Canadian Interprofessional Health Collaborative, 2010) at https://www.cihc.ca/files/CIHC_IPCompetencies_Feb1210.pdf.

Bibliography

Canadian Interprofessional Health Collaborative. (2010). A National Interprofessional Competency Framework. Retrieved from https://www.cihc.ca/files/CIHC_IPCompetencies_Feb1210.pdf

Canadian Nurses Association, Canadian Medical Association, & Health Action Lobby. (2013). Integration: A new direction for Canadian health care. Retrieved from https://www.cna-aiic.ca/-/media/cna/files/en/cna_cma_heal_provider_summit_transformation_to_integrated_care_e.pdf?la=en&hash=094811D94F0487A196901715B5FE14516ACA194E

Hamilton, N., & Bhatti, T. (1996). *Population health promotion: An integrated model of population health and health promotion*. Ottawa, ON, Canada: Government of Canada. Retrieved from https://www.canada.ca/en/public-health/services/health-promotion/population-health/population-health-promotion-integrated-model-population-health-health-promotion.html

EXHIBIT 1-3 ParMed-X Questionnaire

2018 PAR-Q+

The Physical Activity Readiness Questionnaire for Everyone

The health benefits of regular physical activity are clear; more people should engage in physical activity every day of the week. Participating in physical activity is very safe for MOST people. This questionnaire will tell you whether it is necessary for you to seek further advice from your doctor OR a qualified exercise professional before becoming more physically active.

GENERAL HEALTH QUESTIONS

Please read the 7 questions below carefully and answer each one honestly: check YES or NO.	YES	NO
1) Has your doctor ever said that you have a heart condition ☐ OR high blood pressure ☐?	☐	☐
2) Do you feel pain in your chest at rest, during your daily activities of living, **OR** when you do physical activity?	☐	☐
3) Do you lose balance because of dizziness **OR** have you lost consciousness in the last 12 months? Please answer **NO** if your dizziness was associated with over-breathing (including during vigorous exercise).	☐	☐
4) Have you ever been diagnosed with another chronic medical condition (other than heart disease or high blood pressure)? **PLEASE LIST CONDITION(S) HERE:** _____	☐	☐
5) Are you currently taking prescribed medications for a chronic medical condition? **PLEASE LIST CONDITION(S) AND MEDICATIONS HERE:** _____	☐	☐
6) Do you currently have (or have had within the past 12 months) a bone, joint, or soft tissue (muscle, ligament, or tendon) problem that could be made worse by becoming more physically active? Please answer **NO** if you had a problem in the past, but it *does not limit your current ability* to be physically active. **PLEASE LIST CONDITION(S) HERE:** _____	☐	☐
7) Has your doctor ever said that you should only do medically supervised physical activity?	☐	☐

☑ **If you answered NO to all of the questions above, you are cleared for physical activity.**
Please sign the PARTICIPANT DECLARATION. You do not need to complete Pages 2 and 3.

- Start becoming much more physically active – start slowly and build up gradually.
- Follow International Physical Activity Guidelines for your age (www.who.int/dietphysicalactivity/en/).
- You may take part in a health and fitness appraisal.
- If you are over the age of 45 yr and NOT accustomed to regular vigorous to maximal effort exercise, consult a qualified exercise professional before engaging in this intensity of exercise.
- If you have any further questions, contact a qualified exercise professional.

PARTICIPANT DECLARATION
If you are less than the legal age required for consent or require the assent of a care provider, your parent, guardian or care provider must also sign this form.

I, the undersigned, have read, understood to my full satisfaction and completed this questionnaire. I acknowledge that this physical activity clearance is valid for a maximum of 12 months from the date it is completed and becomes invalid if my condition changes. I also acknowledge that the community/fitness centre may retain a copy of this form for records. In these instances, it will maintain the confidentiality of the same, complying with applicable law.

NAME _____ DATE _____

SIGNATURE _____ WITNESS _____

SIGNATURE OF PARENT/GUARDIAN/CARE PROVIDER _____

● **If you answered YES to one or more of the questions above, COMPLETE PAGES 2 AND 3.**

⚠ **Delay becoming more active if:**
- You have a temporary illness such as a cold or fever; it is best to wait until you feel better.
- You are pregnant - talk to your health care practitioner, your physician, a qualified exercise professional, and/or complete the ePARmed-X+ at **www.eparmedx.com** before becoming more physically active.
- Your health changes - answer the questions on Pages 2 and 3 of this document and/or talk to your doctor or a qualified exercise professional before continuing with any physical activity program.

(continued)

EXHIBIT 1.3 ParMed-X Questionnaire (*continued*)

2018 PAR-Q+

FOLLOW-UP QUESTIONS ABOUT YOUR MEDICAL CONDITION(S)

1.	**Do you have Arthritis, Osteoporosis, or Back Problems?**	
	If the above condition(s) is/are present, answer questions 1a-1c If **NO** ☐ go to question 2	
1a.	Do you have difficulty controlling your condition with medications or other physician-prescribed therapies? (Answer **NO** if you are not currently taking medications or other treatments)	YES ☐ NO ☐
1b.	Do you have joint problems causing pain, a recent fracture or fracture caused by osteoporosis or cancer, displaced vertebra (e.g., spondylolisthesis), and/or spondylolysis/pars defect (a crack in the bony ring on the back of the spinal column)?	YES ☐ NO ☐
1c.	Have you had steroid injections or taken steroid tablets regularly for more than 3 months?	YES ☐ NO ☐
2.	**Do you currently have Cancer of any kind?**	
	If the above condition(s) is/are present, answer questions 2a-2b If **NO** ☐ go to question 3	
2a.	Does your cancer diagnosis include any of the following types: lung/bronchogenic, multiple myeloma (cancer of plasma cells), head, and/or neck?	YES ☐ NO ☐
2b.	Are you currently receiving cancer therapy (such as chemotheraphy or radiotherapy)?	YES ☐ NO ☐
3.	**Do you have a Heart or Cardiovascular Condition?** *This includes Coronary Artery Disease, Heart Failure, Diagnosed Abnormality of Heart Rhythm*	
	If the above condition(s) is/are present, answer questions 3a-3d If **NO** ☐ go to question 4	
3a.	Do you have difficulty controlling your condition with medications or other physician-prescribed therapies? (Answer **NO** if you are not currently taking medications or other treatments)	YES ☐ NO ☐
3b.	Do you have an irregular heart beat that requires medical management? (e.g., atrial fibrillation, premature ventricular contraction)	YES ☐ NO ☐
3c.	Do you have chronic heart failure?	YES ☐ NO ☐
3d.	Do you have diagnosed coronary artery (cardiovascular) disease and have not participated in regular physical activity in the last 2 months?	YES ☐ NO ☐
4.	**Do you have High Blood Pressure?**	
	If the above condition(s) is/are present, answer questions 4a-4b If **NO** ☐ go to question 5	
4a.	Do you have difficulty controlling your condition with medications or other physician-prescribed therapies? (Answer **NO** if you are not currently taking medications or other treatments)	YES ☐ NO ☐
4b.	Do you have a resting blood pressure equal to or greater than 160/90 mmHg with or without medication? (Answer **YES** if you do not know your resting blood pressure)	YES ☐ NO ☐
5.	**Do you have any Metabolic Conditions?** *This includes Type 1 Diabetes, Type 2 Diabetes, Pre-Diabetes*	
	If the above condition(s) is/are present, answer questions 5a-5e If **NO** ☐ go to question 6	
5a.	Do you often have difficulty controlling your blood sugar levels with foods, medications, or other physician-prescribed therapies?	YES ☐ NO ☐
5b.	Do you often suffer from signs and symptoms of low blood sugar (hypoglycemia) following exercise and/or during activities of daily living? Signs of hypoglycemia may include shakiness, nervousness, unusual irritability, abnormal sweating, dizziness or light-headedness, mental confusion, difficulty speaking, weakness, or sleepiness.	YES ☐ NO ☐
5c.	Do you have any signs or symptoms of diabetes complications such as heart or vascular disease and/or complications affecting your eyes, kidneys, **OR** the sensation in your toes and feet?	YES ☐ NO ☐
5d.	Do you have other metabolic conditions (such as current pregnancy-related diabetes, chronic kidney disease, or liver problems)?	YES ☐ NO ☐
5e.	Are you planning to engage in what for you is unusually high (or vigorous) intensity exercise in the near future?	YES ☐ NO ☐

EXHIBIT 1.3 ParMed-X Questionnaire (*continued*)

2018 PAR-Q+

6.	**Do you have any Mental Health Problems or Learning Difficulties?** *This includes Alzheimer's, Dementia, Depression, Anxiety Disorder, Eating Disorder, Psychotic Disorder, Intellectual Disability, Down Syndrome*	
	If the above condition(s) is/are present, answer questions 6a-6b If **NO** ☐ go to question 7	
6a.	Do you have difficulty controlling your condition with medications or other physician-prescribed therapies? (Answer **NO** if you are not currently taking medications or other treatments)	YES ☐ NO ☐
6b.	Do you have Down Syndrome **AND** back problems affecting nerves or muscles?	YES ☐ NO ☐
7.	**Do you have a Respiratory Disease?** *This includes Chronic Obstructive Pulmonary Disease, Asthma, Pulmonary High Blood Pressure*	
	If the above condition(s) is/are present, answer questions 7a-7d If **NO** ☐ go to question 8	
7a.	Do you have difficulty controlling your condition with medications or other physician-prescribed therapies? (Answer **NO** if you are not currently taking medications or other treatments)	YES ☐ NO ☐
7b.	Has your doctor ever said your blood oxygen level is low at rest or during exercise and/or that you require supplemental oxygen therapy?	YES ☐ NO ☐
7c.	If asthmatic, do you currently have symptoms of chest tightness, wheezing, laboured breathing, consistent cough (more than 2 days/week), or have you used your rescue medication more than twice in the last week?	YES ☐ NO ☐
7d.	Has your doctor ever said you have high blood pressure in the blood vessels of your lungs?	YES ☐ NO ☐
8.	**Do you have a Spinal Cord Injury?** *This includes Tetraplegia and Paraplegia*	
	If the above condition(s) is/are present, answer questions 8a-8c If **NO** ☐ go to question 9	
8a.	Do you have difficulty controlling your condition with medications or other physician-prescribed therapies? (Answer **NO** if you are not currently taking medications or other treatments)	YES ☐ NO ☐
8b.	Do you commonly exhibit low resting blood pressure significant enough to cause dizziness, light-headedness, and/or fainting?	YES ☐ NO ☐
8c.	Has your physician indicated that you exhibit sudden bouts of high blood pressure (known as Autonomic Dysreflexia)?	YES ☐ NO ☐
9.	**Have you had a Stroke?** *This includes Transient Ischemic Attack (TIA) or Cerebrovascular Event*	
	If the above condition(s) is/are present, answer questions 9a-9c If **NO** ☐ go to question 10	
9a.	Do you have difficulty controlling your condition with medications or other physician-prescribed therapies? (Answer **NO** if you are not currently taking medications or other treatments)	YES ☐ NO ☐
9b.	Do you have any impairment in walking or mobility?	YES ☐ NO ☐
9c.	Have you experienced a stroke or impairment in nerves or muscles in the past 6 months?	YES ☐ NO ☐
10.	**Do you have any other medical condition not listed above or do you have two or more medical conditions?**	
	If you have other medical conditions, answer questions 10a-10c If **NO** ☐ read the Page 4 recommendations	
10a.	Have you experienced a blackout, fainted, or lost consciousness as a result of a head injury within the last 12 months **OR** have you had a diagnosed concussion within the last 12 months?	YES ☐ NO ☐
10b.	Do you have a medical condition that is not listed (such as epilepsy, neurological conditions, kidney problems)?	YES ☐ NO ☐
10c.	Do you currently live with two or more medical conditions?	YES ☐ NO ☐
	PLEASE LIST YOUR MEDICAL CONDITION(S) AND ANY RELATED MEDICATIONS HERE: _____	

GO to Page 4 for recommendations about your current medical condition(s) and sign the PARTICIPANT DECLARATION.

EXHIBIT 1.3 ParMed-X Questionnaire (*continued*)

2018 PAR-Q+

 If you answered NO to all of the FOLLOW-UP questions (pgs. 2-3) about your medical condition, you are ready to become more physically active - sign the PARTICIPANT DECLARATION below:

- ▶ It is advised that you consult a qualified exercise professional to help you develop a safe and effective physical activity plan to meet your health needs.
- ▶ You are encouraged to start slowly and build up gradually - 20 to 60 minutes of low to moderate intensity exercise, 3-5 days per week including aerobic and muscle strengthening exercises.
- ▶ As you progress, you should aim to accumulate 150 minutes or more of moderate intensity physical activity per week.
- ▶ If you are over the age of 45 yr and **NOT** accustomed to regular vigorous to maximal effort exercise, consult a qualified exercise professional before engaging in this intensity of exercise.

 If you answered YES to one or more of the follow-up questions about your medical condition:
You should seek further information before becoming more physically active or engaging in a fitness appraisal. You should complete the specially designed online screening and exercise recommendations program - the **ePARmed-X+ at www.eparmedx.com** and/or visit a qualified exercise professional to work through the ePARmed-X+ and for further information.

⚠ **Delay becoming more active if:**

- You have a temporary illness such as a cold or fever; it is best to wait until you feel better.
- You are pregnant - talk to your health care practitioner, your physician, a qualified exercise professional, and/or complete the ePARmed-X+ **at www.eparmedx.com** before becoming more physically active.
- Your health changes - talk to your doctor or qualified exercise professional before continuing with any physical activity program.

- You are encouraged to photocopy the PAR-Q+. You must use the entire questionnaire and NO changes are permitted.
- The authors, the PAR-Q+ Collaboration, partner organizations, and their agents assume no liability for persons who undertake physical activity and/or make use of the PAR-Q+ or ePARmed-X+. If in doubt after completing the questionnaire, consult your doctor prior to physical activity.

PARTICIPANT DECLARATION

- All persons who have completed the PAR-Q+ please read and sign the declaration below.
- If you are less than the legal age required for consent or require the assent of a care provider, your parent, guardian or care provider must also sign this form.

I, the undersigned, have read, understood to my full satisfaction and completed this questionnaire. I acknowledge that this physical activity clearance is valid for a maximum of 12 months from the date it is completed and becomes invalid if my condition changes. I also acknowledge that the community/fitness center may retain a copy of this form for records. In these instances, it will maintain the confidentiality of the same, complying with applicable law.

NAME _____ DATE _____

SIGNATURE _____ WITNESS _____

SIGNATURE OF PARENT/GUARDIAN/CARE PROVIDER _____

For more information, please contact
www.eparmedx.com
Email: eparmedx@gmail.com

Citation for PAR-Q+
Warburton DER, Jamnik VK, Bredin SSD, and Gledhill N on behalf of the PAR-Q+ Collaboration. The Physical Activity Readiness Questionnaire for Everyone (PAR-Q+) and Electronic Physical Activity Readiness Medical Examination (ePARmed-X+). Health & Fitness Journal of Canada 4(2):3-23, 2011.

Key References
1. Jamnik VK, Warburton DER, Makarski J, McKenzie DC, Shephard RJ, Stone J, and Gledhill N. Enhancing the effectiveness of clearance for physical activity participation; background and overall process. APNM 36(S1):S3-S13, 2011.
2. Warburton DER, Gledhill N, Jamnik VK, Bredin SSD, McKenzie DC, Stone J, Charlesworth S, and Shephard RJ. Evidence-based risk assessment and recommendations for physical activity clearance; Consensus Document. APNM 36(S1):S266-s298, 2011.
3. Chisholm DM, Collis ML, Kulak LL, Davenport W, and Gruber N. Physical activity readiness. British Columbia Medical Journal. 1975;17:375-378.
4. Thomas S, Reading J, and Shephard RJ. Revision of the Physical Activity Readiness Questionnaire (PAR-Q). Canadian Journal of Sport Science 1992;17:4 338-345.

The PAR-Q+ was created using the evidence-based AGREE process (1) by the PAR-Q+ Collaboration chaired by Dr. Darren E. R. Warburton with Dr. Norman Gledhill, Dr. Veronica Jamnik, and Dr. Donald C. McKenzie (2). Production of this document has been made possible through financial contributions from the Public Health Agency of Canada and the BC Ministry of Health Services. The views expressed herein do not necessarily represent the views of the Public Health Agency of Canada or the BC Ministry of Health Services.

EXHIBIT 1.4 Adult Risk Assessment Form

Name _____ DOB _____ Chart # _____
Allergies _____
Occupation _____

Assess the client for the following risk factors:

Family History	
First-degree relatives with remarkable diseases (e.g., hypertension, diabetes mellitus, CAD, cancer, and thyroid)	
1.	6.
2.	7.
3.	8.
4.	9.
5.	10.

CAD, coronary artery disease.

A. Coronary heart disease:
 1. High-fat/high-cholesterol diet.
 2. Obese.
 3. Elevated cholesterol level.
 4. Stroke.
 5. Hypertension.
 6. Tobacco use.
B. Lung cancer:
 1. High-fat/high-cholesterol diet.
 2. Tobacco use.
C. Cervical cancer:
 1. Early age of first intercourse.
 2. Multiple sexual partners.
D. Breast cancer:
 1. Nulliparous.
 2. Primigravida after age 35 years.
 3. High-fat diet.
E. Colon cancer:
 1. History of polyps.
 2. High-fat diet.
F. Osteoporosis:
 1. <1 g of calcium daily.
 2. History of tobacco or alcohol use.
 3. Sedentary lifestyle.
 4. Thin, Caucasian.
 5. Female gender.
G. Glaucoma/visual impairment:
 1. Family history of glaucoma.
 2. Diabetes mellitus.
H. Sexually transmitted infections (STIs)/HIV:
 1. Alcohol and drug use or abuse.
 2. Multiple sexual partners.
 3. Homosexual or bisexual partner.
 4. History of intravenous drug use.
 5. History of blood transfusion.
 6. Exposed to or past history of STI.
I. Substance abuse:
 1. Alcohol or drug use history.
 2. Family history of substance abuse.
 3. Stress or poor coping mechanisms.
 4. Administer the *CAGE* assessment:
 Have you ever tried to **C**ut down on your alcohol/drug use?
 Do you get **A**nnoyed if someone mentions your use is a problem?
 Do you ever feel **G**uilty about your use?
 Do you ever have an "**E**ye-opener" first thing in the morning after you have been drinking or using the night before?
J. Accidents and suicide:
 1. Family history of suicide.
 2. Alcohol or tobacco use.
 3. History of depression.
 4. High-stress or "hot reactor" personality.
 5. Male gender.
 6. Alcohol use.
 7. Previous suicide attempt.
 8. Poor coping mechanisms or stress.
K. Safety:
 1. Does not use seat belt or car seat.
 2. Drinks and drives.
 3. Drives over the speed limit.
 4. Does not wear safety helmet if driving motorcycle.
 5. Inadequate number of smoke detectors or none in the home.
 6. Firearms in the home.
 7. Feels safe at home/at risk for domestic violence.

2 Public Health Guidelines

Homelessness

Robertson Nash and Erin Ziegler

Overview
Homelessness is a multifaceted structural problem that has a syndemic effect on people. The term "syndemic" refers to situations in which the net effect of multiple physical and social comorbidities is worse than the sum of the individual effects. In the case of people experiencing homelessness, consider all the possible interactions among unmanaged chronic diseases (e.g., diabetes mellitus type 2, hypertension, hyperlipidemia), multiple caries and gingival abscesses, chronic soft-tissue infections, and untreated depression and anxiety. For people without the support of stable housing and nutrition, these interactions can be overwhelming. Data show that, on average, people who are chronically homeless live approximately 20 years less than their housed peers.

Definition (Federal)
The Homelessness Partnering Strategy defines individuals who are episodically or chronically homeless. The criteria for the determination of homelessness include the following:
A. Episodically homeless refers to individuals who are currently homeless and have experienced three or more episodes of homelessness in the last year.
B. Chronically homeless refers to individuals who are currently homeless and have been homeless for six months or more in the last year.

Incidence/Prevalence
According to the Canadian National Shelter study, 13,857 Canadians used an emergency shelter on an average night in 2014, using over 90% of Canada's 15,000 shelter beds. The annual number of individual shelter users has decreased from 156,000 in 2005 to 136,000 in 2014. Over 5 million emergency shelter beds were used in 2014, an increase of 300,000 since 2005, which shows that although there are fewer individuals accessing shelters, they are using shelters more often.

Pathogenesis
Homelessness is a catastrophic experience at the individual level. Homelessness is usually the result of multiple factors, including structural, system, and individual factors.
A. Structural factors include lack of adequate income, access to affordable housing, and/or experiences of discrimination. Discrimination can interfere with access to employment and housing.
B. System factors result from the failure of systems of care or support, such as inadequate discharge planning from an institution or lack of support for immigrants and refugees.
C. Individual factors iInclude traumatic events, personal crisis, violence, and health issues.

Predisposing Factors
Chronic illnesses: People who are homeless suffer from chronic illnesses at rates that exceed those in the general population. In many cases, overlapping and negatively interacting manifestations of illness exacerbate each other, leading to several complicated comorbidities whose management may tax the resources available to both client and provider.

Common Findings
A. Cough/upper respiratory infection.
B. Sinusitis.
C. Soft-tissue infections.
D. Dental abscesses/gingivitis.
E. Tinea pedis.
F. Pest infestations.
G. Mental health–related complaints.

Other Signs and Symptoms
A. Does the client smell of smoke, as if he or she has been sleeping outdoors by a fire? If so, this would trigger a detailed pulmonary examination and a chest x-ray.
B. Does the client smell of urine, suggesting a possible urinary tract infection? If so, this would trigger a genitourinary skin examination, urinalysis, and social work consult regarding access to clean clothing.
C. Unilateral lower extremity pitting oedema, pain, and tenderness suggest the presence of a deep vein thrombosis, which is considered a medical emergency.
D. Bilateral lower extremity pitting edema may be a sign of heart failure. This finding would trigger a thorough clinical examination for the following: S3, S4 heart sounds, jugular venous pulse, and jugular venous distension.
E. Brawny edema and venous stasis ulcerations would trigger a thorough peripheral vascular examination and a sensory examination of the plantar surfaces of both feet.
F. Itchiness suggests pest infestation, which needs treatment including a shower, new clothes, and contact with the shelter to treat the environment.
G. Unusual behaviour (e.g., hallucinations, visible depression, intoxication); refer to mental health resources.

Subjective Data:
Factors to Consider When Evaluating People Experiencing Homelessness
A. Where did the client sleep last night? Does the client have a safe place to sleep tonight?
B. When was the last time the client was able to bathe?
C. When was the last time the client ate?
D. Is the client able to find bathrooms when needed?
E. Are symptoms of depression and anxiety interfering with survival?
F. Is the client being physically, sexually, or emotionally abused?
G. Is the client being forced to engage in behaviours against his or her will in exchange for food and shelter?
H. Does the client have a safe way to manage medications on the street, such as insulin?
I. Assess/discuss current substance abuse.

Physical Examination
As with any clinical encounters, the physical examination should be guided by the concerns generated in the history and from general observations. Providers should be aware that, due to past trauma, many people experiencing homelessness are reluctant to touch. Take time with the physical examination. Ask permission for each step of the physical examination. Explain what is being done and why it is being done.
A. Check temperature, pulse, respirations, and blood pressure.
B. Inspect:
  1. Scalp: Assess for nits.
  2. Oral cavity: Assess for caries or active oral abscesses.
  3. Skin: Assess for burns, abrasions, trauma, and evidence of accidental or intentional injury; assess both feet for infection and trauma.
C. Palpate the abdomen for tenderness or masses. Perform pelvic examination as appropriate. This may not be possible on the first examination. For some females, intentionally poor hygiene is viewed as protection against male assault.
D. Auscultate heart, lungs, and abdomen.
E. Neurologic examination:
  1. Assess for neuropathy in feet.
  2. Assess hearing and vision, as these faculties are central to survival when living on the street.
F. Mental health examination:
  1. Perform depression/anxiety screening. See Chapter 22, Psychiatric Guidelines, for screening.
  2. Evaluate suicidal ideation. See Chapter 22, Psychiatric Guidelines, for assessment/screening.
  3. Assess for active audio/visual hallucinations.
  4. Assess for paranoia.

Diagnostic Tests
The following is a list of laboratory tests for consideration based on client history and physical examination. All tests may not be necessary.
A. Complete blood count (CBC).
B. Electrolytes (sodium, potassium, chloride).
C. Alanine amino transferase (ALT).
D. Creatine.
E. B_{12}.
F. Urinalysis for protein/glucose and *Neisseria gonorrhoeae*/chlamydia.
G. Venereal Disease Research Laboratory (VDRL) test for syphilis.
H. HIV.
I. Hepatitis A virus (HAV)/Hepatitis B virus (HBV) profile, hepatitis C virus (HCV) antibody.
J. Glycosylated haemoglobin A1C.
K. Purified protein derivative (PPD)/tuberculin skin test.

Differential Diagnoses
A. Substance use/abuse.
B. Depression.
C. Malnutrition.
D. Schizophrenia.

Plan
A. General interventions:
  1. There are no disease-based standards of care that specifically address people who are homeless. Rather, providers must be creative and resourceful, working with clients toward higher levels of self-efficacy within the resource bounds imposed on the situation by society at large.
  2. Community-based care: No single provider or community service organization can provide all of the care needed for people experiencing homelessness. To maximize care, providers should try to identify and engage community service organizations before a crisis, so that resources can be coordinated and maximized when acute issues arise.
  3. Identifying and assisting the client with current health needs is imperative. In addition to addressing homelessness, the client may have other acute and chronic health conditions that should be addressed and treated as appropriate.
B. Immunization:
  1. Given the preponderance of communicable diseases among homeless individuals, it is important to consider the following immunizations:
     a. Influenzas.
     b. Pneumococcus.
     c. Tetanus, diptheria, pertussis (Tdap).
     d. HAV and/or HBV.
C. Client teaching:
  1. Lifestyle modifications, focusing on diet, exercise, and smoking cessation, form the cornerstone of primary care provider client teaching for chronic disease management. The following principles should be used to guide the teaching of these principles in this population:
     a. People experiencing homelessness rarely have access to exercise facilities. In addition, they often lack a safe place to store their belongings while they exercise.
     b. People experiencing homelessness have little to no control over their food selection. Dependence on volunteer-driven, charity-led food banks and meal programs is a significant impediment to healthy eating, as many of these programs assume that a high-carbohydrate, calorie-dense meal, such as spaghetti and bread, is what people experiencing homelessness like and want to eat.
     c. The prevalence of poor dentition among the homeless greatly exceeds that of the stably housed, employed population. Accordingly, people experiencing homelessness may not be able to eat fresh fruits and vegetables.
     d. The rates of substance abuse among the chronically homeless exceed those of the general population. Some people may be successfully sober from alcohol, yet continue to smoke tobacco. Although this is not ideal, focus on client strengths, praise sobriety, and acknowledge that smoking cessation is perceived as

being more difficult than sobriety from alcohol and may need to have a lower priority in a client's overall plan of care.

e. Blanket dietary and exercise recommendations developed around stably housed, fully employed people will likely not translate well to people experiencing homelessness. Failure to account for the unique challenges of people experiencing homelessness will exacerbate feelings of depression, low self-worth, and decreased self-efficacy.

f. Caring for individuals experiencing homelessness requires a team approach. Successful teams include clinicians, social workers, behavioural health providers, psychiatric providers, and nursing staff. No one provider or discipline can address all the needs of people experiencing homelessness. It is also critical that the care team work well together and prioritize the work of building rapport with the client, whose life experiences have likely reinforced his or her distrust of the systems that we all depend on to deliver care.

Follow-Up

One of the primary challenges facing providers of those experiencing homelessness is the deep-seated lack of trust that these people have in the healthcare system within which most providers operate. To encourage people to return to the clinic for appropriate follow-up care, every effort must be made during the first visit to establish a true therapeutic relationship with the client. Providers should attempt to work with clients to identify and address concerns that are important to the client. Providers should remember that topics such as smoking cessation and sobriety from alcohol may best be deferred during an initial visit. All clinic staff should be trained to treat all clients with a professional, welcoming, and empathetic manner.

Consultation/Referral

Referring clients to specialists is an everyday part of primary care, and primary care providers serve important screening and gatekeeper functions in this role. Effective providers will identify specialists in their local communities and seek to build relationships that will facilitate referrals. Given the lack of access to transportation in this population, it is important to set an expectation that a missed appointment does not mean that the client does not want or need care, and that specialists may need to be flexible regarding missed appointments with people in this population.

Individual Considerations

A. Paediatrics/minors: Forty percent of homeless youth were under 16 years of age when they first experienced homelessness. Young people (ages 13–24) make up approximately 20% of the homeless population in Canada, and on any night there may be up to 7,000 homeless youth. Sixty percent of homeless youth have been the victims of a violent crime. Homeless youth are likely to be extremely mistrustful of medical, social work, and law enforcement professionals.

B. Pregnancy: Providers should screen for homelessness or risk of becoming homeless in pregnant women. Prenatal care should include referral to available resources and community support. In cases where abuse is suspected, law enforcement must be notified.

C. Elderly: All people older than 60 years who are experiencing homelessness and present for care should be connected to resources and community supports. In cases where abuse is suspected, law enforcement must be notified.

Resources

The state of homelessness in Canada 2016: http://homelesshub.ca/sites/default/files/SOHC16_final_20Oct2016.pdf

Without a home: The national youth homelessness survey: https://www.homelesshub.ca/sites/default/files/attachments/WithoutAHome-final.pdf

Bibliography

Gaetz, S., Dje, E., Richter, T., & Redman, M. (2016). *The state of homelessness in Canada 2016*. Toronto, ON, Canada: Canadian Observatory on Homelessness Press. Retrieved from http://homelesshub.ca/sites/default/files/SOHC16_final_20Oct2016.pdf

Gaetz, S., O'Grady, B., Kidd, S., & Schwan, K. (2016). *Without a home: The national youth homelessness survey*. Toronto, ON, Canada: Canadian Observatory on Homelessness Press. Retrieved from https://www.homelesshub.ca/sites/default/files/attachments/WithoutAHome-final.pdf

Government of Canada. (2016). *Homelessness partnering strategy directives 2014–2019*. Retrieved from https://www.canada.ca/en/employment-social-development/services/funding/homeless/homeless-directives.html

Henry, M., Cortes, A., & Morris, S. (2013). *The 2013 Annual Homeless Assessment Report (AHAR) to congress*. Washington, DC: U.S. Department of Housing and Urban Development.

Merrill, S. (2009). *Introducing syndemics: A critical systems approach to public and community health*. San Francisco, CA: Jossey-Bass.

Segaert, A. (2016). *The national shelter study 2005–2014: Emergency shelter use in Canada*. Gatineau, QC: Employment and Social Development Canada. Retrieved from http://publications.gc.ca/collections/collection_2017/edsc-esdc/Em12-17-2017-eng.pdf

U.S. Department of Housing and Urban Development. (2011). *Homeless emergency assistance and rapid transition to housing*. Retrieved from https://www.hudexchange.info/homelessness-assistance/hearth-act

Obesity

Angelito Tacderas, Bunny Pounds, and Erin Ziegler

Definition

A. Obesity is a multifactorial disease with physical, psychological, and social consequences. Body mass index (BMI) is a standard measuring tool. BMI is calculated by using this formula: weight in kilograms divided by height in metres squared (weight [kg]/height [m]^2). In adults, obesity is defined as a BMI >30 kg/m^2.

B. BMI for children is calculated the same way as for adults but is interpreted using age- and gender-specific percentages (BMI-for-age) clinical charts (see Tables 2.1 and 2.2). The Canadian Task Force on Preventive Health Care recommends using the World Health

TABLE 2.1 Childhood Obesity by Percentiles

Childhood Obesity Category	BMI Definitions by Percentiles
Underweight	<5th percentile
Healthy weight	5th to <85th percentile
Overweight	85th to <95th percentile
Obese	≥95th percentile

BMI, body mass index.

Table 2.2 Adult Obesity by BMI

Classification of Adult Obesity by BMI	BMI (kg/m²)
Underweight	<18.5
Normal	18.5–24.9
Overweight (preobese)	25.0–29.9
Obesity	30.0–34.9
Severely obese	>40.0
Morbidly obese	40.0–49.9
Super obese	>50.0
Super-super obese	≥60.0

BMI, body mass index.

Organization (WHO) Growth Charts for Canada. Charts are available at www.dietitians.ca/Dietitians-Views/Prenatal-and-Infant/WHO-Growth-Charts.aspx.

Incidence/Prevalence

In Canada, 67% of adult men and 54% of adult women are overweight or obese. Approximately two-thirds of adults who are overweight or obese were a healthy weight as adolescents. Obesity rates in Indigenous people are 1.6 times higher than the Canadian average. One-third of Canadian youth aged 5 to 17 are as classified as overweight or obese. Obesity rates cross all groups in society, regardless of age, gender, race, ethnicity, socioeconomic status, educational level, or geographic group.

Pathogenesis

Numerous factors contribute to the development of obesity, including the following:
A. Imbalance between energy intake and energy output.
B. Genetics (40%–70% presumed explanation).
C. Environmental factors.
D. Drug-induced obesity:
   1. Antidepressants (amitriptyline, doxepin, imipramine, mirtazapine, nortriptyline, paroxetine, phenelzine).
   2. Antihistamines (cyproheptadine).
   3. Antipsychotics (clozapine, haloperidol, olanzapine, quetiapine, risperidone).
   4. Antidiabetics (insulin, sulfonylureas, thiazolidinediones).
   5. Anticonvulsants (sodium valproate, carbamazepine, gabapentin).
   6. Steroids (glucocorticoids, progestational steroids).
   7. Beta- or alpha-adrenergic blockers (propranolol, doxazosin).
E. Sleep disturbance–induced obesity.

Predisposing Factors

A. Consuming too many calories/high-fat diet.
B. Poor dietary choices.
C. Readily available food sources, especially fast foods.
D. Lack of exercise/sedentary lifestyle.
E. Decrease/elimination of physical education requirements in public schools.
F. Television, computer, and handheld game use of more than three hours a day.
G. Increased leisure time.
H. Lack of funding and planning for community parks and recreation areas.
I. Ethnic background: African American, Hispanic, East and Southeast Asian, Indigenous.
J. Family history of obesity.
K. Poverty.
L. Insomnia, difficulty staying asleep, and frequent wakefulness.

Common Findings

A. Difficulties with activities of daily living (ADLs) or functional impairment.
B. Lack of interest/inability to tolerate exercise.
C. Shortness of breath and/or asthma exacerbations.
D. Difficulty with personal hygiene.
E. Urinary incontinence.
F. Desire to lose weight.

Other Signs and Symptoms

A. Obstructive sleep apnea (OSA).
B. Increased asthma symptoms.
C. Infertility/polycystic ovary syndrome (PCOS).
D. Symptoms associated with cholelithiasis.
E. Hypertension.
F. Early sexual maturity in girls.
G. Joint pain, osteoarthritis (OA).

Subjective Data

A. Review the onset of weight gain and duration of obesity. Identify when the client first noticed the weight gain.
B. Ask the client about other symptoms secondary to obesity.
C. Review full medical history.
D. Review medications, including over-the-counter (OTC) herbal and diet products.
E. Review the client's previous history of weight loss attempts.
F. Assess ADLs and functional limitations and the presence of exercise intolerance.
G. Elicit history of sleep disorders (e.g., snoring and obstruction, sleep apnea).
H. Review 24-hour dietary recall. Review the client's normal average meals per day, including snacks.
I. Review consumption of high-calorie drinks and alcohol intake.
J. Assess for history of binge eating, purging, night eating syndrome, lack of satiety, food-seeking behaviours, and other abnormal feeding habits.
K. Assess for depression.
L. Assess for readiness and commitment for weight loss. People who voluntarily enroll in a weight loss program generally lose weight.
M. Ask the client to describe his or her activity level, exercise routine, and daily activity (work activity).
N. Ask about screen time.
O. Ask about family history of obesity.
P. Ask about possible biopsychosocial and behavioural risk factors for weight gain, such as starting a new medication, change in occupation or marital status, recent illness, pregnancy, menopause, stressful events, or smoking cessation.

Physical Examination

A. Check pulse, respirations, and blood pressure: supine, sitting, and standing.
B. Measurements:
   1. Determine height and weight to calculate BMI.

2. Measure waist and hip circumferences to calculate the waist-to-hip circumference ratio. The waist-to-hip ratio is the strongest anthropometric measure that is associated with myocardial infarction risk and is a better predictor than BMI. A waist-to-hip ratio that is >0.8% usually has some form of premetabolic syndrome or insulin resistance.
C. Inspect:
  1. Observe the overall appearance and note body fat distribution.
  2. Examine the skin.
  3. Mouth and teeth: Assess dental enamel for signs of purging.
D. Auscultate heart, lungs, carotid arteries, and abdomen.
E. Palpate:
  1. Neck and thyroid.
  2. Extremities, noting oedema.
  3. Abdomen for masses, tenderness, rebound tenderness.

Diagnostic Tests
The following is a list of laboratory tests for consideration based on client history and physical examination. All tests may not be necessary.
A. Glycosylated haemoglobin A1C.
B. Thyroid function.
C. Lipid panel.
D. Liver enzymes.
E. Complete blood count (CBC).
F. Pregnancy test (if indicated).
G. Sleep study (if indicated).
H. Consider genetic testing.

Differential Diagnoses
A. Pseudo tumour cerebri.
B. Binge eating.
C. Genetic syndrome (e.g., Prader–Willi syndrome).
D. Cushing's syndrome.
E. Diabetes mellitus.
F. Metabolic syndrome.
G. Primary pulmonary hypertension.

Plan
Manage obesity as a chronic relapsing disease, including the comanagement of other diseases secondary to obesity (e.g., diabetes, hypertension).
A. General interventions:
  1. Treat any underlying cause of obesity.
  2. Reinforce the positive impact that weight loss measures (diet, exercise) can have and the overall health benefits of weight loss. Weight loss of even 5% to 15% can provide a significant reduction in obesity-related complications.
  3. Identify and monitor any cardiovascular complications.
  4. Behaviour modification: Intensive behaviour therapy has been shown to lead to better success with weight loss and sustainable weight loss for longer periods of time. Behaviour therapy includes weekly meetings with healthcare professionals for at least six to eight weeks.
    a. Dietary plan:
      i. Consume 500 to 1,000 fewer calories per day for 0.5 to 1 kg weight loss per week.
      ii. Most diets have good short-term efficacy but limited sustainability.
      iii. Diets shown to be effective include portion control, low-fat, Mediterranean, low-carbohydrate, low glycemic index, and commercial weight loss diets.
      iv. Increase water intake, particularly drinking 500 mL of water before meals.
      v. Protein-dense and high-fiber foods increase satiety with fewer calories.
    b. Exercise:
      i. Approximately 150 minutes of moderate-intensity exercise is recommended per week for adults, 155 to 180 minutes per week for children.
      ii. Multiple short sessions (four 10-minute sessions per day, five days per week) may have the same benefit as fewer longer sessions (one 40-minute session, five days per week).
      iii. Add endurance exercise training.
      iv. Walking 30 minutes per day has been shown to prevent weight gain; higher amounts of exercise promote weight loss.
      v. The combination of exercise and diet is more effective than either alone.
    c. Range of benefits of exercise and weight loss:
      i. Helps lower blood pressure.
      ii. Improves cholesterol count.
      iii. Helps lower haemoglobin A1C in diabetes.
      iv. Helps strengthen bones.
      v. Promotes weight loss.
      vi. Improves depression.
      vii. Boosts immune system.
      viii. Reduces stress.
      ix. Improves sense of well-being.
      x. Believed to be a major driving force in lifestyle change.
      xi. Improves joint pain.
    d. Obtain cognitive-based therapy on stimulus control, goal setting, self-monitoring, and contracts that reward behaviours.
    e. There are several contraindications for beginning exercise.
      i. Individuals with recent myocardial infarction (two weeks).
      ii. Unstable angina.
      iii. Severe aortic stenosis.
      iv. Decompensated congestive heart failure (low ejection fraction).
      v. Left ventricular outflow obstruction.
      vi. Uncontrolled dysrhythmias.
      vii. Uncontrolled diabetes or diabetic complications.
      viii. Uncontrolled hypertension.
      ix. Uncontrolled respiratory conditions (e.g., asthma, chronic obstructive pulmonary disorder).
B. Client teaching on obesity treatment modalities:
  1. Advise the client to keep a food diary to identify food triggers and for accountability. Clients who maintain a food diary have been shown to have as much as 90% more weight loss than those who do not keep a diary.
  2. If drug therapy is indicated, counsel clients about drug's side effects and the lack of long-term safety data. Stress to the client the temporary nature of the weight loss medication. Typical weight loss is modest, <5 kg at one year.
  3. Teach clients how to read food labels.

C. Pharmacological therapy:
  1. The Canadian Task Force on Preventive Health Care does not recommend pharmacological therapy for individuals who are overweight and obese. However, some clients may prefer medication and be a good candidate. After an adequate trial (minimum of six months) of diet and exercise therapy, consider adding pharmacological therapy for individuals with a BMI >30, or >27 with risk factors.
  2. Pharmacological therapy is associated with adverse effects and not indicated for use beyond two years in adults. Orlistat is the only appetite suppressant that is available in Canada.
  3. Lipase inhibitor: Orlistat is for use with a low-fat diet. Recommend 30% of calories spread over three main meals.
     a. May decrease absorption of fat-soluble vitamins and beta-carotene.
     b. Orlistat carries a warning regarding safety and efficacy for use in clients younger than 12 years and in pregnancy and lactation, as it interferes with the absorption of fat-soluble vitamins.
     c. Supplement diet with a multivitamin.
     d. Not approved for use longer than two years.
     e. Gastrointestinal side effects include fatty/oily stools, oily spotting, flatus with discharge, faecal urgency, and faecal incontinence.
     f. Contraindicated in chronic malabsorption syndrome and cholestasis.
     g. May affect doses for antidiabetic medications.
     h. Monitor warfarin and cyclosporine levels.

Follow-Up

A. Reevaluate the client every week for six to eight weeks, then monthly if pharmacological therapy is used until goal is achieved.
B. Maintain the recommended schedule for comorbid conditions.
C. Clients with a BMI >40, or >35 with risk factors, are candidates for bariatric surgery.

Consultation/Referral

A. Refer to a nutritionist/registered dietitian for consultation.
B. Consider a referral to a bariatric center/surgical consultation and evaluation of bariatric surgery.
C. Consider a psychology consultation (may be required before bariatric surgery).

Individual Considerations

A. Pregnancy:
  1. Weight loss should never be a goal during pregnancy.
  2. Counsel clients regarding appropriate weight gain and healthy eating habits during pregnancy.
B. Paediatrics:
  1. The cornerstone for management of obesity in children is modification of dietary and exercise habits.
  2. The first step for overweight children older than 2 years is maintenance of baseline weight if there is no secondary complication of obesity (e.g., diabetes and hypertension). Any dietary modification must ensure adequate nutrients for the growing child.
  3. Do not encourage weight loss, instead allow for linear growth to catch up to weight.
  4. Decrease sedentary behaviours (e.g., watching TV, surfing the internet, and playing video games).
  5. Increase physical activity and incorporate exercise into family time.
  6. Long-term safety and effectiveness of low-carbohydrate, high-protein diets, such as the Atkins diet, have not been adequately studied in children. Special diets used by adults are not recommended in children.
  7. Use of pharmacotherapies in children and adolescents requires further research, unless previously noted under drug therapies.
C. Geriatrics: All adults should avoid inactivity. Some exercise is better than none. Any dietary modification must ensure adequate nutrients for the aging adult.

Resources

Canadian Task Force on Preventative Health–Obesity: https://canadiantaskforce.ca/?s=obesity+&search-type=default
Heart and Stroke Foundation of Canada: http://www.heartandstroke.ca/
Obesity Canada: https://obesitycanada.ca/
SickKids Healthy Eating & Active Living Resources: http://www.sickkids.ca/Research/Obesity-in-Youth-Healthy-Weight-Program/Readings/Great-Resources/index.html

Bibliography

Brauer, P., Grober, S., Shaw, E., Signh, H., Bell, N., Shane, A., . . . Canadian Task Force on Previtive Health Care. (2015). Recommendations for prevention of weight gain and use of behavioural and pharmacological interventions to manage overweight and obesity in adults in primary care. *Canadian Medical Association Journal, 187*(3), 184–195. doi:10.1503/cmaj.140887
Centers for Disease Control and Prevention. (2014). *Adult obesity facts*. Retrieved from https://www.cdc.gov/obesity/data/adult.html
Centers for Disease Control and Prevention. (2015). *Overweight & obesity*. Retrieved from https://www.cdc.gov/obesity/index.html
DynaMed Plus. (2016, March 8). *Obesity in adults*. Ipswich, MA: EBSCO Information Services. Retrieved from https://www.dynamed.com/topics/dmp-AN-T115009/Obesity-in-adults
Gupta, A. K. (2016, February 19). Obesity and weight loss (adult). *Essentials evidence plus*. Retrieved from www.essentialevidenceplus.com
Jensen, M. D., Ryan, D. H., Donato, K. A., Apovian, C. M., Ard, J. D., Comuzzie, A. G., & Yanovski, S. Z. (2014). Special issue: Guidelines for managing overweight and obesity in adults. *Obesity, 22*(S2), i–xvi. S1–S410. doi:10.1002/oby.20818
Roberts, K., Sheilds, M., de Groh, M., Aziz, A., & Gilbert, J. (2012). Overweight and obesity in children and adolescents: Results from the 2009–2011 Canadian health measures survey. *Health Reports, 23*(3), 37–41. Retrieved from https://www150.statcan.gc.ca/n1/pub/82-003-x/2012003/article/11706-eng.htm
Smith, B. R., Schauer, P., & Nguyen, N. T. (2008). Surgical approaches to the treatment of obesity: Bariatric surgery. *Endocrinology & Metabolism Clinics of North America Journal, 37*(4), 943–964.
Statistics Canada. (2013). *Overweight and obese adults (Self-reported), 2012*. Retrieved from https://www150.statcan.gc.ca/n1/pub/82-625-x/2013001/article/11840-eng.htm
U.S. Department of Health and Human Services, National Institute of Diabetes and Digestive and Kidney Diseases. (2012). *Overweight and obesity statistics* (NIH Publication No. 04-4158). Retrieved from win.niddk.nih.gov/statistics

Postbariatric Surgery Long-Term Follow-Up

Cheryl A. Glass, Bunny Pounds, and Erin Ziegler

Definition

A. The traditional management of obesity, which is a combination of diet, exercise, and behavioural modification, often results in moderate success with limited sustainability. The increasing prevalence of obesity combined with improvements in surgical weight loss procedures have resulted in exponential growth of the number of people opting for surgical management. Bariatric surgery is an effective long-term tool for weight loss for individuals with moderate to severe obesity. Clients who undergo surgical weight loss procedures have unique healthcare needs and require lifelong follow-up.

Although the bariatric treatment team is the ideal source of follow-up and monitoring, primary care providers can play a critical role and need to be cognizant of the unique needs of this population.

B. The primary mechanism of action for surgical weight loss procedures is either restriction or a combination of restriction and malabsorption (see Table 2.3). All procedures have some form of restriction that reduces the volume of food that can be ingested. Restriction can occur by means of a physical barrier such as a laparoscopic adjustable gastric band (LAGB; see Figure 2.1) or by removing a portion of the digestive tract such as with the gastric sleeve (GS; see Figure 2.2). Malabsorptive procedures cause weight loss by changing the way nutrients are absorbed, which is accomplished by removing portions of the stomach and/or small intestine and sometimes by rerouting the digestive tract (Roux-en-Y; see Figure 2.3). The success of surgical weight loss is defined by initial weight loss, maintenance of weight loss, and prevention of complications. Success is directly related to the aftercare a person receives.

Incidence/Prevalence

A. One in five adults are obese (body mass index [BMI] >30). The Canadian Institute for Health Information (2014) reported that 6,000 bariatric surgeries were performed in Canadian hospitals, with an additional 1,000 performed in private clinics in 2012. About 90% of surgical weight loss procedures are now performed laparoscopically. The most common procedures performed today include the gastric bypass, GS, adjustable gastric band, and biliopancreatic diversion with duodenal switch.

Pathogenesis

The pathogenesis of obesity is reviewed under the section "Obesity" this chapter. Significant improvements in the safety of surgical weight loss procedures in recent years result from improved surgical techniques, accreditation, and the use of laparoscopy. The overall mortality rate is about 0.1% and the risk of major complications about 4.3%. The incidence of complications vary by surgical procedure. Postoperative complications may occur immediately or may occur many

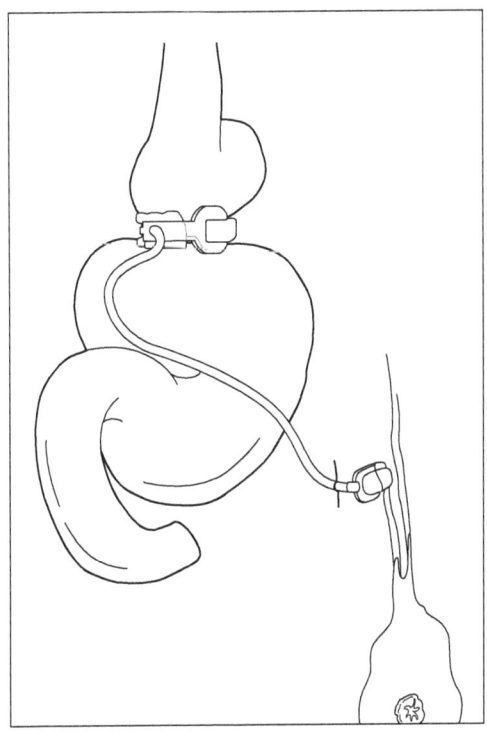

FIGURE 2.1 Laparoscopic adjustable gastric band.

TABLE 2.3 Surgical Weight Loss Procedures and Mechanism of Action

Procedure	Mechanism of Action	Advantages	Disadvantages
Laparoscopic adjustable gastric band (LAGB); Figure 2.1	Restriction	No cutting or rerouting of digestive tract Reversible and adjustable Lowest risk of nutritional deficiencies	Slower (more gradual) weight loss Greater chance of failure to lose 50% of excess weight Foreign device in body; slippage and erosion possible Highest rate of reoperation
Gastric sleeve (GS); Figure 2.2	Restriction and some malabsorption	No rerouting Hormonal hunger suppression, appetite reduction, and increased satiety	Not reversible Potential for nutrient deficiencies Higher complication rate than LAGB
Roux-en-Y gastric bypass (RYGB); Figure 2.3	Restriction and malabsorption	Reduces appetite, enhances satiety Better initial and long-term weight loss compared with LAGB	Long-term nutritional-deficiency risk Lifelong adherence to diet and supplementation required Higher complication rate compared with LAGB and GS
Biliopancreatic diversion with duodenal switch (BPD/DS);	Malabsorption and some restriction	Greatest weight loss overall Reduces appetite, improves satiety Most effective for treatment of diabetes mellitus	Greatest risk of nutritional deficiencies Strict lifetime adherence to diet and supplements Highest complication rate
Vertical banded gastroplasty	No longer performed		

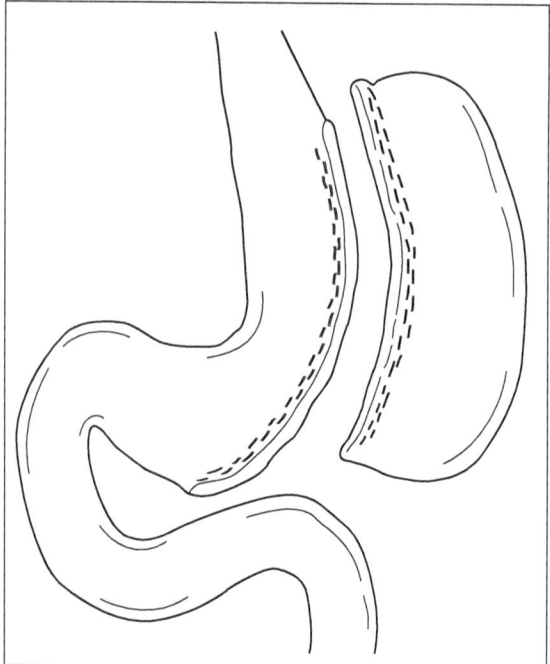

FIGURE 2.2 Sleeve bypass procedure with stomach resection.

years after surgery. Nutritional deficiencies are the most common long-term complication.

Predisposing Factors
A. Higher BMI.
B. Noncompliance with bariatric diet and exercise.
C. Lack of follow-up with healthcare professionals.
D. Obesity-related health problem:
   1. Sleep apnea.
   2. Diabetes.
   3. Arthritis.
   4. Hypertension.
   5. Gastroesophageal reflux disease (GERD).
E. Complexity and type of surgery.

Common Findings
Functional and Nutritional
A. Dumping syndrome usually occurs within 30 minutes of eating high-fat/high-sugar foods and involves flushing, sweating, light-headedness, tachycardia, palpitations, nausea, diarrhoea, and cramping.
B. Hypoglycemia occurs one to three hours after eating high-carb meals and involves shakiness, anxiety, sweating, chills, clamminess, confusion, rapid heart rate, dizziness, hunger, and nausea.
C. New or exacerbated reflux is more common with a GS.
D. Vitamin deficiencies or toxicities (refer to Table 2.4):
   1. Most common:
      a. Iron deficiency: fatigue, lethargy, pica, food cravings.
      b. Iron toxicity: gastrointestinal irritation, nausea, vomiting, indigestion, constipation, diarrhoea.
      c. Protein deficiency: weakness, decreased muscle mass, brittle hair, generalized edema.
      d. Folate deficiency: fatigue, palpitations, sore tongue, diarrhoea, restless legs.
      e. Calcium deficiency: usually silent, hyperparathyroidism.
      f. Calcium toxicity: constipation, nausea, vomiting, dry mouth, loss of appetite.

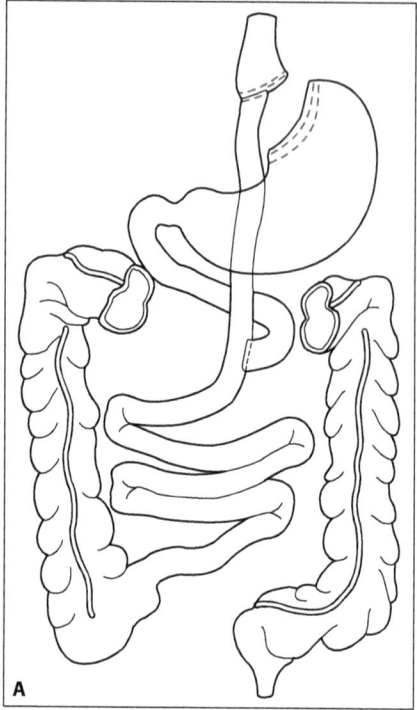

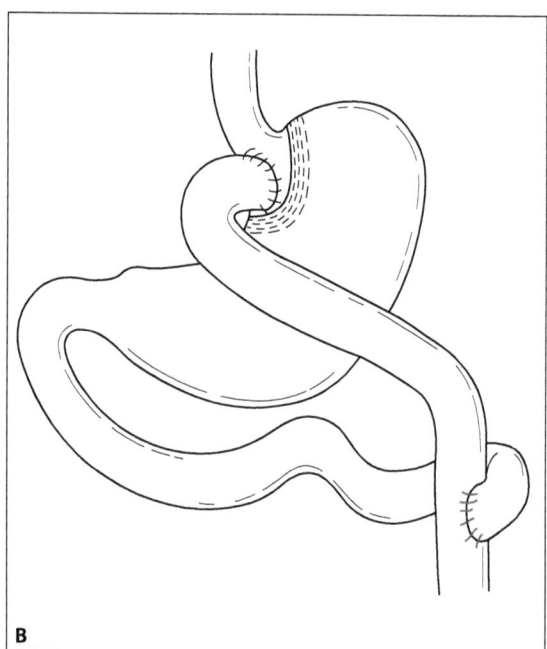

FIGURE 2.3 **(A and B)** Roux-en-Y gastric bypass.

   g. Vitamin D deficiency: spasms/twitching of eyes, burning in mouth, sweating, weakness.
   h. Vitamin B12 deficiency: fatigue, burning lips/mouth, rapid heart rate, palpitations, sore tongue, weakness, mood changes, neurologic changes.
   2. Less common:
      a. Thiamine (B_1) deficiency: usually in first three months postop, often a result of vomiting, blurred or double vision, difficulty swallowing, rapid heart rate, fatigue, confusion, memory loss, burning feet, leg weakness, amnesia.
      b. Zinc deficiency: loss of smell, diminished sense of taste, poor wound healing, skin rashes or roughness, hair loss, poor appetite, lethargy, grooved or deformed nails, canker sores.

TABLE 2-1 Most Common Nutrient Deficiencies Post-Bariatric Surgery

Nutrient	Protein	Iron	Folate	Calcium	Vitamin B12	Vitamin D
Assay	Serum albumin <3.5 mg/dL May need prealbumin and serum creatinine levels also	Iron saturation <10% Serum ferritin <10 ng/mL or iron saturation <7% regardless of ferritin value	Serum folic acid	Total and ionized calcium Phosphorus 24-hr urinary calcium excretion Intact serum parathyroid hormone Bone density	Serum B12 level May need methylmalonic acid level also	25 $(OH)D_3$ <30 nmol/L
Incidence	18%–25% after malabsorptive procedures	6%–50%	1%–10%	10%–25%	5%–25%	Up to 63%
Complications and symptoms	Anaemia Oedema Alopecia Asthenia (weakness, decreased muscle mass, brittle hair, generalized oedema)	Microcytic, hypochromic anaemia (pallor, fatigue, poor capillary refill, palpitations, pica, brittle hair)	Megaloblastic or macrocytic anaemia (palpitations; fatigue; diarrhoea; smooth, sore tongue) Neural tube defects May aggravate B12 deficiency	Secondary hyperparathyroidism Enhanced bone loss Metabolic bone disease (tetany, tingling, cramping)	Megaloblastic anaemia with macrocytosis Neuropathy Cognitive dysfunction (glossitis, constipation, diarrhoea, neurologic changes, depression, dementia)	Myopathy Secondary hypocalcaemia
Recommended daily amount for prevention	1.1–1.5 g/kg ideal body weight/d 10%–35% of total energy intake should be from protein	45–60 mg/d from multivitamins and iron supplements for malabsorptive procedures Menstruating women may need more	400 mcg/d	1,200–1,500 mg/d of calcium citrate from food and supplements	500 mcg/d oral for band 1,000 mcg/d oral for malabsorptive procedures; may need 500–1,000 mcg/mo intramuscular	At least 3,000 IU of oral D_3 daily, better to titrate to therapeutic level
Treatment dosing	If previous options are not effective, may need parenteral nutrition	150–200 mg of elemental iron twice daily, preferably with vitamin C	1,000 mcg/d for three months	2,000 mg/d with adequate vitamin D supplementation	Depends on the level of deficiency Recheck levels after three to six months of repletion	6,000–10,000 IU/d or 50,000 IU/wk up to 50,000 IU/d Recheck level every three months

Source: Adapted from Becker, D. A., Balcer, L. J., & Galetta, S. L. (2012). The neurological complications of nutritional deficiency following bariatric surgery. *Journal of Obesity, 2012*. doi:10.1155/2012/608534; Handzlik-Orlik, G., Holecki, M., Orlik, B., Wylezol, M., & Dulawa, J. (2015). Nutrition management of the post-bariatric surgery client. *Nutrition in Clinical Practice: Official Publication of the American Society for Parenteral and Enteral Nutrition, 30*(3), 383–392. doi:10.1177/0884533614564995; Kerner, J. (2014). Nutrition support after bariatric surgery. *Support Line, 36*(3), 9–20.

c. Magnesium deficiency: hyperexcitability, cramps, tremors, fasciculation, spasms, fatigue, loss of appetite, apathy, confusion, insomnia, irritability, poor memory.

d. Selenium deficiency (very rare): signs of hypothyroidism (selenium is necessary for conversion of thyroxine into its active form, triiodothyronine).

e. Selenium toxicity (rare): hair loss, abnormal nails, dermatitis, peripheral neuropathy, nausea, diarrhoea, fatigue, irritability, garlic odour of breath.

E. Surgical complications:
1. Short term:
   a. Anastomic leak: <4.4% with RYGB, but has a mortality of up to 30% when it does happen; presenting symptom is tachycardia.
   b. Bleeding: <4% after RYGB, 0.1% after LAGB.
   c. Wound infection: 2.9% of laparoscopic cases, 6.6% of open cases.
   d. Thromboembolism: deep vein thrombosis up to 1.3%, pulmonary embolism up to 1.1% after RYGB, lower with LAGB.

e. Anastomotic strictures: 2% to 16% after RYGB, typically within first three months, nausea and/or vomiting.
2. Long term:
   a. Band slippage: 15% to 20% of LAGB clients; abdominal pain, acid reflux, regurgitation, or dysphagia.
   b. Band erosion: up to 4% of LAGB clients; may be asymptomatic, abdominal pain, gastrointestinal bleeding, weight loss, abdominal sepsis.
   c. Intestinal obstruction: 4.4% after RYGB, caused by internal hernias, adhesions, and anastomotic stenosis; colicky central abdominal pain, nausea, vomiting, abdominal distention, absolute constipation.
   d. Hepatobiliary complications: rapid weight loss is associated with gallstone formation; 13% to 36% of clients develop this within six months of surgery.
   e. Gastrointestinal bleeding: rare and usually caused by ulceration.
   f. Marginal ulcers: 0.7% to 5.1% after RYGB; abdominal pain, vomiting, bleeding, or anaemia.

Other Signs and Symptoms
A. Expected weight loss:
   1. LAGB: Initial loss of 40% to 50% of excess body weight in three to five years. Expected maintenance <50%.
   2. GS: Initial loss of >50% of excess body weight in three to five years. Expected maintenance >50%.
   3. RYGB: Initial loss of 60% to 80% of excess body weight in one year. Expected maintenance >50%.
   4. Biliopancreatic diversion with duodenal switch (BPD/DS): Initial loss of 60% to 70% of excess body weight in one year. Expected maintenance of 60% to 70%.
B. Weight regain of up to 9 kilograms is common after two years.
C. Constipation and/or diarrhoea may occur, depending on the procedure.
D. Weight loss of <25% of excess body weight is considered a surgical failure and may be revised.
E. Even if weight loss is adequate, clients may express disappointment and/or depression related to rate or amount of weight lost.
F. Nausea and vomiting after LAGB may indicate need for band adjustment.

Subjective Data
A. Review onset and duration of symptoms.
B. Elicit the date of surgery, type of surgery, and any reoperations or complications.
C. Review previous highest weight and amount of excess weight lost since surgery.
D. Evaluate the location and level of pain/discomfort.
E. Evaluate the overall psychosocial changes since surgery.
F. Review a 24-hour food recall, choices of healthy foods, skipping meals, food aversion (e.g., red meat), and intolerance.
G. Review medications and supplement use.

Physical Examination
A. Check height, weight, and waist and hip circumference. Calculate BMI, waist-to-hip ratio, pulse, respirations, and blood pressure. Check temperature if infection is suspected.
B. Inspect:
   1. Examine the skin, evaluate surgical site(s), and evaluate redness and tenderness.
   2. Oral/dental examination.
   3. Evaluate for dehydration.
   4. Eye examination: Evaluate eye movement (thiamine deficiency).
   5. Evaluate gait.
   6. General overview of personal presence and affect.
C. Auscultate:
   1. Heart and lungs.
   2. Abdomen for bowel sounds.
D. Palpate abdomen:
   1. Evaluate for the presence of tenderness.
   2. Evaluate for masses.
E. Neurologic examination: Perform neurologic examination, including checking deep tendon reflexes (DTRs), sense of smell, and Babinski reflex (vitamin B12 deficiency).

Diagnostic Tests
A. Annual recommended laboratory testing for all procedures:
   1. Complete blood count (CBC) with differential.
   2. Liver function tests.
   3. Glucose.
   4. Creatinine.
   5. Electrolytes.
B. Annual laboratory testing suggested for LAGB, recommended for all other procedures:
   1. Iron/ferritin.
   2. Vitamin B12.
   3. Folate.
   4. Calcium.
   5. Intact parathyroid hormone (PTH).
   6. 25-hydroxy vitamin D.
   7. Albumin/prealbumin.
C. Optional labs that may be required based on symptoms:
   1. Zinc.
   2. Copper.
   3. Vitamin B1.
   4. Vitamin B6.
   5. Vitamin A.
D. Other labs as appropriate for condition and prevention:
   1. Monitor haemoglobin A1C and blood glucose closely in clients with diabetes. Diabetes has resolved after bariatric surgery in some clients.
   2. Lipid profile.
E. Other testing as appropriate for condition and prevention:
   1. Abdominal ultrasound.
   2. CT scan abdomen.
   3. Doppler ultrasound of limb for suspected deep vein thrombosis (DVT).
   4. Bone mineral density (dual-energy x-ray absorptiometry [DEXA]) scan: Recommended annually until stable after malabsorptive procedures.
   5. Endoscopy as needed for abdominal complaints.

Differential Diagnoses
A. Postoperative surgical complication(s).
B. Infection.
C. Abdominal pain.
D. Fascial dehiscence.
E. DVT.
F. Bowel obstruction.
G. Band slippage.
H. Anastomosis leakage.

I. Stomal stenosis/stricture.
J. Cholecystitis.
K. Dumping syndrome.
L. Food intolerance.
M. Gastric ulcer.
N. Gastroenteritis.
O. Vitamin deficiency.
P. Malnutrition/protein deficiency.
Q. Incisional hernia.
R. Osteoporosis.

Plan

A. General interventions: Lifelong follow-up is required after bariatric surgery. Ideally, clients should follow up with their surgical group, but many do not. Primary care providers are well positioned to capture those lost to follow up. Continuous reinforcement of good nutritional habits is important.

B. Client teaching:
Many complications can be prevented by adhering to diet and lifestyle recommendations:
  1. Supplements are required lifelong; strict adherence will prevent deficiencies.
  2. Dumping syndrome can be prevented by avoiding foods that trigger it, such as high-sugar and high-fat foods. Clients can keep food diaries to identify triggers.
  3. Hypoglycemia can usually be prevented by careful monitoring of carbohydrate intake.
  4. Surgery does not replace the need for a balanced diet or exercise. Approximately 150 minutes of moderate activity each week is recommended, though safety and tolerance differ so exercise recommendations should be individualized. Any activity is better than none.
  5. Food should be chewed thoroughly and consumed slowly. Liquids should be avoided 30 minutes before and after meals. Avoid eating and drinking liquids simultaneously.
  6. Protein is important for maintaining muscle mass during rapid weight loss and avoiding hunger during maintenance. Between 60 g and 100 g of protein daily is recommended. Limit carbohydrate intake to 50 g per day or less. Limiting carbohydrate intake reduces risk of weight regain by preventing rebound hunger.
  7. To prevent dehydration, as well as to reduce the risk of kidney stones and constipation, encourage 2 L of fluids daily.
  8. Stress, boredom, and emotions often affect eating habits. Identifying problems and seeking help early are important.
  9. Support groups can be a vital source of education and social support, both of which are key to weight loss and maintenance.
  10. Weight plateaus are common and normal. This is the body's way of trying to establish a new set point. Do not be discouraged by plateaus. Consistency is key to overcoming them.
  11. Adequate sleep and successful stress management are also key to successful weight loss and maintenance.

C. Pharmacological therapy:
  1. Medication absorption can be altered after bariatric surgery. Evaluate need for adjustments of medication dosing, especially diabetic, psychiatric, and antihypertensive medications, as well as any medication with a narrow therapeutic window.
  2. Clients may require alternate formulations of medications, including crushed, chewable, liquid, patches, intramuscular, or subcutaneous. Long-acting, extended-release, or enteric-coated medications may not be absorbed as well and may need to be switched to immediate release.
  3. Refer to Table 2.5.
  4. Recommended supplementations:
    a. Multivitamin plus mineral:
      i. LAGB: One daily.
      ii. All other procedures: Two daily.
    b. Calcium (all procedures): 1,200 mg to 1,500 mg daily from food and from calcium citrate in divided doses.
    c. Vitamin D (all procedures): 3,000 IU daily, titrate to therapeutic level.
    d. Iron:
      i. LAGB: Not usually necessary.

TABLE 2.5 Routine Supplementation Based on Type of Gastric Bypass Surgery

Supplement	Gastric Band	Gastric Sleeve	Gastric Bypass	BPD/DS
Multivitamin plus mineral	One daily	Two daily	Two daily	Two daily
Calcium	1,200–1,500 mg daily from food and from calcium citrate in divided doses	1,200–1,500 mg daily from food and from calcium citrate in divided doses	1,200–1,500 mg daily from food and from calcium citrate in divided doses	1,200–1,500 mg daily from food and from calcium citrate in divided doses
Vitamin D	3,000 IU daily Titrate to therapeutic level	3,000 IU daily Titrate to therapeutic level	3,000 IU daily Titrate to therapeutic level	3,000 IU daily Titrate to therapeutic level
Iron	Not usually necessary	45–60 mg/d from multivitamin plus additional supplement	45–60 mg/d from multivitamin plus additional supplement	45–60 mg/d from multivitamin plus additional supplement
Vitamin B12	Not usually necessary	As needed to maintain levels in the form best tolerated	As needed to maintain levels in the form best tolerated	As needed to maintain levels in the form best tolerated

BPD/DS, biliopancreatic diversion with duodenal switch.
Source: Adapted from Kerner, J. (2014). Nutrition support after bariatric surgery. *Support Line, 36*(3), 9–20; Shannon, C., Gervasoni, A., & Williams, T. (2013). The bariatric surgery client–nutrition considerations. *Australian Family Physician, 42*(8), 547–552. Retrieved from https://www.racgp.org.au/afp.

    ii. All other procedures: 45 mg to 60 mg daily from multivitamin plus additional supplementation.
  e. Vitamin B12:
    i. LAGB: Not usually necessary.
    ii. All other procedures: As needed to maintain levels in the form best tolerated.
  f. Long-term anticoagulation may be needed for DVT/pulmonary embolism (PE) prophylaxis.
  g. Nonsteroidal anti-inflammatory drugs (NSAIDs) and corticosteroids should be avoided to reduce the risk of marginal ulcers.
D. Psychosocial changes: Bariatric surgery often results in dramatic lifestyle and body changes and may require significant psychosocial adjustments for the client as well as his or her friends and family.
  1. Monitor for depression/anxiety, body image concerns, and social support.
  2. Alcoholism can be a concern after bariatric surgery. Less alcohol is needed to elevate blood alcohol levels and blood alcohol levels are sustained longer after bariatric surgery.

Follow-Up
A. Bariatric surgery requires lifelong follow-up, ideally by a multidisciplinary team of healthcare providers. Initial follow-up schedules are set by the surgeon. Long-term follow-up (after the first two years) is usually provided for by the bariatric surgery program, but research has shown that follow-up is often poor, which leads to poor outcomes and substandard client care.
B. Laboratory and diagnostic testing are required as listed in Table 2.6. Early recognition of nutritional deficiencies can prevent permanent damage and even death.

C. Chronic disease management (particularly diabetes, lipids, and bone disease) can be simpler or more complex after bariatric surgery, depending on the client's adherence to lifestyle and nutritional recommendations.

Consultation/Referral
A. Bariatric surgeon for surgical complications, revisions.
B. Surgeon for cholecystectomy (preferably bariatric surgeon or general/gastrointestinal [GI] surgeon experienced in the care of bariatric clients).
C. Gastroenterology consult.
D. Nutrition consultation and/or counselling.
E. Psychologist consultation.
F. Physical therapy/exercise specialist.
G. Support group.

Individual Considerations
A. Women:
  1. All women of childbearing age should receive adequate folate supplementation and be given contraception and preconception counselling.
  2. Oral contraceptives (OCPs) may not be as effective after bariatric surgery because of changes in absorption.
B. Pregnancy:
  1. Pregnancy should be delayed for 12 to 18 months after bariatric surgery or however long it takes for weight loss to stabilize.
  2. Bariatric surgeon consult may be required.
  3. Increased folic acid may be needed preconception to reduce risk of neural tube defects.
  4. Increased vitamin supplementation may be necessary during pregnancy. Vitamin A should be limited to 5,000 IU daily.

Recommended Annual Laboratory Monitoring for Bypass Clients

	Gastric Band	Gastric Sleeve	Gastric Bypass	BPD/DS
Complete blood count	X	X	X	X
Liver function tests	X	X	X	X
Glucose	X	X	X	X
Creatinine	X	X	X	X
Electrolytes	X	X	X	X
Iron/ferritin	Suggested	X	X	X
Vitamin B12	Suggested	X	X	X
Folate	Suggested	X	X	X
Calcium	Suggested	X	X	X
Intact PTH	Suggested	X	X	X
Vitamin D 25-OH	Suggested	X	X	X
Albumin/prealbumin	Suggested	X	X	X
Bone mineral density		X	X	X
Zinc		Optional	Optional	Optional
Vitamin B1		Optional	Optional	Optional
Vitamin A		Optional 24 months and beyond	Optional 24 months and beyond	Optional 24 months and beyond

BPD/DS, biliopancreatic diversion with duodenal switch; PTH, parathyroid hormone.
Source: Adapted from Heber, D., Greenway, F. L., Kaplan, L. M., Livingston, E., Salvador, J., Still, C., . . . Endocrine Society. (2010). Endocrine and nutritional management of the post-bariatric surgery client: An Endocrine Society clinical practice guideline. Journal of Clinical Endocrinology and Metabolism, 95(11), 4823–4843. doi:10.1210/jc.2009-2128.

5. Gastric band may need to be adjusted during pregnancy.
6. Serial ultrasounds may need to be done to follow fetal growth.

Bibliography

American Society for Metabolic and Bariatric Surgery. (2014). *Approved procedures*. Retrieved from https://asmbs.org

Becker, D. A., Balcer, L. J., & Galetta, S. L. (2012). The neurological complications of nutritional deficiency following bariatric surgery. *Journal of Obesity, 2012*, 1–8. doi:10.1155/2012/608534

Canadian Institute for Health Information. (2014). *Bariatric surgery in Canada*. Retrieved from https://secure.cihi.ca/free_products/Bariatric_Surgery_in_Canada_EN.pdf

Hamdan, K., Somers, S., & Chand, M. (2011). Management of late postoperative complications of bariatric surgery. *British Journal of Surgery, 98*(10), 1345–1355. doi:10.1002/bjs.7568

Handzlik-Orlik, G., Holecki, M., Orlik, B., Wylezol, M., & Dulawa, J. (2015). Nutrition management of the post-bariatric surgery client. *Nutrition in Clinical Practice: Official Publication of the American Society for Parenteral and Enteral Nutrition, 30*(3), 383–392. doi:10.1177/0884533614564995

Heber, D., Greenway, F. L., Kaplan, L. M., Livingston, E., Salvador, J., Still, C., . . . Endocrine Society. (2010). Endocrine and nutritional management of the post-bariatric surgery client: An endocrine society clinical practice guideline. *Endocrine Society, 95*(11), 4823–4843. doi:10.1210/jc.2009-2128

Kerner, J. (2014). Nutrition support after bariatric surgery. *Support Line, 36*(3), 9–20.

Pounds, B. P. (2015). *Improving primary care provider knowledge regarding malabsorptive nutritional deficiencies after bariatric surgery*. Hyden, KY: Frontier Nursing University. Unpublished manuscript

Shannon, C., Gervasoni, A., & Williams, T. (2013). The bariatric surgery client–nutrition considerations. *Australian Family Physician, 42*(8), 547–552. Retrieved from https://www.racgp.org.au/afp

Substance Use Disorders

Moya Cook, Robertson Nash, and Erin Ziegler

Definition

With the publication of the fifth edition of the *Diagnostic and Statistical Manual of Mental Disorders (DSM-5)*, there has been a significant shift in the classification of substance use disorders and their categorization. Previously, the *Diagnostic and Statistical Manual of Mental Disorders*, fourth edition *(DSM–IV)* provided distinct groups of substance use, listed as follows:

A. Substance abuse: A maladaptive pattern of substance use leading to clinically significant impairment or distress, as manifested by one or more specific symptoms, occurring within a 12-month period.
B. Substance intoxication: The development of a reversible substance-specific syndrome caused by recent ingestion of (or exposure to) a substance.
C. Substance dependence: A maladaptive pattern of substance use, leading to clinically significant impairment or distress, as manifested by three (or more) specific symptoms, occurring at any time in the same 12-month period.
D. Substance withdrawal: The development of a substance-specific syndrome caused by the cessation of (or reduction in) substance use that has been heavy and prolonged.

The *DSM-5* states that diagnosis of a substance use disorder should be based on a pathologic pattern of behaviours related to the use of the substance. The *DSM-5* notes that an underlying characteristic of substance use disorders is changes in brain circuitry that may persist beyond detoxification. Manifestations of those changes include intense drug craving and relapse. Those patterns of behaviour have been categorized into four groups, listed as follows:
E. Impaired control:
   1. Use of a substance in larger amounts or for a longer time than originally intended.
   2. Repeated unsuccessful attempts to cut down use of the substance.
   3. A great deal of time spent obtaining, using, and recovering from the substance.
   4. Intense desire for the substance, especially in an environment in which it was previously used.
F. Social impairment:
   1. Recurrent substance use leading to a failure to meet personal and social obligations.
   2. Continued substance use, despite significant, ongoing social problems caused or exacerbated by the substance.
   3. Abandoning important personal and social goals because of substance use.
G. Risky use:
   1. Recurrent substance use in environments in which it is dangerous to use the substance.
   2. Continued substance use despite knowledge of persistent/recurrent physical/psychological problems caused by the substance.
H. Pharmacological criteria:
   1. Requirement for a markedly increased dose to achieve desired effect or markedly reduced effect at standard dose.
   2. Desire to consume the substance to mitigate withdrawal symptoms.

As a modifier, use severity is assessed across three categories, listed as follows. It is important to note that the word "addiction" has been removed from the *DSM-5* because of its vague definition and possible negative connotation.
A. Mild: Two or three of the preceding symptoms listed are present.
B. Moderate: Four to five of the preceding symptoms listed are present.
C. Severe: Six or more of the preceding symptoms listed are present.

Incidence/Prevalence

A. Statistics indicate that the most commonly used legal substances are caffeine, alcohol, and nicotine. The Canadian Tobacco, Alcohol and Drugs Survey (CTADS) reported that in 2015, the prevalence of current cigarette smoking was 13% of the population, equaling 3.9 million smokers. Approximately 10% of Canadians aged 15 to 19 are regular smokers. Smoking is the most preventable cause of premature illness and death.
B. In 2015, 22.7 million Canadians reported consuming an alcoholic beverage in the last year. Twenty percent of alcohol consumption was above *Canada's Low Risk Alcohol Drinking Guidelines*. In 2015 to 2016, alcohol was directly related to approximately 77,000 hospitalizations. Underage drinking among youth in grades 7 to 12 has been reported at 44% by the 2016 to 2017 CTADS, with the average age of onset at 13.4 years.
C. The most commonly used drugs are cannabis and opioid pain relievers. The CTADS reported the prevalence of cannabis use was 12% of the population, an increase from 11% in 2013. The median age of initiating use of cannabis for males and females was 17 years. Twenty-four percent of cannabis users reported using it for medical purposes. See Table 2.7 for information regarding commonly abused drugs.
D. Opioid pain relievers were used by 13% of Canadians aged 15 years and older in 2015. Among the 13%, abuse rates were reported in 2% of the population. Use of psychoactive pharmacological substances, including stimulants and sedatives, among Canadians aged 15 years and older was 22%,

with abuse rates reported in 3% of the population. Canada's illegal drug supply is being contaminated with fentanyl and other fentanyl-like drugs (e.g., carfentanil). Fentanyl is 20 to 40 times more potent than heroin and 100 times more potent than morphine. Fentanyl mixed with other drugs is causing high rates of overdoses and overdose deaths in Canada. See Table 2.8 for commonly abused prescription drugs.

E. Youth aged 15 to 24 years old have the highest self-reported use of illicit substances and are five times more likely than adults to report harm due to drug use.

A substance abuse problem is recognized in as few as one in 20 substance-abusing clients seeking medical attention.

Principles of Drug Addiction Treatment

More than three decades of scientific research show that treatment can help drug-addicted individuals stop drug use, avoid relapse, and successfully recover their lives. Based on this research, 13 fundamental principles that characterize effective drug-abuse treatment have been developed. These principles are detailed in NIDA's *Principles of Drug Addiction Treatment: A Research-Based Guide*. The guide also describes different types of science-based treatments and provides answers to commonly asked questions.

A. Addiction is a complex but treatable disease that affects brain function and behaviour. Drugs alter the brain's structure and how it functions, resulting in changes that persist long after drug use has ceased. This may help explain why abusers are at risk of relapse even after long periods of abstinence.

B. No single treatment is appropriate for everyone. Matching treatment settings, interventions, and services to an individual's particular problems and needs is critical to his or her ultimate success.

C. Treatment needs to be readily available. Because drug-addicted individuals may be uncertain about entering treatment, taking advantage of available services the moment people are ready for treatment is critical. Potential clients can be lost if treatment is not immediately available or readily accessible.

D. Effective treatment attends to multiple needs of the individual, not just his or her drug abuse. To be effective, treatment must address the individual's drug abuse and any associated medical, psychological, social, vocational, and legal problems.

E. Remaining in treatment for an adequate period of time is critical. The appropriate duration for an individual depends on the type and degree of his or her problems and needs. Research indicates that most addicted individuals need at least 3 months in treatment to significantly reduce or stop their drug use and that the best outcomes occur with longer durations of treatment.

F. Counselling—individual and/or group—and other behavioural therapies are the most commonly used forms of drug-abuse treatment. Behavioural therapies vary in their focus and may involve addressing a client's motivations to change, building skills to resist drug use, replacing drug-using activities with constructive and rewarding activities, improving problem-solving skills, and facilitating better interpersonal relationships.

G. Medications are an important element of treatment for many clients, especially when combined with counselling and other behavioural therapies. For example, methadone and buprenorphine are effective in helping individuals addicted to heroin or other opioids stabilize their lives and reduce their illicit drug use. Also, for persons addicted to nicotine, a nicotine replacement product (nicotine patches or gum) or an oral medication (bupropion or varenicline), can be an effective component of treatment when part of a comprehensive behavioural treatment program.

H. An individual's treatment and services plan must be assessed continually and modified as necessary to ensure it meets his or her changing needs. A client may require varying combinations of services and treatment components during the course of treatment and recovery. In addition to counselling or psychotherapy, a client may require medication, medical services, family therapy, parenting instruction, vocational rehabilitation, and/or social and legal services. For many clients, a continuing care approach provides the best results, with treatment intensity varying according to a person's changing needs.

I. Many drug-addicted individuals also have other mental disorders. Because drug abuse and addiction—both of which are mental disorders—often co-occur with other mental illnesses, clients presenting with one condition should be assessed for the other(s). And when these problems co-occur, treatment should address both (or all), including the use of medications as appropriate.

J. Medically assisted detoxification is only the first stage of addiction treatment and by itself does little to change long-term drug abuse. Although medically assisted detoxification can safely manage the acute physical symptoms of withdrawal, detoxification alone is rarely sufficient to help addicted individuals achieve long-term abstinence. Thus, clients should be encouraged to continue drug treatment following detoxification.

K. Treatment does not need to be voluntary to be effective. Sanctions or enticements from family, employment settings, and/or the criminal justice system can significantly increase treatment entry, retention rates, and the ultimate success of drug treatment interventions.

L. Drug use during treatment must be monitored continuously, as lapses during treatment do occur. Knowing their drug use is being monitored can be a powerful incentive for clients and can help them withstand urges to use drugs. Monitoring also provides an early indication of a return to drug use, signaling a possible need to adjust an individual's treatment plan to better meet his or her needs.

M. Treatment programs should assess clients for the presence of HIV/AIDS, hepatitis B and C, tuberculosis, and other infectious diseases, as well as provide targeted risk-reduction counselling to help clients modify or change behaviours that place them at risk of contracting or spreading infectious diseases. Targeted counselling specifically focused on reducing infectious-disease risk can help clients further reduce or avoid substance-related and other high-risk behaviours. Treatment providers should encourage and support HIV screening and inform clients in whom highly active antiretroviral therapy (HAART) has proven effective in combating HIV, including among drug-abusing populations.

Pathogenesis

A. No single gene has been identified in the predisposition to substance dependence. Certain biological features seem to be inherited by first-degree relatives (particularly males) of alcoholics, for example, a resistance to intoxication, a subnormal cortisol rise after drinking, and a subnormal epinephrine release following stress.

TABLE 2.7 Commonly Abused Drugs

Substances: Category and Name	Examples of Commercial and Street Names	How Administered[a]	Acute Effects/Health Risks
Tobacco			Increased blood pressure and heart rate/chronic lung disease; cardiovascular disease; stroke; cancers of the mouth, pharynx, larynx, oesophagus, stomach, pancreas, cervix, kidney, bladder, and acute myeloid leukaemia; adverse pregnancy outcomes; addiction
Nicotine	Found in cigarettes, cigars, bidis, and smokeless tobacco (snuff, spit tobacco, chew)	Smoked, snorted, chewed	
Alcohol			In low doses, euphoria, mild stimulation, relaxation, lowered inhibitions; in higher doses, drowsiness, slurred speech, nausea, emotional volatility, loss of coordination, visual distortions, impaired memory, sexual dysfunction, loss of consciousness/increased risk of injuries, violence, foetal damage (in pregnant women); depression; neurologic deficits; hypertension; liver and heart disease; addiction; fatal overdose
Alcohol (ethyl alcohol)	Found in liquor, beer, and wine	Swallowed	
Cannabinoids			Euphoria, relaxation; slowed reaction time, distorted sensory perception, impaired balance and coordination, increased heart rate and appetite, impaired learning and memory, anxiety, panic attacks, psychosis/cough, frequent respiratory infections, possible mental health decline, addiction
Marijuana	Blunt, dope, ganja, grass, herb, joint, bud, Mary Jane, pot, reefer, green, trees, smoke, sinsemilla, skunk, weed	Smoked, swallowed	
Hashish	Boom, gangster, hash, hash oil, hemp	Smoked, swallowed	
Opioids			Euphoria, drowsiness, impaired coordination, dizziness, confusion, nausea, sedation, feeling of heaviness in the body, slowed or arrested breathing, constipation, endocarditis, hepatitis, HIV, addiction, fatal overdose
Heroin	Diacetylmorphine: Smack, horse, brown sugar, dope, H, junk, skag, skunk, white horse, China white; cheese (with OTC cold medicine and antihistamine)	Injected, smoked, snorted	
Opium	Laudanum, paregoric: Big O, black stuff, block, gum, hop	Swallowed, smoked	
Stimulants			Increased heart rate, blood pressure, body temperature, metabolism; feelings of exhilaration; increased energy, mental alertness; tremors; reduced appetite; irritability; anxiety; panic; paranoia; violent behaviour; psychosis/weight loss; insomnia; cardiac or cardiovascular complications; stroke; seizures; addiction Also, for cocaine—nasal damage from snorting Also, for methamphetamine—severe dental problems
Cocaine	Cocaine hydrochloride: Blow, bump, C, candy, Charlie, coke, crack, flake, rock, snow, toot	Snorted, smoked, injected	
Amphetamine	Biphetamine, dexedrine: Bennies, black beauties, crosses, hearts, LA turnaround speed, truck drivers, uppers	Swallowed, snorted, smoked, injected	
Methamphetamine	Desoxyn: Meth, ice, crank, chalk, crystal, fire, glass, go fast, speed	Swallowed, snorted, smoked, injected	
Club Drugs			MDMA—mild hallucinogenic effects; increased tactile sensitivity, empathic feelings; lowered inhibition; anxiety; chills; sweating; teeth clenching; muscle cramping/sleep disturbances; depression; impaired memory; hyperthermia; addiction Flunitrazepam—sedation; muscle relaxation; confusion; memory loss; dizziness; impaired coordination/addiction
MDMA	Ecstasy, Adam, clarity, Eve, lover's speed, peace, uppers	Swallowed, snorted, injected	
Flunitrazepam	Rohypnol: Forget-me pill, Mexican Valium, R2, roach, Roche, roofies, roofinol, rope, rophies	Swallowed, snorted	

(continued)

TABLE 2.7 Commonly Abused Drugs (continued)

Substances: Category and Name	Examples of Commercial and Street Names	How Administered[a]	Acute Effects/Health Risks
GHB[b]	G, Georgia home boy, grievous bodily harm, liquid ecstasy, soap, scoop, goop, liquid X	Swallowed	GHB—drowsiness; nausea; headache; disorientation; loss of coordination; memory loss/unconsciousness; seizures; coma
Dissociative Drugs			Feelings of being separate from one's body and environment, impaired motor function/anxiety, tremors, numbness, memory loss, nausea
Ketamine	Ketalar SV: cat Valium, K, special K, vitamin K	Injected, snorted, smoked	Also, for ketamine—analgesia, impaired memory, delirium, respiratory depression and arrest, death
PCP and analogs	Phencyclidine: Angel dust, boat, hog, love boat, peace pill	Swallowed, smoked, injected	Also, for PCP and analogs—analgesia, psychosis, aggression, violence, slurred speech, loss of coordination, hallucinations
Salvia divinorum	Salvia, shepherdess's herb, Maria Pastora, magic mint, Sally-D	Chewed, swallowed, smoked	Also, for DXM—euphoria, slurred speech, confusion, dizziness, distorted visual perceptions
DXM	Found in some cough and cold medications: Robotripping, robo, triple C	Swallowed	
Hallucinogens			Altered states of perception and feeling; hallucinations; nausea
LSD	Acid, blotter, cubes, microdot, yellow sunshine, blue heaven	Swallowed, absorbed through mouth tissues	Also, for LSD and mescaline—increased body temperature, heart rate, blood pressure; loss of appetite; sweating; sleeplessness; numbness; dizziness; weakness; tremors; impulsive behaviour; rapid shifts in emotion
Mescaline	Buttons, cactus, mesc, peyote	Swallowed, smoked	Also, for LSD—flashbacks, hallucinogen persisting perception disorder
Psilocybin	Magic mushrooms, purple passion, shrooms, little smoke	Swallowed	Also, for psilocybin—nervousness, paranoia, panic
Other Compounds			Steroids—no intoxicating effects/hypertension; blood clotting and cholesterol changes, liver cysts, hostility and aggression, acne; in adolescents—premature stoppage of growth; in males—prostate cancer, reduced sperm production, shrunken testicles, breast enlargement; in females—menstrual irregularities, development of beard and other masculine characteristics
Anabolic steroids	Anadrol, Oxandrin, Durabolin, Depo-Testosterone, Equipoise: Roids, juice, gym candy, pumpers	Injected, swallowed, applied to skin	
Inhalants	Solvents (paint thinners, gasoline, glues); gases (butane, propane, aerosol propellants, nitrous oxide); nitrites (isoamyl, isobutyl, cyclohexyl): Laughing gas, poppers, snappers, whippets	Inhaled through nose or mouth	Inhalants (varies by chemical)—stimulation, loss of inhibition, headache, nausea or vomiting, slurred speech, loss of motor coordination, wheezing/cramps, muscle weakness, depression, memory impairment, damage to cardiovascular and nervous systems, unconsciousness, sudden death
Prescription Medications			
CNS depressants	For more information on prescription medications, please visit publications.gc.ca/collections/Collection/H39-65-2000E.pdf		
Stimulants			
Opioid pain relievers			

[a] Some of the health risks are directly related to the route of drug administration. For example, injection drug use can increase the risk of infection through needle contamination with staphylococci, HIV, hepatitis, and other organisms.
[b] Associated with sexual assaults.
CNS, central nervous system; DXM, dextromethorphan; GHB, gamma-hydroxybutyric acid; LSD, lysergic acid diethylamide; MDMA, methylenedioxymethamphetamine; OTC, over the counter; PCP, phencyclidine.
Source: National Institute on Drug Abuse (NIDA): Visit NIDA at www.drugabuse.gov; National Institutes of Health (NIH); U.S. Department of Health and Human Services; NIH: Turning Discovery Into Health.

TABLE 2.8 Commonly Abused Prescription Drugs

Substances: Category and Name	Examples of Commercial and Street Names	How Administered	Intoxication Effects/Health Risks
Depressants			Sedation/drowsiness, reduced anxiety, feelings of well-being, lowered inhibitions, slurred speech, poor concentration; confusion, dizziness, impaired coordination and memory/slowed pulse, lowered blood pressure, slowed breathing, tolerance, withdrawal, addiction, increased risk of respiratory distress and death when combined with alcohol For barbiturates—euphoria, unusual excitement, fever, irritability/life-threatening withdrawal in chronic users
Barbiturates	Nembutal, Phenobarbital: Barbs, reds, red birds, phennies, tooies, yellows, yellow jackets	Injected, swallowed	
Benzodiazepines	Ativan, Valium, Xanax, Rivotril: Candy, downers, sleeping pills, tranks	Swallowed	
Sleep medications	Sublinox, zopiclone	Swallowed	
Opioids and Morphine Derivatives[a]			Pain relief, euphoria, drowsiness, sedation, weakness, dizziness, nausea, impaired coordination, confusion, dry mouth, itching, sweating, clammy skin, constipation/slowed or arrested breathing, lowered pulse and blood pressure, tolerance, addiction, unconsciousness, coma, death; risk of death increased when combined with alcohol or other CNS depressants For fentanyl—80–100 times more potent analgesic than morphine For oxycodone—muscle relaxation/twice as potent analgesic as morphine; high abuse potential For codeine—less analgesia, sedation, and respiratory depression than morphine For methadone—used to treat opioid addiction and pain; significant overdose risk when used improperly
Codeine	Fiorinal with Codeine, Tylenol with Codeine: Captain Cody, Cody, schoolboy; (with glutethimide: Doors & fours, loads, pancakes, and syrup)	Injected, swallowed	
Morphine	Doloral, MS Contin, Statex, M-Eslon: M, Miss Emma, monkey, white stuff	Injected, swallowed, smoked	
Methadone	Methadose, Metadol: Fizzies, amidone (with MDMA: Chocolate chip cookies)	Swallowed, injected	
Fentanyl and analogs	Abstral, Duragesic, Fentora: Apache, China girl, dance fever, friend, good-fella, jackpot, murder 8, TNT, Tango and Cash	Injected, smoked, snorted	
Other opioid pain relievers: Oxycodone HCL, hydrocodone bitartrate, hydromorphone, oxymorphone, meperidine, propoxyphene	Oxycontin, OxyNEO, Percocet, Endocet, Rivacocet, Percocet: Oxy, O.C., oxycet, hillbilly heroin, percs; Dilaudid: Juice, smack, D, footballs, dillies; Demerol, meperidine hydrochloride: Demmies, pain killer	Chewed, swallowed, snorted, injected, suppositories	
Stimulants			Feelings of exhilaration; increased energy; mental alertness/increased heart rate, blood pressure, and metabolism; reduced appetite; weight loss; nervousness; insomnia; seizures; heart attack; stroke For amphetamines—rapid breathing, tremor, loss of coordination, irritability, anxiousness, restlessness/delirium, panic, paranoia, hallucinations, impulsive behaviour, aggressiveness, tolerance, addiction For methylphenidate—increase or decrease in blood pressure, digestive problems, loss of appetite, weight loss
Amphetamines	Biphentin, Foquest, Dexedrine, Adderall: Bennies, black beauties, crosses, hearts, LA turnaround, speed, truck drivers, uppers	Injected, swallowed, smoked, snorted	
Methylphenidate	Concerta, Ritalin: JIF, MPH, R-ball, skippy, the smart drug, vitamin R	Injected, swallowed, snorted	
Other Compounds			Euphoria, slurred speech/increased heart rate and blood pressure, dizziness, nausea, vomiting, confusion, paranoia, distorted visual perceptions, impaired motor function
DXM	Found in some cough and cold medications: Robotripping, robo, triple C	Swallowed	

[a] Taking drugs by injection can increase the risk of infection through needle contamination with staphylococci, HIV, hepatitis, and other organisms. Injection is a more common practice for opioids, but risks apply to any medication taken by injection.
CNS, central nervous system; DXM, dextromethorphan; HCL, hydrochloride; MDMA, methylenedioxymethamphetamine.
Source: National Institute on Drug Abuse (NIDA): Visit NIDA at www.drugabuse.gov; National Institutes of Health (NIH); U.S. Department of Health and Human Services; NIH: Turning Discovery Into Health.

B. Some theories postulate alterations in metabolism of alcohol and drugs in people who are dependent. Studies pertaining to alcohol have included research into genetic heritability, faulty metabolism of alcohol by alcoholics, insensitivity to alcohol inherited by alcoholics (thus tending to increase tolerance or ability to know when to stop), and alterations in brain waves in alcoholics.

C. Although much of the research is specific to only one drug, much of what we know about the research can be applied to other drugs. There appears to be a higher rate of substance dependence, not limited to alcohol, in children of alcoholics.

Predisposing Factors

Factors vary among individuals, and no one factor can account entirely for the risk of substance abuse. Studies indicate a high correlation between substance use and the presence of psychiatric disorders, especially anxiety disorders, depression, schizophrenia, and, in women, eating disorders.

A. Genetic.
B. Familial.
C. Environmental.
D. Occupational.
E. Socioeconomic.
F. Cultural.
G. Personality.
H. Life stress.
I. Psychiatric comorbidity.
J. Biological.
K. Social learning and behavioural conditioning.

Common Findings

Clients' complaints will be focused on the symptoms of the problem rather than the substance dependence. The problem itself will be avoided using denial, minimization, blaming, and projection (all signs of the disease of substance dependence).

A. Chronic anxiety and tension.
B. Insomnia.
C. Chronic depression.
D. Headaches and/or back pain.

Consider clients who present frequently with somatic complaints, such as back pain or headache, as "drug seeking," especially when the client knows what drugs work best or asks for specific narcotic analgesics.

E. Blackouts.
F. Gastrointestinal problems.
G. Tachycardia/palpitations.
H. Frequent falls or minor injuries.

Substance abuse should be suspected in all clients who present with accidents or signs of repeated trauma, especially to the head.

I. Problems with a loved one, at work, or with friends.

Other Signs and Symptoms

A. Defensiveness about alcohol/drug use or vagueness with answers.
B. History of problems with family life, marital relationships, work, finances, and physical health.
C. Change in spiritual beliefs (stops attending religious services).
D. Unexplained job changes and multiple traffic accidents.
E. History of impulsive behaviour, fighting, or unexplained falls.
F. Arrest for public drunkenness, driving under the influence, or illegal activity when alcohol/drugs were involved.
G. Tremours (shakes).
H. Delirium tremens (DTs).
I. Seizures related to drugs.
J. Hallucinations.
K. History of chronic family chaos and instability.
L. Physical indications of chronic alcohol/drug use include spider angiomas, ruddy nose and face, nasal lesions, bruxism, swollen features, bruises, needle marks/tracks, cutaneous abscesses, malnourishment, anaemia, jaundice, and severe dental problems such as "meth mouth."
M. Active withdrawal symptoms include nausea and vomiting, malaise, weakness, tachycardia, diaphoresis, tremors, light-headedness or dizziness, insomnia, irritability, confusion, perceptual abnormalities or hallucinations (auditory, visual, or tactile), paraesthesia, blurred vision, diarrhoea, anorexia, abdominal cramps, severe depression, severe anxiety, piloerection, fasciculation (muscle twitching), rhinorrhoea, fever, elevated blood pressure and pulse, tinnitus, nystagmus, delirium, or seizures.
N. Overdose symptoms related to drug(s) include seizures, cardiovascular depression/collapse, and respiratory depression/collapse. Be prepared to provide cardiovascular and respiratory support and supportive care until transport.

Subjective Data

A. Review the onset, duration, and course of presenting complaints.
B. Question the client regarding relatives with a history of alcohol, tobacco, or drug use or problems pertaining to use.
C. When questioning the client, assume some use: for example, "At what age did you first start drinking?" Start with the least invasive questions first: cigarettes, OTC medications, prescription medications, followed by alcohol, marijuana, stimulants, opiates, sedatives, hypnotics, benzodiazepines, barbiturates, hallucinogens, inhalants, steroids, and other drugs.
D. Review use of the following drugs concerning quantity and type (if cigarettes, brand smoked; if alcohol, type of alcohol [e.g., beer, wine, or hard liquor]), and age at initiation. Query regarding previous attempts to stop use.
E. Start with the past and proceed to the present with use; include first use of the mood-altering substance, amounts, and the last use of the substance and amount.
F. Follow the CAGE (cut down, annoyed, guilty, eye opener) test. The **CAGE** (two out of four) is highly predictive of addiction.

   1. Have you ever tried to **cut** down on your alcohol/drug use?
   2. Do you get **annoyed** if someone mentions your use is a problem?
   3. Do you ever feel **guilty** about your use?
   4. Do you ever have an **"eye-opener"** first thing in the morning after you've been drinking or using the night before?

G. If client admits drinking or drug use, ascertain specific amounts and last use of each substance.
H. Establish usual weight and recent loss and in what length of time.

I. Determine whether client experiences suicidal ideation and whether there is a history of past attempts (see the section "Suicide" in Chapter 22, Psychiatric Guidelines).

Physical Examination
A. Check temperature, pulse, respirations, blood pressure, and weight.
B. Inspect:
   1. Observe general appearance, dress, grooming, breath odour, wasted appearance, attitude, sad affect, impaired psychomotor ability, or tremors.
   2. Conduct a dermal examination for spider angiomas, bruises, track marks, colour, pallor, rash, jaundice, petechiae, and gynecomastia in men (hallucinogens).
   3. Examine the eyes for sclera colour and features, pupil size, and reactivity.
   4. Inspect the nasal mucosa for erythema, oedema, spider telangiectasis, and discharge; look for septal lesions or perforation, deviation, and polyps.
   5. Inspect the mouth/pharynx: oral lesions, poor dental hygiene, erythema, teeth for uneven surfaces and decay, and gum erosion.
C. Palpate:
   1. Palpate the neck and thyroid.
   2. Axilla and groin for lymphadenopathy.
   3. Abdomen; note hepatomegaly/tenderness.
D. Percuss:
   1. Percuss the chest; note pulmonary consolidation.
   2. Abdomen for hepatosplenomegaly.
E. Auscultate:
   1. Heart for murmur, new S4 gallop, single S2, and arrhythmias.
   2. Lungs for rales, effusion, and consolidation.
F. Perform neurologic examination/mental status.

Diagnostic Tests
The following is a list of laboratory tests for consideration based on client history and physical examination. All laboratory tests may not be necessary.
A. Blood alcohol level.
B. Urine drug screen.
C. Complete blood count (CBC) with differential.
D. Platelet count.
E. HIV or hepatitis.

Intravenous drug use contributes strongly to the spread of AIDS, hepatitis B and hepatitis C, and other infectious diseases. Consider evaluation for sexually transmitted infections.

F. Antinuclear antibody, erythrocyte sedimentation rate, and rheumatoid factor.
G. Electrolytes.
H. Liver panel: Elevated liver enzymes can also be attributed to overuse of acetaminophen, found in combination with opiates.
I. Blood cultures (fever).
J. Bone density studies: Clients who have been drinking for years should have bone density studies done because alcohol increases the risk for osteoporosis.

Differential Diagnoses
A. Chronic pain syndrome.
B. Anxiety.
C. Depression.

Plan
A. General interventions:
   1. Discuss your concerns about alcohol, nicotine, or drug use and discuss addiction treatment with the client. (Refer to the NIDA Principles of Drug Addiction Treatment earlier in this chapter.)
   2. At each office visit, provide support to help prevent relapse. If relapse occurs, encourage the client to try again immediately.
   3. Consider signing a contract with the client to stop smoking, drinking, or using drugs.
   4. Assess potential for suicide with every office visit.
   5. If possible, obtain confirmation of the client's abstinence from a family member.
   6. Stress the importance of 12-step meetings such as Alcoholics Anonymous (AA), Cocaine Anonymous (CA), and Narcotics Anonymous (NA).
   7. Have the client sign a written release of information so that you can speak with a rehabilitation counsellor. If the client is willing, refer to an alcohol and drug treatment facility or smoking-cessation program after initial assessment and differential diagnosis is made.
   8. Treat physical/laboratory findings as indicated.
   9. Identify potential withdrawal symptoms from the cessation of stimulants, such as caffeine intake reduction, alcohol, and drug use.
   10. If malnourished, discuss dietary needs and treatment.
B. Client teaching: Educate the client about the impact of alcohol, tobacco, and drugs on physical/emotional health. Provide information for the client to read at home.
C. Pharmacological therapy:
   1. Consider nicotine replacement for those who smoke more than one pack of cigarettes per day or who smoke their first cigarette within 30 minutes of waking. Stress that there is *no smoking* while using the nicotine patch.
   2. Nonnicotine therapy: Adults—Bupropion. Treat for seven to 12 weeks. The client may continue to smoke during the first two weeks of starting medication. This medication should not be given to clients with seizure disorders.
   3. Varenicline:
      a. Encourage the client to choose a stop date for smoking and start the drug one to two weeks before this stop date.
      b. Clients should be encouraged to quit even if they have relapses.
      c. Instruct clients that the most common side effects are insomnia, vivid or strange dreams, and nausea. Advise that side effects are usually transient.
      d. Warn the client regarding potential side effects of mood swings, aggression, homicidal thoughts, psychosis, anxiety, and panic disorder, which may occur on rare occasions.
      e. See package insert for detailed instructions.
   4. Detoxification and methadone maintenance: Should be performed by specially licensed and trained professionals.
   5. Disulfiram therapy is not recommended. Clients who consume alcohol after taking this drug can become extremely ill.
   6. If the client is experiencing withdrawal, consider referring to a specialist or admission to a rehabilitation center for detoxification and treatment.

Follow-Up
A. Make a follow-up appointment weekly. Contact the referral source (smoking cessation program, alcohol/drug rehabilitation program) before the next follow-up visit to check on the client's progress. At the weekly visit, question the client regarding compliance.
B. Order blood alcohol or urine drug screen with every office visit while in outpatient treatment and throughout the year following treatment.
C. Once positive change is seen, the client can be seen monthly. Discuss changes the client has made, past relapses, circumstances under which they occurred, and any special concerns.
D. Refer to the medical diagnosis for other applicable follow-up recommendations.

Consultation/Referral
A. Refer clients with drug and/or alcohol dependence to a community mental health center that has an outpatient alcohol/drug rehabilitation program or to a specialist in the community who deals frequently with substance abuse/dependence.
B. Planning a family meeting to confront the client is best done with the help of an experienced mental health professional.
C. Have referral numbers at close hand, so that the client's moment of motivation is not lost.

Individual Considerations
A. Pregnancy:
  1. Substance-dependent pregnant women frequently avoid early prenatal care for fear of identification and reprisal.
  2. Cocaine use is associated with abruptio placenta and preterm labor. Consider drug screen for emergent admissions for clients in preterm labor and abruption.
  3. Notify the hospital nursery personnel/neonatologist before delivery to closely monitor the newborn for withdrawal and seizure precautions.
  4. Nicotine/smoking use is associated with intrauterine growth restriction, preterm delivery, and bleeding in pregnancy.
  5. Nicotine-dependent pregnant women should be encouraged to stop smoking without pharmacological treatment. The nicotine patch should be used during pregnancy only if the increased likelihood of smoking cessation, with its potential benefits, outweighs the risk of nicotine replacement and potential concomitant smoking. Similar factors should be considered in lactating women.
  6. Pregnant women who use alcohol, tobacco, or drugs should always be classified as substance dependent rather than substance abusive.
B. Paediatrics:
  1. Infants of smokers have increased risk of sudden infant death syndrome (SIDS).
  2. The diagnosis of substance dependence is more difficult to make in children younger than 18 years. If there is any indication of substance dependence, children should be referred to a paediatrician who deals specifically with this problem.
  3. Consider drug use when alienation of friends and family, falling grades, and isolation occur.
  4. "Huffing" is common with gasoline, glues, aerosol sprays, and spray paints.
  5. The use of synthetic cannabinoid products is on the rise in the adolescent population. K2, Spice, bath salts and other such products are available in tobacco stores, gas stations, over the internet, and in other small shops. These products can be very harmful and are not detected on routine toxicology drug screens. Be aware of illicit drug use if clients present with change in behaviour, depression, paranoid delusion, and aggressive behaviours. Educate the client and family regarding the toxic use of these OTC substances. Stress to the client that these are abusive substances that can potentially be fatal. Stress cessation of use and refer to specialist.
C. Adults:
  1. With women, tolerance can be established by asking the question, "How many drinks does it take to make you high?" More than two drinks indicate some tolerance.
  2. In considering a diagnosis of alcohol dependence, consider the following diagnostic findings: hypertension; nonspecific EKG changes; cardiomyopathy; palpitations; increased mean cell volume; decreased red blood cell count; low platelet count; increased alanine aminotransferase (ALT), aspartate aminotransferase (AST), lactic dehydrogenase, gamma-glutamyl transpeptidase, and alkaline phosphatase; type IV hyperlipoproteinemia; gout; and adult-onset diabetes mellitus.
D. Geriatrics:
  1. In this population, alcohol consumption as little as 30 mL daily can indicate a problem.
  2. Pain medications and benzodiazepines, along with multiple medications for health problems, may create a substance abuse problem.
E. Partners/family members:
  1. For fear of retribution, the family may remain silent about the problem, even if accompanying the client to the healthcare visit.
  2. Some studies by corporate business show that, per capita, business spends more money on the care of family members of substance-dependent clients than on the employee.
  3. Refer family members of alcoholics/drug addicts to Al-Anon, Nar-Anon, Co-dependents Anonymous, or Adult Children of Alcoholics (ACOA) meetings.

Resources
Canada's Low Risk Alcohol Drinking Guidelines: http://www.ccdus.ca/Resource%20Library/2012-Canada-Low-Risk-Alcohol-Drinking-Guidelines-Brochure-en.pdf
Canadian Center on Substance Use and Addiction: http://www.ccdus.ca/eng/Pages/default.aspx

Bibliography
Angstman, K. B., Pietruszewski, P., Rasmussen, N. H., Wilkinson, J. M., & Katzelnick, D. J. (2012). Depression remission after six months of collaborative care management: Role of initial severity of depression in outcome. *Mental Health in Family Medicine, 9*(2), 99–106. Retrieved from https://www.mhfmjournal.com/
Canadian Action Network for the Advancement, Dissemination and Adoption of Practice-informed Tobacco Treatment. (2011). *Canadian smoking cessation clinical practice guidelines.* Toronto, ON, Canada: Canadian Action Network for the Advancement, Dissemination and Adoption of Practice-informed Tobacco Treatment, Centre for Addiction and Mental Health. Retrieved from https://www.nicotinedependenceclinic.com/english/canadaptt/guideline/introduction.aspx
Ewing, J. A. (1984). Detecting alcoholism. The CAGE questionnaire. *Journal of the American Medical Association, 252*(14), 1905–1907. doi:10.1001/jama.1984.03350140051025
Government of Canada. (2017). *Canadian tobacco alcohol and drugs (CTADS): 2015 summary.* Retrieved from https://www.canada.ca/en/health-canada/services/canadian-tobacco-alcohol-drugs-survey/2015-summary.html

Government of Canada. (2018). *Summary of results for the Canadian student tobacco, alcohol and drug survey 2016–2017*. Retrieved from https://www.canada.ca/en/health-canada/services/canadian-student-tobacco-alcohol-drugs-survey/2016-2017-summary.html

Hardy, S. (2013). Prevention and management of depression in primary care. *Nursing Standard, 27*(26), 51–56; quiz 58. Retrieved from https://rcni.com/nursing-standard/evidence-and-practice/clinical

National Institute on Drug Abuse. (2011, March). *Commonly abused drugs chart*. Retrieved from www.drugabuse.gov/drugs-abuse/commonly-abused-drugs/commonly-abused-drugs-chart

National Institute on Drug Abuse. (2016, January). *Commonly abused prescription drug chart*. Retrieved from www.drugabuse.gov/drugs-abuse/commonly-abused-drugs-charts

O'Malley, P. A. (2012). Baby boomers and substance abuse: The curse of youth again in old age: Implications for the clinical nurse specialist. *Clinical Nurse Specialist, 26*(6), 305–307. doi:10.1097/NUR.0b013e318272f7a6

Saha, S., Wilson Deanne, J., & Adger, R. J. (2012). K2, spice, and bath salts drugs of abuse commercially available. *Contemporary Pediatrics, 29*(10), 22–28. Retrieved from http://www.contemporarypediatrics.com/

Smith, M. (2013). Care of adolescents who have mental health and substance misuse problems. *Mental Health Practice, 1*(5), 32–36. Retrieved from https://journals.rcni.com/mental-health-practice

Richardson, L., & Puskar, K. (2012, June). Screening assessment for anxiety and depression in primary care. *Journal for Nurse Practitioners, 8*(6), 475–481. doi:10.1016/j.nurpra.2011.10.005

U.S. Food and Administration Drug. (2016). *Find information about a drug*. Retrieved from www.fda.gov/Drugs/ResourcesForYou/Consumers/ucm450624.htm

Wendell, A. D. (2013). Overview and epidemiology of substance abuse in pregnancy. *Clinical Obstetrics and Gynecology, 56*(1), 91–96.

Violence: Children

Moya Cook, Robertson Nash, and Erin Ziegler

Definition

Child maltreatment incorporates any harm or risk of harm to a child while in the care of a person they care for or depend on. This can include parents, siblings, relatives, teachers, and caregivers. Harm can occur through direct actions or neglect.

A. Physical abuse (assault): Infliction of pain/harm producing injuries, including skeletal fractures, skin (e.g., burns), and central nervous system (CNS) injuries (e.g., abusive head trauma [AHT] and shaken baby syndrome [SBS]/shaking-impact syndrome).

B. Sexual abuse: Inappropriate exposure; fondling; sexual stimulation; coercion; oral, genital, buttock, or breast contact; anal or vaginal penetration; foreign-body insertion; and child pornography.
　1. Canada's age of consent for youth is aimed to protect youth from sexual abuse. Age of consent for sexual activity is 16 years. Children under the age of 12 years cannot consent to any sexual activity. Youth aged 12 to 13 years can consent to sexual activity with a partner who is up to 2 years older than they are. Youth aged 14 to 15 years can consent to sexual activity with a partner who is up to 5 years older than they are. Any youth under the age of 18 years cannot consent to sexual activity with a partner in a position of authority or trust.

C. Emotional harm: Rejection, lack of affection or stimulation, ignoring, dominating, intimidating, describing the child negatively, blaming the child, and verbal abuse (e.g., belittle, yell, threats of severe punishment), abuse resulting in impaired psychological growth and development.

D. Child neglect: Isolation; starvation; lack of medical care; inadequate supervision; failure to provide love, affection, and emotional support; and failure to enroll/attend school.

E. Exposure to family violence: Allowing an infant or child to see, hear, or be exposed to signs of violence in the family.

Incidence/Prevalence

A. Childhood abuse occurs worldwide; the exact incidence is not known. It occurs across all cultures and all racial, socioeconomic, and educational groups.

B. Thirty percent of Canadians reported experiencing physical and/or sexual abuse at the hands of an adult before the age of 15.

C. Sexual abuse is underreported, underrecognized, and undertreated.

D. Childhood physical and/or sexual abuse is more common among males.

E. Seventy percent of children who witness abuse are also victims of physical and/or sexual abuse. Witnessing domestic violence is associated with experiencing physical abuse and witnessing physical abuse of a sibling.

Pathogenesis

Society, lack of parenting skills, the home environment, substance abuse, and untreated mental illness are all factors that contribute to abuse.

Predisposing Factors

A. Child victims:
　1. Minority children.
　2. Disabled or medically fragile children:
　　a. Congenital anomalies.
　　b. Intellectual disabilities.
　　c. Physical disabilities.
　　d. Chronic medical illness.
　　e. Hyperactivity.
　　f. Adopted children/stepchildren.
　　g. Poor bonding.
　3. Age of children (physical abuse):
　　a. Younger than 1 year (67%).
　　b. Younger than 3 years (80%).

B. Parental factors:
　1. Young or single parents.
　2. Distant or absent extended family.
　3. Low formal educational level.
　4. Diffuse or rigid boundaries.
　5. Acute or chronic instability and stress in the family:
　　a. Loss of employment.
　　b. Divorce/death.
　　c. Drug/alcohol abuse.
　　d. Parents with a history of abuse/neglect as a child (learned behaviour).
　　e. Presence of psychiatric illness.
　　f. Poverty.
　　g. Criminal history.

C. Sexual-abuse risk factors:
　1. Male:
　　a. Younger than 13 years of age.
　　b. Ethnic minority.
　　c. Low socioeconomic status.
　　d. Not living with biological father.
　　e. Intellectual or physical disability.
　2. Female:
　　a. Age between 7 and 14 years.
　　b. Absence of a parent.
　　c. Appearance of isolation, depression, or loneliness.

Common Findings
A. Oral/facial injuries:
 1. Oropharyngeal sexually transmitted infections: sexual abuse.
 2. Black eyes.
 3. Nasal perforation/septal deviation.
 4. Skull fracture.
 5. Traumatic alopecia.
 6. Retinal haemorrhage.
 7. Hearing loss/tympanic injury.
B. Burns (6%–20% of injuries):
 1. Cigarette burns (pathognomonic for child abuse).
 2. Scalding/immersion.
 3. Caustic exposure.
 4. Branding.
 5. Microwave burns.
C. Fractures (second most common injury).
D. Bruises (most common type of injury).
E. Lacerations.
F. Bites.
G. Force feeding "bottle jamming"/forced ingestion (water, salt, pepper, poisons).
H. Starvation.
I. Sexual abuse:
 1. Difficulty with bowel movements.
 2. Urinary tract infections.
 3. Vaginal infections, itching, or discharge.
 4. Complaints of stomachaches.
 5. Headaches.
 6. Vaginal or rectal bleeding.
 7. Difficulty walking or sitting.
J. Behavioural signs:
 1. Loss of appetite/eating disorder.
 2. Clinging, withdrawn, or aggressive.
 3. Nightmares, disturbed sleep pattern, and fear of the dark.
 4. Regression (e.g., bedwetting, thumb sucking, crying).
 5. Poor grades/school attendance.
 6. Expression of interest or affection inappropriate for the child's age.
 7. Intercourse, masturbation or other sexual acting out.
 8. Self-injurious behaviour (e.g., cutting, biting, pulling out hair).

Other Signs and Symptoms
A. A caregiver's refusal to allow an interview of the child alone in the examination room is considered a "red flag" for abuse.
B. The history is inconsistent, changes with repeated questioning, conflicts with other family members/caregivers who are interviewed, is implausible, or there is a total lack of history (e.g., "I don't know how it happened").
C. History is inconsistent with the child's developmental ability/stage.
D. Caregiver behaviours that may indicate abuse include delay in seeking care, argumentativeness, lack of emotional response, inappropriateness, or violence.
E. x-Rays should be obtained for a history of "soft," easily broken bones.
F. The child exhibits inappropriate behaviour for his or her developmental age.

Subjective Data
A. Use open-ended questions during the history to evaluate how injuries were sustained. As the interview continues, ask specific questions related to responses. If the child can talk, direct questions to him or her before the caregiver.
B. If this is the first clinic visit, ask whether the child had routine health care, including immunizations.

Physical Examination
Primary care practitioners concerned with suspected abuse need to document a detailed description of their concerns and make a report to the appropriate Child Protection Services authorities in the locality, province, or territory such as Child Welfare, Children's Services, Children's Aid Society, and/or the police. The detailed physical examination including collection of physical evidence will be coordinated and completed as per the policies and procedures of these authorities.

The physical examination should be performed with the child totally unclothed; however, clothing can be removed as the physical examination progresses from head to toe (e.g., upper body, torso, lower body, lastly perineum/rectum). Detailed documentation of history is essential. Formal investigations of suspected child abuse are conducted by Child Protection Services and police. Forensic examination, including photographs and collecting evidence, should be done when possible under the direction of Child Protection Services and the police.

A. Check blood pressure, pulse, and respirations, and temperature if indicated.
B. A forensic examination requires thorough documentation of injuries:
 1. Use colour photographs before any treatment is started.
 2. Photograph damaged clothing.
 3. Take at least one full-body photograph and a facial photograph.
 4. Take close-up photographs of all injuries.
 5. Use a ruler to identify/document the size of injuries.
 6. Documentation on the back of the photographs should include the client's name, date, photographer's name, and any witnesses to the examination. The photographer should also sign each photograph.
C. General observation:
 1. Observe the interactions between the caregiver and the child. Is the child fearful or reluctant to have the examination? Are there signs of discomfort during the examination with movement such as range of motion (ROM)?
 2. Evaluate the child's overall appearance: Is the child clean and are his or her clothes appropriate for the season? Observe for poor hygiene, body odour, malnourishment, dehydration, depression, violence, withdrawal, behavioural compliance even during a painful examination of the rectum/genitalia, and level of consciousness.
 3. Dermal examination: Evaluate from head to toe, including the palms, soles of the feet, and between toes; observe for injuries in different stages of healing and new trauma, including burns, lesions, swelling, bruises, and signs of pinching. Evaluate the corner of the mouth for signs of being gagged. Examine the head for alopecia from hair pulling. Evaluate bruises and burns for the characteristics of shapes (e.g., iron, handprints, long belt marks, loops, bite marks, ligature marks).
 4. Eye examination: Observe for retinal haemorrhages, black eyes, periorbital oedema, and papilledema (indicates increased intracranial pressure).

5. Ear examination: Evaluate hearing, haemotympanum or possible laceration to the external canal, and insertion of foreign objects.
   6. Nasal examination: Evaluate the presence of blood, swelling, and foreign objects.
   7. Mouth and throat: Evaluate the presence of caustic ingestion; observe for ligature marks and cry/voice quality.
D. Auscultate:
   1. Heart.
   2. Lungs.
   3. Abdomen in all four quadrants.
   4. Over the globes of the eyes if warranted (bruit may indicate traumatic carotid cavernous fistula).
   5. The carotid arteries bilaterally if warranted (bruit may indicate carotid dissection).
E. Palpate:
   1. Examine for facial fractures; palpate for instability of the facial bones, including the zygomatic arch.
   2. Palpate abdomen in all four quadrants for guarding, tenderness, and masses (haematoma).
   3. Examine for any trauma to the spine.
F. Neurologic examination:
   1. Assess mental status and memory: Determine whether the client is awake, alert, cooperative, and oriented (to person, place, time, and situation). Temporary impairment of memory is one of the most common deficits after a head injury.
   2. Assess cranial nerve function:
      a. Ophthalmoscopic/visual examination (cranial nerve II).
      b. Pupillary response (cranial nerve III).
      c. Extraocular movements (cranial nerves III, IV, and VI).
      d. Facial sensation and muscles of mastication (cranial nerve V).
      e. Facial expression and taste (cranial nerve VII).
   3. Perform a motor examination on all four extremities.
   4. Perform a sensory examination on all four extremities.
G. Genital/rectal examination:
   1. Evaluate genitals/anal area for redness, swelling, bruising, haematomas, abrasions, or lacerations.
   2. Evaluate for evidence of sperm.
   3. Evaluate for presence of condyloma.
   4. Evaluate for presence of foreign bodies.

Diagnostic Tests

Diagnostic tests and x-rays are ordered dependent on the type of presenting complaints and physical examination.
A. Complete blood count (CBC) with differential and peripheral smear; bleeding evaluation, including prothrombin time/partial thromboplastin time (PT/PTT), alanine aminotransferase (ALT), and aspartate aminotransferase (AST), to evaluate injury to the liver, serum amylase, or lipase to rule out pancreatic injury.
B. Urinalysis.
C. Drug screen/toxicology (urine and serum).
D. Obtain forensic DNA samples from the skin, under nails, vagina, rectum, and saliva from bite marks using sterile cotton-tipped applicators that have been moistened with sterile saline. These should be sent to a crime laboratory as soon as possible.
E. Test for sexually transmitted infections/HIV.
F. Pregnancy test (age appropriate).
G. x-Rays: facial injury, anteroposterior (AP) and lateral radiograph for any areas of bone tenderness, swelling, deformity, or limited (ROM).
H. Neuroimaging CT/MRI for any suspected nonaccidental head injury (e.g., head trauma, history of shaking, scalp haematoma).

Differential Diagnoses
A. Congenital syphilis.
B. Rickets.
C. Osteogenesis imperfecta (OI).
D. Mongolian spots.
E. Impetigo.
F. Dermatitis herpetiformis.
G. Folk-healing practices.
H. Immune thrombocytopaenia (ITP).
I. Malignancy.
J. Meningitis: neurologic signs.

Plan
A. General interventions:
   1. Duty to report: Everyone has a duty to report child abuse and neglect under Canadian child welfare laws. Known or suspected child abuse must be reported to the local Child Protection Services.
B. Safety planning is the first priority. Contact local Child Protection Services.
C. Increase public awareness.
D. Failure to report a suspected case of sexual abuse may incur criminal charges.

Client Teaching
A. Listen to the child. Believe the child.
B. Reinforce that abuse/neglect is not the child's fault.
C. Tell the child that help is available.

Pharmacological Therapy
A. Prescribe antibiotics to treat sexually transmitted infections or wounds.
B. Antidepressant therapy may be appropriate.

Follow-Up
A. Canadian child welfare law mandates reporting of child abuse. Professionals who work with children have added responsibility and duty to report. Refer to your provincial/territorial laws for the reporting procedure. Child Protection Services is responsible for investigations. Depending on your location, police involvement may be mandatory.
B. Hospitalization may be required, depending on physical findings, child safety, and parental observation.
C. Child clients are at high risk of depression, anxiety, eating disorders, discipline problems, drug/alcohol use, runaway tendencies, and low self-esteem. Therapy and follow-up vary for each individual child. Family participation in a recommended treatment program is helpful. The goal of treatment is to help children regain their prior state of mental and psychological health. Neglect is the major reason that children are removed from a home, especially when the parents have drug/alcohol problems.

Consultation/Referral
A. Consult with other healthcare providers who have expertise with abuse (e.g., Child Protection Services, psychiatrist, psychologist, social worker).

B. Report all suspicions of abuse to Child Protection Services.
C. Specialty consultations:
1. Genetic consultation: OI.
2. Orthopaedic consultation.
3. Plastic surgeon.
4. Child psychiatrist.
5. Ophthalmology.

Resources

Canadian Centre for Child Protection: https://www.protectchildren.ca/en/
Canadian Child Welfare Research Portal: http://cwrp.ca/
Childhelp Prevention and Treatment of Child Abuse: www.childhelp.org
Kids Help Line: 1-800-668-6868

Bibliography

Burczycka, M. (2016). *Statistics Canada. Family violence in Canada: A statistical profile, 2016*. Retrieved from https://www150.statcan.gc.ca/n1/pub/85-002-x/2018001/article/54893-eng.htm

Domestic Abuse Intervention Project. (n.d.). *Abuse of children wheel*. Retrieved from www.theduluthmodel.org/pdf/Abuse%20of%20Children.pdf

Giardino, A. P. (2013, April 1). *Physical child abuse. Medscape*. Retrieved from http://emedicine.medscape.com/article/915664-overview

HelpGuide.org. (n.d.). *Child abuse and neglect: Recognizing, preventing, and reporting child abuse*. Retrieved from www.helpguide.org/mental_abuse_physical_emoional_sexual_neglect.htm

Prevent Child Abuse America. (2016a, February). *Fact sheet: Emotional child-abuse*. Retrieved from www.preventchildabuse.org/images/docs/emotionalchildabuse.pdf

Prevent Child Abuse America. (2016b, February). *Fact sheet: Maltreatment of children with disabilities*. Retrieved from http://www.preventchildabuse.org/images/docs/maltreatmentofchildrenwithdisabilities.pdf

Prevent Child Abuse America. (2016c, February). *Fact sheet: Sexual abuse of children*. Retrieved from www.preventchildabuse.org/resource/sexual-abuse-of-children-fact-sheet

Prevent Child Abuse America. (2016d, February). *Recognizing child abuse: What parents should know*. Retrieved from www.preventchildabuse.org/images/docs/recognizingchildabuse-whatparentsshouldknow.pdf

Prevent Child Abuse America. (n.d.-a). *Fact sheet: The relationship between parental alcohol or other drug problems and child maltreatment*. Retrieved from www.preventchildabuse.org/images/docs/therelationshipbetweenparentalalcoholandotherdrugproblemsandchildmaltreatment.pdf

Prevent Child Abuse America. (n.d.-b). *Fact sheet: Sexual abuse of boys*. Retrieved from www.preventchildabuse.org/images/docs/sexualabuseofboys.pdf

Rape, Abuse & Incest National Network (RAINN). (n.d.). *Victims of sexual violence: Statistics*. Retrieved from http://www.rainn.org/get-information/statistics/sexual-assault-victims

Sinha, M. (2017). *Family violence in Canada: A statistical profile*. Statistics Canada. Retrieved from https://www150.statcan.gc.ca/n1/daily-quotidien/170216/dq170216b-eng.htm

Violence: Intimate Partner

Definition

A. Intimate partner violence (IPV) is defined as the intentional control or victimization of a person with whom the abuser has had or is currently in an intimate, romantic, or spousal relationship. IPV crosses all cultures and economic boundaries; it encompasses violence between all genders in all types of intimate partner relationships. Abusive behaviours can occur in a single event, sporadically, or continually. The following is a list of the many forms through which IPV may manifest itself:
B. Physical abuse, sexual assault, coercion, social isolation, emotional abuse, economic control, and deprivation are associated with IPV.
C. Forms of physical violence include threatening or assaulting with weapons, pushing, shoving, slapping, punching, choking, kicking, holding, throwing objects, and binding.
D. Psychological abuse includes threats of physical harm to the victim or others, humiliations, intimidation, degradation, ridicule, false accusation, isolation, and deprivation of food, money, access to health care, and transportation.
E. Psychological abuse in LGBTQ relationships includes the threat to "out" the partner and threats related to custody of co-parented children.
F. Cyberstalking is psychological abuse. It occurs online on social media platforms (e.g., Facebook, Snapchat, Instagram) and/or with texting. Intimate partner stalking can occur during a relationship or when a relationship ends:
1. Monitoring cellphone and online activity/social media accounts.
2. Posting photographs or any content with an intent to humiliate a partner or former partner on social media.
G. Sexual abuse includes being exposed to unwanted sexual behaviour or being forced to take part in nonconsensual sexual activity (e.g., touching, kissing, or any type of intercourse without consent).
H. Reproductive coercion is another form of IPV:
1. Partner sabotage of safe-sex practices (e.g., refusal to use condoms, exposing the client to sexually transmitted infections [STIs]).
2. Refusal/control of contraception.
3. Forcing the woman to have an abortion, or utilizing physical violence to endanger a pregnancy.
4. Controlling access to healthcare.

Incidence/Prevalence

The exact incidence of IPV is unknown. The United Nations estimates that more than 600 million women live in countries where domestic violence is not considered a crime. The most significant reason for missing the diagnosis of IPV is failure to ask the client or screen for IPV.

A. Globally, IPV is the leading cause of homicide of women.
B. IPV often occurs after separation; women are most likely to be murdered when reporting abuse or attempting to leave an abusive relationship.
C. Stalking is repeated and unwanted attention that causes a person to fear for their personal safety or for the safety of someone they know. This definition qualifies stalking as criminal harassment under the *Criminal Code* of Canada. According to the 2014 General Social Survey, 48% of stalking victims were between 15 and 34 years of age; most victims (62%) were women. With intimate partner stalking, women are overrepresented as victims, there is a greater association with violence, and it is reported to the police at higher levels.
D. Women presenting in ED may have experienced IPV. According to a study reported by Statistics Canada (2016), 31% of those experiencing spousal violence in Canada reported sustaining physical injuries (e.g., bruises, cuts, broken bones) during the previous five years as a result of this violence. Women are more likely than men to report physical injuries. Bruises were the most common injury, followed by cuts, scratches, and burns. Fractures and internal injuries were less common. Hospitalization was required by 16% of spousal violence victims who reported an injury.
E. Women who separate have a risk of violence approximately three times that of divorced women More than half of children who witness domestic violence intervene in some way, including yelling at the abuser to stop, calling for help, and trying to get away.

F. Men can also be victims of sexual assault.
G. Pregnancy is a risk factor for IPV:
1. 53% of young women have experienced birth control sabotage.
2. It is estimated that up to 20% of intimate partner abuse occurs against pregnant women.
H. Results from a Statistics Canada study in 2014 showed that individuals who described themselves as gay, lesbian, or bisexual were twice as likely as heterosexuals to report having been the victim of spousal violence during the previous five years. This difference was pronounced for lesbian or bisexual women compared with heterosexual women.
I. Indigenous people are particularly vulnerable to IPV. Spousal abuse against Indigenous women is more than three times higher than that of non-Indigenous women and men.

Pathogenesis
IPV is not associated with an underlying medical condition. The cycle of abuse has three phases:
A. Tension building, in which the victim tries to avoid violence and is described as "walking on eggshells," unsure what will trigger an abusive incident.
B. Explosion and acute battering occur.
C. The "Loving Contrition" or "Honeymoon Phase" is noted for the absence of tension and gestures of reconciliation.
D. Clients stay with their partners for multiple reasons, including fear, shame, denial, religious beliefs, lack of resources, child custody and other legal issues, fear of being "outed," and family pressures.

Predisposing Factors
A. Gender: Victims are predominantly female.
B. Pregnancy.
C. History of violence:
1. Violence present in family of origin.
2. Abuse as a child: 50% report abuse as an adult.
D. History of drug use.
E. Posttraumatic stress disorder (PTSD).
F. Lack of social support systems.
G. Impulse control disorders.
H. Poor economic status.
I. LGBTQ.

Common Findings
A. Vague complaints.
B. Sexual problems.
C. Depression.
D. Chronic pain inconsistent with organic disease.
E. Chronic headaches/migraines.
F. Stress:
1. Anxiety.
2. Panic attacks.
G. Alcohol or drug abuse (e.g., perpetrator, victim, or both).
H. Current or past self-mutilation.
I. Gynecologic and obstetric complaints:
1. Dyspareunia.
2. Frequent vaginal or urinary tract infections.
3. Pelvic pain/infection.
4. Recurrent STIs.
5. Unintended pregnancy.
6. Late prenatal care.
7. Miscarriage.
8. Preterm bleeding/delivery.
J. Complaints of falls and other recurrent accidents.
K. Eating disorders.
L. Gastrointestinal complaints/irritable bowel syndrome.
M. Musculoskeletal complaints.

Other Signs and Symptoms
A. Multiple visits to the ED for traumatic and nontraumatic complaints.
B. A delay between injury and office visits (may result from lack of transportation or the inability to leave the house).
C. Noncompliance with the treatment or missed appointments (lack of access to money or telephones).
D. Suicide attempt (25% higher in women with IPV).
E. A partner who accompanies the client at all visits.

Subjective Data
It is important to document the person's exposure to violence by conducting the interview one on one and in private, and asking open-ended questions to develop rapport followed by specific direct questions.
A. The perpetrator often refuses to leave the client alone and may answer questions for the client. Translators should not be a member of the client's or suspected abuser's family.
B. Use direct questions: women-validated Partner Violence Screen (PVS).
1. Have you been hit, punched, kicked, or otherwise hurt by someone in the past year? If yes, by whom and were you injured?
2. Do you feel safe in your current relationship?
3. Is a partner from a previous relationship making you feel unsafe now?
4. Are you here today because of injuries from a partner?
5. Are you here today because of illness or stress related to threats, violent behaviour, or fears of a partner?
C. Assess whether the client has ever reported abuse to family or friends, accessed resources, or attempted to leave the abuser.
D. Has the client sought help with law enforcement or legal help, that is, filed a criminal complaint or got an order of protection?
E. Are there any weapons in the home?
1. Has the abuser ever threatened or tried to kill you?
2. Are you thinking of suicide? Have you ever considered or attempted to commit suicide because of problems in your relationship?
3. Have you ever considered or attempted killing the person perpetrating the abuse?
4. Do you have a safety plan?

Physical Examination
Primary care practitioners concerned with IPV need to document a detailed description of their concerns. It is possible that a report may be made to the appropriate authorities in the locality, province, or territory such as the police or the Royal Canadian Mounted Police (RCMP). The detailed physical examination including collection of physical evidence will be coordinated and completed as per the policies and procedures of the authorities:
A. Explain the importance of interviewing and conducting the physical examinations in private. Do a full-body examination, including the head/scalp:
1. Most injuries are to the central (e.g., breast, chest, and abdomen) area, which is easily concealed by clothing.
2. Other frequent sites of injury include the head, face, throat, and genitals.
3. Explain the physical examination; touch during the physical examination with permission.

4. Forensic examinations need thorough documentation of injuries. Note, photographs may be taken at the request of the police after receiving written consent:
   a. Use colour photographs before any treatment is started.
   b. Photograph damaged clothing.
   c. Take at least one full-body photograph and a facial photograph.
   d. Take close-up photographs of all injuries.
   e. Use a ruler to identify/document the size of injuries.
   f. Documentation on the back of the photographs should include the client's name, date, and photographer's name, as well as any witnesses to the examination. The photographer should also sign each photograph.
   g. Use direct quotes of the client's history of the violence.
B. Check blood pressure, pulse, and respirations.
C. General observation: Observe for depression/withdrawal, or flat affect, anxiousness, fearfulness, evasiveness, poor eye contact, and wearing heavy makeup or clothing to conceal signs of abuse. Evaluate voice changes (e.g., dysphonia and aphonia). Observe for difficulty breathing.
D. Inspect:
   1. Dermal examination for the presence of cigarette burns, impression marks, rope burns, welts, abrasions, scratch marks, claw marks, bite marks, ligature marks, petechiae, and contusions at multiple sites (e.g., back, legs, and buttocks).

ABUSE ASSESSMENT SCREEN

1. Have you ever been emotionally or physically abused by your partner or someone important to you?
   Yes ☐   No ☐
   If yes, by whom? _____
   Total number of times _____

2. Within the last year, have you been hit, slapped, kicked, or otherwise physically hurt by someone?
   Yes ☐   No ☐
   If yes, by whom? _____
   Total number of times _____

3. Since you've been pregnant, have you been hit, slapped, kicked, or otherwise physically hurt by someone?
   Yes ☐   No ☐
   If yes, by whom? _____
   Total number of times _____

4. Within the last year, has anyone forced you to engage in sexual activity?
   Yes ☐   No ☐
   If yes, by whom? _____
   Total number of times _____

5. Are you afraid of your partner or anyone you listed previously?
   Yes ☐   No ☐

MARK THE AREA OF INJURY ON A BODY MAP AND SCORE EACH INCIDENT ACCORDING TO THE FOLLOWING SCALE

If any of the descriptions for the higher number apply, use the higher number.

1 = Threats of abuse, including use of a weapon
2 = Slapping, pushing; no injury and/or lasting pain
3 = Punching, kicking, bruises, cuts, and/or continuing pain
4 = Beating up, severe contusions, burns, broken bones
5 = Head injury, internal injury, permanent injury
6 = Use of weapon; wound from weapon

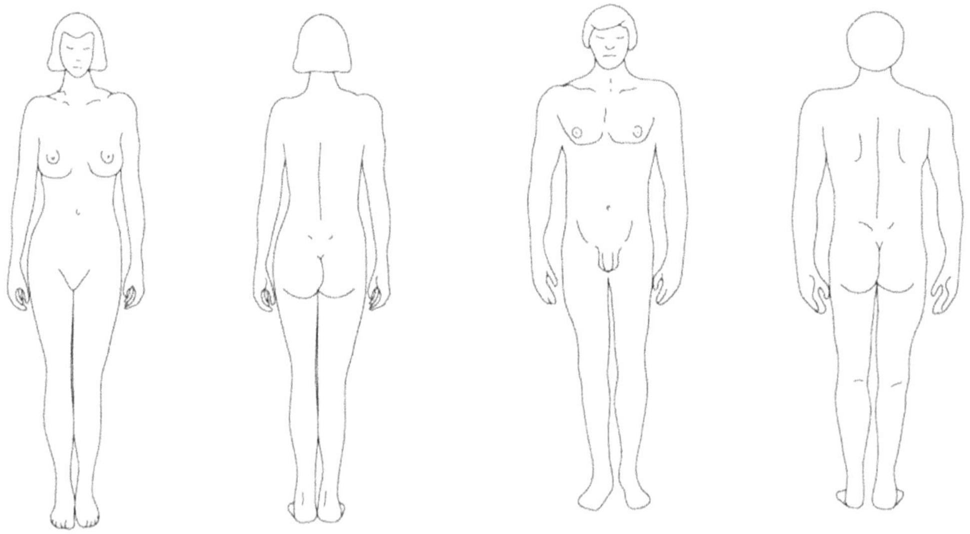

FIGURE 2.4 Abuse assessment screening tool with body map.
Source: This resource was adapted from material developed and produced by Futures Without Violence. www.futureswithoutviolence.org.

2. Eye examination:
      a. Observe subconjunctival haemorrhages from strangulation/struggle.
      b. Perform a funduscopic examination (if indicated secondary to trauma).
   3. Evaluate the genitals for lacerations and haematomas of the vagina or labia.
E. Auscultate:
   1. All lung fields.
   2. The bowel sounds in all four quadrants of the abdomen.
F. Palpate:
   1. Evaluate skull/facial trauma to the maxillofacial area, eye orbits, mandible, and nasal bones. Facial injuries are common.
   2. Evaluate for dislocations, fractures (including spiral fractures), sprains, and contusions to the wrists, forearms, and shoulders.
G. Percuss abdomen, chest, and areas of injury (if indicated secondary to trauma).
H. Perform a neurologic examination (if indicated secondary to trauma).
I. Genital/rectal examination:
   1. Evaluate genitals/anus area for redness, swelling, bruising, haematomas, abrasions, or lacerations.
   2. Perform bimanual examination (females).
   3. Order an anoscopy (if indicated).
   4. Evaluate for evidence of sperm (recto/vaginal).
   5. Evaluate for the presence of condyloma (perineum, rectum, vagina).
   6. Evaluate for the presence of foreign bodies (recto/vaginal).

Diagnostic Tests
Diagnostic tests and x-rays are ordered dependent on the type of presenting complaints and physical examination:
A. Administer a domestic abuse assessment screening tool and have the client mark a body map of injuries (see Figure 2.4).
B. Complete blood count (CBC) with differential and peripheral smear, bleeding evaluation, including prothrombin time/partial thromboplastin time (PT/PTT), alanine aminotransferase (ALT), and aspartate aminotransferase (AST), to evaluate injury to the liver, serum amylase, or lipase to rule out pancreatic injury.
C. Urinalysis.
D. Drug/toxicology screen (urine and blood).
E. Obtain forensic DNA samples from the skin, under nails, vagina, rectum, and saliva from bite marks using sterile cotton-tipped applicators that have been moistened with sterile saline. These should be sent to a crime laboratory as soon as possible.
F. Test for STIs/HIV.
G. Pregnancy test (if indicated).
H. x-Rays: Facial injury, anteroposterior (AP), and lateral x-ray for any areas of bone tenderness, swelling, deformity, or limited range of motion (ROM).
I. Ultrasounds as indicated.
J. Neuroimaging (e.g., CT/MRI) may be used for any suspected nonaccidental head injury (e.g., head trauma, scalp haematoma).

Differential Diagnoses
A. Rape.
B. Other: Related to presenting symptoms.

Plan
A. Provide a safe environment. Assess for immediate danger. Listen to the client. Believe what the client is reporting; maintain a nonjudgmental attitude.
B. Clearly document the history, physical findings, and interventions.
C. Determine the risk to the client and any children.
D. Evaluate the need for ED/hospital admission.
E. Assault is a crime; assess the client's readiness for police intervention and need for a court order of protection.
F. Help develop a safety plan.
G. Assess the client's potential readiness to leave the relationship. Signs include collection of important papers and documents (e.g., birth certificates, custody papers, divorce papers, legal agreements, address book, copies of restraining orders), having access to money/credit cards in the client's name, and telling family and friends.
H. Provide contact numbers for resources, including shelters. Have the client store information in a secure place.
I. Counsel that violence is an ongoing pattern of behaviour; it will likely escalate in frequency and severity over time.

Client Teaching
A. Listen to the client. Believe what the client is reporting.
B. Reinforce that the violence is not the client's fault.
C. Discuss the cycle of violence.
D. Violence almost always increases in frequency and severity over time.
E. Help and supports are available.

Pharmacological Therapy
A. Prescriptions are related to physical injuries.
B. Provide treatment may be offered for STIs in the oral, anal, and genital areas.
C. Tranquilizers may impair the client's ability to flee or defend herself or himself and should not be prescribed.
D. Provide tetanus vaccine update, if needed, with any open wounds or cuts.

Follow-Up
A. Develop a follow-up plan:
   1. What type of help does the client want? Based on the client's response to this question, make referrals.
   2. Provide contact information for resources and shelters, if needed.
B. Screen the client for abuse at all subsequent visits.
C. Mandatory reporting:
   1. Canada's duty to report requires reporting when domestic violence involves a child younger than 16 years and abuse or neglect of the child is suspected.
   2. Reporting elder abuse may be mandatory in your province or territory.

Consultation/Referral
A. Facilitate referrals to shelters, counselling, and legal services.
B. Refer to community or private support groups and agencies.
C. Refer for a consultation with a psychiatrist if the client is homicidal or suicidal.
D. Refer for a neurologic or neurosurgical consultation for intracranial injuries or focal neurologic findings.
E. Refer for an orthopaedic consultation for fractures.

Individual Considerations

A. Pregnancy is a risk factor for initiation of and/or increased frequency/severity of IPV:
 1. The genitals, breasts, and abdomen are common sites targeted for trauma.
 2. Women may present with a miscarriage or premature labor.
 3. Blunt trauma is a common injury in pregnancy.
 4. Perform universal screening at each trimester and postpartum, as abuse often begins during pregnancy.

Resources

Amnesty International: https://www.amnesty.ca/our-work/issues/womens-human-rights
Break the Cycle: http://www.breakthecycle.org/
Centers for Disease Control & Prevention. Violence Prevention Intimate Partner Violence: https://www.cdc.gov/ViolencePrevention/intimatepartnerviolence/index.html
Ending Violence Association of Canada: http://endingviolencecanada.org/
Family violence in Canada, a statistical profile, 2016: https://www150.statcan.gc.ca/n1/pub/85-002-x/2018001/article/54893-eng.htm
National Aboriginal Circle Against Family Violence: http://nacafv.ca/
Public Health Agency of Canada. Just Facts. Research and Statistics Division Intimate partner violence: https://justice.gc.ca/eng/rp-pr/jr/jf-pf/2017/may01.html
World Health Organization Intimate partner and sexual violence (violence against women): https://www.who.int/violence_injury_prevention/violence/sexual/en/

Bibliography

American College of Obstetricians and Gynecologists. American College of Obstetricians and Gynecologists. (2012, February). Intimate partner violence. *Committee Opinion, 518*, 1–5. Retrieved from https://www.acog.org/Clinical-Guidance-and-Publications/Committee-Opinions/Committee-on-Health-Care-for-Underserved-Women/Intimate-Partner-Violence?IsMobileSet=false

Burczycka, M. (2016). *Statistics Canada. Family violence in Canada: A statistical profile, 2016*. Retrieved from https://www150.statcan.gc.ca/n1/pub/85-002-x/2018001/article/54893-eng.htm

Dating Abuse Stops Here. (n.d.-a). *Create a safety plan*. Retrieved from www.datingabusestopshere.com/create-a-safety-plan/

Dating Abuse Stops Here. (n.d.-b). *Warning signs in depth*. Retrieved from www.datingabusestopshere.com/warning-signs/warning-signs-in-depth

Devries, K. M., Mak, J. Y. T., Garcia-Moreno, C., Petzold, M., Child, J. C., Falder, G., & Watts, C. H. (2013, June 30). The global prevalence of intimate partner violence against women. *Science, 340*(6140), 1527–1528. doi:10.1126/science.1240937. Retrieved from http://www.sciencemag.org/content/early/recent

Domestic Abuse Intervention Project. (n.d.). *Power and control wheel*. Retrieved from www.theduluthmodel.org/pdf/powerandcontrol.pdf

Ending Violence Association of BC. (2016). *Sexual assault workers handbook*. Retrieved from http://endingviolencecanada.org/wp-content/uploads/2016/12/EVABC_SexualAssault_Support-Worker-Handbook_2016_vF.pdf

Ending Violence Association of Canada. (n.d.). *Find help across Canada*. Retrieved from http://endingviolencecanada.org/getting-help/

Futures Without Violence, Formerly Family Violence Prevention Fund. (n.d.-a). *The facts on children's exposure to intimate partner violence*. Retrieved from https://www.futureswithoutviolence.org/the-facts-on-childrens-exposure-to-intimate-partner-violence

Futures Without Violence, Formerly Family Violence Prevention Fund. (n.d.-b). *The facts on the military and violence against women*. Retrieved from https://www.futureswithoutviolence.org/userfiles/file/Children_and_Families/Military.pdf

Healthy Place America's Mental Health Channel. (n.d.). *Abuse test: Woman abuse screening tool*. Retrieved from http://www.healthyplace.com/psychological-tests/woman-abuse-screening-tool

HelpGuide.org. (n.d.-a). *Help for abused men: Escaping domestic violence by women or domestic partners*. Retrieved from www.helpguide.org/mental/domestic-violence-men-abused-by-women.htm

HelpGuide.org. (n.d.-b). *Domestic violence and abuse: Signs of abuse and abusive relationships*. Retrieved from www.helpguide.org/mental/domestic_violence_abuse_types_signs_causes_effects.htm

Moyer, V. A. (2013). U.S. Preventive Services Task Force. *Annals of Internal Medicine, 158*(6), 478–486. doi:10.7326/0003-4819-158-6-201303190-00588

Ross, R., Roller, C., Rusk, T., Martsolf, D., & Draucker, C. (2009). The SATELLITE sexual violence assessment and care guide for perinatal clients. *Women's Health Care: A Practical Journal for Nurse Practitioners, 8*(11), 25–31. Retrieved from https://www.ncbi.nlm.nih.gov/pmc/articles/PMC3324818/pdf/nihms316342.pdf

Statistics Canada. (2016). Trends in self-reported spousal violence in Canada, 2014. Retrieved from https://www150.statcan.gc.ca/n1/pub/85-002-x/2016001/article/14303/01-eng.htm

U.S. Department of Justice, Office on Violence Against Women. (2013). *A national protocol for sexual assault medical forensic examinations: Adults/adolescents* (2nd ed.). Washington, DC: Author. Retrieved from https://www.ncjrs.gov/pdffiles1/ovw/241903.pdf

Walker, L. E. A. (2009). *The battered woman syndrome* (3rd ed.). New York, NY: Springer Publishing Company.

World Health Organization. (2011). *Intimate partner violence during pregnancy*. Retrieved from http://apps.who.int/iris/bitstream/10665/70764/1/WHO_RHR_11.35_eng.pdf

World Health Organization. (2013a). *Gender and women's mental health*. Retrieved from www.who.int/mental_health/prevention/genderwomen/en

World Health Organization. (2013b). *Global and regional estimates of violence against women: Prevalence and health effects of intimate partner violence and non-partner sexual violence*. Retrieved from http://apps.who.int/iris/bitstream/handle/10665/85239/?sequence=1

Violence: Older Adults

Definition

Abuse in older individuals, defined as older than age 65, is associated with loss of functional capacity, depression, cognitive impairment, and increased morbidity and mortality. Perpetrators include partners, and family members (of all ages), as well as strangers. There are several types of maltreatment in this population:

A. Physical abuse: Willful unnecessary restraint, the infliction of physical pain, or injury.
B. Sexual abuse: Nonconsensual sexual contact.
C. Psychological abuse: Infliction of emotional harm, bullying, ridicule, verbal abuse, and terrorizing.
D. Neglect: Failing to provide for needs and protection of a vulnerable adult.
E. Self-neglect: Failure to thrive (FTT) of the elder as a subset of neglect.
F. Abandonment: Desertion.
G. Financial exploitation: Misappropriation of resources.
H. Health care fraud and abuse: Not providing care, but charging for services, overmedicating, or under-medicating.

Incidence/Prevalence

A. In 2010, the population of Canadians over the age of 65 was estimated to be 4.8 million. Within this total, 1.3 million individuals were 80 and older, while 6,500 individuals were over the age 100. By 2036, the population of Canadians older than 65 is projected to be between 9.9 and 10.9 million people.
B. The exact incidence of elder abuse, neglect, exploitation, and self-neglect is unknown; however, it is believed to be common. Abuse of older adults is underreported because of the reluctance to report abuse, fear of implicating family members, and fear of being removed from the home.
C. Abuse occurs in institutional settings.
D. The highest rate of abuse is among elderly women older than age 80, with the abuser being the spouse or adult child. In the case of cognitive impairment, the client may not remember or recognize abuse.

Pathogenesis

Maltreatment of vulnerable adults occurs by people who have an ongoing relationship with the older person when there is an expectation of responsibility; these include sons/daughters, spouses/intimate partners, other family members, such as grandchildren; and others, including paid and unpaid caregivers. There have been several identifying psychopathologies in the abuser:

A. Physical frailty and mental impairment of the client plays an indirect role. The client may have a decreased ability to defend or escape.
B. Caregiver stressors from caring for the elderly client, including the client's physical and verbal demands. Psychosocial factors of the caregiver, mental illness, and alcohol or drug abuse contribute.
C. The child who was once abused may continue the cycle of violence transferred to the parent.

Predisposing Factors
A. Age: 65 years and older (some studies indicate age 60 years).
B. Institutionalized.
C. Cognitive impairment/diminished capacity.
D. Decreased capacity for performing activities of daily living (ADLs):
   1. Difficulty feeding themselves.
   2. Difficulty bathing and dressing themselves.
   3. Difficulty going to the toilet and performing personal hygiene.
E. Decreased capacity performing instrumental activities of daily living (IADLs):
   1. Ability to prepare meals.
   2. Ability to do household chores.
   3. Ability to use the telephone.
   4. Ability to manage personal finances.
F. Females have a higher incidence of physical/sexual abuse.
G. Male gender is associated with self-neglect associated with impaired ADLs and IADLs.
H. Family stressors involving the caretaker.

Common Findings
A. Depression.
B. Falls.
C. History of hip fracture.
D. Pressure ulcers.
E. Bruises, lacerations, and burns.

Other Signs and Symptoms
A. Indications of healing spiral fractures on x-ray.
B. Poor nutrition: Lack of resources/transportation to obtain food, caregiver not providing adequate nutrition/withholding food.
C. Multiple hospitalizations.
D. Recurrent urinary tract infections.
E. Noncompliance: May not be able to pay for medications; medications may be withheld or even given in excess by the caregiver.
F. Reports of sexual abuse:
   1. Pain or soreness in the genital area.
   2. Bruises or lacerations on the perineum/rectum.
   3. Vaginal or rectal bleeding.
G. Traumatic tooth and/or hair loss.
H. Sedation from overmedicating.
I. Changes in personality.

Subjective Data
A. The caregiver often refuses to leave the client alone and may answer questions for the client.
B. The caregiver has a different explanation of the injury.
C. Ask the client directly about abuse, neglect, or exploitation:
   1. Has anyone at home threatened or ever hurt you?
   2. Are you afraid of anyone at home?
   3. Are you left alone for long periods of time?
   4. Who cooks your meals? How often and what amounts of food do you eat?
   5. Who handles your financial business? Have you signed any documents that you did not understand?
D. Assess the client's living arrangements. Has the client ever told family or friends of his or her concerns, called hotlines, or attempted to leave the caregiver?

Physical Examination
Primary care practitioners concerned with abuse of older adults need to document a detailed description of their concerns. When reporting to the appropriate authorities in the locality, province, or territory such as the police or the Royal Canadian Mounted Police (RCMP), a detailed physical examination including collection of physical evidence will be coordinated and completed as per the policies and procedures of the authorities.

A. Assessment:
   1. Observation: If abuse is suspected, enforce the need to do the physical examination in private. Do a full-body examination:
      a. Forensic examinations need thorough documentation of injuries. Note, forensic examination should be conducted under direction by police:
         i. Use colour photographs before any treatment is started.
         ii. Take at least one full-body photograph and a facial photograph.
         iii. Take close-up photographs of all injuries.
         iv. Use a ruler to identify/document the size of the injuries.
         v. Documentation on the back of the photographs should include the client's name, date, and photographer's name, as well as any witness to the examination. The photographer should also sign each photograph.
         vi. Use direct quotes of the client's history.
   2. Check blood pressure, pulse, respirations, and weight.
   3. General observation: Observe for depression, withdrawal demeanor, flat affect, fearfulness, poor eye contact, inappropriate dress, and signs of malnutrition.
   4. Observe for poor hygiene, presence of urine and faeces, matted or lice-infected hair, odours, dirty nails and skin, and soiled clothing.
   5. Assess cognitive abilities, depression, and functional ability of ADLs and IADLs.

B. Inspect:
   1. Dermal examination for signs of burns, tears, lacerations, impression marks, and bruises in different stages of healing. Frequent areas of the body involved are the neck, arms, and/or legs. Evaluate for the presence of decubitus/pressure ulcers. Signs of dehydration include dry fragile skin, dry sore mouth, and mental confusion.
   2. Oral examination for poor oral hygiene, absence of dentures, and dry mucous membranes.
   3. Evaluate breasts and genitals for lacerations, and haematomas of the vagina or labia.

C. Auscultate:
   1. All lung fields.
   2. Bowel sounds in all four quadrants of the abdomen.

D. Palpate: Evaluate for dislocation, fractures, sprains, and contusions to the wrists, forearms, and shoulders.
E. Percuss abdomen and chest (if indicated).
F. Genital/rectal examination:
  1. Evaluate genitals/anus for redness, swelling, bruising, haematomas, abrasions, or lacerations.
  2. Evaluate for evidence of sperm.
  3. Evaluate for the presence of foreign bodies.

Diagnostic Tests
A. Diagnostic tests and x-rays are ordered dependent on the type of presenting complaints.
B. Obtain a CT for evaluation of injuries to the head and assault to the face, neck, or head. A CT or Doppler ultrasound may be ordered for abdominal injuries.
C. Order laboratory testing to evaluate dehydration, malnutrition, electrolyte imbalance, and medication/substance abuse:
  1. Complete blood count (CBC).
  2. Chemistry.
  3. Urinalysis.
  4. Calcium, magnesium, and phosphorus.
  5. Drug/alcohol screen.
  6. Serum levels for relevant medications.
D. Obtain DNA samples if sexual abuse is present.

Differential Diagnoses
A. Depression.
B. Abdominal trauma.
C. Sexual assault.
D. Gait disturbance/fall.
E. Pathologic fracture.
F. Epidural/subdural haematoma.

Plan
A. Provide a safe environment.
B. Clearly document the history, physical findings, and interventions.
C. Determine the perpetrator(s).
D. Evaluate the need for ED/hospital admission.

Client Teaching
A. Listen to the client. Believe what the client is reporting.
B. Reinforce that the violence is not the client's fault.
C. Help and supports are available.

Pharmacological Therapy
A. Ensure prescriptions are related to physical injuries.
B. Recommend treatment for sexually transmitted infections in the oral, anal, and genital areas.

Follow-Up
A. Develop a follow-up plan. Legislation protecting against abuse, neglect, and exploitation of the older population is different among provinces/territories in Canada.
B. Know whether your province or territory has mandatory requirements to report any suspicion of elder mistreatment.
C. At the present time, there is no recommendation for universal screening of all older adult clients except in nursing facilities.

Consultation/Referral
A. Schedule a social work consultation to coordinate an in-home geriatric assessment visit.
B. Facilitate referrals to a shelter, counselling, and legal services.
C. Refer to the community resources for assistance.
D. Refer for a psychiatric consultation if indicated.
E. Refer for a neurologic or neurosurgical consultation for intracranial injuries or focal neurologic findings.
F. Refer for an orthopedic consultation for fractures.

Resources
Canadian Network for the Prevention of Elder Abuse (CNPEA): https://cnpea.ca/en/
Elder Abuse Awareness: https://www.canada.ca/en/employment-social-development/campaigns/elder-abuse.html
Government of Canada - Aging and Seniors: https://www.canada.ca/en/public-health/services/health-promotion/aging-seniors.html
World Health Organization – Elder Abuse: http://www.who.int/ageing/projects/elder_abuse/en/

Bibliography
Cahoo, C. G. (2012). Depression in older adults. *American Journal of Nursing, 112*(11), 22–31. doi:10.1097/01.NAJ.0000422251.65212.4b
HelpGuide.org. (n.d.). *Elder abuse and neglect: Warning signs, risk factors, prevention, help*. Retrieved from www.helpguide.org/mental/elder_abuse_physical_emotional_sexual_neglect.htm
Moyer, V. A. (2013). U.S. Preventive Services Task Force. *Annals of Internal Medicine, 158*(6), 478–486. doi:10.7326/0003-4819-158-6-201303190-00588
National Committee for the Prevention of Elder Abuse. (2008). *Elder abuse*. Retrieved from www.preventelderabuse.org/elderabuse
National Committee for the Prevention of Elder Abuse. (n.d.-a). *Domestic violence*. Retrieved from http://www.preventelderabuse.org/elderabuse/domestic.html
National Committee for the Prevention of Elder Abuse. (n.d.-b). *Financial abuse*. Retrieved from http://www.preventelderabuse.org/elderabuse/fin_abuse.html
National Committee for the Prevention of Elder Abuse. (n.d.-c). *Neglect*. Retrieved from http://www.preventelderabuse.org/elderabuse/neglect.html
National Committee for the Prevention of Elder Abuse. (n.d.-d). *Physical abuse*. Retrieved from http://www.preventelderabuse.org/elderabuse/physical.html
National Committee for the Prevention of Elder Abuse. (n.d.-e). *Psychological abuse*. Retrieved from http://www.preventelderabuse.org/elderabuse/psychological.html
National Committee for the Prevention of Elder Abuse. (n.d.-f). *Sexual abuse*. Retrieved from http://www.preventelderabuse.org/elderabuse/s_abuse.html
Public Health Agency of Canada. (2011). *Elder abuse in Canada: A gender-based analysis*. Retrieved from http://publications.gc.ca/collections/collection_2012/aspc-phac/HP10-21-2012-eng.pdf
Statistics Canada. (2011). *Seniors. Statistics Canada*. Retrieved from https://www150.statcan.gc.ca/n1/pub/11-402-x/2011000/chap/seniors-aines/seniors-aines-eng.htm

3 Pain Management Guidelines

Pain

Monakshi Sawhney and Roger Pilon

Definition
A. *Pain* is a subjective experience associated with actual or potential tissue damage.
B. *Nociceptive pain* is caused by direct stimulation of peripheral nociceptors. It is usually associated with tissue damage as well as inflammatory processes. It is usually well localized, but it can be more diffuse if deeper structures or viscera are involved. It can be classified as somatic nociceptive pain (involving skin, muscle, and bone), or visceral nociceptive pain (involving organs). Descriptors include aching, sharp, or dull.
C. *Neuropathic pain* is initiated or caused by a damage or dysfunction in the nervous system. This may include the central or peripheral nervous system. Descriptors include burning, shooting, numbness/tingling, electric shocks, allodynia (due to a stimulus that does not normally cause pain), and hyperalgesia (exaggerated pain response from a stimulus that normally causes pain).

Acute Pain

Moya Ook, Mona Sawhney, and Roger Pilon

Definition
A. *Acute pain* is defined as the physiologic response to and experience of unpleasant or noxious (unpleasant) stimuli that can be related to disease or injury.
B. It is a pain that normally has a sudden onset, is of short duration, and is associated with tissue injury (such as surgery, trauma, or medical illness/procedures). It usually resolves as tissue healing takes place. It lasts between seven and 30 days, with subacute pain lasting 90 days.

Incidence/Prevalence
A. Acute pain is the most common reason for presentation for treatment in the healthcare system. Clients experiencing acute pain will often self-medicate to relieve the pain. Acute pain is subjective and, if not treated effectively, can have devastating physiological and psychological effects and lead to chronic, long-term pain. Due to the subjective nature of acute pain, the client care plan needs to be individualized to meet the client's needs.

Pathogenesis
A. Acute pain is usually the result of stimulation of peripheral nociceptors (pain-sensing nerves), which are activated by noxious stimuli associated with tissue injury or damage. The message of pain travels along these peripheral nociceptors to the dorsal horn of the spinal cord and up the spinothalamic tract, where the sensation of pain is interpreted. In response, the brain sends a message to the periphery along the corticospinal tract, and the sympathetic nervous system is activated. Although the sympathetic nervous system may be activated, the signs of sympathetic response should be used very cautiously as a positive indicator of pain, as other pathology may cause or modify these symptoms.

Common Findings
A. Pain at the specific site of injury.
B. Increased heart rate.
C. Increased respiratory rate.
D. Elevated blood pressure (BP).
E. Sweating.
F. Nausea.

Other Signs and Symptoms
A. Urinary retention.
B. Dilated pupils.
C. Pallor.

Subjective Data
A. *Onset*: When did the pain begin?
B. *Precipitating* or *palliative* factors. What makes the pain better or worse?
C. *Quality* of the pain: What does the pain feel like?
D. *Region* or location of pain: Does the pain *radiate* to other body parts?
E. *Severity* of the pain: This can be assessed using a pain-rating scale (e.g., 0–10 scale, where 0 is no pain and 10 is the worst pain).
F. *Timing*: When does the pain occur (e.g., at rest or movement, daytime or nighttime)?
G. *Understanding*: What does the client believe is causing the pain?
H. *Values*: Does the pain hold any value for the client, or are there any personal, cultural, or religious beliefs or values that influence pain or pain management?
I. *Impact* of pain on activities of daily living (ADLs).

Valid and reliable tools are available and should be used to assess pain in infants, children, nonverbal clients, critically ill clients, and clients with dementia. Examples include the COMORT/COMFORT scale for infants, The Face, Legs, Activity, Cry, Consolability (r-FLACC) Scale for infants and cognitively impaired children, the PAINAD, and the CPOT.

Physical Examination
A. Clients experiencing acute pain require a comprehensive physical examination. Start with the assessment of vital signs, including temperature, pulse, respiration, oxygen saturation and B/P.
B. Inspect:
  1. Observe overall appearance.
  2. Level of consciousness.
  3. Note affect and ability to express self and pain.
  4. Note facial grimaces with movement.
  5. Note gait, stance, and movements.
  6. Inspect area at pain site.
C. Auscultate:
  1. Heart and lungs.
  2. Neck and abdomen.
D. Palpate: Palpate affected area of pain.
E. Percuss:
  1. Chest.
  2. Abdomen.
F. Perform musculoskeletal examination:

When performing a musculoskeletal examination, identify the location of pain, presence of trigger points, evidence of injury or trauma, edema, erythema, warmth, heat, lesions, petechiae, tenderness, decreased range of motion, pain with movement, crepitus, laxity of ligaments or cords, spasms, or guarding.

  1. Perform complete musculoskeletal examination, concentrating on the area of pain.
G. Neurologic examination:
  1. Perform complete neurologic examination.
  2. Identify change in sensory function, skin tenderness, weakness, muscle atrophy, and/or loss of deep tendon reflexes (DTRs).

Diagnostic Tests
A. **Diagnostic testing may be required to rule out organic cause of pain.** If organic disease is suspected, diagnostic testing may include the following, based on the suspected cause:
  1. CT imaging.
  2. MRI.
  3. Blood chemistries.
  4. Radiographic x-ray.
  5. Lumbar puncture.
  6. Ultrasound.
  7. ECG/echocardiogram.
  8. Electromyogram (EMG).

Differential Diagnoses
The differential diagnoses depend on the location of the acute pain and may include any of the following:
A. Head:
  1. Cluster headache/migraine headache.
  2. Temporal arteritis.
  3. Intracranial bleeding or stroke.
  4. Sinusitis.
  5. Dental abscess.
B. Neck:
  1. Meningitis.
  2. Muscle strain/sprain.
  3. Whiplash injury.
  4. Thyroiditis.
C. Chest:
  1. Pulmonary emboli.
  2. Myocardial infarction.
  3. Pneumonia.
  4. Costochondritis.
  5. Angina.
  6. Gastro-oesophageal reflux disease/oesophagitis.
  7. Fractured ribs.
  8. Pleurisy (pleuritic chest pain).
D. Abdomen:
  1. Peritonitis.
  2. Appendicitis.
  3. Ectopic pregnancy/uterine pregnancy.
  4. Endometriosis.
  5. Pelvic inflammatory disease.
  6. Peptic ulcer.
  7. Cholelithiasis.
  8. Colitis, Crohn's, diverticulitis.
  9. Constipation.
  10. Gastroenteritis.
  11. Irritable bowel syndrome.
  12. Urinary tract infection, kidney stone, pyelonephritis.
  13. Prostatitis.
  14. Malignancies.
E. Musculoskeletal:
  1. Muscle sprain/strain/tear.
  2. Skeletal fracture.
  3. Viral infection.
  4. Gout.
  5. Vitamin D deficiency.

Plan
A. General interventions:
  1. Acute pain is a symptom, not a diagnosis.
  2. Identify the cause or source of the acute pain depending on the location. If the pain is organic in nature, make the appropriate referral.
  3. Overall goal is to treat the acute pain appropriately.
B. Client teaching:
  1. The pain management plan must include client and family education regarding preventing and controlling pain, potential medication side effects, and how to prevent the side effects.
  2. Explain that complete pain relief may not be achievable initially, but the overall goal is to decrease the pain and improve function, thus allowing some daily activities at home to begin recovery.
  3. Management will include nonopioid therapy, nonpharmacological treatments, and, if appropriate, opioids. The recommendation from Health Quality Ontario regarding opioid prescribing for acute pain indicates that people who require opioids for acute pain should receive the lowest effective dose of an immediate release opioid. A prescription duration of three to seven days should be sufficient, and if opioids are needed for longer periods of time the client should be reevaluated.
  4. Provide information about the benefits and harms of all treatments. This includes the benefits and harms of

opioid therapy, addiction and overdose risk, and safe storage and safe disposal of medication.

C. Pharmacological therapy:
1. Multimodal analgesia is recommended to manage acute pain. This includes nonopioid pain medicines with physical interventions and psychological interventions if needed. Use opioids if indicated for the pain the client is experiencing.
2. *Visceral nociceptive pain*: Depending on the origin of the pain, treatments can include acetaminophen, nonsteroidal anti-inflammatory drugs (NSAIDs), steroids, opioids, and epidural or spinal local anaesthetics.
3. *Somatic nociceptive pain*: Treatments can include acetaminophen, cold packs, corticosteroids, peripheral local anesthetics, NSAIDs, and opioids.
4. *Neuropathic pain*: Gabapentionoids (gabapentin and pregabalin), tricyclic antidepressants (TCAs), and serotonin reuptake inhibitors. Other treatments include local anesthetics, tramadol, and glucocorticoids.

Know each medication's mechanism of action, potential adverse side effects, half-life, and drug–drug interaction potential. Always document that you have advised on the potential for sedation, suggested no driving/machinery use, or no alcohol while taking medication with these potential adverse side effects. Use caution when using NSAIDs with clients with cardiovascular disease due to the increased risk of heart attack and stroke.

Follow-Up

A. Once the organic cause of pain has been investigated, the initial follow-up is recommended as 48 to 72 hours after onset.
B. Ensure that the client has access to care on a regular schedule.

Individual Considerations

A. Geriatrics:
1. Physiologic changes that occur in the elderly, such as decreased body mass, hepatic dysfunction, and renal dysfunction, may cause increased serum drug concentrations of pain medication. Use caution when prescribing pain medication to this population.
2. Anti-inflammatories should be used cautiously and should be prescribed in a time-limited fashion (7–14 days) in persons who are frail or elderly due to the potential adverse gastrointestinal and renal effects.

Bibliography

Andersen, R. D., Langius-Eklof, A., Nakstad, B., Bernkler, T., & Jylli, L. (2017). The measurement properties of pediatric observational pain scales: A systematic review of reviews. *International Journal of Nursing Studies, 73*, 93–101. doi:10.1016/j.ijnurstu.2017.05.010

Choiniere, M., Watt, B., Watson, C., Victor, R. J. F., Baskett, J. S., Bussieres, C. C. J., & Taillefer, C. (2014). Prevalence of and risk factors for persistent postoperative nonanginal pain after cardiac surgery: A 2 year prospective multicenter study. *CMAJ, 186*, E213–E223. doi:10.1503/cmaj.114-0057

Chou, R., Gordon, D., de Leon-Cassola, O., Rosenberg, J. M., Bickler, S., Brennan, T., . . . Wu, C. L. (2016). Management of postoperative pain: A clinical practice guideline from the American Pain Society, the American Society of Regional Anesthesia and Pain Medicine, the American Society of Anesthesiology's Committee on Regional Anesthesia, Executive Committee and Administrative Council. *The Journal of Pain, 17*(2), 131–157. doi:10.1016/j.jpain.2015.12.008

Furlan, A. D., Hassan, S., Famiyeh, I. M., Wang, W., & Dhanju, J. (2016). Long-term opioid use after discharge from inpatient musculoskeletal rehabilitation. *Journal of Rehabilitation Medicine, 48*, 464–468. doi:10.2340/16501977-2080

Gelinas, C. (2016). Pain assessment in the critically ill adult: Recent evidence and new trends. *Intensive and Critical Care Nursing, 34*, 1–11. doi:10.1016/j.iccn.2016.03.001

Health Quality Ontario. (2018). *Opioid prescribing for acute pain.* Toronto, ON, Canada: Queen's Printer for Ontario.

Horgas, A. L. (2017). Pain assessment in older adults. *Nursing Clinics of North America, 52*, 375–385. doi:10.1016/j.cnur.2017.04.006

Kent, M. L., Tighe, P. J., Belfer, I., Brennan, T. J., Bruehl, S., Brummett, C. M., . . . Terman, G. (2017). The ACTTION-APS-AAPM Pain Taxonomy (AAAPT) mulitdimensional approach to classifying acute pain conditions. *Journal of Pain, 18*(5), 479–489. doi:10.1016/j.jpain.2017.02.421

Webster, L. R., & Webster, R. M. (2005). Predicting aberrant behaviours in opioid-treated patients: Preliminary validation of the opioid risk tool. *American Academy of Pain Medicine, 6*(6), 432–442. doi:10.1111/j.1526-4637.2005.00072.x

Chronic Pain

Moya Cook, Mona Sawhney, and Roger Pilon

Definition

A. *Chronic pain* is defined as pain that lasts longer than three months or past the time of normal tissue healing. The pain may be continuous or recurrent and of sufficient duration and intensity. Chronic pain interferes with a client's ability to function with normal daily activities and decreases quality of life.

Incidence/Prevalence

It is estimated that 19% of the population report some form of chronic pain and the prevalence of chronic pain increases with age. The cost of chronic pain in Canada is estimated at $7.2 billion, based on provincial health benefits paid to provide care and not including private health insurance coverage, loss of wages, or loss of quality of life. Chronic pain impacts quality of life more significantly than other chronic conditions such as chronic lung or heart disease. Clients with chronic pain have double the risk of suicide as compared to the general population.

A. Women are affected more than men.
B. Onset is usually in the fifth decade and is often associated with marked functional disability.

Pathogenesis

A. *Skeletal muscle pain* occurs in the soft tissue involving the neck, shoulders, trunk, arms, low back, hips, and lower extremities. *Myofascial pain syndrome* relates to the fascia surrounding the muscle tissue.
B. *Inflammatory pain* is caused by chemicals, such as prostaglandins, leading to the stimulation of the pain receptors. Examples include arthritis, infection, tissue injury, and postoperative pain.
C. *Mechanical/compressive pain* is the direct result of the muscle, ligament, and tendon causing strain, leading to the stimulation of the pain receptors. Diagnosis may be based on diagnostic imaging results, which may include fracture, obstruction, dislocation, or compression of tissue by a tumour, cyst, or bony structure.
D. *Central sensitization.* According to Ingraham (2018), "Pain itself often modifies the way the central nervous system works, so that a client actually becomes more sensitive and gets more pain with less provocation. Sensitized clients are not only more sensitive to things that should hurt, but also to ordinary touch and pressure as well. Their pain also 'echoes,' fading more slowly than in other people" (p. 1).

Predisposing Factors
A. Age 50 years or more.
B. Female gender.
C. History of having seen many providers.
D. Frequent use of several nonspecific medications.
E. Depression.
F. Personality, including moods, fears, expectations, coping efforts, and resources.

Common Findings
A. Specific to site of pain.
B. Emotional distress related to fear, maladaptive or inadequate support systems, and other coping resources.
C. Treatment-induced complications.
D. Overuse of drugs.
E. Inability to work.
F. Financial complications.
G. Disruption of usual activities.
H. Sleep disturbances.
I. Pain becomes primary life focus.

Other Signs and Symptoms
A. Pain lasts longer than three to six months.
B. There may be anger and loss of faith or trust in the healthcare system. This type of client frequently takes too many medications, spends a great deal of time in bed, sees many care providers, and experiences little joy in either work or play.

Subjective Data
A. Elicit a clear description of the onset, location, quality, intensity, and time course of pain and any factor that aggravates or relieves it. Use the acronym OPQRSTUV: O = onset, P = palliative (relieving), provoke (aggravating), Q = quality, R = region/radiating (location), S = severity, T = timing, U = understanding, V = value. Also examine past and current treatments and impact on function and quality of life.
B. *Self-reporting pain assessment tools* should be used early in the process of client evaluation. Use the tool at each office visit to see progression or regression. Lack of pain assessment is a barrier to good pain control. Consider the age of the client; his or her physical, emotional, and cognitive status; and preference when choosing the self-reporting pain assessment tool.
   1. Brief Pain Inventory Short Form (www.npcrc.org/files/news/briefpain_short.pdf).
   2. Severity of pain, using the following:
      a. Numeric rating scales rate pain intensity from 0 to 10.
      b. Verbal rating scales rate pain as none, mild, moderate, or severe.
      c. The Faces scale is useful for paediatric and cognitively impaired clients. Multicultural translations may be downloaded at www.wongbakerfaces.org or www.iasp-pain.org/Education/Content.aspx?ItemNumber=1519.
C. Determine the extent to which the client is suffering, disabled, and unable to enjoy usual activity. It is important to inquire about activities of daily living (ADLs) and functional limitations.
D. Obtain a complete review of systems, including nausea, numbness, weakness, insomnia, loss of appetite, dysphoria, malaise, fatigue, or depression signs and symptoms.
E. Obtain a complete family and social history. Address spiritual and cultural issues. History of chemical dependency is of interest in this client population.
F. Obtain the client's medical history relevant to the pain, including diagnosis, testing, treatments, and outcomes.
G. Obtain a pain history to identify the client's attitudes, beliefs, level of knowledge, and previous experiences with pain. Are previously used methods for pain control helpful? What is the client's attitude toward the use of certain pain medications? Often, the client discusses certain adverse side effects or allergies from undesired pain medication.

Physical Examination
A. Clients experiencing chronic pain require a comprehensive physical examination to identify physical and/or psychological diagnoses utilizing valid tools. This includes assessment of functional status, quality of life, and pain.
B. Assess vital signs, including temperature, pulse, respirations, oxygen saturation, and blood pressure.
C. Inspect:
   1. Observe overall appearance.
   2. Assess level of consciousness or signs of lethargy.
   3. Note affect and ability to express self and pain.
   4. Note facial grimaces with movement.
   5. Note gait, stance, and movements.
   6. Inspect area at pain site.
D. Auscultate:
   1. Heart and lungs.
   2. Neck and abdomen.
E. Palpate the affected area of pain.
F. Percuss:
   1. Chest.
   2. Abdomen.
G. Perform musculoskeletal examination.

When performing musculoskeletal examination, identify the location of pain, presence of trigger points, evidence of injury or trauma, edema, erythema, warmth, heat, lesions, petechiae, tenderness, decreased range of motion, pain with movement, crepitus, laxity of ligaments or cords, spasms, or guarding.

   1. Perform a complete musculoskeletal examination, concentrating on the area of pain.
   2. Note limitations in range of motion.
H. Neurologic examination:
   1. Perform complete neurologic examination.
   2. Note the client's affect and mood. Is the client cooperative during examination?
   3. Identify change in sensory function, skin tenderness, weakness, muscle atrophy, and/or loss of deep tendon reflexes (DTRs).
I. Functional assessment:
   1. The baseline functional assessment provides objective measurable data on a client's physical abilities and limitations. It can be used to determine whether the client's efforts are valid and complaints are reliable.
   2. The information may be used to identify areas of impairment, establish specific functional goals, and measure the effectiveness of treatment interventions.
   3. These objective data may be used in worker compensation cases, returning-to-work status, federal disability, and motor vehicle accident lawsuits.

4. Know the resources in your area who are trained to perform functional assessments. Physical therapists and occupational therapists are the best qualified to perform the assessments.

Diagnostic Tests
Remember that pain previously diagnosed as chronic pain syndrome can be organic and vice versa. Organic causes must always be evaluated and excluded.
A. **Diagnostic testing may be required to rule out organic cause of pain.** If organic disease is suspected, diagnostic testing may include the following:
  1. Plain radiography should be ordered first for muscle, inflammatory, or skeletal pain. Plain radiography will diagnose a fracture. Additional studies may be recommended by the radiologist if a lesion/abnormality is seen on plain radiography.
  2. MRI and CT are ordered if the plain radiograph is negative and the client continues to complain of pain.
  3. Electromyography and nerve conduction studies are used to evaluate neuropathic pain. Numerous serum and urine studies should also be considered if the neuropathic pain is undiagnosed.
B. Depression screening tool: Consider using a depression assessment tool such as the Beck Depression Inventory or Patient Health Questionnaire 9 (PHQ9). These tools can be administered at a subsequent appointment to follow the client's symptoms.

Differential Diagnoses
A. Pain disorder.
B. Pain related to a disease with no cure/malignancy.
C. Somatization disorder.
D. Conversion disorder.
E. Hypochondriasis.
F. Depression.
G. Chemical dependency.
H. Fibromyalgia.

Plan
A. General interventions:
  1. Treatment is multidimensional and should not be focused on pharmacological treatment alone.
  2. Offer hope and potential for improvement of pain control and improvement of function but *not* cure.
  3. The pain is real to the client, and acceptance of the problem must occur before a mutually agreed-on treatment plan can be initiated.
  4. Depression is a common emotional disturbance in chronic pain clients and is treatable.
  5. Identify specific and realistic goals for therapy such as having a good night's sleep, going shopping, or returning to work. Client discussion needs to include the idea that the goal may be decreasing pain intensity, not eliminating pain.
  6. Carefully assess the level of pain using available tools such as a daily pain diary or other pain assessment scales.
  7. Avoid pain reinforcement such as sympathy and attention to pain. Provide positive response to productive activities. Improving activity tolerance assists in desensitizing the client to pain.
  8. Shift the focus from pain to accomplishing daily assigned self-help tasks. The accomplishment of these tasks functions as positive reinforcement.
B. Client teaching.

C. Pharmacological interventions:
Nonopioid pharmacotherapies and nonpharmacological therapies should be optimized before considering an opioid for the management of chronic noncancer pain.
  1. Skeletal muscle pain: Treatment should focus on physical rehabilitation and behavioural management. Tricyclic antidepressants (TCAs) and muscle relaxants (cyclobenzaprine) may be used. Research is lacking regarding the need for opioids.
  2. Inflammatory pain: Nonsteroidal anti-inflammatory drugs (NSAIDs) and corticosteroids are first-line pharmacological interventions. Topical creams and solutions have been used in treating arthritis pain.
  3. Mechanical/compressive pain: Opioids may be used to manage these symptoms while other measures are being taken.
  4. Neuropathic pain:
     a. Gabapentin and pregabalin are the first-line treatments for diabetic neuropathy and postherpetic neuralgia.
     b. TCAs are extremely useful. Clients who are not depressed obtain excellent pain relief with TCAs such as amitriptyline and doxepin.
     c. Selective serotonin reuptake inhibitors (SSRIs) are also effective for chronic pain control. Duloxetine has been approved for chronic pain as monotherapy or in conjunction with TCAs.
     d. Anticonvulsants are useful in controlling some neuropathic pain: carbamazepine, phenytoin, and valproic acid. **Clients need to be monitored monthly for hepatic dysfunction and hematopoietic suppression**.
     e. Topical agents: Capsaicin can reduce pain without significant systemic effects. Topical lidocaine patches are approved for postherpetic neuralgia.
     f. Carbamazepine is used as the first-line treatment for trigeminal neuralgia.
     g. Opioids: Tramadol may be effective for neuropathic pain control; tramadol also causes serotonin reuptake inhibition similar to that seen with the TCAs. It should be used cautiously as it has many drug–drug interactions.
  5. All therapies need a two- to three-week trial period to adequately evaluate therapy. Some medications take longer than that to evaluate.
  6. NSAIDs should be used for flare-ups of mild to moderate inflammatory or nonneuropathic pain.
  7. Benzodiazepines and barbiturates should not be used for treatment of chronic pain due to the high risk of substance abuse.
  8. Opioids require careful client selection, titration, and monitoring. Avoid long-term, daily treatment with short-acting opioids. For as-needed use, prescribe small quantities.
     a. Clients already receiving high-dose opioid therapy should be encouraged to gradually taper dose, and multidisciplinary support should be offered where available to those who experience challenges. A resource to help clinicians with tapering from the Center for Effective Practice can be found at thewellhealth.ca/opioidtaperingtool/.
  9. Perform addiction risk screening interventions when considering opioids: Urine drug screen and a risk of misuse assessment should be completed prior to initiating this class of medications.

a. The Opioid Risk Tool will generate a score that identifies individuals found to be at low, moderate, or high risk for addiction. Clients with a current diagnosis of anxiety, depression, and trauma (i.e., posttraumatic stress disorder [PTSD]) or with a current or past history of problematic alcohol or drug use should be monitored closely if opioids are prescribed, as they may be at risk of opioid misuse.
b. Perform urine drug screen before prescribing controlled substances initially, as needed, and annually. The enzyme immunoassay (EIA) and gas chromatography/mass spectroscopy urine screen can be used. Depending on the results of urine drug screening, the provider may seek additional consultation, change medication therapy, refer for substance misuse treatment, or discharge the client to another healthcare provider.
c. A written controlled substance treatment agreement among the client, provider, and clinic is recommended. Incorporate expectations of the client, including that no other controlled substances will be prescribed by any other provider. Only one pharmacy should be used. Medication must be taken as prescribed. These are no early refills on controlled substances. The client must agree to random drug screens and may be called to report to the clinic for random drug screens and/or pill counts.
10. For clients with active substance use disorder, there is a strong recommendation against the use of opioids.
D. Nonpharmacological interventions:
1. Cognitive behavioural training and mindfulness-based stress reduction: Examples of cognitive behavioural training include problem-solving, guided imagery, hypnosis, controlled breathing exercises, attention diversion, meditation, and yoga exercises; progressive muscle relaxation (PMR) is recommended to help relax major muscle groups. Randomized controlled trials showed significant reduction in pain with alternative interventions such as music, relaxation, distraction, and massage use.
2. Exercise: Examples of exercise include yoga exercises and PMR. PMR is recommended to help relax major muscle groups. Research indicates that yoga decreases bothersome pain after 12 weeks of regular exercise. The benefits of yoga exercise include improved strength, balance, coordination, range of motion, and reduced anxiety. Yoga instruction by a qualified teacher is a low-cost intervention. Yoga is an effective form of self-care and is an affordable way to alleviate pain. Always advise clients to start slowly and be prepared for an approach to pain management that may take several weeks of therapy.
3. Alternative therapies: Randomized controlled trials have demonstrated a significant reduction in pain with alternative interventions such as music, relaxation, distraction, acupuncture, myofascial release treatments, and massage.
4. Occupational therapy.
5. Vocational therapy.
6. Physical therapy, including noninvasive techniques, transcutaneous electrical nerve stimulation, hot or cold therapy, hydrotherapy, traction, massage, bracing, and exercise.
7. Individual and family therapy or counseling.
8. Aesthetic or neurosurgical procedures.
9. Clients may inquire about the use of herbal products to treat chronic pain. Advise clients of the following:
a. Herbal products are generally not regulated.
b. Herbal products may interact with current medications and cause complications; all herbal products should be researched on reputable medically based websites, not blogs or chat rooms.
c. Devil's claw, feverfew, willow bark, glucosamine, and chondroitin should be avoided.
d. Any use of dimethylsulfoxide is discouraged.

Follow-Up
A. See clients every four to six weeks for evaluation.
B. Ensure that the client has access to care on a regular schedule.
C. These brief visits should be regular so that care is not perceived to be dependent on escalation of symptoms.

Consultation/Referral
A. Consider client referral to a pain management clinic if pain control is not adequate. Interventions commonly performed at the specialty clinic include facet joint injections, percutaneous radiofrequency neurotomy, epidural corticosteroid injections, transforaminal epidural injections, and sacroiliac joint injections.
B. Refer for psychological counseling if substance abuse is suspected.
C. Refer to a certified pain specialist if the client is taking high doses of opioids and detoxification is indicated. Buprenorphine is the most common medication prescribed by a certified pain specialist.
D. Consider rheumatology consult if indicated.

Resources
Many patient resources on pain are available at your local library, bookstores, and on the Internet. Look for a local support group in your area to join and learn how other people are coping with your same condition.
There are many pain organizations available to assist patients. Below are a sample of website that contain information for patients and families that may be helpful to provide further information.
Canadian Arthritis Society: https://arthritis.ca/
Canadian Pain Society: www.canadianpainsociety.ca
Choosing Wisely Canada: https://choosingwiselycanada.org/
Choosing Wisely Canada, Low back Pain: https://choosingwisely canada.org/treating-lower-back-pain/
Choosing Wisely Canada, Opioid Wisely: https://choosingwisely canada.org/campaign/opioid-wisely/
Health Quality Ontario, Quality Standards, patient resources: https://www.hqontario.ca/Evidence-to-Improve-Care/Quality-Standards/View-all-Quality-Standards
Pain BC: https://www.painbc.ca/

Bibliography
Busse, J. W., Craigie, S., Juurlink, D. N., Buckley, D. N., Wang, L., Couban, R. J., . . . Guyatt, G. H. (2017). Guideline for opioid therapy and chronic noncancer pain. *Canadian Medical Association Journal, 189*(18), E659–E666. doi:10.1503/cmaj.170363
Center for Effective Practice. (2018). *Opioid tapering template*. Retrieved from https://thewellhealth.ca/opioidtaperingtool/
Furlan, A. D., Hassan, S., Famiyeh, I. M., Wang, W., & Dhanju, J. (2016). Long-term opioid use after discharge from inpatient musculoskeletal rehabilitation. *Journal of Rehabilitation Medicine, 48*, 464–468. doi:10.2340/16501977-2080
Health Quality Ontario. (2018a). *Opioid prescribing for chronic pain*. Toronto, ON, Canada: Queen's Printer for Ontario.
Health Quality Ontario. (2018b). *Opioid use disorder*. Toronto, ON, Canada: Queen's Printer for Ontario.
Hogan, M. E., Taddio, A., Katz, J., Shah, V., & Krahn, M. (2016). Incremental health care costs for chronic pain in Ontario, Canada: A population-based matched cohort study of adolescents and adults using administrative data. *Pain, 156*(8), 1626–1633. doi:10.1097/j.pain.0000000000000561
Hooten, W. M., Timming, R., Belgrade, M., Gaul, J., Goertz, M., Haake, B., & Walker, N. (2013). *Health care guideline: Assessment and*

management of chronic pain (6th ed.). Bloomington, MN: Institute for Clinical Systems Improvement. Retrieved from https://pdfs.semanticscholar.org/e1f7/c26a36d83686607ad89ee835daa3c9db3f4c.pdf

Horgas, A. L. (2017). Pain assessment in older adults. *Nursing Clinics of North America, 52*, 375–385. doi:10.1016/j.cnur.2017.04.006

Ingraham, P. (2018). *Central Sensitization in Chronic Pain: Pain itself can change how pain works, resulting in more pain with less provocation*. Retrieved from https://www.painscience.com/articles/central-sensitization.php

Lynch, M. E. (2011). The need for a Canadian pain strategy. *Pain Research and Management, 16*(2), 77–80. doi:10.1155/2011/654651. Retrieved from https://www.ncbi.nlm.nih.gov/pmc/articles/PMC3084407/

Merskey, H. & Bogduk, N. (Eds.). (1994). *Classification of chronic pain: Descriptions of chronic pain syndromes and definitions of pain terms* (2nd ed.). Seattle, WA: IASP Press.

Moulin, D. E., Boulanger, A., Clark, A. J., Clarke, H., Dao, T., Finley, G. A., ... Williamson, O. D. (2014). Pharmacological management of chronic neuropathic pain: Revised consensus statement from the Canadian Pain Society. *Pain Research and Management, 19*(6), 328–335. doi:10.1155/2014/754693

Reitsma, M. L., Tranmer, J. E., Buchanan, D. M., & Vandenkerkhof, E. G. (2011). The prevalence of chronic pain and pain-related interference in the Canadian population from 1994 to 2008. *Chronic Diseases and Injuries in Canada, 31*(4), 157–164. Retrieved from http://www.phac-aspc.gc.ca/publicat/hpcdp-pspmc/31-4/assets/pdf/cdic-mcbc-31-4-ar-04-eng.pdf

Schopflocher, D., Jovey, R., & Taenzer, P. (2011). The prevalence of chronic pain in Canada. *Pain and Research Management, 16*(6), 445–450. doi:10.1155/2011/876306

Tang, N., & Crane, C. (2006). Suicidality in chronic pain: Review of the prevalence, risk factors and psychological links. *Psychological Medicine, 36*, 575–586. doi:10.1017/S0033291705006859

Webster, L. R., & Webster, R. M. (2005). Predicting aberrant behaviours in opioid-treated patients: Preliminary validation of the opioid risk tool. *American Academy of Pain Medicine, 6*(6), 432–442. doi:10.1111/j.1526-4637.2005.00072.x

Lower Back Pain

Moya Cook, Mona Sawheny, and Roger Pilon

The Core Back Tool is a resource that outlines the assessment of low back pain and can be accessed at thewellhealth.ca/low-back-pain/.

Definition
Painful conditions of the lower back may be categorized as follows:
A. Potentially serious disorders: acute fractures, tumour, progressive neurologic deficit, nerve root compression, and cauda equina syndrome.
B. Degenerative disorders: aging or repetitive use, degenerative disease, and osteoarthritis.
C. Nonspecific disorders: benign and self-limiting with unclear aetiology.

Incidence/Prevalence
A. Lower back pain is commonly seen in clients from ages 20 to 40 years.
B. Approximately 70% to 80% of people experience back pain at some point in their lifetime.

Pathogenesis
A. Pain arises from fracture, tumour, nerve root compression, a degenerative disc, osteoarthritis, and strain of the ligaments and musculature of the lumbosacral area.

Predisposing Factors
A. Trauma causing ligament tearing; stretching of vertebra, muscles, tendons, ligaments, or fascia.
B. Repetitive mechanical stress.
C. Tumour.
D. Exaggerated lumbar lordosis.
E. Abnormal, forward-tipped pelvis.
F. Uneven leg length.
G. Chronic poor posture due to inadequate conditioning of muscle strength and flexibility, improper lifting techniques causing excessive strain, and poor body mechanics.
H. Inadequate rest.
I. Emotional depression.

Common Findings
A. Pain in the lower back area may range from discomfort to severe back pain, with or without radiation.

Other Signs and Symptoms
A. Ambulating with a limp.
B. Limited range of motion.
C. Posture normal to guarded.

Subjective Data
A. Ask the client to discuss the origin of pain. How has the pain progressed or changed since the initial injury?
B. Ask the client to point to an area where pain is felt.
C. Have the client describe the pain. Is it radiating, with sharp, shooting pain down to the lower leg and feet?
D. Ask, What makes the pain worse or better? Does activity make the pain worse or better? Have the client list current medications or therapies used for pain, noting results of treatment.
E. Investigate occurrence of systemic symptoms such as fever and weight loss.
F. Explore the client's past medical history. Note previous trauma or overuse, tuberculosis, arthritis, cancer, and osteoporosis.
G. Inquire about symptoms such as dysuria, bowel or bladder incontinence, muscle weakness, paresthesia, and loss of sensation. **Bowel or bladder dysfunction, bilateral sciatica, and saddle compression may be symptoms of severe compression of the cauda equina that necessitate an urgent workup and referral.**
H. Ask the client about precipitating factors such as athletics, heavy lifting, driving, yard work, occupation, sleep habits, or systemic disease.
I. Use a pain scale to describe the worst pain and the best pain levels.

Physical Examination
A. Check temperature, pulse, blood pressure, and respiration.
B. Inspect:
  1. Observe general appearance: Note discomfort and grimacing on movement and/or examination.
  2. Distraction may distinguish pain behaviour from actual pathology.
  3. Note evidence of trauma with bruises, cuts, and fractures.
  4. Note posture and gait.
C. Palpate:
  1. Palpate spine and paravertebral structures, noting point tenderness and muscle spasm. Palpation elicits paravertebral tenderness and generalized tenderness over the lower back to upper buttocks.
  2. Examine abdomen for masses.
  3. Extremities: Palpate peripheral pulses.
D. Perform neurologic examination:
  1. Identify sensation and pain distribution.

2. Determine motor strength and evaluate whether muscle strength is symmetrical: Upper extremity resistance is equal bilaterally.
   3. Test deep tendon reflexes (DTRs) and dorsiflexion of the big toes.
E. Check sensation of perineum to rule out cauda equina syndrome.
F. Perform traction tests: straight leg raises, crossed leg raises, Yeoman Guying, and Patrick's test. Musculoskeletal findings include the following:
   1. Straight leg raising and dorsiflexion of foot on the affected side may reduce lower back discomfort.
   2. Elevate each leg passively with flexion at the hip and extension of the knee. Positive straight leg raise gives radicular pain when the leg is raised 30 to 60 degrees.
   3. Crossed leg raises: Test is positive when pain occurs in the leg not being raised.
   4. Yeoman Guying: Unilateral hyperextension in prone position identifies lumbosacral mechanical disorder.
   5. Patrick's test: Place heel on opposite knee and apply lateral force; check for hip or sacroiliac disease.
   6. Range of motion: Increased pain with extension often indicates osteoarthritis. Increased pain with flexion often indicates strain or injured disc.
G. Pelvic examination: Consider pelvic and rectal examination, if indicated. If the client has fallen on the coccyx, a rectal examination is needed to check for stability.

Diagnostic Tests
A. Laboratory: Complete blood count, erythrocyte sedimentation rate, serum calcium, alkaline phosphatase, urinalysis, and serum immunoelectrophoresis when inflammatory, neoplastic, diffuse bone disease, or renal disease is suspected.
B. Radiography of spine.
C. Consider the following tests:
   1. MRI to rule out disc disease and tumours.
   2. Bone scan to rule out cancer.

Differential Diagnoses
A. Back pain secondary to musculoskeletal pain.
B. Herniated intervertebral disease.
C. Sciatica.
D. Fracture.
E. Ankylosing spondylitis.
F. Malignancy/tumour.
G. Abdominal aneurysm.
H. Pyelonephritis.
I. Metabolic bone disease.
J. Gynecologic disease.
K. Peripheral neuropathy.
L. Depression.
M. Prostatitis.
N. Spinal stenosis.
O. Osteoarthritis.
P. Osteoporosis.

Plan
A. General interventions:
   1. The client should continue physical activity as tolerated.
   2. For acute muscle strain, have the client apply local cold packs 20 to 30 minutes several times a day for the first 24 hours. Heat packs are recommended after the initial 24 hours of injury.
   3. Chronic or recurrent pain may be treated with either ice or heat applications, whichever gives relief.
B. Client teaching:
   1. Give accurate information on the prognosis for quick recovery, such as continuing light physical activity, performing back-strengthening exercises, and avoiding overuse of medications.
   2. Improvement occurs in most cases in a few weeks, although mild symptoms may persist.
   3. Several Canadian guidelines recommend rehabilitative therapies for clients who do not improve after medications and self-care recommendations. Rehabilitative therapies include exercise therapy, acupuncture, massage therapy, spinal manipulation, cognitive behavioural therapy, and yoga.
   4. Provide educational handouts on back exercises.
   5. After intense pain abates, the client may perform low-back exercises for range of motion and strengthening, and isometric tightening exercises of abdominal and gluteal muscles.
   6. Teach client knee–chest exercises. Recommend to the client to place his or her back against the wall and contract abdominal and gluteal muscles with five to 10 repetitions, four to six times per day.
   7. Research indicates that yoga is beneficial for many types of back pain. Types of back pain benefited by yoga include musculoskeletal injury, herniated disc, spinal stenosis, spondylolisthesis, piriformis syndrome, arthritis, and sacroiliac joint derangement.
   8. Encourage the client to perform walking exercise daily.
   9. Teach relaxation techniques.
   10. Encourage the client to modify work hours and job tasks.
   11. Refer the client for therapeutic massage or physical therapy as needed.
   12. Obesity is often related to decreased exercise and poor physical fitness with reduced trunk muscle strength and endurance. Obese clients may experience back pain with normal activity.
C. Pharmacological therapy:
   1. Analgesics: acetaminophen.
   Inquire of any other current medications and/or over-the-counter preparations containing acetaminophen.
   2. Nonsteroidal anti-inflammatory drugs (NSAIDs), unless contraindicated due to gastrointestinal symptoms or cardiovascular disease:
      a. ASA: do not use if the patient has an allergy or contradiction (such as GI bleed). Use with caution in the presence of renal and hepatic dysfunction.
      b. Ibuprofen: Use with caution in the presence of renal or hepatic dysfunction.
      c. Naproxen: Use with caution in the presence of renal and hepatic dysfunction.
      d. Celecoxib: Note to use lowest possible dose and for short duration.
   3. Muscle relaxants:
      a. Cyclobenzaprine HCl: Use with caution in the presence of renal and hepatic dysfunction and in geriatric clients. Note to use lowest possible dose and for short duration.
      b. Methocarbamol: Use with caution in the presence of renal dysfunction or cirrhosis and caution with EtOH use as the combination of methocarbamol and alcohol consumption can increase the side effect of sedation.
      c. Orphenadrine citrate: Do not use with a patient who has an allergy or contradiction to ASA. This medication can cause drowsiness; use cautiously with medications that cause sedation and avoid alcohol use.

Follow-Up
A. If pain is severe or unimproved, follow up in 24 hours.
B. If pain is moderate, reevaluate the client in seven to 10 days.
C. See the client in two to four weeks to reevaluate his or her condition and behavioural changes.
D. Recurrences are not uncommon but do not indicate a chronic or worsening case.

Consultation/Referral
A. Consult with a neurologist when considering red-flag diagnoses such as cauda equina syndrome, herniated disc, widespread neurologic involvement, carcinoma, or significant trauma.
B. Referral to a rheumatology specialist is needed for clients who note significant morning stiffness with a gradual onset prior to age 40 years, with continuing spinal movements in all directions, and involving some peripheral joints, iritis, skin rashes indicating inflammatory disorders such as ankylosing spondylitis, and related disorders.

Individual Considerations
A. Pregnancy: Pregnancy is often associated with low-back discomfort. This is due to the redistribution of body weight. As weight increases in the abdominal area with the growing fetus, clients tend to compensate by changing posture and tilting the spine back.
B. Adults:
   1. For clients older than 50 years presenting with no prior history of backache, consider a differential diagnosis of neoplasm. The most common metastasis seen is secondary to the primary site of breast cancer, prostate cancer, or multiple myeloma. Pain most prominent in a recumbent position rarely radiates into the buttock or leg.
   2. Men and women in their early adulthood (ages 20–45 years) who present with chronic back pain that improves with activity should be further evaluated for ankylosing spondylitis.

Bibliography
Center for Effective Practice. (2016). *Core back tool*. Retrieved from https://thewellhealth.ca/low-back-pain/

Chang, D. G., Holt, J.A., Sklar, M., & Groessl, E.J. (2016). Yoga as treatment for chronic low back pain: A systematic review of the literature. *Journal Orthopedics and Rheumatology, 3*(1), 1–8. PMID: 27231715 https://www.ncbi.nlm.nih.gov/pmc/articles/PMC4878447/

Cherkin, D. C., Sherman, K. J., Balderson, B. H., Cook, A. J., Anderson, M. L., Hawkes, R. J., . . . Turner, A. (2016). Effect of mindfulness-based stress reduction vs cognitive behavioural therapy or usual care on back pain and functional limitations in adults with chronic low back pain: A randomized clinical trial. *JAMA, 315*(12), 1240–1249. doi:10.1001/jama.2016.2323

Goertz, M., Thorson, D., Bonsell, J., Bonte, B., Campbell, R., Haake, B., & Timming, R. (2012). *Health care guideline: Adult acute and subacute low back pain* (15th ed.). Bloomington, MN: Institute for Clinical Systems Improvement. Retrieved from https://www.icsi.org/_asset/bjvqrj/LBP.pdf

Michigan Quality Improvement Consortium. (n.d.). *Management of acute low back pain*. Retrieved from https://www.guidelines.gov

4 Dermatology Guidelines

Acne Rosacea

Jill C. Cash, Amy C. Bruggemann, Elsie Duff, and Cindy Fehr

Definition
A. A multifactorial vascular skin disorder, acne rosacea is characterized by chronic inflammatory processes in which flushing and dilation of the blood vessels occur on the face. It is manifested in four stages of pathologic events.

Incidence/Prevalence
A. Acne rosacea affects approximately two million people, 6% of the population in Canada.

Pathogenesis
A. Rosacea is a functional vascular anomaly with a tendency toward recurrent dilation and flushing of the face. This results in inflammatory mediator release, extravasation of inflammatory cells, and the formation of inflammatory papules and pustules.

Predisposing Factors
A. Tendency to flush frequently.
B. Exposure to heat, cold, or sunlight.
C. Consumption of hot or spicy foods and alcoholic beverages.
D. Some topical medications, astringents, or toners.

Common Findings
A. Papules, pustules, and nodules. Hallmarks for diagnosis are the small papules and papulopustules. Many presenting erythematous papules have a tiny pustule at the crest. No comedones are present.
B. Periodic reddening or flushing of face.
C. Increase in skin temperature of face.
D. Face flushing in response to heat stimuli (hot liquids) in mouth.

Other Signs and Symptoms
A. Periorbital erythema.
B. Telangiectasia, paranasally and on cheeks.
C. Rhinophyma.
D. Blepharoconjunctivitis with erythematous eyelid margins.
E. Conjunctivitis —diffuse hyperemic type or nodular.
F. Keratitis—lower portion of cornea, associated with pain, photophobia, and foreign-body sensation.

Subjective Data
A. Ask the client to describe the location and the onset. Was the onset sudden or gradual? How have the symptoms continued to develop?
B. Assess whether the skin is itchy or painful.
C. Assess for any associated discharge (blood or pus).
D. Complete a drug history. Has the client recently taken any antibiotics or other medications?
E. Determine whether the client has used any topical medications, astringents, toners, or new skin-care products.
F. Rule out any possible exposure to industrial or domestic toxins, insect bites, and possible contact with venereal disease or HIV.
G. Ask the client about close contact with others with skin disorders.
H. Identify whether exposure to heat, cold, or sunlight provokes the symptoms.
I. Ask whether eating or drinking hot or spicy foods or consumption of alcoholic beverages provokes the symptoms.

Physical Examination
A. Check temperature, pulse, and blood pressure.
B. Inspect:
    1. Skin, focusing on face and scalp.
    2. Nose and paranasal structures.
    3. Eyes, eyelids, conjunctiva, and cornea. **An ocular manifestation, rosacea keratitis, may cause corneal ulcers to develop.**

Diagnostic Tests
Consider a skin biopsy to rule out lupus, sarcoidosis, or other possible causes if history and physical exam findings warrant further testing.

Differential Diagnoses
A. Acne vulgaris.
B. Steroid-induced acne.
C. Perioral dermatitis.
D. Seborrhoeic dermatitis.
E. Lupus erythematosus.
F. Cutaneous sarcoidosis.

Plan
A. General interventions: Identify any causative or provocative factors—heat, cold, hot or spicy foods, alcoholic beverages, sunlight:
    1. Advise washing face with a mild skin cleanser in the morning and at night.

2. Avoid direct sunlight exposure by wearing protective clothing/hats when outdoors. Suggest using a sunscreen of sun protection factor (SPF)-30 when exposed to sunlight.
▶ **B.** Client teaching: *Refer to Client Teaching Guide: Acne Rosacea.*
C. Pharmacological therapy:
  1. First-line treatment: Tetracycline.
  2. Others: Erythromycin, minocycline, doxycycline, amoxicillin, and metronidazole. Start at a higher dose and taper to the maintenance dose.
    a. Topical antibiotics. Apply topical antibiotic/steroid combinations twice daily after cleansing skin.
  3. Refractory cases may respond to isotretinoin.

Follow-Up
A. Follow up in two weeks to evaluate therapy.
B. See clients monthly for evaluation until maintenance is reached.
C. Relapses are common following discontinuance of antibiotics; repeat treatment.

Consultation/Referral
A. Consult or refer the client to a dermatologist if there is no improvement, or if the client is unable to reach maintenance.
B. Provide an immediate referral to an ophthalmologist for treatment and follow up if the eye is involved.

Individual Consideration
A. Adults: Sodium sulfacetamide and sulfur topical may be used to treat erythema.
B. Laser and light therapies may be used to treat erythema.

Bibliography
Canadian Skin Client Alliance. (2016b). *Skin Conditions: Rosacea*. Retrieved from http://www.skinclientalliance.ca/skin-conditions-and-diseases#fast-facts-11
Habif, T. P. (Ed.). (2011). *Skin disease diagnosis and treatment* (3rd ed.). Philadelphia, PA: Saunders Elsevier.
Oge, L. K., Muncie, L. H., & Phillips, A. R. (2015). Rosacea: Diagnosis and treatment. *American Family Physician, 92*(3), 187–196.
Van Onselen, J. (2012). Rosacea: Symptoms and support. *British Journal of Nursing (Mark Allen Publishing), 21*(21), 1252–1255. doi:10.12968/bjon.2012.21.21.1252

Acne Vulgaris

Jill C. Cash, Amy C. Bruggemann, Elsie Duff, and Cindy Fehr

Definition
A. Acne vulgaris is a disorder of the sebaceous glands and hair follicles of the skin that are most numerous on the face, back, and chest. The sebaceous glands become inflamed and form papules, pustules, cysts, open or closed comedones, and/or nodules on an erythemic base. In severe cases, scarring can result.

Incidence/Prevalence
A. Acne is the most common skin disorder in the United States, affecting 5.6 million Canadians. Nearly 85% age 12 to 24 years experience acne during their lifetime. Acne vulgaris, commonly seen in adolescence, may even extend into the third or fourth decade of life.

Pathogenesis
A. Sebum is overproduced and collects in the sebaceous gland. Sebum, keratinized cells, and hair collect in the follicle. With *Propionibacterium acnes* present, the duct becomes clogged and lesions (noninflammatory and/or inflammatory) evolve.

Predisposing Factors
A. Age (adolescence).
B. External irritants to skin (make-up, oils, equipment contact on skin).
C. Hormones (oral contraceptives with high progestin content).
D. Medications (lithium, halides, hydantoin derivatives, rifampin).
E. Hot, humid weather.

Common Findings
A. Outbreak of pimples on face, chest, shoulders, and back that do not resolve with over-the-counter (OTC) treatment.
B. Acne rosacea: Telangiectasia, flushing, and rhinophyma present.

Other Signs and Symptoms
A. Mild: Comedones open (blackhead) and closed (whitehead).
B. Moderate: Comedones with papules and pustules.
C. Severe: Nodules, cysts, and scars.

Subjective Data
A. Elicit the age of onset of outbreak, duration, and course of symptoms.
B. Determine what makes the lesions worse or better.
C. Ask whether there are certain times of the month or year when lesions are better or worse.
D. Identify the client's current method of cleanser or moisturizer treatment.
E. Ask whether the client has ever been treated by a provider for this problem. If so, determine the treatment and results of the treatment.
F. Assess whether other family members have this same problem.
G. Ask the client for a description of his or her environment and occupation.
H. Explore with the client any current stress factors in his or her life.

Physical Examination
A. Inspect:
  1. Observe skin for location and severity of lesions.
  2. Rate severity of lesions as mild, moderate, or severe:
    a. Mild: Few papules/pustules, no nodules.
    b. Moderate: Several papules/pustules, rare nodules.
    c. Severe: Many papules/pustules with many nodules.
  3. Take a picture of areas of affected skin for chart and document date. Use this for future appointments as a reference to compare results for follow-up visits.

Diagnostic Tests
A. No tests are generally required.

▶ Client Teaching Guides are available at https://connect.springerpub.com/content/reference-book/978-0-8261-9498-5

B. Culture lesions to rule out Gram-negative folliculitis with clients on antibiotics.
C. Consider hormone testing if other primary causes of acne are taken into account (follicle-stimulating hormone, luteinizing hormone, testosterone levels).

Differential Diagnoses
A. Acne rosacea.
B. Steroid rosacea.
C. Folliculitis.
D. Perioral acne.
E. Drug-induced acne.

Plan
A. General interventions:
  1. Document location and severity of lesions. Assess quality of improvement at each office visit.
  2. The primary goal of treatment is prevention of scarring. Good control of lesions during puberty and early adulthood is required for best results. Anticipate ups and downs during the normal course of treatment.
▶ B. Client teaching: *Refer to Client Teaching Guide: Acne Vulgaris*. Instruct the client on proper cleansing routine. The client should wash affected areas with a mild soap or soapless cleanser twice a day and apply medications as directed.
  1. Warn the client that washing the face more than two to three times a day can decrease oil production and cause drying.
  2. Discuss current stressors in the client's life and discuss treatment options.
  3. Recommend an exercise routine three to five days a week.
  4. Recommend oil-free sunscreens.
C. Pharmacological therapy: **It may take one to three months before results are visible when using these medications:**
  1. Mild: First-line treatment is topical. Use one of the following:
    a. Benzoyl peroxide.
    b. Topical retinoid:
      i. With retinoid use, the client may see rapid turnover of keratin plugs.
      ii. Instruct the client to avoid abrasive soaps.
      iii. Warn the client regarding photosensitivity.
      iv. Warn the client regarding increased dryness.
      v. May apply a moisturizer such as if needed.
  2. Moderate: Use one of the aforementioned topical medications in addition to one of the following oral medications:
    a. Tetracycline:
      i. Instruct the client to take tetracycline on an empty stomach and to avoid dairy products, antacids, and iron.
      ii. Warn the client about photosensitivity. This medication may be used as a maintenance dose for those clients who break out after discontinuing antibiotic therapy. No drug resistance is seen with tetracycline.
    b. Erythromycin or topical erythromycin 2%, solution or gel, or clindamycin solution, pads, or gel, twice daily. Erythromycin resistance has been seen.
    c. Minocycline:
      i. Have the client drink plenty of fluids?
      ii. Central nervous system side effects (headaches) have been seen.
    d. Bactrim single strength twice daily if the aforementioned regimens do not work well. Bactrim works well if others fail because it is effective for Gram-negative folliculitis.
    e. Oral contraceptives with higher doses of estrogen have also been effective for girls.
    f. Doxycycline.
    g. Spironolactone.
  3. Severe: Medications as prescribed by the dermatologist.

Follow-Up
See clients every six to eight weeks for evaluation:
A. Mild: Adjust dose depending on local irritation.
B. Moderate (oral and topical medications):
  1. Adjust dose according to irritation.
  2. Taper oral antibiotics with discretion and/or continue topical medications.
  3. Oral antibiotics may be tapered and discontinued when inflammatory lesions have resolved.
C. Severe: Recommend referral to dermatology and follow up with the specialty.

Consultation/Referral
A. Consult with a physician if treatment is unsuccessful after 10 to 12 weeks of therapy or if acne is severe.
B. The client may need dermatology consultation.

Individual Considerations
A. Pregnancy:
  1. Acne may flare up or improve during pregnancy.
  2. Medications preferred during pregnancy are topical agents.
  3. **Teratogens include tretinoin, tetracycline, and minocycline:**
    a. **When using teratogenic medications, contraception must be practiced to avoid pregnancy to prevent severe fetal malformations.**
    b. **Begin contraception one month before starting the medication and continue contraception one month after finishing the medication.**

Bibliography
Brackenbury, J. (2016). Recommended topical treatments for managing adult acne in women. *Nurse Prescribing, 14*(3), 126–129. doi:10.12968/npre.2016.14.3.126

Canadian Skin Client Alliance. (2016a). *Skin conditions: Acne*. Retrieved from http://www.skinclientalliance.ca/skin-conditions-and-diseases#fast-facts

Habif, T. P. (Ed.). (2011). *Skin disease diagnosis and treatment* (3rd ed.). Philadelphia, PA: Saunders Elsevier.

Lee, M., Jensen, B., & Regier, L., (2017). Acne treatment. *RxFiles drug comparison charts* (11th ed., pp. 33–34). Saskatoon, SK: Saskatoon Health Region. Available from: www.RxFiles.ca

Radley, K. (2015). The management and treatment of acnes. *Primary Health Care, 25*(4), 34–41. doi:10.7748/phc.25.4.34.e996

Titus, S., & Hodge, J. (2012). Diagnosis and treatment of acne. *American Family Physician, 86*(8), 734–740.

Watkins, J. (2012). Problems with acne vulgaris in adolescence. *Practice Nursing, 23*(11), 562–565. doi:10.12968/pnur.2012.23.11.562

Williams, H. C., Dellavalle, R. P., & Garner, S. (2012). Acne vulgaris. *Lancet (London, England), 379*(9813), 361–372. doi:10.1016/S0140-6736(11)60321-8

▶ Client Teaching Guides are available at https://connect.springerpub.com/content/reference-book/978-0-8261-9498-5

Animal Bites, Mammalian

Jill C. Cash, Amy C. Bruggemann, Elsie Duff, and Cindy Fehr

Definition
A. Bites of any mammalian animal to the human can be potentially dangerous. Human bites are included.

Incidence/Prevalence
A. One to two human deaths per year are attributed to dog bites.
B. About 80% to 90% of bites are dog bites.
C. About 3% to 28% of dog bites result in infection.
D. About 28% to 80% of cat bites result in infection.
E. From 1% to 15% of bites are human bites.
F. Children and the elderly are especially prone.

Pathogenesis
A. Mechanical trauma and break to skin and/or underlying structures.
B. Infection from transmission of bacteria:
   1. *Pasteurella multocida* is primarily associated with cat bites but may also be associated with dog bites.
   2. *Staphylococcus aureus, Staphylococcus epidermis*, and *Enterobacter* species can be transmitted by dog and cat bites.
   3. *Streptobacillus moniliformis* can be transmitted by rat and mice bites.
   4. *Streptococcus, Staphylococcus*, and *Eikenella* can be transmitted by human bites.
   5. Human bites can transmit diseases: Actinomycosis, syphilis, tuberculosis, hepatitis B, and potentially HIV.
C. Rabies, an acute viral infection, may be transmitted by means of infected saliva or by an infected animal licking mucosa of an open wound. It is rarely contracted by means of airborne transmission, but this has been reported to occur in bat-infested caves.

Predisposing Factors
A. Entering an animal's territorial space and/or surprising an animal.

Common Findings
A. Bitten.
B. Pain.
C. Redness.
D. Swelling.

Other Signs and Symptoms
A. Normal: Mild redness and swelling, serosanguineous oozing, discomfort.
B. Abnormal: Erythema, fever, pus, red streaks, pain, loss of sensation.

Subjective Data
A. What person or type of animal bit the client?
B. Was this a provoked or an unprovoked attack?
C. Did the client identify and contact the owner of the animal?
D. What was the behaviour of the animal: unusual, strange, or ill appearing?
E. How much time elapsed from being bitten to seeking treatment?
F. Did the client start any self-treatment?
G. What is the client's tetanus immunization status?
H. Review history for any prior rabies immunizations.
I. Does the client know if the animal was a domestic animal? Is the animal's vaccination status known?
J. If the bite is of human origin, determine if it is a closed-fist injury or plain bite.

Physical Examination
A. Check blood pressure, pulse, and respirations, and observe overall respiratory status.
B. See Table 4.1.

Diagnostic Test
A. Refer to Table 4.1.

Differential Diagnoses
A. Animal bite—dog, cat, human, and so forth:
   1. Cat bites more frequently become infected.
   2. Bites on the hand have the highest infection rates. Bites on the face have the lowest infection rates.
B. Cellulitis and abscesses.
C. Risk potential for rabies:
   1. Skunks, foxes, raccoons, and bats are primary carriers.
   2. Rabbits, squirrels, chipmunks, rats, and mice are seldom infective for rabies.
   3. Properly vaccinated animals seldom are infective.

Plan
A. General interventions:
   1. Control bleeding.
   2. Perform wound care:
      a. Immediately wash wound copiously with soap and water.
      b. Irrigate wound copiously with saline using a 20-gauge or larger catheter.
      c. Use 150 to 1,000 mL of solution.
      d. Direct saline stream on the entire wound surface.
      e. Scrub entire surrounding area.
      f. Debride all wounds.
      g. Trim any jagged edges to prevent cosmetic and/or functional complications.
      h. Cover with dry dressing.
   3. Do not suture wounds with high risk of infection:
      a. Hand bites, closed-fist injuries.
      b. Bites older than six hours.
      c. Deep or puncture wounds.
      d. Bites with extensive injury of surface or underlying structures.
   4. Rabies control measures:
      a. Consult with the local health department regarding the risk of rabies in the area.
      b. The domestic animal should be identified, caught, and confined for 10 days of observation. If the animal develops any signs of rabies, it should be destroyed and its brain tissue should be analyzed. No treatment is necessary if results are negative.
      c. The wild animal should be caught and destroyed for brain tissue analysis. No treatment is necessary if results are negative.
      d. If the bat or wild carnivore cannot be found, rabies prophylaxis is instituted.
B. Client teaching:
   1. Stress the importance of keeping the site free from infection. Instruct the client on how to keep the site

TABLE 4.1 Bites

Animal	Signs and Symptoms	Physical Examination: Check Client Temperature for All Animal Bites	Diagnostic Tests
Dog	Crush injury, lacerations, abrasions	Inspect site, underlying structures, and distal neurovascular, motor, and sensory functions. Palpate area. If wound is more than 24 hours old, check for any signs of cellulitis or lymphangitis.	If infected—Laboratory: CBC, culture and sensitivity for anaerobes and aerobes
Cat	Puncture wounds; may be deep	Determine depth and extent of wound. Check for foreign bodies. If wound is more than 24 hours old, check for any signs of cellulitis or lymphangitis.	If sepsis suspected—Laboratory: CBC, culture and sensitivity of abscess/tissue site
Rat or squirrel	Laceration, abrasions; more superficial in nature	Check for signs of infection if wound is more than 24 hours old. Check for any signs of cellulitis or lymphangitis.	
Human	Crush injury, laceration; wound of hand (closed-fist wound)	Check for signs of infection if wound is more than 24 hours old. Check for any signs of cellulitis or lymphangitis. Also, examine for fractures, air in the joint, subchondral bone defects, and osteomyelitis. Examine for full range of interphalangeal and metacarpophalangeal joints.	If infected—Laboratory: CBC, culture, and sensitivity. Also, take an x-ray film of structures underlying the bite.

CBC, complete blood count.

free from infection, such as teaching cleaning techniques, good handwashing, and using medications as prescribed.
2. Discuss symptoms to report to the provider if signs of infection begin (erythema, swelling, drainage, and tenderness).
C. Pharmacological therapy:
  1. Antibiotic prophylaxis is controversial, but it is generally recommended for wounds involving subcutaneous tissues and deeper structures:
    a. Amoxicillin/clavulanate.
    b. Alternatively, prescribe doxycycline.
    c. Metronidazole is important in human bites for anaerobic coverage.
  2. Tetanus prophylaxis.
  3. Rabies prophylaxis.

Follow-Up
A. Evaluate wound and change dressing in 24 to 48 hours.
B. Reevaluate as indicated. If the client is on immunoprophylaxis and has no signs of infection, see the client in one week.
C. Instruct the client to return immediately in case of any signs of infection.

Consultation/Referral
A. Refer all clients with bites of the ears, face, genitalia, hands, and feet.
B. Refer to agency guidelines for management and reporting to public health officials.
C. Wounds involving tendon, joint, or bone require hospitalization and surgical consultation.

Individual Consideration
A. Pregnancy: Use appropriate antibiotic management.
B. Paediatrics: Children are more prone to animal bites.
C. Geriatrics: The elderly population is more prone to animal bites.

Bibliography
Anti-infective Review Panel. (2019). *Anti-infective guidelines for community-acquired infections.* Toronto: MUMS Guideline Clearinghouse.
Aziz, H., Rhee, P., Pandit, V., Tang, A., Gries, L., & Joseph, B. (2015). The current concepts in management of animal (dog, cat, snake, scorpion) and human bite wounds. *Journal of Trauma and Acute Care Surgery*, 78(3), 641–648. doi:10.1097/TA.0000000000000531
Ellis, R., & Ellis, C. (2014). Dog and cat bites. *American Family Physician*, 90(4), 239–243.
Habif, T. P. (Ed.). (2011). *Skin disease diagnosis and treatment* (3rd ed.). Philadelphia, PA: Saunders Elsevier.
Gaston, R., & Lewis, D. R. (2010). Animal bites to the hand. *Current Orthopaedic Practice*, 21(6), 559–563. doi:10.1097/BCO.0b013e3181f7a08f

Benign Skin Lesions

Jill C. Cash, Amy C. Bruggemann, Elsie Duff, and Cindy Fehr

Definition
A benign skin lesion is a cutaneous growth with no harmful effects to the body. Benign lesions must be distinguished from the following:
A. Basal cell carcinoma (BCC): Nodular tumour with pearly surface, telangiectasia on surface, and depressed center or rolled edge.
B. Squamous cell carcinoma (SCC): Irregular papule with scaly, friable, bleeding surface.
C. Malignant melanoma: Asymmetric papule with irregular border and of two or more colours; size varies.

Incidence/Prevalence
A. Benign lesions are common to all races, and they are seen primarily in the adult and elderly populations.

Pathogenesis
A. The course varies, depending on the specific type of lesion.

Predisposing Factors
A. Sun exposure in the adult and elderly populations.
B. Dermatosis papulosa nigra: Common in those of African or Asian descent.

Common Findings
A. New lesion of the skin.

Other Signs and Symptoms
A. Seborrhoeic keratosis: Waxy papule with a stuck-on appearance is seen in adults; they appear symmetric, 0.2 to 3.0 cm in size, with a well-demarcated border, and in a variety of colours (tan, black, and brown).
B. Dermatosis papulosa nigra: Hyperpigmented mole located on face or neck; a pedunculated papule that is symmetric, 1 to 3 mm in diameter.
C. Cherry angioma: Vascular papule, red to purple, located on trunk in adults; begins in early adulthood; 1- to 3-mm diameter papules that do not blanch.
D. Solar lentigines (liver spots): Tan maculae on sun-exposed areas in elders, especially on face and hands; border is irregular, and the size varies.
E. Sebaceous hyperplasia: Enlarged sebaceous glands that appear as yellow papules on sun-exposed areas, especially on the face in elders; papules have central umbilication, and their size varies.
F. Actinic keratoses: Rough, scaly patch on skin that develops from years of exposure to sun. They are most commonly found on face, lips, ears, back of the hands, forearms, scalp, or neck. These areas should be monitored closely as they can become cancerous.

Subjective Data
A. Identify when the client first discovered the lesion.
B. Determine whether the lesion has changed in size, shape, or colour.
C. Ask whether the client has discovered more lesions.
D. Elicit information regarding a family history of skin lesions or cancer.

Physical Examination
A. Inspect skin: Note all lesions and evaluate each for asymmetry, border, colour, diameter, evolving changes, and/or elevation change. Note client's skin type.

Diagnostic Tests
A. Benign lesions do not require any tests.
B. If unsure regarding possible malignancy, a biopsy is recommended.

Differential Diagnoses
A. Benign skin lesion:
 1. Seborrhoeic keratosis.
 2. Dermatosis papulosa nigra.
 3. Cherry angioma.
 4. Solar lentigines.
 5. Senile sebaceous hyperplasia.
 6. Keratoacanthoma.

Plan
A. General interventions:
 1. Reassure the client that lesions are benign. No treatment is required unless the client chooses to have the lesion removed for cosmetic purposes.
 2. Benign skin lesions may be removed using cryotherapy if they are bothersome for the client.
B. Client teaching: *Refer to Client Teaching Guide: Skin Care Assessment.*
C. Pharmacological therapy: Medications are not recommended for treatment.

Follow-Up
A. Routine skin examinations should be performed yearly.

Consultation/Referral
A. Immediately refer the client to a dermatologist if malignancy is suspected or confirmed by biopsy.

Individual Considerations
A. Adults: Skin lesions begin to appear in early adulthood. Encourage clients to monitor lesions over time.
B. Geriatrics: Benign lesions are commonly seen in the elderly population.

Bibliography
Habif, T. P. (Ed.). (2011). *Skin disease diagnosis and treatment* (3rd ed.). Philadelphia, PA: Saunders Elsevier.
Higgins, J.C., Maher, M.H., Douglas, M.S. (2015). Diagnosing common benign skin tumors. *American Family Physician, 92*(7), 601–607.
Huynh, L., & Esho, D. (2013). Benign skin lesions. *Family and Community Medicine*, University of Toronto. Retrieved from https://dfcmopen.com/item/benign-skin-lesion-one-page-primer/
No Author. (2011). Skin disorders in older adults: Benign growths and neoplasms. *Consultant 360, 51*(9). Retrieved from https://www.consultant360.com/content/skin-disorders-older-adults-benign-growths-and-neoplasms

Candidiasis

Jill C. Cash, Amy C. Bruggemann, Elsie Duff, and Cindy Fehr

Definition
A. A fungal infection of the mucous membranes and/or skin; candidiasis is caused by the *Candida albicans* fungus.

Incidence/Prevalence
A. It occurs frequently in women, children, and the elderly population.

Pathogenesis
A. An overgrowth of *C. albicans* occurs when mucous membranes and/or skin are exposed to moisture, warmth, and an alteration in the membrane barrier.

Predisposing Factors
A. Immunosuppression.
B. Use of antibiotics.
C. Hyperglycaemia.
D. Chronic use of steroid.
E. Frequent douching by women.
F. Use of dentures.

Common Findings
A. Oral: A persistent white patch on the tongue or roof of mouth may be slightly reddened with or without crevices on the tongue.
B. Vaginal: Thick, white, "cottage cheese-like" vaginal discharge with or without vaginal itching.
C. Genital: Bright red rash with well-demarcated satellite lesions advancing to pustules or erosions in genital or diaper area.
D. Males: Erythemic rash that may advance to erosions seen on male genitalia; scrotum is perhaps involved.

Subjective Data
A. Question the client about onset, duration, and location of lesions.
B. Determine whether the client has a history of previous infections.
C. Inquire into medical history and current medications.
D. Rule out the presence of any other current medical conditions.

Physical Examination
A. Inspect:
  1. Assess skin and mucous membranes for discharge and lesions.
  2. Observe location and severity of lesions.
B. Palpate: Palpate lymph nodes in neck and groin.

Diagnostic Tests
A. Vaginal or genital wet preparation/potassium hydroxide (KOH) 10% solution, Gram stain culture for *Candida*.

Differential Diagnoses
A. Oral candidiasis:
  1. Leukoplakia.
  2. Stomatitis.
  3. Formula (for newborns).
B. Diaper area:
  1. Candidiasis.
  2. Contact dermatitis.
  3. Bacterial infection.
C. Genital area.
  1. Candidiasis.
  2. Bacterial infection.
  3. Bacterial vaginosis.
  4. Chlamydia.
  5. Gonorrhoea.
  6. Trichomoniasis.

Plan
A. General interventions:
  1. Treatment can be successful with good hygiene and medications.
  2. Stress to the client to keep the affected area cool and dry. Frequent changes of moisture-wicking, breathable clothing may be necessary to keep the area cool and dry.
  3. Diaper area will need to be changed more frequently; suggest using cotton diapers and allowing skin to be exposed to air for short periods.
B. Client teaching:
  1. Use medication on the skin to help with symptoms.
  2. Do not scratch. Keep fingernails short.
C. Pharmacological therapy—choose *one* of the following pharmacological therapies:
  1. Oral:
    a. Nystatin oral suspension.
    b. Gentian violet aqueous solution.
  2. Diaper: Nystatin cream.
  3. Vaginal:
    a. Clotrimazole 1% cream; safe in pregnancy and breastfeeding.
    b. Miconazole 2% cream; caution with use when breastfeeding.
    c. Fluconazole; contraindicated in pregnancy.
    d. In recurrent resistant cases, three to four weeks of therapy may be needed.
  4. Recurrent:
    a. Fluconazole (contraindicated in pregnancy).
    b. Topical azole.
    c. Boric acid gelatin capsule intravaginally (contraindicated in pregnancy).

Follow-Up
A. None indicated unless not resolved or complications arise.

Consultation/Referral
A. None.

Individual Considerations
A. Pregnancy:
  1. Most effective medications for pregnant women are clotrimazole and miconazole.
  2. Recommend a full seven-day course of treatment during pregnancy.
B. Adults:
  1. Consider immunosuppression in all adults with oral candidiasis (HIV, diabetes, chemotherapy, leukemia).
  2. Adults with oral lesions need to be assessed for leukoplakia, especially if the client has a history of smoking or chewing tobacco.
  3. Oil-based ovules and creams may cause latex condoms or diaphragms to fail.

Bibliography
Bortolussi, R., Martin, S., & Canadian Pediatric Society. (2007 reaffirmed 2018). Antifungal agents for common outpatient paediatric infections. *Paediatric Child Health*, 12(10), 875–878. doi:10.1093/pch/12.10.875

Clancy, C. J., & Nguyen, M. H. (2012). The end of an era in defining the optimal treatment of invasive candidiasis. *Clinical Infectious Diseases*, 54(8), 1123–1125. doi:10.1093/cid/cis023

Expert Working Group. (2016). *Canadian guidelines on sexually transmitted infections*. Retrieve from https://www.canada.ca/en/public-health/services/infectious-diseases/sexual-health-sexually-transmitted-infections/canadian-guidelines/sexually-transmitted-infections/canadian-guidelines-sexually-transmitted-infections-26.html

Government of Canada. (2013). *Canadian guidelines on sexually transmitted infections—Management and treatment of specific infections—Ectoparasitic infestations (Section 5–3)*. Retrieved from https://www.canada.ca/en/public-health/services/infectious-diseases/sexual-health-sexually-transmitted-infections/canadian-guidelines/sexually-transmitted-infections/canadian-guidelines-sexually-transmitted-infections-31.html

Habif, T. P. (Ed.). (2011). *Skin disease diagnosis and treatment* (3rd ed.). Philadelphia, PA: Saunders Elsevier.

Iavazzo, C., Gkegkes, I. D., Zarkada, I. M., & Falagas, M. E. (2011). Boric acid for recurrent vulvovaginal candidiasis: The clinical evidence. *Journal of Women's Health (2002)*, 20(8), 1245–1255.

Contact Dermatitis

Jill C. Cash, Amy C. Bruggemann, Elsie Duff, and Cindy Fehr

Definition
A. Contact dermatitis is a cutaneous response to direct exposure of the skin to irritants (irritant contact dermatitis) or allergens (allergic contact dermatitis):
  1. Irritant contact dermatitis is a nonimmunologic response of the epidermis.
  2. Allergic contact dermatitis is an immunologic response after one or more exposures to a particular agent.

Incidence/Prevalence
A. Occurs in all ages. People who work with chemicals daily and wash their hands numerous times a day have a higher incidence of irritant dermatitis. Irritant contact dermatitis is seen in the elderly because of dry skin.

Pathogenesis
A. Irritant contact dermatitis is caused by an alteration of the outer layer of the dermis caused by exposure to chemicals; lotions; cold, dry air; soaps; detergents; or organic solvents.
B. Allergic contact dermatitis is caused by an alteration in the epidermis when, after exposure to an allergen, the immune system responds by producing inflammation of the cutaneous tissue. Common allergens include poison ivy, poison oak, sumac, nickel jewellery, hair dye, rubber and leather chemicals (latex gloves), cleaning supplies, harsh soaps, detergents, and topical medicines.

Predisposing Factors
A. Occupation (hairdresser, nurse, housecleaner, etc.).
B. Jewellery.
C. Activities in yard or woods or contact with pets that have been active in woods.

Common Findings
A. Irritation of the skin, ranging from redness to pruritic inflammation, with possible progression of blisters:
  1. Poison oak, ivy, and sumac induce classic presentation—lesions (vesicles) and papules on an erythemic base presenting in a linear fashion with sharp margins.
  2. Diffuse pattern with erythema may be seen when oleoresin is contacted from pets or smoke from burning fire.
B. Exposure to some type of irritant known to the client. Round or annular lesions may have an internal cause, such as a drug reaction.

Other Signs and Symptoms
A. Chronic:
  1. Erythema with thickening.
  2. Scaling.
  3. Fissures.
  4. Inflammation; with chronic dermatitis, lichenification may occur with scales and fissures.
B. Diaper dermatitis: Prominent red, shiny rash on buttocks and genitalia.
C. Candidiasis diaper rash:
  1. Bright red rash with satellite lesions at margins.
  2. Inflammation and excoriations present.
  3. Creases may be involved.

Subjective Data
A. Ask the client when irritation began and how it has progressed.
B. Elicit history of exposure to allergens.
C. Question the client regarding activity and skin contact with irritants before outbreak (cleaning agents, walking in woods, hobbies, change in soap/laundry detergent, shaving cream, lotions, etc.).
D. List occupation and family history of allergens.
E. Review medication list, including prescription, over-the-counter (OTC), and herbal medicines, to evaluate an interaction.
F. List medications used to relieve symptoms and results.

Physical Examination
A. Check temperature (if indicated).
B. Inspect:
  1. Skin, noting types of lesions and location of lesions. **Note the pattern of inflammation. The shape of irritation may mimic the shape of the irritant, such as the skin under a ring or watch.**
  2. Determine progression of lesions.
  3. Differentiate between primary and secondary lesions.

Diagnostic Tests
A. Consider none if source is known.
B. Wet mount (potassium hydroxide [KOH], saline) to rule out fungal infection if candida is suspected.
C. Culture/sensitivity of pustules.
D. Patch test to rule out allergic contact dermatitis.

Differential Diagnoses
A. Irritant contact dermatitis.
B. Allergic contact dermatitis.
C. Diaper dermatitis.
D. Candida.
E. Tinea pedis, corporis, cruris.
F. Drug reactions.
G. Pityriasis rosea.
H. Scabies.

Plan
A. General interventions:
  1. Irritant contact dermatitis—removal of irritating agent:
    a. Use topical soaks with saline or Burow's solution (1:40 dilution) for weeping areas.
    b. Suggest lukewarm baths (not hot) or oatmeal baths, as needed.
    c. For dry, erythematous skin, use recommend moisturizing emollient creams/ointments to rehydrate skin.
    d. Remind the client to avoid scratching skin and to keep nails short.
    e. Suggest use of mild soaps and cleansers.
    f. If dermatitis is a result of exposure to poison ivy, oak, or sumac, use a soap to dissolve and emulsify urushiol oil (plant based oils in poison ivy, oak, or sumac), leave the soap on the site for about five minutes, and then rinse off; wash all clothing and bedding. Wash pets with soap if needed.
  2. Allergic contact dermatitis:
    a. Instruct the client to avoid contact with the causative agent.

b. Have the client wash the affected area with cool water immediately after exposure.
  c. Recommend lukewarm baths with oatmeal three to four times per day.
  d. Apply calamine lotion after baths.
  3. Diaper dermatitis:
  a. Instruct the caretaker to change the client's diaper frequently, clean with water only, and allow skin to air dry 15 to 30 minutes four times a day. Discuss with the parent not to use lotions or powders, but to apply zinc oxide with each diaper change.
  b. If candidiasis diaper rash presents, for treatment refer to the section "Candidiasis" in this chapter.
▶ **B.** Client teaching: *Refer to Client Teaching Guide: Dermatitis.*
C. Pharmacological therapy:
  1. Irritant contact dermatitis: Hydrocortisone ointment.
  2. Allergic contact dermatitis:
    a. Low-dose topical steroids—hydrocortisone ointment.
    b. Intermediate-dose topical steroids—triamcinolone acetonide cream.
    c. High-potent topical steroids—fluocinonide ointment.
    d. Hydroxyzine or diphenhydramine.
    e. If the rash is severe (face, eyes, genitalia, mucous membranes), consider prednisone.
  3. Secondary bacterial infections—erythromycin or amoxicillin/clavulanate.
  4. Candidiasis:
    a. Use clotrimazole 1%, miconazole 2% cream, miconazole powder, or nystatin cream.
    b. If inflammation is present along with yeast, use a compound prescription with an antifungal and a hydrocortisone 2.5%.
    c. If secondary bacterial infection is present, use mupirocin ointment.

Follow-Up
A. None required if case is mild.
B. See the client again in two to three days for severe cases, or phone to assess progress.

Consultation/Referral
A. Consult with a physician when steroid treatment is necessary or if worsening symptoms develop despite adequate therapy.

Individual Considerations
A. Pregnancy: If medications are necessary during pregnancy, consider the gestational age of the fetus and category of medication.
B. Paediatrics: For infants and children, consider hydroxyzine for severe pruritus.
C. Elderly: Clients may only exhibit scaling as the prominent irritation rather than erythema and inflammation. Topical medications (neomycin, vitamin E, lanolin) and acrylate adhesives are common causes of contact dermatitis.

Bibliography
Canadian Dermatology Association. (2019). Eczema. Author. Retrieved from https://dermatology.ca/public-patients/skin/eczema/
Habif, T. P. (Ed.). (2011). *Skin disease diagnosis and treatment* (3rd ed.). Philadelphia, PA: Saunders Elsevier.
Sampson, O. & Galbraith, L. (2017). Diagnosing and treating contact dermatitis. *BC Medical Journal, 59*(6), 317.
Sandomirsky, L. (2017). Atopic dermatitis – Guidelines for prescribing topical corticosteroids. MedSask, *University of Saskatchewan*. Retrieved from https://medsask.usask.ca/professional/guidelines/atopic-dermatitis.php

Eczema or Atopic Dermatitis

Jill C. Cash, Amy C. Bruggemann, Elsie Duff, and Cindy Fehr

Definition
A. This pattern of skin inflammation has clinical features of erythema, itching, scaling, lichenification, papules, and vesicles in various combinations. Currently, the term "eczema" is used interchangeably with "dermatitis." Most common variants are atopic dermatitis and atopic eczema. Classification is done by cause, either endogenous or exogenous.

Incidence/Prevalence
A. Atopic dermatitis affects all ages and is more frequent in children.

Pathogenesis
A. Eczema is characterized by a lymphohistiocytic infiltration around the upper dermal vessels. Epidermal spongiosis or intercellular epidermal edema and inflammation are seen.

Predisposing Factors
A. Family history of atopic triad: Dermatitis, asthma, and allergic rhinitis.
B. Exposure to allergens:
  1. Common foods: Cow's milk, nuts, wheat, soy, and fish.
  2. Common environmental allergens: Dust, mold, cat dander, and low humidity (dry air).
C. Exposure to topical medications, most commonly neomycin, lanolin, and topical anesthetics like benzocaine.
D. Skin irritants: Harsh soaps; skin-care products with perfumes, chemicals, and alcohol; fabrics containing wool; and tight clothing.
E. Stress.

Common Findings
A. Skin changes:
  1. Itching, impossible to relieve.
  2. Dryness.
  3. Discolouration, lichenification, and scaling.
  4. Skin thickening.
  5. Associated bleeding and oozing skin.

Other Signs and Symptoms
A. Primary lesions, papules, and pustules that may lead to excoriation.
B. Lesions commonly seen on trunk, face, and antecubital and popliteal fossae of children. Adults will have lesions on the face, trunk, neck, and genital area.
C. Other common features include infraorbital fold (Dennie sign), increased palmar creases, facial erythema, and scaling.

▶ Client Teaching Guides are available at https://connect.springerpub.com/content/reference-book/978-0-8261-9498-5

Subjective Data

A. Determine whether the onset was sudden or gradual.
B. Ask the client whether the skin is itchy or painful.
C. Assess whether there is any associated discharge (blood or pus).
D. Ask whether the client has recently taken any antibiotics, other oral drugs, or topical medications.
E. Ask the client about use of soaps, creams, or lotions.
F. Assess for any preceding systemic symptoms (fever, sore throat, anorexia, vaginal discharge).
G. Ask the client about recent travel abroad.
H. Rule out insect bites.
I. Rule out any possible exposure to industrial or domestic toxins.
J. Elicit what precipitates itching.
K. Evaluate for increased stress level at home, work, in relationships, and so on.

Physical Examination

A. Check temperature (if indicated).
B. Inspect skin for lesions: Recognize bacteria-infected eczema—*Staphylococcus aureus* is the most common pathogen. It appears with acute weeping dermatitis, crusted and small superficial pustules.

Diagnostic Tests

A. Culture skin lesions to determine viral, bacterial, or fungal etiology.
B. Blood work: Serum immunoglobulin E (IgE) is elevated with atopic dermatitis.

Differential Diagnoses

A. Contact dermatitis, acute or chronic.
B. Seborrhoeic dermatitis.
C. Ichthyosis vulgaris.
D. Bacterial/fungal infections.
E. Neoplastic disease.
F. Immunologic and metabolic disorders.

Plan

A. General interventions:
  1. Frequently treat the dry skin with emollients (four times a day or more).
  2. Pat skin; do not rub.
  3. Children: Only bathe every two to three nights. Avoid excessive use of soap and water when bathing; use gentle cleansers.
  4. Avoid wool products and lanolin preparations.
  5. Keep fingernails cut short to prevent scratching/scarring skin.
  6. May need to treat secondary bacterial infections as appropriate.
  7. Eliminate trigger foods one at a time for one month at a time to see improvement. Begin with eliminating cow's milk products. Consider soy-based foods instead.
  8. Allergy testing may be considered if symptoms continue.
  9. Ointments are usually recommended over creams for moisturizing.
▶ B. Client teaching: *Refer to Client Teaching Guide: Eczema.*
C. Pharmacological therapy:
  1. Atopic: Acute, adult:
    a. Wet dressings with Burow's solution and change every two to three hours.
    b. Potent topical corticosteroid—betamethasone valerate.
    c. First-line antihistamine—cetirizine HCl or diphenhydramine HCl.
    d. For severe cases—oral steroid (prednisone).
  2. Atopic—acute; occurs in infants and children:
    a. Hydrocortisone.
    b. Adolescents—triamcinolone acetonide 0.1% ointment. **Precautions should be given regarding possibility of hypopigmentation of skin with even short-term use of steroids on skin.**
    c. Antihistamines for itching:
      i. Infants and children: May use hydroxyzine or diphenhydramine.
      ii. Adolescents: May use hydroxyzine or diphenhydramine.
      iii. Atopic: Chronic, adult—short course of potent topical corticosteroid betamethasone dipropionate glycol or clobetasol propionate.
  3. Antibacterial treatments for secondary bacterial infections: *S. aureus*:
    a. Adults:
      i. Cloxaciilin.
      ii. Cephalexin.
      iii. Erythromycin.
    b. Children:
      i. Cephalexin.
      ii. Erythromycin.
      iii. Azithromycin.

Follow-Up

A. See client in office in one to two weeks and then every month until condition is stabilized.
B. Monitor the client for superimposed staphylococcal infection.
C. Client may be seen every three to six months thereafter for client education updates.

Consultation/Referral

A. Eczema herpeticum (herpes simplex type 1) may progress rapidly. Refer the client to a dermatologist.
B. Refer the client to a dermatologist if skin eruptions are severe or fail to respond to conservative treatment.

Individual Considerations

A. Pregnancy: Avoid oral steroids.
B. Children: Teach clients to apply emollients when they have an itching rather than scratching. The goal is to control the rash and symptoms.
C. Young adults and elderly: Nummular eczema is commonly seen, characterized by coin-shaped vesicles and papules seen on extremities and/or trunk.

Bibliography

Anti-infective Review Panel. (2019). Anti-infective guidelines for community-acquired infections. Toronto: MUMS Guideline Clearinghouse.

Eichenfield, L. F., Tom, W. L., Berger, T. G., Krol, A., Paller, A. S., Schwarzenberger, K., & Sidbury, R. (2014). Guidelines of care for the management of atopic dermatitis: Section 2. Management and treatment of atopic dermatitis with topical therapies. *Journal of the American Academy of Dermatology*, *71*(1), 116–132. doi:10.1016/j.jaad.2014.03.023

▶ Client Teaching Guides are available at https://connect.springerpub.com/content/reference-book/978-0-8261-9498-5

Habif, T. P. (Ed.). (2011). *Skin disease diagnosis and treatment* (3rd ed.). Philadelphia, PA: Saunders Elsevier.

Nutten, S. (2015). Atopic dermatitis: Global epidemiology and risk factors. *Annals of Nutrition & Metabolism, 66* (Suppl. 1), 8–16. doi:10.1159/000370220

Thompson, D. L., & Thompson, M. J. (2014). Knowledge, instruction and behavioural change: Building a framework for effective eczema education in clinical practice. *Journal of Advanced Nursing, 70*(11), 2483–2494. doi:10.1111/jan.12439

Vandiver, A., & Cohe, B. A. (2016). Vesicular rash in an infant with eczema. *Contemporary Pediatrics, 33*(6), 38–40.

Watkins, J. (2011). Eczema diagnosis and management in the community. *British Journal of Community Nursing, 16*(9), 418, 420, 422. doi:10.12968/bjcn.2011.16.9.418

Weinstein, M., Drucker, A. M., Lynde, C., Marcoux, D., Rehmus, W., & Cresswell-Melville, A. (2016). *Atopic dermatitis: A practical guide to management.* Keswick, Ontario, Canada: Exzema Society of Canada.

Erythema Multiforme

Jill C. Cash, Amy C. Bruggemann, Elsie Duff, and Cindy Fehr

Definition
A. This dermal and epidermal inflammatory process is characterized by symmetric eruption of erythematous, iris-shaped papules ("target" lesions), and vesiculobullous lesions.

Incidence/Prevalence
A. Erythema multiforme accounts for up to 1% of dermatology outpatient visits.
B. Children younger than 3 years and adults older than 50 years are rarely affected.
C. It may occur in seasonal epidemics.
D. Approximately 90% of cases of erythema multiforme minor follow a recent outbreak of herpes simplex virus (HSV)-1 or mycoplasma infection.

Pathogenesis
A. The disorder is thought to be an immunologic reaction in the skin, possibly triggered by circulating immune complexes.

Predisposing Factors
A. Infections: Recurrent HSV, mycoplasmal infections, and adenoviral infections.
B. Drugs: Sulphonamides, phenytoin, barbiturates, phenylbutazone, penicillin.
C. Idiopathic: >50%, consider occult malignancy.

Common Findings
A. Rash with intense pruritus.
B. Nonspecific upper respiratory infection followed by rash.
C. General malaise, body aches, and joint pain.
D. Fever.

Other Signs and Symptoms
A. Primary: Macules, papules, and plaques.
B. Secondary: Erythema, dull red target-like lesions blanch to pressure; distribution is symmetric, primarily on flexor surfaces. **Classic target lesions develop abruptly and symmetrically and are heaviest peripherally; they often involve palms and soles.**
C. Swelling of hands and feet.
D. Painful oral lesions.
E. Eye discomfort (redness, itching, burning, pain, changes in vision).

Subjective Data
A. Ask whether the client has ever been diagnosed with erythema multiforme.
B. Determine whether the onset of symptoms was sudden or gradual.
C. Assess for any associated discharge (blood or pus).
D. Identify the location of the symptoms.
E. Complete a drug history. Has the client recently taken any antibiotics or other drugs? Question the client regarding use of any topical medications.
F. Determine the presence of any preceding systemic symptoms (fever, sore throat, anorexia, or vaginal discharge).
G. Rule out any possible exposure to industrial or domestic toxins.
H. Question the client concerning any possible contact with venereal disease.
I. Ask the client about any close physical contact with others with skin disorders.
J. Elicit information concerning any possible exposure to HIV.
K. Rule out sources of chronic infection, neoplasia, or connective tissue disease.

Physical Examination
A. Check temperature, pulse, respirations, and blood pressure.
B. Inspect:
  1. Skin for lesions.
  2. Mouth and mucous membranes for lesions.
C. Palpate abdomen for masses and tenderness.
D. Auscultate heart, lungs, and abdomen.
E. Neurologic examination.

Diagnostic Tests
A. Punch biopsy of skin.
B. Complete blood count (CBC).
C. Urinalysis.

Differential Diagnoses
A. Erythema multiforme:
  1. Erythema multiforme minor: Pruritus, swelling of hands and feet, painful oral lesions.
  2. Erythema multiforme major: Fever, arthralgias, myalgias, cough, oral erosions with severe pain.
B. Urticaria.
C. Viral exanthems.
D. Stevens–Johnson syndrome (SJS): **SJS is a severe, life-threatening, systemic reaction with fever, malaise, cough, sore throat, chest pain, vomiting, diarrhoea, myalgia, arthralgia, and severe skin manifestations with painful bullous lesions on mucous membranes.**
E. Pemphigus vulgaris.
F. Bullous pemphigoid.
G. Other bullous diseases.
H. Staphylococcal scalded skin syndrome.
I. Vasculitis.

Plan
A. General interventions:
  1. Identify and treat precipitating causes or triggers.
  2. Burow's solution or warm compresses may be used for mild cases as needed.
  3. Oral lesions may be treated with saline solution, warm salt water, and/or compound mouthwash.

4. Discontinue any medications suspected of precipitating symptoms.
   5. Provide adequate pain relief if skin or oral lesions are painful. Lesions remain fixed at least seven days.
   6. Maintain nutrition and fluid replacement for this hypercatabolic state.
   7. Consider chronic viral suppression therapy for recurrent herpes simplex viral infections.
▶ **B.** Client teaching: *Refer to Client Teaching Guide: Erythema Multiforme.*
C. Pharmacological therapy:
   1. Antihistamines may be used for itching.
   2. Acetaminophen may be used to reduce fever and for general discomfort/pain.
   3. Potent topical corticosteroids: Betamethasone dipropionate glycol 0.05% or clobetasol propionate 0.05%. Avoid use on face and groin.
   4. Open lesions should be treated like open burn wounds. Stop offending medications that may cause blistering of wounds and treat with steroids.
   5. Oral antibiotics may be needed to control secondary bacterial skin infection.
   6. Hospitalization for severe cases. Intravenous immunoglobulins may be needed.

Follow-Up
A. See the client in the office in one to two days to evaluate initial treatment.

Consultation/Referral
A. Immediate consultation and/or hospital admission is critical if SJS is suspected.

Individual Consideration
A. Paediatrics: Systemic corticosteroids may increase the risk of infection and prolong healing. Use low- to mid-potency topical corticosteroids.

Bibliography
Habif, T. P. (Ed.). (2011). *Skin disease diagnosis and treatment* (3rd ed.). Philadelphia, PA: Saunders Elsevier.
Plaza, J. A., & Prieto, V. G. (2013). Erythema multiforme. *Medscape*. Retrieved from http://emedicine.medscape.com/article/1122915-overview.
Sokumbi, O., & Wetter, D. A. (2012). Clinical features, diagnosis, and treatment of erythema multiforme: A review for the practicing dermatologist. *International Journal of Dermatology*, 51(8), 889–902. doi:10.1111/j.1365-4632.2011.05348.x

Folliculitis

Jill C. Cash, Amy C. Bruggemann, Elsie Duff, and Cindy Fehr

Definition
A. Folliculitis is a bacterial infection of the hair follicle.
B. Malassezia folliculitis, also known as pityrosporum, is an inflammatory skin disorder of the hair follicle triggered by yeast. This is often confused with acne vulgaris; the defining difference is itching.

Incidence/Prevalence
A. A very common disorder, folliculitis occurs in all ages and is seen more frequently in males.
B. Malassezia folliculitis is commonly seen in clients with immunosuppression, diabetes, and antibiotic use.

Pathogenesis
A. Bacterial organisms (most commonly *Staphylococcus aureus*) invade the follicle wall and cause an infectious process.
B. For malassezia folliculitis, fungal organisms invade the follicle walls and cause a fungal infection, which causes a pruritic rash.

Predisposing Factors
A. Break in the skin tissue.
B. Use of razors on skin.
C. Poor hygiene.
D. Diabetes.

Common Findings
A. Outbreak of pustules on the face, scalp, or extremities that do not resolve despite proper hygiene and care.

Other Signs and Symptoms
A. Tenderness and itching at the site.
B. Furuncle (abscess): A deep pustule, tender, firm, or fluctuant, found in groin, axilla, waistline, or buttocks.
C. Carbuncle: A group of follicles coalescing into one larger, painful, infected area; fever and chills possible.
D. Excoriated folliculitis: Chronic thickened, excoriated papules or nodules.

Subjective Data
A. Elicit the initial outbreak of lesions and onset and progression of lesions.
B. Identify what makes the lesions better or worse.
C. Ask the client what medications, soaps, or lotions have been used on the lesions.
D. Complete a medical history. Ask whether the client has had an outbreak similar to this before.
E. Describe systemic symptoms if they have occurred (fever, chills, etc.).
F. Does the client have a beard, shave his face, or use a razor frequently?
G. Is there a recent history of use of a hot tub? (Commonly seen one to four days after use of hot tub, whirlpool, or swimming pool.)
H. Does the client wear tight pants/jeans or use oils that clog pores in the groin area?
I. Is the client currently being treated with antibiotics for acne? (May see flare of Gram-negative folliculitis with chronic use of antibiotics.)

Physical Examination
A. Check temperature, pulse, respirations, and blood pressure.
B. Inspect skin for lesions and describe.
C. Palpate lesions and associated lymph nodes.

Diagnostic Tests
A. Culture and sensitivity to verify appropriate antibiotic coverage.
B. Gram stain.

C. Potassium hydroxide (KOH)/wet preparation.
D. Fungal culture hair if fungi suspected (tinea of scalp).
E. Skin biopsy for the diagnosis of malassezia folliculitis.

Differential Diagnoses
A. Acne vulgaris.
B. Ingrown hair follicle.
C. Keratosis pilaris.
D. Contact dermatitis.

Plan
A. General interventions: Apply warm, moist compresses to site for comfort.
▶ B. Client teaching: *Refer to Client Teaching Guide: Folliculitis*. If razors are used on the area, have the client use clean, sharp razors, throw old razors away, and not share razors. Avoid use of irritating creams or lotions on affected area.
  1. Encourage proper hygiene, with frequent washing of hands and skin with an antibacterial soap.
  2. Warm compresses three to four times a day are encouraged at the site for 15 to 20 minutes.
  3. Bleach bath (0.5–1 cu of bleach to 20 L water) reduces spread of *Staphylococcus* infection.
C. Pharmacological therapy:
  1. Mild cases: Apply mupirocin ointment to the affected area three times daily until resolved:
    a. Adults:
      i. Cloxaciilin.
      ii. Cephalexin.
      iii. Erythromycin.
    b. Children:
      i. Cephalexin.
      ii. Erythromycin.
      iii. Azithromycin.
  2. Bacterial infections caused by organisms other than *Staphylococcus* may be treated for an extended period, four to eight weeks. These areas may include axilla, chest, back, beard, and groin.
  3. Methicillin-resistant *S. aureus* (MRSA):
    a. Co-trimoxazole.
    b. Doxycycline.
  4. Severe cases may be treated with oral antibiotics with topical permethrin or itraconazole, isotretinoin with ultraviolet B (UVB) light therapy. Consider dermatology referral for severe cases.
  5. Antifungal treatment: Oral antifungal medications should be prescribed for at least four weeks for treatment.

Follow-Up
A. If not resolved in two weeks, further evaluation is needed.
B. Severe cases, in which carbuncles are not improved with antibiotic therapy, warrant incision and drainage and referral to dermatology.
C. Continue to follow every two weeks until resolved.
D. Test for diabetes mellitus in severe cases.

Consultation/Referral
A. Refer the client to a physician for testing for immunodeficiency if severe cases occur or if resistance is seen.
B. Dermatology referral.

Bibliography
Anti-infective Review Panel. (2019). Anti-infective guidelines for community-acquired infections. Toronto: MUMS Guideline Clearinghouse.
Blereau, R. P. (2012). Acneiform folliculitis. *Consultant (00107069)*, 52(6), 469.
Habif, T. P. (Ed.). (2011). *Skin disease diagnosis and treatment* (3rd ed.). Philadelphia, PA: Saunders Elsevier.

Hand, Foot, and Mouth Syndrome

Jill C. Cash, Amy C. Bruggemann, Elsie Duff, and Cindy Fehr

Definition
A. This is a viral infection caused by coxsackievirus A16, with vesicular lesions present on the hands, feet, and oral mucosa.

Incidence/Prevalence
A. Hand, foot, and mouth syndrome is most commonly seen in preschool children.

Pathogenesis
A. Enteroviruses invade the intestinal tract of humans and are spread to others by fecal–oral and/or oral–oral (respiratory) routes. The incubation period is approximately four to six days.

Predisposing Factors
A. Childhood.
B. Confined households or day-care centers, camps.
C. Seasonal: Summer and fall most common.

Common Findings
A. Generalized rash, with lesions on the tongue, gums, and roof of the mouth.
B. Lesions (vesicles) also present on the hands, feet, and buttocks.

Other Signs and Symptoms
A. Fever.
B. Sore throat.
C. Some enteroviruses have been associated with severe consequences, such as meningitis and encephalitis. The family should monitor symptoms carefully.

Subjective Data
A. Question the client regarding onset, duration, and progression of symptoms and lesions.
B. Determine whether any family member or other contact person had similar symptoms.
C. Identify areas where the child comes in contact with numerous children (childcare facility; nurseries at church, school, etc.).
D. If not noted in the presenting symptoms, ask the client about his or her upper respiratory symptoms (sore throat, fever, headache, runny nose, cough, etc.).

Physical Examination
A. Check temperature, pulse, respirations, and blood pressure.

▶ Client Teaching Guides are available at https://connect.springerpub.com/content/reference-book/978-0-8261-9498-5

B. Inspect skin, ears, nose, and oral cavity for lesions.
C. Palpate abdomen and lymph nodes in neck, assess for meningism.
D. Auscultate lungs and heart.

Diagnostic Test
A. Usually none; consider cultures of oral lesions if secondary bacterial infection is suspected.

Differential Diagnoses
A. Pharyngitis.
B. Pneumonia.
C. Meningitis.
D. Meningococcaemia: Exanthem, petechial rash.

Plan
A. General interventions: Supportive treatment—warm saline gargles, acetaminophen as needed for discomfort, and increased fluids. Popsicles are useful to soothe oral lesions, especially for small children.
B. Client teaching: Reinforce good oral and body hygiene. The virus may be harboured in the gastrointestinal tract for long periods.
C. Pharmacological therapy:
   1. None is recommended.
   2. Acetaminophen as needed for fever and malaise.

Follow-Up
A. None is recommended unless symptoms worsen or do not resolve in seven to 10 days.

Consultation/Referral
A. Refer to specialist for any symptoms related to meningitis or encephalitis.

Individual Consideration
A. Paediatrics: Seen primarily in the paediatric population.

Bibliography
Government of Canada. (2019). Hand, foot and mouth disease (Enterovirus 71, EV 71). Retrieved from https://www.canada.ca/en/public-health/services/diseases/hand-foot-mouth-disease.html

Habif, T. P. (Ed.). (2011). *Skin disease diagnosis and treatment* (3rd ed.). Philadelphia, PA: Saunders Elsevier.

HealthLinkBC. (2015). Hand, foot and mouth disease. Retrieved from https://www.healthlinkbc.ca/healthlinkbc-files/hand-foot-and-mouth-disease

Renda, S., & Sanchez, M. (2017). Hand-foot-and-mouth disease in adults. Clinical Advisor. Retrieved from https://www.clinicaladvisor.com/home/features/hand-foot-and-mouth-disease-in-adults/

Herpes Simplex Virus Type 1

Jill C. Cash, Amy C. Bruggemann, Elsie Duff, and Cindy Fehr

Definition
Herpes simplex virus (HSV)-1 viral infection of the cutaneous tissue manifests itself by vesicular lesions on the mucous membranes and skin. HSV-1 is most often associated with oral lesions (mouth and lips), and HSV-2 is associated with genital lesions. The virus appears in three stages:
A. Primary.
B. Latent.
C. Recurrent infections.

Incidence/Prevalence
A. HSV-1 is seen in clients of all ages and in equal numbers of males and females.

Pathogenesis
A. Viral infection can be transmitted from a vesicular lesion or fluid (saliva) containing the virus to the skin or mucosa of another person by direct contact, with an incubation period of two to 14 days. Trigeminal ganglia are the host of the oral virus. The virus can be reactivated, whereupon it travels along the affected nerve route and produces recurrent lesions. Common sites of infection are the lips, face, buccal mucosa, and throat.

Predisposing Factors
A. Immunocompromised clients.
B. Prior HSV infections.
C. Exposure to virus.

Common Findings
A. Painful lips, gums, and oral mucosa.

Other Signs and Symptoms
A. Primary lesion: Fever, blisters on lips, malaise, and tender gums.
B. Recurrent episodes: Fever blisters with prodrome of itching, burning, and tingling sensation at the site before vesicles appear.

Subjective Data
A. Ask questions regarding location, onset, and duration of lesions.
B. Elicit description of prodromal symptoms.
C. Ask the client whether systemic symptoms occur with vesicular outbreak.
D. Determine when the initial outbreak of lesions occurred (commonly seen in childhood).
E. Inquire whether the client has been exposed to anyone with similar lesions.
F. If the lesion(s) is/are recurrent, ask the client whether stress, skin trauma, or sun exposure stimulates an outbreak of fever blisters.

Physical Examination
A. Inspect the skin and note location, appearance, and stage of vesicles.
B. Palpate lymph nodes for lymphadenopathy.

Diagnostic Test
A. Viral cultures.

Differential Diagnoses
A. Impetigo: Appears as amber-coloured vesicular lesions with crusting.
B. Stomatitis: Appears as erythemic or erosion lesions in the mouth and lips.
C. Herpes zoster: Causes vesicles that run along a single dermatome.
D. Stevens–Johnson syndrome (SJS).
E. Herpangina: Vesicles can be noted on the soft palate, tonsillary area, and uvula area; usually caused by the coxsackievirus.

Plan

A. General interventions:
1. Comfort measures. Ice may be used to reduce swelling as needed.
2. Vaseline or other lip ointments may be applied as needed and lip ointment with sun protection factor (SPF) 30 or greater may be applied when exposed to sunlight.

B. Client teaching:
1. Educate the client regarding the disease process of HSV-1.
2. Instruct the client to wash hands frequently.
3. Suggest proper care of lips to prevent drying and to reduce pain.
4. Educate regarding transmission of virus to others.
5. Teach the client to expect recurrences at variable times.

C. Pharmacological therapy—precautions should be used when administering medication to clients who are immunocompromised and who have a history of renal insufficiency:
1. Lidocaine 2% as needed for comfort.
2. Diphenhydramine elixir may be used to rinse mouth as needed.
3. Acetaminophen as needed for pain.
4. Campho-Phenique application as needed.
5. Initial episode: If mild or occasional, no treatment is required. If severe symptoms, begin antiviral treatment within 12 hours of prodrome tingling/burning or within 2 days of onset of lesions to decrease symptoms.
6. Recurrent episodes of 3 or greater per year, provide antiviral treatment:
    a. Valacyclovir.
    b. Acyclovir.
7. Chronic suppressive therapy of six or greater episodes a year provide continuous antiviral treatment:
    a. Valacyclovir.
    b. Acyclovir.

Follow-Up

A. None needed if resolved without complications.

Consultation/Referral

A. Refer the client to a physician if treatment is unsuccessful or further complications arise.

Individual Considerations

A. Paediatrics: Initial outbreak commonly occurs in childhood.

B. Adolescents/adults:
1. HSV-1 can also be transmitted sexually when having oral sex. Educate teens/adults regarding transmitting the virus during sexual contact. Transmission is possible if having sexual relations with partners; avoid contact when lesions are present.
2. Advise using a dental dam during oral sex to prevent transmission.
3. Avoid sharing eating utensils and toothbrushes.

Bibliography

Centers for Disease Control and Prevention. (2013). *Genital herpes—CDC fact sheet*. Retrieved from https://www.cdc.gov/std/herpes/STDFact-Herpes.htm

Expert Working Group. (2016). *Canadian guidelines on sexually transmitted infections*. Retrieved from https://www.canada.ca/en/public-health/services/infectious-diseases/sexual-health-sexually-transmitted-infections/canadian-guidelines/sexually-transmitted-infections/canadian-guidelines-sexually-transmitted-infections-26.html

Habif, T. P. (Ed.). (2011). *Skin disease diagnosis and treatment* (3rd ed.). Philadelphia, PA: Saunders Elsevier.

Herpes Zoster or Shingles

Jill C. Cash, Amy C. Bruggemann, Elsie Duff, and Cindy Fehr

Definition

A. Herpes zoster is a viral infection manifested by painful, vesicular lesions on the skin, limited to one side of the body, following one body dermatome.

Incidence/Prevalence

A. Infection may occur at any age; however, it is more common in older adults and the elderly.

Pathogenesis

A. After the primary episode of chickenpox (varicella zoster), the virus remains dormant in the body. Herpes zoster occurs when the varicella virus has been stimulated and reactivated in the dorsal root ganglia, producing the clinical manifestations of herpes zoster as discussed in the following. Duration of infection usually lasts 14 to 21 days, but may be longer in elderly or debilitated clients.

Predisposing Factors

A. Adulthood.
B. Immunocompromised clients.
C. Spinal cord trauma or injury.

Common Findings

A. Prodrome: Itching, burning, tingling, or painful sensation at lesion sites.
B. Active: Malaise, fever, headache, or pruritic rash on the skin.

Other Signs and Symptoms

A. Lesions: Clusters of vesicles on an erythemic base that burst and produce crusted lesions. These are most commonly found on the chest and back area, but they may also occur on the head and neck area or extremities. Distribution of lesions typically appears along a single dermatome.
B. Motor weakness (may be seen in approximately 5% of clients).

Subjective Data

A. Determine onset, location, and progression of rash.
B. Ask the client about prodromal symptoms—burning, itching, tingling, or painful sensation at the site before lesions break out.
C. Evaluate client status regarding immunosuppressive agents, diseases, and so forth.

Physical Examination

A. Check temperature, pulse, respiration, and blood pressure.
B. Inspect:
1. Observe skin for lesions, noting characteristics and distribution.
2. Examine ears, nose, and throat.

C. Auscultate heart and lungs.

Diagnostic Tests

A. Usually none.
B. Culture vesicular lesions.
C. Young clients with herpes zoster—consider test for HIV.

Differential Diagnoses
A. Varicella.
B. Poison ivy.
C. Herpes simplex virus (HSV).
D. Contact dermatitis.
E. Coxsackievirus.
F. Postherpetic neuralgia.

Plan
A. General interventions:—comfort measures: Instruct the client to apply wet dressings (Burow's solution) on the site for 30 to 60 minutes at least four times a day. Calamine lotions may be used as needed; oatmeal (Aveeno) bath may be used for comfort; acetaminophen is taken as needed for malaise, temperature, and comfort.
▶ B. Client teaching: *Refer to Client Teaching Guide: Herpes Zoster or Shingles.* Discuss with the client that the rash usually lasts approximately two to three weeks.
   1. Instruct the client to monitor for signs/symptoms of postherpetic neuralgia.
   2. Instruct the client to call if symptoms worsen or do not improve, or signs of bacterial infection occur.
   3. Emphasize to the client that the virus is easily transmitted to vulnerable persons.
C. Pharmacological therapy (Anti-infective Review Panel, 2019):
   1. Antiviral medications should be initiated within 24 to 48 hours after outbreak:
      a. Famciclovir.
      b. Valacyclovir.
      c. Acyclovir.
   2. Acetaminophen or ibuprofen as needed for pain or discomfort.
   3. Narcotics may be used for severe pain as needed.
   4. Postherpetic neuralgia:
      a. Postherpetic neuralgia may be treated with narcotics or other pain-relieving medications.
      b. Long-term medications may be needed for control of pain:
         i. Gabapentin.
         ii. Amitriptyline or other low-dose tricyclic antidepressants.
         iii. Pregabalin.
   5. If secondary bacterial infection of the skin occurs, apply silver sulphadiazine topically to the site until resolved.
   6. Use of steroids is controversial. Corticosteroids may be used with caution. May increase risk of dissemination.

Follow-Up
A. As needed for complications.
B. Monitor the client for complications—postherpetic neuralgia, Guillain–Barré syndrome, motor weakness, secondary infection, meningoencephalitis, ophthalmic and facial palsy, corneal ulceration, and so forth.

Consultation/Referral
A. Ramsay Hunt syndrome occurs when a shingles outbreak affects the facial nerve near one of the ears. This can cause facial paralysis and hearing loss in the affected ear.
B. Hutchinson's sign refers to vesicles in the periorbital region. These clients require an ophthamologist referral.

Individual Considerations
A. Pregnancy: The safety and efficacy of the use of the antiviral medications during pregnancy need to be considered.
B. Paediatrics: Shingles is rarely seen in children.
C. Elderly:
   1. Postherpetic neuralgia occurs in approximately 15% of clients. It is commonly seen in elderly clients.
   2. The shingles vaccine for all clients 50 years of age and older, irrespective of whether they have had the chickenpox or shingles infection in the past. For those who have had a recent shingles outbreak, it is recommended that resolution of the rash be complete before administering the vaccination.
   3. The virus is contagious for those who have not had chickenpox.

Bibliography
Centers for Disease Control and Prevention. (2016, August 19). *Shingles (herpes zoster)*. Retrieved from https://www.cdc.gov/shingles
Gagliardi, A. M. Z., Andriolo, B. N. G., Torloni, M. R., & Soares, B. G. O. (2016). Vaccines for preventing herpes zoster in older adults. *Cochrane Database of Systematic Reviews, 3*, CD008858. doi:10.1002/14651858.CD008858.pub3
Habif, T. P. (Ed.). (2011). *Skin disease diagnosis and treatment* (3rd ed.). Philadelphia, PA: Saunders Elsevier.
Watkins, J. (2010). Treating shingles (herpes zoster) in the older person. *British Journal of Community Nursing, 15*(9), 420, 422, 424 passim. doi:10.12968/bjcn.2010.15.9.78097
Wilson, J. F. (2011). In the clinic. Herpes zoster. *Annals of Internal Medicine, 154*(5), ITC31–ITC15; quiz ITC316

Impetigo

Jill C. Cash, Amy C. Bruggemann, Elsie Duff, and Cindy Fehr

Definition
A. Impetigo is a bacterial infection of the skin, most commonly caused by *Staphylococcus aureus* or *Streptococcus pyogenes*, or both.

Incidence/Prevalence
A. It occurs equally in males and females and is most commonly seen in children, especially those 3 to 5 years of age.

Pathogenesis
A. An alteration in the skin integrity allows bacterial invasion into the epidermis, causing an infection. Small, moist vesicles ranging from red macules to honey-coloured crusts or erosions occur singly or grouped together. Most common organisms are *S. aureus* and Group A beta-haemolytic *S. pyogenes*.

Predisposing Factors
A. Poor hygiene.
B. Warm climate.
C. Break in the skin.

Common Findings
A. Tender sores around the mouth and nose area in which the lesions continue to spread and worsen, despite over-the-counter (OTC) medication treatment.

Subjective Data
A. Elicit onset, progression, duration, and location of lesions.
B. Ask the client whether he or she has had contact with any other child or person with similar lesions.
C. Assess whether the client exhibits any other symptoms, especially systemic symptoms (fever, malaise, etc.).
D. Elicit what treatment has been tried, if any.

Physical Examination
A. Check temperature.
B. Inspect:
  1. Skin, noting types of lesions and skin involvement.
  2. Ears, nose, mouth, and throat.
C. Auscultate lungs and heart.

Diagnostic Tests
A. None required.
B. May perform culture if recurrent or resistant to treatment.

Differential Diagnoses
A. Varicella.
B. Folliculitis.
C. Erysipelas.
D. Herpes simplex.
E. Second-degree burns.
F. Pharyngitis or tonsillitis—throat erythema, with tonsillary hypertrophy and exudate present; lymph nodes—adenopathy of anterior cervical chain.
G. Ecthyma—severe case of impetigo with lymphadenitis.
H. Insect bites.
I. Necrotizing fasciitis.
J. Contact dermatitis.
K. Scabies.

Plan
A. General interventions:
  1. Crusted lesions may be removed with thorough, gentle washing with mild soap three to four times daily.
  2. Impetigo must be adequately treated and resolved to prevent postinfection complications such as poststreptococcal acute glomerulonephritis, cellulitis, ecthyma, and bacteraemia.
B. Client teaching: Encourage good handwashing and hygiene to reduce spreading infection.
C. Pharmacological therapy:
  1. If few lesions are noted without involvement of face or cellulitis, mupirocin ointment—to site three times daily for seven to 10 days.
  2. Systemic antibiotics:
    a. Children older than 3 months—cephalexin or erythormycin.
    b. Adults—cloxacillin or cephalexin.
  3. Other effective antibiotics include clarithromycin, clindamycin, and azithromycin.

Follow-Up
A. Schedule appointment in 10 to 14 days to determine resolution of infection.

Consultation/Referral
A. Consult a physician if complications arise or if resolution is not complete with antibiotic therapy.

Bibliography
Anti-infective Review Panel. (2019). *Anti-infective guidelines for community-acquired infections.* Toronto: MUMS Guideline Clearinghouse.
Habif, T. P. (Ed.). (2011). *Skin disease diagnosis and treatment* (3rd ed.). Philadelphia, PA: Saunders Elsevier.
Hartman-Adams, H., Banvard, C., & Juckett, G. (2014). Impetigo: Diagnosis and treatment. *American Family Physician, 90*(4), 229–235.

Insect Bites and Stings

Jill C. Cash, Amy C. Bruggemann, Elsie Duff, and Cindy Fehr

Definition
A. Bites and/or stings on the skin come from commonly encountered insects: bees, hornets, wasps, mosquitoes, chiggers, ticks, fleas, fire ants, and bedbugs.

Incidence/Prevalence
A. Bites are seen in all age groups, more common in summer months.

Pathogenesis
A. Some bites elicit local tissue inflammation and destruction because of proteins and enzymes in the poison or venom of the insect.
B. Immunoglobulin E (IgE)-mediated allergic reactions (immediate or delayed) may occur.
C. Serum sickness reaction may appear 10 to 14 days after a sting with venom. Toxic reactions can also occur from multiple stings yielding large inoculation of poison or venom.
D. With tick bites, exposure to Rocky Mountain spotted fever, Lyme disease, ehrlichiosis, and babesiosis disease may occur.

Predisposing Factors
A. Exposure to areas of heavy insect infestations.
B. Warm-weather months.
C. Outdoor exposure with bare feet, bright clothes.
D. Use of perfumes and/or colognes.
E. Previous sensitization.

Common Findings
A. Local reaction—pain, swelling, and redness at the site after insect bite.
B. Toxic reaction—local reaction plus headache, vertigo, gastrointestinal symptoms (nausea, vomiting, and diarrhoea), syncope, convulsions, and/or fever.

Subjective Data
A. Did the client see what bit or stung him or her?
B. If the client felt the bite or sting, was he or she bitten or stung once or multiple times?
C. How long ago did it occur?
D. Where was the client when the injury occurred (environment)?
E. Has the client ever been bitten or stung before? If so, did he or she have any reaction then? If so, what was the treatment?

Physical Examination
A. Check temperature, pulse, respiration, and blood pressure. Observe overall respiratory status.

B. Inspect:
1. Site of injury for local reaction; note erythema, rash, or oedema.
2. Ear, nose, and throat.
C. Auscultate: Assess heart and lungs.
D. Palpate:
1. Palpate injured site.
2. Assess nodes for lymphadenopathy.
3. Perform abdominal examination, if appropriate.

Diagnostic Tests
A. None is required.
B. Consider taking skin scrapings to evaluate under a microscope.
C. Consider culture if infection is suspected.
D. In endemic tick geographical areas, consider drawing Lyme disease bacterium antibodies at 2 to 4 weeks and then a 6 week interval for either an acute or convalecent stage. A two-tiered serological testing incubation period (3–30 days) requires: (1) an enzyme-linked immunosorbent assay (ELISA) screening test; (2) a confirmatory immunoblot (IB) test (if the ELISA is positive or equivocal).

Differential Diagnoses
A. Insect bite:
1. Bees, hornets, wasps, bedbugs: Local pain, redness, pruritus, and swelling occur at the site. Red papules and wheals appear, enlarge, and then subside within hours. Delayed hypersensitivity occurs within seven days with enlarged, local reaction, with fever, malaise, headache, arthralgias, and lymphadenopathy. Toxicity can occur. Anaphylaxis may be seen with generalized warmth and urticaria, erythema, angio-oedema, intestinal cramping, bronchospasm, laryngospasm, shock, and collapse.
2. Ticks: Local redness, swelling, itching. Enlarged area of redness and swelling may occur.
3. Mosquitoes and chiggers: Local redness, swelling, and itching occur. Delayed reaction can include oedema and burning sensation.
4. Fleas: Local redness, swelling, and itching occur. Usually papules noted in a zigzag pattern, especially on legs and waist. Note haemorrhagic puncta surrounded by erythematous and urticarial patches.
5. Body lice: Small noninflammatory red spots, intensely pruritic, are found on waist, shoulders, axilla, and neck. Note linear scratch marks. Note secondary infection.
6. Scabies: Pruritus is the dominant symptom. Note inflammation and burrows in skin with papules and vesicles, especially in the webs of the hands and feet.
7. Fire ants: Papules appear and turn to pustules within six to 24 hours after bite. Watch for localized necrosis with scarring. Urticaria and angio-oedema can occur.
B. Allergic reaction.

Plan
A. General interventions: Anaphylaxis—activate emergency medical services (EMS) immediately.
1. With all bites and stings, treat anaphylaxis first.
2. Local reactions—treat with analgesic of choice. Apply ice packs to the site for approximately 10 minutes. Elevate affected extremities.
3. Delayed reactions—administer antihistamines as needed. Consider corticosteroid use.
4. Routine wound care—cleanse wound. Remove stinger. If it is a painful sting, apply a cotton ball soaked in meat tenderizer or sodium bicarbonate paste.
5. Debride as necessary.
6. For embedded insects, apply petroleum jelly, nail polish, or alcohol over site for 30 minutes and wait for insect or tick to withdraw.
7. Referral to allergist–immunologist is recommended for clients with a severe systemic reaction for skin testing and to evaluate for candidacy of venom immunotherapy treatment.
8. Hospitalize the client for severe reactions.
B. *Refer to Client Teaching Guide: Insect Bites and Stings.*
C. Pharmacological therapy:
1. Antihistamines: Diphenhydramine.
2. Mild anaphylaxis: Epinephrine.
3. Oral antihistamines for next 24 hours.
4. Severe anaphylaxis:
   a. Epinephrine.
   b. Oxygen.
   c. Salbutemol.
5. Self-treatment for anaphylaxis (emergency treatment kits): Epinephrine autoinjector.
6. Early lyme disease treatment should be initiated without waiting for laboratory confirmation in high endemic areas. A single dose of doxycycline (200mg) may be offered to adults patients or children over age 8 or under 45kg (4.0mg/kg up to a maximum of 200mg).
7. Encourage use of permethrin-treated clothing (repels crawling and flying insects, which may carry diseases), that is effective for up to 70 washings, such as, No Fly Zone™. This clothing is not recommended for children.

Follow-Up
A. Follow up in two weeks to evaluate effectiveness of treatment. If symptoms worsen before this, reevaluation is needed.

Consultation/Referral
A. Consult with a physician when anaphylaxis occurs.

Individual Considerations
A. Paediatrics: Children are at a higher risk than adults for complications of a reaction.
B. Geriatrics: Elderly adults are at high risk for complications of reactions.

Bibliography
Habif, T. P. (Ed.). (2011). *Skin disease diagnosis and treatment* (3rd ed.). Philadelphia, PA: Saunders Elsevier.
Health Canada. (2018). Lyme Disease. Retrieve from https://www.canada.ca/en/public-health/services/diseases/lyme-disease/health-professionals-lyme-disease.html
Moore, S. J., Luntz, Mordue., J, A., & Logan, J. G. (2012). Insect bite prevention. *Infectious Disease Clinics of North America, 26*(3), 655–673. doi:10.1016/j.idc.2012.07.002

Lice (Pediculosis)

Jill C. Cash, Amy C. Bruggemann, Elsie Duff, and Cindy Fehr

Definition
Pediculosis (lice) is an infestation of the louse on human beings in one of three areas:
A. Head (*Pediculosis capitis*).

B. Pubic area (*Pthirus pubis*).
C. Body (*Pediculosis corporis*).

Incidence/Prevalence
A. *Pediculosis capitis* is most common in children. It is estimated that head lice infestations occur in the school systems anywhere from 10% to 40% of the time.
B. They are more commonly found in girls than boys.
C. *Phthirus pubis* infestation is more common in adults.
D. Lice affect all demographics; all social, racial, and economic groups get lice.

Pathogenesis
A. Head and body lice are transmitted by direct contact from person to person, that is, through sharing hats, combs, brushes, and so forth. The parasite hatches from an egg, or nit. Once hatched, the lice live on humans by sucking blood through the skin. The average adult louse lives nine to 10 days. The nits appear as small white eggs on the hair shaft. Nits are very difficult to remove and survive up to three weeks after removal from the host. Body lice lay nits in the seams of clothing.
B. Pubic lice are found at the base of the hair shaft, where they lay nits. Pubic lice are transmitted through sexual contact.

Predisposing Factors
A. Head and body lice: Exposure to crowded public areas, such as schools; inability to clean and launder clothing, bed linens, and so forth.
B. Pubic lice: Sexual contact with infected people.
C. Poor hygiene.

Common Findings
A. Head lice: Severe itching and scratching of the head, neck area, and, commonly, behind the ears.
B. Body lice: Severe itching on the body, which may lead to secondary infections of the skin.
C. Pubic lice: Severe itching of genital area.

Other Signs and Symptoms
A. Excoriated skin from intense scratching.
B. Visible lice or nits in hair, body, or clothing.
C. Papules with an erythemic base may develop on the genital area, axilla, chest, beard, or eyelashes.
D. *Phthirus pubis* or nits or lice are found on eyelashes of children.

Subjective Data
A. Inquire as to exposure to anyone known to have lice.
B. Identify whether the client attends a crowded environment such as school, day care, and so forth.
C. Ask whether lice and nits have been seen by the client or guardian.
D. Determine onset, duration, and course of symptoms. Ask when were lice or nits first discovered.
E. Assess whether the client has been symptomatic (itching, scratching).
F. Inquire about social habits of cleaning, laundry, and so forth.

Physical Examination
A. Check temperature to rule out any secondary infection.
B. Inspect:
　1. Inspect hair, body, pubic area, and clothing seams for nits or lice.
　2. Note excoriation of skin.
　3. Examine eyelashes of children.
　4. Examine skin for secondary bacterial infection.

Diagnostic Tests
A. None.
B. Culture excoriated area if secondary bacterial infection suspected.

Differential Diagnoses
A. Scabies.

Plan
A. General interventions:
　1. Treat immediately with appropriate pediculicides (see section "Pharmacological therapy," in the following).
　2. After treatment, it is imperative to remove each nit and louse; use fine-tooth comb for nit removal.
　3. Evaluate entire family for lice.
　4. Treat secondary bacterial infection as needed.
B. Client teaching: *Refer to Client Teaching Guide: Lice (Pediculosis)*. Specific instructions need to be given to clients on how to get rid of lice and nits.
　1. Reinforce good hygiene; teach children not to share combs, brushes, hats, and hair accessories.
C. Pharmacological therapy:
　1. Pyrethrins and permethrin are first-line treatment in Canada for those 2 months of age or older: pediculicidal.
　　a. In pregnancy, permethrin is the only recommended treatment.
　　b. Application: Soak hair and scalp. Let sit 10 minutes, work lather into hair and rinse with cool water. Re-treat in seven to 10 days.
　2. Noninsecticidal treatments approved by Health Canada include the following:
　　a. Isopropyl myristate/ST-cyclomethicone for those 4 years of age or older: pediculicidal. Application: Treat dry scalp and hair, keep eyes closed throughout procedure and wait time, let sit in hair/scalp for 10 minutes, rinse with warm water, and repeat in seven days.
　　b. Dimeticone solution for those 2 years of age or older: pediculicidal and ovicidal. Application: Spray and massage into hair, let sit at least 30 minutes, then comb through hair, leave in overnight and wash as usual, re-treat in eight to 10 days.
　　c. Benzyl alcohol lotion 5% for those 6 months to 60 years of age: pediculicidal. Application: Must retreat after nine days.
　3. Oral ivermectin is available in Canada only through Health Canada's Special Access Programme: antihelminthic. Due to potential neurotoxicity, only for those >15 kg.
　4. Home remedies and homeopathics—There are no published trials supporting the safety, toxicity, or efficacy of home remedies such as wet combing, vinegar, mayonnaise, petroleum jelly, olive oil, margarine, or thick hair gel, or homeopathic treatments such as tea tree oil or peppermint oil.
　5. Topical lice treatments: Do not use a shampoo/conditioner or conditioner before using head lice treatments.

▶ Client Teaching Guides are available at https://connect.springerpub.com/content/reference-book/978-0-8261-9498-5

Do not wash hair for one to two days after using lice treatment regimen.

6. *Pthirus pubis:* Permethrin; apply to pubic area as directed.

7. Eyelash manifestation: After removing nits, apply petroleum jelly to lashes three to four times a day for eight to 10 days. **Eyelashes should never be treated with pediculicides.**

Follow-Up

A. None recommended, but it is important to note that there are increasing resistance rates across Canada to a variety of treatment options.

B. Some schools and institutions require follow-up to evaluate whether infestation is resolved before admitting the child back into the classroom. However, exclusion policies are discouraged as there is no medical reason to exclude children with nits or lice from school or day care. Likewise, research supporting environmental decontamination is lacking, but washing of items having been in close contact with scalp in hot water or placed in a hot dryer for 15 minutes may be warranted. Alternatively, items can be sealed in a plastic bag for two weeks to kill lice and nits.

Consultation/Referral

A. If lice are a repeated problem, contact social services or the public health department to have a visiting nurse or aide visit the home to evaluate home conditions and to teach the family how to prevent infestations.

Individual Considerations

A. Pregnancy: Lindane is contraindicated during pregnancy.
B. Paediatrics:
   1. Head lice is commonly seen in school-aged children.
   2. Lindane should not be used in infants. The American Academy of Pediatrics does not recommend lindane as a first-line treatment for head lice in children secondary to the toxic effects of the brain and central nervous system.

Bibliography

Cummings, C., Finlay, J. C., & MacDonald, N. E. (2018). Head lice infestations: A clinical update. *Pediatrics & Child Health, 2391*, e18–e24. doi:10.1093/pch/pxx165

Government of Canada. (2013). *Canadian guidelines on sexually transmitted infections—Management and treatment of specific infections—Ectoparasitic infestations (Section 5–3).* Retrieved from https://www.canada.ca/en/public-health/services/infectious-diseases/sexual-health-sexually-transmitted-infections/canadian-guidelines/sexually-transmitted-infections/canadian-guidelines-sexually-transmitted-infections-31.html

Gunning, K., Pippitt, K., Kiraly, B., & Sayler, M. (2012). Pediculosis and scabies: Treatment update. *American Family Physician, 86*(6), 535–541.

Habif, T. P. (Ed.). (2011). *Skin disease diagnosis and treatment* (3rd ed.). Philadelphia, PA: Saunders Elsevier.

Martinez-Diaz, G., & Mancini, A. (2010). CNE series. Head lice: Diagnosis and therapy. *Dermatology Nursing, 22*(4), 2–8.

Lichen Planus

Jill C. Cash, Amy C. Bruggemann, Elsie Duff, and Cindy Fehr

Definition

A. Lichen planus is a relatively common acute or chronic inflammatory dermatosis. It affects skin and mucous membranes with characteristic flat-topped, shiny, violaceous (purplish colour) pruritic papules with lacy lines on the skin, and milky-white papules in the mouth.

Incidence/Prevalence

A. Lichen planus accounts for 0.1% to 1.2% of office visits to dermatologists and is estimated to affect approximately 1% of the population. It is estimated that up to 50% have oral involvement, which can be more persistent in nature.

B. It exhibits no racial preference.

Pathogenesis

A. Aetiology is unknown, although it is possibly a cell-mediated immune response. Most cases remit within seven years. Lesions may heal with significant postinflammatory hyperpigmentation.

Predisposing Factors

A. Severe emotional stress.
B. Drugs may induce lichenoid plaques.

Common Findings

A. Rash with or without pruritus.
B. Primary lesions: Small, flat-topped papules that are polygonal, lightly scaly, and violaceous.
C. Secondary lesions: Erythema, scales, and erosions.
D. Oral lesions: White lines/patches, erythema, ulcers, dryness, pain, metallic/burning taste.

Other Signs and Symptoms

A. Distribution: Volar aspect of wrists, ankles, mouth, genitalia, and lumbar region.
B. Wickham's striae (white, lacelike pattern on surface).
C. Scalp: Atrophic skin with alopecia.
D. Nails: Destruction of nail fold and bed, especially in the large toe.
E. Men: Lesions of glans penis.
F. Women: Erosive lesions of labia and vulva.

Subjective Data

A. Determine whether the onset was sudden or gradual.
B. Ask the client to describe whether the skin is itchy or painful.
C. Assess lesions for any associated discharge (blood or pus).
D. Identify the location(s) of the problem.
E. Complete a drug history. Ask the client whether he or she has recently taken any antibiotics or other drugs. Ask whether he or she has used any topical medications, lotions, or other creams.
F. Determine the presence of any preceding systemic symptoms (fever, sore throat, anorexia, or vaginal discharge).
G. Rule out insect bites.
H. Identify any possible exposure to industrial toxins, domestic toxins, or colour-film developing chemicals.
I. Ask whether the client has had any possible sexual contact with persons with HIV or sexually transmitted infections.
J. Ask whether the client has had close physical contact with others with skin disorders.

Physical Examination

A. Inspect:
   1. Skin; note lesion distribution.
   2. Mucous membranes: Buccal mucosa, tongue, and lips.
   3. Hair and nails.
   4. Genitalia.

Diagnostic Tests
A. A drop of mineral oil accentuates the papule.
B. If necessary to confirm diagnosis, deep shave or punch biopsy of developed lesions.
C. HIV or sexually transmitted infection (STI) testing if indicated.
D. Hepatitis testing should be completed to assess for hepatitis C, as lichen planus has been shown to have a correlation.

Differential Diagnoses
A. Lichenoid drug eruptions.
B. Leukoplakia.
C. Chronic graft-versus-host disease.
D. Candidiasis (thrush).
E. Lupus erythematosus.
F. Contact dermatitis.
G. Bite trauma.
H. Secondary syphilis.

Plan
A. General interventions: Discontinue any suspected drug agent.
▶ **B.** Client teaching: *Refer to Client Teaching Guide: Lichen Planus.*
  1. Instruct clients that the disease may be chronic; most cases resolve spontaneously.
  2. Encourage the client to avoid severe emotional stress.
  3. Encourage the client to avoid scratching and prevent secondary infection.
  4. Reassure the client that lichen planus is not contagious.
C. Pharmacological therapy:
  1. Oral antihistamines: Hydroxyzine hydrochloride or cetirizine.
  2. Medium- to high-potency topical corticosteroids:
    a. Mouth lesions: Fluocinonide 0.05%, ointment or gel.
    b. Body lesions: Betamethasone dipropionate 0.05%, triamcinolone, clobetasol 0.05%, or other class 1 cream or ointment. **Caution clients about steroid atrophy.**
    c. Genital lesions: Desonide cream 0.05%, although higher potency creams may be necessary. Topical corticosteroids should be used on genitalia in short bursts only.
    d. Hypertrophic lesions: Intralesional injections, such as injecting triamcinolone, are helpful for pruritus relief. Use cautiously in dark-skinned clients because of risk of hypopigmentation.
  3. Oral prednisone is rarely used, but if necessary, use with a short course only and taper.

Follow-Up
A. See the client in one week for evaluation of treatment.

Consultation/Referral
A. Refer the client to a dermatologist if there is no response to initial treatment.

Individual Considerations
A. Pregnancy: Use caution with medications prescribed.
B. Paediatrics: For severe itching, consider oral antihistamine.

Bibliography
College of Dental Hygienists of Ontario. (2017). *Lichen planus.* Retrieved from http://www.cdho.org/Advisories/CDHO_Factsheet_Lichen_Planus.pdf
Habif, T. P. (Ed.). (2011). *Skin disease diagnosis and treatment* (3rd ed.). Philadelphia, PA: Saunders Elsevier.
Nordqvist, C., & Felman, A. (2017). *Everything you need to know about lichen planus. Medical News Today.* Reviewed by the University of Illinois-Chicago, School of Medicine. Retrieved from https://www.medicalnewstoday.com/articles/184866.php
Oakley, A. (2015). *Lichen planus.* DermNet NZ. Retrieved from https://www.dermnetnz.org/topics/lichen-planus/

Pityriasis Rosea
Jill C. Cash, Amy C. Bruggemann, Elsie Duff, and Cindy Fehr

Definition
A. Pityriasis rosea is an acute, self-limiting, benign skin eruption characterized by a preceding "herald patch" that is followed by widespread papulosquamous lesions.

Incidence/Prevalence
A. Pityriasis rosea is relatively common, with more than 75% of cases in individuals from 10 to 35 years of age.
B. Incidence is slightly higher in women than in men.
C. Incidence is higher during the spring and autumn.

Pathogenesis
A. Disease is idiopathic; some evidence exists to support a viral origin or autoimmune disorder.

Predisposing Factor
A. Recent acute infection.

Common Findings
A. Rash: Salmon, pink, or tawny-coloured lesions generally are concentrated in the trunk, but may develop on arms, legs, and, rarely, on the face.
B. Mild pruritus.

Other Signs and Symptoms
A. Earliest lesions may be papular but may progress to 1- to 2-cm oval plaques.
B. Long axes of oval lesions run parallel to each other, hence the term "Christmas tree distribution."
C. Preceding herald patch (2–10 cm with central clearing) closely resembles ringworm; usually appears abruptly a few days to several weeks before the generalized eruptive phase.

Subjective Data
A. Elicit information about occurrence of initial, single, 2- to 10-cm round to oval lesion.
B. Question the client as to known contact with similar symptoms. Small epidemics have been identified in fraternity houses and military bases.

Physical Examination
A. Check temperature to rule out any infection.
B. Inspect:
  1. All body surfaces with client unclothed; look for characteristic lesions and distribution.
  2. The mucous surfaces, palms, and soles, which are usually spared by pityriasis rosea.

▶ Client Teaching Guides are available at https://connect.springerpub.com/content/reference-book/978-0-8261-9498-5

Diagnostic Tests

A. Generally none required; however, potassium hydroxide (KOH) wet preparation may be useful to distinguish a herald patch from tinea corporis.
B. Serology to rule out syphilis, if applicable.
C. If unable to identify herald patch, a serologic test for syphilis should be ordered because syphilis may be clinically indistinguishable from pityriasis rosea.
D. White blood count (WBC) normal; no specific laboratory markers for pityriasis rosea.

Differential Diagnoses

A. Nummular eczema.
B. Tinea corporis.
C. Tinea versicolour.
D. Viral exanthems.
E. Drug eruptions.
  1. Captopril.
  2. Bismuth.
  3. Barbiturates.
  4. Clonidine.
  5. Metronidazole.
F. Secondary syphilis.
G. Lichen planus.

Plan

A. General interventions:
  1. Direct sunlight to the point of minimal erythema hastens the disappearance of lesions and decreases itching. Ultraviolet B (UVB) light in five consecutive daily exposures can decrease pruritus and shorten rash, particularly if administered within the first week of eruption.
  2. Not proven to be contagious and relatively harmless, so isolation is not required.
▶ **B.** Client teaching: *Refer to Client Teaching Guide: Pityriasis Rosea.* Advise clients that the disease is self-limiting and clears spontaneously in one to three months.
C. Pharmacological therapy:
  1. Generally none is required, but for itching the following recommendations exist: Group V topical steroids and oral antihistamines as per usual dosing.
  2. Prednisone in rare cases of intense itching.

Follow-Up

A. None is required unless secondary infection (impetigo) develops. Disease may recur in approximately 2% of clients.

Consultation/Referral

A. Consult or refer the client to a physician when disease persists beyond three months.

Individual Considerations

A. Pregnancy: Disease has not been shown to affect fetus.
B. Paediatrics: Rash more frequently affects face and distal extremities. Impetigo may result from scratching or poor hygiene.
C. Geriatrics: Disease is rarely seen in geriatric clients. Strongly consider other differential diagnoses, particularly drug reactions.

Bibliography

Habif, T. P. (Ed.). (2011). *Skin disease diagnosis and treatment* (3rd ed.). Philadelphia, PA: Saunders Elsevier.
Sankararaman, S., & Velayuthan, S. (2014). Multiple recurrences in pityriasis rosea—A case report with review of the literature. *Indian Journal of Dermatology, 59*(3), 316. doi:10.4103/0019-5154.131457
Wyndham, M. (2011). Pityriasis rosea. *Practice Nurse, 41*(1), 41.

Precancerous or Cancerous Skin Lesions

Jill C. Cash, Amy C. Bruggemann, Elsie Duff, and Cindy Fehr

Definition

A. Potentially malignant or malignant cutaneous cells form precancerous or cancerous skin lesions, respectively.

Incidence/Prevalence

Skin cancer is the most common cancer diagnosed in Canada each year, accounting for over 80,000 new cases annually and is the second most common cancer in those 15 to 34 years of age.
A. Nonmelanoma types of skin cancer, including squamous cell carcinomas (SCC), basal cell carcinomas (BCC), Merkel cell carcinoma, and cutaneous T-cell lymphoma. Specific statistical reporting of nonmelanoma skin cancer types is not tracked in Canada. BCC is believed to make up 75% to 80% of all skin cancers in Canada, and is two to four times more frequent than SCC.
B. Melanoma impacts more than 7,000 Canadians each year; one in 73 women and one in 59 men will develop melanoma. Greater than 80% of skin cancers are thought to be directly related to ultraviolet (UV) radiation, and those using tanning beds before 30 years of age have a 75% greater risk of developing melanoma.

Pathogenesis

A. SCC: Abnormal cells of the epidermis penetrate the basement membrane of the epidermis and move into the dermis, producing SCC. This often begins as actinic keratosis that undergoes malignant change.
B. BCC: Abnormal cells of the basal layer of the epidermis expand. The surrounding stroma supports the basal cell growth. UV rays (sunlight) are the major contributor to BCC. BCC is a slow-growing tumour that rarely metastasizes.
C. Malignant melanoma: Abnormal cells proliferate from the melanocyte system. Initially, the cells grow superficially and laterally into the epidermis and papillary dermis. After a period, the cells begin growing up into the reticular dermis and subcutaneous fat. Malignant tumours occur because of the inability of the damaged cells to protect themselves from the long-term exposure to UV rays.
D. Keratoacanthoma: Sun-exposed area lesion that at first appears as a smooth, skin-coloured, or reddish, dome-shaped papule, which may then grow to 1 to 2 cm in a few weeks, with crusted interior.

Predisposing Factors

A. Advanced age (older than age 50 years),
B. Median age of 40 years for malignant melanoma,
C. Exposure to UV light (sun exposure),
D. Fair complexion,
E. Smokers (damaged lips),
F. Skin damaged by burns and/or chronic inflammation,
G. History of blistering sunburns before 18 years of age increases risk.

▶ Client Teaching Guides are available at https://connect.springerpub.com/content/reference-book/978-0-8261-9498-5

Common Findings
A. New lesions found on the skin.
B. Ulcer that does not heal.

Other Signs and Symptoms
A. SCC: Skin lesions seen in sun-exposed areas or skin damaged by burns or chronic inflammation; lower lip lesions common; firm, irregular papules with scaly, bleeding, friable surface like sandpaper; grows rapidly.
B. BCC: Tumour seen on face and neck; nodules >1 cm that appear shiny; pearly colour with telangiectasia; center caves in.
C. Malignant melanoma: Asymmetrical tumour of skin with irregular border, variation in colour, and >6 mm in diameter; can metastasize to any organ.
D. Bowen's disease (SCC in situ): Chronic, nonhealing erythemic patch with sharp, irregular borders; occurs on skin and/or the mucocutaneous tissue; resembles eczema but does not respond to steroids.

Subjective Data
A. Have the client identify when lesion was first noted.
B. Ask the client to describe any changes in size, colour, or shape of the lesion.
C. Determine whether the client has noted any new lesions.
D. Ascertain any family history of malignant melanoma.
E. Determine the client's history of skin exposure to the sun or any other UV rays.
F. Ask the client about smoking history. If the client smokes, ask how many packs per day.
G. Ask whether the client is up to date on routine cancer screenings.

Physical Examination
A. Inspect:
  1. Perform full body exam of the skin for lesions.
  2. Note surface, size, shape, border, colour, and diameter of lesion(s).

Diagnostic Test
A. Biopsy suspicious lesions.

Differential Diagnoses
A. SCC.
B. BCC.
C. Malignant melanoma.
D. Actinic keratosis.
E. Solar lentigo.
F. Seborrhoeic keratosis.
G. Common nevus.
H. Leukoplakia.

Plan
A. General interventions:
  1. Monitor progress/change of lesions detected.
  2. Biopsy any suspicious lesions. Excise lesion with narrow margins, making sure to include all margins. If biopsy results of specimen are inadequate for accurate histologic diagnosis or staging, repeat biopsy. Include all clinical history information on the pathology report with the specimen when sending to pathology.
B. Client teaching: *Refer to Client Teaching Guide: Skin Care Assessment.* Educate clients regarding importance of early identification of lesions and monthly assessment of skin.
C. Pharmacological therapy: None indicated.

Follow-Up
A. If diagnosis is made, follow up with examination every month for three months, twice a year for five years, then yearly.

Consultation/Referral
A. Refer all clients to the dermatologist if skin cancer is suspected.

Individual Considerations
A. Paediatrics: Teach parents to use sun protection factor (SPF) 30 or greater on paediatric clients exposed to the sun.
B. Geriatrics: The elderly are at high risk of skin lesions. Monitor them closely.

Bibliography
Canadian Cancer Society. (2018). *What is non-melanoma skin cancer?* Retrieved from http://www.cancer.ca/en/cancer-information/cancer-type/skin-non-melanoma/non-melanoma-skin-cancer/?region=on

Canadian Cancer Society, Statistics Canada, Public Health Agency of Canada, Provincial/Territorial Cancer Registries. (2017). *Canadian cancer statistics 2017.* Retrieved from http://www.cancer.ca/~/media/cancer.ca/CW/cancer%20information/cancer%20101/Canadian%20cancer%20statistics/Canadian-Cancer-Statistics-2017-EN.pdf?la=en

Canadian Dermatology Association. (2017). *2017 skin cancer fact sheet.* Retrieved from https://dermatology.ca/wp-content/uploads/2017/11/2017-Skin-Cancer-Fact-Sheet.pdf

Canadian Skin Cancer Foundation. (n.d.). *About skin cancer.* Retrieved from http://www.canadianskincancerfoundation.com/about-skin-cancer.html

Government of Canada. (2018). *Skin cancer.* Retrieved from https://www.canada.ca/en/public-health/services/sun-safety/skin-cancer.html

Habif, T. P. (Ed.). (2011). *Skin disease diagnosis and treatment* (3rd ed.). Philadelphia, PA: Saunders Elsevier.

National Clearing House Guidelines. (2001). *Guidelines of care for the management of primary cutaneous melanoma (revised 2011 November)* NGC: 009038. Rockville, MD: American Academy of Dermatology-Medical Specialty Society.

Pinault, L., Bushnik, T., Fioletov, V., Peters, C.E., King, W.D., & Tjepkema, M. (2017). The risk of melanoma associated with ambient summer ultraviolet radiation. *Health Reports, 28*(5), 3–11. Statistics Canada, Catalogue no. 82-003-X

Psoriasis

Jill C. Cash, Amy C. Bruggemann, Elsie Duff, and Cindy Fehr

Definition
A. A common benign, chronic, inflammatory skin disorder, psoriasis is characterized by whitish scaly patches commonly seen on the scalp, knees, and elbows.

Incidence/Prevalence
A. Disease occurs in about 2% of the world population.
B. Psoriasis affects 1 million people in Canada.
C. It occurs at any age:
  1. Peaks of onset seen in young adults aged 15 to 30 years.
  2. May also be seen in adults aged 57 to 60 years.

▶ Client Teaching Guides are available at https://connect.springerpub.com/content/reference-book/978-0-8261-9498-5

Pathogenesis

A. Aetiology is unknown; this is a multifactorial disease with a definite genetic component. Hyperproliferation of the epidermis and inflammation of the epidermis and dermis are seen, with epidermal transit time rapidly increased (six- to ninefold). A T-lymphocyte-mediated dermal immune response may occur because of microbial antigen or autoimmune process.

Predisposing Factors

A. Family history.
B. Drugs that exacerbate condition:
  1. Lithium.
  2. Beta-blockers.
  3. Nonsteroidal anti-inflammatory drugs.
  4. Antimalarial drugs.
  5. Sudden withdrawal of systemic or potent topical corticosteroids.
C. Stress (common triggering factor).
D. Local trauma or irritation.
E. Recent streptococcal infection.
F. Alcohol use.
G. Tobacco use.
H. HIV association; suspected if onset is abrupt.

Common Findings

A. Dry scaly rash.

Other Signs and Symptoms

A. Pruritic and/or painful lesions.
B. Silvery scales on discrete erythematous plaques:
  1. Onset commonly occurs as a guttate form with small, scattered, teardrop-shaped papules and plaques after a streptococcal infection in a child or young adult.
  2. Larger, chronic plaques occur later in life.
C. Lesions commonly seen on the scalp, elbows, and knees, but may involve any area of the body.
D. Glossitis or geographic tongue: Small pits or yellow-brown spots (oil spots).
E. Positive Auspitz sign: Punctate bleeding points with removal of scale.
F. Onycholysis.
G. Stippled nails and pitting; approximately 50% of clients have nail involvement.
H. Periarticular swelling of small joints of fingers and toes. **Joint pain and involvement signals psoriatic arthritis.**
I. Pustular variant with predominant involvement of hands and/or feet, including nails.

Subjective Data

A. Question the client regarding any predisposing factors listed earlier to identify risk factors.
B. Ask the client whether there have been changes in the course of symptoms.
C. Ascertain whether the symptoms worsen in winter and improve in summer.
D. Determine the site of the lesion and whether the onset is sudden and/or painful.
E. Ask the client to describe the skin, whether it is itchy or painful.
F. Assess lesions for any associated discharge (blood or pus).
G. Ask whether the client is using any new soaps, creams, or lotions.
H. Rule out any exposure to industrial or domestic toxins.
I. Ask the client about any possible contact with venereal disease (sexually transmitted diseases [STDs]).
J. Review whether there has been any close physical contact with others with skin disorders.
K. Elicit information regarding any preceding systemic symptoms (fever, sore throat, and anorexia).

Physical Examination

A. Check temperature (if indicated).
B. Inspect:
  1. Skin; note type of lesion and distribution. Assess oral mucosa, nails, and nail beds.
  2. Joints.
C. Palpate joints for tenderness.

Diagnostic Tests

A. None is indicated unless HIV infection is suspected; if so, order HIV test.
B. If joint inflammation is present, consider rheumatoid factor, erythrocyte sedimentation rate, and uric acid.
C. If there is a history of streptococcal infection, order antistreptolysin O titer.

Differential Diagnoses

A. Scalp: Seborrhoeic dermatitis.
B. Body folds: Candidiasis.
C. Trunk: Pityriasis rosea, tinea corporis.
D. Hand dermatitis.
E. Squamous cell carcinoma (SCC).
F. Cutaneous lupus erythematosus.

Plan

A. General interventions:
  1. This is a chronic disorder that requires long-term treatment, a high degree of client involvement, and therapy that is simple and inexpensive.
  2. Aim of treatment is control, not cure.
  3. Exposure to sunlight may be beneficial. However, symptoms worsen in a small percentage of clients with exposure to sunlight.
  4. Mild to moderate disease may be treated with phototherapy if allowable because of cost.
  5. Sequence of agents for involvement of <20% body surface is as follows:
    a. Emollients.
    b. Keratolytic agents (salicylic acid gel or ointment).
    c. Topical corticosteroids: Use lowest potency to control disease.
    d. Calcipotriol and calcitriol topical formulations: Vitamin D analogue calciprotinol, calcipotriol-steroid, calcitriol topical.
    e. Coal tar: Use in conjunction with topical steroids or anthralin. May apply at bedtime, or in the morning for 15 minutes and then shower off.
    f. Medicated shampoos: Useful for scalp psoriasis in conjunction with topical steroids and other treatments.
B. Client teaching: *Refer to Client Teaching Guide: Psoriasis.* ◀ Help the client understand the chronic nature of this disease, characterized by flares and remission. Teach stress monitoring and control. Assist with coping techniques.
  1. A trial of a gluten-free diet may be tried to help symptoms. See Appendix B: "Gluten-Free Diet."

2. If phototherapy is not effective, systemic agents are recommended.
C. Pharmacological therapy: If the disease is not controlled with the first agent, then an alternative agent may be tried:
   1. Mild to moderate disease: Topical steroids as first-line therapy.
   2. Emollients to start treatment.
   3. Scalp: Use coal tar shampoo in place of regular shampoo two times per week.
      a. Apply lather to scalp, allow to soak for five minutes, and then rinse.
      b. If plaques are very thick, use P and S Liquid (over the counter [OTC]). Massage in at night and wash out in the morning.
   4. For additional treatment as needed, apply triamcinolone acetonide 0.1% lotion or equivalent to scaly, stubborn areas once or twice daily until controlled. **Avoid face.**
   5. Dovonex scalp solution: Apply on dry scalp as directed.
   6. Face and skin folds: Hydrocortisone cream.
   7. Body, arms, and legs: Use triamcinolone topical cream twice. **Avoid normal skin.**
   8. For thick plaques, try salicylic acid or salicylic acid–corticosteroid combination therapy.
   9. Use coal tar once or twice daily in combination with corticosteroids.
   10. Anthralin is beneficial as an alternate to steroid lotion for scalp psoriasis. **Avoid sunlight.**
   11. Vitamin D3 analogue is comparable to mid-potency corticosteroids. **Avoid face and skin folds.**
   12. Systemic agents for moderate to severe psoriasis may be used if other measures fail. Systemic agents should be prescribed by a dermatology specialist; these medications include retinoids, methotrexate, cyclosporine, and apremilast. These medications should be monitored closely for liver/kidney function changes.

Follow-Up
A. See clients in two to three weeks to evaluate treatment.
B. Follow up in two months to monitor side effects.
C. Follow-up must be individualized for each client.

Consultation/Referral
A. Medical management: For involvement >20% of body, refer the client to a dermatologist for the following:
   1. Light therapy with ultraviolet A (UVA) or UVB. UVB light therapy is often used in conjunction with keratolytic agents.
   2. Synthetic retinoids: Etretinate or acitretin are options.
   3. Low-dose cyclosporine or sulfasalazine can be effective.
B. Refer clients with extensive disease, psoriatic arthritis, or inflammatory disease to a rheumatologist. New medications, called biologics, are used to suppress the immune system's response; they include adalimumab, alefacept, etanercept, infliximab, and ustekinumab.
C. Cases of generalized pustular psoriasis of exfoliative erythroderma should be referred immediately to a dermatologist.
D. All systemic therapies should be given under supervision of a dermatologist or rheumatologist.

Individual Considerations
A. Adults: Clients with moderate to severe disease that is not well controlled should be referred to a dermatology specialist for systemic treatment.

Bibliography
Canadian Dermatology Association. (2018b). *Psoriasis*. Retrieved from https://dermatology.ca/public-clients/skin/psoriasis/
Habif, T. P. (Ed.). (2011). *Skin disease diagnosis and treatment* (3rd ed.). Philadelphia, PA: Saunders Elsevier.
Kim, W.B., Jerome, D., & Yeund, J. (2017, April). Diagnosis and management of psoriasis. *Canadian Family Physician, 63*, 278–285.
Monroe, J. (2012). Papules and plaques from head to foot. *Journal of the American Academy of Physician Assistants, 25*(9), 16. doi:10.1097/01720610-201209000-00003
Weigle, N., & McBane, S. (2013). *Psoriasis. American Family Physician, 87*(9), 626–633.

Scabies

Jill C. Cash, Amy C. Bruggemann, Elsie Duff, and Cindy Fehr

Definition
A. Scabies is a contagious skin infestation by the mite *Sarcoptes scabiei*.

Incidence/Prevalence
A. Scabies occurs mainly in individuals in close contact with many other individuals, such as schoolchildren or nursing-home residents. It is estimated that 300 million cases globally occur annually across individuals of varying socioeconomic levels. In Canada, incidence is disproportionally higher in those living in overcrowded situations and Indigenous communities with preexisting risk factors.

Pathogenesis
A. Scabies is transmitted through close contact with an individual who is infested with the mite *S. scabiei*. Transmission may occur through sexual contact or contact with mite-infested clothing or sheets. The fertilized female mite burrows into the stratum corneum of a host and deposits eggs and faecal pellets. Larvae hatch, mature, and repeat the cycle.
B. A hypersensitivity reaction is responsible for the intense pruritus.

Predisposing Factors
A. Close contact with large numbers of individuals.
B. Institutionalization.
C. Poverty.
D. Sexual promiscuity.

Common Findings
A. Intense itching, worse at night.
B. Skin excoriation.
C. Generalized pruritus.
D. Rash.

Other Signs and Symptoms
A. Mites burrow in finger webs, at wrists, in the sides of hands and feet, at the axilla buttocks, and in the penis and scrotum in males.
B. Discrete vesicles and papules, distributed in linear fashion.
C. Erythema is a symptom.

D. Secondary infections caused by scratching or infection (pustules and pinpoint erosions).
E. Nodules in covered areas (buttocks, groin, scrotum, penis, and axilla), which may have slightly eroded surfaces that persist for months after mites have been eradicated.
F. Diffuse eruption that spares the face.

Subjective Data
A. Elicit information regarding housing conditions, close contact, or sexual contact with potentially infected individuals.
B. Question the client regarding onset, duration, and location of itching.

Physical Examination
A. Check temperature.
B. Inspect:
   1. Examine all body surfaces with client unclothed.
   2. Use a magnifying lens to identify characteristic burrows in finger webs, wrists, and penis.
   3. Inspect adult pubic area for lesions.

Diagnostic Tests
A. Three findings are diagnostic of scabies:
   1. Microscopic identification of *S. scabiei* mites.
   2. Eggs.
   3. Faecal pellets (scybala).
B. Burrow identification: Ink the suspected area with a blue or black felt-tipped pen, then wipe with an alcohol swab. The burrow absorbs the ink, while the surface ink is wiped clean.
C. A tiny black dot may be seen at the end of a burrow, which represents the mite, ova, or faeces, and can be transferred by means of a 25-gauge hypodermic needle to immersion oil on a slide for microscopic identification.
D. Place a drop of mineral oil on a suspected lesion, scrape the lesion with a no. 15 blade, and transfer the shaved material to a microscope slide for direct examination of the mite under low power.

Differential Diagnoses
A. Atopic dermatitis.
B. Insect bites.
C. Pityriasis rosea.
D. Eczema.
E. Seborrhoeic dermatitis.
F. Syphilis.
G. Pediculosis.
H. Allergic or irritant contact dermatitis.

Plan
A. General interventions:
   1. Implement comfort measures to reduce pruritus.
   2. Treat secondary infection(s) with antibiotics.
   3. Household members should be treated simultaneously as a prophylactic measure and to reduce the chance of reinfection. Individuals can return to work, school, or day care after first treatment cycle.
   4. All bed linens and clothing worn next to skin should be laundered in hot water and dry cycles or stored in sealed plastic bags for five to seven days.
   5. The client should be advised that pruritus may continue for up to a week even with a successful treatment because of local irritation.
B. Client teaching: *Refer to Client Teaching Guide: Scabies.*
C. Pharmacological therapy:
   1. First line of therapy, because of its low toxicity (safe in those over 3 months of age), is 5% permethrin applied to all body areas from the neck down and washed off in eight to 14 hours. One application is highly effective, but some dermatologists recommend retreatment in one week.
   2. Alternative therapy is lindane 1% cream, applied to all skin surfaces from the neck down and washed off in eight to 12 hours. Some dermatologists retreat in one week.
   3. Another alternative treatment is sulphur compounded in petroleum jelly, which is safe in pregnancy and with infants, but messy and malodourous.
   4. A single oral dose of the anthelmintic agent ivermectin has been shown to be effective and to rapidly control pruritus in healthy clients and HIV clients. Only available through Health Canada's Special Access Programme.
   5. Diphenhydramine if indicated for pruritus. Other nonsedating antihistamines may be used. Toxicity is usually a result of client overtreatment (failure to follow prescribed regimen). Advise the client of this danger.

Follow-Up
A. Follow up in two weeks to assess treatment response.

Consultation/Referral
A. Consult or refer the client to the physician if, at two-week follow-up, pharmacological therapy has been ineffective.

Individual Considerations
A. Pregnancy:
   1. Permethrin is preferred to lindane in pregnant and/or lactating women because of decreased toxicity.
   2. Client should be warned of its potential to cause neurotoxicity and convulsions with overuse (more than two treatments).
B. Paediatrics:
   1. Infants and toddlers often have more widespread involvement that can include the face and scalp.
   2. Vesicular lesions on palms and soles are more commonly seen.
   3. First-line treatment is permethrin 5% cream; apply over the head, neck, and body, avoiding the eyes. The cream should be removed by bathing within eight to 14 hours.
   4. Lindane should not be used in infants and toddlers.
   5. Infants and children with underlying cutaneous disease, malnutrition, prematurity, or a history of seizure disorders should be treated with special caution because of their increased risk of toxicity.
C. Partners: All intimate contacts within the past month and close household and family members should be treated to avoid transmission and reinfestation.
D. Geriatrics:
   1. The elderly tend to have more severe pruritus despite fewer lesions.
   2. They are at risk of extensive infections because of age-related decline in immunity.
   3. The excoriations may become severe and may be complicated by cellulitis.

Bibliography

Canadian Paediatric Society. (2015). *Position statement: Scabies*. Retrieved from https://www.cps.ca/en/documents/position/scabies

Government of Canada. (2013). Canadian guidelines on sexually transmitted infections—Management and treatment of specific infections—Ectoparasitic infestations (Section 5–3). Retrieved from https://www.canada.ca/en/public-health/services/infectious-diseases/sexual-health-sexually-transmitted-infections/canadian-guidelines/sexually-transmitted-infections/canadian-guidelines-sexually-transmitted-infections-31.html

Gunning, K., Pippitt, K., Kiraly, B., & Sayler, M. (2012). Pediculosis and scabies: Treatment update. American Family Physician, 86 (6), 535–541.

Habif, T. P. (Ed.). (2011). *Skin disease diagnosis and treatment* (3rd ed.). Philadelphia, PA: Saunders Elsevier.

Mounsey, K. E., & McCarthy, J. S. (2013). Treatment and control of scabies. *Current Opinion in Infectious Diseases, 26*(2), 133–139. doi:10.1097/QCO.0b013e32835e1d57

Seborrhoeic Dermatitis

Jill C. Cash, Amy C. Bruggemann, Elsie Duff, and Cindy Fehr

Definition
A. A common chronic, erythematous, scaling dermatosis, seborrhoeic dermatitis occurs in areas of the most active sebaceous glands such as the face and scalp, body folds, and presternal region.

Incidence/Prevalence
A. Seborrhoeic dermatitis is very common.
B. Incidence is higher in HIV-infected individuals.

Pathogenesis
A. Aetiology is unknown. There is a possibility that it is hormonally dependent, has a fungal (*Pityrosporum ovale* or *Candida albicans*) component, is neurogenic, or may reflect a nutritional deficiency.
B. Currently, it is identified as an inflammatory disorder that most probably results from a dysfunction of sebaceous glands.

Predisposing Factors
A. Possible link between infantile and adult forms.
B. Possible familial trend.
C. High association with HIV-infected individuals.

Common Findings
A. Infants: "Cradle cap."
B. Adults: "Dandruff," dry flaky scalp.
C. Rash with "sticky flakes."

Often no presenting complaints are found on a routine physical examination.

Other Signs and Symptoms
A. Variable pruritus, often increasing with perspiration and in winter.
B. Oily, flaking skin on erythemic base around ears, nose, eyebrows, and eyelids.
C. Red, cracking skin in body folds; axilla; groin; or anogenital, submammary, or umbilical areas.
D. Primary lesions: Plaques.
E. Secondary lesions: Erythema, scales, fissures, exudate, and symmetric eyelid involvement.
F. Lesions with drainage or crusting may indicate secondary bacterial infection.
G. Distribution pattern in infants: Scalp and diaper area.
H. Distribution area in adults: Scalp, eyebrows, paranasal area, nasolabial fold, chin, behind ears, chest, and groin.
I. Secondary impetigo in children.

Subjective Data
A. Identify location, onset, and progression of symptoms.
B. Ask the client to describe symptoms. Ask whether the skin is itchy or painful.
C. Assess lesions for any associated discharge (blood or pus).
D. Elicit information regarding use of topical medications, soaps, creams, or lotions. Quiz the client regarding any oral medications being taken.
E. Determine whether there were any preceding systemic symptoms (fever, sore throat, anorexia, or vaginal discharge).
F. Rule out any possible exposure to industrial or domestic toxins.
G. Ask the client to identify what improves or worsens this condition.

Physical Examination
A. Inspect:
  1. Skin; note areas of lesions and distribution.
  2. Eyes, for blepharitis.
  3. Ears and nose.
B. Palpate skin, noting texture and moisture.

Diagnostic Tests
A. None required.
B. Consider fungal culture in children and adolescents to rule out a fungal infection.
C. Consider possible skin biopsy to rule out other conditions.

Differential Diagnoses
A. Atopic dermatitis.
B. Candidiasis.
C. Dermatophytosis.
D. Histiocytosis X.
E. Psoriasis vulgaris.
F. Rosacea.
G. Systemic lupus erythematosus.
H. Tinea capitis.
I. Tinea versicolour.
J. Vitamin deficiency.
K. Impetigo.
L. Eczema.

Plan
A. General interventions:
  1. Shampooing is the foundation of treatment:
     a. Infants: Rub petroleum jelly into scalp to soften crusts 20 to 30 minutes before shampooing.
     b. Shampoo daily with baby shampoo using a soft brush.
     c. Toddlers or adolescents: Shampoo every other day with antiseborrhoeic shampoo.
  2. If skin does not clear after one to two weeks of treatment, it is appropriate to use ketoconazole 2% cream.
  3. Seborrhoeic blepharitis:
     a. Hot compresses plus gentle debridement with cotton-tipped applicator and baby shampoo twice a day.
     b. For secondary bacterial infection, sulfacetamide sodium 10%.

    4. Continue treatment for several days after lesions disappear.
B. Client teaching: *Refer to Client Teaching Guide: Seborrhoeic Dermatitis.*
C. Pharmacological therapy:
    1. Most shampoos should be used two times per week. Those with coal tar can be used three times per week.
    2. Medicated shampoos:
        a. Coal tar shampoo, apply as directed.
        b. Salicylic acid shampoo, apply as directed.
        c. Selenium sulphide shampoo, use daily.
        d. Ketoconazole 2% cream.
        e. Combination shampoos: Coal tar and salicylic acid; salicylic acid and sulphur. These shampoos may be used one to two times a week, alternating with other shampoos during the week. Always apply corticosteroids in a thin layer only; avoid the eyes.
        f. Ciclopirox olamine prescription-strength antifungal shampoo.
    3. Topical corticosteroid lotions or solutions: Use in combination with medicated shampoo if two to three weeks of treatment with shampoo alone fails.
    4. Adults: Scalp:
        a. Start with medium potency; for example, betamethasone valerate 0.1% lotion.
        b. If treatment is not effective in two weeks, increase potency; for example, fluocinonide 0.05% or fluocinolone acetonide 0.01% oil.
        c. As dermatitis is controlled, decrease to mild potency; for example, hydrocortisone 1% to 2.5%.
    5. Adults: Face or groin:
        a. Low-potency agents; for example, hydrocortisone 1% cream or desonide 0.05% cream.
        b. Consider lotion for eyebrows for easier application.
        c. Metronidazole 1% gel on face once or twice daily.
    6. Recalcitrant disease:
        a. Add ketoconazole 2% cream (15, 30, or 60 g) every day.
        b. Use sulfacetamide sodium 10%, with sulfur 5%.

Follow-Up
A. Have the client to call the office in five to six days to report progress.
B. Have the client return to the office if no improvement is seen.

Consultation/Referral
A. Refer the client to a dermatologist if the condition does not clear in 10 to 14 days.

Individual Considerations
A. Pregnancy: Ketoconazole is not recommended.
B. Paediatrics:
    1. Avoid using tar preparations on infants.
    2. Use baby shampoo only.
    3. If lesions are inflammatory, use topical steroids no stronger than hydrocortisone 0.5% to 1.0% twice daily.
    4. Betamethasone valerate lotion may be used daily for scalp only if other treatments fail.
    5. Be aware of potential for emotional distress in adolescents.
    6. Treat with antiseborrhoeic shampoo every other day for adolescents.

Bibliography
Canadian Dermatology Association. (2018). *Dandruff*. Retrieved from https://dermatology.ca/public-clients/hair/dandruff/
Habif, T. P. (Ed.). (2011). *Skin disease diagnosis and treatment* (3rd ed.). Philadelphia, PA: Saunders Elsevier.
Selden, S. (2012). Seborrheic dermatitis. *Medscape*. Retrieved from http://emedicine.medscape.com/article/1108312-overview.

Tinea Corporis (Ringworm)

Jill C. Cash, Amy C. Bruggemann, Elsie Duff, and Cindy Fehr

Definition
A. Tinea corporis (ringworm) is a fungal infection of the skin tissue (keratin) commonly seen on the face, trunk, and extremities.

Incidence/Prevalence
A. Ringworm is a fairly common fungal infection seen in adults and children. Affecting 10% to 20% of the general population at some point in their lifetime.

Pathogenesis
A. The causative fungal species varies, depending on the location of the infection. Three common organisms are *Epidermophyton*, *Microsporum*, and *Trichophyton*.
B. The infection can be obtained from other people, animals (puppies, kittens), and the soil.

Predisposing Factors
A. Exposure to person or facilities (e.g., locker rooms) infected with the fungus.
B. Poor nutrition.
C. Poor health.
D. Poor hygiene.
E. Warm climates.
F. Immunosuppression.

Common Findings
A. Scaly, itchy patch of skin, often circular in shape.

Other Signs and Symptoms
A. Tinea capitis: Erythema, scaling of scalp, with hair loss at site asymptomatic (usually pediatric).
B. Tinea corporis: Circular, erythematous, well-demarcated lesion on the skin with hypopigmentation in center of lesion; usually pruritic.
C. Tinea cruris: Well-demarcated scaling lesions on groin (not scrotum) or thigh; usually pruritic.
D. Tinea pedis: Scaly, erythemic vesicles on feet, between toes, and in arch, with extreme pruritus.
E. Tinea unguium (onychomycosis): Thickening and yellowing of toenail or fingernail, often with other fungal infection or alone.

Subjective Data
A. Ask the client about onset, duration, and progression of the patch or rash on the skin.
B. Assess the client about other areas of skin involvement.
C. Ask whether the lesion is pruritic.
D. Inquire as to the client's exposure to anyone with similar symptoms.

▶ Client Teaching Guides are available at https://connect.springerpub.com/content/reference-book/978-0-8261-9498-5

E. Determine whether the client has a history of similar lesions.
F. Query the client regarding predisposing factors.
G. Review with the client what remedies were used and with what results.

Physical Examination
A. Check temperature (if indicated).
B. Inspect all areas of skin; note type of lesions present.

Diagnostic Tests
A. Obtain scrapings of the border of the lesion for evaluation:
   1. Potassium hydroxide (KOH).
   2. Wet preparation.
   3. Fungal cultures.

Differential Diagnoses
A. Dermatitis.
B. Alopecia areata.
C. Psoriasis.
D. Contact dermatitis.
E. Atopic eczema.

Plan
A. General interventions:
   1. Identify type of lesion.
   2. Identify other infected family members or sexual partners for treatment.
▶ B. Client teaching: *Refer to Client Teaching Guide: Ringworm Tinea*. Reinforce medication regimen for four- to eight-week period for resolution.
C. Pharmacological therapy:
   1. Tinea capitis.
      a. Adults: Terbinafine or Itraconzaole tablets or oral fluconazole.
      b. Children: Griseofulvin, which is best absorbed with high-fat foods; terbinafine, itraconazole tablets, or fluconazole oral solution.
      c. Ketoconazole may also be used.
   2. Tinea corporis, pedis, and cruris: Use wet dressings with Burow's solution along with one of the following:
      a. Clotrimazole 1% cream, or miconazole 2% topical cream.
      b. Terbinafine 1% cream. Not recommended for children.
   3. Onychomycosis: Successful treatment is difficult.
      a. Itraconazole.

Monitor LFTs at six weeks after starting medication.
LFT, liver function tests.

      b. Terbinafine oral.
      c. Topical efinaconazole.
      d. Home cure: Apply a camphor/eucalyptus/menthol ointment on toenail bed every night at bedtime for approximately four to six months or until resolved. This treatment offers a safe, cost-effective alternative to oral medications.

Follow-Up
A. A two- to four-week follow-up is recommended to evaluate progress.

B. Monitor LFT at six weeks and if itraconazole is continued longer.

Consultation/Referral
A. Consult a physician if the infection has not improved.

Individual Considerations
A. Pregnancy: Oral antifungal medications are not recommended during pregnancy.
B. Paediatrics:
   1. Tinea capitis is common in children 2 to 10 years old. When hair has been lost, regrowth takes time.
   2. Tinea pedis is common in adolescents.
   3. Tinea unguium is common in adolescents, but rare in children.
C. Adults:
   1. Tinea capitis is rare in adults.
   2. Tinea cruris is more common in obese males, but rare in females.
   3. Tinea pedis is common in adults.
   4. Tinea unguium is seen in adults.

Bibliography
Derby, R., Rohal, P., Jackson, C., Beutler, A., & Olsen, C. (2011). Novel treatment of onychomycosis using over-the-counter mentholated ointment: A clinical case series. *Journal of the American Board of Family Medicine, 24*(1), 69–74. doi:10.3122/jabfm.2011.01.100124

Ely, J. W., Rosenfeld, S., & Seabury Stone, M. (2014). Diagnosis and management of tinea infections. *American Family Physician, 90*(10), 702–710.

Habif, T. P. (Ed.). (2011). *Skin disease diagnosis and treatment* (3rd ed.). Philadelphia, PA: Saunders Elsevier.

Janssen Inc. (2002, Rev. 2017). *Product monograph: PrSoranox®*. Retrieved from https://www.janssen.com/canada/sites/www_janssen_com_canada/files/prod_files/live/sporanox_caps_cpm.pdf

Lee, M., Jensen, B., & Regier, L., (2017). Acne treatment. *RxFiles drug comparison charts* (11th ed., pp. 33-34). Saskatoon, SK: Saskatoon Health Region. Available from: www. RxFiles.ca

medSask. (2017). *Tinea corporis infection–Guidelines for prescribing topical antifungals*. Retrieved from http://m.medsask.usask.ca/professional/guidelines/tinea-corporis-infection.php

Turchin, I., Barankin, B., Alanen, K. W., & Saxinger, L. (2005, April). Dermacase. *Canadian Family Physician, 51*, 499–501.

Tinea Versicolour

Jill C. Cash, Amy C. Bruggemann, Elsie Duff, and Cindy Fehr

Definition
A. Tinea versicolour is a fungal infection of the skin, and may be chronic in nature. It is most commonly seen on the upper trunk; however, it may spread to extremities.

Incidence/Prevalence
A. Tinea versicolour is seen most frequently in adolescents and young adults.

Pathogenesis
A. Tinea versicolour is a fungal infection of the skin caused by an overgrowth of *Pityrosporum orbiculare*, part of the normal skin flora.
B. Discolouration of the skin is seen, forming round or oval maculae, which may become confluent.
C. Maculae range from 1 cm to very large, >30 cm.

▶ Client Teaching Guides are available at https://connect.springerpub.com/content/reference-book/978-0-8261-9498-5

Predisposing Factors
A. Immunosuppressive therapy.
B. Pregnancy.
C. Warm temperatures.
D. Corticosteroid therapy.

Common Findings
A. Scaly rash on the upper trunk with occasional mild itching.

Other Signs and Symptoms
A. Annular maculae with mild scaling.
B. Asymptomatic or pruritic.
C. Pink-, white-, or brown-coloured rash.

Subjective Data
A. Ascertain when and where the rash began.
B. Have the client describe how the rash has changed.
C. Assess the client for any associated symptoms with the rash, such as itching and burning.
D. Identify what products the client has used on the skin to treat rash, and with what results.
E. Elicit information regarding a history of similar rashes.
F. Query the client regarding current medications.
G. Review any medical history for comorbid conditions.

Physical Examination
A. Inspect:
  1. Skin, note type of lesion.
  2. Other areas of skin, for similar lesions.

Diagnostic Tests
A. Wet preparation/potassium hydroxide (KOH).
B. Wood's lamp: Wood's lamp is useful in examining skin to determine the extent of infection. Inspection of fine scales with Wood's lamp reveals scales with a pale yellow-green fluorescence that contains the fungus.
C. Culture lesion: When obtaining a sample scraping, obtain the sample from the edge of the lesion for the best sample of hyphae. (Hyphae and spores have a "spaghetti and meatball" appearance.).

Differential Diagnoses
A. Tinea corporis.
B. Pityriasis alba.
C. Pityriasis rosea: Herald patch is clue to diagnosis.
D. Seborrhoeic dermatitis.
E. Vitiligo.

Plan
A. General interventions: Apply medication as directed.
▶ B. Client teaching: *Refer to Client Teaching Guide: Tinea Versicolour.* These causative species are a normal inhabitant of skin flora; recurrence is possible.
  1. Skin pigmentation returns after infection is cleared up. This may take several months to resolve.
C. Pharmacological therapy:
  1. Selenium sulphide 2.5%.
     a. Apply to skin at bedtime one time. Shower off in the morning.
     b. For 12 days, apply Selsun Blue to skin lesions, wait 30 minutes, and then shower off.
     c. Treatment may be needed monthly until desired results are obtained. Encourage use of Selsun Blue on entire body surface except for face and head.
  2. Other medications used:
     a. Clotrimazole 1% cream.
     b. Ketoconazole cream, for adults only. When using ketoconazole as treatment, caution the client regarding liver damage with toxicity.

Follow-Up
A. None is required if resolution occurs.
B. Monitor liver function tests (LFTs) every six weeks if client is on ketoconazole.

Consultation/Referral
A. Consult with a physician if current treatment is unsuccessful.

Individual Considerations
A. Paediatrics: Commonly seen in adolescents.
B. Adults: Commonly seen in young adults.

Bibliography
Ely, J. W., Rosenfeld, S., & Seabury Stone, M. (2014). Diagnosis and management of tinea infections. *American Family Physician, 90*(10), 702–710.
Habif, T. P. (Ed.). (2011). *Skin disease diagnosis and treatment* (3rd ed.). Philadelphia, PA: Saunders Elsevier.

Warts
Jill C. Cash, Amy C. Bruggemann, Elsie Duff, and Cindy Fehr

Definition
A. A wart is an elevation of the epidermal layer of the skin (skin tumour). Warts are caused by the papillomavirus.

Incidence/Prevalence
A. Warts occur in people of all ages, more common in children and during early adulthood.
B. By adulthood, 90% of all people have positive antibodies to the virus.
C. Warts are seen more frequently in females than in males.

Pathogenesis
A. A circumscribed mass develops on the skin that is limited to the epidermal layer. The virus, papillomavirus, is located within the nucleus of the cell.
B. The virus may be transmitted by touch and is commonly seen on the hands and feet.
C. Most warts resolve without treatment within 12 to 24 months.

Predisposing Factors
A. Skin trauma.
B. Immunosuppression.
C. Exposure to public showers, pools, locker rooms, and so forth.

Common Findings
A. Bump on the skin or specific area of the body (hands, feet, arms, and legs).
B. Usually painless unless present on the bottom of the foot.

▶ Client Teaching Guides are available at https://connect.springerpub.com/content/reference-book/978-0-8261-9498-5

Other Signs and Symptoms
A. Common wart (verruca vulgaris): Flesh-coloured, irregular lesion with rough surface; black dots in center of lesion occasionally seen, which are thrombosed capillaries; can occur on any body part.
B. Filiform wart (verruca filiformis): Thin, threadlike, projected papule on face, lips, nose, or eyelids.
C. Flat wart (verruca plana): Flat-topped, flesh-coloured papule, 1 to 3 mm in diameter, with smooth surface, seen in clusters or in a line, on face and extremities.
D. Plantar wart (verruca plantaris): Firm papula, 2 to 3 cm in diameter, indented into skin with verrucous surface; painful with ambulation when placed on ball or heel of foot.
E. Genital warts: See Chapter 15, "Sexually Transmitted Infections Guidelines."

Subjective Data
A. Determine onset, location, and duration of tumour.
B. Elicit information regarding a history of previous warts.
C. Identify with the client what treatment has been used in the past and what the results were. Question the client regarding length of time over-the-counter (OTC) medications were used, and how aggressive he or she was with the treatment.

Physical Examination
A. Inspect:
　1. Assess skin for lesions, noting location, appearance, size, and surface texture of tumour(s).
　2. Examine the entire body for other lesions.

Diagnostic Test
A. None indicated.

Differential Diagnoses
A. Wart:
　1. Verruca vulgaris.
　2. Verruca filiformis.
　3. Verruca plana.
　4. Verruca plantaris.
B. Seborrhoeic keratosis.
C. Callus.
D. Molluscum contagiosum: Flesh-coloured group of firm papules found on the face, trunk, and/or extremities. A white core may be expressed from the lesion. Lesion may be successfully removed by curettage or cryotherapy.

Plan
A. General interventions:
　1. Identify the type of wart.
　2. Conservative treatment is recommended for children.
▶ **B.** Client teaching: *Refer to Client Teaching Guide: Warts.*
C. Pharmacological therapy:
　1. Common wart: After soaking and filing wart with a nail file, apply one of these.
　　a. Salicylic acid 17% gel twice daily for up to 12 weeks if needed. Keep site covered with adhesive.
　　b. Apply duct tape to site after treatment. Repeat this treatment every night for up to 12 weeks or until resolved.
　　c. Cryotherapy with liquid nitrogen to site. Repeat every three to four weeks until resolved. Apply adhesive tape over site and keep covered.
　2. Flat wart or filiform wart:
　　a. Retinoic acid: Apply to site twice daily for four to six weeks.
　　b. Imiquimod 5% cream may be applied by the client at home. Although the labeled use is for genital warts, the client may consider off-label use at bedtime and wash off after six to eight hours every other day until resolved. Precautions should be stressed regarding the caustic nature of the cream to healthy skin.
　3. Plantar wart: Salicylic acid 40%, apply over wart. Remove in 24 to 48 hours, and remove dead skin with a pumice stone or by scraping or using a nail file. Repeat every 24 to 48 hours until wart is removed. May take up to six to eight weeks.
　4. Educate the client to throw away the emory board nail file after each use. If using a nail file, after each use, cleanse with alcohol.

Follow-Up
A. Follow the client every four to six weeks until resolved.

Consultation/Referral
A. If diagnosis is unclear, refer the client to a dermatologist for surgical excision and biopsy.

Individual Consideration
A. Paediatrics: Warts are commonly seen in young school-aged children.

Bibliography
Dinulos, J.G.H. (2018). *Warts*. Merck Manual Professional Version. Retrieved from https://www.merckmanuals.com/professional/dermatologic-disorders/viral-skin-diseases/warts
Finley, C., Korownyk, C., & Kolber, M. R. (2016). What works best for nongenital warts? *Canadian Family Physician, 62*(12), 997.
Habif, T. P. (Ed.). (2011). *Skin disease diagnosis and treatment* (3rd ed.). Philadelphia, PA: Saunders Elsevier.

Wound Care

Lower Extremity Ulcer
Amy C. Bruggemann, Elsie Duff, and Cindy Fehr

Definition
A. Vascular ulcer:
　1. Arterial/ischaemic ulcer: Skin ulcers usually found on the medial or lateral foot or ankle; ulcers are nonhealing because of inadequate arterial flow.
　2. Venous ulcer: Chronic skin and subcutaneous lesions are usually found on the lower extremity between the ankle and knee, thought to occur from intracellular oedema or inflammatory processes.
B. Diabetic foot ulcer: Skin ulcers are usually found on the plantar surface of the foot, most commonly occurring from trauma or plantar pressure.

Incidence/Prevalence
A. Diabetic foot ulcer prevalence in Canada is estimated at 75 per 100,000 population, with a male dominance of 63%. The economic burden is estimated at over $21,000 annual cost per case, or more than $540 million nationally. Amputations related to diabetic ulcers increase mortality rate to 50% in five years.

▶ Client Teaching Guides are available at https://connect.springerpub.com/content/reference-book/978-0-8261-9498-5

B. The estimated prevalence of venous ulcers in Canada is approximately one per 1,000 population and a recurrence rate of up to 34% at 12 months.
C. Up to 20% of lower extremity ulcers have been shown to have mixed aetiology disease.

Pathogenesis
A. An ulcer that is found between the knees and toes constitutes a lower extremity ulcer, and guidelines are based according to the aetiology. The thing to remember with lower extremity ulcers is that they may have more than one cause. The most common aetiologies are venous insufficiency, arterial insufficiency, diabetic foot ulcer, and/or pressure of time.

Predisposing Factors
A. Arterial insufficiency.
B. Congestive heart failure.
C. Coronary artery disease.
D. Diabetes.
E. Oedema.
F. Hyperlipidaemia.
G. Obesity.
H. Age: Older than 65 years.
I. Venous insufficiency.
J. Peripheral neuropathy.

Common Findings
A. Lower extremity or foot pain.
B. Bleeding.
C. Drainage.
D. Hyperglycaemia.

Subjective Data
A. Ask the client to describe the location and onset. What does he or she think may have been the cause? Was the onset sudden or gradual? How have the symptoms continued to develop?
B. Assess whether the area is itchy or painful. Does the client feel the area?
C. Assess for any associated drainage. Ask about the colour and whether any odour is noted.
D. Complete a drug history. Ask the client whether he or she is taking any steroids or anticoagulants.
E. Has the client been treated in this location before? If so, describe.
F. Determine whether the client has attempted to treat this at home. If yes, with what?
G. Does the client have any numbness or tingling in the lower extremities? Does the client wake up at night with pain? Does he or she have any pain with ambulation? Does he or she have sensation in the feet?
H. Rule out any possible exposure to industrial or domestic toxins or insect bites.
I. Assess for iodine and sulfa allergies before starting treatment.

Physical Examination
A. Check temperature, pulse, respiration, and blood pressure.
B. Inspect:
  1. Assess the lower extremities, feet, and toes:
    a. Colour of the skin:
      i. Assess skin: Begin at the top of the legs, move down the legs to the toes looking for changes in colour that may exhibit signs of ischaemia.
      ii. Haemosiderin staining may exhibit venous insufficiency.
  2. Inspect the ulcer:
    a. Measure length × width × depth:
      i. Undermining: Measure and note location, using the face of a clock to document the site of undermining: 12 o'clock, 3 o'clock, 6 o'clock, or 9 o'clock.
      ii. Tunneling: Measure and note the location, using the face of a clock to document the site of tunneling: 12 o'clock, 3 o'clock, 6 o'clock, or 9 o'clock.
    b. Describe the wound bed:
      i. Tissue in the wound bed: Necrotic tissue, granulation tissue, or epithelial tissue.
      ii. Colour of the tissue (percentage to equal 100%, i.e., 80% pink, 20% yellow): Red, pink, yellow, brown, tan, or black.
      iii. Drainage:
        1) Amount: None, scant, moderate, or copious.
        2) Colour: Serous, sanguineous, purulent, yellow, serosanguineous, or green.
      iv. Odour.
      v. Periwound:
        1) Intact.
        2) Not intact: Describe periwound—Note erythema, fever, induration, maceration, excoriation, calloused, or epiboly.
C. Palpate:
  1. Note temperature of the skin.
  2. Assess sensation of the skin.
  3. Check capillary refill.
  4. Assess pulses in bilateral extremities.

Diagnostic Tests
A. Ankle brachial index (ABI).
B. Arterial Doppler.
C. Bone scan.
D. Complete blood count (CBC).
E. Haemoglobin A1C.
F. MRI.
G. Wound culture.
H. Wound biopsy.
I. Venous Doppler.
J. X-ray.

Differential Diagnoses
A. Vascular ulcer:
  1. Arterial/ischaemic ulcer.
  2. Venous ulcer.
B. Diabetic foot ulcer.
C. Abscess.
D. Atypical ulcers.
E. Dermatological disorder.
F. Necrotizing fasciitis.
G. Skin cancers.
H. Pressure ulcer.
I. Trauma.
J. Pyoderma gangrenosum.

Plan
A. General interventions:
  1. Vascular ulcers:
    a. Arterial ulcer:

i. Refer to vascular surgery for assessment to improve arterial flow.
ii. Refer to wound care specialist.
b. Venous ulcer:
  i. Establish arterial flow, refer to vascular surgeon if deficiency found.
  ii. For signs and symptoms of infection, treat the infection first with tissue culture and sensitivity. Treat per pharmacological recommendations. Treat with silver alginate to the site for moderate drainage and silver gel to the site for scant drainage.
  iii. Once arterial flow has been established as sufficient and infection has been ruled out, compression therapy is the mainstay of treatment for venous ulcers. Compression therapy recommendations:
    1) ABI: 0.8 to 1.0 full compression:
      a) High compression: Change in three to seven days; if tolerating, then change weekly.
    2) ABI: 0.6 to 0.8 Light compression:
      a) Moderate compression: Change in two to seven days; if tolerating well, then change weekly.
2. Diabetic foot ulcer:
  a. Establish arterial flow, refer to a vascular surgeon if deficiency found.
  b. For signs and symptoms of infection, use a sterile culturette to obtain a tissue culture and sensitivity first to assess what organism is present and to determine sensitivities. Treat per pharmacological recommendations. Treat with silver alginate to the site for moderate drainage and silver gel to the site for scant drainage.
  c. Initiate offloading to site, refer to an orthotist for assessment if devices are required.
  d. Treatment options:
    i. To debride: Cleanse with normal saline (NS), apply gel and change dressing daily and as needed.
    ii. To granulate an ulcer with scant drainage: Cleanse with NS, apply hydrogel, and change dressing daily and as needed.
    iii. To granulate an ulcer with moderate drainage: Cleanse with NS, apply calcium alginate, and change dressing daily as needed.
▶ B. Client teaching: *Refer to Client Teaching Guide: Wound Care: Lower Extremity Ulcers*.
C. Pharmacological therapy: If culture and sensitivity are performed, antibiotics may be used as recommended per sensitivity.

Follow-Up
A. Follow up in one to two weeks to evaluate therapy.
B. See clients every one to two weeks until healing well; then client may reduce to two- to four-week evaluation until complete closure.

Consultation/Referral
A. Consult or refer the client to a wound care specialist when the client has the following:
1. Extensive ulcer that you are not comfortable with (visible bone, muscle, or tendon).
2. Multiple medical comorbidities (especially diabetes).
3. Unresponsive to treatment of two to four weeks.
4. Ulcer showing decline on follow-up visit.
5. Infection present.

Individual Considerations
A. Adults:
1. Ischaemic ulcers warrant immediate referral.
2. Complaints of severe pain, lack of pulse, cool digit, or new onset of purplish/bluish discolourations to the feet require immediate workup for arterial clot to lower extremity.

Pressure Ulcers
Amy C. Bruggemann

Definition
A. "A pressure ulcer is localized damage to the skin and/or underlying soft tissue, usually over a bony prominence, or related to a medical or other device. The injury can present as intact skin or related to a medical or other device. The injury occurs as a result of intense pressure in combination with shear. The tolerance of soft tissue for pressure and shear may also be affected by microclimate, nutrition, perfusion, comorbidities and condition of the soft tissue" (Diagnosis; used with permission from the National Pressure Ulcer Advisory Panel [NPUAP], 2016).

Incidence/Prevalence
A. Acute care: 0.4% to 38%.
B. Long-term care: 2.2% to 23.9%.
C. Home care: 0% to 17%.

Pathogenesis
A. Pressure ulcers occur when an area of tissue remains in surface contact for a period of time. This contact causes occlusion of microvascular vessels, which leads to tissue hypoxia and eventually may cause ischaemia. Over time, a pressure ulcer develops. The amount of time this takes is client dependent and can be altered by physical and/or environmental factors of time.

Predisposing Factors
A. Acute illness.
B. Faecal/urinary incontinence.
C. Malnutrition.
D. Weight loss.
E. Failure or inability to offload; for example, fracture, elevation of head of bed (HOB), lack of education, or noncompliance.

Common Findings
A. Pain.
B. Bleeding.

Subjective Data
A. Ask the client to describe the location and onset. What did he or she think may have been the cause? Was the onset sudden or gradual? How have the symptoms continued to develop?

▶ Client Teaching Guides are available at https://connect.springerpub.com/content/reference-book/978-0-8261-9498-5

B. Assess whether the area is itchy or painful.
C. Assess for any associated drainage. Ask about the colour and whether any odour is noted.
D. Complete a drug history. Ask the client whether he or she is taking any steroids or anticoagulants.
E. Has the client been treated in this location before? If so, describe.
F. Determine whether the client has attempted to treat this problem at home. If yes, ask with what.
G. Rule out any possible exposure to industrial or domestic toxins or insect bites.
H. Assess for iodine and sulpha allergies before starting treatment.

Physical Examination
A. Check temperature, pulse, respirations, and blood pressure.
B. Inspect the pressure ulcer:
　1. Measure length × width × depth:
　　a. Undermining: Measure and note location, using the face of a clock to document the site of undermining: 12 o'clock, 3 o'clock, 6 o'clock, or 9 o'clock. Undermining is documented as from one time to another.
　　b. Tunneling: Measure and note location, using the face of a clock to document the site of tunneling. Tunneling is documented at one point of time per the clock face.
　2. Describe the wound bed:
　　a. Tissue in the wound bed— necrotic tissue, slough tissue, granulation tissue, or epithelial tissue.
　　b. Colour of the tissue (percentage to equal 100%, i.e., 80% pink, 20% yellow): red, pink, yellow, brown, tan, or black.
　　c. Drainage:
　　　i. Amount: none, scant, moderate, or copious.
　　　ii. Colour: serous, sanguineous, purulent, yellow, serosanguineous, or green.
　　d. Odour.
　　e. Periwound:
　　　i. Intact.
　　　ii. Not intact: erythema, fever, induration, maceration, excoriation, calloused, or epiboly.

Diagnostic Tests
A. CBC.
B. Wound culture.
C. Wound biopsy.
D. X-ray.
E. MRI.
F. Bone scan.

Diagnosis
A. Stage 1: Pressure injury—Nonblanchable erythema of intact skin:
　1. Definition: Intact skin with localized area of nonblanchable erythema, which may appear differently in darkly pigmented skin. Presence of blanchable erythema or changes in sensation, temperature, or firmness may precede visual changes. Colour changes do not include purple or maroon discolouration; these may indicate deep tissue injury.
B. Stage 2: Pressure injury—Partial-thickness skin loss with exposed dermis:
　1. Definition: Partial-thickness loss of skin with exposed dermis. The wound bed is visible, pink or red, moist, and may also present as an intact or ruptured serum-filled blister. Adipose (fat) is not visible and deeper tissues are not visible. Granulation tissue, slough, and eschar are not present. These injuries commonly result from adverse microclimate and shear in the skin over the pelvis and shear in the heel. This stage should not be used to describe moisture-associated skin damage (MASD) including incontinence-associated dermatitis (IAD), intertriginous dermatitis (ITD), medical adhesive–related skin injury (MARSI), or traumatic wounds (skin tears, burns, abrasions).
C. Stage 3: Pressure injury—Full-thickness skin loss:
　1. Definition: Full-thickness loss of skin, in which adipose (fat) is visible in the ulcer and granulation tissue and epibole (rolled wound edges) are often present. Slough and/or eschar may be visible. The depth of tissue damage varies by anatomical location; areas of significant adiposity can develop deep wounds. Undermining and tunneling may occur. Fascia, muscle, tendon, ligament, cartilage, and/or bone are not exposed. If slough or eschar obscures the extent of tissue loss, this is an unstageable pressure injury.
D. Stage 4: Pressure injury—Full-thickness skin and tissue loss:
　1. Definition: Full-thickness skin and tissue loss with exposed or directly palpable fascia, muscle, tendon, ligament, cartilage, or bone in the ulcer. Slough and/or eschar may be visible. Epibole (rolled edges), undermining, and/or tunneling often occur. Depth varies by anatomical location. If slough or eschar obscures the extent of tissue loss, this is an unstageable pressure injury.
E. Unstageable pressure injury: Obscured full-thickness skin and tissue loss:
　1. Definition: Full-thickness skin and tissue loss in which the extent of tissue damage within the ulcer cannot be confirmed because it is obscured by slough or eschar. If slough or eschar is removed, a Stage 3 or Stage 4 pressure injury will be revealed. Stable eschar (i.e., dry, adherent, intact without erythema, or fluctuance) on an ischaemic limb or the heel(s) should not be removed.
F. Deep tissue pressure injury (DTPI): Persistent nonblanchable deep-red, maroon, or purple discolouration.
　1. Definition: Intact or nonintact skin with localized area of persistent nonblanchable deep-red, maroon, purple discolouration, or epidermal separation revealing a dark wound bed or blood-filled blister. Pain and temperature change of skin precede skin colour changes. Discolouration may appear differently in darkly pigmented skin. This injury results from intense and/or prolonged pressure and shear forces at the bone–muscle interface. The wound may evolve rapidly to reveal the actual extent of tissue injury, or may resolve without tissue loss. If necrotic tissue, subcutaneous tissue, granulation tissue, fascia, muscle, or other underlying structures are visible, this indicates a full-thickness pressure injury (unstageable, Stage 3, or Stage 4). Do not use DTPI to describe vascular, traumatic, neuropathic, or dermatologic conditions.
G. Additional pressure injury definitions: This describes an aetiology. Use the staging system to stage:
　1. Medical device–related pressure injury: This describes the aetiology of the injury. Medical devicerelated pressure injuries result from the use of devices designed and applied for diagnostic or therapeutic purposes. The resultant pressure injury generally conforms to the pattern or shape of the device. The injury should be staged using the staging system.

2. **Mucosal membrane pressure injury:** Mucosal membrane pressure injury is found on mucous membranes with a history of a medical device in use at the location of the injury. Due to the anatomy of the tissue, these injuries cannot be staged.

Differential Diagnoses
A. Abscess.
B. Trauma.
C. Skin cancer.
D. Vascular ulcer.
E. Diabetic foot ulcers.
F. Dermatological disorder.
G. Venous ulcer.

Plan
A. General interventions:
  1. Identify the cause of pressure and alleviate.
  2. Steps taken to debride ulcer: Cleanse with normal saline (NS), apply ointment, and change dressing daily and as needed.
  3. Steps taken to granulate an ulcer with scant drainage: Cleanse with NS, apply hydrogel, and change dressing daily and as needed.
  4. Steps taken to granulate an ulcer with moderate drainage: Cleanse with NS, apply calcium alginate, and change dressing daily as needed.
B. Client teaching:
  1. Educate client and family regarding the treatment plans for the pressure ulcer.
  2. Stress importance of alleviating pressure to the site. Depending on location of the ulcer, provide suggestions to alleviate/offload pressure to the area.
C. Pharmacological therapy: Unless bacterial infection is present, oral antibiotics are not indicated with initial wound treatment.

Follow-Up
A. Follow up in one to two weeks to evaluate therapy.
B. See clients every one to two weeks until healing well; then client may reduce to two- to four-week evaluation until complete closure.

Consultation/Referral
A. Consult or refer the client to a wound care specialist for the following:
  1. Extensive ulcer that you are not comfortable treating.
  2. Client with multiple medical comorbidities (especially diabetes).
  3. Client not responding to treatment of two to four weeks.
  4. Ulcer showing decline on follow-up visit.
  5. Infection present needing alternative treatment.

Individual Consideration
A. Adults: Clients at end of life may develop pressure ulcers related to the dying process, referred to as Kennedy terminal ulcers. These clients are treated for comfort.

Bibliography
Baranoski, S., & Ayello, E. (2015). *Wound care essentials: Practice principle.* Philadelphia, PA: Lippincott Williams, and Wilkins.
Collins, L., & Seraj, S. (2010). Diagnosis and treatment of venous ulcers. *American Family Physician, 81*(8), 989–996.
Habif, T. P. (Ed.). (2011). *Skin disease diagnosis and treatment* (3rd ed.). Philadelphia, PA: Saunders Elsevier.
Hopkins, R. B., Burke, N., Harlock, J., Jegathisawaran, J., & Goeree, R. (2015). Economic burden of illness associated with diabetic foot ulcers in Canada. *BioMed Central health Services Research, 15*(13). doi:10.1186/s12913-015-0687-5
Hopman, W. M., Buchanan, M., VanDenKerkhof, E. G., & Harrison, M. B. (2013). Pain and health-related quality of life in people with chronic leg ulcers. *Health Canada Chronic Diseases and Injuries in Canada, 33*(3), 167–174. Retrieved from https://www.canada.ca/en/public-health/services/reports-publications/health-promotion-chronic-disease-prevention-canada-research-policy-practice/vol-33-no-3-2013/pain-health-related-quality-life-people-with-chronic-leg-ulcers.html
Kennedy, K. (2016). *Understanding the Kennedy terminal ulcer.* Retrieved from http://www.kennedyterminalulcer.com
National Pressure Ulcer Advisory Panel. (2016, April 13). *Pressure injury staging.* Retrieved from http://www.npuap.org/resources/educational-and-clinical-resources/npuap-pressure-injury-stages
National Pressure Ulcer Advisory Panel and European Pressure Ulcer Advisory Panel. (2009). *Prevention and treatment of pressure ulcers; clinical practice guideline.* Washington, DC: Author.
Reddy, M., Gill, S. S., & Rochon, P. A. (2006). Preventing pressure ulcers: A systematic review. *Journal of the American Medical Association, 296*(8), 974–984. doi:10.1001/jama.296.8.974
Shah, J., Sheffield, P., & Fife, C. (2011). *Wound care certification: Study guide.* Flagstaff, AZ: Best Publishing.
Thakral, G., LaFontaine, J., Kim, P., Najafi, B., Nichols, A., & Lavery, L. A. (2015). Treatment options for venous leg ulcers: Effectiveness of vascular surgery, bioengineered tissue, and electrical stimulation. *Advances in Skin & Wound Care, 28*(4), 164–172. doi:10.1097/01.ASW.0000462328.60670.c3
Winnipeg Regional Health Region. (2011, Rev. 2016). *Regional wound care clinical practice guidelines: Venous, arterial, and mixed lower leg ulcers.* Retrieved from http://www.wrha.mb.ca/extranet/eipt/files/EIPT-013-005.pdf

Wounds of the Skin

Jill C. Cash, Amy C. Bruggemann, Elsie Duff, and Cindy Fehr

Definition
A. Wounds are breaks in the external surface of the body.

Pathogenesis
A. Wounds can be caused by any one of the innumerable objects that breach the skin. Lacerations and abrasions typically heal by a three-stage process of clotting, inflammation, and skin cell proliferation. The most common pathogens of wound infections are *Staphylococcus aureus* and beta-haemolytic streptococcus.

Predisposing Factors
A. Exposure to accidental or intentional injury.
B. Accident prevention failure.
C. High-risk behaviours.
D. Conditions that predispose to poor wound healing:
  1. Diabetes.
  2. Corticosteroid therapy.
  3. Immunodeficiency.
  4. Advanced age.
  5. Undernourishment.

Common Findings
A. Bleeding.
B. Pain.
C. "Cut" in the skin integrity.

Other Signs and Symptoms
A. Infection: Deep wounds and dirty wounds have increased risk for infection.
B. Soft-tissue damage: Wounds with tissue necrosis have increased risk for infection.

Subjective Data

A. Elicit the client's description of how the wound occurred, including where and when the injury was sustained.
B. Ascertain how much time elapsed until treatment. If six hours have elapsed, bacterial multiplication is likely.
C. Ask whether the client is currently immunized for tetanus.
D. Complete a drug history; include any allergies to medications, anesthetics, or dressings.
E. Ask whether the client is taking any medications, especially steroids, or anticoagulants.
F. Assess iodine and sulpha drug allergies before starting treatment.
G. Review with the client whether anything significant in the past medical history may interfere with the healing process (immunodeficiency, diabetes, etc.).

Physical Examination

A. Check temperature, pulse, respirations, and blood pressure.
B. Inspect:
  1. Inspect wound.
  2. Measure wound for size: Length, width, and depth. Wounds with untidy edges may heal more slowly and with disfigurement.
  3. Assess underlying bony structures.
  4. Inspect for foreign objects.
C. Palpate:
  1. Extremities for neurovascular function and sensation.
  2. Tissue distal to wound.
  3. Lymph nodes surrounding injured area.
D. Neurologic examination: Assess motor function distal to wound.

Diagnostic Tests

A. Culture wound site if suspicious of infection.
B. Take x-ray films for deep or crushing wounds.

Differential Diagnoses

A. Wound, minor.
B. Nonaccidental self-inflicted injury.
C. Self-inflicted injury.
D. Domestic violence.

Plan

A. General interventions:
  1. Wounds that require open-wound management:
    a. Abrasions and superficial lacerations.
    b. Wounds with great amount of tissue damage.
    c. Wounds more than six hours old.
    d. Contaminated wounds.
    e. Large area of superficial skin denudation.
    f. Puncture wounds.
  2. For wounds that do not require sutures:
    a. Cleanse wound well with normal saline (NS); remove all dirt and foreign bodies.
    b. Forceful irrigation may be needed; use fine-pore sponge with a surfactant such as poloxamer 188. If wound edges easily approximate, apply Steri-Strips.
    c. Dry, sterile dressings may be used.
  3. If inflammation is present, soak and wash for 15 to 20 minutes three to four times per day. Cover with clean, dry dressing. **Do not use wound closure strips.**
  4. For wounds that require sutures:
    a. Irrigate with sterile saline solution.
    b. Anesthetize with 1% to 2% lidocaine. Do not use solution with epinephrine at fingertips, nose, or ears. Probe wound for any remaining foreign bodies. Approximate wound edges.
    c. Suture with technique appropriate to site:
      i. Skin sutures: Nonabsorbable material (e.g., nylon or silk).
      ii. Subcutaneous and mucosal sutures: Absorbable material (e.g., plain or chromic gut).
      iii. Extremities: 4–0 nylon.
      iv. Soles of feet: 2–0 nylon.
    d. Cover with clean, dry dressing; change after first 24 hours.
    e. Suture removal is based on location:
      i. Head and trunk: Five to seven days.
      ii. Extremities: Seven to 10 days.
      iii. Soles and palms: Seven to 10 days.
      iv. Distal extremities: 10 to 14 days.
    f. Tetanus prophylaxis (see Chapter 1, "Health Maintenance Guidelines").
B. Client teaching: ◄ *Refer to Client Teaching Guide: Wound Care: Pressure Ulcers.*
C. Pharmacological therapy:
  1. Control pain with acetaminophen as needed.
  2. Topical antibiotic ointments: Bacitracin and mupirocin.
  3. Oral antibiotics for prophylaxis:
    a. Amoxicillin/clavulanate.
    b. With penicillin allergy, use erythromycin.
  4. Other alternatives: Cephalexin, ciprofloxacin.
  5. Tetanus toxoid if no booster has been administered in the last five years.

Follow-Up

A. Have the client return for evaluation and dressing change in 24 to 48 hours.

Consultation/Referral

Refer the client to a physician for wounds of the type listed here:
A. Facial wounds.
B. Subcutaneous tissue penetration.
C. Functional disturbance of tendons, ligaments, vessels, or nerves.
D. Grossly contaminated wounds.
E. Wounds requiring hospitalization or aggressive antimicrobial therapy for evidence of pyogenic abscess, cellulitis, and ascending lymphangitis.
F. Wounds diagnosed with methicillin-resistant *S. aureus* should be treated with the following oral antibiotics: trimethoprim sulfamethoxazole, doxycycline, clindamycin, rifampin (should be used in combination with one of the previous antibiotics), and linezolid. Antibiotics that are not recommended because of high resistance include beta lactams, fluoroquinolones, cloxacillin, and cephalexin. Treating the nares with mupirocin 2% ointment twice a day and having the client use skin-cleansing antiseptic soap for showering will help to prevent recurrent infections. For severe cases of infection, the client requires hospitalization for aggressive antibiotic treatment.

▶ Client Teaching Guides are available at https://connect.springerpub.com/content/reference-book/978-0-8261-9498-5

Individual Consideration
A. Adults with chronic conditions, such as diabetes or immune deficiency, should be monitored closely for infection and delayed wound healing.

Bibliography
British Columbia Provincial Nursing Skin and Wound Committee. (2014). *Guideline : Assessment and treatment of lower leg ulcers (arterial, venous & mixed) in adults.* Retrieved from https://www.clwk.ca/buddydrive/file/guideline-lower-limb-venous-arterial/

Habif, T. P. (Ed.). (2011). *Skin disease diagnosis and treatment* (3rd ed.). Philadelphia, PA: Saunders Elsevier.

O'Rourke, D., et al. (2016). *Regional wound care clinical practice guidelines: Venous, arterial, and mixed lower leg ulcers.* Winnipeg Regional Health Authority. Retrieved from http://www.wrha.mb.ca/extranet/eipt/files/EIPT-013-005.pdf

Xerosis (Winter Itch)

Jill C. Cash, Amy C. Bruggemann, Elsie Duff, and Cindy Fehr

Definition
A. Xerosis, often called "winter itch," is dry skin.

Incidence/Prevalence
A. Xerosis occurs in 48% to 98% of clients with atopic dermatitis.
B. It occurs more frequently in elderly clients.

Pathogenesis
A. Dry skin may fissure, appear shiny and cracked, and leave subsequent inflammatory changes.

Predisposing Factors
A. Frequent bathing with hot water and harsh soaps.
B. Cold air.
C. Low humidity.
D. Central heating or cooling.
E. Alcohol use.
F. Poor nutrition.
G. Cholesterol-lowering drugs.
H. Systemic disease manifested by thyroid, renal, or hepatic disease; anaemia; diabetes; or malignancy.

Common Findings
A. Dry, rough skin, especially on legs.

Other Signs and Symptoms
A. Pruritic, scaling skin, particularly on legs, with cracks and/or fissures.
B. Pruritus may be associated with systematic disorders or other infections. **Itching of scabies is particularly intense at night.**
C. Plaques 2 to 5 cm in diameter.
D. Erythema.
E. Wheal-and-flare response typical of urticaria.

Subjective Data
A. Obtain the client's description of the onset of symptoms and whether it was sudden or gradual.
B. Ask the client to identify any discomfort. Ask whether the skin is itchy or painful.
C. Assess lesions for any associated discharge (blood or pus).
D. Determine whether the client has recently ingested any new medicines (antibiotics, cholesterol-lowering medications, or other drugs), alcohol, or new foods.
E. Ask the client about use of any topical medications.
F. Identify any preceding systemic symptoms (fever, sore throat, anorexia, or vaginal discharge).
G. Ask the client about bathing in hot water and whether the client is bathing regularly.
H. Review the client's full medication history for comorbid conditions.

Physical Examination
A. Inspect: Skin for lesions, noting texture of skin.
B. Palpate:
  1. Abdomen for masses and hepatosplenomegaly.
  2. Lymph nodes.

Diagnostic Test
A. There are no diagnostic tests for xerosis.

Differential Diagnoses
A. Scabies.
B. Atopic dermatitis.

Plan
A. General interventions:
  1. Hydrate and lubricate the skin.
  2. Assess for and treat secondary infection.
B. Client teaching: *Refer to Client Teaching Guide Xerosis ◀ (Winter Itch).* Advise client to avoid alkaline soaps and to use mild soap or soap substitute.
C. Pharmacological therapy:
  1. Apply emollient cream or lotion.
  2. Use over-the-counter (OTC) skin lubricants (petroleum jelly, mineral oil, or cold cream).
  3. Topical corticosteroid:
     a. Triamcinolone 0.025% two to four times daily or 0.1% two to three times daily; apply sparingly.
     b. Hydrocortisone 1% or 2.5% two to four times daily; apply thin film, avoid face.
  4. Systemic antihistamine is used to control pruritus, such as diphenhydramine.

Follow-Up
A. Follow up as indicated until resolved.

Consultation/Referral
A. Consult or refer the client to a dermatologist if no improvement is seen.

Individual Considerations
A. Paediatrics: Avoid corticosteroid preparation or use low-potency corticosteroid only.
B. Geriatrics: Monitor the client for possible skin breakdown and/or ulceration.

Bibliography
Habif, T. P. (Ed.). (2011). *Skin disease diagnosis and treatment* (3rd ed.). Philadelphia, PA: Saunders Elsevier.

Lee, M., Jensen, B., & Regier, L., (2017). *Acne treatment. RxFiles drug comparison charts* (11th ed., pp. 33–34). Saskatoon, SK: Saskatoon Health Region. Available from: www. RxFiles.ca

Nowak, D., & Yeung, J. (2017). Diagnosis and treatment of pruritus. *Canadian Family Physician*, 63, 918–24.

Oakley, A. (2015). *Dry skin.* DermNet NZ. Retrieved from https://www.dermnetnz.org/topics/dry-skin/

▶ Client Teaching Guides are available at https://connect.springerpub.com/content/reference-book/978-0-8261-9498-5

5 Eye Guidelines

Amblyopia

Jill C. Cash, Nancy Pesta Walsh, and Krista A. Bradley

Definition
A. Amblyopia is a deficiency in the visual acuity of one eye. It is commonly seen in young children and cannot be corrected with either glasses or contact lenses. There are three classifications of amblyopia based on the underlying cause:
  1. Strabismic amblyopia: Abnormal eye alignment.
  2. Refractive: Unequal focus between eyes.
  3. Deprivational: Structural abnormalities of the eye causing blurred vision.

Incidence/Prevalence
A. Amblyopia is most commonly diagnosed in children and occurs in approximately 2.5% of the population.
B. Most common cause of childhood vision loss.

Pathogenesis
Amblyopia has numerous causes, including the following:
A. Congenital defect.
B. Corneal scar or cataract.
C. Uncorrected high refractive error.
D. Strabismic amblyopia may also occur due to the loss of vision in the eye that turns inward or outward.

Predisposing Factors
A. One parent with amblyopia.
B. Prematurity.
C. Small for gestational dates.
D. Maternal smoking or alcohol use.

Common Findings
A. Decreased vision—complaints of sitting close to the TV, sitting in the front row of a classroom, having trouble seeing the ball in sports, and so on.
B. Vision that is not corrected with either glasses or contact lenses.
C. Wandering eye and frequent eye squinting.

Other Signs and Symptoms
A. Frequent rubbing of the eyes.
B. Tired eyes.

Subjective Data
A. Elicit the onset of visual changes, noting course of symptoms and severity.
B. Assess for pain or any new injury or trauma to the eye.
C. Inquire about new events or changes in health history, including contact lenses, glasses, illnesses, and cataracts.
D. Review client and family history of amblyopia.

Physical Examination
A. Inspect eyes:
  1. Note extraocular movements (EOMs) of eyes.
  2. Examine sclera, pupil, iris, and fundus.
  3. Examine eyes for red reflex.
B. Assess vision based on age, using LEA SYMBOLS®, Sloan letters, Sloan numerals, Tumbling E, and the HOTV. The Kindergarten Eye Chart and the Snellen chart are less preferred methods, as they do not meet the World Health Organization/Committee on Vision Standards.
C. Visual fields may be assessed with a parent holding the child in his or her lap.

Diagnostic Test
A. None.

Differential Diagnoses
A. Organic brain, retinal, or optic nerve lesion.
B. Psychogenic.

Plan
A. General interventions:
  1. All children need to have a visual examination prior to starting school.
  2. Recommend examination by an ophthalmologist for children with strabismus, any other abnormality found, and for those with a family history of amblyopia.
  3. Measures for refractive correction or patching of the stronger eye are usually performed to encourage the weak eye to develop.
  4. Surgery may be required for abnormal positioning of the eye.

Follow-Up
A. Follow up with an ophthalmologist.

Consultation/Referral
A. Refer the client to an ophthalmologist for evaluation and treatment.

Individual Consideration
A. None.

Bibliography

Centers for Disease Control and Prevention. (2015, September). *Vision quest initiative*. Retrieved from https://www.cdc.gov/visionhealth/faq.htm

Blepharitis

Jill C. Cash, Nancy Pesta Walsh, and Krista A. Bradley

Definition

A. Blepharitis is redness, swelling, and itching that may be accompanied by dryness and flaking of the eyelid margin, resulting from an inflammatory response of the eyelid.

Incidence/Prevalence

A. The exact incidence is not known; however, blepharitis is one of the most commonly seen eye conditions.

Pathogenesis

A. Seborrhoeic: Excessive shedding of skin cells and blockage of glands.
B. *Staphylococcus:* Most common colonizing bacteria, responsible for bacterial infection of lid margin.
C. Commonly seen with inadequate flow of oil and mucus into the tear duct.

Predisposing Factors

A. Diabetes.
B. Candida.
C. Seborrhoeic dermatitis.
D. Acne rosacea.

Common Findings

A. Burning and itching.
B. Lacrimal tearing.
C. Photophobia.
D. Recurrent eye infections, styes, or chalazions.
E. Dry, flaky secretions on lid margins and eyelashes.
F. Dry eyes.

Other Signs and Symptoms

A. Seborrhoeic blepharitis: Lid margin swelling and erythema, flaking, nasolabial erythema, and scaling.
B. *Staphylococcus aureus* blepharitis: Erythema/oedema, scaling, burning, tearing, itching, and recurrent stye or chalazia.
C. Meibomian gland dysfunction: Prominent blood vessels crossing the mucocutaneous junction, frothy discharge along eyelid margin, thick discharge, and chalazion; may have rosacea or seborrhoeic dermatitis.
D. May have dandruff on scalp and eyebrows.

Subjective Data

A. Elicit onset and duration of signs and symptoms.
B. Note sensations of itching, burning, or pain in the eye.
C. Ask, What makes signs and symptoms worse? What makes signs and symptoms better?
D. Any change in soaps, creams, lotions, or shampoos?
E. Has the client had similar signs and symptoms in the past?
F. Note any visual change or pain since the last eye examination.
G. Note contributing factors involved, if present.

Physical Examination

A. Inspection:
   1. Inspect eyes, noting extraocular movements (EOMs) of eyes.
   2. Examine sclera, pupil, iris, and fundus.
   3. Examine eyes for red reflex.
   4. Note erythema or oedema on lid margin; note dryness, scaling, and flakes.
   5. Assess vision based on age, using Snellen chart for children older than 3 years.
   6. Visual fields may be assessed with a parent holding the child in his or her lap.

Diagnostic Test

A. None.

Differential Diagnoses

A. Blepharitis:
   1. Bacterial infection.
   2. Inflammatory skin conditions/diseases.
   3. Meibomian gland dysfunction.
B. Conjunctivitis.
C. Eyelid malignancy.
D. Hordeolum (stye) or chalazion.
E. Upper respiratory infection, sinusitis.

Plan

A. General interventions:
   1. Assess client and rule out conjunctivitis and vision changes.
   2. When examining a child, notify the parent of diagnosis and educate the parent regarding the findings.
   3. Clients with recurrent blepharitis need further follow-up with an ophthalmologist.
B. Client teaching: The most important intervention is eyelid hygiene:
   1. Wash eye with antibacterial soap and water. May use gentle baby shampoo.
   2. Apply warm compresses to the eye for comfort and to liquify secretions.
   3. Lid massage in a circular motion toward to the eye after warm compresses.
   4. Using a clean washcloth, gauze, or other, clean along each lash line. Very dilute baby shampoo or commercial eyelid wash may be used.
   5. Stop use of contacts until the eye is healed.
C. Pharmacological therapy: For mild to moderate blepharitis, good eyelid hygiene may be all that is needed. For severe/chronic blepharitis or if hygienic measures are not effective, antibiotics may be considered:
   1. Apply bacitracin or erythromycin ophthalmic ointment to the margin of the eye at bedtime, taking care not to contaminate the medication bottle.
   2. Oral antibiotics: Tetracycline or doxycycline. Alternative: Erythromycin or azithromycin.

Follow-Up

A. Recommend follow-up with a primary provider in one to two weeks.
B. Consider referral to an eye specialist for recurrent episodes of blepharitis.

Individual Considerations
A. Paediatrics: Tetracycline is not recommended for children younger than eight years.
B. Pregnant or lactating women: Tetracycline is not recommended.
C. Azithromycin may lead to abnormalities of heart electrical rhythm; use with caution in clients with a high risk of cardiovascular disease.

Bibliography
American Academy of Ophthalmology. (2018, November). *Blepharitis PPP 2018*. Retrieved from https://www.aao.org/preferred-practice-pattern/blepharitis-ppp-2018

Carlisle, R. T., & Digiovanni, J. (2015). Differential diagnosis of the swollen red eyelid. *American Family Physician*, *15*(92), 106–112.

Cataracts

Jill C. Cash and Nancy Pesta Walsh

Definition
A. A cataract, opacity of the crystalline lens of the eye, causes progressive, painless loss of vision (functional impairment). Presenile and senile cataract formation is painless and progresses throughout months and years. Cataracts are frequently associated with intraocular inflammation and glaucoma.

Incidence/Prevalence
A. Cataracts are the most common cause of blindness in the world.
B. Ninety-five percent of people older than 60 years have cataracts without visual disturbance.
C. Fifty percent of people older than 40 years have significant visual loss due to cataracts.

Pathogenesis
A. Age-related changes of the lens of the eye result from protein accumulation, which produces a fibrous thickened lens that obscures vision.

Predisposing Factors
A. Age.
B. Trauma.
C. Medications (e.g., topical or systemic steroids, major tranquilizers, or some diuretics).
D. Medical diseases (e.g., diabetes mellitus, Wilson's disease, hypoparathyroidism, glaucoma, congenital rubella syndrome, chronic anterior uveitis).
E. Chronic exposure to ultraviolet (UV) B light.
F. Alcohol use.
G. Family history.
H. Prior intraocular surgery.
I. Obesity.
J. Smoking.

Common Findings
A. Decreased vision.
B. Blurred or foggy vision, "ghost" images.
C. Inability to drive at night.

Other Signs and Symptoms
A. Initial visual event can be a shift toward nearsightedness.
B. Visual impairment can be more marked at distances, with abnormal visual acuity examinations.
C. Severe difficulty with glare can occur.
D. Altered colour perception may be noticed.
E. Frequent falls or injuries may occur.

Subjective Data
A. Review the onset, course, and duration of visual changes including altered day or night vision and nearsighted versus farsighted vision.
B. Assess whether involvement is in one or both eyes.
C. Determine what improves vision—use of glasses or use of extra light.
D. Review the client's medical history and current medications.
E. Review the client's history for traumatic injury.
F. Discuss the client's occupation and leisure activities to determine exposure to UV rays.

Physical Examination
A. Inspect.
   1. Conduct a funduscopic examination:
      a. Check red reflex and opacity:
         i. A bright red reflex is seen in the normal eye.
         ii. Cataract formation is seen by the disruption of the red reflex.
         iii. Lens opacities appear as dark areas against the background of the red–orange reflex.
      b. Examine colour of opacity. For brunescent cataracts, the nucleus acquires a yellow–brown colouration and becomes progressively more opaque.
      c. Check retinal abnormalities, haemorrhage, scarring, and drusen (small yellow deposits).

Diagnostic Tests
A. Perform visual acuity examination.
B. Perform peripheral vision examination.

Differential Diagnoses
A. Glaucoma.
B. Age-related macular degeneration (macular degeneration causes vision loss that is symptomatically similar to cataracts).
C. Diabetic retinopathy.
D. Temporal arteritis.

Plan
A. General intervention:.
   1. Monitor the client for increased interference of visual impairment on his or her lifestyle.
   2. Cataracts do not need to be removed unless there is impairment of normal, everyday activities.
   3. Surgery is the definitive treatment; however, modification of glasses may improve vision adequately to defer surgery. Contact lenses are optically superior to glasses.
B. Client teaching:
   1. Prevention is important. Teach the client to use protective eyewear to prevent trauma.
   2. Use sunglasses to prevent the penetration of UVB rays.
   3. Wear a hat with a visor to protect eyes when outdoors.

Follow-Up
A. Surgical removal is indicated if the visual disturbance is interfering with the client's life, such as causing falls or prohibiting reading.

Consultation/Referral
A. Refer client for ophthalmologic consultation.
B. Clients should be followed by an ophthalmologist to monitor the cataract for increased size and progressive visual impairment.
C. Contact a social worker or community resources as needed.

Bibliography
Chang, R. T. (2018). Cataracts. BMJ Best Practices. Retrieved from https://bestpractice.bmj.com/topics/en-us/499

Chalazion

Jill C. Cash and Nancy Pesta Walsh

Definition
A. Chalazion is a chronic lipogranulomatous inflammation of a meibomian gland located in the eyelid margin. Inflammation occurs from occlusion of the ducts.

Incidence/Prevalence
A. Commonly seen, though the incidence is unknown.

Pathogenesis
A. Meibomian glands secrete the oil layer of the tear film that covers the eye. When the glands become blocked, the oil or lipid extrudes into the surrounding tissue, causing the formation of a nodule.

Predisposing Factor
A. Chalazion may occur as a result of infection of the surrounding tissues.

Common Findings
A. Swelling, nontender palpable nodule, usually pea-sized, inside lid margin or eye.
B. Discomfort or irritation due to swelling.

Other Signs and Symptoms
A. Tearing.
B. Feeling of a foreign body in the eye.
C. If infection is present, the entire lid becomes painfully swollen.

Subjective Data
A. Review the onset of symptoms, their course and duration, and any concurrent visual disturbance.
B. Question the client regarding possible foreign body or trauma to the eye.
C. Elicit the quality of pain or tenderness of the eyelid.
D. Review the past eye problems and the treatment received.

Physical Examination
A. Temperature.
B. Inspect:
  1. Inspect the eye, sclera, and conjunctiva for a foreign body.
  2. Check for red- or gray-coloured subconjunctival mass.
C. Palpate:
  1. Palpate the eyelid for masses and tenderness. Usually a hard, nontender nodule is found on the middle portion of the tarsus, away from the lid border; it may develop on the lid margin if the opening of the duct is involved. Some chalazia continue to increase in size and can cause astigmatism by putting pressure on the eye globe.
  2. Chalazia may become acutely tender; however, note the difference between the chalazia and the hordeolum (stye), which is found on the lid margin.
  3. Check for preauricular adenopathy.

Diagnostic Test
A. Perform visual acuity examination.

Differential Diagnoses
A. Chronic dacryocystitis.
B. Hordeolum (Stye).
C. Blepharitis.
D. Xanthelasma.
E. Cellulitis of the eyelid.

Plan
A. General interventions:
  1. Small chalazia, usually, do not require treatment.
  2. Warm, moist compresses may be applied for 15 minutes 4 times a day.
B. Client teaching: Instruct client regarding compresses and handwashing.
C. Pharmacological therapy:
  1. Erythromycin ophthalmic ointment.
  2. Tobradex ophthalmic drops. Not recommended in children younger than 2 years.
  3. Intrachalazion corticosteroid injection is performed by an ophthalmologist.

Follow-Up
A. For large infected chalazia, follow up with client in one week and then evaluate the client every two to four weeks.

Consultation/Referral
A. If the chalazion does not resolve spontaneously, incision and curettage by an ophthalmologist may be necessary.

Bibliography
Maurer, K. (2015). Chalazion Treatment. Kellogg Eye Center. Retrieved from http://www.med.umich.edu/1libr/Ophthalmology/comprehensive/ChalazionTreatment.pdf

Conjunctivitis

Jill C. Cash and Nancy Pesta Walsh

Definition
A. Conjunctivitis is inflammation of the conjunctiva.

Incidence/Prevalence
A. Viral conjunctivitis is the most common type; conjunctivitis occurs in 1% to 12% of newborns.

Pathogenesis
Primarily three types of conjunctivitis are seen:
A. Bacterial (*Haemophilus influenzae, Streptococcus pneumoniae, Streptococcus aureus, Neisseria gonorrhoeae*, and *Chlamydia*).
B. Viral (adenovirus, coxsackievirus, and enteric cytopathic human orphan [ECHO] viruses).
C. Allergic (seasonal pollens or allergic exposure).

Predisposing Factors
A. Contact with another person with the diagnosis of conjunctivitis.
B. Exposure to sexually transmitted infection (STI).
C. Other atopic conditions (allergies).

Common Findings
A. Red eyes.
B. Eye drainage.
C. Itching (with allergic conjunctivitis).

Other Signs and Symptoms
A. Bacterial:
   1. Fast onset, 12 to 24 hours of copious purulent or mucopurulent discharge.
   2. Burning, stinging, or gritty sensation in eyes.
   3. Crusted eyelids upon awakening, with swelling of eyelid.
   4. Usually starts out unilateral; may progress to bilateral.
   5. Bacterial conjunctivitis may present as beefy-red conjunctiva.
B. Viral:
   1. Symptoms may begin in one eye and progress to both eyes.
   2. Tearing of eyes.
   3. Sensation of foreign body.
   4. Systemic symptoms of upper respiratory infection (runny nose, sore throat, sneezing, and fever).
   5. Preauricular or submandibular lymphadenopathy.
   6. Photophobia, impaired vision.
   7. Primary herpetic infection: Vesicular skin lesion, corneal epithelial defect in form of dendrite, uveitis.
C. Allergic:
   1. Itchy, watery eyes, bilateral.
   2. Seasonal symptoms.
   3. Oedema of eyelids without visual change.
   4. With allergic conjunctivitis, hyperaemia of eyes is always bilateral and giant papillae on tarsa may be seen.
   5. May also see eczema, urticaria, and asthma flare.

Subjective Data
A. Elicit the onset, duration, and course of symptoms.
B. Question client regarding the presence of discharge upon awakening.
C. Elicit changes in vision since symptoms began.
D. Determine whether there has been any injury or trauma to the eye.
E. Assess whether these symptoms have appeared before.
F. Rule out exposure to anyone with conjunctivitis.
G. Ask client about any new events, such as use of contact lenses, change in contact lenses or solutions, or cosmetic products.
H. Review client and family history of allergies.

Physical Examination
A. Check temperature.
B. Inspect:
   1. Observe eyes for colour and foreign objects. Perform complete eye examination.
   2. Note lid oedema.
   3. Assess pupillary reflexes.
   4. Examine skin.
   5. Inspect ears, nose, and throat.
C. Auscultate heart and lungs.
D. Palpate:
   1. Palpate preauricular lymph nodes and anterior and posterior cervical chain lymph nodes.

Diagnostic Tests
A. Gram stain testing for discharge/exudate extracted from eyes if gonococcal infection is suspected and/or all neonates.
B. Culture for chlamydia, if suspected.
C. Perform fluorescein stain of eye if foreign body or corneal abrasion/ulceration is suspected.
D. Test visual acuity with the Snellen chart. Assess peripheral vision and extraocular movements (EOMs).

Differential Diagnoses
A. Conjunctivitis:
   1. Viral: Consider herpetic keratoconjunctivitis.
   2. Bacterial: Consider gonorrhoea, chlamydia.
B. Corneal abrasion.
C. Blepharitis.
D. Drug-related conjunctivitis.
E. Iritis.

Plan
A. General interventions:
   1. Distinguish among bacterial, allergic, or viral infection.
   2. Consider other diagnoses if eye pain is noted.
B. Client education: *Refer to Client Teaching Guides: Eye Medication Administration* and *Conjunctivitis*.
   1. Cool compresses to the affected eye should be applied several times a day.
   2. Clean eyes with warm, moist cloth from inner to outer canthus to prevent spreading infection.
   3. Encourage good handwashing technique with antibacterial soap.
   4. Instruct on the proper method of instilling medication into eye. Give client the teaching guide on "How to Administer Eye Medications."
   5. Instruct the female client to discard all eye makeup, including mascara, eyeliner, and eye shadow, worn at the time of the infection.
   6. Teach the client/parent the difference among bacterial, allergic, and viral infections. Educate according to appropriate diagnosis.
   7. If using aminoglycoside or neomycin ointments or drops, use caution and monitor closely for reactive keratoconjunctivitis.
   8. Bacterial conjunctivitis is contagious until 24 hours after beginning medication.
   9. Viral conjunctivitis is contagious for 48 to 72 hours, but it may last up to two weeks. This is typically self-limiting, and does not require antibiotic treatment.
C. Pharmacological therapy:
   1. Bacterial:
      a. Polymyxin B: Trimethoprim/polymyxin B sulfate ophthalmic ointment; Polymyxin B/bacitracin drops may also be used.
      b. Macrolides: Erythromycin (Ilotycin) ophthalmic ointment 0.5%.
      c. Fluoroquinolones: Ciprofloxacin 0.3% and Moxifloxacin 0.5%.

▶ Client Teaching Guides are available at https://connect.springerpub.com/content/reference-book/978-0-8261-9498-5

d. Other medications include bacitracin, sulfacetamide or bacitracin/polymyxin B ointment, fluoroquinolone or azithromycin drops. These cover the most common pathogens.
2. Viral (herpetic):
   a. Antiviral medications:
      i. Trifluridine 1% drops.
      ii. Oral antiviral medications (valacyclovir, famcyclovir) may be used for herpes simplex keratitis. Herpes zoster ophthalmicus is often treated with acyclovir, famciclovir, or valacyclovir and lessens symptoms if started within 72 hours of onset of symptoms.
3. Allergic:
   a. Topical antihistamines/mast cell stabilizer:
      i. Olopatadine HCl 0.2%: Not recommended for those younger than 3 years.
      ii. Olopatadine HCl 0.1%: Not recommended for those younger than 3 years.
   b. Mast cell stabilizer.
      i. Cromolyn sodium ophthalmic solution for children older than 4 years.
   c. Topical nonsteroidal anti-inflammatory drug (NSAID):
      i. Ketorolac tromethamine 0.5%: Not for use in children younger than 3 years. This is used for severe symptoms of atopic keratoconjunctivitis.
   d. Artificial tears four to five times daily.
   e. Oral antihistamines may be used in severe cases (loratadine or diphenhydramine HCl).
4. Concurrent conjunctivitis and otitis media should be treated with a systemic antibiotic; no topical eye antibiotic is needed.

Follow-Up
A. If resolution occurs within five to seven days after proper treatment, follow-up is not needed.
B. If client continues to have symptoms or if different symptoms appear, then follow up with the primary provider is recommended.

Consultation/Referral
A. Refer if client is suspected of having periorbital cellulitis, herpes virus infection, vision change, eye pain or if not responding to treatment.

Individual Considerations
A. Paediatrics: In neonates, consider gonococcal and chlamydial conjunctivitis. Perform culture if suspected.
B. Partners: Check partners for gonorrhoea and chlamydia when adolescent or adult presents with gonococcal or chlamydial conjunctivitis.

Bibliography
American Academy of Ophthalmology. (2013, October). *Conjunctivitis PPP 2013*. Retrieved from https://www.aao.org/preferred-practice-pattern/conjunctivitis-ppp–2013

American Academy of Ophthalmology. (2015, November). *Conjunctivitis summary benchmark 2015*. Retrieved from https://one.aao.org/summary-benchmark-detail/conjunctivitis-summary-benchmark-october-2012

Carlisle, R. T., & Digiovanni, J. (2015). Differential diagnosis of the swollen red eyelid. *American Family Physician, 15*(92), 106–112.

Corneal Abrasion

Jill C. Cash and Nancy Pesta Walsh

Definition
A. A corneal abrasion is the loss of epithelial tissue, either superficial or deep, from trauma to the eye.

Incidence/Prevalence
A. In the United States, approximately 2.4 million eye injuries occur annually.
B. Corneal abrasions account for approximately 10% of new admissions to eye emergency units.

Pathogenesis
A. Trauma occurs to the epithelial tissue of the cornea.

Predisposing Factors
A. Trauma to the eye caused by a human fingernail, tree branches, wood particles, children's toys, and sports injuries.
B. A history of surgical trauma, causing globe weakening.

Common Findings
A. Sudden onset of eye pain.
B. Foreign-body sensation in the eye.
C. Watery eye.
D. Mild photophobia.
E. Blurred vision.
F. Headache.

Other Signs and Symptoms
A. Change in vision.
B. Redness, swelling, and inability to open the eye.

Subjective Data
A. Elicit the onset, duration, and course of symptoms; note any past history of similar symptoms.
B. Question the client regarding visual changes (blurred, double, or lost vision, or loss of a portion of the visual field).
C. Question the client regarding the mechanism of injury and how much time has elapsed since the injury (minutes, hours, or days). Ask, What is his or her occupation, and what sports or activities are involved? Were goggles being worn and are they routinely worn during the sport or activity?
D. Review the client's history of exposure to herpetic outbreaks.
E. Determine the degree of pain, if any; headache, photophobia, redness, itching, or tearing.
F. Ascertain whether the client wears contact lenses or glasses and for what length of time.
G. Ask whether the client has tried any treatments before presentation to the office. If so, what?
H. Rule out the presence of any other infections, such as sinus infection. **Conjunctival discharge signifies an infectious aetiology.**

Physical Examination
A. Vital signs: Temperature.
B. Inspect:
   1. Observe *both* eyes.
   2. Test visual acuity and pupil reactivity and symmetry.

3. Observe the corneal surface with direct illumination, noting any shadow on the surface of the iris.
4. Perform funduscopic examination.
5. Evert eyelids for cornea inspection.
6. Inspect for foreign body and remove if indicated.
7. Fluorescein stain to visualize changes in epithelial lining. Cobalt blue light or Wood's lamp should be used for visualization.

Diagnostic Test
A. Perform fluorescein stain test: An epithelial defect that stains with fluorescein is the hallmark sign.

Differential Diagnoses
A. Corneal foreign body.
B. Acute-angle glaucoma.
C. Herpetic infection (herpes simplex virus [HSV]): HSV is associated with decreased corneal sensation.
D. Recurrent corneal ulceration.
E. Ulcerative keratitis.
F. Corneal erosion.

Plan
A. General interventions:
1. Superficial corneal abrasions do not need patching.
2. For deeper abrasions, apply a patch that prevents lid motion for 24 to 48 hours.
3. Pressure patch is no longer recommended.
B. Client teaching:
1. Discuss the use of protective eyewear and prevention of future ocular trauma for the client with a history of use of power tools or hammering.
2. *Refer to Client Teaching Guide: Eye Medication Administration.* Advise that the client should not use/wear contact lenses until the eye is completely healed.
C. Pharmacological therapy:
1. Antibiotic drops or ointment. Ointments are suggested over drops as they provide lubrication for the eye. Never instill antibiotic ointment if there is a possibility of a perforation. Patch the eye.
2. Adults and children: Polymyxin B sulfate or bacitracin zinc ophthalmic ointment.
3. Adults and children: Erythromycin ophthalmic ointment 0.5%.
4. Bacitracin ointment.
5. Contact lens wearers are often colonized with *Pseudomonas*, and should be treated with either a fluoroquinolone or an aminoglycoside: ciprofloxacin 0.3%, gentamycin 0.3%, or tobramycin ointment or drops.
6. Analgesics: Topical analgesics should be used sparingly: diclofenac 0.1% or ketorolac 0.5% solution.
7. Avoid use of home prescriptions, which will interfere with the healing process.
8. Avoid the use of medications containing steroids. These products may increase the risk of superinfection and may slow down the healing process.

Follow-Up
A. Reevaluate the client within 24 hours. The cornea usually heals within 24 to 48 hours.
B. Ophthalmic ointment or drops should be continued for four days after reepithelialization occurs to help in the healing process.
C. If the client is still symptomatic in 48 hours, consider referral to an ophthalmologist.

Consultation/Referral
Immediate referral to an ophthalmologist is required for large or central lesions, or deep or penetrating wounds.

Individual Considerations
A. Pregnancy: Retinal detachment should be considered as a source of eye pain and visual loss, especially in a woman with severe pregnancy-induced hypertension.
B. Paediatrics: The use of ointments is suggested over the use of eye drops due to the lubricating effect. Blurry vision may be experienced; therefore, apply the ointment at nap time and bedtime. Eye drops commonly burn/sting.
1. Pressure patches are not recommended.
2. Preventive precautions include encouraging the use of protective eyewear for contact sports, including hockey, soccer, baseball, and basketball.

Bibliography
Swaminathan, A., Otterness, K., Milne, K., & Rezaie, S. (2015). The safety of topical anesthetics in the treatment of corneal abrasions: A review. *Journal of Emergency Medicine, 49*(5), 810–815. doi:10.1016/j.jemermed.2015.06.069
Wipperman, J. L., & Dorsch, J. N. (2015). Evaluation and management of corneal abrasions. *American Family Physician, 87*(2), 114–120.

Dacryocystitis

Jill C. Cash and Nancy Pesta Walsh

Definition
A. Infection or inflammation of the lacrimal sac, or dacryocystitis, can be acute or chronic.
B. Dacryocystitis is usually secondary to obstruction.

Incidence/Prevalence
A. The incidence is unknown.

Pathogenesis
A. Bacterial infection of the lacrimal sac usually is caused by *Staphylococcus* or *Streptococcus.*

Predisposing Factors
A. Nasal trauma.
B. Deviated septum.
C. Nasal polyps.
D. Congenital dacryostenosis.
E. Inferior turbinate hypertrophy.

Common Findings
A. Pain in the eye.
B. Redness.
C. Swelling.
D. Fever.
E. Tearing.

Other Signs and Symptoms
A. Purulent exudate may be expressed from the lacrimal duct.

Subjective Data

A. Elicit the onset, course, and duration of symptoms. Are symptoms bilateral or unilateral?
B. Review the client's activity when the symptoms began to determine if aetiology is chemical, traumatic, or infectious.
C. Review other presenting symptoms such as fever and discharge.
D. Review the client's history for previous episodes. Note treatments used in past.
E. Review history for a recent herpes simplex virus (HSV) or fever blister.
F. Review ophthalmologic history.
G. Review medications.

Physical Examination

A. Check temperature, pulse, and blood pressure.
B. Inspect:
  1. Assess both eyes.
  2. Check peripheral fields of vision and sclera.
  3. Evaluate conjunctiva for distribution of redness, ciliary flush, and foreign bodies.
  4. Inspect lid margins: Evaluate for crusting, ulceration, and masses.
C. Palpate: Lacrimal duct. Discharge can be expressed from the tear duct with the application of pressure.

Diagnostic Tests

A. Check visual acuity.
B. Culture discharge for *Neisseria* if suspected.

Differential Diagnoses

A. Chalazion.
B. Blepharitis.
C. Xanthoma.
D. Bacterial conjunctivitis.
E. Hordeolum.
F. Foreign body.
G. Cellulitis.

Plan

A. General interventions:
  1. Apply warm, moist compresses at least four times per day.
  2. Instruct female clients to discard old makeup, including mascara, eyeliner, and eye shadow, used before infection.
B. Client teaching: Application of compresses, handwashing, and proper cleaning. *Refer to Client Teaching Guide: Eye Medication Administration.* See Figure 5.1.
C. Pharmacological therapy:
  1. Cloxacillin.
  2. Erythromycin.

Follow-Up

A. Follow up in two weeks if symptoms are not resolved.

Consultation/Referral

A. Refer the client to an ophthalmologist for irrigation and probing if needed.
B. Lab studies are generally performed by an ophthalmologist.

Bibliography

Carlisle, R. T., & Digiovanni, J. (2015). Differential diagnosis of the swollen red eyelid. *American Family Physician, 15*(92), 106–112.

Dry Eyes

Jill C. Cash and Nancy Pesta Walsh

Definition

A. Insufficient lubrication of the eye, or dry eyes, is caused by a deficiency of any one of the major components of the tear film.
B. Defects in tear production are uncommon but may occur in conjunction with systemic disease. Presence of systemic disease should be evaluated.

Incidence/Prevalence

A. Increased incidence of dry eyes in the elderly is due to decreased rate of lacrimal gland secretions.

Pathogenesis

A. Decreased production of one or more components of the tear film results in dry eyes. The tear film comprises three layers:
  1. An outermost lipid layer, secreted by the lid meibomian glands.
  2. A middle aqueous layer, secreted by the main and accessory lacrimal glands.
  3. An innermost mucinous layer, secreted by conjunctival goblet cells.
B. A defect in production of the aqueous phase by lacrimal glands causes dry eyes or keratoconjunctivitis sicca. The condition most often occurs as a physiological consequence of aging, and it is commonly exacerbated by dry environmental factors. It may also develop in clients with connective tissue disease.
C. In Sjögren's syndrome, the lacrimal glands become involved in immune-mediated inflammation.
D. Mucin production may decline with vitamin A deficiency.
E. Loss of goblet cells can occur secondary to chemical burns.

Predisposing Factors

A. History of severe conjunctivitis.
B. Eyelid defects such as fifth or seventh cranial nerve palsy, incomplete blinking, exophthalmos, and lid movement hindered by scar formation.
C. Drug-induced conditions, including the use of anticholinergic agents:
  1. Phenothiazine.
  2. Tricyclic antidepressants.
  3. Antihistamines.
  4. Diuretics.
  5. Isotretinoin.
D. Systemic disease such as rheumatoid disease, Sjögren's syndrome, and neurologic disease.
E. Environmental factors such as heat (wood, coal, and gas), air conditioners, winter air, and tobacco smoke.
F. Use of contacts.
G. Increasing age.
H. Lipid abnormalities.
I. Prolonged computer use.

Common Findings

A. Ocular fatigue.
B. Foreign-body sensation in the eye.

C. Itching, burning, irritation, or dry sensation in the eye.
D. Redness.
E. Eye discharge.

Other Signs and Symptoms
A. Photophobia.
B. Cloudy, blurred vision.
C. Rainbow of colour around lights. Acute angle-closure glaucoma can present with a red, painful eye; cloudy, blurred vision and a rainbow of colour around lights; dilatation of the pupil; nausea and vomiting.
D. Bell's palsy, signs of stroke, or other conditions that affect the blinking mechanism.

Subjective Data
A. Elicit the onset, duration, and frequency of symptoms.
B. Note factors that worsen or alleviate symptoms.
C. Note medical history for systemic conditions and strokes.
D. List current medications, noting anticholinergic drugs and isotretinoin use.
E. Note whether the client wears contact lenses or glasses, and ask for what length of time.
F. Review occupational and home exposure to irritants and allergens.
G. Assess whether the client produces tears. Note eye drainage amount, colour, and frequency.
H. Review history of any previous ocular disease, surgeries, and so forth.

Physical Examination
A. Check temperature, pulse, respirations, and blood pressure.
B. Inspect:
  1. Observe and evaluate *both* eyes.
  2. Conduct a detailed eye examination: Check the eye, lid, and conjunctiva for masses and redness.
  3. Check pupil reactivity and corneal clarity. The corneal reflex should be checked if there is concern about a neuroparalytic keratitis or facial nerve palsy.
  4. Complete a funduscopic examination. Check for completeness of lid closure as well as position of eyelashes.
  5. Examine mouth for dryness.
  6. Inspect skin for butterfly rash.
C. Palpate:
  1. Palpate lacrimal ducts for drainage.
  2. Invert upper lid and check for foreign body or chalazion.
  3. Check sinuses for tenderness.
  4. Palpate thyroid.
  5. Palpate joints for warmth and redness or inflammation.

Diagnostic Test
A. Diagnosis is generally based on client symptoms supported by clinical eye exam.

Differential Diagnoses
A. Stevens–Johnson syndrome.
B. Sjögren's syndrome: Chronic dry mouth, dry eyes, and arthritis triad suggest Sjögren's syndrome. Facial telangiectasias, parotid enlargement, Raynaud's phenomenon, and dental caries are associated features. Clients complain first of burning and a sandy, gritty, foreign-body sensation, particularly later in the day.

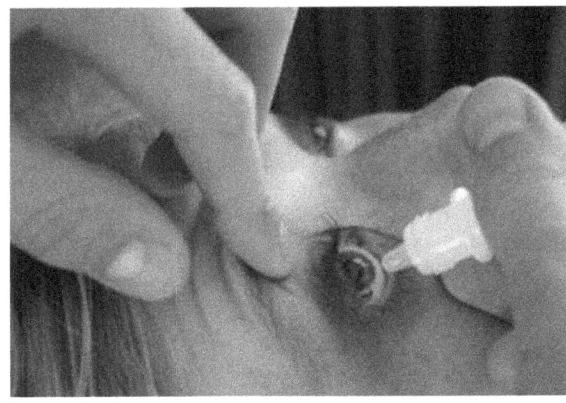

FIGURE 5.1 How to instill eye drops into the eye.

C. Systemic lupus erythematosus.
D. Scleroderma.
E. Ocular pterygium.
F. Superficial pemphigoid.
G. Vitamin A deficiency.

Plan
A. General interventions:
  1. If no ocular disease is present, reduce environmental dryness by use of a room humidifier for a two-week trial.
  2. Apply artificial tear substitutes.
  3. Consider stopping medications being used that may be contributing to the source of dry eye symptoms.
  4. Caution should be used when using over-the-counter (OTC) allergy medications if allergy is a contributing cause. Topical antihistamines may exacerbate the condition over time.
B. Client teaching: *Refer to Client Teaching Guide: Eye Medication Administration.*
C. Pharmacological therapy:
  1. Topical artificial tears.
  2. Drops may be instilled as often as desired.

Follow-Up
A. Determined by the severity of the issue. Reevaluate the client in two weeks.

Consultation/Referral
A. Refer the client to an ophthalmologist if symptoms are unrelieved at the two-week follow-up.
B. Make an immediate referral for red eye, visual disturbance, or eye pain.

Individual Consideration
A. Geriatrics: The rate of lacrimal gland secretions diminishes with age; therefore, the elderly are at an increased risk for developing dry eye.
B. Acute concussion evaluation (ACE) inhibitors may reduce the risk of dry eye syndrome in some clients. Consider treatment with ACE inhibitors for hypertension as appropriate.

Bibliography
American Academy of Ophthalmology. (2013, October). Dry eye syndrome. *PPP 2013*. Retrieved from https://www.aao.org/preferred-practice-pattern/dry-eye-syndrome-ppp-2013

▶ Client Teaching Guides are available at https://connect.springerpub.com/content/reference-book/978-0-8261-9498-5

Excessive Tears

Jill C. Cash and Nancy Pesta Walsh

Definition
A. Excessive tears is an overproduction of tears. Complaints vary from watery eyes to overflowing tears that run down the cheeks, a condition known as *epiphora*.

Incidence/Prevalence
A. The incidence is unknown.

Pathogenesis
A. The most common cause is reflex overproduction of tears (as occurs in the elderly) due to a deficiency of the tear film.
B. Lacrimal pump failure and obstruction of the nasolacrimal outflow system are other causes of excessive tears.
C. Canalicular infections may be caused by *Actinomyces israelii* (Streptothrix) and *Candida*.

Predisposing Factors
A. Blepharitis (inflammation of the eyelid).
B. Allergic conjunctivitis (infectious or foreign body).
C. Exposure to cold, air conditioning, or dry environment.
D. Lid problems: Impaired pumping action of the lid motion due to seventh nerve palsy or conditions that stiffen the lids such as scars or scleroderma.
E. Lid laxity from aging or ectropion (sagging of the lower lid).
F. Sinusitis.
G. Atopy.
H. Age: Increased incidence in the elderly due to an overproduction of tears by the lacrimal gland.
I. Congenital obstruction.

Common Findings
A. Watery eyes or tears running down cheeks are common complaints.

Other Signs and Symptoms
A. Unilateral tearing: Obstructive aetiology.
B. Bilateral tearing: Environmental irritants.

Subjective Data
A. Inquire about onset, course, and duration of symptoms. Note frequency of excessive tearing.
B. Ascertain whether this is a new symptom or whether the client has a past history of similar complaints. Ask how it was treated, and what was the response to treatment(s).
C. Determine severity. Do the tears run down the cheek?
D. Ascertain whether tearing is unilateral or bilateral.
E. Review common environmental predisposing factors.
F. Question the client regarding vision changes.
G. Review medical history.
H. Review recent history for sinus infections or drainage, facial fractures, and surgery.

Physical Examination
A. Inspect:
  1. Evaluate *both* eyes.
  2. Observe the lid structure and motion.
  3. Conduct a dermal examination to rule out butterfly rash.

B. Palpate:
  1. Apply gentle pressure over the lacrimal sac to check drainage.
  2. Invert upper lid to check for foreign body.
  3. Palpate face for sinus tenderness.

Diagnostic Test
A. Culture any drainage expressed from the lacrimal sacs.

Differential Diagnoses
A. Dendritic ulcer: Early symptoms are tears running down cheeks associated with a foreign-body sensation.
B. Congenital glaucoma.
C. Dacryocystitis (purulent discharge).
D. Reflex tearing caused by dry eye.
E. Blepharitis.

Plan
A. General interventions:
  1. Eliminate identifiable irritants.
  2. Treatment is mainly aimed at the underlying condition (i.e., ocular infection).
  3. Dacryocystitis is treated with hot compresses at least four times a day and systemic antibiotics.
B. Client teaching: Instruct the client on the application of compresses.
C. Pharmacological therapy:
  1. None is required for diagnosis of excessive tears without infectious pathology.
  2. Dacryocystitis:
     a. Erythromycin.
     b. Cloxacillin.

Follow-Up
A. See client in 48 to 72 hours to evaluate symptoms, especially if antibiotic therapy was needed.

Consultation/Referral
A. Clients unresponsive to treatment should be promptly referred to an ophthalmologist.
B. Consider referral for lid malposition or nasolacrimal duct obstructions.

Individual Consideration
A. Paediatrics: Nasolacrimal duct obstruction. Approximately 6% of newborns are diagnosed with a congenital obstruction within the first weeks of life. With moist heat and massage, many resolve spontaneously.

Bibliography
Price, K. M., & Richard, M. J. (2009). The tearing patient: Diagnosis and management. EyeNet Magazine. Retrieved from https://www.aao.org/eyenet/article/tearing-patient-diagnosis-management?

Eye Pain

Jill C. Cash and Nancy Pesta Walsh

Definition
A. Sensation of pain may affect the eyelid, conjunctiva, or cornea.

Incidence/Prevalence
A. Unknown. Pain in the eye is most often produced by conditions that do not threaten vision.

Pathogenesis
A. The external ocular surfaces and the uveal tract are richly innervated with pain receptors. As a result, lesions or disease processes affecting these surfaces can be acutely painful.
B. Pathology confined to the vitreous, retina, or optic nerve is rarely a source of pain.

Predisposing Factors
A. Eyelids: Inflammation such as hordeolum (stye), trichiasis (in-turned lash), and tarsal foreign bodies.
B. Conjunctiva: Viral and bacterial conjunctivitis or allergic conjunctivitis; toxic, chemical, and mechanical injuries.
C. Cornea: Keratitis (inflammation of the cornea) accompanying trauma, infection, exposure, vascular disease, or decreased lacrimation; microbial keratitis from contact use. If blood vessels invade the normally avascular corneal stroma, vision may become cloudy. Severe pain is a prominent symptom; movement of the lid typically exacerbates symptoms.

Common Findings
A. Eye pain (sharp, dull, deep): The quality of the pain needs to be considered. Deep pain is suggestive of an intraocular problem. Inflammation and rapidly expanding mass lesions may cause deep pain. Displacement of the globe and diplopia may ensue.
B. Eye movement may cause sharp pain due to meningeal inflammation (the extraocular rectus muscles insert along the dura of the nerve sheath at the orbital apex). Most cases are idiopathic, but 10% to 15% are associated with multiple sclerosis.
C. Headache.

Other Signs and Symptoms
These symptoms may be unilateral or bilateral.
A. Eyelids:
  1. Tenderness.
  2. Sensation of foreign body.
  3. Redness.
  4. Oedema.
B. Conjunctiva:
  1. Mild burning.
  2. Sensation of foreign body.
  3. Itching (allergic).
C. Cornea:
  1. Burning.
  2. Foreign-body sensation.
  3. Considerable discomfort.
  4. Reflex photophobic tearing.
  5. Blinking exacerbates pain.
  6. Pain relieved with pressure (i.e., holding the lid shut). With a foreign body or a corneal lesion, pain is exacerbated by lid movement and relieved by cessation of lid motion.
D. Sclera: Redness.
E. Uveal tract (uveitis or iritis):
  1. Dull, deep-seated ache and photophobia.
  2. Profound ocular and orbital pain radiating to the frontal and temporal regions accompanying sudden elevation of pressure (acute angle-closure glaucoma).
  3. Vagal stimulation with high pressure may result in nausea and vomiting.
  4. Usual history of mild intermittent episodes of blurred vision preceding onset of throbbing pain, nausea, vomiting, and decreased visual acuity.
  5. Halos around light.
F. Orbit:
  1. Deep pain with inflammation and rapidly expanding mass lesions.
  2. Eye movement causing sharp pain due to meningeal inflammation.
G. Sinusitis: Secondary orbital inflammation and tenderness on extremes of eye movement.

Subjective Data
A. Review the onset, duration, and course of symptoms. Inquire regarding the quality of pain.
B. Review any predisposing factors such as trauma or a foreign object. Ask, Was the onset sudden or gradual?
C. Note reported changes in visual acuity or colour vision.
D. Note aggravating or alleviating factors.
E. Determine whether the eye pain is bilateral or unilateral.
F. Review history for herpes, infections, and toxic or chemical irritants.
G. Review history for glaucoma and previous eye surgeries or treatments.
H. Assess the client for any other symptoms such as migraine headache, sinusitis, or tooth abscess.
I. Inquire whether the client has lost a large amount of sleep.
J. Inquire whether he or she has been exposed to a large amount of ultraviolet (UV) light or sunlight (vacation, tanning beds).
K. Review history for any other medical problems such as lupus, sarcoidosis, or inflammatory bowel disease.

Physical Examination
A. Inspect:
  1. Evaluate *both* eyes.
  2. Test visual acuity and colour vision.
  3. Observe for extraocular movements (EOMs).
  4. Check the eye, lid, and conjunctiva for masses and redness.
  5. Check pupil reactivity and corneal clarity.
  6. Conduct a funduscopic examination for disc abnormalities.
  7. Perform ear, nose, and throat examination.
B. Palpate:
  1. Palpate lacrimal ducts for drainage.
  2. Palpate sinuses for tenderness.
  3. Invert upper lid and check for foreign body or chalazion.

Diagnostic Tests
A. Fluorescein stain.
B. Measurement of intraocular pressure (IOP).

Differential Diagnoses
A. Hordeolum.
B. Chalazion.
C. Acute dacryocystitis.
D. Irritant exposure.
E. Conjunctival infection.
F. Corneal abrasion.
G. Foreign body.
H. Ulcers.
I. Ingrown lashes.
J. Contact lens abuse.

K. Scleritis.
L. Acute angle-closure glaucoma; may present with fixed, midposition pupil, redness, and a hazy cornea.
M. Uveitis.
N. Referred pain from extraocular sources such as sinusitis, tooth abscess, tension headache, temporal arteritis, and prodrome of herpes zoster.

Plan
A. General interventions:
   1. The initial task is to be sure that there is no threat to vision.
   2. Treatment modality depends on the underlying cause of eye pain.
▶ **B.** Client teaching: *Refer to Client Teaching Guide: Eye Medication Administration.* See Figure 5.1.
C. Pharmacological therapy: Medication depends on the underlying cause.

Follow-Up
A. Follow-up depends on the underlying cause.

Consultation/Referral
A. Any change in visual acuity or colour vision requires an urgent ophthalmologic consultation.

Bibliography
Philips, P. (2008). Pain in the eye. Eyenet Magazine. Retrieved from https://www.aao.org/eyenet/article/pain-in-eye

Glaucoma, Acute Angle-Closure

Jill C. Cash and Nancy Pesta Walsh

Definition
A. This ocular emergency is caused by elevations in intraocular pressure (IOP) that damage the optic nerve, leading to loss of peripheral fields of vision; it can lead to loss of central vision and result in blindness.

Incidence/Prevalence
A. Acute angle-closure glaucoma is the fourth leading cause of blindness in Canada with approximately 300,000 people affected.

Pathogenesis
A. The essential pathophysiologic feature of glaucoma is an IOP that is too high for the optic nerve. Increased IOP increases vascular resistance, causing decreased vascular perfusion of the optic nerve and ischemia. Light dilates the pupil, causing the iris to relax and bow forward. As the iris bows forward, it comes into contact with the trabecular meshwork and occludes the outflow of aqueous humour, resulting in increased IOP.

Predisposing Factors
A. Narrow anterior ocular chamber.
B. Prolonged periods of darkness.
C. Drugs that dilate the pupils (i.e., anticholinergics).
D. Advancing age: Older than 60 years.
E. African American heritage.
F. Family history.
G. Trauma.
H. Neoplasm.
I. Corticosteroid therapy.
J. Neovascularization.
K. Female sex.

Common Findings
A. Ocular pain.
B. Blurred vision, decreased visual acuity, "cloudiness" of vision.
C. "Halos" around lights at night.
D. Neurologic complaints (headache, nausea, or vomiting).

Other Signs and Symptoms
A. Red eye with ciliary flush.
B. "Silent blinder" causes extensive damage before the client is aware of visual field loss.
C. Dilated pupil.
D. Hard orbital globe.
E. No pupillary response to light.
F. Increased IOP (normal IOP is 10–20 mmHg).

Subjective Data
A. Review the onset, course, and duration of symptoms; note visual changes in one or both eyes.
B. Review medical history and medications.
C. Review family history of glaucoma.
D. Determine whether there has been any difficulty with peripheral vision, any headache photophobia, or any visual blurring.
E. In children, ask about rubbing of eyes, refusal to open eyes, and tearing.
F. Rule out presence of any chemical, trauma, or foreign bodies in the eye.
G. Review any recent history of herpes outbreak.
H. Ask the client whether this has ever occurred before, and if so, how it was treated.

Physical Examination
A. Blood pressure.
B. Inspect:
   1. Examine both eyes.
   2. Rule out foreign body.
   3. Inspect for redness, inflammation, and discharge.
   4. Check pupillary response to light.
   5. Redness noted around iris, pupil is dilated, and cornea appears cloudy.
   6. Inspect anterior chamber of eye by holding penlight laterally and direct toward nasal area. Shallow chamber will cast a shadow on the nasal side of the iris.
C. Palpate: Palpate the globe of the eye, which will feel firm on palpation.
D. Funduscopic examination: This may reveal notching of the cup and a difference in cup-to-disc ratio between the two eyes.

Diagnostic Tests
A. Check visual acuity and peripheral fields of vision.
B. Measure IOP with a tonometer. Normal level is 10 to 21 mmHg; acute angle-closure glaucoma IOP is >50 mmHg. Tonometer examination is not recommended if external infection is present.

▶ Client Teaching Guides are available at https://connect.springerpub.com/content/reference-book/978-0-8261-9498-5

C. Slit-lamp examination: Oedematous and/or cloudy cornea.

Differential Diagnoses
A. Acute iritis.
B. Acute bacterial conjunctivitis.
C. Iridocyclitis.
D. Corneal injury.
E. Foreign body.
F. Herpetic keratitis.

Plan
A. General interventions:
   1. Severe attacks can cause blindness in two to three days. Seek medical attention immediately to prevent permanent vision loss.
   2. Frequency of attacks is unpredictable.
▶ B. Client teaching: *Refer to Client Teaching Guide: Eye Medication Administration.*
C. Pharmacological therapy: Must be instituted by an ophthalmologist:
   1. Acetazolamide.
   2. Pilocarpine during acute attack.
D. Surgical intervention:
   1. Surgery is indicated if IOP is not maintained within normal limits with medications or if there is progressive visual field loss with optic nerve damage.
   2. Surgical treatment of choice is peripheral iridectomy—excision of a small portion of the iris whereby the aqueous humour can bypass the pupil.

Follow-Up
A. Annual eye examinations by an ophthalmologist are necessary to monitor IOP and treatment efficacy.

Consultation/Referral
A. All clients should be referred to an ophthalmologist *immediately* for measurement of IOP, acute management, and possible surgical intervention (laser peripheral iridectomy).

Individual Considerations
A. Paediatrics: Infants with tearing, rubbing of eyes, and refusal to open eyes should be referred to a paediatric ophthalmologist for immediate care.
B. Adults:
   1. Women normally have slightly higher IOPs than men.
   2. Asians may have higher IOPs than African Americans and Caucasians.
   3. Individuals older than age 40 years should have their IOP measured periodically. Every three to five years is sufficient after a stable baseline is established for the client.
C. Geriatrics: Incidence increases with age, usually in those older than 60 years.

Bibliography
MacIver, S., McDonald, D., & Prokopich, C. L. (2017). Screening, Diagnosis, and Management of Open Angle Glaucoma: An Evidence-Based Guideline for Canadian Optometrists. *Canadian Journal of Optometry, 79*(S1), 4–71.

Hordeolum (Stye)

Jill C. Cash and Nancy Pesta Walsh

Definition
A. Hordeolum is an infection of the glands of the eyelids (follicle of an eyelash or the associated gland of Zeis [sebaceous] or Moll's gland [apocrine sweat gland]), usually caused by *Staphylococcus aureus.*
B. If swelling is under the conjunctival side of the eyelid, it is an internal hordeolum.
C. If swelling is under the skin of the eyelid, it is an external hordeolum.

Incidence/Prevalence
A. The incidence is unknown; it is more common in children and adolescents than in adults.

Pathogenesis
A. Acute bacterial infection of the meibomian gland (internal hordeolum) or of the eyelash follicle (external hordeolum) is usually caused by *S. aureus.*

Predisposing Factor
A. Age: More common in the paediatric population.

Common Findings
A. Eye tenderness.
B. Sudden onset of a purulent discharge.

Other Signs and Symptoms
A. Redness and swelling of the eye.

Subjective Data
A. Review the onset, course, and duration of symptoms.
B. Determine whether there is any visual disturbance.
C. Note whether this is the first occurrence. If not, ask how it was treated before.
D. Evaluate how much pain or discomfort the client is experiencing.
E. Review the client's history for chemical, foreign body, and/or trauma aetiology.
F. Review the client's medical history and medications.

Physical Examination
A. Inspect:
   1. Examine both eyes; note redness, site of swelling, and amount and colour of discharge.
   2. Evert the lid and check for pointing.
   3. Assess sclera and conjunctivae for abnormalities.
   4. Inspect ears, nose, and throat.
B. Palpate:
   1. Palpate eye for hardness and expression of discharge.
   2. Evaluate for preauricular adenopathy.

Diagnostic Tests
A. Test visual acuity.
B. Discharge can be cultured but is usually treated presumptively.

▶ Client Teaching Guides are available at https://connect.springerpub.com/content/reference-book/978-0-8261-9498-5

Differential Diagnoses
A. Chalazion: The main differential diagnosis is chalazia, which are on the conjunctival side of the eyelid and do not usually affect the margin of the eyelid.
B. Blepharitis.
C. Xanthoma.
D. Bacterial conjunctivitis.
E. Foreign body.

Plan
A. General interventions: Contain the infecting pathogen. Crops occur when the infectious agent spreads from one hair follicle to another.
B. Client teaching:
  1. *Refer to Client Teaching Guide: Eye Medication Administration.* See Figure 5.1.
  2. Reinforce good handwashing.
  3. Instruct on proper eyelid hygiene.
  4. Clients should discard all eye makeup, including mascara, eyeliner, and eye shadow.
C. Pharmacological therapy:
  1. This is often not needed, as lesions usually resolve without treatment.
  2. Ophthalmic ointment 10%.
  3. Ophthalmic drops.
  4. Polymyxin B sulfate and bacitracin zinc ophthalmic ointment.
  5. If crops of styes occur, some clinicians recommend a course of tetracycline to stop recurrences (consult with a physician).

Follow-Up
A. Have client telephone or visit the office in 48 hours to check response.
B. If crops occur, diabetes mellitus must be excluded. Perform blood glucose evaluation.

Consultation/Referral
A. Hordeolum may produce a diffuse superficial lid infection known as *preseptal cellulitis* that requires referral to an ophthalmologist.
B. If hordeolum does not respond to topical antimicrobial treatment, refer the client to an ophthalmologist.

Individual Consideration
A. None.

Bibliography
Canadian Association of Optometrists. (n.d.). Hordeolum (Styes). Retrieved from https://opto.ca/health-library/hordeolum-styes

Strabismus

Jill C. Cash and Nancy Pesta Walsh

Definition
Strabismus is an eye disorder in which the optic axes cannot be directed toward the same object due to a deficit in muscular coordination. It can be nonparalytic or paralytic:
A. *Esotropia* is a nonparalytic strabismus in which the eyes cross inward.
B. *Exotropia* is a nonparalytic strabismus in which the eyes drift outward. Exotropia may be intermittent or constant.
C. Pseudostrabismus gives a false appearance of deviation in the visual axes.

Incidence/Prevalence
A. Strabismus occurs in approximately 3% of the population.
B. Esotropia (nonparalytic strabismus) is the most common ocular misalignment, representing more than half of all ocular deviations in the paediatric population. Accommodative esotropia typically occurs between one and three years of age, with an average age of 2.5 years, and it may be intermittent or constant.
C. Intermittent exotropia is the most common type of exotropic strabismus and is characterized by an outward drift of one eye, most often occurring when a child is fixating at distance.

Pathogenesis
A. *Paralytic strabismus* is related to paralysis or paresis of a specific extraocular muscle. *Nonparalytic strabismus* is related to a congenital imbalance of normal eye muscle tone, causing focusing difficulties, unilateral refractive error, nonfusion, or anatomical difference in the eyes.

Predisposing Factors
A. Familial tendencies.
B. Congenital defects.

Common Findings
A. Crossing of the eyes.
B. Turning in of the eyes.
C. Photophobia.
D. Diplopia.

Other Signs and Symptoms
A. The client's head or chin tilts or the client closes one eye to focus on objects.

Subjective Data
A. Describe the onset, duration, and progression of symptoms.
B. Review any history of eye problems. Ask, How were they corrected?
C. Determine whether the client, if a child, has reached the age-appropriate milestones in development.
D. Does the client make faces or move his or her head to see better (tilting the head or chin to improve acuity or to correct diplopia)?
E. Rule out any eye damage, surgery, and so forth.

Physical Examination
A. Inspect: Observe alignment of lids, sclera, conjunctiva, and cornea.
B. Check pupillary response to light, size, shape, and equality.
C. Check the red reflex.

Diagnostic Tests
A. Test visual acuity.
B. Perform the cover–uncover test: In this test, the "lazy eye" drifts out of position and snaps back quickly when uncovered.

▶ Client Teaching Guides are available at https://connect.springerpub.com/content/reference-book/978-0-8261-9498-5

C. Corneal light reflex (Hirschberg's) test: Perform the Hirschberg's test for symmetry of the pupillary light reflexes to help detect strabismus. Normally, the light reflexes are in the same position on each pupil, but not with strabismus (positive Hirschberg's test).
D. Test extraocular movements (EOMs): If a nerve supplying an extraocular muscle has been interrupted or the muscle itself has become weakened, the eye fails to move in the direction of the damaged muscle. If the right sixth nerve is damaged, the right eye does not move temporally. This is paralytic strabismus.

Differential Diagnoses
A. Pseudostrabismus.
B. Ocular trauma.
C. Congenital defect.

Plan
A. General interventions:
  1. When poor fixation is present, patch the stronger, dominant eye to promote vision and muscle strengthening in the weaker eye.
B. Client teaching: Reinforce the need to consistently wear an eye patch, especially with children.
C. Pharmacological therapy: None.

Follow-Up
A. Monitor progress with eye patch.
B. Surgical intervention depends on the degree of deviation.

Consultation/Referral
A. Additional testing should be done by an ophthalmologist.
B. Pseudostrabismus (a false appearance of strabismus when visual axes are really in alignment) is one of the most common reasons a paediatric ophthalmologist is asked to evaluate an infant.

Individual Considerations
A. Paediatrics:
  1. Use the tumbling or illiterate E to test children; for preschoolers, use the Allen picture cards.
  2. In very young children, test visual acuity by assessing developmental milestones: Looking at mother's face, responsive smile, reaching for objects. By three to five years of age, most children can cooperate for performance of accurate visual acuity screening tests.
  3. The eyes of the newborn are *rarely aligned* during the first few weeks of life. By the age of three months, normal oculomotor behaviour is usually established, and an experienced examiner may be able to document the existence of abnormal alignment by that time.

Bibliography
Centers for Disease Control and Prevention. (2015, September). *Vision quest initiative*. Retrieved from https://www.cdc.gov/visionhealth/faq.htm
Gunton, W. B., Wasserman, B. N., & DeBenedictis, C. (2015). Strabismus. *Primary Care: Clinics in Office Practice, 2*(3), 393–407. doi:10.1016/j.pop.2015.05.006

Subconjunctival Haemorrhage

Jill C. Cash and Nancy Pesta Walsh

Definition
A. Subconjunctival haemorrhage presents as blood patches in the bulbar conjunctiva.

Incidence/Prevalence
A. Frequently seen in newborns, subconjunctival haemorrhage may also be seen in adults after forceful exertion (coughing, sneezing, childbirth, and strenuous lifting).

Pathogenesis
A. This disorder is believed to be secondary to increased intrathoracic pressure that may occur during labour and delivery or with physical exertion.

Predisposing Factors
A. Local trauma.
B. Systemic hypertension.
C. Acute conjunctivitis.
D. Vaginal delivery (pushing during delivery).
E. Severe coughing.
F. Severe vomiting.

Common Finding
A. Red-eyed appearance without pain.

Other Signs and Symptoms
A. Bright red blood in plane between the conjunctiva and sclera.
B. Usually unilateral.
C. Normal vision.

Subjective Data
A. Identify onset and duration of symptoms.
B. Elicit information about trauma to the eye: Is it due to severe coughing or vomiting?
C. Identify history of conjunctivitis or hypertension.

Physical Examination
A. Check temperature, pulse, respirations, and blood pressure (rule out hypertension).
B. Inspect:
  1. Observe eyes.
  2. Inspect ears, nose, and mouth.
  3. Inspect skin for bruises or other trauma.
  4. Assess for signs of trauma or abuse. Blood in the anterior chamber (hyphaema) can result from injury or abuse.
C. Other physical examination components are dependent on aetiology.

Diagnostic Tests
A. Perform visual screening.
B. Test extraocular movements (EOMs) and peripheral vision.

Differential Diagnoses
A. Systemic hypertension.
B. Blood dyscrasia.
C. Trauma to eye.
D. Conjunctivitis.
E. Hyphema.
F. Abuse.

Plan
A. General interventions: Reassure the client. The haemorrhage is not damaging to the eye or vision, and the blood reabsorbs on its own over several weeks.

B. Teach safety to prevent trauma to the eye.
C. Pharmacological therapy: None.

Follow-Up
A. If subconjunctival haemorrhage recurs, evaluate the client further for systemic hypertension or blood dyscrasia.

Consultation/Referral
A. Consult or refer the client to a physician if hyphema is noted, if glaucoma is suspected, or if the client has additional eye injuries.

Individual Considerations
A. Paediatrics: Haemorrhage is common in newborns after vaginal delivery.
B. Adults: Always measure blood pressure to rule out systemic hypertension.
C. Geriatrics:
   1. Always measure blood pressure to rule out systemic hypertension.
   2. Consider evaluation for blood dyscrasia.
   3. Check clotting times if client is taking warfarin.

Bibliography
College of Optometrists. (2017). Sub-conjunctival haemorrhage. Clinical Practice Guideline. Retrieved from https://www.college-optometrists.org/guidance/clinical-management-guidelines/sub-conjunctival-haemorrhage.html

Uveitis

Jill C. Cash and Nancy Pesta Walsh

Definition
A. Uveitis, also known as *iritis*, is inflammation of the uveal tract (iris, ciliary body, and choroid) and is usually accompanied by a dull ache and photophobia resulting from the irritative spasm of the pupillary sphincter.

Incidence/Prevalence
A. The true incidence is unknown. Approximately 15% of clients with sarcoidosis present with uveitis.

Pathogenesis
A. The cause is unknown. Underlying causes include infections, viruses, and arthritis.

Predisposing Factors
A. Collagen disorders.
B. Autoimmune disorders.
C. Ankylosing spondylitis.
D. Sarcoidosis.
E. Juvenile rheumatoid arthritis.
F. Lupus.
G. Reiter's syndrome.
H. Behcet's syndrome.
I. Syphilis.
J. Tuberculosis.
K. AIDS.
L. Crohn's disease.

Common Findings
A. Eye pain: Painless to deep-seated ache.
B. Photophobia.
C. Blurred vision with decreased visual acuity.
D. Black spots.
E. Eye redness.

Other Signs and Symptoms
A. Unilateral or bilateral symptoms:
   1. Unilateral: The pupil is smaller than that of the other eye because of spasm of the circular muscles of the iris.
B. Ciliary flush.
C. Nausea and vomiting with vagal stimulation.
D. Halos around lights.
E. Hypopyon (pus in anterior chamber).
F. Limbal flush with small pupil.

Subjective Data
A. Elicit the onset, course, duration, and frequency of symptoms. Are symptoms bilateral or unilateral?
B. Identify the possible causal activity or agent (chemical, traumatic, or infectious aetiologies).
C. Review the client's history of previous uveitis and other ophthalmologic disorders.
D. Review any associated fever, rash, weight loss, joint pain, back pain, oral ulcers, or genital ulcers.
E. Review full medical history for comorbid conditions.

Physical Examination
A. Check temperature, pulse, respirations, and blood pressure.
B. Inspect:
   1. Assess both eyes for visual acuity and peripheral fields of vision.
   2. Check sclera and conjunctiva.
C. Other physical components need to be completed related to comorbid conditions.

Diagnostic Tests
These will be done by an ophthalmologist, as the client needs immediate referral:
A. Slit-lamp test: Slit-lamp examination reveals cells in the anterior chamber and "flare," representing increased aqueous humour protein. Inflammatory cells, called *keratic precipitates*, can collect in clusters on the posterior cornea.
B. Penlight examination: Flashlight examination shows a slightly cloudy anterior chamber in the uveitic eye.

Differential Diagnoses
A. Uveitis: Uveitis is usually idiopathic, but it may be associated with many systemic and ocular diseases.
B. Acute angle-closure glaucoma.
C. Retinal detachment.
D. Central retinal artery occlusion.
E. Endophthalmitis.

Plan
A. General interventions:
   1. Treat underlying cause as indicated.
   2. Provide immediate referral to an ophthalmologist due to possible complications of cataracts and blindness.
B. Client teaching: Inform the client that recurrent attacks are common and also require immediate attention.
C. Pharmacological therapy:
   1. Medications are given per ophthalmologist.
   2. Uveitis and colitis often flare simultaneously; oral steroids are effective for both.

Follow-Up
A. The client with uveitis needs a follow-up with an ophthalmologist.

Consultation/Referral
A. The client should be referred *immediately* to an ophthalmologist for evaluation and intervention.

Individual Considerations
A. Recurrent uveitis may be a sign of another systemic condition. Other conditions to consider include infections (bacterial, spirochetal, viral, fungal, and parasitic infections); inflammatory diseases, including spondyloarthropathies (ankylosing spondylitis, psoriatic arthritis, and reactive arthritis); inflammatory bowel disease; multiple sclerosis; and the use of new medications. Further workup should be performed for recurrent uveitis.

Bibliography
Dohm, K. D. (2015, January). Practice pearls for managing anterior uveitis. *Review of Optometry, 2015*(1), 58–63.

6 Ear Guidelines

Acute Otitis Media

Jill C. Cash, Moya Cook, and Paul Jeffrey

Definition
A. Acute otitis media (AOM) is inflammation of the middle ear associated with an acute bacterial infection of the middle ear.

Incidence/Prevalence
A. AOM may occur at any age. It is most commonly seen in children.
B. Over two-thirds of children have had at least one episode of otitis media by three years of age.
C. One-third of children have had three or more episodes by three years of age.
D. One-third of all paediatric visits are for otitis media.

Pathogenesis
A. Obstruction of the eustachian tube can lead to a middle ear effusion and infection. Contamination of this middle ear fluid often results from a backup of nasopharyngeal secretions. The most common bacterial pathogens are *Streptococcus pneumoniae*, *Haemophilus influenzae*, and *Moraxella catarrhalis*.

Predisposing Factors
A. Age <12 months.
B. Recurrent otitis media (three or more episodes in the last six months).
C. Previous episode of otitis media within the last month.
D. Medical condition that predisposes to otitis media (i.e., Down syndrome, AIDS, cystic fibrosis, cleft palate, and craniofacial abnormalities).
E. Indigenous Peoples of Canada.
F. Exposure to tobacco smoke and air pollution.
G. Day care attendance.
H. Bottle propping.
I. Family history of allergies.
J. Pacifier use.

Common Findings
A. Ear pain.
B. Pulling ears.
C. Fever may or may not be present.

Other Signs and Symptoms
A. Sleeplessness within past 48 hours.
B. Decreased appetite.
C. Increased fussiness.
D. Acute hearing loss.
E. Upper respiratory infection (URI) symptoms.
F. Mastoiditis presenting with a swollen and red mastoid.
G. Perforated tympanic membrane (sudden severe pain followed by immediate relief of pain with fluid drainage from the ear).
H. Cholesteatoma (saclike structure in the middle ear accompanied by white, shiny, greasy debris).

Subjective Data
A. Elicit onset and duration of symptoms.
B. Inquire whether the client recently had (or has concurrently) a URI.
C. Determine whether the client has any change in hearing.
D. Assess the client for any drainage from the ear(s).
E. Question the client or his or her caregiver regarding risk factors.
F. Identify the client's history of otitis media.

Physical Examination
A. Check temperature, pulse, respirations, and blood pressure.
B. Inspect:
    1. Observe the canal and auricle for redness, deformity, drainage, or foreign body.
    2. Inspect the tympanic membrane position to determine if it is neutral and whether landmarks are visible, retracted, full, or bulging.
    3. Observe ears for decreased or absent tympanic membrane mobility.
    4. Inspect nose, mouth, and throat.
C. Auscultate heart and lungs.

Diagnostic Tests
A. Tympanogram shows flat or type B curve.
B. Hearing test should be done in clients with persistent otitis media (≥ three months' duration).
C. Consider complete blood count if the client appears toxic with a high fever.

Differential Diagnoses
A. Otitis media with effusion (OME).
B. Red tympanic membrane secondary to crying (differentiated from AOM by mobility with pneumatic otoscopy).
C. URI.
D. Mastoiditis.
E. Foreign body in the ear.
F. Otitis externa.

Plan

A. General intervention: Pain relief with acetaminophen or ibuprofen. Topical pain relief can be used in children older than 3 years.

B. Client teaching:

  1. *Refer to Client Teaching Guide: Acute Otitis Media.* Educate parents and care providers that children should avoid smoke exposure. Smoke-filled rooms increase the risk of frequent ear infections in children.
  2. For young children who use a bottle for feeding, stress the importance of NOT propping bottles at any time for feeding. Propping bottles increases the risk of ear infections.

C. Pharmacological therapy:

  1. First-line treatment: amoxicillin.
  2. For concerns of amoxicillin resistance, treatment failure, recent use of antibiotic in the previous 30 days, and/or concurrent other infections, use an antibiotic with beta-lactamase activity such as amoxicillin-clavulanate. Other alternatives include cefdinir, cefpodoxime, cefuroxime, and ceftriaxone.
  3. For penicillin allergy: cefpodoxime or cefuroxime susp.
  4. Alternative: ceftriaxone. If clinically improved in 48 hours, no further treatment is recommended. If signs/symptoms continue, administer the second dose of ceftriaxone in 48 hours.
  5. Other alternatives: macrolides:
      a. Azithromycin.
      b. Clarithromycin.
      c. Trimethoprim.
  6. Children younger than 2 years should be treated with antibiotic therapy for 10 days. Children older than 2 years without a previous history of otitis media may be treated for five to seven days.
  7. If the client is asymptomatic and AOM is found on examination, consider observation without antibiotics only if child is older than 2 years. Recommend follow-up examination in 48 hours.
  8. Other antibiotics (if first-line treatment fails): amoxicillin and clavulanic acid, cefixime, azithromycin, and cefprozil.
  9. For persistent otitis media (three months or longer), consider using an antibiotic for 21 days. **Residual otitis media may need treatment with additional amoxicillin or beta-lactamase-resistant antibiotic.**

Follow-Up

A. Check the client in two to four weeks or if fever and complaints persist for more than 48 hours after the antibiotic is begun. Documentation of the resolution of the ear infection is valuable information if recurrent infections occur.

Consultation/Referral

A. Consult or refer the client to a specialist if he or she is less than six weeks of age, appears septic, or has mastoiditis.

B. A client with persistent otitis media with a hearing loss of 20 dB or more should be referred to an ear, nose, and throat (ENT) specialist.

Individual Considerations

A. Pregnancy: Do not use sulfa medications (sulfonamides) in pregnant clients.

B. Paediatrics:

  1. Children six weeks old or younger. Consider a blood culture and lumbar puncture if septicemia is suspected. The client may need intravenous (IV) antibiotics depending on culture results. Do not use sulfa medications (sulfonamides) in children younger than 2 months.
  2. Health Canada and the Canadian Paediatric Society conclude that over-the-counter (OTC) medications are not effective in most cases, and should not be given to children less than six years of age. In older children, consider decongestants for nasal congestion. Antihistamines are not recommended.

C. Geriatrics: Elderly clients may present with OME and/or otitis media secondary to a blocked eustachian tube and/or URI.

Bibliography

Bugs and Drugs. (2018). *Acute otitis media.* Retrieved from http://bugsanddrugs.org/Home/Index/bdpage06AE59AE13F340CAA6F3E987054DFEEA

Goldman, R. (2011). *Treating cough and cold: Guidance for caregivers of children and youth.* Retrieved from https://www.cps.ca/en/documents/position/treating-cough-cold

Government of Canada. (2017). *Indigenous peoples and communities.* Retrieved from https://www.rcaanc-cirnac.gc.ca/eng/1100100013785/1529102490303

Government of Canada. (2018). *Concerns about children's medications: Avoiding cough and cold medications.* Retrieved from https://www.canada.ca/en/health-canada/services/drugs-medicaldevices/concerns-about-children-s-medication.html

Indigenous Corporate Training Inc. (2018). *Indigenous peoples terminology guidelines for usage.* Retrieved from https://www.ictinc.ca/blog/indigenous-peoples-terminology-guidelines-for-usage

Klein, J. O., & Pelton, S. (2015). Acute otitis media in children: Treatment. In M. Edwards & G. Isaacson (Eds.), *UptoDate.* Retrieved from http://www.uptodate.com/contents/acute-otitis-media-in-children-treatment

Le Saux, N. & Robinson, J. (2016). Position statement: Management of otitis media in children six months of age and older. *Paediatric Child Health, 21*(3), 39–44. Retrieved from https://www.cps.ca/en/documents/position/acute-otitis-media

Poe, D., & Bassem, M. (2016). Eustachian tube dysfunction. In D. Deschler (Ed.), *UpToDate.* Retrieved from http://www.uptodate.com/contents/eustachian-tube-dysfunction?source=search_result&search=eustachian+tube+dysfunction&selectedTitle=1%7E39

Shevchuk, Y. (2016). *Canadian pharmacists association: Otitis media and otitis externa.* Retrieved from http://www.pharmacists.ca/cpha-ca/assets/File/Sample%20chapters/CTMAChapter-OtitisMediaOtitisExterna.pdf

Toward Optimized Practice. (2016). *Acute otitis media.* Retrieved from http://www.topalbertadoctors.org/cpgs/?sid=15&cpg_cats=54

Cerumen Impaction (Earwax)

Jill C. Cash and Moya Cook

Definition

A. Cerumen impaction, or earwax buildup, can cause conductive hearing loss or discomfort.

Incidence/Prevalence

A. Cerumen impaction occurs in clients of all ages. It is commonly seen in the elderly. The incidence in nursing home clients is 40%.

Pathogenesis

A. Wax builds up in the external canal. With age, the normal self-cleaning mechanisms of the ear fail. Cilia, which have become stiff, cannot remove cerumen and dirt from the ear canal. The pushing of cotton swabs, paper clips, bobby pins, and so forth into the ear canal may also impact cerumen.

Predisposing Factors
A. Aging (decreased function of ear cilia).
B. Use of hearing aids.
C. Use of cotton swabs to clean ear canals.

Common Findings
A. Dryness and itching of ear canal.
B. Dizziness.
C. Ear pain.
D. Hearing loss.

Subjective Data
A. Elicit onset and duration of symptoms.
B. Elicit history of cerumen impaction.
C. Question the client regarding the method of cleaning ears.

Physical Examination
A. Check temperature, pulse, respirations, and blood pressure.
B. Inspect:
   1. Observe ears for thick, light- to dark-brown wax occluding the auditory canal.
   2. Observe the tympanic membrane if possible. A perforated tympanic membrane is associated with otitis media.
   3. Inspect the nose and throat.
C. Auscultate heart and lungs.

Diagnostic Tests
A. Conductive hearing loss of 35 to 40 dB.
B. Perform Rinne and Weber tests.
   1. The Rinne tuning fork test reveals bone conduction greater than air conduction in the affected ear (abnormal). The Rinne test is performed by placing the struck tuning fork against the mastoid bone. Begin counting or timing the interval from the start to when the client can no longer hear. Continue counting or timing the interval to determine the length of time sound is heard by air conduction. Air-conducted sound should be heard twice as long as bone-conducted sound after bone conduction stops.
   2. The Weber test reveals conductive hearing loss when sound travels toward the poor ear. Sensorineural hearing loss is present when sound travels toward the good ear. This is performed by striking a tuning fork and then placing it on the middle of the head. The client should be asked where sound is being heard: from the left ear, the right ear, or equal in both ears. Normal results are reflected by sound being heard equally in both ears.

Differential Diagnoses
A. Foreign body in the ear canal.
B. Otitis externa: white, mucus-like ear discharge associated with otitis externa.

Plan
A. General interventions:
   1. Remove impaction by means of lavage or curettage. Be sure to inspect the canal and tympanic membrane after removal of the cerumen.
   2. Document the client's hearing before and after removal of cerumen.
B. Client teaching: Instruct the client not to clean ears with cotton swabs, bobby pins, and so forth. Using these devices pushes the wax further into the ear canal and can worsen symptoms. *Refer to Client Teaching Guide: Cerumen Impaction (Earwax).*
C. Pharmacological therapy:
   1. First-line treatment: hydrogen peroxide - urea, mineral oil, or olive oil two to three drops in the ear every day for one week to loosen the cerumen before lavage or curettage. **Do not use hydrogen peroxide–urea if perforation of tympanic membrane is suspected.**
   2. For prevention, have the client use the aforementioned softeners for two to three days. Then have him or her use one capful of hydrogen peroxide in the ear twice daily, allow it to bubble for five to 10 minutes, then turn head to allow it to run out.

Follow-Up
A. No follow-up is needed unless indicated. Recurrence is common.

Consultation/Referral
A. No referral is needed unless indicated.

Individual Considerations
A. Geriatrics:
   1. Cerumen impaction is very common in the elderly due to atrophic cilia and dry epithelium in the ear canal.
   2. The use of hearing aids also can contribute to wax buildup and cause wax to be pushed further into the canal. Persons with hearing aids should be evaluated for wax buildup as indicated.

Bibliography
Bird, S. (2008). Ear syringing: Minimizing the risks. *Australian Family Physician*, *37*(4), 359–360. Retrieved from www.racgp.org.au/afp/backissues/2008
Dinces, E. (2015). Cerumen. In D. Deschler (Ed.), *UpToDate*. Retrieved from https://www.uptodate.com/contents/cerumen?source=machine Learning&search=ear+lavage&selectedTitle=1%7E150&sectionRank=1&anchor=H9#H9

Hearing Loss

Jill C. Cash, Moya Cook, and Paul Jeffrey

Definition
Impaired hearing (complete or partial hearing loss) results from interference with the conduction of sound, its conversion to electrical impulses, or its transmission through the nervous system. There are three types of hearing loss:
A. Conductive hearing loss.
B. Sensorineural hearing loss.
C. Combined conductive and sensorineural loss.

Incidence/Prevalence
A. Hearing loss is present in approximately 40% of adults between 20 and 79 years of age, and 8% of children and youth between 6 and 19 years of age.

Pathogenesis
A. *Conductive hearing loss* presents with a diminution of volume, particularly low tones and vowels. It may be caused by one of the following:
  1. Otosclerosis disorder of the architecture of the bony labyrinth, which fixes the footplate of the stapes in the oval window.
  2. Exostoses: bony excrescences of the external auditory canal.
  3. Glomus tumours: benign, highly vascular tumours derived from normally occurring glomera of the middle ear and jugular bulb.
B. *Sensorineural hearing loss* characteristically produces impairment of the high-tone perception. Affected clients can hear people speaking, but they have difficulty deciphering words because discrimination is poor. It may be caused by one of the following:
  1. Presbycusis: hearing loss associated with aging and the most common cause of diminished hearing in the elderly; onset is bilateral, symmetric, and gradual.
  2. Noise: noise-induced hearing loss is due to chronic exposure to sound levels in excess of 85 to 90 dB.
  3. Drugs: drug-induced hearing loss can be caused by aminoglycoside antibiotics, furosemide, ethacrynic acid, quinidine, and ASA.
  4. Ménière's disease, which produces a fluctuating, unilateral, low-frequency impairment usually associated with tinnitus, a sensation of fullness in the ear, and intermittent episodes of vertigo.
  5. Acoustic neuroma: a benign tumour of the eighth cranial nerve (rare).
  6. Genetics: generally bilateral and symmetric, it may be genetically determined.
  7. Sudden onset can derive from head trauma, skull fracture, meningitis, otitis media, scarlet fever, mumps, congenital syphilis, multiple sclerosis, and perilymph leaks or fistulas.

Predisposing Factors
A. Acoustic or physical trauma.
B. Ototoxic medications (such as gentamicin and ASA).
C. Changes in barometric pressures.
D. Recent upper respiratory infection (URI).
E. Pregnancy.
F. Otosclerosis.
G. Nasopharyngeal cancer.
H. Serous otitis media.
I. Cerumen impaction.
J. Foreign body in the ear.

Common Findings
A. Partial hearing loss.
B. Total hearing loss.
C. Difficulty understanding the television, phone conversations, and people talking.

Other Signs and Symptoms
A. Unilateral or bilateral hearing loss.
B. Hearing noises, such as "ringing" or "buzzing."
C. Fullness in ear(s).

Subjective Data
A. Elicit the onset, duration, progression, and severity of symptoms. Note whether symptoms are bilateral or unilateral.
B. Obtain the client's history of past or recent trauma.
C. Review the client's occupational and recreational exposure to risk factors.
D. Review the client's medical history and medications, including over-the-counter (OTC) drugs and prescriptions.
E. Review the client's history for recent URI or ear infections, especially for chronic ear infections.
F. Elicit data about any previous hearing loss, how it was treated, and how it affected daily activities. There is often a history of previous ear disease with conductive hearing loss.
G. Review the client's other symptoms, such as dizziness, fullness or pressure in the ears, and noises.
H. Review what causes difficulty with hearing: high tones versus low frequencies. Can the client hear people talking, television at normal volume, doorbells ringing, telephone ringing, and watch ticking?

Physical Examination
A. Temperature.
B. Inspect:
  1. Examine both ears for comparison.
  2. Externally inspect ears for discharge, note colour and odour. Obstruction of the auditory canal by impacted cerumen, a foreign body, exostoses, external otitis, otitis media with effusion (OME), or scarring or perforation of the eardrum due to chronic otitis may be present.
  3. Conduct otoscopic examination to observe the auditory canal for cerumen impaction or foreign body.
  4. Examine tympanic membrane for colour, landmarks, contour, perforation, and acute otitis media (AOM). A reddish mass visible through the intact tympanic membrane may indicate a high-riding jugular bulb, an aberrant internal carotid artery, or a glomus tumour.
C. Palpate:
  1. Palpate auricle and mastoid area for tenderness, swelling, or nodules.
  2. Check lymph nodes if infection is suspected.
D. Neurologic testing:
  1. Weber test: Perform a Weber screen, which reveals conductive hearing loss when sound travels toward the poor ear. Sensorineural hearing loss is present when sound travels toward the good ear. This is performed by striking a tuning fork and then placing it on the middle of the head. The client should be asked where sound is being heard from: the left ear, the right ear, or equal in both ears. Normal results are reflected by sound being heard equally in both ears.
  2. Rinne screen: The Rinne tuning fork test reveals bone conduction greater than air conduction in the affected ear (abnormal). The Rinne test is performed by placing the struck tuning fork against the mastoid bone. Begin counting or timing the interval from the start to when the client can no longer hear. Continue counting or timing the interval to determine the length of time sound is heard by air conduction. Air-conducted sound should be heard twice as long as bone-conducted sound after bone conduction stops.

Diagnostic Tests
A. Audiogram in primary setting.
B. Air insufflation for tympanic membrane mobility.

C. Tympanometry brainstem-evoked response audiogram.
D. CT scan or MRI after consultation with an otolaryngologist.

Differential Diagnoses
A. Congenital hearing loss.
B. Traumatic hearing loss.
C. Ototoxicity.
D. Presbycusis.
E. Ménière's disease.
F. Acoustic neuroma.
G. Cholesteatoma.
H. Infection.
I. Cerumen impaction.
J. Otitis externa.
K. Foreign body in the ear.
L. Tumours.
M. Otosclerosis.
N. Perforation of tympanic membrane.
O. Serous otitis media.
P. Hypothyroidism.
Q. Paget's disease.

Plan
A. General interventions:
   1. Treat any primary cause (i.e., remove impacted cerumen).
   2. Inform the client regarding results of screening and indications for further testing.
B. Client teaching:
   1. Discuss avoiding loud noises, using earplugs, and so forth.
   2. Instruct the client not to insert small objects into the ear.
C. Pharmacological therapy: Treat primary condition if applicable.

Follow-Up
A. If the primary cause of hearing loss is not identified, refer the client to a hearing specialist.

Consultation/Referral
A. The client should be referred to an otolaryngologist for an extensive workup when the primary cause cannot be identified.
B. Referral should be made to a hearing aid specialist for hearing evaluation and treatment as indicated (i.e., hearing aids).

Individual Considerations
A. Paediatrics:
   1. Most children are able to respond to a test of gross hearing using a small bell. To determine the client's hearing ability, note if the child stops moving when the bell is rung and if the child turns his or her head toward the sound.
   2. When examining children, pull the pinna back and slightly upward to straighten the canal.
B. Adults: The external auditory canal in the adult can best be exposed by pulling the earlobe upward and backward.
C. Geriatrics:
   1. Impaired hearing among the elderly is common and can lower the quality of life.
   2. People with seriously impaired hearing often become withdrawn or appear confused.
   3. Subtle hearing loss may go unrecognized.
   4. Impacted cerumen is very common in the elderly.

Bibliography
Bhattacharyya, N., & Meyers, A. D. (2015). Auditory brainstem response auditometry. *Medscape.* Retrieved from http://emedicine.medscape.com/article/836277-overview#a6

Centers for Disease Control and Prevention, National Institute for Occupational Safety and Health. (2013). *Noise and hearing loss prevention.* DHHS (NIOSH) Pub. No. 2001-103. Retrieved from www.cdc.gov

Mener, D. J., Betz, J., Genther, D. J., Chen, D., & Lin, F. R. (2013). Hearing loss and depression in older adults. *Journal of the American Geriatrics Society, 61*(9), 1627–1629. doi:10.1111/jgs.12429

National Institute on Deafness and Other Communication Disorders. (2016, March). *NIDCD fact sheet: Hearing and balance: Hearing loss and older adults.* NIH Pub. No. 01-4913. Washington, DC: U.S. Department of Health and Human Services. Retrieved from https://www.nidcd.nih.gov/health/hearing-loss-older-adults

National Institutes of Health, National Institute on Deafness and Other Communication Disorders. (2015a). *NIDCD fact sheet: Hearing and balance: Pendred syndrome.* NIH Publication No. 06-5875. November 2012, Reprinted December 2014. Washington, DC: U.S. Department of Health and Human Services. Retrieved from https://www.nidcd.nih.gov/health/pendred-syndrome

National Institutes of Health, National Institute on Deafness and Other Communication Disorders. (2015b). *Quick statistics about hearing.* Retrieved from https://www.nidcd.nih.gov/health/statistics/quick-statistics-hearing

Roland, P. S. (2015). Presbycusis. *Medscape.* Retrieved from www.medscape.comarticle/855989-overview

Statistics Canada. (2016). *Hearing loss of Canadians, 2012 to 2015.* Retrieved from https://www150.statcan.gc.ca/n1/pub/82-625-x/2016001/article/14658-eng.htm

Otitis Externa

Jill C. Cash and Moya Cook

Definition
A. Otitis externa is a common, acute, self-limiting inflammation or infection of the external auditory canal and auricle.

Incidence/Prevalence
A. Otitis externa is seen in clients of all ages. Incidence is higher during summer months. All varieties (with exception of necrotizing otitis externa) are common.

Pathogenesis
A. Acute diffuse otitis externa (swimmer's ear): *Pseudomonas* is the most common bacterial infection (67%), followed by *Staphylococcus* and *Streptococcus*. Infection can also be fungal (*Aspergillus*, 90%). Bacterial or fungal invasion is usually preceded by trauma to the ear canal, aggressive cleaning of the naturally bactericidal cerumen, or frequent submersion in water (swimming).
B. Chronic otitis externa: The condition generally results from a persistent, low-grade infection and inflammation with *Pseudomonas*.
C. Eczematous otitis externa: Otitis externa is associated with a primary coexistent skin disorder such as atopic dermatitis, seborrhoeic dermatitis, and psoriasis.
D. Necrotizing or malignant otitis externa: Invasive *Pseudomonas* infection results in skull base osteomyelitis. It is most commonly seen in the immunocompromised or diabetic geriatric client.

Predisposing Factors
A. Ear trauma from scratching with a foreign object or fingernail, overly vigorous cleaning of cerumen from canal.
B. Humid climate.
C. Frequent swimming.
D. Use of a hearing aid.
E. Eczema (eczematous otitis externa).
F. Debilitating disease (necrotizing otitis externa).

Common Findings
A. Otalgia.
B. Itching.
C. Erythematous and swollen external canal.
D. Purulent discharge.
E. Hearing loss from edema and obstruction of canal with drainage.

Other Signs and Symptoms
A. Plugged ear sensation (aural fullness).
B. Tenderness to palpation (tragus).

Subjective Data
A. Elicit the onset, duration, and intensity of ear discomfort.
B. Inquire into the client's history of previous ear infections.
C. Determine whether the client notes any degree of hearing loss.
D. Question the client about recent exposure to immersion in water (swimming).
E. Question the client as to ear canal cleaning practices and any recent trauma to the canal.

Physical Examination
A. Temperature.
B. Inspect:
  1. Carefully examine the ear with an otoscope for extreme tenderness.
  2. Observe the ear for erythematous and edematous external canal; look for otorrhoea and debris.
  3. Observe the tympanic membrane, which may appear normal.
  4. Inspect nose and throat.
C. Auscultate heart and lungs.
D. Palpate:
  1. Apply gentle pressure to tragus and manipulate pinna to assess for tenderness.
  2. Palpate cervical lymph nodes.

Diagnostic Tests
A. Examine ear canal scrapings and drainage under a microscope for hyphae (if fungal infection is suspected from previous history or ineffective topical therapy).
B. Culture vesicular lesions for viruses.

Differential Diagnoses
A. Otitis media.
B. Foreign body.
C. Mastoiditis.
D. Hearing loss.
E. Wisdom tooth eruption.
F. Herpetic otitis externa (vesicular eruptions in the ear canal are associated with herpetic otitis externa).
G. Necrotizing or malignant otitis externa (life-threatening condition that occurs in diabetic or immunocompromised clients). Cranial nerve palsies (of the seventh, eighth, and 12th cranial nerves) and periostitis of the skull base have been associated with necrotizing otitis externa.

Plan
A. General interventions:
  1. When the client's ear canal is sufficiently blocked by edema or drainage, preventing passage of ear drops, cautiously irrigate the canal and insert a cotton wick to allow passage of drops.
  2. Insert the wick by gently rotating it while inserting it into the ear. The client then places ear drops on the wick. The drops are absorbed through the wick, which allows medicine to reach the external canal. The provider may need to change the wick daily or several times per week.
B. Client teaching:
  1. *Refer to Client Teaching Guide: Otitis Externa.* The client should be advised to keep water out of the ear for four to six weeks. The client should not swim until symptoms are completely resolved and the wick is removed.
  2. Bathing or showering is permitted with a cotton ball coated with petroleum jelly inserted into the ear to block water passage into the ear canal.
C. Pharmacological therapy:
  1. For early, mild cases associated with swimming in which the primary symptom is pruritus, homemade preparations of 50% isopropyl alcohol and 50% vinegar can be used as a drying agent and to create an unsatisfactory environment for *Pseudomonas* growth. A compound of 95% isopropyl alcohol and glycerin or acetic acid 2% solution can also be used.
  2. Mild infection: Topical therapy with acidifying agent such as aluminum acetate (otic solution). Apply two to three drops, three to four times a day (no duration stated).
  3. Moderate infection: Use of an acidifying agent, antibiotic and glucocorticoid therapy, and cortisporin is suggested. Other alternatives include iprofloxacin, ofloxacin, polymyxin B, and neomycin suspension or solution. Adults should apply four drops to the canal four times daily for seven days; children should apply three drops to the canal four times daily for seven days. The suspension is recommended rather than the solution if the integrity of the tympanic membrane is in question. If fungal infection is suspected, Nystatin or clotrimazole topical solutions may be used for candidal or yeast infections.
  4. Severe or resistant infections may require additional management with oral antibiotics and antifungals:
    a. Ciprofloxacin for pseudomonal infections; dicloxacillin or cephalexin for staphylococcal infections.
    b. Itraconazole for treatment of otomycosis (fungal otitis externa).
  5. For analgesia, use acetaminophen or ibuprofen. Short-term use of opiates may be necessary when acetaminophen and ibuprofen fail to control pain.

Follow-Up
A. Usual follow-up is within 48 hours to assess improvement. Recheck in one to two weeks.
B. In severe cases requiring antibiotic drops instilled by means of a wick, follow-up may be required daily or several times per week to remove and replace the wick.

▶ Client Teaching Guides are available at https://connect.springerpub.com/content/reference-book/978-0-8261-9498-5

Consultation/Referral
A. Parenteral antibiotics are required for necrotizing otitis externa.
B. Consult or refer the client if osteomyelitis is suspected.

Individual Considerations
A. Geriatrics:
  1. Persistent otitis externa in the geriatric client (especially those who are immunocompromised or diabetic) may evolve into osteomyelitis of the skull base. The external ear is painful and edematous, and a foul, green discharge is usually present. Treatment may require parenteral gentamicin with a beta-lactam agent. Surgery may be necessary. Oral fluoroquinolones may be useful if infection has not progressed to osteomyelitis.

Bibliography
Bugs and Drugs. (2018). *Swimmers ear*. Retrieved from http://bugsanddrugs.org/Home/Index/bdpage001044B8CBCC459896042D4DD7E2B814

Hui, C. (2013). Acute otitis externa: Canadian paediatric society. *Paediatric Child Health*, *18*(2), 96–98. doi:10.1093/pch/18.2.96. Retrieved from https://www.cps.ca/en/documents/position/acute-otitis-externa

Medscape. (2018). *Aluminum acetate solution (OTC)*. Retrieved from https://reference.medscape.com/drug/domeboro-astringent-solution-powder-packets-burows-solution-aluminum-acetate-solution-999353

Schaefer, P., & Baugh, R. (2012). Acute otitis externa: An update. *American Family Physician*, *86*(11), 1055–1061.

Shevchuk, Y. (2016). *Canadian pharmacists association: Otitis media and otitis externa*. Retrieved from http://www.pharmacists.ca/cpha-ca/assets/File/Sample%20chapters/CTMAChapter-OtitisMediaOtitisExterna.pdf

Otitis Media With Effusion

Jill C. Cash, Moya Cook, and Paul Jeffrey

Definition
A. Otitis media with effusion (OME) is asymptomatic middle ear fluid without signs of bacterial infection.

Incidence/Prevalence
A. OME is seen in clients of all ages.
B. After the onset of acute otitis media (AOM), approximately 70% of children have fluid present at two weeks.
  1. 40% have fluid present at one month.
  2. 20% have fluid present at two months.
  3. 10% have an effusion at three months.

Pathogenesis
A. The effusion may be sterile fluid secondary to upper respiratory infection (URI) and Eustachian tube dysfunction. It may be residual fluid after an episode of AOM.

Predisposing Factors
A. Recent otitis media.
B. Concurrent URI.

Common Findings
A. Ear pain.
B. Increased pressure sensation in the ears.
C. Recent hearing loss.

Other Signs and Symptoms
A. The client has a sense of fullness in the ears.

Subjective Data
A. Elicit the onset and duration of symptoms.
B. Question the client about recent history of otitis media or URI.
C. Question the client about hearing loss.
D. Determine if the client has a past history of frequent otitis media.

Physical Examination
A. Check temperature, pulse, respirations, and blood pressure.
B. Inspect:
  1. Ears, noting fluid level, serous middle fluid, and a translucent, amber, gray membrane with decreased mobility.
  2. Nose, mouth, and throat.
C. Auscultate heart and lungs.
D. Palpate head, neck, and lymph nodes.
E. Neurologic examination:
  1. Perform the Rinne test. This test is performed by placing the struck tuning fork against the mastoid bone. Begin counting or timing the interval from the start to when the client can no longer hear. Continue counting or timing the interval to determine the length of time sound is heard by air conduction. Air-conducted sound should be heard twice as long as bone-conducted sound after bone conduction stops.
  2. Perform the Weber test.

Diagnostic Tests
A. Pneumatic otoscopy reveals decreased mobility. **Assessment with pneumatic otoscopy is strongly recommended.**
B. Negative pressure on tympanogram.

Differential Diagnoses
A. Cerumen impaction.
B. AOM.
C. Foreign body in the ear.

Plan
A. General interventions:
  1. Client should be monitored closely for resolution of effusion without treatment within several weeks.
  2. Clients who have persistent effusion are at risk for hearing loss and speech, language, and learning disorders.
  3. Children with persistent OME should be referred to an ear, nose, and throat specialist for a hearing evaluation and possible tympanostomy tubes as indicated.
  4. Speech and language evaluation or documentation of hearing loss is recommended for children with OME older than 3 months.
B. Client teaching:
  1. *Refer to Client Teaching Guide: Otitis Media With Effusion.* Educate parents that OME is not treated with antibiotics, since no infection is present.
  2. If symptoms change, infection should be suspected and the primary care provider should be notified of new symptoms and that reevaluation is needed.
  3. Teach the parents/care provider that routine use of antihistamines and decongestants is not recommended.
C. Pharmacological therapy:
  1. Both Health Canada and Speech-Language and Audiology Canada do not recommend routine use of

antibiotic therapy for OME. However, in certain situations, a course of antibiotics (amoxil) for 10 to 14 days is recommended.
2. Intranasal glucocorticoids are not recommended for routine use for OME in children.
3. Antihistamines and decongestants are not recommended for routine use for OME in children.

Follow-Up
A. Recheck the client's ears after four to six weeks to evaluate effectiveness of treatment.

Consultation/Referral
A. Consider referring the client to an ear, nose, and throat specialist, especially in the face of recurrent infections.

Individual Considerations
A. Geriatrics:
  1. OME may be present in the elderly, usually unilaterally, and usually associated with a URI or allergies due to a blocked eustachian tube.
  2. If there is no accompanying URI, a nasopharyngeal mass must be ruled out.

Bibliography
Bugs and Drugs. (2018). *Persistent otitis media*. Retrieved from http://bugsanddrugs.org/Home/Index/bdpage001044B8CBCC459896042D4DD7E2B814

Government of Canada. (2017b). *Adult care - chapter 2 - ears, nose, throat and mouth*. Retrieved from https://www.canada.ca/en/indigenousservices-canada/services/first-nations-inuit-health/healthcareservices/nursing/clinical-practice-guidelines-nurses-primary-care/adultcare/chapter-2-ears-nose-throat-mouth.html#a15

Klein, J. O., & Pelton, S. (2016). Management of otitis media with effusion (serous otitis media) in children. In S. Kaplan & G. Isaacson (Eds.), *UpToDate*. Retrieved from http://www.uptodate.com/contents/management-of-otitis-media-with-effusion-serous-otitis-media-in-children?source=search_result&search=otitis+meda+with+effusion&selectedTitle=1 48

Lustig, L. R., Limb, C. J., Baden, R., & LaSalvia, M. T. (2015). Chronic otitis media, cholesteatoma, and mastoiditis in adults. In D. Deschler (Ed.), *UpToDate*. Retrieved from http://www.uptodate.com/contents/chronic-otitis-media-cholesteatoma-and-mastoiditis-in-adults?source=search_result&search=otitis+media+adult&selectedTitle=2%7E150

Poe, D., & Bassem, M. (2016). Eustachian tube dysfunction. In D. Deschler (Ed.), *UpToDate*. Retrieved from http://www.uptodate.com/contents/eustachian-tube-dysfunction?source=search_result&search=eustachian+tube+dysfunction&selectedTitle=1%7E39

Shevchuk, Y. (2016). *Canadian pharmacists association: Otitis media and otitis externa*. Retrieved from http://www.pharmacists.ca/cpha-ca/assets/File/Sample%20chapters/CTMAChapter-OtitisMediaOtitisExterna.pdf

Speech-Language & Audiology Canada. (2016). *AAO-HNSF updated clinical practice guideline: Otitis media with effusion (American Academy of Otolaryngology – Head and Neck Surgery)*. Retrieved from https://www.sac-oac.ca/news-events/news/aao-hnsf-updated-clinical-practice-guideline-otitis-media-effusion-american-academy

Tinnitus

Jill C. Cash and Moya Cook

Definition
A. The word *tinnitus* comes from the Latin *tinnire*, which means "to ring." It refers to any sound heard in the ears or head.

Incidence/Prevalence
A. Over 40% of Canadians are affected by tinnitus at least once in their lifetime.

Pathogenesis
A. Tinnitus is poorly understood. It is best described as a nonspecific manifestation of pathology of the inner ear, eighth cranial nerve, or the central auditory mechanism.

Predisposing Factors
A. Cerumen impaction.
B. Tympanic membrane perforation.
C. Fluid in the middle ear.
D. Acute otitis media (AOM).
E. Acoustic trauma.
F. Ototoxic drugs:
  1. Sulfas.
  2. Aminoglycosides.
  3. Salicylate.
  4. Indomethacin.
  5. Propranolol.
  6. Levodopa.
  7. Carbamazepine.
G. Vascular aneurysm.
H. Jugular bulb anomaly. Compression of the ipsilateral jugular vein abolishes the objective tinnitus of a jugular megabulb anomaly.
I. Anemia.
J. Temporomandibular joint syndrome.
K. Hypertension.

Common Findings
A. Ringing.
B. Roaring.
C. Buzzing.
D. Clicking.
E. Hissing.
F. Hearing loss.

Other Signs and Symptoms
A. "Muffled" hearing.
B. Change in own voice, lower pitch.

Subjective Data
A. Review the onset, duration, course, and type of symptoms; note whether they are bilateral or unilateral.
B. Determine the frequency and quality of sound; is the ringing constant, intermittent, or pulsating?
C. Review all medications, including over-the-counter (OTC) drugs and prescriptions.
D. Determine whether the client has experienced trauma (domestic violence, motor vehicle accident, and so forth).
E. Rule out a recent sinus, oral, or ear infection.
F. Review any previous occurrences. Ask, How was it treated?
G. Review work, hobbies, and music habits for noise levels (potential damage).
H. Assess the date of last hearing examination and determine whether there was any known hearing loss.
I. Review whether the client uses cotton-tipped swabs or other small objects for ear cleaning.

Physical Examination
A. Take temperature if infectious cause is suspected.
B. Inspect:
  1. Observe the external ear for discharge; note colour and odour.
  2. Conduct otoscopic examination of the auditory canal for cerumen impaction or foreign body.

3. Inspect tympanic membrane for colour, landmarks, contour, perforation, and AOM:
   a. The landmarks (umbo, handle of malleus, and the light reflex) should be visible on a normal examination.
   b. The tympanic membrane should be pearly gray in colour and translucent.
   c. A bulging tympanic membrane is more conical, usually with a loss of bony landmarks and a distorted light reflex.
   d. A retracted tympanic membrane is more concave, usually with accentuated bony landmarks and a distorted light reflex (pathologic conditions in the middle ear may be reflected by characteristics of the tympanic membrane).

C. Auscultation: The skull should be auscultated for a bruit if the origin of the problem remains obscure.
D. Palpate:
   1. Auricle and mastoid area for tenderness, swelling, or nodules.
   2. Lymph nodes if infection is suspected.
E. Visual examination: Check for nystagmus if vertigo is reported.
F. Neurologic examination:
   1. The eighth cranial nerve is tested by evaluating hearing.
   2. First evaluate how the client responds to your questions.
   3. Clients who speak in a monotone or with erratic volume may have hearing loss.
   4. Check the client's response to a soft whisper (should respond at least 50% of the time).
   5. Perform the Rinne test: Place the struck tuning fork against the mastoid bone. Begin counting or timing the interval from the start to when the client can no longer hear. Continue counting or timing the interval to determine the length of time sound is heard by air conduction. Air-conducted sound should be heard twice as long as bone-conducted sound after bone conduction stops.
   6. Perform the Weber test.

Diagnostic Tests
A. Audiogram is performed in the primary care setting; other testing is performed by an otolaryngologist. Any association of the sound with respiration, drug use, vertigo, noise trauma, or ear infection should be checked. When the problem is present only at night, it suggests increased awareness of normal head sounds.
B. CT scan or MRI after referral to an ear, nose, and throat (ENT) specialist.
C. Posterior fossa myelography.

Differential Diagnoses
A. Cerumen impaction.
B. Foreign body in the ear.
C. AOM.
D. Otitis externa.
E. Acoustic traumas.
F. Vascular aneurysm.
G. Temporomandibular joint syndrome.
H. Otosclerosis.
I. Ototoxicity.
J. Ménière's disease.
K. Presbycusis.
L. Central nervous system lesion.

Plan
A. General interventions:
   1. Stress the importance of not placing small objects in the ear and of using cotton-tipped applicators to clean external ear only.
   2. Suggest to the client that keeping a radio on for background noise often facilitates sleep or work.
   3. Address underlying conditions if present (depression, insomnia, hearing loss, drug toxicity).
   4. Consider behavioural therapy, such as biofeedback or cognitive behavioural therapy, to teach client coping strategies.
B. Client teaching: *Refer to Client Teaching Guide: Tinnitus.* ◀
   1. Educate the client regarding techniques/therapies to improve symptoms of tinnitus.
   2. Encourage the client to attend therapy sessions as indicated.
C. Pharmacological therapy:
   1. No medication "cures" tinnitus.
   2. Vasodilators, tranquilizers, antidepressants, and seizure medications have been shown to reduce symptoms.
   3. Placebos are also of therapeutic value.

Follow-Up
A. No specific follow-up is required for tinnitus unless a treatable problem is identified.

Consultation/Referral
A. Consult with an ENT specialist as indicated.
B. Referral of an anxious client to the ENT specialist may be necessary to satisfy the client that everything has been explored and that there is no serious or correctable underlying condition.
C. Any client with a history of head trauma should be referred because tinnitus may be associated with an arteriovenous fistula or an aneurysm of the intrapetrous portion of the internal carotid artery.

Bibliography
Tunkel, D. E., Bauer, C. A., Sun, G. H., Rosenfeld, R. M., Chandrasekhar, S. S., Cunningham, E. R., . . . Whamond, E. J. (2014). Clinical guidelines: Tinnitus. *Otolaryngology Head Neck Surgery, 151*(Suppl. 2), S1–40. doi:10.1177/0194599814547475. Retrieved from https://www.guideline.gov/content.aspx?id=48751&search=tinnitus

Wu, V., Cooke, B., Eitutis, S., Simpson, M., & Beyea, J. (2018). Approach to tinnitus management. *Canadian Family Physician, 64*(7), 491–495.

7 Nasal Guidelines

Allergic Rhinitis

Jill C. Cash, Moya Cook, and Valda Duke

Definition
A. Allergic rhinitis is a chronic or recurrent condition characterized by nasal congestion, clear nasal discharge, sneezing, nasal and oropharynx itching, conjunctival itching, and can be accompanied by excessive tearing. It usually occurs seasonally after exposure to allergens (same time every year, associated with pollen count), or it may be perennial (year-round, related to indoor inhalants, animal dander, and mould). "Allergic" suggests that a specific immunoglobulin E (IgE) antibody mediates the condition.

Incidence/Prevalence
A. Prevalence varies according to geographic region; 40% of the population have allergic rhinitis.

Pathogenesis
A. This is an IgE-mediated inflammatory disease involving nasal mucosa; IgE antibodies bind to mast cells in the respiratory epithelium, and histamine is released. This results in immediate local vasodilatation, mucosal oedema, and increased mucus production.

Predisposing Factors
A. Genetic predisposition to allergy.
B. Exposure to allergic stimuli: Pollens, moulds, animal dander, dust mites, and indoor inhalants.

Common Findings
A. Nasal congestion.
B. Sneezing.
C. Clear rhinorrhoea.
D. Coughing from postnasal drip.
E. Sore throat.
F. Itchy, puffy eyes with tearing.
G. Often associated with asthma and atopic dermatitis.

Other Signs and Symptoms
A. Dry mouth from mouth breathing, snoring.
B. Itchy nose.
C. Loss of smell and taste.
D. Eczema rash.
E. Shortness of breath, difficulty breathing, and wheezing.
F. Headache.
G. Halitosis.

Subjective Data
A. Ask about onset, course, frequency, and duration of symptoms.
B. Inquire about characteristics of nasal discharge.
C. Inquire about exposure to people with similar symptoms.
D. Ask about seasonal impact on symptoms.
E. Inquire about other diseases caused by allergens, such as asthma, eczema, and urticaria or family history of same.
F. Rule out pregnancy.
G. Ask female clients about their birth control method, specifically birth control pills.
H. Review exposure to irritants.
I. Ask about any past or recent nasal or facial trauma.
J. Interference with activities of daily living (ADL; sleep, work, and school) and degree of severity.
K. Ask about smoking history.
L. Inquire about recent swimming or diving.
M. Ask about presence of other associated symptoms such as fever, weight loss, myalgias, or cough.
N. Inquire about the current use of medications and recreational drugs.

Physical Examination
A. Vital signs: Temperature, blood pressure, pulse, and respirations.
B. Inspect:
  1. Examine face: Note Dennie's lines (skin folds under eyes) and allergic salute (transverse crease on nose from chronic rubbing of nose).
  2. Examine eyes and conjunctivae:
    a. Tearing; red, swollen eyelids; and "allergic shiners" (dark circles under eyes from venous congestion in maxillary sinuses) are seen with allergies.
    b. Palpebral conjunctiva pale and swollen, bulbar conjunctiva is injected.
  3. Examine ears, nose, and throat:
    a. Red, dull, bulging, perforated tympanic membrane is seen with otitis media.
    b. Nasal redness, swelling, polyps, and enlarged turbinates are seen with upper respiratory infection (URI). Mucosa appears pale blue, and boggy with clear discharge in chronic allergy.
    c. Cobblestone appearance in posterior pharynx, tonsils, and adenoids seen in chronic allergies.

d. Use otoscope light to transilluminate under superior orbital ridge of frontal sinus cavity and also maxillary sinus cavity to assess for fluid in sinus cavity. Healthy sinuses contain air and light up symmetrically.
C. Palpate:
  1. Palpate face and frontal maxillary sinuses for tenderness.
  2. Examine the head and neck for enlarged lymph nodes.
D. Percuss:
  1. Sinus cavities and mastoid bone.
  2. Chest for consolidation.
  3. Teeth for dental abcesses.
E. Auscultate heart and lungs.

Diagnostic Tests

Diagnosis may be made from history and physical. Other diagnostic tests include the following:
A. Complete blood count (CBC) with increased eosinophils (confirm allergy).
B. Skin testing for allergies.
C. Enzyme-linked immunosorbent assay (ELISA) test.

Differential Diagnoses

A. URI.
B. Medication-induced rhinitis.
C. Sinusitis.
D. Otitis media.
E. Deviated septum.
F. Nasal polyps.
G. Endocrine conditions such as hypothyroidism.
H. Influenza.
I. Substance induced (cocaine).
J. Nonallergic rhinitis.

Plan

A. General interventions:
  1. Avoid allergens (most effective treatment).
  2. Keep bedroom as allergen free as possible.
  3. Saline nose rinse.
▶ B. Client teaching: *Refer to Client Teaching Guide: Allergic Rhinitis.*
C. Pharmacological therapy:
Decongestants and first-generation antihistamines not to be used in children under the age of 6.
  1. Second-generation antihistamines (H_1 receptor antagonists) are first-line treatment. Several may need to be tried before an effective one is found. Drugs may also need to be switched occasionally to prevent tolerance:
    a. Loratadine.
    b. Fexofenadine.
    c. Cetirizine.
    d. Desloratadine.
    e. Montelukast.
  2. Decongestants for significant congestion of the mucous membranes. These drugs may also stimulate the sympathetic nervous system and cause insomnia, nervousness, and palpitations. **Use no longer than three to five days. Discontinuing these drugs after five days may result in a rebound effect. NOT for children <6 years of age**:
    a. Oxymetazoline hydrochloride.
    b. Phenylephrine.
  3. Steroid sprays may be used to decrease nasal inflammation. Steroid sprays are not recommended in children younger than 6 years old unless there is an allergic component. Sprays do not cause significant systemic absorption in usual doses, but occasionally they may cause pharyngeal fungal infections:
    a. Beclomethasone dipropionate.
    b. Fluticasone propionate.
    c. Triamcinolone acetonide.
    d. Mometasone furoate.
    e. Fluticasone furoate.
    f. Budesonide.
    g. Beclomethasone dipropionate.
  4. Saline spray:
    a. Saline spray is effective in liquefying thick secretions and helps keep mucosa moist.
    b. Use neti pot to cleanse inside of nasal mucosa; daily use suggested.
  5. Petroleum jelly applied with Q-tip to inside mucosa of nares three to four times a day helps to provide lubrication and hold in moisture to prevent nasal dryness and bleeding.

Follow-Up

A. Client should return for follow-up visit in two to three weeks if necessary; earlier if symptoms worsen after three days of treatment.

Consultation/Referral

A. Refer the client to an allergist if symptoms continue and interfere with daily activities.
B. Allergist may prescribe immunotherapy following identification of offending allergens.

Individual Considerations

A. Pregnancy:
  1. Over-the-counter (OTC) antihistamines, such as diphenhydramine HCl, limited human data in relation to lactation.
  2. OTC decongestants, AVOID.
  3. **Saline nasal spray is safe for use in pregnancy and with lactation**.

Bibliography

Dains, J. E., Baumann, L. C., & Scheibel, P. (2016). *Advanced health assessment and clinical diagnosis in primary care* (5th ed.). St. Louis, MO: Elsevier.

deShazo, R., & Kemp, S. (2016). Pharmacotherapy of allergic rhinitis. In J. Corren (Ed.), *UpToDate*. Waltham, MA: Wolters Kluwer. Retrieved from http://www.uptodate.com/contents/pharmacotherapy-of-allergic-rhinitis?source=search_result&search=Pharmacotherapy+of+allergic+rhinitis&selectedTitle=1%7E150

Canadian Pharmacists Association. (2011). *Therapeutic choices* (6th ed.). Ottawa, ON, Canada: Canadian Pharmacists Association.

Ramavaram, S., & Jones, S. M. (2012). Natural course and comorbidities of allergic and nonallergic rhinitis in children. *Pediatrics, 130*(Suppl. 1), S23–S24. doi:10.1542/peds.2012-2183KK

Regier, L. (2014). *RxFiles drug comparison charts* (10th ed.). Saskatoon, SK, Canada: Saskatchewan Health.

Sandomirsky, L., & Taylor, J. (2017). *Allergic rhinitis: Guidelines for prescribing intranasal corticosteroids.* Retrieved from http://m.medsask.usask.ca/professional/guidelines/allergic-rhinitis.php

Thompson, E. G., O'Brien, B. D., Husney, A., & Katial, R. K. (2017). Allergy and immunology. *HealthLinkBC*. Retrieved from https://www.healthlinkbc.ca/medical-tests/hw198350

▶ Client Teaching Guides are available at https://connect.springerpub.com/content/reference-book/978-0-8261-9498-5

Epistaxis

Jill C. Cash, Moya Cook, and Valda Duke

Definition
A. Epistaxis is a nosebleed or haemorrhage from the nose.

Incidence/Prevalence
A. About 60% of the population have had at least one nosebleed in their lifetime.

Pathogenesis
A. Epistaxis is caused by disruption of the nasal mucosa. More than 90% of nosebleeds are related to local irritation rather than underlying anatomic lesions and are self-limiting. Most start in the anterior nasal cavity (Kisselbach's plexus).
B. Posterior nasal bleeding usually originates from the turbinates or lateral nasal wall and is more serious.

Predisposing Factors
A. Local trauma, usually from nose picking.
B. Acute inflammation from an upper respiratory infection (URI; e.g., common cold, acute sinusitis, and allergic rhinitis).
C. Vigorous nose blowing.
D. Inhalation of chemical irritants.
E. Drying and crusting of nasal septum.
F. Trauma.
G. Cocaine use.
H. Pregnancy.
I. Neoplasm.
J. Systemic causes:
   1. Bleeding disorders (most common).
   2. Hypertension.
   3. Arteriosclerosis.
   4. Renal disease.

Common Findings
A. Common complaint is unusually severe or frequent nosebleeds.

Other Signs and Symptoms
A. Anterior epistaxis:
   1. Unilateral.
   2. Continuous, moderate bleeding from septum of nose.
B. Posterior epistaxis:
   1. Brisk (arterial) bleeding.
   2. Blood flowing into pharynx (indicates a more serious problem).

Subjective Data
A. Inquire about amount, duration, and frequency of bleeding.
B. Ask about use of oral anticoagulants, ASA, or ASA-containing compounds.
C. Ask about recent or current URIs, family history of abnormal bleeding, recent surgery, or trauma.
D. Ask about the first day of female client's last menstrual period (if appropriate). Determine if the client is pregnant.
E. Ask about a possible foreign body in the nose.
F. Ask about cocaine use or occupational exposure to irritants or chemicals.
G. If the client has a history of nosebleeds, how did the client treat previous nosebleeds?
H. Has the client ever been evaluated for a blood clotting abnormality, such as thrombocytopenia or platelet dysfunction or conditions that can affect coagulations, such as cancer, cirrhosis of the liver, and HIV?
I. Does the client complain of bruising or bleeding easily, melena, tarry stools, haemoptysis, or heavy menstrual periods?
J. Ask about family history of bleeding disorders such as hemophilia or von Willebrand's disease.
K. Ask about the use of nasal sprays.

Physical Examination
A. Check temperature, blood pressure (check for orthostatic hypertension), pulse, and respirations. **If nasal packing is required, take precaution and monitor client closely for vasovagal episode during insertion of nasal packing.**
B. Inspect:
   1. Check airway patency with client sitting and leaning forward.
   2. Observe skin, mucous membranes, and conjunctiva for rash, pallor, purpura, petechiae, and oral mucosal telangiectasias.
   3. Perform full eye examination, noting pupillary response.
   4. Examine nose for septal perforation and ulcerations, which indicate cocaine use. Collagen diseases (such as lupus) are occasionally responsible for ulceration. Epistaxis is rare in haemophiliacs without trauma but is characteristic of von Willebrand's disease.
   5. Examine nasal discharge: A unilateral foul discharge with blood indicates a foreign body in the nose.
   6. After bleeding has stopped:
      a. Inspect nasal mucosa for colour, discharge, masses, lesions, and swelling of turbinates.
      b. Inspect nasal septum for alignment, septal perforation, and crusting.
C. Auscultate heart and lungs.
D. Palpate: Check for enlarged lymph nodes in the neck to rule out sarcoidosis, tuberculosis, or malignancy.
E. Percuss sinuses.
F. Assess for red flags such as signs of hypovolemia or haemorrhagic shock, anticoagulant drug use.

Diagnostic Tests
A. **None is required unless the client has recurrent or severe blood loss.**
B. Perform drug screen, if indicated.
C. Haematocrit and haemoglobin, if bleeding is severe.
D. Complete blood count (CBC) with differential.
E. Platelets, prothrombin time (PT), and partial thromboplastin time (PTT) if bleeding disorder is suspected.
F. Sinus films if recurrent sinus pain, tenderness, and bleeding.

Differential Diagnoses
A. Foreign body.
B. Septal deformity.
C. Perforated nasal septum.
D. Coagulation disorder (von Willebrand's disease).
E. Nasal tumours.
F. Drug-induced coagulopathy.
G. Hypertension.
H. Pregnancy.

Plan

A. General interventions: Main goal is to control episodes of bleeding.
B. Client teaching: *Refer to Client Teaching Guide: Nosebleeds.*
C. Pharmacological therapy/medical/surgical management:
  1. To control *anterior septal bleeding*:
     a. Have client sit and lean forward, apply pressure by pinching nasal alae to reduce venous pressure, and prevent swallowing of blood.
     b. Visualize the bleed and soak a cotton pledget with 1:1 mix oxymetazoline HCl and lidocaine 2% and apply with pressure against bleeding site for 5 to 10 minutes.
     c. Remove and check for bleeding after 10 minutes.
     d. Then apply a silver nitrate stick to the bleeding site maximum 5 to 10 seconds and any prominent vessels, until gray eschar appears. Warn the client that this is painful.
     e. If bleeding still does not stop (rare), repeat last two steps. Then place a small amount of oxidized regenerated cellulose against the bleeding artery, or pack a small petroleum gauze strip in the nasal vestibule for 24 hours. Monitor the client for vasovagal episode during the insertion of packing. Apply ice to the palate (popsicles, ice in the mouth) to reduce nasal blood flow.
  2. To control *posterior* septal bleeding:
     a. Have the client sit and lean forward.
     b. Control bleeding: Spray nose with topical anaesthetic and vasoconstrictor, and apply pressure to the bleeding site.
     c. **The client needs ED care immediately because of rapid blood loss.**
     d. Take blood pressure and pulse; order haematocrit; blood type and crossmatch may be needed.

Follow-Up

A. Anterior septal bleeding: Referral to otolaryngologist is recommended for unsuccessful cessation of haemorrhage.
B. For posterior nosebleeds, admission to hospital and referral to otolaryngologist is recommended.

Consultation/Referral

A. Posterior epistaxis: Refer to an otolaryngologist immediately.

Individual Considerations

A. Pregnancy:
  1. Nosebleeds are common.
  2. Suggest use of saline spray to keep mucous membranes moist and use humidifier at bedtime.
  3. Follow use of saline spray with petroleum jelly applied with Q-tip daily to prevent recurrent nosebleeds.
B. Paediatrics:
  1. The most common cause of nosebleeds is trauma from nose picking or rubbing.
  2. Advise parents to keep fingernails short.
  3. Applying water-based lubricant on rims of nostrils to maintain mucosal moisture may cause lipoid pneumonia in infants and children.
C. Geriatrics:
  1. Spontaneous posterior haemorrhage is more common in elderly clients.
  2. Epistaxis is classically associated with hypertension or arteriosclerosis.
  3. Airway obstruction from posterior packing is especially risky in the elderly.
  4. Applying water-based lubricant on rims of nostrils to maintain mucosal moisture may cause lipoid pneumonia in the elderly.

Bibliography

Fried, M. P. (2018). *Epistaxis. Approach to the patient with nasal and pharyngeal symptoms*. Retrieved from https://www.merckmanuals.com/en-ca/professional/ear,-nose,-and-throat-disorders/approach-to-the-patient-with-nasal-and-pharyngeal-symptoms/epistaxis

Messner, M. D. (2014). Management of epistaxis in children. In A. Stack & G. Isaacson (Eds.), *UpToDate*. Waltham, MA: Wolters Kluwer. Retrieved from http://www.uptodate.com/contents/management-of-epistaxis-in-children?source=search_result&search=epistaxis&selectedTitle=2%7E150

Newton, E., Lasso, A., Petrich, W., & Kilty, S. J. (2016). An outcomes analysis of anterior epistaxis management in the emergency department. *Journal of Otolaryngology- Head Neck Surgery, 45*, 24. doi:10.1186/s40463-016-0138-2

Nonallergic Rhinitis

Jill C. Cash, Moya Cook, and Valda Duke

Definition

A. Nonallergic rhinitis is an inflammation of nasal mucous membranes, usually accompanied by a nasal discharge and mucosal oedema. Nonallergic rhinitis disorder has no correlation to specific allergen exposures. It is classified in several ways: vasomotor, perennial, atrophic, geriatric, drug induced, or rhinitis of pregnancy.

Pathogenesis

A. Vasomotor and perennial nonallergic rhinitis results from hyperreactive nasal mucosa.
B. Atrophic and geriatric rhinitis results from progressive degeneration and atrophy of the mucous membranes and bones of the nose.
C. Overuse of topical nasal decongestants can worsen symptoms and cause severe rebound congestion.
D. Cocaine abuse causes nasal congestion and discharge.
E. Rhinitis in pregnancy results from hormonal increase; congestion abates with delivery.

Predisposing Factors

A. Adulthood.
B. Abrupt changes in temperature, odours, and emotional stress.
C. Other predisposing factors depend on type of cause.

Common Findings

A. Nasal congestion.
B. Sneezing.
C. Clear rhinorrhaea.
D. Coughing.
E. Sore throat.
F. Itchy, puffy eyes.

Subjective Data
A. Ask about the onset, duration, and course of symptoms.
B. Inquire about the colour and other characteristics of nasal discharge.
C. Ask about other discomforts and exposure to people with similar symptoms.
D. Inquire about seasonal impact on symptoms, previous treatments, and results.
E. Rule out pregnancy. Ask female clients about birth control method, specifically contraceptives.
F. Ask about use of prescription drugs, over-the-counter (OTC) drugs (especially ASA), and illicit drugs (cocaine).
G. Review medical history for other respiratory problems such as asthma, emphysema, or chronic bronchitis.
H. With children, investigate possibility of a foreign object in nostrils.

Physical Examination
A. Check temperature and blood pressure.
B. Inspect:
   1. Observe general appearance.
   2. Inspect conjunctivae for "allergic shiners" (dark circles under eyes), tearing, and eyelid swelling.
   3. Examine ears for signs of otitis media (red, bulging, perforated tympanic membrane, and purulent drainage).
   4. Examine nose for redness, swelling, polyps (soft, pedunculated, nontender, pale-gray smooth structures), enlarged turbinates, foreign objects, septal deviation, septal perforation (sign of cocaine abuse), ischaemia, mucosal injury, atrophy, and "cobblestoned" pharyngeal mucosa (sign of allergy).
C. Auscultate heart and lungs.
D. Percuss:
   1. Sinus cavities and mastoid process.
   2. Chest for consolidation.
E. Palpate:
   1. Face for sinus tenderness.
   2. Head and neck for enlarged lymph nodes.

Diagnostic Test
A. Referral for skin testing for allergies may be done if rhinitis persists.

Differential Diagnoses
A. Allergic rhinitis.
B. Upper respiratory infection (URI).
C. Foreign body.
D. Sinusitis.
E. Otitis media.
F. Deviated septum.
G. Nasal polyps.
H. Endocrine conditions, such as hypothyroidism and pregnancy.
I. Drug use: Oral contraceptives, ASA, alpha-adrenergic blockers, cocaine, and nasal decongestant overuse.

Plan
A. General interventions:
   1. Avoid changes in temperature, odours, and emotional stress.
   2. Identify triggers for condition and address alleviating triggers.
B. Client teaching:
   1. Teach the client the significance of individual triggers for nonallergic rhinitis. Encourage use of a journal to learn personal triggers.
   2. Avoid triggers, such as smoking, smoke-filled rooms, wood-burning stoves/fireplaces, sprays, and perfumes.
   3. Other triggers may include weather changes, hormonal changes, and medications.
   4. Teach methods of treatment and identify treatments that work best for the client.
   5. Encourage use of neti pot daily to cleanse sinus cavity. Cleansing sinus cavity daily will help to remove foreign materials inhaled and will also help with tissue oedema. Clean pot after each use and allow to air dry.
   6. Viral rhinitis cause of symptoms typically resolve untreated in seven to 10 days.
C. Pharmacological therapy:
   1. Vasomotor rhinitis: Inhaled ipratropium bromide.
   2. Atrophic rhinitis: Dextromethorphan.
   3. Physiological saline nasal spray to nares three times a day.
   4. Decongestants: These should not be used longer than two to three days at a time for congestion due to the effects of rebound congestion with long-term use.

Follow-Up
A. Have the client return in two to three weeks and for biannual examinations and/or as needed.

Consultation/Referral
A. If treatment fails, refer the client to the allergist for testing.

Individual Consideration
A. Pregnancy: Reassure pregnant clients that rhinitis is a common hormonal response. Nonallergic rhinitis is not contagious and cannot cross the placenta.

Bibliography
Canadian Pharmacists Association. (2011). *Therapeutic choices* (6th ed.). Ottawa, ON, Canada: Canadian Pharmacists Association.
Ramavaram, S., & Jones, S. M. (2012). Natural course and comorbidities of allergic and nonallergic rhinitis in children. *Pediatrics, 130*(Suppl. 1), S23–S24. doi:10.1542/peds.2012-2183KK

Acute Sinusitis/Rhinosinusitis

Jill C. Cash, Moya Cook, and Valda Duke

Definition
Sinusitis is the inflammation of mucous membranes lining paranasal sinuses. Sinusitis is often referred to as rhinosinusitis due to the inflammation of the nasal mucosa that almost always accompanies the inflammation of the sinus cavity. It may be acute bacterial, subacute, or chronic rhinosinusitis.
A. Acute sinusitis: Abrupt onset of infection with symptom resolution after therapy. Acute sinusitis lasts less than four weeks.
B. Subacute sinusitis: Persistent purulent nasal discharge despite therapy.
C. Chronic sinusitis: Episodes of prolonged (greater than three months) inflammation and/or repeated or inadequately treated acute infections.

Incidence/Prevalence

A. Sinusitis is very prevalent. However, true incidence is unknown because people with frontal headaches or congestion self-medicate with over-the-counter (OTC) decongestants and then request antibiotics if symptoms persist. Most cases of acute sinusitis are viral and last <10 days. Incidence increases in spring and fall (allergy seasons) and in winter (cold season).

Pathogenesis

A. One cause is obstruction of mucus flow due to oedema of nasal mucosa from allergies and upper respiratory infections (URIs).
B. Another cause is anatomical abnormalities that interfere with the normal mucocilliary clearance mechanism.
C. Exposure to pathogens following URI also causes sinusitis. Pathogens include *Staphylococcus aureus, Haemophilus influenzae*, pneumococci, streptococci, and bacteroides. Incubation period depends on the pathogen.
D. Dental abscess is a cause in 10% of cases.
E. Fungi such as *Mucor, Rhizopus*, and *Aspergillus* can produce invasive sinusitis in poorly controlled diabetics or people with leukaemia.
F. Common cold is a cause in 0.5% to 5.0% of cases.

Predisposing Factors

A. Recent URI.
B. Allergens (pollens, moulds, smoking, occupational exposure such as coal mining, and animal dander).
C. Nicotine/smoke exposure (first- or secondhand smoke).
D. Air pollutants.
E. Deviated septum.
F. Adenoidal hypertrophy.
G. Dental abscess.
H. Diving and swimming.
I. Neoplasms.
J. Cystic fibrosis.
K. Trauma.
L. Medical disorders (diabetes, immune disorders, inflammatory disorders, mucosal disorders, cystic fibrosis, and asthma).
M. Flying or rapid changes in altitude.

Common Findings

A. Yellow or green nasal discharge.
B. Fever.
C. Sore throat.
D. Facial pain, frontal pain, or pressure that worsens when client bends forward.
E. Headache.
F. Toothache.

Other Signs and Symptoms

A. Anosmia (loss of sense of smell).
B. Nasal congestion.
C. Cough (worse when lying down); may be chronic.
D. Periorbital oedema (especially early morning).
E. Malaise or fatigue.
F. Halitosis.
G. Snoring, mouth breathing.
H. Nasal-sounding speech.

Potential Complications to Consider: Immediate Ear, Nose, and Throat Referral

A. Meningitis (symptoms are increased fever, stiff neck).
B. Subdural and epidural purulent drainage.
C. Brain abscess.
D. Cavernous sinus thrombosis (acute thrombophlebitis due to infection in the area where veins drain into cavernous sinus).
E. Tender periorbital oedema (orbital cellulitis).
F. Altered mental status.
G. Limitation of ocular motion and diminished visual acuity.
H. Frontal or retro-orbital headache.

Subjective Data

A. Elicit the onset, duration, and course of symptoms.
B. Inquire whether seasons affect symptoms.
C. Ask the client about recent URI and how it was treated:
  1. Did the client receive antibiotics?
  2. Did the client finish the full course of antibiotics?
D. Ask about allergies.
E. Inquire about recent dental problems, especially dental abscesses.
F. Find out what home therapies and OTC medications the client tried before the office visit.
G. Ask whether the client took a trip recently, especially by airplane.
H. With a child, look for a foreign object up the nose.
I. Inquire whether the client was swimming or diving recently.
J. Ask whether the symptoms change with position change.
K. Inquire whether the client has other symptoms such as halitosis, eye pain, fatigue, fever, headache, and weight loss.
L. Ask about recent exposures to infections.
M. Ask about recent trauma to the head or face.
N. Review the client's medical history for cystic fibrosis, asthma, nasal abnormalities (e.g., deviated septum), and other respiratory problems.

Physical Examination

A. Check temperature, blood pressure, pulse, and respirations.
B. Inspect:
  1. Observe eyes for periorbital swelling, "allergic shiners" (dark circles under eyes), tearing, and signs of orbital cellulitis (conjunctival oedema, drooping lid, decreased extraocular motion, and vision loss).
  2. Examine ears.
  3. Inspect the nose for erythema, oedema, discharge, lack of nostril patency, septal deviation and polyps, and presence of a foreign body.
  4. Transilluminate maxillary and frontal sinuses in a darkened room. Absence of light reflection is not definitive.
  5. Examine the mouth and pharynx for erythema and tonsillar enlargement, check teeth for uneven surfaces (sign of grinding), and check retropharynx for evidence of postnasal drip.
C. Auscultate heart and lungs.
D. Palpate:
  1. Neck for lymphadenopathy.
  2. Sinuses (do not press on eyes):
     a. Frontal sinusitis: Pain and tenderness over lower forehead (worse when bending forward) and purulent drainage from middle meatus of nasal turbinates.
     b. Maxillary sinusitis: Pain and tenderness over cheeks from inner canthus to teeth (referred pain), oedematous hard palate (severe cases), and purulent drainage in middle meatus.

c. Ethmoid sinusitis: Frontal or orbital headache, tenderness, and erythema over upper lateral aspect of nose, drainage from anterior ethmoid cells through middle meatus, drainage of posterior cells through superior meatus.
  d. Sphenoid sinusitis (uncommon): Frontal or orbital headache or facial pain (headache referred to top of head and deep into eyes), purulent drainage from superior meatus.
E. Percuss:
  1. Tap maxillary teeth to rule out dental cause.
  2. Percussion maxillary and frontal sinuses and do chest percussion, if indicated.
  3. Percussion over affected area exacerbates pain.
F. Neurologic examination:
  1. Evaluate for signs of meningeal irritation, assessing for Brudzinski's sign, Kernig's sign, and nuchal rigidity.

Diagnostic Tests
A. **Diagnosis is usually made through history and physical.**
B. Consider sinus x-ray films that show air-fluid level and thickening of sinus mucous membranes with sinusitis for chronic or recurrent sinusitis or complicated cases. Consider three-view plain sinus x-ray.
C. CT of sinuses if indications include chronic sinusitis, recurrent sinusitis, allergic fungal sinusitis, or osteomeatal complex occlusion.

Differential Diagnoses
A. Headache (cluster, migraine).
B. Rhinitis (allergic, medicamentosa, or vasomotor).
C. Nasal polyps.
D. Tumour.
E. URI.
F. Trigeminal neuralgia.
G. Pregnancy.

Plan
A. General interventions:
  1. Preventive techniques suggested to avoid sinus infections.
  2. Clients with frequent sinus infections should be encouraged to keep a log of triggers, if present. Avoiding these triggers helps to prevent the onset of infection. Avoid smoking and secondhand smoke; use of nasal saline, neti pot, and increased fluids also help prevent the onset of infection.
  3. Recurrent frequent sinus infections should be further investigated for other causes, such as autoimmune diseases.
B. Client teaching:
  1. Teach client to avoid smoking and secondhand smoke.
  2. Drinking extra fluids helps to loosen secretions and hydrate the body.
  3. Encourage the client to use medications as prescribed. OTC medications, such as antihistamines and decongestants, should be used with caution.
  4. Application of warm, moist compresses to the face several times a day will help with discomfort.
  5. Humidifiers should be used daily.
  6. Nasal saline to the nares three times a day will help to keep nasal passages moist. *Refer to Client Teaching Guide: Sinusitis.*
C. Pharmacological therapy:
  1. Although clients are often prescribed antibiotics for disorders such as sinus infections, hay fever, and other respiratory allergies, most do not need the drugs.
    a. Sinus infections almost always stem from a viral infection. Sinus infections often clear up on their own in a week or so.
    b. About one in four people who take antibiotics have side effects such as stomach problems, dizziness, or rashes. Such problems often disappear after stopping the drugs, but antibiotics can cause severe allergic reactions in rare cases. Overuse of antibiotics can make clients more vulnerable to antibiotic-resistant infections and undermines the good that antibiotics can do.
    c. Antibiotics are required only when symptoms persist longer than one week, start to improve but then worsen again, or are very severe. Worrisome symptoms warranting immediate antibiotic treatment include fever over 38.6°C, extreme pain, tenderness over the sinus area, or signs of a skin infection When antibiotics are needed, the best choice often is amoxicillin.
      i. Clients should use over-the-counter remedies with caution.
      ii. Rest is especially important in the first few days of the virus. Tell clients to elevate the head when lying down to ease postnasal drip.
      iii. Warm fluids can help thin nasal secretions and loosen phlegm.
      iv. Warm, moist air from a bath, shower, or a pan of boiled water can loosen phlegm and soothe the throat.
      v. Recommend that clients gargle with half a teaspoon of salt dissolved in a glass of warm water.
      vi. Saltwater sprays or nasal irrigation kits (such as neti pot) can help.
        1) Nasal drops or sprays containing oxymetazoline (such as otrivin, drixoral, and generic) can cause rebound congestion if used for longer than three days.
        2) The benefits of oral decongestants (such as pseudoephedrine) rarely outweigh the risks or side effects.
        3) Unless significant allergies are present, it is best to skip antihistamines, since they do not ease cold symptoms and have side effects.
  2. Antibiotics for infection:
    a. Drugs of choice for acute sinusitis:
      i. Children:
        1) First-line treatment: Amoxicillin. Second-line treatment: Amoxicillin/clavulanate or cefprozil.
        2) Beta-lactam allergy: Type I hypersensitivity: Cefuroxime. Non-type I hypersensitivity: Clarithromycin or Azithromycin:
          a) TMP/SMX trimethoprim.
        3) Risk for antibiotic resistance or failed initial therapy:

▶ Client Teaching Guides are available at https://connect.springerpub.com/content/reference-book/978-0-8261-9498-5

a) Amoxicillin for children older than 2 years, in daycare or antibiotic treatment within past 3 months; treatment failure, community resistance TMP/SMX less desirable with *H. influenzae* and pneumococcal increased resisitance rates. **Antimicrobial resisitance rates change according to community regions and choice of antibiotic section should reflect same.**

  ii. Adults:
  1) First-line treatment: Intranasal corticosteroids can be considered: ampicillin or amox/clav.
  2) Beta-lactam allergy:
     a) Doxycycline.
     b) Levofloxacin.
     c) Moxifloxacin.
     d) Clarithromycin.
     e) Azithromycin.
  3) Risk for antibiotic resistance or failed initial therapy: TMP/SMX less desirable with *H. influenzae* and pneumococcal increased resisitance rates. **Antimicrobial resistance rates change according to community regions and choice of antibiotic section shold reflect same.**

  b. The same antibiotics can be used for chronic sinusitis, but treatment should last three to four weeks.
     i. If failure of treatment after second course then referral to a specialist is warrented. Fluroquinolones should be reserved for those who do not benefit from other medication treatment, as the risks associated with these antibiotics outweigh the benefits; also consider leukotriene receptor antagonist (LRA); allergy testing and other specialty referral and should be reserved for severe cases.

D. Oral and topical decongestants to correct the underlying edematous mucosa (use cautiously with hypertension):
  1. Adults: Xylometazoline.
  2. Adults and children older than 6 years.
     a. Phenylephrine.
  3. Pseudoephedrin for congestion for adults.
  4. Nasal saline to nares for hydrating nasal mucosa.

E. Steroid sprays may be used to decrease nasal inflammation. Steroid nasal sprays should only be used on children younger than 6 years of age if there is an allergic component:
  1. Beclomethasone dipropionate.
  2. Mometasone furoate monohydrate.

F. Antihistamines are not recommended.

G. **Paediatric doses are available for all products.**

Follow-Up

A. Recheck the client in three to four days if signs and symptoms are not improving with the use of treatment prescribed.

B. Recommend treatment can vary from five to 10 or 10 to 14 days but improved symptoms should be seen in three days. Clients not improving may be resistant to antibiotics and may be switched to a different antibiotic and will be dependent on antibiotic resistance rates.

Consultation/Referral

A. Admission to hospital is needed if the client has fever with facial orbital cellulitis and mental changes.

B. Refer chronic sinusitis clients to an otolaryngologist if they do not improve in four weeks.

C. Refer clients to a physician or pertinent specialist for suspected neoplasm, abscess, osteomyelitis, meningitis, or sinus thrombosis.

Individual Considerations

A. Paediatrics: Sinusitis may be considered for children who present with symptoms of low-grade temperature lasting longer than 10 days but <30 with the following: any colour nasal discharge; day and night-time cough; halitosis, facial pain, headache, and fatigue are seen less common. Severe symptoms are considered to be purulent nasal discharge and fever >39°C.

B. Geriatrics:
  1. Precautionary measures should be used for clients with long-term nasogastric tubes. These clients are at higher risk for the development of occult sinusitis.
  2. Precautions should be used with clients currently prescribed warfarin.
  3. Avoid use of TMP-SMX with warfarin because the medication can cause a significant increase in prothrombin time/international normalized ratio (PT/INR).

Bibliography

Adelson, R. T., & Adappa, N. D. (2013). What is the proper role of oral antibiotics in the treatment of patients with chronic sinusitis? *Current Opinion in Otolaryngology & Head and Neck Surgery, 21*(1), 61–68. doi:10.1097/MOO.0b013e32835ac625

Anti-infective Review Panel. (2013). *Anti-infective guidelines for community-acquired infections*. Toronto, ON, Canada: MUMS Guideline Clearinghouse.

Choosing Wisely Canada. (n.d.). *Sinusitis*. Retrieved from https://choosingwiselycanada.org/treating-sinusitis/

Dains, J. E., Baumann, L. C., & Scheibel, P. (2016). *Advanced health assessment and clinical diagnosis in primary care* (5th ed.). St. Louis, MO: Elsevier.

DeMuri, G. P., & Wald, E. R. (2012). Clinical practice. Acute bacterial sinusitis in children. *New England Journal of Medicine, 367*(12), 1128–1134. doi:10.1056/NEJMcp1106638

Health Canada. (2008). *Health releases decision on the labelling of cough and cold products for children*. Retrieved from: https://www.healthycanadians.gc.ca/recall-alert-rappel-avis/hc-sc/2008/13267a-eng.php

Kaplan, A. (2013). Canadian guidelines for chronic rhinosinusitis. *Canadian Family Physician, 59*, 1275–1281.

Kaplan, A. (2014). Canadian guidelines for acute bacterial rhinosinusitis. *Canadian Family Physician, 60*, 227–234.

Patel, Z., & Hwang, P. (2016). Acute sinusitis and rhinosinusitis in adults: Treatment. In D. Deschler & S. Calderwood (Eds.), *UpToDate*. Waltham, MA: Wolters Kluwer. Retrieved from http://www.uptodate.com/contents/uncomplicated-acute-sinusitis-and-rhinosinusitis-in-adults-treatment?source=search_result&search=sinusitis&selectedTitle=1%7E150

Rosenfeld, R. M., Piccirillo, J. F., Chandrasekhar, S. S., Brook, I., Kumar, K. A., Kramper, M., . . . Corrigan, M. D. (2015). Clinical practice guideline (update): Adult sinusitis executive summary. *Otolaryngology—Head and Neck Surgery, 152*(4), 598–609. doi:10.1177/0194599815574247. Retrieved from https://www.guideline.gov/content.aspx?id=49207&search=acute+rhinitis

Wald, E. (2016). Acute bacterial rhinosinusitis in children: Microbiology and treatment. In S. Kaplan, G. Isaacson, & R. Wood (Eds.), *UpToDate*. Waltham, MA: Wolters Kluwer Retrieved from http://www.uptodate.com/contents/acute-bacterialrhinosinusitis-in-children-microbiology-and-treatment? source=search_result&search=sinusitis+children+treatment&selectedTitle=3%7E150

8 Throat and Mouth Guidelines

Avulsed Tooth

Jill C. Cash, Moya Cook, and Lynn Miller

Definition
A. A tooth that has been completely displaced from its alveolar socket.

Incidence/Prevalence
A. Avulsion accounts for 0.5% to 16% of all dental injuries to the permanent teeth. It occurs predominantly in children between ages 7 and 10 years. The upper central incisor is the tooth most frequently avulsed.

Pathogenesis
A. Trauma causes a tooth to be completely displaced from its alveolar socket.

Predisposing Factor
A. Erupting teeth are most susceptible to avulsion due to immature periodontal ligaments.

Common Findings
A. Tooth displaced.
B. Pain.
C. Bleeding.

Subjective Data
A. Ascertain the client's age, and note whether the avulsed tooth is primary or permanent.
B. Determine how long the tooth has been avulsed (minutes or hours).
C. Ask the client about the underlying cause or trauma. Are there any other injuries that need assessment, such as lacerations or concussion?
D. Did the tooth fall out of the mouth or remain in the mouth?

Physical Examination
A. Check temperature, pulse, respirations, and blood pressure.
B. Inspect:
   1. Observe general appearance:
      a. Check for signs that are secondary to traumatic etiology, such as lacerations, concussion, facial injury, and eye injury.
      b. Keep the client calm. Check to be sure that the client is not in respiratory distress and has not aspirated the tooth.
   2. Inspect gums and avulsed tooth, noting poor dental hygiene. **Do not touch the root surface.**

Diagnostic Tests
A. Dental x-ray should be considered to assess for fracture.

Differential Diagnoses
A. Luxation injuries: concussion and subluxation.

Plan
A. General interventions: **If the tooth is not in the mouth, rinse it off briefly under cold running water** (<10 seconds) and attempt to reposition the tooth into the socket if there is no concern that the child will swallow or drop it.
B. Client teaching:
   1. Instruct the client not to let the tooth air dry; it may cause permanent destruction of periodontal cells.
   2. Instruct the client to transport the tooth in the tooth socket and bite on gauze or a small handkerchief to help hold the tooth in position.
   3. If unable to transport inside the tooth socket, use another medium to transport the tooth (e.g., saline, Hanks balanced storage medium, milk). If the client is conscious, the tooth can be transported in the cheek pocket or inside the lip. If this is not possible, the client can spit in a container and transport the tooth in saliva.
C. Pharmacological therapy:
   1. Use of oral antibiotics is not routinely required but can be considered for prophylaxis. Consider amoxicillin or clindamycin (if penicillin allergy) for adults. Amoxicillin may be used for children.
   2. If the tooth had contact with soil, determine tetanus status and administer tetanus booster if necessary.

Follow-Up
A. Follow-up is done with the dentist until stabilization is complete.

Consultation/Referral
A. Immediately refer the client to a dentist or an emergency department. Teeth replanted within 30 minutes have the best prognosis. Teeth avulsed longer than two hours have a poor prognosis.

Individual Consideration
A. Paediatrics: Primary teeth do not need to be replaced.

Bibliography
Anti-infective Review Panel. (2013). *Anti-infective guidelines for community-acquired infections.* Toronto, ON, Canada: MUMS Guidelines Clearinghouse.

Casis, M. J. (2014). Immediate replantation of avulsed permanent incisor. *Journal of the Canadian Dental Association, 80,* e56.

Doshi, D. (2009). Bet 3. Avulsed tooth brought in milk for replantation. *Emergency Medicine Journal, 26*(10), 736–737.

International Association of Dental Traumatology. (2013). *Dental trauma guidelines.* Retrieved from https://www.iadt-dentaltrauma.org/1-9%20%20iadt%20guidelines%20combined%20-%20lr%20-%2011-5-2013.pdf

Dental Abscess
Jill C. Cash, Moya Cook, and Lynn Miller

Definition
A. A dental abscess is a space infection of the gingival or periodontal tissues.

Incidence/Prevalence
A. Unknown.

Pathogenesis
A. An abscess occurs when bacteria gain access into the gingiva or periodontal tissues.

Predisposing Factors
A. Poor dental hygiene.
B. Dental caries.
C. Trauma.

Common Findings
A. Constant, severe jaw pain.
B. Swelling.
C. Difficulty in chewing with tooth due to pain.

Other Signs and Symptoms
A. Fever.
B. Warmth, redness.
C. Loss of appetite.
D. Heat and cold sensitivity.
E. Halitosis.

Potential Complications
Risk of complications increases with valvular disease. The following are complications:
A. Sepsis.
B. Leukocytosis associated with facial cellulitis.

Subjective Data
A. Elicit information from the client regarding the onset, duration, location, and quality of pain.
B. Note the radiation of pain as well as alleviating or aggravating factors.
C. Note if pain is brought on by contact with hot, cold, or sweet substances; this may indicate periapical abscess or dental caries.
D. Ask whether the client has a fever. If so, how high and for how long?
E. Inquire about the history of mitral valve prolapse or rheumatic fever.

Physical Examination
A. Check temperature, pulse, respirations, and blood pressure.
B. Inspect:
  1. Inspect teeth for caries, mobility of teeth, or protrusion from sockets, signs of trauma, and gum disease.
  2. Examine the teeth for erosion, enamel decalcification, diminished tooth size, discolouration, and sensitivity to temperature changes.
C. Palpate neck and submental area for enlarged, tender lymph nodes.
D. Percuss all teeth. Tenderness is diagnostic of an abscess.
E. Auscultate heart, if indicated.

Diagnostic Tests
A. None usually required.
B. White blood cell (WBC) count, if cellulitis is suspected.

Differential Diagnoses
A. Periodontal disease.
B. Cellulitis.

Plan
A. General interventions:
  1. Treat immediate infection.
  2. Refer to the dentist for immediate evaluation and treatment.
B. Client teaching:
  1. Advise the client to apply a source of moist heat to the painful facial area for comfort.
  2. Advise soft diet until pain resolves.
  3. Review daily dental care and hygiene with the client.
C. Pharmacological therapy:
  1. First-line treatment while the client awaits dental consultation: penicillin V potassium.
  2. Other medications:
    a. Amoxicillin.
    b. Cephalexin.
    c. Clindamycin.
  3. For discomfort and fever: acetaminophen.

Follow-Up
A. Follow up two to three days after dental examination to evaluate results.

Consultation/Referral
A. Advise the client to see a dentist promptly, even if pain resolves.

Individual Considerations
A. Pregnancy:
  1. It is safe for clients to have dental procedures during pregnancy.
  2. X-ray films may be taken if a lead shield is placed over client's abdomen.
  3. Epinephrine and nitrous oxide should not be used during dental procedures.
  4. Tetracycline should not be used; it causes staining of fetal bones and teeth.

Bibliography

Anti-infective Review Panel. (2013). *Anti-infective guidelines for community-acquired infections*. Toronto, ON, Canada: MUMS Guidelines Clearinghouse.

Gregoire, C. (2010). How are odontogenic infections best managed? *Journal of the Canadian Dental Association, 76*, a37.

Jensen, B., & Regier, L. D. (2017). *RxFiles drug comparison charts*. Saskatoon Health Region, Saskatoon, SK: Author. Retrieved from https://www.rxfiles.ca/rxfiles/uploads/documents/ChartsTitlePage-11th-edition-2017-book-references.pdf

Epiglottitis

Jill C. Cash, Moya Cook, and Lynn Miller

Definition
A. Epiglottitis is the inflammation and swelling of the epiglottis and is a medical emergency.

Incidence/Prevalence
A. Epiglottitis usually occurs in children between ages 2 and 8 years, but it may also occur in adults. Incidence has decreased dramatically since the *Haemophilus influenzae* vaccine was introduced.

Pathogenesis
A. Epiglottitis is almost always caused by *H. influenzae*, although *Streptococcus pneumoniae* and *Streptococcus pyogenes* have also been implicated.

Predisposing Factor
A. Upper respiratory infection (URI).

Common Findings
A. Sudden onset of fever.
B. Sudden onset of dysphagia.
C. Sudden onset of drooling.
D. Sudden onset of muffled voice.

Other Signs and Symptoms
A. Respiratory distress.
B. Stridor.
C. Very ill appearance.

Subjective Data
A. Determine the onset, duration, and course of illness.
B. Is the child's breathing laboured?
C. Are the child's breathing problems affecting his or her ability to eat or drink?
D. Has he or she had a fever?
E. Has he or she had trouble swallowing or talking?

Physical Examination
A. Check temperature, pulse, respirations, and blood pressure.
B. Inspect:
   1. Observe overall appearance.
   2. Check nail beds and lips for cyanosis.
   3. Note drooling or difficulty in swallowing.
   4. Note breathing pattern and rhythm.
   5. Note cough if present.
   6. Do not examine the throat — airway occlusion may result.
C. Auscultate heart and lungs.

Diagnostic Test
A. Lateral neck radiograph confirms diagnosis. However, this test may delay the establishment of an airway.
B. Obtain blood and epiglottis cultures before starting antibiotics.

Differential Diagnoses
A. Bacterial tracheitis (a paediatric emergency).
B. Viral croup.
C. Foreign-body aspiration.
D. Retropharyngeal abscess.

Plan
A. General interventions:
   1. Immediate transport to hospital.
   2. While awaiting transport to hospital, establish patent airway, start oxygen, and assemble airway equipment. Move the child as little as possible.
   3. Insert intravenous (IV) access for fluids and antibiotic administration.
   4. If a respiratory arrest occurs, you may not be able to see the airway to intubate. A bag and mask may work temporarily, but nasogastric (NG) tube insertion may be necessary to prevent gastric distension.
   5. Prompt recognition and appropriate treatment usually result in rapid resolution of swelling and inflammation.
B. Client teaching:
   1. Educate the child and the family that epiglottitis is a medical emergency.
   2. If client has drooling and no cough, diagnosis is most likely epiglottitis. If the child has cough and no drooling, then diagnosis is most likely croup.
C. Pharmacological therapy (in-hospital treatment):
   1. IV fluids.
   2. Antibiotics; IV antibiotics after physician consultation:
      a. Cefotaxime.
      b. Ceftriaxone.
      c. Cefuroxime.
      d. Amoxicillin/clavulanic acid.
   3. May give acetaminophen as needed.

Follow-Up
A. Follow-up care occurs in the hospital.
B. An airway specialist should evaluate the client.

Consultation/Referral
A. If you suspect epiglottitis, refer the client to the ED.

Individual Considerations
A. Paediatrics:
   1. Never place a child in supine position, because respiratory arrest has been reported.
   2. All close contacts (children and adults) exposed to a child diagnosed with epiglottitis should be treated with prophylactic antibiotics.

Bibliography
Anti-infective Review Panel. (2013). *Anti-infective guidelines for community-acquired infections*. Toronto, ON, Canada: MUMS Guidelines Clearinghouse.

Jensen, B., & Regier, L. D. (2017). *RxFiles drug comparison charts*. Saskatoon Health Region. Saskatoon, SK: Author. Retrieved from https://www.rxfiles.ca/rxfiles/uploads/documents/ChartsTitlePage-11th-edition-2017-book-references.pdf

Richards, A. M. (2016). Pediatric respiratory emergencies. *Emergency Medicine Clinics of North America, 34*(1), 77–96. doi:10.1016/j.emc.2015.08.006

Udeani, J. (2016). Pediatric epiglottitis treatment & management. *Medscape*. Retrieved from http://emedicine.medscape.com/article/963773-treatment#d13

Oral Cancer

Jill C. Cash, Moya Cook, and Lynn Miller

Definition

A. Oral cancer is the cancer of the buccal mucosa, tongue, gingiva, hard palate, soft palate, or lips. White patches, known as *leukoplakia*, or red, velvety patches, known as *erythroplakia*, on the buccal mucosa may indicate premalignant lesions.

Incidence/Prevalence

A. Oral cancer is primarily seen in the elderly. Male-to-female predominance is two to one. The death rate is fairly high for oral cancer secondary to the cancer being diagnosed in the late stages of development.
B. In 2017, 4,700 Canadians were diagnosed with oral cancer and 1,250 Canadians died from oral cancer.
C. Frequency of oral cancer of cheek and gum rises among long-term users of smokeless tobacco.
D. Clients diagnosed with oral cancer are at greater risk of developing cancer in another part of the body, such as the lung, larynx, esophagus, or liver.

Pathogenesis

Pathogenesis is unknown; 50% of oral cancers have already been metastasized by the time of diagnosis. The following factors are involved:
A. Use of tobacco in all its forms is highly correlated with the risk of oral cancer.
B. Risk of oral cancer also is high with heavy alcohol consumption. Whether this is due to a direct effect of alcohol on the oral mucosa or associated smoking or vitamin deficiency remains unclear.
C. Chronic iron deficiency leading to Plummer–Vinson syndrome is known to alter mucosal tissues, and this change may be related to increased oral cancer. Research has shown that a diet low in fruits and vegetables contributes to oral cancer.
D. Epstein–Barr virus and papillomavirus have been found in the cells of the tongue manifesting in oral hairy leukoplakia, a hyperplastic change found in AIDS clients. Human papillomavirus (HPV) is found in approximately 20% to 30% of cases of oral cancer.
E. Occupational hazards also exist from sun exposure. It is estimated that 30% of those with oral cancer worked outdoors.

Predisposing Factors

A. Male gender.
B. Age >45 years.
C. Smoking or use of other tobacco products, including smokeless products such as snuff and dip.
D. Alcohol consumption.
E. Sun exposure.
F. Poor diet: deficient in vitamins A, C, and E, and high in salted or smoked meats, fats, and oils.
G. Previous cancer.

Common Findings

A. Oral sores that do not heal, which is the primary reason clients seek medical care.
B. Poorly fitting dentures.
C. Bleeding mucosa or gingiva without apparent cause.
D. Difficulty swallowing, usually indicating more advanced disease.
E. Altered sensations: burning or numbness, usually indicating more advanced disease.
F. Leukoplakia or erythroplakia.

Other Signs and Symptoms

A. No symptoms, possibly.
B. Decreased appetite related to altered taste.
C. Increased salivation.
D. Sore throat.
E. Foul breath odour.
F. Neck mass.

Subjective Data

A. Review the onset, course, and duration of symptoms. Question the client regarding altered taste, sensations, difficulty swallowing, and foul breath.
B. Evaluate for risk factors. See section "Predisposing Factors."
C. Ask the client about previous history of cancer and treatments.
D. Review the client's use of tobacco products (including cannabis), including age of onset, amount of daily use, and quit dates.
E. Evaluate amount of alcohol intake, including age of onset, amount of daily use, and quit dates.
F. Review the client's general health history for other chronic conditions.
G. Review medication history, including prescription and over-the-counter (OTC) drug use, especially ASA.
H. Take dental history, including previous gum surgery, how long ago dentures were fitted, and whether they always fit well.
I. Establish usual weight. Is there any weight loss related to altered taste, and, if so, how much and during what length of time?

Physical Examination

A. Check temperature, pulse, respirations, blood pressure, and weight.
B. Inspect:
   1. Observe general appearance.
   2. Note quality of voice patterns.
   3. Note odour of breath.
   4. Inspect lips, gums, tongue, and buccal mucosa for swelling, discolouration, bleeding, asymmetry, texture, limited movement of tongue, abnormal ulcerations, leukoplakia, and erythroplasia. Take out dentures first.
   5. Assess for tenderness or pain in mouth/tongue:
      a. Leukoplakia ranges from slightly raised, white, translucent areas to dense, white, opaque plaques, with or without adjacent ulceration. Normal intraoral mucosa is pinkish or salmon coloured.
      b. Mucosal erythroplasia is red, inflammatory, or shows erythroplastic mucosal changes. It appears

smooth, granular, and minimally elevated, with or without leukoplakia, and it persists more than 14 days.

   c. Erythroplakia may mimic inflammatory lesions, but it can be differentiated by failure of the affected area to blanch with light pressure. Erythroplakia is a malignant change seen as a red, velvety, plaque-like lesion on the mucous membrane.
   d. Other oral lesions appear black, blue, or brown.
   e. Approximately 90% of cancers are squamous cell carcinomas and most occur in sites accessible by clinical examination: tongue, oropharynx (soft palate, lingual aspect of retromolar trigone, anterior tonsillar pillar), and floor of mouth.
   f. Cancer of the lip is a lesion that fails to heal.
   g. Signs and symptoms of cancer of the tongue are swelling, ulceration, areas of tenderness or bleeding, abnormal texture, and limited movement.
C. Palpate:
   1. Palpate mouth for masses. Try to remove or scrape patches.
   2. Palpate lymph nodes: Cervical (anterior/posterior chain), submandibular, sublingual, and submental, pre/postauricular; check nodes for size, firmness, and tenderness.
D. Auscultate lungs and heart. The lungs are the most frequently involved extranodal metastatic site.

Diagnostic Tests
A. Check for HIV, if indicated.
B. Staining of oral lesion with toluidine blue: lesion stains dark blue after rinsing with acetic acid. Normal tissue does not absorb the stain.
C. Biopsy for persistent lesions (more than two weeks): It is essential to differentiate blue–black lesion of malignant melanoma.
D. Perform chest radiography to rule out metastasis.
E. Consider CT scan, MRI, or bone scan to rule out metastasis.

Differential Diagnoses
A. Oral leukoplakia.
B. Pulpitis.
C. Periapical abscess.
D. Gingivitis.
E. Periodontitis.
F. Lichen planus.
G. Oral candidiasis.
H. Discoid lupus.
I. Pemphigus vulgaris.

Plan
A. General interventions:
   1. If oral cancer is suspected, refer to an otolaryngologist/dentist for evaluation.
   2. Suspicious lesions should be biopsied.
B. Client teaching:
   1. Advise the client to stop smoking and stop using oral tobacco products.
   2. Advise the client to decrease/eliminate alcohol consumption.
   3. Encourage routine dental care and examinations.
   4. Review dietary intake and educate the client regarding benefits of increasing dietary intake of vitamins A, C, and E. Encourage the client to decrease dietary intake of foods that are high in salt, smoked meats, fats, and oils.
   5. Recommend wearing sunscreen/lip balm with sun protection factor (SPF) of 15 or greater.
   6. Review strategies to avoid contracting the HPV infection. Recommend HPV vaccination for females between the ages of 9 and 45 years and males 9 to 26 years of age.
C. Pharmacological therapy:
   1. Erythroplakia does not respond to antifungal therapy.
   2. Treatment is based on diagnosis.

Follow-Up
A. If immediate biopsy is not indicated, ask the client to return for reevaluation in two weeks, after eliminating irritants and noxious agents.

Consultation/Referral
A. Refer the client to an otolaryngologist and/or a dentist for immediate biopsy for deeply ulcerative or fungating lesions. Follow-up treatment may include one or more of the following: wide excision, radical neck dissection, radiation, and chemotherapy.

Individual Considerations
A. Paediatrics:
   1. Currently, the highest rate is in smokeless tobacco use.
   2. Oral screening should be considered annually in adolescents who use tobacco and/or alcohol.
B. Adults: The Canadian Cancer Society recommends that people between ages 20 and 40 years undergo an oral cancer screening every three years, and that those older than 40 years be screened every year. Oral screening should be considered annually in adults who use tobacco and/or alcohol.

Resources
Canadian Cancer Society: www.cancer.ca
College of Family Physicians of Canada: https://www.cfpc.ca/Home/

Bibliography
Canadian Cancer Society. (2018a). *All about HPV vaccines*. Retrieved from http://www.cancer.ca/en/prevention-and-screening/reduce-cancerrisk/make-informed-decisions/get-vaccinated/all-about-hpv-vaccines/?region=on
Canadian Cancer Society. (2018b). *Oral cancers*. Retrieved from http://www.cancer.ca/en/cancer-information/cancer-type/oral/oralcancer/?region=on
Truong Lam, B., O'Sullivan, B., Gullan, P., & Huong, S. H. (2016). Challenges in establishing the diagnosis of human papillomavirus-related oropharyngeal carcinoma. *The Laryngoscope, 126*(10), 2270–2275. doi:10.1002/lary.25985

Pharyngitis

Jill C. Cash, Moya Cook, and Lynn Miller

Definition
A. Pharyngitis is the inflammation of the pharynx and the surrounding lymph tissue.

Incidence/Prevalence
A. Pharyngitis accounts for 2% to 4% of visits to family practice clinics in Canada.

Pathogenesis
Pharyngitis may be due to viral, bacterial, and fungal agents; environmental irritants; and other atypical agents.

A. Viral agents include coxsackievirus, enteric cytopathic human orphan (ECHO) viruses, and Epstein–Barr virus.
B. Bacterial agents include Group A beta-hemolytic *Streptococcus*, *Neisseria gonorrhoeae*, and *Corynebacterium diphtheriae*.
C. The fungal source is *Candida albicans*.
D. Atypical agents include *Mycoplasma pneumoniae* and *Chlamydia trachomatis* (rare).
E. Noninfectious causes include allergic rhinitis, postnasal drip, mouth breathing, and trauma.

Predisposing Factors
A. Cigarette smoking.
B. Allergies.
C. Upper respiratory infections (URI).
D. Oral sex.
E. Drugs (antibiotics and immunosuppressants).
F. Debilitating illnesses (such as cancer) that can cause *C. albicans* to proliferate.

Common Findings
A. Sore and/or scratchy throat.
B. Fever.
C. Headache.
D. Malaise.

Other Signs and Symptoms
A. Oral vesicles.
B. Exudate on throat or "beefy" red throat without exudate.
C. Lymphadenopathy.
D. Fatigue.
E. Dysphasia.
F. Abdominal pain.
G. Vomiting.

Potential Complications
Without proper antimicrobial treatment, streptococcal pharyngitis can lead to serious complications, such as the following:
A. Suppurative adenitis with tender, enlarged lymph nodes.
B. Scarlet fever.
C. Peritonsillar abscess.
D. Glomerulonephritis.
E. Rheumatic fever.

Subjective Data
A. Ask the client about the onset, course, and duration of symptoms. Ask about dyspnoea or dysphagia.
B. Inquire about mouth lesions, rhinorrhoea, cough, drooling, and fever.
C. Ask about malaise, headache, fatigue, and fever; these are symptoms of mononucleosis.
D. Take a sexual history, if indicated. Ask whether family members or sexual partners have the same signs and symptoms. Pharyngeal gonorrhoea has no symptoms, so high-risk clients should be tested.
E. Ask whether symptoms have caused decreased intake of food and fluid.
F. Determine history of heart disease; previous strep pharyngitis; rheumatic fever; and other respiratory diseases such as asthma, emphysema, and chronic allergies.
G. If rash is present, find out when it first occurred and whether it has spread.
H. Ask about signs and symptoms of urinary tract infection and pyelonephritis.
I. Ask about a history of herpes, immunosuppressive disorders, and steroid use.
J. Review immunization history.

Physical Examination
A. Temperature and blood pressure, if indicated.
B. Inspect:
   1. Observe general appearance.
   2. Examine the mouth, pharynx, tonsils, and hard and soft palate for vesicles and ulcers, candidal patches, erythema, hypertrophy, exudate, and stomatitis. Check gum and palate for petechiae and tongue for colour and inflammation.
      a. Herpangina are small oral vesicles on the fauces and soft palate caused by the coxsackie A virus.
      b. Herpes causes vesicles and small ulcers (stomatitis) of the buccal mucosa, tongue, and pharynx.
      c. Trench mouth (gingivitis) and necrotic tonsillar ulcers (Vincent's angina) cause foul breath, pain, pharyngeal exudate, and a gray membranous inflammation that bleeds easily.
      d. *C. albicans* (thrush) may be painful and causes cheesy, white exudate.
      e. Oral candidiasis may be the first symptom of HIV.
      f. Peritonsillar cellulitis causes inflamed, oedematous tonsils; grayish white exudate; high fever; rigors; and leukocytosis. Peritonsillar abscess (palpable mass) may also develop.
      g. Mononucleosis causes tonsillar exudates in 50% of clients; 33% develop petechiae at junction of the hard and soft palate.
      h. *C. diphtheriae* causes a whitish blue pharyngeal exudate "pseudomembrane," which covers the pharynx and bleeds if removal is attempted.
   3. Examine the ears, nose, and throat. Assess patency of airway if tonsils are enlarged.
   4. Inspect skin for rashes:
      a. Pastia's lines are petechiae present in a linear pattern along major skin folds in axillae and antecubital fossa that are seen with Group A *Streptococcus*.
      b. Erythema marginatum, caused by Group A *Streptococcus*, is an evanescent, nonpruritic, pink rash mainly on the trunk and extremities. It may be brought out by heat application.
C. Auscultate heart and lungs.
D. Percuss:
   1. Abdomen, especially spleen area.
   2. Chest.
E. Palpate:
   1. Palpate lymph nodes, especially of the anterior and posterior cervical chains, axilla, and groin.
   2. Palpate abdomen for organomegaly and suprapubic tenderness.
   3. Palpate back for costovertebral angle (CVA) tenderness.
F. Neurologic examination: Check for nuchal rigidity and meningeal irritation.

Diagnostic Tests
A. Rapid strep test; if negative, then perform throat culture and sensitivity. **Throat culture and sensitivity are the gold standard for diagnosis.**
B. Modified Centor Score.
C. Monospot test, if mononucleosis is suspected.
D. Complete blood count with differential.
E. Gonorrhoea culture.

F. Blood cultures if sepsis is suspected.
G. Radiograph of neck if possible trauma.

Differential Diagnoses
A. Stomatitis.
B. Rhinitis.
C. Sinusitis with postnasal drip.
D. Epiglottis.
E. Peritonsillar abscess.
F. Mononucleosis.
G. Herpes simplex.
H. Coxsackie A virus.
I. *C. diphtheriae.*
J. Trench mouth.
K. Vincent's angina.
L. *C. albicans.*
M. HIV.

Plan
A. General interventions:
   1. Clients with a history of rheumatic fever and those who have a household member with a documented Group A streptococcal infection need immediate treatment without prior testing.
   2. Do not put instruments in the airway if you suspect epiglottitis.
▶ B. Client teaching. *Refer to Client Teaching Guide: Pharyngitis.*
C. Pharmacological therapy.
   1. First-line treatment:
      a. Penicillin V potassium.
      b. Amoxicillin.
   2. If the client is allergic to penicillin:
      a. **Type IV hypersensitivity** (e.g., rash): Cephalexin.
      b. **Type I hypersensitivity** (e.g., anaphylaxis) and only if Group A Strep infection is confirmed:
         i. Clindamycin.
         ii. Clarithromycin.
         iii. Erythromycin.
         iv. Azithromycin.
   3. Recurrent bacterial pharyngitis: —Consider and manage potential for either carrier state or failure to eradicate organism with first course of treatment, but avoid prolonged treatment with antibiotics without confirmation of causative organism using appropriate laboratory tests.
   4. For pharyngeal gonorrhoea: a. Ceftriaxone.
   5. For *M. pneumoniae* and *C. trachomatis*: doxycycline or azithromycin.
   6. For *M. pneumoniae:* azithromycin is the first-line treatment.
   7. For pharyngeal candidiasis in the immunocompromised client:
      a. Oral nystatin suspension by swish-and-swallow method four times a day.
      b. Clotrimazole troche held in mouth 15 to 30 minutes 3 times daily.

Follow-Up
A. If symptoms do not improve in three to four days, recheck client.

B. Treat sexual partners of clients with pharyngeal gonorrhoea.

Consultation/Referral
A. Refer the client to an otolaryngologist if peritonsillar abscess is noted or if client has severe dysphagia or dyspnoea, signaling possible airway obstruction.

Individual Considerations
A. Paediatrics:
   1. Rheumatic fever follows between 0.5% and 3% of ineffectively treated cases of Group A streptococcal URI.
   2. Approximately 20% of children ages 5 to 15 years who are diagnosed with rheumatic fever had pharyngitis in the preceding 3 months.

Bibliography
Anti-infective Review Panel. (2013). *Anti-infective guidelines for community-acquired infections.* Toronto, ON, Canada: MUMS Guidelines Clearinghouse.

Jensen, B., & Regier, L. D. (2017). *RxFiles drug comparison charts.* Saskatoon Health Region. Saskatoon, SK: Author. Retrieved from https://www.rxfiles.ca/rxfiles/uploads/documents/ChartsTitlePage-11th-edition-2017-book-references.pdf

Little, P., Hobbs, F. D., Moore, M., Mant, D., Williamson, I., McNulty, C., . . . PRISM investigators. (2013). Clinical score and rapid antigen detection test to guide antibiotic use for sore throats: randomized controlled trial of PRISM (primary care streptococcal management). *BMJ, 347,* f5806. doi:10.1136/bmj.f5806

Luzuriaga, K., & Sullivan, J. L. (2010). Infectious mononucleosis. *New England Journal of Medicine, 362,* 1993–2000. doi:10.1056/NEJMcp1001116. Retrieved from https://www.nejm.org/doi/full/10.1056/NEJMcp1001116

Shulman, S. T., Bisno, A. L., Clegg, H. W., Gerber, M. A., Kaplan, E. L., Lee, G., . . . Van Beneden, C. (2012). Clinical practice guideline for the diagnosis and management of Group A Streptococcal Pharyngitis: 2012 Update by the Infectious Diseases Society of America. *Clinical Infectious Diseases, 55*(10), e86–e102. https://doi.org/10.1093/cid/cis629

Toward Optimized Practice. (2008). *Guideline for the diagnosis and management of acute pharyngitis.* Retrieved from http://www.topalbertadoctors.org/download/368/acute_pharyngitis_guideline.pdf

Stomatitis, Minor Recurrent Aphthous Stomatitis

Jill C. Cash, Moya Cook, and Lynn Miller

Definition
A. Stomatitis is tender, round, discrete, oval, shallow, 1- to 5-mm ulcers in the oral cavity. The ulcers are gray, white, or yellow; on nonkeratinized skin; and surrounded by erythematous halos. They typically involve the labial and buccal mucosa and tongue, and adjacent tissue appears healthy.
B. Major recurrent aphthous stomatitis (RAS) has larger, deeper ulcers; lasts a longer period of time; usually recurs up to four times a year; and frequently leaves scars. It can cause significant dysphagia.

Incidence/Prevalence
A. Stomatitis affects 20% to 50% of the population. It is very common in North America.

Pathogenesis
A. Cause is poorly understood. Genetic, immunologic, viral, or nutritional causes are possible.

▶ Client Teaching Guides are available at https://connect.springerpub.com/content/reference-book/978-0-8261-9498-5

Predisposing Factors
A. Minor trauma.
B. History of RAS.
C. Possible nutritional deficiency of iron, folic acid, or zinc.
D. Hormonal changes.

Common Finding
A. Painful sore in mouth.

Other Signs and Symptoms
A. Burning sensation in mouth for 24 to 48 hours before lesions appear.

Subjective Data
A. Elicit history of aphthous stomatitis.
B. Ask the client about prodrome of burning or stinging in the mouth.
C. Elicit information regarding previous illness and trauma.

Physical Examination
A. Check temperature, pulse, respirations, and blood pressure.
B. Inspect:
   1. Mouth for ulcers.
   2. Ears, nose, and throat.
   3. Skin, especially palms and soles, for lesions: indicates hand, foot, and mouth disease.
C. Auscultate heart and lungs.

Diagnostic Tests
A. Specific diagnostic testing for stomatitis is not needed.
B. Consider herpes simplex virus (HSV) culture if herpes simplex virus is considered for diagnosis.
C. If syphillis is of concern, order serum rapid plasma reagin (RPR).

Differential Diagnoses
A. Herpetic stomatitis.
B. Behçet's disease.
C. Crohn's disease.
D. HIV.
E. Kawasaki syndrome.
F. Hand, foot, and mouth disease.

Plan
A. General interventions:
   1. Avoid spicy, salty, or hot foods.
   2. Encourage cold foods, such as fluids and ice pops, to help with pain.
   3. Avoid hard, sharp food that is difficult to chew.
   4. Recommend use of a soft-bristle toothbrush.
B. Client teaching.
C. Pharmacological therapy:
   1. Mouthwash made of diphenhydramine, with bismuth subsalicylate, or sucralfate, and viscous lidocaine three to four times a day. Leave out lidocaine when using in children. Instruct the client not to swallow medication.
   2. Sucralfate suspension may be used to swish in mouth and spit out for oral comfort.
   3. Glucocorticoid gel, such as fluocinonide gel.
   4. Orabase with or without triamcinolone acetonide.

Follow-Up
A. Follow up as needed for treatment of recurrences.

Consultation/Referral
A. Refer the client to or consult with a physician if ulcers are deeper or larger than 1 to 5 mm, if Kawasaki disease is suspected, or if no improvement is seen with adequate treatment.
B. Any lesion lasting longer than three weeks should be evaluated by a dentist or oral surgeon to rule out cancer.

Individual Considerations
A. Pregnancy: Avoid use of fluocinonide and triamcinolone acetonide in pregnant or nursing women.
B. Paediatrics:
   1. Avoid use of fluocinonide and triamcinolone acetonide.
   2. Do not use viscous lidocaine.

Bibliography
Hennessy, B. J. (2018). *Recurrent aphthous stomatitis*. Merck Manual. Retrieved from https://www.merckmanuals.com/en-ca/professional/dental-disorders/symptoms-of-dental-and-oral-disorders/recurrent-aphthous-stomatitis

International Association of Dental Traumatology. (2013). *Dental trauma guidelines*. Retrieved from https://www.iadt-dentaltrauma.org/1-9%20%20iadt%20guidelines%20combined%20-%20lr%20-%2011-5-2013.pdf

Thrush

Jill C. Cash, Moya Cook, and Lynn Miller

Definition
A. Thrush is a fungal infection of the oral cavity and/or the pharynx caused by *Candida*.

Incidence/Prevalence
A. It is estimated that 5% to 7% of babies younger than 1 month, both bottle-fed and breastfed infants, will develop oral candidiasis. Approximately 9% to 31% of AIDS clients and 20% of clients diagnosed with cancer will have thrush.

Pathogenesis
A. Thrush is an overgrowth of yeast cells, *Candida albicans*, on the oral mucosa, which leads to desquamation of the epithelial cells, creating a psuedomembrane over the normal oral mucosa.

Predisposing Factors
A. Use of broad-spectrum antibiotics.
B. Adults:
   1. HIV.
   2. Prolonged steroid use (systemic or inhaled corticosteroids).
   3. Cancer treatments (radiation/chemotherapy).
   4. Dentures.
   5. Malnutrition.
C. Children.
   1. Endocrine disorders (thyroid disease, diabetes mellitus, and Addison's disease).
   2. HIV.
   3. Cancer.

Common Findings
A. Soreness, pain of the mouth.

Other Signs and Symptoms
A. Irritability in infants.
B. Refusal to eat in infants.
C. White plaques coating buccal mucosa.

Subjective Data
A. Determine the onset, duration, and course of illness.
B. Ask whether the child refuses to eat.
C. Has the client used antibiotics or other medications in the previous weeks?
D. Does the client use inhaled or systemic steroids on a daily basis?

Physical Examination
A. Check temperature, pulse, respirations, and blood pressure.
B. Inspect:
  1. Oral cavity for white, curd-like plaques that cannot be removed.
  2. Ears, nose, and throat.
  3. Genital area for red rash and satellite papular lesions.

Diagnostic Tests
A. If diagnosis is certain, no testing recommended.
B. If uncertain of diagnosis, swab lesion for KOH testing.
C. If treatment prescribed is not working, fungal culture should be sent for diagnosis.

Differential Diagnoses
A. Milk deposits on tongue or buccal mucosa.
B. Stomatitis.
C. Aphthous ulcer.
D. Hairy leukoplakia.

Plan
A. General interventions:
  1. If the infant is breastfeeding, instruct the mother to clean breasts and nipples well with warm water between feedings to prevent contamination. Consider prescribing antifungal cream to be applied to breasts; this should be washed off before feedings.
  2. If bottle-feeding, boil all bottles, nipples, and pacifiers to kill the organism.
  3. Instruct caregiver to attempt removal of large plaques with a moistened, cotton-tipped applicator and/or small, moist gauze pad before inserting medication in mouth.
  4. If thrush is recurrent or resistant, consider checking the mother for candidal vaginitis.
  5. For adults, instruct the client/family on proper use and cleaning/rinsing of inhalers/dentures to prevent reoccurrence of thrush.
  6. Mother and infant should both be treated to reduce reinfection or cross-infection.
B. Client teaching
C. Pharmacological therapy:
  1. Oral candidiasis:
     a. Paediatrics: nystatin oral suspension. Place medication in front of mouth on each side. Rub directly on plaques with a cotton swab.
     b. Adults: pastilles or swish-and-swallow or tablets.
  2. Clotrimazole troche: Monitor for side effects.
  3. Fluconazole.
  4. Genital candidal dermatitis: nystatin cream. Have caregiver discontinue use of all baby wipes, lotions, powders, and creams.

Follow-Up
A. Instruct caregiver to telephone the office if the child refuses to eat, if there is no improvement, if thrush lasts more than 10 days, or if there is unexplained fever.

Consultation/Referral
A. Consult a physician if thrush does not resolve with adequate antifungal treatment.

Bibliography
Jensen, B., & Regier, L. D. (2017). *RxFiles drug comparison charts.* Saskatoon Health Region. Saskatoon, SK: Author. Retrieved from https://www.rxfiles.ca/rxfiles/uploads/documents/ChartsTitlePage-11th-edition-2017-book-references.pdf

Pappas, P. G., Kauffman, C. A., Andes, D. R., Clancy, C. J., Marr, K. A., Ostrosky-Zeichner, L., . . . Sobel, J. D. (2016). Executive summary: Clinical practice guideline for the management of candidiasis: 2016 Update by the Infectious Diseases Society of America. *Clinical Infectious Diseases, 62*(4), 409–417. doi:10.1093/cid/civ1194

9 Respiratory Guidelines

Asthma

Cheryl A. Glass, Melissa A. Hall, and Shelley Ann Walkerley

Definition
Pathophysiologically, asthma is defined by airway inflammation, intermittent airflow obstruction secondary to increased smooth muscle tone, and bronchial hyperresponsiveness. Episodes are associated with widespread, variable, often reversible airflow obstruction and bronchial hyperresponsiveness when airways are exposed to various stimuli or triggers. Asthma is responsible for lost school days, lost productivity, and presenteeism.
Asthma is classified into four categories:

A. *Step 1—Mild intermittent*: Symptoms less than or equal to two per week; asymptomatic with normal peak expiratory flow rate (PEFR) between attacks; nighttime symptoms less than or equal to two per month; PEFR >80% is predicted with a variability of <20%.
B. *Step 2—Mild persistent*: Symptoms greater than two per week but less than one per day; exacerbations may affect activity; nighttime symptoms greater than two per month; PEFR ≥80% is predicted with variability of 20% to 30%.
C. *Step 3—Moderate persistent*: Daily symptoms require beta 2 agonist use; attacks affect activity; exacerbations greater than or equal to two per week; nighttime symptoms greater than one per week; PEFRs between 60% and 80% with a variability >30%.
D. *Step 4—Severe persistent*: Continuous symptoms with limited physical activity; frequent exacerbations; frequent nighttime symptoms; PEFR ≤60% is predicted with >30% variability.

Incidence/Prevalence
A. Asthma affects 3.8 million people in Canada, or 300 million worldwide.
B. Asthma is the most common chronic disease of childhood, affecting 12.5% of children.
C. Up to 95% of clients with asthma also suffer from persistent rhinitis.
D. Asthma is often associated with other comorbid conditions, including gastroesophageal reflux disease (GERD) and obesity.
E. Asthma can present at any age and should be considered between the ages of one and five years if key symptoms are present.

Pathogenesis
A. Asthma arises from a complex cycle of processes initiated by airway inflammation resulting from physical, chemical, and pharmacological agents (such as environmental irritants, allergens, furry animals, cockroaches, dust mites, pollen and mold, cold air, viral respiratory infections, and exercise). It progresses to airway hyperresponsiveness, bronchoconstriction, airway wall oedema, chronic mucus plug formation, and chronic airway remodelling.

Predisposing Factors
A. In children:
  1. Allergy or family history of allergy.
  2. Atopy.
  3. Male gender.
B. In adults:
  1. Family history.
  2. Coexisting sinusitis, nasal polyps, and sensitivity to ASA or other nonsteroidal anti-inflammatory drugs (NSAIDs).
  3. Exposure in workplace to wood dust, metals, and animal products.
  4. Premenstrual asthma (PMA).
  5. Female gender.
  6. Occupational exposures.
  7. Comorbidities in older adults.
C. In all ages:
  1. Inhalation of irritants such as tobacco smoke.
  2. Viral respiratory infections.
  3. Gastroesophageal reflux.
  4. Obesity.
D. Triggers:
  1. Allergen exposure.
  2. Viral infections of the upper airways.
  3. Medication (potential risk with beta-blockers, angiotensin-converting enzyme [ACE] inhibitors, ASA, cyclooxygenase [COX] inhibitors).
  4. Exercise.
  5. Situational factors: Cold air, laughter, strong odours, air pollution, smoke exposure, pregnancy.
  6. Foods.
  7. Hormones.
  8. Gastrointestinal (GI) reflux.
  9. Stress.

Common Findings
A. Recurrent cough (worse at night and early morning).
B. Recurrent wheezing.
C. Recurrent shortness of breath (SOB).
D. Dyspnea (less likely to be reported in the elderly).
E. Recurrent chest tightness (may worsen with moderate activity).

Other Signs and Symptoms
A. Nocturnal awakening from symptoms.
B. Variation of symptoms with seasons or environment.
C. Chest discomfort, tightness with moderate activity.

Subjective Data
A. Ask about the onset, duration, and course of symptoms.
B. Inquire about sudden severe episodes of coughing, wheezing, and SOB and whether precipitating factors can be identified.
C. Ask whether the client has chest colds that take more than 10 days to resolve.
D. Ask if the client is a smoker, how much, and for how long he or she has smoked.
E. Ask whether symptoms seem to occur during certain seasons or during exposure to the following environmental irritants:
   1. Tobacco smoke.
   2. Perfume.
   3. Household pets.
   4. Fireplaces.
   5. Woodburning stoves.
   6. Mold.
   7. Dust mites.
   8. Cockroaches.
F. Find out how often coughing, wheezing, or SOB awakens the client.
G. Ask whether symptoms are caused or exacerbated by moderate exercise or physical activity.
H. Determine the family history of asthma, allergies, and eczema.
I. Determine whether the client is pregnant or has medical problems. If so, do not prescribe long-term beta2 adrenergics or NSAIDs. The safest medications are short-acting beta2 agonists (SABA), cromolyn sodium, and anticholinergic drugs.
J. Administer the asthma control test for adults or children. This test is for self-report (or parent-report) to determine whether asthma symptoms are under control. The Asthma Control Check is available online from lungontario.ca/protect-your-breathing/are-you-at-risk/take-asthma-control-check. If the client answers YES to any of these questions they are advised to speak to their health-care provider about the right medications to take control of their asthma symptoms. (Canadian Lung Association)
K. Evaluate whether the client has ever been tested for allergies.
L. Ask whether the client has ever needed to go to the ED or had to be hospitalized for an asthma attack.
M. Review all medications, including over-the-counter (OTC) and herbal supplements.

Physical Examination
A. Check temperature (if indicated), blood pressure, pulse, respirations, and pulse oximetry. Measure the client's height and weight to calculate body mass index (BMI) because obesity is associated with asthma, and evaluate failure to thrive if suspected.
B. Inspect:
   1. Especially in children, observe for hyperexpansion of thorax and signs that accessory muscles are being used (retractions, nasal flaring) or stridor.
   2. Note appearance of hunched shoulders and/or chest deformity.
   3. In children, inspect the nose for a foreign body.
   4. In all clients, inspect ears, nose, and throat. Evaluate the presence of enlarged tonsils and adenoids, and nasal polyps.
   5. Inspect skin for eczema, dermatitis, or other irritation that might signal allergy.
   6. Observe for allergic shiners and pebbled conjunctiva.
   7. Observe for digital clubbing.
C. Auscultate.
   1. Auscultate lung sounds. Note wheezing during normal expiration and prolonged expiration, which is seen with asthma.
   2. Listen to all lung fields for an asymmetric wheeze.
   3. Auscultate heart.
D. Percuss lung fields.

Diagnostic Tests
A. **Spirometry is the gold standard.** Peak flow meter measurements can be used as a substitute when spirometry is not available or client is under six years of age. Evaluate the forced vital capacity (FVC) and forced expiratory volume in one second (FEV_1) before and after the client inhales a short-acting bronchodilator (SABD, SABA). Diagnosis is confirmed if FEV_1 is improved by $\geq 12\%$.
B. Evaluate chest radiograph (CXR) and complete blood count (CBC) to exclude other diagnoses and infection.
C. Allergy testing is recommended for children with persistent asthma.
D. Check PEFR after inhalation of SABA. Diagnosis is confirmed if:
   1. There is a 20% increase in PEFR after 15 to 20 minutes.
   2. PEFR varies >20% between arising and 12 hours later in clients taking bronchodilators.
   3. There is a >10% to 15% decrease in FEV_1 post exercise.
E. Consider a bronchial provocation test with histamine or methacholine for nondiagnostic spirometry.

Differential Diagnoses
A. In infants and children:
   1. Asthma.
   2. Pulmonary infections:
      a. Pneumonia.
      b. Respiratory syncytial virus (RSV).
      c. Viral bronchiolitis.
      d. Tuberculosis (TB).
   3. Allergic rhinitis and sinusitis.
   4. Foreign body in the nose, trachea, or bronchus.
   5. GERD.
   6. Cystic fibrosis (CF).
   7. Bronchopulmonary dysplasia.
   8. Vocal cord dysfunction.
   9. Enlarged lymph nodes or tumours.
B. In adults:
   1. Asthma.
   2. Chronic obstructive pulmonary disease (COPD).
   3. GERD.
   4. Congestive heart failure (CHF).
   5. Cough secondary to medications such as ACE inhibitors or beta-blockers.
   6. Pneumonia, including aspiration pneumonia in elderly or post-cerebrovascular accident (CVA).
   7. Pulmonary embolism.
   8. Laryngeal dysfunction.
   9. Benign and malignant tumours.
   10. Vocal cord dysfunction.

Plan

A. General interventions:
  1. Review proper medication dosages. Short- and long-term agents come in several formulations, such as nebulizer, metered-dose inhaler (MDI), and a dry powder inhaler (DPI). Young children should have medication via a MDI inhaler using a spacer with an appropriate-size face mask.
  2. Demonstrate correct use of inhalers, spacers, and nebulizers. If the client does not use correct technique when using these devices, medication does not get delivered to the bronchioles, and therefore the client may believe that the medication does not work. Most often, the medication works well when delivered to the bronchioles correctly. *Refer to Client Teaching Guide: Asthma: How to Use a Metered-Dose Inhaler.*
  3. Stress the importance of using a peak flow monitor at home to monitor progress of the disease. *Refer to Client Teaching Guide: Asthma: Action Plan and Peak Flow Monitoring.*
  4. SABAs are used for rescue from acute symptoms.
  5. Use of a SABA more than twice a week for symptom relief indicates that the client has inadequate asthma control and needs an inhaled corticosteroid (ICS) as controller therapy.
  6. Stress the need for an asthma action plan. *Refer to Client Teaching Guide: Asthma: Action Plan and Peak Flow Monitoring.*

B. Client teaching: *Refer to Client Teaching Guide: Asthma.*

C. Pharmacological therapy: Drugs are prescribed in a stepwise fashion for the type of asthma. The amount of medication used depends on the severity of the asthma (Steps 1–5 in the following list). **Before any medication/dosage changes, monitor the client's compliance** (see Table 9.1). The following treatments are recommended for children aged five years and older and for adults (see note re: children under four years of age):
  1. Step 1: Mild:
     a. No long-term preventive medications are needed.
     b. SABA/ prn.
     c. Consider a low-dose inhaled corticosteroid (ICS).
  2. Step 2: Mild to moderate:
     a. Low-dose ICSs are used daily as a long-term preventive medication.
     b. Budesonide inhalation suspension and fluticasone propionate (MDI) are approved by Health Canada for use in infants and children younger than four years. Mometasone furoate and fluticasone/salmeteral are available by MDI and approved for children four years and older.
     c. Alternative medications include an ICS plus either a leukotriene modifier or low dose theophylline.
  3. Step 3: Moderate:
     a. Low-dose ICS plus a long-acting beta2 agonist (LABA) *or* a medium/high-dose ICS.
     b. Low-dose ICS plus LTRA.
     c. Use SABA prn or low-dose ICS/fometerol prn as reliever medication for Steps 3, 4, and 5.
  4. Step 4: Moderate to severe:
     a. Medium- to high-dose ICS plus a LABA.
     b. Add a muscarinic antagonist (LAMA) (anticholinergic: tiotropium), high-dose ICS plus LTRA or theophylline.
  5. Step 5: Severe:
     a. Refer for add-on treatment such as tiotropium, anti-IgE (omalizumab) or anti-IL5 (mepolizumab).
     b. Add low-dose OCS.
  6. Acute exacerbations in paediatrics: Salbutamol pMDI 6–10 puffs Q20 mins x 3 (use a spacer with an appropriately sized facial mask) or nebulized salbutamol (wt 10 kg: 1.25–2.5 mg/dose, 11–20 kg: 2.5mg does, 20 kg: 5mg dose).
  7. Exercise-induced bronchospasm:
     a. Short-acting inhaled beta 2 agonist: One inhalation 15 minutes before exercise.
  8. Hypertension and asthma: First-line treatment is a calcium channel blocker. Asthmatics also tolerate diuretics well. Avoid beta-blockers (beta-adrenergic antagonists). ACE inhibitors can cause dry cough.
  9. Theophylline can cause cardiac arrhythmias; therefore, use it with caution and monitor serum theophylline levels.
  10. Vaccinations:
      a. Inhaled flu vaccine is not used in children with asthma. Inactivated influenza vaccine is safe, including for children with severe asthma.
      b. Pneumococcal vaccine is recommended for children with asthma.

D. Goal of asthma therapy:
  1. Minimal to no chronic symptoms, including night-time symptoms.
  2. Minimal exacerbations.
  3. No ED visits.
  4. Minimal use of SABA.
  5. No limitations of activities.
  6. Peak expiratory flow maintained in normal range.
  7. Minimal adverse effects of medications.
  8. Prevent asthma-related mortality.

Follow-Up

A. After acute episodes, follow up within one to two hours or next day to monitor improvement until client is stable.

B. For clients with mild intermittent or mild persistent asthma under control for at least three months, assess and follow up at least every six months to provide education and reinforce positive behaviors. Step-down therapy: reduce medication (ICS, other agents) dosage gradually in three-month intervals. If control is not achieved, consider increasing the dosage after reviewing medication technique, compliance, and environmental control.

Consultation/Referral

A. Consider hospitalization for clients with acute episodes who do not completely respond to treatment within one to two hours.

B. Refer to an asthma specialist if asthma is severe, or there is inadequate response to standard care, for add-on therapy.

C. Consult with a specialist when the client is pregnant or has other medical problems, or when standard treatment is ineffective.

Individual Considerations

Inhaled budesonide is the preferred ICS for treatment of asthma in pregnancy.

A. Pregnancy:
  1. Risks of uncontrolled asthma far outweigh risks to mother or foetus from drugs used to control the disease.

▸ Client Teaching Guides are available at https://connect.springerpub.com/content/reference-book/978-0-8261-9498-5

TABLE 9.1 Medications for Asthma and COPD

Brand	Generic	Drug Classification	Availability
SABA, for Rescue/Fast-Acting Rescue			
Ventolin, Ventolin HFA, Airomir, Ventolin Diskus	salbutamol	Beta2 agonist; SABA	Nebules, inhaler solution
			pMDI, diskus
Bricanyl	turbuhaler	SABA	Turbuhaler
LABA, for Maintenance/Long-Acting Control			
Oxeze Turbuhaler	formoterol fumarate dihydrate	LABA	Turbuhaler
Onbrez Breezhaler	indacaterol	LABA	Breezhaler
Foradil	formoterol fumarate		DPI
Serevent Diskus	salmeterol	LABA	Diskhaler, diskus
Duaklir Genuair	aclidinium/formoterol	Long-acting muscarinic antagonist + long-acting beta 2-adrenergic agonist (LAMA/LABA)	DPI
Ultibro Breezhaler	glycopyrronium/indacaterol	LAMA/LABA	DPI
Inspiolto Respimat	tiotropium/olodaterol	LAMA/LABA	DPI
Anoro Ellipta	umeclidinium/vilanterol	LAMA/LABA	DPI
ICS Anti-inflammatory, for Maintenance or Long-Term Control			
Alvesco	ciclesonide	ICS	pMDI
Asmanex	mometasone furoate	ICS	Twisthaler dry powder
generics	beclomethasone dipropionate	ICS	pMDI
Flovent HFA Flovent Diskus	fluticasone proionate	ICS	pMDI, diskus
Pulmicort	budesonide	ICS	Turbuhaler, nebuamp
QVAR	beclomethasone	ICS	pMDI
Arnuity Ellipta	fluticasone furoate	ICS	DPI
Symbicort	budesonide + formoterol fumerate dihydrate	Combination corticosteroid + long-acting beta2 agonist (ICS/LABA); not approved for relief of acute bronchospasm in COPD	DPI
Breo Ellipta	fluticasone furoate/vilanterol	ICS + LABA	DPI
Advair Diskus	fluticasone + salmeterol	ICS/LABA	pMDI, diskus
Zenhale	mometasone/formoteral fumarate dihydrate	ICS/LABA	pMDI
LTRA			pMDI–HFA inhaler
Singulair	montelukast	LTRA	Chewable tablets
			Tablets, granules
IL-5 inhibitor			
Nucala	mepolizumab	IL-5 inhibitor	Subcutaneous injection
Anticholinergics (Muscarinic Antagonists; Long-Acting [LAMA] and Short-Acting [SAMA])			
Atrovent HFA	ipratropium	Muscarinic antagonist, short-acting (SAMA)	pMDI and nebules
Combivent UDV	ipratropium/salbutamol	SAMA/SABA	pMDI and nebules
Combivent Respimat	ipratropium/salbutamol	SAMA/SABA	SMI
Spiriva Respimat	tiotropium	Muscarinic antagonist, long-acting (LAMA)	Soft mist inhaler
Spiriva	tiotropium	LAMA	DPI
Tudorza Genuair	aclidinium	LAMA	DPI

(continued)

TABLE 9-1 Medications for Asthma and COPD (*continued*)

Brand	Generic	Drug Classification	Availability
Seebri Breezhaler	glycopyrronium	LAMA	DPI
Incruse Ellipta	umeclidinium	LAMA	DPI
Methylxanthine			
Uniphyl, generics	theophylline	Methylxanthines	Tablet
Apo-Theo LA	theophylline sustained-release	Methylxanthines	Tablet
IgE-Neutralizing Antibody			
Xolair	omalizumab	IgE-Neutralizing antibody	Subcutaneous injection
Systemic Corticosteroids			
Prednisone (generics)	prednisone	Systemic corticosteroid	Tablet
PDE4			
Daliresp	roflumilast	Selective PDE4	Tablet
Mucolytics	N-acetylcysteine	Mucolytic	Oral

COPD, chronic obstructive pulmonary disease; DPI, dry powder inhaler; HFA, hydrofluoroalkanes; ICS, inhaled corticosteroid; IL, interleukin; LABA, long-acting beta2-adrenergic agonist; LTRA, leukotriene receptor antagonists; PDE4, phosphodiesterase-4 Inhibitors; pMDI, pressurized metered-dose inhaler; SABA, short-acting beta2-adrenergic agonist. (CPhA, RxTx, 2018)

2. Most drugs used to treat asthma and rhinitis, with the exception of brompheniramine and epinephrine, pose little increased risk to the foetus.
3. Classes of drugs that are associated with risk include decongestants, antibiotics (tetracycline, sulfonamides, and ciprofloxacin), live virus vaccines, immunotherapy (if doses are increased), and iodides. Always weigh benefits against risks, because adequate foetal oxygen supply is essential.
4. If corticosteroids are necessary, recommend aerosolized forms due to their lower systemic effects. Prednisone or methylprednisolone are preferred and should be prescribed at minimum effective doses.
5. Do not prescribe inhaled triamcinolone (synthetic glucocorticoid) because it is teratogenic.
6. Drugs recommended during pregnancy:
   a. A beta 2 agonist (SABA), such as salbutamol and terbutaline, are preferred. Regular daily use suggests a need for additional medications.
   b. Regular ICS is indicated if asthma symptoms are not well controlled (more than twice per week).
   c. Add oral theophylline if ICS is not effective. May increase symptoms of GERD or cause nausea. Tachycardia has been noted in the foetus. Avoid if possible. Referral to a specialist is recommended.
   d. Oral prednisone if all other therapies fail. Recommend obstetric consult before prescribing. Associated with increased risk of oral cleft.
7. Leukotrine inhibitors should be prescribed in pregnancy only if clearly needed.
   a. Montelukast has not been studied in pregnancy. Some rare congenital abnormalities have been reported. Referral to a specialist is recommended.

B. Geriatrics:
1. Asthma in the elderly is often associated with comorbidities such as cardiac conditions, COPD, or dementia.
2. The onset of asthma in seniors is usually in childhood or early adulthood. Less commonly, some have the first onset after age 65.
3. Triggers and symptoms are similar to those experienced by younger people with asthma.
4. Treatment is the same as with younger clients, with inhaled steroids the mainstay and oral steroids reserved for severe episodes. The elderly have more adverse effects from inhaled ICS.
5. If steroids are prescribed, carefully monitor the client for complications, including cataracts, increased intraocular pressure, hyperglycaemia, and accelerated loss of bone mass.
6. Inhaled anticholinergics and beta 2 agonists are second-line treatments.
7. The elderly may have difficulty with inhaling medications and may require a spacer or nebulizer.
8. Theophylline is rarely effective in the elderly. Asthma medications may have increased adverse effects in the elderly or may aggravate coexisting medical conditions, requiring medication adjustments. Also consider drug interactions and drug-and-disease interactions.

C. Paediatrics:
1. Spacing chambers are recommended to assist in proper delivery of medication.

Resources

AboutKidsHealth Asthma resources https://www.aboutkidshealth.ca/Article?contentid=1491&language=English
Asthma Canada www.asthma.ca
Adult and Children Asthma Control tests: www.asthmacontrol.com
Asthma & Allergy Foundation of America: www.aafa.org
BREATHE. The Canadian Lung Association www.lung.ca/asthma
Global Initiative for Asthma (GINA) Instructions for Inhaler and Spacer Use: www.ginasthma.com

Bibliography

Barnes, P. J. (2015). Asthma. In D. L. Kasper, A. S. Fauci, S. L. Hauser, D. L. Longo, & J. L. Jameson (Eds.), *Harrison's principles of internal medicine* (19th ed.). New York, NY: McGraw-Hill.
Canadian Lung Association. *Asthma control check*. Retrieved from https://lungontario.ca/protect-your-breathing/are-you-at-risk/take-asthma-control-check

Centers for Disease Control and Prevention. (2015b, August 7). *Prevention and control of influenza with vaccines: Recommendations of the advisory committee on immunization practices, United States, 2015–16 Influenza season*. Retrieved from https://www.cdc.gov/mmwr/preview/mmwrhtml/mm6430a3.htm

Centers for Disease Control and Prevention. (2015c, August 31). *Pertussis (whooping cough) surveillance & reporting*. Retrieved from www.cdc.gov/pertussis/surv-reporting.html

Centers for Disease Control and Prevention. (2016b, February 16). *FastStats asthma*. Retrieved from www.cdc.gov/nchs/fastats/asthma.htm

Ducharme, F., Dell, S., Radhakrishnan, D., Grad, R. M., Watson, W. T. A., . . . Zelman, M. (2015). Diagnosis and management of asthma in preschoolers: A Canadian Thoracic Society and Canadian Paediatric Society position paper. *Canadian Respiratory Journal, 22*(3), 135–143. doi:10.1155/2015/101572

Fanta, H. (2014, July). Diagnosis of asthma in adolescents and adults. *UpToDate*. Retrieved from http://www.uptodate.com/contents/diagnosis-of-asthma-in-adolescents-and-adults

Flaherty, E., & Resnick, R (Eds.). (2014). *Geriatric nursing review syllabus: A core curriculum in advanced practice geriatric nursing* (4th ed.). New York, NY: American Geriatrics Society.

Harding, S. M. (2015, August 11). Gastroesophageal reflux and asthma. *UpToDate*. Retrieved from http://www.uptodate.com/online/contents/gastroesophageal-reflux-and-asthma

Koren, G., Sarkar, M., & Einarson, A. (2010). Safety of using montelukast during pregnancy. *Canadian Family Physician, 56*(9), 881–882.

Lougheed, M., Lemiere, C., Dell, S., Ducharme, F. M., Fitzgerald, J. M., Leigh, R., . . . Boulet, L. P. (2010). Canadian Thoracic Society Asthma Management Continuum–2010 Consensus Summary for children six years of age and over, and adults. *Canadian Respiratory Journal, 17*(1), 15–24. doi:10.1155/2010/827281

Lougheed, M., Lemiere, C., Ducharme, F. M., Licskai, C., Dell, S., Row, B. H., . . . Boulet, L. P. (2012). Canadian Thoracic Society 2012 guideline update: Diagnosis and management of asthma in preschoolers, children and adults. *Canadian Respiratory Journal, 19*(2), 127–164. doi:10.1155/2012/635624

Medscape Drug Reference. (n.d.ï»¿). Theophylline oral. *Medscape*. Retrieved from http://www.medscape.com/druginfo/dosage?drugid=3591&drugname=Theophylline+Oral&monotype=default

Ortiz-Alvarez, O., Mikrogianakis, A., & Canadian Paediatric Society, Acute Care Committee. (2012). Managing the paediatric client with acute asthma exacerbation. *Paediatr Child Health, 17*(5), 251–255. doi:10.1093/pch/17.5.251

Park-Wyllie, L., Mazzotta, P., Pastuszak, A., Moretti, M.E., Beique, L., Hunnisett, L., . . . Koren, G. (2010). Birth defects after maternal exposure to corticosteroids: prospective cohort study and meta-analysis of epidemiological studies. *Canadian Family Physician, 56*(9), 881–882.

Prescriber's Letter. (2013, May). *Appropriate med use* (Vol. 29). Retrieved from http://prescribersletter.therapeuticresearch.com/pl/ArticleDD.aspx?cs=&s=PRL&pt=6&fpt=31&dd=290501&pb=PRL&searchid=55980185

Prescriber's Letter. (2016a, January). *Asthma* (Vol. 23). Retrieved from prescribersletter.therapeuticresearch.com

Public Health Agency of Canada. (2018).*Canadian immunization guide*. Ottawa, Ontario, Canada https://www.canada.ca/en/public-health/services/canadian-immunization-guide.html

Rains, S. G. (2013). Fifteen-to-eighteen-month visit. In B. Richardson (Ed.), *Pediatric primary care: Practice guidelines for nurses* (2nd ed., pp. 113–124). Burlington, MA: Jones & Bartlett.

Sawicki, G., & Haver, K. (2015, December 9). Acute asthma exacerbations in children: Outpatient management. *UpToDate*. Retrieved from http://www.uptodate.com/contents/acute-asthma-exacerbations-in-children-home-office-management-and-severity-assessment?source=search_result&search=acute+asthma+exacerbations+in+children&selectedTitle=3%7E150

Schatz, M., & Weinberger, S. E. (2015, December). Management of asthma during pregnancy. *UpToDate*. Retrieved from http://www.uptodate.com/contents/management-of-asthma-during-pregnancy

Schwartzstein, R. M., & Adams, L. (2016). *Murray & Nadel's textbook of respiratory medicine* (6th ed.). Philadelphia, PA: Elsevier-Saunders.

Terry, E. G. (2017). Seven-to-ten-year visit (school age. In B. Richardson (Ed.), *Pediatric primary care: Practice guidelines for nurses* (3rd ed., pp. 143–158). Burlington, MA: Jones & Bartlett.

Valentine, N. (2017). Respiratory disorders. In B. Richardson (Ed.), *Pediatric primary care: Practice guidelines for nurses* (3rd ed., pp. 143–158). Burlington, MA: Jones & Bartlett.

Vaz Fragoso, C. (2016). Diagnosis and managment of asthma in older adults. *UpToDate*. Retrieved from http://www.uptodate.com/contents/diagnosis-and-management-of-asthma-in-older-adults?source=search_result&search=diagnosis+and+management+in+older+adults&selectedTitle=1%7E150

Zachary, K. C. (2015, December). Treatment of seasonal influenza in adults. *UpToDate*. Retrieved from http://www.uptodate.com/contents/treatment-of-seasonal-influenza-in-adults

Bronchiolitis: Child

Cheryl A. Glass, Melissa A. Hall, and Shelley Ann Walkerley

Definition

A. Bronchiolitis is a narrowing and inflammation of the bronchioles, causing wheezing and mild to severe respiratory distress. Infants are affected most often because of their small airways and insufficient collateral ventilation. It is one of the most common causes of acute hospitalizations in infants, especially in the fall and winter. A small decrease in a bronchiole's already small airway will have a fourfold increase in airway resistance and accounts for this pathologic manifestation in this age group.

B. The average length of illness with bronchiolitis is 12 days.

Incidence/Prevalence

A. Respiratory infection is seen in one-third of children in the first two years of life, with one in ten requiring hospitalization.

B. Bronchiolitis occurs most often in infants and children aged one to two years. Approximately two to four percent of adults with respiratory illnesses, comorbidity of immunosuppression, and the elderly will also be diagnosed with bronchiolitis.

Pathogenesis

The pathology results in obstruction of bronchioles from inflammation, oedema, and debris, leading to hyperinflation of the lungs, increased airway resistance, atelectasis, and ventilation–perfusion mismatching.

A. Respiratory syncytial virus (RSV) is the most common cause (50%–80%) of bronchiolitis.

B. Human metapneumovirus (hMPV) is the second most common cause (3%–19%).

C. Other causes include parainfluenza virus, adenovirus, influenza, *Chlamydia pneumoniae*, *Mycoplasma pneumoniae*, and human bocavirus (hBoV).

Predisposing Factors

A. Low birth weight, particularly in premature infants.
B. Chronic lung disease (CLD; formerly bronchopulmonary dysplasia).
C. Parental smoking.
D. Congenital heart disease.
E. Immunodeficiency.
F. Lower socioeconomic group.
G. Crowded living conditions and day care.
H. Gender: Bronchiolitis occurs in males 1.25 times more frequently than in females.

Common Findings

Clinical manifestations are initially subtle:
A. Infants who become increasingly fussy.
B. Difficulty feeding during the two- to five-day incubation period. This is because infants prefer to breathe through their nose (obligate nasal breathing) as opposed to their mouths and significant nasal oedema and/or rhinorrhoea may force mouth breathing and disturb feedings.
C. Low-grade fever (usually <38.6°C).
D. Cough.

E. Tachypnoea.
F. Wheezing.
G. Retractions.
H. Nasal flaring and grunting.

Other Signs and Symptoms
A. Coryza.
B. Irritability.
C. Lethargy.
D. Respiratory distress.
E. Nasal flaring and grunting.
F. Hypothermia, apnoea and cyanosis (infants younger than one month).

Subjective Data
A. Determine the onset, course, and duration of illness.
B. Are breathing problems affecting the ability to eat and drink? Is the baby able to be breastfed?
C. Evaluate a history of fever, nausea, vomiting, or diarrhoea.
D. Does the client or any family members have asthma?
E. Are there any other family members who are ill?
F. Are there smokers in the family environment?

Physical Examination
A. Check temperature, blood pressure, oxygen saturation, and respirations. **Count respirations for a full minute. Respirations >60 breaths per minute in an infant may be associated with risk for severe disease and warrant further evaluation for pneumonia. Tachypnoea at any age is a concern for severe lower respiratory illness.**
B. Inspect:
  1. Observe overall appearance.
  2. Note respiratory pattern and nasal flaring.
  3. Note the use of accessory muscles for breathing.
  4. Check for tachypnoea, which differentiates bronchiolitis from upper respiratory infections and bronchitis.
  5. Examine eyes, ears, and throat, noting other potential infections.
  6. Inspect nose for nasal flaring.
  7. Assess for signs of dehydration.
C. Auscultate:
  1. Heart.
  2. **Lungs. On examination there are fine inspiratory crackles and/or high-pitched expiratory wheezes. A prolonged expiration phase is seen with bronchiolitis.**
D. Palpate liver and spleen.
E. Percuss chest/lungs for hyperresonance.
F. Neurologic examination: Assess for irritability and lethargy.

Diagnostic Tests
A. **Diagnosis is made based on age and seasonal occurrence, tachypnea, and the presence of profuse coryza and fine rales, wheezes, or both on auscultation.**
B. Viral isolation from nasopharyngeal secretions or rapid antigen detection (enzyme-linked immunosorbent assay [ELISA], immunofluorescence) for RSV can confirm diagnosis.
  Note: RSV testing is not normally done outside of a hospital setting or for infection control purposes.
C. Consider pulse oximetry.
D. Routine use of a chest radiograph (CXR) is not recommended.

Differential Diagnoses
A. Asthma.
B. Viral or bacterial pneumonia.
C. Aspiration syndromes.
D. Pertussis.
E. Cystic fibrosis (CF).
F. Cardiac disease.
G. Reflux.
H. Aspiration including foreign body.
I. Tracheo-oesophageal fistula.

Plan
A. General interventions:
  1. Use a humidifier in the client's bedroom.
  2. Clear stuffy nose with saline solution drops and suction out nares with bulb syringe.
  3. Infants should not be exposed to second-hand smoke.
  4. Monitor respiratory pattern.
  5. Use good hygiene practices—handwashing.
B. Client teaching: *Refer to Client Teaching Guide: Bronchiolitis: Child.*
C. Dietary management:
  1. Encourage fluids, such as juice and water. Dilute juice for younger infants.
  2. Offer small, frequent feedings.
  3. Breastfeeding should continue.
D. Medical/surgical management:
  1. Clients may only require supportive care. Clients with respiratory distress require hospitalization.
  2. Hypoxaemic clients need oxygen therapy and possibly mechanical ventilation.
  3. Chest physiotherapy is not recommended.
E. Pharmacological therapy:
  1. Bronchodilators should not be routinely used. They do not improve the duration of illness or lessen hospitalization.
  2. Corticosteroids should not be routinely used. They do not improve the duration of illness or lessen hospitalization.
  3. Antibiotics should be used only with proven coexistence of a bacterial infection.
  4. There is no vaccine against bronchiolitis. Palivizumab (Synagis) is a humanized monoclonal antibody used in the prevention of serious respiratory diseases such as bronchiolitis in infants and children at high risk of RSV disease. It has been shown to prevent infection and reduce hospitalizations due to RSV in these paediatric clients, and should be administered to high-risk children during RSV season (CPhA, CPS, 2018). A vaccine against human metapneumovirus (hMPV) is currently in the early stages of development. hMPV has been in existence in humans for >60 years, but is only newly categorized. hMPV is most closely related to avian metapneumovirus. The virus most frequently infects young children and the elderly. hMPV is most common in late winter and early spring, and is associated with up to 25% of respiratory infections. hMPV is responsible for the majority of viral upper respiratory infections in children and adults. The

▶ Client Teaching Guides are available at https://connect.springerpub.com/content/reference-book/978-0-8261-9498-5

virus has a worldwide distribution and is most prevalent in late winter and early spring. Guidelines for the administration of Palivizumab vary from province to province. Consult provincial guidelines.

5. Use of montelukast has not proven beneficial in resolution of symptoms.

Follow-Up
A. Contact the client/family within 12 to 24 hours for evaluation.

Consultation/Referral
A. Consider hospitalization if the client's breathing becomes laboured, his or her wheezing becomes worse, and/or respiratory distress is suspected.
B. Refer clients with RSV to the ED if moderate respiratory distress, dehydration, or hypoxaemia occurs.
C. Younger clients in moderate to severe respiratory distress require hospitalization.
D. Infants less than two months of age require hospitalization.
E. Clients with pulmonary hypertension, chronic lung disease (CLD; formerly bronchopulmonary dysplasia), or CF need hospitalization if their respiratory rate is >60, their pulse oximetry is <92%, or they eat poorly.

Individual Considerations
A. Clients with pulmonary hypertension, bronchopulmonary dysplasia, or CF may have prolonged courses with high morbidity and mortality. Some may have reactive airway diseases in the future.
B. Young children and the elderly are most susceptible to hMPV infection. The majority of children are seropositive for hMPV infection by age five. History of prematurity and asthma increase risk for hospitalization in children.
C. Human pneumovirus was identified in 8% of adults requiring hospitalization for lower respiratory infections.

Bibliography
Crow, J. E. (2015, November). *Human metapneumovirus infections*. Retrieved from http://www.uptodate.com/contents/human-metapneumovirus-infections

Friedman, J. N., Rieder, M. J., Walton, J. M., & Canadian Paediatric Society Acute Care Committee, & Drug Therapy and Hazardous Substances Committee. (2014). *Bronchiolitis: Recommendations for diagnosis, monitoring and management of children one to 24 months of age*. Retrieved from https://www.cps.ca/en/documents/position/bronchiolitis

Munoz, F. M., & Flomenberg, P. (2015, June). Diagnosis, treatment, and prevention of adenovirus infection. *UpToDate*. Retrieved from http://www.uptodate.com

Piedra, P. A. (2016, February 23). Bronchiolitis in infants and children: Clinical features and diagnosis. *UpToDate*. Retrieved from http://www.uptodate.com/contents/bronchiolitis-in-infants-and-children-clinical-features-and-diagnosis

Prescriber's Letter. (2013, May). *Appropriate med use* (Vol. 29). Retrieved from http://prescribersletter.therapeuticresearch.com/pl/ArticleDD.aspx?cs=&s=PRL&pt=6&fpt=31&dd=290501&pb=PRL&searchid=55980185

Prescriber's Letter. (2015a, January). *Pediatrics* (Vol. 3). Retrieved from http://prescribersletter.therapeuticresearch.com/pl/ArticleDD.aspx?cs=&s=PRL&pt=6&fpt=31&dd=310118&pb=PRL&searchid=55978611

Schwartzstein, R. M., & Adams, L. (2016). *Murray & Nadel's textbook of respiratory medicine* (6th ed.). Philadelphia, PA: Elsevier-Saunders.

Valentine, N. (2017). Respiratory disorders. In B. Richardson (Ed.), *Pediatric primary care: Practice guidelines for nurses* (3rd ed., pp. 143–158). Burlington, MA: Jones & Bartlett.

Weiner, D. L. (2014, November). Causes of acute respiratory distress in children. *UpToDate*. Retrieved from http://www.uptodate.com/contents/causes-of-acute-respiratory-distress-in-children

Bronchitis, Acute

Cheryl A. Glass, Melissa A. Hall, and Shelley Ann Walkerley

Definition
A. Acute bronchitis is inflammation of the tracheobronchial tree. Bronchitis is nearly always self-limited in the otherwise healthy individual. Generally, the clinical course of acute bronchitis lasts 10 to 14 days. The cause is usually infectious, but allergens and irritants may also produce a similar clinical profile. Asthma can be mistaken as acute bronchitis if the client has no prior history of asthma.

Incidence/Prevalence
A. Bronchitis is more common in fall and winter in relation to common cold or other respiratory illness. It occurs in both children (younger than five years of age) and adults and is diagnosed in men more frequently than in women. Fewer than five percent of clients with bronchitis develop pneumonia.

Pathogenesis
A. Most attacks are caused by viral agents, such as adenovirus, influenza, parainfluenza viruses, and respiratory syncytial virus (RSV).
B. Bacterial causes include *Bordetella pertussis, Mycobacterium tuberculosis, Corynebacterium diphtheriae*, and *Mycoplasma pneumoniae. B. pertussis* should be considered in children who are incompletely vaccinated.

Predisposing Factors
A. Viral infection.
B. Upper respiratory infection.
C. Smoking.
D. Exposure to cigarette smoke.
E. Exposure to other irritants.
F. Allergens.
G. Chronic aspiration/gastro-oesophageal reflux disease (GERD).

Common Findings/Presenting Signs
A. The most common symptom initially is a dry, hacking, or raspy-sounding cough. The cough then loosens and becomes productive. Prolonged cough (>3 weeks) is common in cases of viral bronchitis.

Other Signs and Symptoms
A. Sore throat.
B. Rhinorrhoea or nasal congestion.
C. Rhonchi during respiration.
D. Low-grade fever.
E. Malaise.
F. Retrosternal pain during deep breathing and coughing.
G. Decreased/lack of appetite.

Subjective Data
A. Ask about the onset, duration, and course of symptoms.
B. Is the cough productive?
C. Is there substernal discomfort?
D. Is there malaise or fatigue?
E. Has the client had a fever?
F. Does the client smoke or is the client exposed to secondhand smoke? (smoking aggravates bronchitis).

G. A review of occupational history may be important in determining whether irritants play a role in symptoms.
H. Assess for symptoms of gastroesophageal reflux.

Physical Examination
Examinations of children may best be completed with the child sitting on the parent's lap.
A. Check temperature, pulse, and blood pressure. Always check a pulse oximeter.
B. Inspect:
  1. Observe overall appearance.
  2. Inspect eyes, ears, nose, and throat (pharynx may be injected).
  3. Transilluminate sinuses.
C. Palpate lymph nodes, maxillary, and frontal sinuses.
D. Auscultate all lung fields for adventitious breath sounds, i.e., crackles and wheezes.

Diagnostic Test
A. Consider chest x-ray to exclude pneumonia.

Differential Diagnoses
A. Pneumonia.
B. Upper respiratory infection.
C. Asthma.
D. Sinusitis.
E. Cystic fibrosis (CF).
F. Aspiration.
G. Respiratory tract anomalies.
H. Foreign-body aspiration.
I. Pneumonia.
J. Chronic obstructive pulmonary disease (COPD) and emphysema.
K. Paediatrics: Pertussis.

Plan
A. General interventions are primarily supportive and should ensure the client is adequately oxygenating.
  1. Discuss with the client to increase fluid intake.
  2. Suggest humidity and mist therapy.
  3. Avoid irritants, such as smoke.
▶ B. Client teaching: *Refer to Client Teaching Guide: Bronchitis, Acute.*
C. Pharmacological therapy:
  1. Acetaminophen or Ibuprofen for fever and malaise.
  2. There is fair evidence that antitussives can sometimes be useful for short-term symptomatic relief of cough. The evidence is poor for the use of over-the-counter cough and cold remedies.

  In 2016, the American College of Chest Physicians released clinical practice guidelines for the management of cough. Health-care providers should refrain from recommending cough suppressants and OTC cough medicines for young children because of associated morbidity and mortality. The American Academy of Pediatrics and Canadian Paediatric Society both remind consumers to avoid the use of OTC cough and cold products in children younger than four years.
  3. Among otherwise healthy individuals, antibiotics have **not demonstrated** benefit for acute bronchitis as the aetiology is usually viral.
  4. Can use Salbutamol for clients with wheeze, FEV_1 80%, or for clients experiencing bronchial hyper-responsiveness.

Follow-Up
A. Follow up if client does not improve in 48 hours.
B. Recommend yearly influenza vaccinations.

Consultation/Referral
A. In uncomplicated cases, mucus production decreases and cough disappears in seven to ten days.
B. Refer the client if you note respiratory distress or if he or she appears ill and you suspect pneumonia.

Individual Considerations
A. Paediatrics:
  1. Children who have repeated episodes of bronchitis or episodes that last more than four weeks despite treatment can be considered **chronic** although there is no consensus as to specific diagnostic criteria. This is complicated in children by the significant clinical overlay with asthma. As well as asthma, children with prolonged productive cough should be evaluated for asthma, CF, dyskinetic cilla, foreign body aspiration, protracted bacterial bronchitis, and exposure to airway irritants.
  2. Chronic bronchitis in adults are characterized by excessive mucus secretion with chronic or recurrent productive cough occurring three successive months a year for two consecutive years. Symptoms are often related to smoking and will be discussed under si»¿ection "Chronic Obstructive Pulmonary Disease."
  3. Instruct clients regarding the need for immunization against pertussis, diphtheria, and influenza, which reduces the risk of bronchitis.
  4. Children may attend school or day care without restrictions except during acute bronchitis with fever.
B. Geriatrics: Monitor elderly clients for complications such as pneumonia. The elderly have a greater morbidity and mortality rate.

Bibliography
American Academy of Pediatrics. (2016). *Cough and cold medicine—Not for children*. Retrieved from https://www.aap.org/en-us/about-the-aap/aap-press-room/aap-press-room-media-center/Pages/Cough-and-Cold-Medicine-Not-for-Children.aspx?nfstatus=401&nftoken=00000000-0000-0000-0000-000000000000&nfstatusdescription=ERROR:+No+local+token

Centers for Disease Control and Prevention. (2010). Infant deaths associated with cough and cold medications: Two states, 2005. *Morbidity and Mortality Weekly Report, 56*(1), 1–4. Retrieved from https://www.cdc.gov/mmwr/preview/mmwrhtml/mm5601a1.htm

Centers for Disease Control and Prevention. (n.d.). *Bronchitis (chest cold)*. Retrieved from https://www.cdc.gov/getsmart/antibiotic-use/url/bronchitis.html

Chang, A., Oppenheimer, J., Weinberger, M., Rubin, B. K., Grant, C. C., Weir, K., ... CHEST Expert Cough Panel. (2017). Management of children with chronic wet cough and protracted bacterial bronchitis. *Chest, 151*(4), 884–890. doi:10.1016/j.chest.2017.01.025

CNBC News. (2016, March 17). Cold remedies and kids: Study finds some parents ignoring warnings against use. Retrieved from http://www.cbc.ca/news/health/cold-medicines-children-1.3496164

File, T. M. (2016, February 24). Acute bronchitis in adults. *UpToDate*. Retrieved from http://www.uptodate.com/contents/acute-bronchitis-in-adults

Flaherty, E., & Resnick, R (Eds.). (2014). *Geriatric nursing review syllabus: A core curriculum in advanced practice geriatric nursing* (4th ed.). New York, NY: American Geriatrics Society.

▶ Client Teaching Guides are available at https://connect.springerpub.com/content/reference-book/978-0-8261-9498-5

Krawczyk, J., Gharahbaghian, L., & Rutkowski, A. (2006, July 14). Toxicity, cough and cold preparation. *emedicine*. Retrieved from http://emedicine.medscape.com/article/1010513-print

Prescriber's Letter. (2013, May). *Appropriate med use* (Vol. 29). Retrieved from http://prescribersletter.therapeuticresearch.com/pl/ArticleDD.aspx?cs=&s=PRL&pt=6&fpt=31&dd=290501&pb=PRL&searchid=55980185

Schwartzstein, R. M., & Adams, L. (2016). *Murray & Nadel's textbook of respiratory medicine* (6th ed.). Philadelphia, PA: Elsevier-Saunders.

Valentine, N. (2017). Respiratory disorders. In B. Richardson (Ed.), *Pediatric primary care: Practice guidelines for nurses* (3rd ed., pp. 143–158). Burlington, MA: Jones & Bartlett.

Weiner, D. L. (2014, November). Causes of acute respiratory distress in children. *UpToDate*. Retrieved from http://www.uptodate.com/contents/causes-of-acute-respiratory-distress-in-children

Zachary, K. C. (2015, December). Treatment of seasonal influenza in adults. *UpToDate*. Retrieved from http://www.uptodate.com/contents/treatment-of-seasonal-influenza-in-adults

Chronic Obstructive Pulmonary Disease (COPD)

Cheryl A. Glass, Melissa A. Hall, and Shelley Ann Walkerley

Definition

Chronic obstructive pulmonary disease (COPD) is progressive, chronic, expiratory airway obstruction. The relief of bronchoconstriction due to inflammation has some reversibility. Chronic bronchitis is a chronic productive cough lasting three months during two consecutive years, after all causes of chronic cough have been excluded. Emphysema is an abnormal, permanent enlargement (hyperinflation) and destruction of the alveoli air sacs, as well as the destruction of the elastic recoil. Many clients have both types of air-obstruction symptoms of chronic bronchitis and emphysematous destruction leading to COPD. Clients with asthma whose airflow obstruction is completely reversible are not considered to have COPD. When clients with asthma do not have complete reversal of airflow obstruction as confirmed by spirometry, their condition may be described as Asthma/COPD overlap (ACO). Figure 9.1

Irreversible airflow obstruction is a key factor in the client's disability. The goal of COPD management is to improve daily quality of life (QOL) and reduce the recurrence of exacerbations. Smoking cessation continues to be the most important therapeutic intervention for clients who smoke.

Management of COPD is based on an approach that matches treatment with symptom burden and risk of future exacerbations (Figure 9.1). This can be accomplished by including accurate assessment of dyspnea and activity limitations as well as tracking exacerbations. Dyspnea can be measured using the Modified Medical Research Council (mMRC) Questionnaire for Assessing the Severity of Breathlessness (www.thermh.org.au/sites/default/files/media/documents/mrc_dyspnoea_scale.pdf). Symptoms can be assessed using the COPD Assess test: www.catestonline.org/images/pdfs/CATest.pdf

Comorbidities commonly seen with COPD include hypertension; cardiac disorders, including atrial fibrillation and heart failure; diabetes/metabolic syndrome; gastrointestinal (GI) disorders; lung cancer; depression; and osteoporosis.

Incidence/Prevalence

A. Approximately 4.4% of the Canadian population aged >35 years has been diagnosed with COPD. It is still an underrecognized diagnosis although it is the third leading cause of death in Canada, and the number one reason for hospitalization. Prevalence is higher in women than men except for those aged ≥75 years.

Pathogenesis

It is estimated that 90% of cases of COPD are the result of prolonged exposure to tobacco smoke.

A. Chronic bronchitis leads to the narrowing of the airway caliber and increase in airway resistance. Mucous gland enlargement is the histologic hallmark of chronic bronchitis.

B. In emphysema, loss of the air sac's elastic recoil and alveoli destruction causes air limitation. Emphysema caused by smoking is the most severe in the upper lobes.

C. **Stages:** COPD severity is classified by symptoms and disability.

　1. **Mild:** Shortness of breath (SOB) when hurrying on the level or walking up a slight hill (mMCR 2). FEV_1 80% predicted, $FEV_1/FVC < 0.7$.

　2. **Moderate:** SOB from COPD causing the client to stop after walking approximately 100 metres (or after a few minutes) on the level (mMCR 3 to 4). 50% FEV_1 < 80% predicted, $FEV_1/FVC < 0.7$

　3. **Severe–Very Severe:** SOB from COPD resulting in the client being too breathless to leave

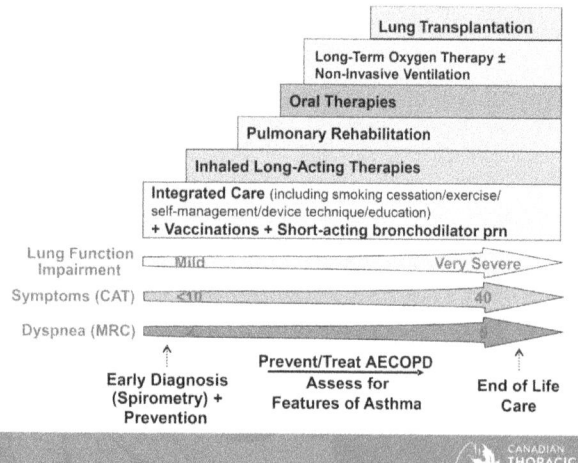

FIGURE 9.1 Comprehensive management of COPD.
COPD, chronic obstructive pulmonary disease.
Source: From the Canadian Thoracic Society, 2010, 2017, with permission.

the house, breathless when dressing or undressing (mMCR 5), or the presence of chronic respiratory failure or clinical signs of right heart failure. 30% FEV_1 < 50% predicted, FEV_1/FVC < 0.7 (severe); FEV_1 < 30% predicted, FEV_1/FVC < 0.7 (very severe).

Predisposing/Risk Factors
A. Cigarette smoking.
B. Occupational, environmental, or atmospheric pollutants.
   1. Dust.
   2. Chemical fumes.
   3. Second-hand smoke.
   4. Air pollution.
C. Genetic factor: Alpha 1-antitrypsin (AAT) deficiency.

Common Findings
A. Chronic cough and sputum, usually worse in morning.
B. Dyspnea with exertion, progressing to dyspnea at rest.
C. Wheezing.
D. Difficulty speaking or performing tasks.
E. Weight loss (decrease in fat-free mass).

Other Signs and Symptoms
A. Pursed-lip breathing: induces auto peeping and hence helps keep alveoli open.
B. Use of accessory muscles.
C. Tripod position.
D. Barrel chest (increased anteroposterior chest diameter).
E. Cyanosis (fingertips, tip of nose, around lips).
F. Tachypnoea.
G. Tachycardia.
H. Difficulty speaking or performing tasks.
I. Distended neck veins.
J. Abnormal, diminished, or absent lung sounds.
K. Mental status changes.
L. Anxiety and depression.
M. Pulmonary hypertension.
N. Cor pulmonale.
O. Left-sided heart failure.

Subjective Data
A. Ask the client about past respiratory problems and infections. Does he or she currently have fever, chills, or other signs of infection?
B. Ask about the onset of cough and characteristics of sputum (amount, colour, and presence of blood).
C. Determine tobacco (smoking) pack-year history (pack/day × number of years smoked).
D. Inquire about exposure to occupational or environmental irritants.
E. How far can the client walk before becoming breathless? Is there more breathlessness when the client walks on a slight incline? (See mMRC).
F. Does the client become breathless or tired when performing activities of daily living (ADLs)? (See mMRC).
G. Ask about insomnia, anxiety, restlessness, oedema, and weight change.
H. How many pillows does the client sleep on? Does he or she have to sleep in a recliner or sitting up?
I. Assess the client's ability to perform ADLs and instrumental ADLs (IADLs), including grooming and personal hygiene, performing chores around the house, shopping, cooking, and driving.
J. Ask about alcohol use.
K. Review all medications, including over-the-counter (OTC) and herbal products.
L. Review review pattern of symptom development; history of exacerbations or hospitalizations for resp conditions; social and family support available; review possibilities for reducing risk factors/smoking cessation.

Physical Examination
A. Record temperature (if indicated), blood pressure, pulse, respirations, and pulse oximetry. The respiratory rate increases proportionally to disease severity. Take height and weight to calculate the body mass index (BMI). **The client may have a fairly normal examination early in the disease.**
B. Inspect:
   1. Observe general appearance: Skin colour, affect, posture, gait, amount of respiratory effort when walking; note increased anteroposterior chest diameter.
   2. Examine sputum: Frothy pink signals pulmonary oedema. Haemoptysis as seen in tuberculosis (TB).
   3. Examine lips, fingertips, and nose for cyanosis. (Finger clubbing is not characteristic of COPD.)
   4. Observe the neck for distended veins and peripheral oedema (advanced disease).
   5. Check for pursed-lip breathing and use of accessory muscles.
C. Auscultate:
   1. Auscultate the heart.
   2. Auscultate the lungs for wheezes, crackles, decreased breath sounds, and prolonged forced expiratory rate.
   3. Assess for vocal fremitus (vibration) and egophony (increased resonance and high-pitched bleating quality). Air trapping causes air pockets that don't transmit sound well. Absent ventricular lung sounds are a distinctive characteristic of COPD.
   4. Auscultate the carotid arteries.
D. Percuss the chest for the presence of hyperresonance and for signs of consolidation.
E. Palpation:
   1. Palpate the neck for lymphadenopathy.
   2. Palpate the chest.
   3. Evaluate the abdomen for organomegaly.
   4. Evaluate pedal eodema.
F. Mental status: Assess for decreased level of consciousness.
G. Six-minute walking distance (6MWD) test to evaluate oxygen desaturation.
H. Further physical examinations are dependent on comorbidities.

Diagnostic Tests
A. **Spirometry is the gold standard for diagnosing COPD. Pulmonary function tests (PFTs) are used to diagnose, determine severity, and follow the disease progression of COPD. Spirometry should be performed before and after using a short-acting bronchodilator (SABA/SABD) to determine airway restriction reversibility:**
   1. FEV_1 is used as an index to airflow obstruction and evaluates the prognosis in emphysema.
   2. Forced vital capacity (FVC).
   3. FEV_1/FVC ratio <0.70 indicates COPD.
B. Chest radiograph (CXR; not required to diagnose COPD but rules out other diagnoses).
C. Complete blood count (CBC)—evaluate polycythaemia due to chronic hypoxia.
D. Sputum specimen for culture (generally not required).

E. If the client is younger than age 40 years or has a family history of early onset of emphysema, measure AAT levels. Clients with a family history of AAT deficiencies are at risk of lung damage early in life as AAT serves to protect lower lung tissue from damage by proteolytic enzymes.
F. Arterial blood gas (ABG).
G. ECG: Note sinus tachycardia, atrial arrhythmias.
H. Two-dimensional echocardiogram is used to evaluate secondary pulmonary hypertension.
I. Chest CT is an alternative imaging study for emphysema; however, it is not required as a diagnostic tool.
J. Perform a purified protein derivative (PPD) test if TB is suspected.
K. Brain natriuretic peptide (BNP) as a predictor of heart failure.
L. Theophylline level (if applicable).

Differential Diagnoses

A. Asthma.
B. Heart failure.
C. Bronchiectasis.
D. Pulmonary oedema.
E. TB.
F. AAT deficiency.
G. Pneumonia.
H. Pulmonary embolism.
I. CF.
J. Cancer.

Plan

A. General interventions:
  1. Educate and encourage active participation in the plan of care, including medication adherence.
  2. A smoking-cessation plan is an essential part of a comprehensive treatment plan. Develop a smoking-cessation plan; assess readiness to quit. Set a quit date; encourage a group smoking-cessation program. **Discuss smoking at every subsequent visit.** (*Refer to Client Teaching Guide: Nicotine Dependence*)
  3. Advise to stay away from secondhand smoke and limit exposure to other pulmonary irritants, including extreme temperature changes.
  4. Advise regular physical activity, include strength training, as tolerated.
  5. Educate and counsel clients regarding advance directives.
  6. Refer for pulmonary rehabilitation for all stages of COPD.
  7. The selection of inhalers is dependent on the client's age and ability to use the inhaler. Clients should be evaluated as to their coordination and inspiration abilities necessary to use inhalers; otherwise, aerosol medication via nebulizer is the best delivery method.
  8. Have clients bring in their medication/spacers to demonstrate correct use.
  9. Consider group visits for teaching sessions.
  10. Encourage influenza and pneumococcal vaccines to decrease the risk of lower respiratory tract infections.
B. Client teaching: *Refer to Client Teaching Guide: Chronic Obstructive Pulmonary Disease.*
C. Dietary management:
  1. About 25% of COPD clients are malnourished because of coexisting medical conditions, depression, and inability to shop for or prepare food.
  2. Suggest a low-carbohydrate diet. High-carbohydrate intake may increase respiratory work by increasing CO_2 production.
D. **Pharmacological therapy: Treatment guidelines are based on spirometry and functional capacity.**

Peak flow meters should not be used to diagnose or monitor COPD.

  1. **Mild: CAT <10, mMRC 1–2.** The client may be unaware that he or she has COPD. Give influenza vaccine and use short-acting beta 2 agonist bronchodilators (SABA/SABD) as needed. Add a long-acting muscarinic acid antagonist (LAMA) or long-acting $beta_2$-adrenergic agonist (LABA) as monotherapy if client becomes symptomatic.
  2. **Moderate: COPD Assessment Test (CAT) (greater than or equal to 10), mMRC 3–5 with infrequent acute exacerbations of COPD (AECOPD).** Give influenza vaccine. Treat with LAMA or LABA as monotherapy. Add combined LAMA/LABA if symptoms or disability persist. If progression continues step up to LAMA + ICS/LABA.
  3. **Severe or Very Severe: COPD Assessment Test (CAT) (greater than or equal to 10), mMRC 3–5 with frequent AECOPD or severe symptoms.** Give influenza vaccine. Treat with LAMA/LABA. Step up to LAMA + ICS/LABA if symptoms or disability persist. If progression continues add phosphodiesterase-4 inhibitor (PDE_4). A referral to a Respirologist is indicated at this stage. Add Home Oxygen if client meets criteria (each province has specific criteria bases on PaO_2 (partial pressure of oxygen), resting O_2 saturation and co-morbidities (Can Respir J. 2015 Nov-Dec; 22(6): 324–330. doi: [10.1155/2015/280604]) (Figure 9.2). See Table 9.1 *Medications for Asthma and COPD* for a list of available pharmacological products for the treatment of COPD.
  4. Utilization of a spacer/holding chamber for inhalers should be encouraged.
  5. Administer pneumonia vaccines for clients 65 years and older according to Canadian Immunization Guidelines recommendations and based on the individual client's vaccine history.
  6. Tobacco (smoking) cessation:
    a. Counselling using a variety of different formats is effective. Multiple sessions increase the chances of prolonged cessation.
    b. Nicotine replacement therapy (NRT) comes in a variety of delivery methods including patches, inhalers, lozenges, sprays and gum. All have been shown to be effective in managing cravings for tobacco. Vaping products have been recognized as smoking cessation aids but research is limited at this time.
    c. Use of an antidepressant such as bupropion has been shown to be effective for smoking cessation.
    d. Combined treatment with counselling and smoking cessation medication is more effective than either approach alone.
    e. Varenalcine is a partial agonist selective for alpha 4, beta 2-nicotinic acetylcholine receptors. NRT and antidepressants are contraindicated with varenicline.

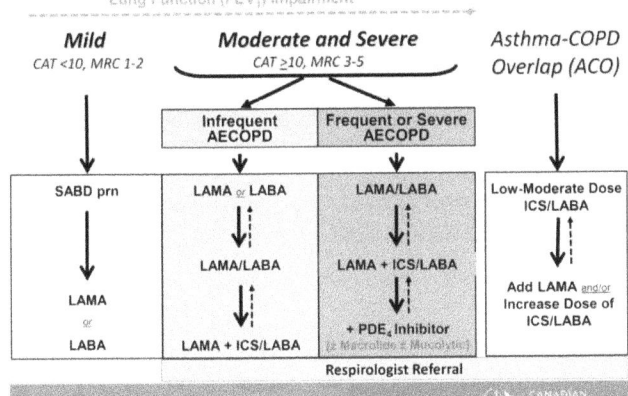

FIGURE 9.2 COPD pharmacology.
COPD, chronic obstructive pulmonary disease.
Source: From the Canadian Thoracic Society, 2010, 2017, with permission.

7. Antibiotics are recommended for clients with COPD experiencing acute exacerbations (AECOPD), with symptoms of increased dyspnea, increased sputum volume, and increased sputum purulence, changes in cough, fever, or other evidence of an infection such as an infiltrate on Chest x-ray. Commonly used antibiotics include cephalosporins, fluoroquinolones, macrolides, penicillins, sulfonamide combinations, and tetracyclines.
8. Mucolytic agents (N-acetylcysteine) may reduce AECOPD in people with moderate to severe COPD with at least two exacerbations over the previous two years.
9. Antitussives are not recommended.
10. Alpha-1 antitrypsin therapy may slow the progression of the disease.
11. **Cardioselective beta-blockers are not contraindicated in COPD. Cardioselective beta-blockers at low dosages do not cause bronchospasm. A noncardioselective beta-blocker or a cardioselective beta-blocker (B1 blocker) at higher dosages may contribute to bronchospasms.**

Follow-Up

A. For acute exacerbations, follow up same day or following day.
B. Follow up stable, chronic COPD every one to three months, depending on the client's needs.
C. Serial PFTs or spirometry may help guide therapy and offer prognostic information.
D. Monitor serum theophylline levels for clients taking theophylline. Theophylline has a narrow therapeutic window and the potential for toxicity. Adverse effects, including nausea and nervousness, are the most common. Other adverse effects include abdominal pain with cramps, anorexia, tremors, insomnia, cardiac arrhythmia, and seizures.
E. Re-evaluate clients on oxygen therapy one to three months after starting oxygen.
F. Evaluate for osteoporosis; bone mineral density is lower in COPD clients, and they are at risk for vertebral fractures.
G. Monitor the client's body weight.

Consultation/Referral

A. Consult with a specialist or MD if the client has acute respiratory decompensation, or severe cor pulmonale (distended neck veins, hepatomegaly, dependent peripheral oedema, ascites, and pleural effusion).
B. Refer the client for pulmonary rehabilitation, if available:
 1. Outpatient education for the client and family.
 2. Exercise training.
 3. Breathing retraining, that is, pursed-lip breathing, huff coughing.
 4. Correct administration of medications.
C. Refer to a registered dietitian (RD) for nutritional planning and support. RDs focus on the prevention and treatment of weight and muscle loss associated with COPD and other comorbidities.
D. Refer to a respirologist for consultation and management of clients with severe disease (including surgical interventions, lung transplantation).

Individual Considerations

A. Pregnancy:
 1. COPD is rare except in AAT deficiency (age of onset is generally aged >50 years).
 2. Monitor drug treatment for potential teratogenic effects.
B. Adults: Sexual dysfunction (secondary to disability) is common in clients with COPD; encourage other ways to display affection/intimacy.
C. Geriatrics:
 1. Presentation may be atypical.
 2. Clients should have annual flu vaccinations and pneumococcal vaccinations.
 3. Clients may not have the ability to use inhaler devices because of tremors, muscle weakness, poor hand–eye coordination, and/or poor memory.
 4. Theophylline is on the Beers list of drugs to use with caution in the geriatric population related to cardiovascular, renal, and hepatic concerns; insomnia; and peptic ulcers.
 5. Discuss the course of disease, living wills, advanced directives, and resuscitation status early, before a crisis occurs. Plan for End-of-Life Care.

Resources

The Global Initiative for Chronic Obstructive Lung Disease (GOLD) guidelines: www.goldcopd.org

Bibliography

Bartlett, J. G., & Sethi, S. (2016, March). Management of infection in exacerbations of chronic obstructive pulmonary disease.

UpToDate. Retrieved from http://www.uptodate.com/contents/management-of-infection-in-exacerbations-of-chronic-obstructive-pulmonary-disease?source=search_result&search=Management+of+infection+in+exacerbations+of+chronic+obstructive+pulmonary+disease&selectedTitle=1 150

Bourbeau, J., Bhutani, M., Hernandez, P., Marciniuk, D. C., Aaron, S. D., Balter, M., & Sin, D. D. (2017). CTS position statement: Pharmacotherapy in clients with COPD: An update. *Canadian Journal of Respiratory, Critical Care, and Sleep Medicine*, *1*(4), 222–241. doi:10.1080/24745332.2017.1395588

Centers for Disease Control and Prevention. (2015b, August 7). *Prevention and control of influenza with vaccines: Recommendations of the advisory committee on immunization practices, United States, 2015–16 Influenza season*. Retrieved from https://www.cdc.gov/mmwr/preview/mmwrhtml/mm6430a3.htm

Centers for Disease Control and Prevention. (2016a, February 10). *FastStats chronic obstructive pulmonary disease (COPD) includes: Chronic bronchitis and emphysema*. Retrieved from www.cdc.gov/nchs/fastats/copd.htm

Chronic Respiratory Disease Working Group of the Canadian Chronic Disease Surveillance System. (2018). *Report from the Canadian chronic disease surveillance system: Asthma and chronic obstructive pulmonary disease (COPD) in Canada*. Public Health Agency of Canada. https://www.canada.ca/en/public-health/services/publications/diseases-conditions/asthma-chronic-obstructive-pulmonary-disease-canada-2018.html

Ferguson, E., & Make, B. (2016, January 21). Management of stable chronic obstructive pulmonary disease. *UpToDate*. Retrieved from http://www.uptodate.com/contents/management-of-stable-chronic-obstructive-pulmonary-disease

Flaherty, E., & Resnick, R (Eds.). (2014). *Geriatric nursing review syllabus: A core curriculum in advanced practice geriatric nursing* (4th ed.). New York, NY: American Geriatrics Society.

GlaxoSmithKline. *COPD assessment test*. Retrieved from http://www.catestonline.org/US_residents.htm

Global Initiative for Chronic Obstructive Lung Disease. (2016). *Global strategy for the diagnosis, management, and prevention of COPD*. Retrieved from http://goldcopd.org/global-strategy-diagnosis-management-prevention-copd-2016

Han, M. K., Dransfield, M. T., & Martinez, F. J. (2015, September 29). Chronic obstructive pulmonary disease: Definition, clinical manifestations, diagnosis, and staging. *UpToDate*. Retrieved from http://www.uptodate.com/contents/chronic-obstructive-pulmonary-disease-definition-clinical-manifestations-diagnosis-and-staging

King-Han, M., Dransfield, M. T., & Martinez, F. J. (2015, September 29). Chronic obstructive pulmonary disease: Definition, clinical manifestations, diagnosis, and staging. *UpToDate*. Retrieved from http://www.uptodate.com/contents/chronic-obstructive-pulmonary-disease-definition-clinical-manifestations-diagnosis-and-staging

Long-Term Oxygen Treatment Trial Research Group, Albert, R. K., Au, D. H., Blackford, A. L., Casaburi, R., & Cooper, J. A., Jr. (2016). A randomized trial of long-term oxygen for COPD with moderate desaturation. *New England Journal of Medicine*, *375*(17), 1617–1627. doi:10.1056/NEJMoa1604344

Medscape Drug Reference. (n.d.). Theophylline oral. *Medscape*. Retrieved from http://www.medscape.com/druginfo/dosage?drugid=3591&drugname=Theophylline+Oral&monotype=default

Prescriber's Letter. (2013, May). *Appropriate med use* (Vol. 29). Retrieved from http://prescribersletter.therapeuticresearch.com/pl/ArticleDD.aspx?cs=&s=PRL&pt=6&fpt=31&dd=290501&pb=PRL&searchid=55980185

Public Health Agency of Canada. (2018). *Canadian immunization guide*. Ottawa, Ontario, Canada https://www.canada.ca/en/public-health/services/canadian-immunization-guide.html

Rains, S. G. (2013). Fifteen-to-eighteen-month visit. In B. Richardson (Ed.), *Pediatric primary care: Practice guidelines for nurses* (2nd ed., pp. 113–124). Burlington, MA: Jones & Bartlett.

Reilly, J. J., Silverman, E. K., & Shapiro, S. D. (2015). Chronic obstructive pulmonary disease. In D. L. Kasper, A. S. Fauci, S. L. Hauser, D. L. Longo, & J. L. Jameson (Eds.), *Harrison's principles of internal medicine* (19th ed.). New York, NY: McGraw-Hill.

Schwartzstein, R. M., & Adams, L. (2016). *Murray & Nadel's textbook of respiratory medicine* (6th ed.). Philadelphia, PA: Elsevier-Saunders.

Selby, P., Brosky, G., Cote-Meek, S., & Canadian Action Network for the Advancement, Dissemination and Adoption of Practice-informed Tobacco Treatment (CAN-ADAPTT). (2012). *Guideline for smoking cessation*.

Terry, E. G. (2017). Seven-to-ten-year visit (school age. In B. Richardson (Ed.), *Pediatric primary care: Practice guidelines for nurses* (3rd ed., pp. 143–158). Burlington, MA: Jones & Bartlett.

Valentine, N. (2017). Respiratory disorders. In B. Richardson (Ed.), *Pediatric primary care: Practice guidelines for nurses* (3rd ed., pp. 143–158). Burlington, MA: Jones & Bartlett.

Weiss, S. T. (2016, March 17). Chronic obstructive pulmonary disease: Risk factors and risk reduction. *UpToDate*. Retrieved from http://www.uptodate.com/contents/chronic-obstructive-pulmonary-disease-risk-factors-and-risk-reduction

Zachary, K. C. (2015, December). Treatment of seasonal influenza in adults. *UpToDate*. Retrieved from http://www.uptodate.com/contents/treatment-of-seasonal-influenza-in-adults

Common Cold/Upper Respiratory Infection

Cheryl A. Glass, Melissa A. Hall, and Shelley Ann Walkerley

Definition

A. The common cold is a self-limiting acute upper respiratory tract infection (URTI) resulting from viral infection of the upper respiratory tract. It is also called *acute nasopharyngitis*. URTI is characterized by mild coryzal symptoms, rhinorrhoea, nasal obstruction, and sneezing.

Incidence/Prevalence

A. URTIs are among the most frequent reasons for office visits. However, the true incidence is not known because clients treat themselves with over-the-counter (OTC) and home remedies, as well as seasonal and locational variability. Most children have six to eight colds a year; most adults have two to four.

Pathogenesis

A. About 50% of URTIs are caused by a rhinovirus (>100 antigenic serotypes). Other viral agents include coronaviruses (10%–20%), RSV, adenoviruses (5%), influenza viruses (10%–15%), and parainfluenza viruses. Incubation period is one to five days with viral shedding lasting up to two weeks.

B. Rhinoviral infections are chiefly limited to the upper respiratory tract and may cause otitis media and sinusitis.

Predisposing Factors

A. Exposure to airborne droplets.
B. Direct contact with virus by touching hands or skin of infected people, or by touching surfaces they touched, and then touching eyes or nose.
C. Very young or old ages.
D. Smoking.
E. Crowded conditions such as day-care centers and schools.

Common Findings

A. Low-grade fever.
B. Generalized malaise.
C. Nasal congestion and discharge (initially clear, then yellow and thick).
D. Sneezing.
E. Sore throat or hoarseness.
F. Watery and/or inflamed eyes.

Other Signs and Symptoms

A. Headache.
B. Cough.

Subjective Data

A. Elicit the onset, course, and duration of symptoms.
B. Inquire about colour and other characteristics of nasal discharge and sputum. **Purulent nasal discharge after 14 days may signal bacterial sinusitis.**

C. Inquire about other discomforts and exposure to people with similar symptoms.
D. Review allergens, seasonal problems, and exposure to irritants and smoke.
E. Review history for other respiratory problems, such as asthma, chronic bronchitis, and emphysema.

Physical Examination
A. Check temperature, pulse, respirations, and blood pressure. Carry out pulse oximetry if difficult respiratory symptoms are noted.
B. Inspect:
   1. Observe general appearance.
   2. Inspect eyes. **Note "allergic shiners," tearing, and eyelid swelling.**
   3. Observe ears, throat, and mouth. **Otitis media is indicated by redness and bulging of tympanic membrane, or by membrane perforation with drainage.**
   4. Inspect nose for nasal redness, swelling, polyps, enlarged turbinates, septal deviation, and foreign bodies:
      a. Group A *Streptococcus*: Tonsillar enlargement, exudate, petechiae.
      b. Allergies: "Cobblestoned" pharyngeal mucosa.
      c. Mononucleosis: About half of clients with mononucleosis develop tonsillar exudates, and about one-third develop petechiae at the junction of the hard and soft palates, which is highly suggestive of the disease.
   5. Transilluminate sinuses.
C. Auscultate:
   1. All lung fields.
   2. Heart.
D. Percuss:
   1. Sinus cavities and mastoid process of temporal bone to rule out otitis media.
   2. Chest for consolidation.
E. Palpate:
   1. Palpate face for sinus tenderness.
   2. Examine head and neck for enlarged, tender lymph nodes.

Diagnostic Tests
A. Diagnosis may be made from history and physical. Because common cold manifestations are so prevalent, an aggressive workup is rarely necessary.
B. Consider rapid strep test if the client has symptoms or was exposed to Group A *Streptococcus*. This is not a reliable test in young children.
C. Consider throat culture if negative rapid strep test and symptomatic, or if a young child.

Differential Diagnoses
A. Allergic rhinitis.
B. Foreign body.
C. Sinusitis.
D. Influenza.
E. Group A strep pharyngitis.
F. Otitis media.
G. Pneumonia.

Plan
A. General interventions:
   1. Controlled trials reveal minimal therapeutic benefits of vitamin C for the treatment and prevention of colds. Zinc lozenges can shorten the average duration of a cold but the appropriate dosage has not been determined and the product may cause nausea. Echinacea has not shown any clinically relevant differences in rates of infection or severity of symptoms when compared with placebo. Validation and standardization of herbal products have not been completed.
B. Client teaching: *Refer to Client Teaching Guide: Common Cold.*
C. Pharmacological therapy.
   1. **In 2016, the American College of Chest Physicians released clinical practice guidelines for the management of cough. Healthcare providers should refrain from recommending cough suppressants and OTC cough medicines for young children because of associated morbidity and mortality. The American Academy of Pediatrics and Canadian Paediatric Society both remind consumers to avoid the use of OTC cough and cold products in children younger than four years.**
   2. **Antibiotics are ineffective in treating viral infection.**
   3. Corticosteroids may actually increase viral replication and have no impact on cold symptoms.
   4. Topical decongestants for rhinorrhoea and nasal congestion:
      a. Adults and children aged 12 years:
         - Topical decongestants or topical anticholinergic.
      b. Children <12 years"
         - saline nasal drops.
         - consider clearing nasal congestion in infants with a rubber suction bulb; secretions can be softened with saline nose drops or a cool-mist humidifier.
   5. Oral decongestants are available such as pseudoephedrine:
      a. Adults and children aged 12 years: Oral decongestants or antihistamine/decongestant combinations. Pseudoephedrine is contraindicated in people with hypertension.
      b. Children aged 6–11 years: Oral antihistamine/decongestant combinations × 3 days.
      c. Children under six years: Oral OTC products are not recommended.
   6. Analgesics, such as acetaminophen and ibuprofen, may be used for symptomatic relief.
   7. Cough Preparations: Health Canada recommends no cough or cold drugs for children under six years due to questionable efficacy and potential harm. Generally, the evidence for the use of OTC products for acute cough is limited and lacks consensus.
      a. Dextromethorphan: Cough suppressant.
      b. Guiafisin: Decreases viscosity of secretions.
      c. Codeine: Cough suppressant. Contraindicated in persons aged <18 years. Dosage in OTC products is subtherapeutic in adults.
      d. Hydrocodone: Cough suppressant. Not approved for use in children aged 12 years and should be avoided in adolescents 12–18 years.
   8. Antihistamines: Colds have no allergic mechanism, so antihistamines are generally ineffective. The atropine-like drying effect from antihistamines may exacerbate congestion and obstruct the upper airway by impairing mucus flow. **Seniors:** use antihistamines with caution

in older adults due anticholinergic side effects and potential adverse effects including confusion, cognitive impairment, delirium, dry mouth, constipation, urinary retention, and sedation. Diphenhydramine may be appropriate in acute treatment of severe allergic reactions. (CPhA, RxTx, 2018)

Follow-Up
A. None is recommended unless symptoms persist longer than seven days from onset.
B. Parents should return to the office if their child's fever exceeds 102°F, if respiratory symptoms increase, or if symptoms do not resolve in 10 to 14 days.

Consultation/Referral
A. Consider consultation with a specialist if symptoms persist or progress over time despite treatment.
B. Refer the client to the ED or urgent consultation with an otolaryngologist if tonsillary abscess is suspected.

Individual Considerations
A. Paediatrics.
 1. Oral decongestants are not recommended for children younger than six years of age.
 2. The most common reported calls reported to poison control centers that involve OTC medications concerning the ingestion of acetaminophen and cough and cold preparations:
  a. Accidental paediatric toxic ingestion is reported in children younger than six years, and intentional toxic ingestion is more common in adolescents aged 13 to 19 years.
  b. Adolescents have used dextromethorphan as a recreational drug.
B. Geriatrics:
 1. Use of antihistamines with anticholinergic properties may cause side effects of confusion and delirium as listed earlier, along with increased rates of hospitalization.

Bibliography
American Academy of Pediatrics. (2016). *Cough and cold medicine—Not for children*. Retrieved from https://www.aap.org/en-us/about-the-aap/aap-press-room/aap-press-room-media-center/Pages/Cough-and-Cold-Medicine-Not-for-Children.aspx?nfstatus=401&nftoken=00000000-0000-0000-0000-000000000000&nfstatusdescription=ERROR:+No+local+token

Centers for Disease Control and Prevention. (2009, September 11). *For parents: Young children and adverse drug events*. Retrieved from https://www.cdc.gov/MedicationSafety/parents_childrenAdverseDrugEvents.html

Dolin, R. (2015). Common viral respiratory infections. In D. L. Kasper, S. L. Hauser, J. L. Jameson, A. S. Fauci, D. L. Longo, & J. Loscalzo (Eds.), *Harrison's principles of internal medicine* (19th ed.). New York, NY: McGraw-Hill.

MPR: Nurse Practitioner's Edition. (2016, Spring). New York, NY: Haymarket Media.

Munoz, F. M., & Flomenberg, P. (2015, June). Diagnosis, treatment, and prevention of adenovirus infection. *UpToDate*. Retrieved from http://www.uptodate.com

Pappas, D. E. (2015, August 4). *Client information: The common cold in children (Beyond the Basics)*. Retrieved from http://www.uptodate.com/contents/the-common-cold-in-children-beyond-the-basics

Prescriber's Letter. (2013, May). *Appropriate med use* (Vol. 29). Retrieved from http://prescribersletter.therapeuticresearch.com/pl/ArticleDD.aspx?cs=&s=PRL&pt=6&fpt=31&dd=290501&pb=PRL&searchid=55980185

Prescriber's Letter. (2016b, March). *Poison prevention* (Vol. 30). Retrieved from http://prescribersletter.therapeuticresearch.com/pl/ArticleDD.aspx?nidchk=1&cs=&s=PRL&pt=6&fpt=31&dd=300305&pb=PRL&searchid=55978305

Schwartzstein, R. M., & Adams, L. (2016). *Murray & Nadel's textbook of respiratory medicine* (6th ed.). Philadelphia, PA: Elsevier-Saunders.

Science, M., Johnstone, J., Roth, D., Guyatt, G., & Loeb, M. (2012). Zinc for the treatment of the common cold: A systematic review and meta-analysis of randomized controlled trials. *CMAJ: Canadian Medical Association Journal, 184*(10), E551–E561. doi:10.1503/cmaj.111990

Valentine, N. (2017). Respiratory disorders. In B. Richardson (Ed.), *Pediatric primary care: Practice guidelines for nurses* (3rd ed., pp. 143–158). Burlington, MA: Jones & Bartlett.

Cough

Cheryl A. Glass, Melissa A. Hall, and Shelley Ann Walkerley

Definition
A. Coughing is a mechanism that clears the airway of secretions and inhaled particles. The act of coughing has the potential to traumatize the upper airway (e.g., vocal cords). A chronic cough is one that lasts longer than eight weeks.
B. Because coughing can be an affective behavior (psychogenic), psychological issues must be considered as a cause or effect of coughing.

Incidence/Prevalence
A. Data on the incidence of coughing are not available. However, most healthy people do not cough, and the main reason for coughing is airway clearance. A chronic cough is a common presenting symptom in adults who seek medical treatment in an ambulatory setting.
B. Pertussis (whooping cough) affects infants and young children; however, the incidence is increasing in adults secondary to the lack of booster vaccination.

Pathogenesis
A. Stimulation of mucosal neural receptors in the nasopharynx, ears, larynx, trachea, and bronchi can produce a cough, as can acute inflammation and/or irritation of the respiratory tract. Cough is a reflex response that is mediated by the medulla but is subject to voluntary control. There is clear evidence that vagal afferent nerves regulate involuntary coughing.
B. Pertussis is caused by the bacterium *Bordetella pertussis*.
C. The **pathogenic triad of chronic cough** responsible for the majority of cases of chronic cough is as follows:
 1. Upper airway cough syndrome (UACS), previously referred to as postnasal drip syndrome.
 2. Asthma.
 3. Generally known as gastroesophageal reflux disease (GERD) in Canada.

Predisposing Factors
A. Pharyngeal irritants.
B. Foreign-body aspiration.
C. Tuberculosis (TB; persons in prisons and nursing homes and immigrants from areas where TB is endemic).
D. Psychogenic factors (more common in children and those with emotional stress).
E. Mediastinal or pulmonary masses.
F. Congestive heart failure (CHF).
G. Cystic fibrosis (CF).
H. Congenital malformations.
I. Viral bronchitis.
J. Asthma (sole symptom in 28%).
K. Mycoplasma infection.
L. UACS, previously referred to as postnasal drip.
M. Chronic sinusitis.
N. Allergic rhinitis.
O. Environmental irritants.
P. GERD.

Q. Chronic bronchitis.
R. Pulmonary oedema.
S. Medications, including angiotensin-converting enzyme (ACE) inhibitors.
T. Impacted cerumen and external otitis.
U. Nonasthmatic eosinohilic bronchitis.

Common Findings
A. Common complaint is a cough that interferes with activities of daily living (ADLs) and sleeping, leading to a decrease in a client's quality of life (QOL).
B. The cough associated with pertussis is uncontrollable and violent. Following coughing, a "whooping" sound follows with a deep breath.

Other Signs and Symptoms
A. Fatigue.
B. Rhinitis.
C. Epistaxis.
D. Tickle in throat.
E. Pharyngitis.
F. Night sweats.
G. Dyspnoea.
H. Fever.
I. Sputum production.
J. Hoarseness.
K. Postnasal drip.

Subjective Data
A. Elicit information about the onset, duration, and course of the cough. Was the onset recent or gradual? Does the cough occur at night? **Nocturnal cough may be caused by GERD, chronic interstitial pulmonary oedema and may signal left-sided heart failure. Cough caused by asthma can be worse at night. Morning cough with sputum suggests bronchitis.**
B. Inquire about the cough's characteristics. For example, is it productive, dry, bronchospastic, brassy, wheezy, strong, or weak? If it is productive, is it bloody or mucoid? Note the colour, consistency, odour, and amount of sputum or mucus.
C. Inquire whether the cough is associated with eating and choking episodes. Wheezing or stridor with coughing may indicate a foreign body or aspiration.
D. Ask whether the cough is associated with postnasal drip, which produces a chronic cough, clear sputum, oedematous nasal mucosa, and a "cobblestoned" pharyngeal mucosa.
E. Find out whether the cough is associated with heartburn or a sour taste in the mouth, indicating GERD.
F. Ask about precipitating factors, such as exercise, cold air, or laughing. Also ask about alleviating factors. **Cough from asthma can be triggered or exacerbated by exposure to environmental irritants, allergens, cold, or exercise.**
G. Ask about current and previous work. Is the client exposed to occupational and environmental irritants, such as dust, fumes, or gases? If so, what are the type, level, and duration of exposures?
H. Ask about family history of respiratory illness, such as CF or asthma.
I. Is the client a smoker? If so, how much does he or she smoke, and how long has he or she smoked? Is he or she exposed to second-hand smoke? How much of the day? **Smoking is the main cause of chronic cough.**
J. Find out the date of the client's last tuberculin skin test. Ask about recent exposure to TB, travel to endemic areas, or occupational exposures.
K. Inquire about any exposure to influenza.
L. Does the client have a history of heart problems?
M. Does the client have a history of respiratory problems or other medical problems? Chronic bronchitis is a major cause of chronic cough and sputum production. Cough may also be an early sign of lung cancer; in late stages, cough occurs along with weight loss, anorexia, and dyspnoea.
N. Review medications such as ACE inhibitors. Cough related to ACE inhibitors can appear within hours of initiation of the drug or may takes weeks or months to appear. Generally, cough will subside within one to four weeks of discontinuing the drug.
O. Common causes of chronic cough in the elderly include postnasal drip, asthma, and gastro-oesophageal reflux (GERD).

Physical Examination
A. Measure and record vital signs.
B. Inspect:
   1. Observe general appearance for cyanosis, difficulty breathing, use of axillary muscles, and finger clubbing.
   2. Examine ears, nose, and throat.
   3. Conduct an abdominal exam if GERD is suspected.
C. Auscultate heart and lungs.
D. Percuss:
   1. Sinus cavities and mastoid process.
   2. Chest and lungs for consolidation.
E. Palpate:
   1. Palpate face for sinus tenderness.
   2. Examine head and neck for lymph nodes, masses, and jugular vein distension (JVD).

Diagnostic Tests
Testing can be held to a minimum by careful review of history and physical examination. Children with chronic cough should undergo, at a minimum, a chest x-ray and spirometry (if age appropriate and considering safety issues).
A. White blood cell (WBC) count if infection suspected.
B. HIV test if indicated.
C. Sputum for eosinophils, Gram's stain, and/or culture.
D. Mantoux test if indicated.
E. Chest radiograph (CXR).
F. Sweat chloride test to rule out CF.
G. Pulmonary function testing/spirometry.
H. Methacholine challenge to rule out asthma.
I. Esophageal pH monitoring to rule out GERD.
J. CT scan if indicated (may require consultation or referral).

Differential Diagnoses
A. Environmental irritants:
   1. Cigarette, cigar, or pipe smoking.
   2. Pollutants (wood smoke, smog, burning leaves, etc.).
   3. Dust.
   4. Lack of humidity.
B. Lower respiratory tract problems.
   1. Lung cancer.
   2. Asthma.
   3. Chronic obstructive lung disease (includes bronchitis).
   4. Interstitial lung disease.
   5. CHF.
   6. Pneumonitis.
   7. Bronchiectasis.
C. Upper respiratory tract problems.
   1. Chronic rhinitis.

2. Chronic sinusitis.
3. Disease of external auditory canal.
4. Pharyngitis.
D. Medication-induced cough from ACE inhibitors.
E. Extrinsic compression lesions:
   1. Adenopathy.
   2. Malignancy.
   3. Aortic aneurysm.
F. Psychogenic factors, more common in children and those with emotional stress.
G. Gastrointestinal (GI) problems such as reflux oesophagitis.
H. Genetic problems such as CF.

Plan

A. General intervention:
   1. If sputum is purulent, obtain a sample for examination if indicated.
   2. Clients with chronic obstructive pulmonary disease (COPD) and CF should be taught huffing as an adjunct to other methods of sputum clearance.
▶ B. Client teaching: *Refer to Client Teaching Guide: Cough.*
C. Pharmacological therapy:
   1. **The American College of Chest Physicians and Canadian Paediatric Society have both published clinical practice guidelines for the management of cough. Health-care providers should refrain from recommending cough suppressants and over-the-counter (OTC) cough medicines for young children because of associated morbidity and mortality.**
   2. Antibiotics should not be prescribed for cough unless a bacterial infection is suspected.
   3. Therapy depends on various acute inflammatory and chronic irritating processes and on the cause of the cough. Refer to applicable sections of this chapter, such as "Asthma," "Tuberculosis," and see Chapter 11, "Gastrointestinal Guidelines."

Follow-Up

A. The client with a normal CXR and no risk factors for lung cancer (e.g., smoking or occupational exposure) can be followed expectantly without further testing.
B. In clients whose cough resolves after the cessation of ACE inhibitors consider switching to an ARB (Angiotensin Receptor Blocker).
C. See applicable sections for specific diagnoses.
D. Pertussis vaccination is available for infants, children, preteens, adults, and the elderly. Pertussis cases are required to be reported to the local health department.

Consultation/Referral

A. Consider consultation or referral if symptoms persist despite treatment.
B. When a cough lasts more than two weeks without another apparent cause and it is accompanied by paroxysms of coughing, post-tussive vomiting, and/or an inspiratory whooping sound, the diagnosis of a *Bordetella pertussis* infection should be made unless another diagnosis is proven.

Individual Considerations

A. Pregnancy: Cough may be an early symptom of pulmonary oedema. Watch intrapartum clients for signs of oedema.

B. Paediatrics:
   1. The most common reported calls to poison control centers involve the ingestion of acetaminophen and cough and cold preparations. Accidental paediatric toxic ingestion is reported in children younger than six years, and intentional toxic ingestion is more common in adolescents aged 13 to 19 years. Adolescents have used dextromethorphan as a recreational drug.
   2. Children with chronic productive purulent cough should always be investigated to document the presence or absence of bronchiectasis and to identify underlying and treatable causes such as CF and immune deficiency.
C. Geriatrics.
   1. Aspiration should be considered in the elderly with chronic cough, as well as heart failure, laryngeal dysfunction, bronchiectasis, or tumours of the central airway.

Bibliography

Centers for Disease Control and Prevention. (2015c, August 31). Pertussis (whooping cough) surveillance & reporting. Retrieved from www.cdc.gov/pertussis/surv-reporting.html

Flaherty, E., & Resnick, R (Eds.). (2014). Geriatric nursing review syllabus: A core curriculum in advanced practice geriatric nursing (4th ed.). New York, NY: American Geriatrics Society

Gibson, P., Wang, G., McGarvey, L., Vertigan, A. E., Altman, K. W., Birring, S. S., & Chest Expert Cough Panel. (2016). Treatment of unexplained chronic cough: CHEST guideline and Expert Panel report. *Chest, 149*, 27–44. doi:10.1378/chest.15-1496

Kritek, P. A., & Fanta, C. H. (2015). Cough and hemoptysis. In D. L. Kasper, A. S. Fauci, S. L. Hauser, D. L. Longo, J. L. Jameson, & J. Loscalzo (Eds.), *Harrison's principles of internal medicine* (19th ed.). New York, NY: McGraw-Hill.

Prescriber's Letter. (2013, May). *Appropriate med use* (Vol. 29). Retrieved from http://prescribersletter.therapeuticresearch.com/pl/ArticleDD.aspx?cs=&s=PRL&pt=6&fpt=31&dd=290501&pb=PRL&searchid=55980185

Prescriber's Letter. (2015b, September). *Infectious disease* (Vol. 22). Retrieved from http://prescribersletter.therapeuticresearch.com/pl/ArticleDD.aspx?cs=&s=PRL&pt=6&fpt=31&dd=310922&pb=PRL&searchid=55978639

Public Health Agency of Canada. (2018). *Canadian immunization guide.* Ottawa, Ontario, Canada https://www.canada.ca/en/public-health/services/canadian-immunization-guide.html

Rains, S. G. (2013). Fifteen-to-eighteen-month visit. In B. Richardson (Ed.), *Pediatric primary care: Practice guidelines for nurses* (2nd ed., pp. 113–124). Burlington, MA: Jones & Bartlett.

Schwartzstein, R. M., & Adams, L. (2016). *Murray & Nadel's textbook of respiratory medicine* (6th ed.). Philadelphia, PA: Elsevier-Saunders.

Terry, E. G. (2017). Seven-to-ten-year visit (school age. In B. Richardson (Ed.), *Pediatric primary care: Practice guidelines for nurses* (3rd ed., pp. 143–158). Burlington, MA: Jones & Bartlett.

Valentine, N. (2017). Respiratory disorders. In B. Richardson (Ed.), *Pediatric primary care: Practice guidelines for nurses* (3rd ed., pp. 143–158). Burlington, MA: Jones & Bartlett.

Zachary, K. C. (2015, December). Treatment of seasonal influenza in adults. *UpToDate.* Retrieved from http://www.uptodate.com/contents/treatment-of-seasonal-influenza-in-adults

Croup, Viral

Cheryl A. Glass, Melissa A. Hall, and Shelley Ann Walkerley

Definition

A. Viral croup is an acute inflammatory disease of the larynx, also called *laryngotracheobronchitis.* Croup is the most common cause of stridor in febrile children. The uncomplicated disease usually wanes in three to five days but may persist up to ten days. Croup is most often self-limited, occasionally severe but rarely fatal. Lethargy, cyanosis, and decreasing retractions are indications of impending respiratory failure.
B. Inspiratory stridor suggests a laryngeal obstruction.

▶ Client Teaching Guides are available at https://connect.springerpub.com/content/reference-book/978-0-8261-9498-5

C. Poiseuille's equation states that flow (air, fluid) is proportional to the radius of the chamber to the fourth power and inversely to the length. Realizing that paediatric airways are relatively small compared to adult counterparts, a twofold decrease in airway radius decreases the airflow by 16-fold. Therefore, airway resistance is exquisitely sensitive to changes in radius in the paediatric population.
D. Expiratory stridor suggests tracheobronchial obstruction.
E. Spasmodic croup may be a noninfectious variant with symptoms always occurring at night and has the hallmark of reoccurring in children. Although viral illness may trigger this variant, the reaction may be allergic.

Incidence/Prevalence
A. The most common form of acute upper airway obstruction, croup generally affects children aged three months to six years. Croup has a peak incidence during the second year of life. It is most prevalent in younger children in fall and early winter.

Pathogenesis
A. Croup is most commonly caused by a virus. Parainfluenza viruses types 1 and 3 cause the majority of cases of croup. The initial port of entry is the nose and nasopharynx. Other viral causes include enterovirus and rhinovirus. Influenza A and B, respiratory syncytial virus (RSV), adenovirus, coronavirus, herpes simplex virus (HSV), and measles are less common causes. In a small number of cases, croup may be caused by *Mycoplasma pneumoniae*. Inflammation usually occurs in the entire airway, and oedema formation in the subglottic space accounts for the predominant signs of upper airway obstruction.

Predisposing Factors
A. Upper respiratory tract infection.
B. Male-to-female ratio of 1.4:1.
C. Incidence is highest in children aged six months to three years (mean onset: 18 months).
D. Hyperactive airway.
E. Anatomic narrowing of the airway.
F. Acquired airway narrowing (from intubation, gastro-oesophageal reflux disease [GERD] scarring, or human papillomavirus [HPV] papillomas).

Common Findings
A. Hoarseness.
B. Cough progressing to a seal-like barking cough.
C. Stridor, especially during sleep.
D. Fever, usually absent or low grade, but may be high.
E. Runny nose.

Subjective Data
A. Determine the onset, duration, and course of illness.
B. Has the child been exposed to respiratory illness?
C. Is the child coughing? Having trouble breathing?
D. Has the child had fever, nausea, vomiting, or diarrhoea?
E. Are immunizations up to date?

Physical Examination
Have the child sit upright in a parent's lap to perform the physical examination. Persistent crying increases oxygen demand and respiratory muscle fatigue.
A. Record temperature, pulse, respirations, oxygen saturation, and blood pressure.

TABLE 9.2   Westley Scoring for Croup

Symptom	Scoring
Inspiratory stridor	No inspiratory stridor = 0 points
	Stridor upon agitation = 1 point
	Stridor at rest = 2 points
Retractions	Mild = 1 point
	Moderate = 2 points
	Severe = 3 points
Air entry	Normal = 1 point
	Mild decrease = 1 point
	Marked decrease = 2 points
Cyanosis	None = 0 points
	Cyanosis upon agitation = 4 points
	Cyanosis at rest = 5 points
Level of consciousness	Normal = 0 points
	Disoriented = 5 points

Mild disease = A score of <2 points. Occasional barking coughs, no stridor at rest, and mild to no suprasternal or subcostal retraction.
Moderate disease = A score of 3 to 7 points. Frequent cough, audible stridor at rest, visible retractions, but little distress or agitation.
Severe disease = A score of ≥8. Frequent cough, prominent inspiratory (occasional expiratory) stridor, obvious retraction, decreased air entry on auscultation, and significant distress and agitation.
Source: Adapted from Westley, C. R., Cotton, E. K., & Brooks, J. G. (1978). Nebulized racemic epinephrine by IPPB for the treatment of croup: A double-blind study. *Am J Dis Child*, 132, 484.

B. Inspect:
  1. Observe overall appearance, noting respiratory pattern, retractions, nasal flaring, and air hunger. Children often sound terrible but do not look very ill.
  2. Check nail beds and lips for cyanosis (ominous sign).
  3. Assess skin and mucous membranes for signs of dehydration.
  4. Observe for drooling or difficulty swallowing.
  5. Inspect throat for foreign body. This needs to be done with great care and is best managed in the ER by experienced practitioners.
  6. Inspect eyes, ears, nose, and throat for infection.
C. Auscultate:
  1. Auscultate heart. Tachycardia is out of proportion to fever.
  2. Auscultate lungs for unequal breath sounds (signals foreign-body aspiration). **Stridor is an audible harsh, high-pitched musical sound that may be noted on inspiration or heard during both inspiration and expiration.** Stridor is audible without a stethoscope.
  3. The Westley score is a way to quantify the severity of respiratory compromise. The severity of croup is evaluated by assessing inspiratory stridor, air entry, retractions, cyanosis, and level of consciousness (see Table 9.2).
D. Percuss chest.
E. Palpate neck to evaluate lymph nodes.
F. Neurologic examination: Assess level of alertness.

Diagnostic Tests
The diagnosis of croup is largely clinical, based on the presenting history and physical examination findings.
A. Pulse oximetry assesses respiratory status.

B. Laboratory testing is usually not needed for croup in a well-hydrated client. However, a complete blood count (CBC) may be indicated.
C. Imaging is not required in mild cases with a typical history that responds appropriately to treatment.
D. Chest radiograph (CXR) may show the "steeple or pencil sign." Not generally required for diagnosis.
E. Anteroposterior (AP) soft tissue neck radiography may show subglottic narrowing.
F. Bronchoscopy or laryngoscopy may be required in unusual circumstances or if a foreign body is present in the airway.
G. Arterial blood gases (ABGs) are unnecessary as they do not indicate hypoxia or hypercarbia unless respiratory fatigue is present.

Differential Diagnoses
A. Bacterial croup.
B. Epiglottitis.
C. Spasmodic croup.
D. Membranous croup.
E. Bacterial tracheitis.
F. Retropharyngeal abscess.
G. Diphtheria.
H. Foreign bodies (gastrointestinal [GI] or trachea).
I. Respiratory syncytial virus (RSV).
J. Measles.
K. Varicella.
L. Influenza A or B.
M. Mechanical trauma or lesions.

Plan
A. General interventions:
  1. Treatment is supportive for clients without stridor at rest.
  2. Stress rest and minimal activity.
  3. Cool-mist therapy has not been shown to be clinically effective.
  4. Hot steam should be avoided due to the potential of scalding.
▶ B. Client teaching: *Refer to Client Teaching Guide: Croup, Viral.*
C. Dietary management: Give plenty of fluids.
D. Medical/surgical management: If pulse oximetry shows desaturation, administer oxygen and monitor carefully.
E. Pharmacological therapy.
  1. Antibiotics are not indicated for the treatment of croup.
  2. Acetaminophen.
  3. In moderate to severe cases requiring hospitalization: Nebulized racemic epinephrine solution may relieve airway obstruction up to two hours. Treatment may be repeated three times.
  4. Corticosteroids are the first line pharmacological treatment for croup. They are used to decrease subglottic oedema by suppressing the local inflammatory process. Corticosteroids should not be given to children with untreated tuberculosis (TB).
    a. Dexamethasone is the first-line treatment.
    b. Budesonide (Pulmicort Respules inhalation suspension) has been shown to be equivalent to oral dexamethasone.
    c. Observation for three to four hours is recommended following the initial treatment.

Follow-Up
A. Call the parent in 12 to 24 hours to evaluate client status.

Consultation/Referral
A. Consultation with an otolaryngologist and anesthetist before rapid sequence induction may be necessary if the client is exhibiting rapid deterioration.
B. Refer the client to the ED or a specialist if the child is severely ill with respiratory distress or dehydration.
C. Clients with stridor at rest should be admitted to the hospital.

Individual Considerations
A. Paediatrics.
  1. Most children improve within a few days.
  2. Virus is most contagious during the first few days of fever.
  3. Children may return to day care or school when temperature is normal and they feel better, even if cough lingers.
  4. Children older than five years of age with recurrent croup should be referred to an otolaryngologist for evaluation.

Bibliography
Dolin, R. (2015). Common viral respiratory infections. In D. L. Kasper, S. L. Hauser, J. L. Jameson, A. S. Fauci, D. L. Longo, & J. Loscalzo (Eds.), *Harrison's principles of internal medicine* (19th ed.). New York, NY: McGraw-Hill.
Munoz, F. M., & Flomenberg, P. (2015, June). Diagnosis, treatment, and prevention of adenovirus infection. *UpToDate.* Retrieved from http://www.uptodate.com
Prescriber's Letter. (2013, May). *Appropriate med use* (Vol. 29). Retrieved from http://prescribersletter.therapeuticresearch.com/pl/ArticleDD.aspx?cs=&s=PRL&pt=6&fpt=31&dd=290501&pb=PRL&searchid=55980185
Schwartzstein, R. M., & Adams, L. (2016). *Murray & Nadel's textbook of respiratory medicine* (6th ed.). Philadelphia, PA: Elsevier-Saunders.
Valentine, N. (2017). Respiratory disorders. In B. Richardson (Ed.), *Pediatric primary care: Practice guidelines for nurses* (3rd ed., pp. 143–158). Burlington, MA: Jones & Bartlett.
Woods, C. R. (2015a, April). Croup: Approach to management. *UpToDate.* Retrieved from http://www.uptodate.com/contents/croup-approach-to-management
Woods, C. R. (2015b, December). Croup: Clinical features, evaluation, and diagnosis. *UpToDate.* Retrieved from http://www.uptodate.com/contents/croup-clinical-features-evaluation-and-diagnosis
Weiner, D. L. (2014, November). Causes of acute respiratory distress in children. *UpToDate.* Retrieved from http://www.uptodate.com/contents/causes-of-acute-respiratory-distress-in-children

Obstructive Sleep Apnoea (OSA)

Cheryl A. Glass, Melissa A. Hall, and Shelley Ann Walkerley

Definition
Obstructive sleep apnoea (OSA) is the periodic reduction (hypopnoea) or cessation (apnoea) of breathing due to a narrowing or occlusion of the upper airway during sleep. OSA has been linked to traffic accidents, cardiac diseases, stroke, diabetes, and visceral obesity. OSA is also associated with nocturnal cardiac arrhythmias and chronic and acute cardiac events, and is a risk factor for strokes. OSA worsens in the supine sleeping position. The following are diagnostic criteria for OSA if either of these two conditions exists:
A. The presence of ≥15 apnoeas, hypopnoeas, or respiratory effort-related arousals per hour of sleep in an asymptomatic

▶ Client Teaching Guides are available at https://connect.springerpub.com/content/reference-book/978-0-8261-9498-5

client. More than 75% of the apnoeas and hypopnoeas must be obstructive (the differentiation between obstructive hypopnoeas and apnoeas is not considered necessary in the Canadian guidelines).
B. The presence of five or more obstructive apnoeas, obstructive hypopnoeas, or respiratory effort-related arousals per hour of sleep in a client with symptoms or signs of disturbed sleep. More than 75% of the apnoeas or hypopnoeas must be obstructive (the differentiation between obstructive hypopnoeas and apnoeas is not considered necessary in the Canadian guidelines).

Incidence/Prevalence
A. The incidence of OSA in the morbidly obese population is between 38% and 88%. Otherwise, incidence in males is between 20% and 30% and females between 10% and 15%.
B. In nonobese and otherwise healthy children younger than eight years, incidence is between 1% and 3%. Obesity adds a fourfold added risk for disordered breathing.
C. Most children with OSA are aged two to ten years, coinciding with adenotonsillar lymphatic tissue growth. (Surgical removal of enlarged tonsils and adenoids usually results in a complete cure.)
D. Most cases in adults are undiagnosed.

Pathogenesis
A. Increased tissue thickness of the structures of the tongue and soft tissues in the pharyngeal cavity, which decreases the passageway for air to the trachea, is thought to be the mechanism of OSA. During the night, the muscles of the oropharynx relax, which result in the relative obstruction of the airway. Obesity and hypertrophy of tonsils and/or adenoids account for most cases of OSA in children. OSA is associated with poor neurocognitive performance and increased risk for mortality, including cardiovascular disease.

Predisposing Factors
A. Obesity.
B. Increased neck circumference.
C. Age: prevalence increases up to age 65 years at which time it appears to plateau.
D. Gender: Males.
E. Postmenopause.
F. Hypothyroidism.
G. Tonsillar hypertrophy.
H. Alcohol.
I. Craniofacial abnormalities.
J. Medications:
  1. Benzodiazepines.
  2. Antipsychotics.
  3. Opioid analgesics.
  4. Beta-blockers.
  5. Barbiturates.
  6. Antihistamines.
  7. Sedative antidepressants.
K. Allergic rhinitis.
L. Genetic conditions (e.g., Down syndrome, Pierre Robin anomalies, Marfan syndrome, etc.).
M. Ethnicity (e.g., Black, Asian, Hispanic).
N. Acromegaly.
O. Family history.
P. Diabetes.
Q. Hypertension.

Common Findings
A. Daytime sleepiness.
B. Loud snoring, gasping, or snorting during sleep.
C. Fatigue.

Other Signs and Symptoms
A. Adults:
  1. Asymptomatic: Clients may not recognize they have OSA because they are able to go to sleep anytime.
  2. Restless sleep.
  3. Dry mouth or sore throat.
  4. Lack of physical or mental energy.
  5. Falling asleep when watching TV, reading, driving/riding in a car.
  6. Morning headaches.
  7. Decreased libido and impotence.
  8. Cognitive deficits.
B. Children:
  1. Short attention span.
  2. Emotional lability.
  3. Behavioral problems.
  4. Enuresis.

Subjective Data
A. Does the client feel sleepy during the day? Is daytime sleepiness a problem?
B. Does the client struggle to stay awake during the day?
C. Does the client take naps? How often and how long does the client sleep?
D. Does the client feel physically and mentally exhausted?
E. Does the client's bed partner complain about snoring, gasping, or snorting?
F. Ask the Epworth Sleepiness Scale questions related to how often the client dozes off or falls asleep (in contrast to just feeling tired). Each situation is scored from 0 = would never doze, to 1 = a slight change of dozing, 2 = moderate chance of dozing, and 3 = a high chance of dozing. There are eight situations to which the client should respond:
  1. Sitting and reading.
  2. Watching TV.
  3. Sitting inactive in a public place (e.g., a theater or meeting).
  4. As a passenger in a car for an hour without a break.
  5. Lying down to rest during the day when circumstances permit.
  6. Sitting and talking to someone.
  7. Sitting quietly after lunch without alcohol.
  8. In a car, while stopped for a few minutes in traffic.
G. Ask the client to list all medications currently being taken, particularly substances not prescribed, including over-the-counter (OTC) and herbal products.
H. Review alcohol use.
I. Men who present with sleep disorders should also be questioned about the presence of erectile dysfunction.

Physical Examination
A. Blood pressure, pulse, respirations, height and weight to calculate BMI, and waist measurement
B. Inspect:
  1. Oropharynx examination for:
    a. Peritonsillar narrowing or hypertrophy.
    b. Tongue (evaluate for macroglossia).
    c. Elongated or enlarged uvula.
    d. Palate (high arch or narrow palate).

2. Nasal examination: look for septal deviation and nasal polyps.
3. Inspect for signs of pulmonary hypertension or cor pulmonale:
   a. Jugular venous distension.
   b. Peripheral oedema.
C. Palpate thyroid gland.
D. Auscultate heart and lungs.
E. Mental status: Assess for confusion.

Diagnostic Tests

A. Polysomnography (PSG) is the standard method of diagnosis. The apnea hypopnoea index (AHI) or the respiratory disturbance index (RDI) is used to quantify hypopneas and classify the degree of sleep disturbance:
1. Full-night PSG.
2. Split-night PSG.
3. Home testing with portable monitors (not recommended for clients with comorbidities).
B. Routine laboratory work is not helpful in the confirmation or exclusion of OSA.

Differential Diagnoses

A. Primary snoring.
B. Narcolepsy.
C. Restless leg syndrome.
D. Swallowing disorder.
E. Nocturnal seizures.
F. Gastro-oesophageal reflux disease (GERD).
G. Obesity hypoventilation syndrome.
H. Sleep deprivation.
I. Neurodegenerative disease (e.g., Parkinson's, dementia, Alzheimer's).
J. Substance abuse.
K. Tonsillar hypertrophy.

Plan

A. General interventions:
   1. **Continuous positive airway pressure (CPAP) or bi-level positive airway pressure (BiPAP) is the mainstay of treatment for moderate to severe OSA.**
▶ B. Client teaching: *Refer to Client Teaching Guide: Sleep Apnea.*
   1. Educate the client about modifying controllable risk factors such as keeping diabetes and hypertension under control, healthy diet, exercise, and stopping smoking.
   2. Treatment with CPAP and BiPAP is required at all times during the night and during naps.
   3. Behavioral strategies include sleeping in a nonsupine position using a positioning device (e.g., alarm, pillow, backpack, tennis ball are used for positional therapy).
   4. Give the client a teaching sheet on sleep apnoea.
C. Dietary management:
   1. Even a modest weight loss of 10% to 20% has been associated with an improvement.
D. Nonsurgical treatment.
   1. Oral appliances (OAs): Require a thorough dental examination.
      a. Custom-made OAs may improve airway patency during sleep by enlarging the upper airway and/or by decreasing the upper airway collapse.
      b. Mandibular repositioning appliances (MRAs) cover the upper and lower teeth and hold the mandible in an advance position.
      c. Tongue-retaining devices (TRDs) hold the tongue in a forward position without mandibular repositioning.
E. Surgical treatment:
   1. Tracheostomy can eliminate OSA but not central hypoventilation syndromes. This procedure should be considered only when other options have failed or when it is considered necessary by clinical urgency.
   2. Maxillomandibular advancement (MMA) is indicated when the client cannot tolerate/refuses CPAP and an OA is not appropriate/effective.
   3. Surgical treatment should be considered after using an OA or positive airway pressure for three months. Surgical treatment has been shown to benefit clients with tonsillar or adenoid hypertrophy, or craniofacial deformities.
   4. Weight loss resulting from bariatric surgery has been effective in improving sleep efficiency and increasing amounts of rapid eye movement (REM) sleep. The severity of presurgical OSA determines the degree to which OSA improves postbariatric surgery.
   5. Radiofrequency ablation (RFA) is for treatment of mild to moderate OSA when the client cannot tolerate/refuses CPAP and an OA is not appropriate/effective.
   6. Laser-assisted uvulopalatoplasty is not recommended for OSA.

Follow-Up

A. There is no standard for recommending repeat PSG testing or a CPAP titration study after significant weight loss.

Consultation/Referral

A. Refer to a dentist for an OA.
B. Refer to a pulmonologist for management of therapy and/or surgical treatment.
C. Refer the client to a cardiologist as needed.

Bibliography

British Columbia. (B.C.), Centre for Palliative Care. (The BC Centre for Palliative Care, Fraser Health, First Nations Health Authority, Interior Health, Island Health, Providence Health, Vancouver Coastal, and Northern Health). (2017). *Inter-professional palliative symptom management guidelines: Dyspnea.*

Fleetham, J., Ayas, N., Bradley, D., Fitzpatrick, M., Oliver, T. K., Morrison, D., & Canadian Thoracic Society Sleep Disordered Breathing Committee. (2011). Canadian Thoracic Society 2011 guideline update: Diagnosis and treatment of sleep disordered breathing. *Canadian Respiratory Journal, 18*(1), 25–47. doi:10.1155/2011/506189

Kline, L. R. (2016, March 23). Clinical presentation and diagnosis of obstructive sleep apnea in adults. *UpToDate.* Retrieved from http://www.uptodate.com/contents/clinical-presentation-and-diagnosis-of-obstructive-sleep-apnea-in-adults

Marciniuk, D., Goodridge, D., Hernandez, P., Rocker, G., Balter, M., Bailey, P., & Canadian Thoracic Society Dyspnea Expert Working Group. (2011). Managing dyspnea in clients with advanced chronic obstructive pulmonary disease: A Canadian Thoracic Society clinical practice guideline. *Canadian Respiratory Journal, 18*(2), 69–78. doi:10.1155/2011/745047

MDCalc. *CURB-65.* Retrieved from https://www.mdcalc.com/curb-65-score-pneumonia-severity

MDCalc. *Modified medical research council dyspnea scale.* Retrieved from https://www.mdcalc.com/mmrc-modified-medical-research-council-dyspnea-scale

MPR: Nurse Practitioner's Edition. (2016, Spring). New York, NY: Haymarket Media.

National Guideline Clearinghouse. (2013, October). *Guideline summary: Management of obstructive sleep apnea in adults: A clinical practice guideline from the American College of Physicians.* Rockville, MD: Agency for Healthcare Research and Quality. Retrieved from https://www.guideline.gov/summaries/summary/47136/management-of-obstructive-sleep-apnea-in-adults-a-clinical-practice-guideline-from-the-american-college-of-physicians

▶ Client Teaching Guides are available at https://connect.springerpub.com/content/reference-book/978-0-8261-9498-5

Prescriber's Letter. (2013, May). *Appropriate med use* (Vol. 29). Retrieved from http://prescribersletter.therapeuticresearch.com/pl/ArticleDD.aspx?cs=&s=PRL&pt=6&fpt=31&dd=290501&pb=PRL&searchid=55980185

Schwartzstein, R. M. (2013, July). Physiology of dyspnea. *UpToDate*. Retrieved from http://www.uptodate.com/contents/physiology-of-dyspnea

Schwartzstein, R. M. (2015, November). Approach to the client with dyspnea. *UpToDate*. Retrieved from http://www.uptodate.com/contents/approach-to-the-client-with-dyspnea

Schwartzstein, R. M., & Adams, L. (2016). *Murray & Nadel's textbook of respiratory medicine* (6th ed.). Philadelphia, PA: Elsevier-Saunders.

Strohl, K. P. (2016, March). An overview of sleep apnea in adults. *UpToDate*. Retrieved from http://www.uptodate.com/contents/overview-of-obstructive-sleep-apnea-in-adults?source=search_result&search=sleep+apnea&selectedTitle=1%7E150

Valentine, N. (2017). Respiratory disorders. In B. Richardson (Ed.), *Pediatric primary care: Practice guidelines for nurses* (3rd ed., pp. 143–158). Burlington, MA: Jones & Bartlett.

Weinburger, S. E. (2015, June). Dyspnea during pregnancy. *UpToDate*. Retrieved from http://www.uptodate.com/contents/dyspnea-during-pregnancy

Wellman, A., & Redline, S. (2015). Sleep apnea. In D. L. Kasper, A. S. Fauci, S. L. Hauser, D. L. Longo, & J. L. Jameson (Eds.), *Harrison's principles of internal medicine* (19th ed.). New York, NY: McGraw-Hill.

Pneumonia (Bacterial)

Cheryl A. Glass, Melissa A. Hall, and Shelley Ann Walkerley

Definition
A. Pneumonia is inflammation and consolidation of lung tissue caused by a bacterial pathogen. The causative agent and the anatomic location classify pneumonia. It is not uncommon to have acute viral and bacterial pneumonia concurrently.
B. Other types of pneumonia and pulmonary inflammation occur secondary to smoking, exposure to chemicals, fungi, near-drowning, mycobacterium tuberculosis complex, and from recurrent aspiration with gastroesophageal reflux.
C. The CURB acronym represents the assessments for confusion, urea, respiratory rate, and blood pressure (BP). The CURB-65 severity score for community-acquired pneumonia (CAP) is a tool to estimate pneumonia mortality and assist in determining whether the client should best be treated in the inpatient or outpatient setting. Each parameter is given a score = 1 if present. There are five parameters: Confusion, urea >19 mg/dL, respiratory rate >30/min, systolic BP <91 mmHg or diastolic BP <60 mmHg, and age >65 years. (www.mdcalc.com/curb-65-score-pneumoniaseverity). (The Pneumonia Severity Index [PSI] can be applied to both men and women of all ages; www.thermh.org.au/sites/default/files/media/documents/pneumonia_severity_scores.pdf)

Incidence/Prevalence
Pneumonia is the second leading cause of death of children worldwide after complications of preterm birth. Pneumonia is also a common cause of death for clients aged >65 years.
A. Pneumonia is more prevalent in the very old and very young.
B. A higher mortality rate occurs in young infants, in persons with immunodeficiency, and in adults with comorbidities.
C. The incidence rate also varies by pathogens.

Pathogenesis
Pneumonia results from inflammation of the alveolar space and anatomically can be thought of as an alveolitis. Lobar pneumonia has four stages:

A. Vascular congestion and alveolar oedema within the first 24 hours of infection.
B. Red hepatization (two to three days), characterized by erythrocytes, neutrophils, and fibrin within the alveoli.
C. Gray hepatization (two to three days), characterized by a gray-brown to yellow colour secondary to exudate.
D. Resorption and restoration of the pulmonary architecture; a rub may still be auscultated due to the fibrinous inflammation.

Bacterial causes include *Streptococcus pneumoniae* (the most common pathogen), *Haemophilus influenzae* type b (Hib; the second most common pathogen), *Staphylococcus aureus*, *Legionella*, *Chlamydia trachomatis*, *Chlamydia pneumoniae*, *Mycoplasma pneumoniae* (most common pathogen in school-age children and adolescents), and *Pneumocystis jiroveci* pneumonia previously known as *Pneumocystis carinii* pneumonia (PCP) in clients with HIV.

Predisposing Factors
A. Age extremes.
B. Chronic obstructive pulmonary disease (COPD).
C. Alcoholism.
D. Cigarette smoking.
E. Aspiration.
F. Heart failure.
G. Diabetes.
H. Heart failure/heart disease.
I. Crowded conditions (day care, dormitories).
J. Immunodeficiency.
K. Congenital anomalies.
L. Abnormal mucus clearance.
M. Lack of immunization.
N. Measles.
O. Indoor air pollutants from cooking or heating with wood.
P. Prematurity.

Common Findings
Acute onset of these symptoms.
A. Fever.
B. Shaking chills.
C. Dyspnea; rapid, laboured breathing.
D. Cough.
E. Rust-coloured sputum.

Other Signs and Symptoms
A. Increased respiratory rate (tachypnoea).
B. Chest pain.
C. Upper respiratory tract infection (URI) symptoms such as pharyngitis.
D. Headache.
E. Nausea.
F. Vomiting.
G. Vague abdominal pain.
H. Diarrhoea.
I. Myalgia.
J. Arthralgias.
K. Poor feeding.
L. Lethargy in infants.
M. New onset confusion in the elderly.

Subjective Data
A. Determine the onset, duration, and course of illness.
B. Has the client had fever or shaking chills?
C. Has there been breathing trouble? Are the breathing problems interfering with eating and drinking?

D. If a child, review the presence of acute onset of fever, cough, tachypnoea, dyspnoea, and grunting.
E. Is there a cough? Is the cough productive? What colour is the sputum?
F. Are any other family members ill?
G. If a child, has he or she been hospitalized for pneumonia or respiratory distress before?
H. Review the history for any chronic diseases.
I. Has the client been immunized for pneumonia?
J. Review all medications, including over-the-counter (OTC) and herbal products. Specifically review whether the client has been on any antibiotics in the past three months. **Recent exposure to an antibiotic is a risk factor for antibiotic resistance. Continued or repeated use of that class of antibiotics is not recommended.**

Physical Examination
A. Temperature, BP, pulse, and weight. Count respirations for a full minute:
 1. Tachypnoea is the single best predictor of pneumonia in children and the elderly.
 2. In the elderly the BP is usually low.
B. Inspect:
 1. Observe overall appearance. Does the client appear ill? Consider the clinical presentation, age of the person, and history.
 2. Observe breathing pattern and the use of accessory muscles, grunting, retractions, and tachypnea.
 3. Obtain a pulse oximetry to assess oxygen saturation. **An oxygen saturation <92% is an indicator of severity and the need for oxygen therapy.**
 4. Check nail beds and lips for cyanosis.
 5. Examine the eyes, nose, ears, and throat.
C. Auscultate:
 1. Heart.
 2. Lungs for the following (auscultate bases first in geriatric clients):
  a. Crackles represent fluid in the alveolar sacs (present in 80% of clients), wheezes, and decreased breath sounds.
  b. Whispered pectoriloquy (increased loudness of whisper during auscultation).
  c. Egophony (client's "e" sounds like "a" during auscultation).
  d. Bronchophony (voice sounds louder than usual).
 3. Abdomen (usually hypoactive bowel sounds).
D. Percuss chest to identify areas of consolidation.
E. Palpate:
 1. Chest for tactile fremitus (increased conduction when client says "99").
 2. Lymph nodes for adenopathy.
 3. Sinuses for tenderness; sinusitis is a sign of *Mycoplasma* infection.

Diagnostic Tests
A. The British Thoracic Society in their 2011 guideline update for CAP in children notes that no diagnostic tests are necessary in the community, but emphasizes the importance of education on management, signs of deterioration, and the need for reassessment.
B. The WHO defines pneumonia solely on the basis of clinical finding observed by inspection and timing of respirations.
C. Chest radiograph (CXR):
 1. Infiltrates confirm diagnosis. False negatives result from dehydration, evaluation in first 24 hours, and infection.
 2. Ordering a posterior, anterior, and lateral CXR ensures adequate visualization for diagnosis.
D. Complete blood count (CBC) with differential.
E. Urea is needed to calculate the CURB-65 score.
F. Cultures:
 1. Blood cultures if critically ill, immunocompromised, or for persistent symptoms.
 2. Sputum cultures are reserved for very ill clients with unusual presentations.
G. Consider rapid viral testing if indicated.
H. Consider skin testing for TB for high-risk exposure.

Differential Diagnoses
A. Pneumonia:
 1. Viral pneumonia.
 2. Aspiration pneumonia.
 3. Chemically induced pneumonia.
B. Asthma.
C. Bronchitis/bronchiolitis.
D. Pertussis.
E. Heart failure.
F. Pulmonary embolus.
G. Empyema and abscess.
H. Aspiration of foreign body.
I. Tuberculosis.

Plan
A. General interventions:
 1. Encourage rest during acute phase.
 2. Encourage clients to avoid smoking/second-hand smoke.
 3. A vaporizer may be used to increase humidity.
 4. Encourage good handwashing or use of hand sanitizer.
 5. Chest physiotherapy is not prescribed for pneumonia.
B. Client teaching: *Refer to Client Teaching Guides: Pneumonia, Bacterial: Adult* and *Child*.
C. Dietary management: Encourage a nutritious diet with increased fluid intake.
D. Pharmacological therapy:
 1. Treatment with antibiotics is empirical for CAP. Oral therapy should continue for seven to 14 days. Clients should be treated for a minimum of five days if afebrile for 48 to 72 hours and clinically stable:
  a. Amoxicillin, amoxicillin/clavulanate, or penicillin are reasonable choices and supported by international guidelines for adults and children with mild to moderate CAP.
  b. Macrolides (clarithromycin or azithromycin) as first line for clients with a PSI 90 with no comorbidities or risks for drug-resistant *S. pnuemoniae* (can be treated as an outpatient). Doxycycline is an alternative.
  c. For outpatients with comorbidities or who have had antibiotics within the last three months, respiratory fluoroquinolones (levofloxacin) orally OR high-dose amoxicillin or amoxicillin/clavulanate + a macrolide orally are the recommendations.
  d. Do not use erythromycin as monotherapy.
  e. For inpatients respiratory fluoroquinolones PO/IV OR beta-lactams + macrolide PO/IV are recommended. It is recommended that clients in ICU be

▶ Client Teaching Guides are available at https://connect.springerpub.com/content/reference-book/978-0-8261-9498-5

treated with a beta-lactam IV either a macrolide IV or a respiratory fluoroquinolone.
2. **Treatment of specific pathogens for CAP:**
   a. *S. pneumonia*: penicillin or third-generation cephalosporin if resistant to penicillin. Alternatives include macrolides, clindamycin, doxycycline, respiratory fluoroquinolone (penicillin sensitive) or vancomycin, linezolid, high-dose amoxicillin (penicillin-resistant).
   b. *H. influenza*: second- or third-generation cephalosporin, amoxicillin/clavulanate, fluoroquinolones, macrolides, or amoxicillin monotherapy if non-beta-lactamase producing.
   c. *Staphylococcus aureus*: methicillin-susceptible: cloxacillin, cefazolin, clindamycin. Methicillin-resistant: vancomycin, linezolid, tigecycline.
   d. *Legionella* species: fluoroquinolones or azithromycin. Alternative: doxycline.
   e. *Mycoplasma pneumoniae, Chlamydophila pneumoniae*: macrolides or tetracyclines. Alternative: fluoroquinolones.
   f. *Coxiella burnetiid* (Q fever): doxycycline or fluoroquinolones. Alternative: macrolides (some strains may be resistant).
   g. Pseudomonas aeruginosa: Antispseudomonal beta-lactam (aztreonam, cefepime, piperacillin, ticarcillin).
3. Administer acetaminophen for fever.
4. Avoid cough suppressants. Suppression of a cough may interfere with airway clearance.
5. Vaccines:
   a. Children: Pneumococcal Conjugate 13 vaccine is recommended for all children in Canada.
   b. Geriatrics: Pneumococcal 13 and 23 vaccines are recommended for the elderly.

Follow-Up
A. Clients/parents should know the signs of increasing respiratory distress and seek immediate medical attention.
B. Follow up with a telephone call in 24 hours.
C. If there is no improvement after 48 hours on antibiotics, the client is advised to return to the office.
D. Schedule a return visit in two weeks for evaluation.
E. Follow up CXR in four to six weeks for clients >60 years and for those who smoke. However, if the client <60 years, a nonsmoker, and feels well at six-week follow-up, there is no need to follow up with a CXR.

Consultation/Referral
A. Clients who are immunocompromised or have signs of toxicity or hypoxia may need hospitalization.
B. If the child is in moderate respiratory distress, dehydrated, or hypoxaemic, consult with or refer the client to a paediatrician/hospital.
C. Poor prognostic signs that require referral are age >65 years, respiration rate ≥30 breaths per minute, systolic BP <90 mmHg or diastolic BP <60 mmHg, temperature >101°F, altered mental status, extrapulmonary infection, and white blood cells (WBC) <4,000 or >30,000.
D. Specialist consultation is needed for suspected PJP.

Individual Considerations
A. Pregnancy:
   1. The annual U.S. rate of antepartum CAP is 0.5 to 1.5 per 1,000 pregnancies.
   2. Perinatal mortality may increase slightly due to an associated increase in prematurity. Pneumonia puts older mothers at high risk of maternal death.
   3. The symptoms of bacterial pneumonia are the same in pregnancy.
   4. CXRs are acceptable in pregnancy to diagnose pneumonia if indicated.
B. Paediatrics.
   1. **Hospitalization is recommended in infants aged six months and younger and also in very severe cases of pneumonia.**
   2. **Immunization against *Haemophilus influenzae* type B (Hib), pneumococcus, measles, and whooping cough (pertussis) is the most effective way to prevent pneumonia.**
C. Geriatrics:
   1. Depending on the frailty status of the client, hospitalization may be required. A calculation to objectively determine client risk has been developed (CURB-65 Severity Score) and is available at: www.mdcalc.com/curb-65-severity-score-community-acquired-pneumonia/

Bibliography
Centers for Disease Control and Prevention. (2016c). *Recommended adult immunization schedule. U.S.–2016*. Retrieved from http://www.cdc.gov/vaccines/schedules/downloads/adult/adult-schedule.pdf
Flaherty, E., & Resnick, R (Eds.). (2014). *Geriatric nursing review syllabus: A core curriculum in advanced practice geriatric nursing* (4th ed.). New York, NY: American Geriatrics Society.
Goldblatt, D., & O'Brien, K. L. (2015). Pneumococcal infections. In D. L. Kasper, A. S. Fauci, S. L. Hauser, D. L. Longo, & J. L. Jameson (Eds.), *Harrison's principles of internal medicine* (19th ed.). New York, NY: McGraw-Hill.
MDCalc. *CURB-65*. Retrieved from https://www.mdcalc.com/curb-65-score-pneumonia-severity
MDCalc. *Pneumonia severity scale*. Retrieved from https://www.mdcalc.com/psi-port-score-pneumonia-severity-index-cap
MPR: Nurse Practitioner's Edition. (2016, Spring). New York, NY: Haymarket Media.
Ottawa, Ontario, Canada https://www.canada.ca/en/public-health/services/canadian-immunization-guide.html
Prescriber's Letter. (2013, May). *Appropriate med use* (Vol. 29). Retrieved from http://prescribersletter.therapeuticresearch.com/pl/ArticleDD.aspx?cs=&s=PRL&pt=6&fpt=31&dd=290501&pb=PRL&searchid=55980185
Public Health Agency of Canada. (2018). *Canadian immunization guide*. Ottawa, Ontario, Canada https://www.canada.ca/en/public-health/services/canadian-immunization-guide.html.
Rains, S. G. (2013). Fifteen-to-eighteen-month visit. In B. Richardson (Ed.), *Pediatric primary care: Practice guidelines for nurses* (2nd ed., pp. 113–124). Burlington, MA: Jones & Bartlett.
Schwartzstein, R. M., & Adams, L. (2016). *Murray & Nadel's textbook of respiratory medicine* (6th ed.). Philadelphia, PA: Elsevier-Saunders.
Terry, E. G. (2017). Seven-to-ten-year visit (school age. In B. Richardson (Ed.), *Pediatric primary care: Practice guidelines for nurses* (3rd ed., pp. 143–158). Burlington, MA: Jones & Bartlett.
Valentine, N. (2017). Respiratory disorders. In B. Richardson (Ed.), *Pediatric primary care: Practice guidelines for nurses* (3rd ed., pp. 143–158). Burlington, MA: Jones & Bartlett.
Weiner, D. L. (2014, November). Causes of acute respiratory distress in children. *UpToDate*. Retrieved from http://www.uptodate.com/contents/causes-of-acute-respiratory-distress-in-children
World Health Organization. (2015, November). *Pneumonia fact sheet N331*. Retrieved from http://www.who.int/mediacentre/factsheets/fs331/en

Pneumonia (Viral)

Cheryl A. Glass, Melissa A. Hall, and Shelley Ann Walkerley

Definition
A. Viral pneumonia is inflammation and consolidation of lung tissue due to a viral pathogen.

Incidence/Prevalence

A. Viral pneumonia is the most common paediatric pulmonary infection. Viral agents account for only 2% to 15% of pneumonia cases in adults. Viruses were documented in up to 45% of pneumonia cases in children. It is not uncommon to have concurrent viral and bacterial infections.
B. Children younger than five years and elderly persons have the highest rate of influenza-associated hospitalizations.
C. Pneumonia is the second leading cause of death of children worldwide after complications of preterm birth.

Pathogenesis

A. Pneumonia results from inflammation of the alveolar space and may compromise air at the alveoli–pulmonary capillary interface. Viral pneumonia is caused by influenza viruses, parainfluenza virus, and adenovirus and respiratory syncytial virus (RSV).
B. Viruses and bacteria are spread from a cough or sneeze.
C. Pneumonia can also be spread via blood, especially during and shortly after birth.

Predisposing Factors

A. Age extremes.
B. Prematurity.
C. Exposure to viral illness.
D. Lack of immunization.

Common Findings

A. Fever.
B. Cough.
C. Dyspnoea.
D. Tachypnoea.
E. Wheezing (more common in viral pneumonia).

Other Signs and Symptoms

A. Upper respiratory prodrome.
B. Poor appetite.
C. Malaise/lethargy in paediatrics.
D. Myalgia.
E. Muscle aches.
F. Headache.
G. Fatigue.
H. Chest pain/tightness.

Subjective Data

A. Determine the onset, duration, and course of illness.
B. Has the client had fever, cough, and upper respiratory infection?
C. Have there been any flu-like symptoms?
D. Has there been any laboured breathing?
E. Has there been a cough? Is it a productive cough? What colour is the sputum?
F. Are the breathing problems affecting the ability to eat or drink?
G. Has the child had nausea, vomiting, or diarrhoea?
H. Review if the client is up to date on immunizations.
I. Review all medications, including over-the-counter (OTC) and herbal products.

Physical Examination

A. Temperature, blood pressure, pulse, and respirations. Count respirations for a full minute. **Tachypnoea is the single best predictor of pneumonia in children.**
B. Inspect:
  1. Observe overall appearance. Does the client appear ill? Consider the clinical presentation, age of person, and history.
  2. Observe respiratory pattern, grunting, nasal flaring, retractions, and use of accessory muscles.
  3. Check pulse oximetry. **An oxygen saturation <92% is an indicator of severity and the need for oxygen therapy.**
  4. Check nail beds and lips for cyanosis.
  5. Examine eyes, ears, nose, and throat.
C. Auscultate:
  1. Heart.
  2. Lungs for the following (auscultate bases first in geriatric clients):
    a. Crackles, decreased breath sounds.
    b. Whispered pectoriloquy (client's whispered sounds are louder than normal).
    c. Egophony (client's "e" sounds like "a").
    d. Bronchophony (voice sounds louder than usual).
D. Percuss chest for dull sound (consolidation).
E. Palpate:
  1. Lymph nodes for swelling.
  2. Chest for tactile fremitus (increased conduction when client says "99").
  3. Sinuses.

Diagnostic Tests

A. Chest radiograph (CXR), which reveals interstitial, perihilar, or diffuse infiltrates.
B. Complete blood count (CBC) with differential.
C. Rapid viral tests per nasal swab.
D. Sputum Gram stain if indicated.

Differential Diagnoses

A. Bacterial pneumonia.
B. Varicella pneumonia.
C. Herpes pneumonia.
D. Cytomegalovirus pneumonia.
E. Pertussis.
F. Asthma.
G. Bronchitis/bronchiolitis.
H. Sinusitis.
I. Foreign body obstruction (usually in small children and the mentally handicapped).
J. Aspiration.

Plan

A. General interventions:
  1. Recommend to the client to rest during acute phase.
  2. Avoid smoking or second-hand smoke.
  3. Respiratory isolation; may use facial masks.
  4. Encourage good handwashing or use of hand sanitizer.
  5. Chest physiotherapy is not recommended for pneumonia.
B. Client teaching: *Refer to Client Teaching Guides: Pneumonia, Viral: Adult* and *Child*.
C. Dietary management: Encourage fluids and a nutritious diet.
D. Pharmacological therapy: Antiviral agents should be considered in immunocompromised clients, those at high risk for complications, or those requiring hospitalization. High risk includes: Age >65 years; pregnancy or up to two weeks postpartum; long-term care residents; pulmonary disease, including asthma; diabetes; cardiovascular disease, excluding hypertension; chronic kidney disease; hepatic dysfunction; and active malignancy:

1. Zanamivir is the recommended first-line treatment when influenza A infection or exposure is suspected. Zanamivir is administered by a metered-dose inhaler (MDI). Zanamivir is only effective if it is started within 24 to 48 hours of onset of fever and symptoms.
2. The combination of oseltamivir and rimantadine, an adamantane, is considered a second-line alternative. Resistance should be considered before antiviral selection.
3. Acyclovir for herpes viruses is administered as an IV infusion.
4. Ribavirin for RSV is administered as an aerosol. Synagis has also been used in conjunction with ribavirin for high-risk clients (generally hospitalized infants and young children).

E. Clients with viral pneumonia who are superinfected with bacterial organisms require antibiotic therapy.
F. Avoid cough suppressants. The suppression of a cough may interfere with airway clearance.
G. Acetaminophen for fever.
H. Immunizations:
1. Recommend the annual influenza vaccine for prevention.
2. Consider RSV vaccine prophylaxis for paediatrics following the Canadian Paediatric Society.
3. The measles vaccine is recommended except during pregnancy and in immunocompromised clients.

Follow-Up

Signs and symptoms may vary greatly according to the viral pathogen, severity of disease, and client's age:
A. Recommend to the client to return to the clinic if no improvement is seen after 48 hours on antiviral agents.
B. Follow up with a phone call in 24 hours.
C. Consider follow-up at two weeks if bronchoconstriction is noted on examination.

Consultation/Referral

A. Consult a specialist if viral pneumonia is suspected in a severely ill client.
B. Consider consultation if the client is pregnant and severely ill.
C. Transfer to the ED if the client is in respiratory distress, dehydrated, or hypoxaemic.
D. All infants younger than three months of age, or premature infants, who exhibit symptoms (fever, dyspnoea, tachypnoea, etc.) need to be assessed urgently by paediatric specialists; transfer to hospital.
E. Consider consultation with a respirologist if client's condition does not improve as expected.

Individual Considerations

A. Pregnancy:
1. **Ribavirin is contraindicated in pregnancy; it is a class X drug.**
2. Acyclovir is given in the third trimester in cases in which herpes pneumonia is suspected, which carries a high mortality rate.
3. The varicella-zoster immune globulin may be considered in pregnancy. Consultation with the specialist is recommended.
4. The measles virus is a live-attenuated virus and should not be given during pregnancy.

B. Paediatrics:
1. **Hospitalization is recommended in infants aged three months and younger and also in very severe cases of pneumonia.**

Bibliography

Centers for Disease Control and Prevention. (2015a, April 20). *Respiratory syncytial virus infection (RSV)*. Retrieved from www.cdc.gov/rsv
Centers for Disease Control and Prevention. (2016c). *Recommended adult immunization schedule. U.S.–2016*. Retrieved from http://www.cdc.gov/vaccines/schedules/downloads/adult/adult-schedule.pdf
Dolin, R. (2015). Common viral respiratory infections. In D. L. Kasper, S. L. Hauser, J. L. Jameson, A. S. Fauci, D. L. Longo, & J. Loscalzo (Eds.), *Harrison's principles of internal medicine* (19th ed.). New York, NY: McGraw-Hill.
MDCalc. *Pneumonia severity scale*. Retrieved from https://www.mdcalc.com/psi-port-score-pneumonia-severity-index-cap
Prescriber's Letter. (2013, May). *Appropriate med use* (Vol. 29). Retrieved from http://prescribersletter.therapeuticresearch.com/pl/ArticleDD.aspx?cs=&s=PRL&pt=6&fpt=31&dd=290501&pb=PRL&searchid=55980185
Public Health Agency of Canada. (2018). *Canadian immunization guide*. Ottawa, Ontario, Canada https://www.canada.ca/en/public-health/services/canadian-immunization-guide.html.
Rains, S. G. (2013). Fifteen-to-eighteen-month visit. In B. Richardson (Ed.), *Pediatric primary care: Practice guidelines for nurses* (2nd ed., pp. 113–124). Burlington, MA: Jones & Bartlett.
Schwartzstein, R. M., & Adams, L. (2016). *Murray & Nadel's textbook of respiratory medicine* (6th ed.). Philadelphia, PA: Elsevier-Saunders.
Terry, E. G. (2017). Seven-to-ten-year visit (school age. In B. Richardson (Ed.), *Pediatric primary care: Practice guidelines for nurses* (3rd ed., pp. 143–158). Burlington, MA: Jones & Bartlett.
Valentine, N. (2017). Respiratory disorders. In B. Richardson (Ed.), *Pediatric primary care: Practice guidelines for nurses* (3rd ed., pp. 143–158). Burlington, MA: Jones & Bartlett.
Weiner, D. L. (2014, November). Causes of acute respiratory distress in children. *UpToDate*. Retrieved from http://www.uptodate.com/contents/causes-of-acute-respiratory-distress-in-children
World Health Organization. (2015, November). *Pneumonia fact sheet N331*. Retrieved from http://www.who.int/mediacentre/factsheets/fs331/en

Respiratory Syncytial Virus (RSV) Bronchiolitis

Cheryl A. Glass, Melissa A. Hall, and Shelley Ann Walkerley

Definition

A. Respiratory syncytial virus (RSV) is the most frequent cause of viral respiratory tract infection in infants. Most infants develop upper respiratory tract symptoms; 20% to 30% develop lower respiratory tract disease with their first infection. Infection with RSV may produce minimal respiratory symptoms. Most previously healthy infants who develop RSV bronchiolitis do not require hospitalization. Preterm infants with respiratory symptoms with lethargy, irritability, and poor feeding may require admission for treatment. There is no specific treatment for RSV infection.

Incidence/Prevalence

A. RSV is prevalent worldwide and affects all age groups. Infants, the elderly, and adults with chronic heart or lung disease or weakened immune systems are at high risk. Annual epidemics occur in winter and early spring, usually in temperate climates. The peak season in North America is between November and April. Most infants are infected during the first year of life. Peak incidence of occurrence of severe RSV disease is observed at ages of two to eight months. Virtually all children have been infected at least once by their third birthday. Reinfection with RSV throughout life is common.

B. The period of viral shedding usually is three to eight days, but shedding may continue up to four weeks. The incubation period ranges from two to eight days.
C. Full recovery from RSV illness occurs in about one to two weeks.

Pathogenesis
A. RSV is an enveloped, nonsegmented, negative-strand RNA virus of the *Paramyxoviridae* family. Two major strains (Groups A and B) have been identified, and strains of both often circulate concurrently.
B. Humans are the only source of infection. Transmission is by direct or close contact with contaminated secretions. RSV can persist on environmental surfaces for several hours and for a half hour or more on hands.

Predisposing Factors
A. Prematurity.
B. Congenital heart disease.
C. Chronic lung disease (CLD).
D. Immunodeficiency.
E. Child-care centers.
F. Two or more siblings younger than five years.
G. Hospitalization.

Common Findings
A. Paediatrics:
  1. Fever (<101°F); 20% of clients have higher temperatures.
  2. Decreased appetite.
  3. Irritability.
  4. Lethargy.
  5. Rapid respirations.
  6. Cough.
  7. Coryza.
  8. Decreased activity.
  9. Wheezing.
B. Adults:
  1. Rhinorrhoea.
  2. Pharyngitis.
  3. Cough.
  4. Headache.
  5. Fatigue.
  6. Fever.

Other Signs and Symptoms
A. Tachypnoea or apnoea.
B. Nasal flaring.
C. Retractions.
D. Crackles.
E. Wheezes.

Subjective Data
A. Ask about the onset, duration, and course of illness.
B. Inquire whether the child is having trouble eating or drinking because of breathing problems.
C. Review other symptoms, including fever, nausea, vomiting, or diarrhoea.
D. Are there any laboured breathing patterns?
E. Calculate the child's age—how old the baby is and birth date—if palivizumab is prescribed.
F. Was the baby born preterm and at what gestational age?
G. Has the client ever been diagnosed with any cardiac or lung problems, including cystic fibrosis (CF)?
H. Do the client's siblings attend day care?

Physical Examination
A. Record temperature, pulse, respirations, blood pressure, and pulse oximetry.
B. Inspect:
  1. Observe general appearance.
  2. Note respiratory pattern, retractions, nasal flaring, grunting, and circumoral cyanosis.
  3. Inspect eyes, ears, nose, and throat. As many as 40% have an associated viral and/or bacterial otitis media.
  4. Assess hydration status: Skin turgor, capillary refill, mucous membranes.
C. Auscultate:
  1. Heart.
  2. Lungs for crackles and mild to moderate respiratory distress with scattered wheezes.
D. Percuss chest.
E. Palpate:
  1. Lymph nodes for adenopathy.
  2. Head and fontanelles (if applicable).

Diagnostic Tests
A. Rapid diagnostic assay of nasopharyngeal secretions are not recommended except for infection control (cohorting of hospitalized clients).
B. Laboratory studies are frequently not indicated in the infant who is comfortable in room air, is well hydrated, and is feeding adequately. Nonspecific laboratory tests may include complete blood count (CBC), serum electrolytes, and urinalysis.
C. Chest radiograph (CXR) may show hyperexpansion, atelectasis, and/or infiltrates in a specific nonlobar (bacterial) viral pattern.
D. Arterial blood gases (ABGs) or pulse oximetry may show hypoxaemia.

Differential Diagnoses
A. Viral or bacterial pneumonia.
B. Asthma.
C. Croup.
D. Influenza.
E. Neonatal sepsis.
F. Foreign body aspiration.

Plan
A. General interventions:
  1. Most infants require only supportive care, such as nasal suctioning.
  2. Supportive care and supplemental oxygen are recommended for adults as indicated.
  3. Infants should never be exposed to cigarette smoke.
  4. Hydration is important.
  5. Contact precautions are recommended for the duration of RSV-associated illness among infants and young children. Adhere to appropriate hand-hygiene practices.
  6. Prevention includes limiting, when feasible, exposure to contagious settings (e.g., child-care centers).
B. Client teaching: *Refer to Client Teaching Guide: Respiratory Syncytial Virus.*
C. Dietary management:
  1. Discuss with the caregiver to offer oral fluids frequently if infant/child is able to drink safely (RR < 60 bpm). Continue breastfeeding if possible.
  2. Suggest offering small, frequent feedings.
D. Pharmacological therapy:
  1. The use of bronchodilators and corticosteroids is not recommended in infants and children unless they have

preexisting disease (asthma). May be useful in older adults with wheeze and/or preexisting disease (asthma, COPD).
2. Antibiotics are not indicated for RSV bronchiolitis or pneumonia unless there is a secondary bacterial infection.
3. Palivizumab immunoprophylaxis is extremely costly and should be limited to infants at risk of hospitalization related to RSV (See Canadian Paediatric Society Criteria) Immunizations are given from three to five months depending on the gestational age, risk factors, and month that prophylaxis is started. For high-risk infants and children immunization should start before periods of high risk for infection (generally November to April in North America) (CPhA, CPS, 2018). Palivizumab is not indicated for adult use.

Follow-Up
A. Call the client's caregiver in 12 to 24 hours to assess feeding and respiratory status.

Consultation/Referral
A. Refer the client to a specialist or ED if the infant is in moderate respiratory distress, is dehydrated, is hypoxaemic, or is less than six months of age.
B. Admit hypoxaemic infants to the hospital for hydration, oxygen therapy, and, possibly, mechanical ventilation.
C. Age is a significant factor in the severity of infection: The younger the client is, the more severe the infection/hypoxaemia tends to be. Infants younger than six months are most severely affected secondary to their smaller, more easily obstructed airways and their decreased ability to clear secretions.

Individual Considerations
A. Adults: Palivizumab is not approved for adults.
B. Paediatrics:
   1. All high-risk infants six months of age and older and their contacts should be administered the annual influenza vaccine as well as other recommended age-appropriate immunizations.
   2. Palivizumab does not interfere with response to vaccines.
C. Pregnancy: Ribavirin is contraindicated during pregnancy. A negative pregnancy test and assurance of contraception should be obtained before prescribing.

Bibliography
American Academy of Pediatrics. (2015). Respiratory syncytial virus. In Kimberlin, D., Brady, M. T., Jackson, M. A., & Long, S. S (Eds.). *Red book: 2015 Report of the committee on Infectious diseases* (30th ed., pp. 667–676). Elk Grove Village, IL: Author. Retrieved from: http://redbook.solutions.aap.org/chapter.aspx?sectionId=88187226&bookId=1484

Barr, R.G., & Graham, B.S. (2015, July). Respiratory syncytial virus: Treatment. Retrieved from http://www.uptodate.com/contents/respiratory-syncytial-virus-infection-treatment?source=search_result&search=Respiratory+syncytial+virus%3A+Treatment&selectedTitle=1147

Barr, R.G., & Graham, B.S. (2016, March). *Respiratory syncytial virus: Prevention*. Retrieved from http://www.uptodate.com/contents/respiratory-syncytial-virus-infection-prevention?source=search_result&search=Respiratory+syncytial+virus%3A+Treatment&selectedTitle=2147

Centers for Disease Control and Prevention. (2015a, April 20). *Respiratory syncytial virus infection (RSV)*. Retrieved from: file:///Users/swalkerl/Downloads/www.cdc.gov/rsv" www.cdc.gov/rsv

Centers for Disease Control and Prevention. (2015b, August 7). *Prevention and control of influenza with vaccines: Recommendations of the advisory committee on immunization practices, United States, 2015–16 Influenza season*. Retrieved from https://www.cdc.gov/mmwr/preview/mmwrhtml/mm6430a3.htm

MPR: Nurse Practitioner's Edition. (2016, Spring). New York, NY: Haymarket Media.

Prescriber's Letter. (2013, May). *Appropriate med use* (Vol. 29). Retrieved from http://prescribersletter.therapeuticresearch.com/pl/ArticleDD.aspx?cs=&s=PRL&pt=6&fpt=31&dd=290501&pb=PRL&searchid=55980185

Public Health Agency of Canada. (2018). *Canadian immunization guide*. Ottawa, Ontario, Canada https://www.canada.ca/en/public-health/services/canadian-immunization-guide.html

Rains, S. G. (2013). Fifteen-to-eighteen-month visit. In B. Richardson (Ed.), *Pediatric primary care: Practice guidelines for nurses* (2nd ed., pp. 113–124). Burlington, MA: Jones & Bartlett.

Schwartzstein, R. M., & Adams, L. (2016). *Murray & Nadel's textbook of respiratory medicine* (6th ed.). Philadelphia, PA: Elsevier-Saunders.

Terry, E. G. (2017). Seven-to-ten-year visit (school age. In B. Richardson (Ed.), *Pediatric primary care: Practice guidelines for nurses* (3rd ed., pp. 143–158). Burlington, MA: Jones & Bartlett.

Valentine, N. (2017). Respiratory disorders. In B. Richardson (Ed.), *Pediatric primary care: Practice guidelines for nurses* (3rd ed., pp. 143–158). Burlington, MA: Jones & Bartlett.

Weiner, D. L. (2014, November). Causes of acute respiratory distress in children. *UpToDate*. Retrieved from http://www.uptodate.com/contents/causes-of-acute-respiratory-distress-in-children

Zachary, K. C. (2015, December). Treatment of seasonal influenza in adults. *UpToDate*. Retrieved from http://www.uptodate.com/contents/treatment-of-seasonal-influenza-in-adults

Shortness of Breath (SOB)

Cheryl A. Glass, Melissa A. Hall, and Shelley Ann Walkerley

Definition
A. Shortness of breath (SOB; dyspnoea) is derived from the Greek terms for DIFFICULT and BREATH. Dyspnoea may be experienced by clients with or without respiratory disorders. SOB/dyspnoea is clinically significant when it interferes with normal functioning. Dyspnoea is considered chronic when it persists longer than four to eight weeks. SOB is a subjective symptom, reported by the client. As self-reported, SOB may cause greater distress than pain.

Incidence/Prevalence
A. Dyspnoea affects millions of people and is commonly associated with pulmonary disease, cardiovascular disease, anaemia, obesity, and deconditioning. Dyspnoea is reported in more than one-fourth of the elderly. An estimated 25 million people with asthma or chronic obstructive pulmonary disease (COPD) experience SOB during the course of their illness. SOB is reported in >95% of clients in terminal stages of lung cancer, COPD, and heart failure.

Pathogenesis
A. The sensation of SOB can involve psychological, physical, social, and environmental factors. A sensation of SOB is stimulated by chemoreceptors that respond to changes in pH and carbon dioxide. Mechanoreceptors are located in upper airways, lungs, and the chest wall.
B. A sensation of SOB occurs with ventilation–perfusion mismatch, metabolic acidosis, increase in respiratory dead space, or stimulation of chest wall or pulmonary respiratory receptors.
C. SOB is perceived more by clients with existing lung disease.
D. Anaemia and cardiovascular disease compromise the amount of oxygen delivered to tissues, worsening the sensation of dyspnoea.

E. Interstitial lung disease associated with autoimmunity increases dyspnea/SOB, and with disease progression tissue oxygenation is reduced.

Predisposing Factors
A. Exertion.
B. Asthma.
C. COPD.
D. Congestive heart failure (CHF).
E. Cardiac valve disorders.
F. Cardiac anomalies.
G. Pulmonary embolism.
H. High altitudes.
I. Environmental air pollution.
J. Respiratory muscle weakness or paralysis, including neuromuscular disorders.
K. Metabolic acidosis (renal failure).
L. Haemoglobinopathies.
M. Hyperventilation syndrome, anxiety disorder, panic episodes.
N. Reduced vital capacity and thoracic expansion with aging.
O. Severe kyphoscoliosis.
P. Obesity.
Q. Pregnancy.
R. Pleural effusions.
S. Pulmonary hypertension.
T. Foreign body aspiration.
U. Obstructive sleep apnoea.
V. End-stage terminal illness (lung cancer, COPD, CHF).

Common Findings
A. Discomfort with breathing or air hunger, worsening with positioning or activity.

Subjective Data
A. How long have the symptoms been present?
B. How do they interfere with functioning?
C. What worsens and what improves the SOB?
D. Associated with syncope?
E. Associated with palpitations?
F. Increased anxiety before episodes?
G. History of similar symptoms?
H. Associated with odours (including household cleaners)?
I. Associated with certain social environments?
J. Weight changes since symptoms began?
K. History of lung or cardiac disease?
L. Treatments used to relieve the SOB?
M. Family history of similar issues?
N. If using a short-acting beta 2 agonist, how often, and has it helped?
O. Is cough associated?
P. Is it haemoptysis?
Q. Is the client smoking now or ever? Pack years?
R. Did the client use illicit substances? What type? In what amount? When was the most recent use?
S. Has the client taken any new medications, foods, or been stung by an insect?
T. Has the client been injured in the chest or neck?
U. Does the client's chest hurt anywhere?
V. What is the client's history of sickle cell disease?
W. What does the client feel is causing the SOB?
   1. Onset sudden or gradual; what was the client doing before onset of SOB; any associated symptoms such as fever, chest pain, itching, rash, wheezing any recent surgery.
   2. take birth control or estrogen? Serum estrogen receptor modulators? ACE inhibitors or digitalis? Anticoagulants?
   3. History of DVT?
   4. Family hx of clotting disorder?
   5. Any recent pain in the legs, recent travel?
   6. Any history of anaemia?

Physical Examination
A. Record temperature, pulse, respirations, blood pressure, and pulse oximetry.
B. Inspect:
   1. Observe general appearance, including morbid obesity, gravid uterus, skin tones, and use of accessory muscles of breathing, and facial appearance for fear or reduced level of consciousness, as well as tobacco or other chemical odours.
   2. Position in the tripod position for ability to speak in complete sentences.
   3. Assess hydration status: Skin turgor, capillary refill, and mucous membranes. Note distal fingers for clubbing.
   4. Pharynx and tonsils for erythema or hypertrophy.
   5. Trachea for deviation.
   6. Chest for barrel appearance or obvious trauma (measure ratio of anteroposterior chest dimension to lateral dimension).
   7. Spine for scoliosis or kyphosis.
   8. Abdomen for distension.
   9. Infants: Note respiratory pattern, retractions, nasal flaring, grunting, and circumoral cyanosis.
C. Auscultate:
   1. Heart for murmur, rate, irregular rhythm, S3 or S4.
   2. Lungs for crackles and mild to moderate respiratory distress with wheezing.
D. Percuss chest.
E. Palpate:
   1. Palpate lymph nodes for adenopathy.
   2. Palpate the chest for expansion and fremitis.
   3. Perform strength testing against resistance of upper and lower extremities to assess for lethargy/atonia.
F. Neurologic examination:
   1. Assess mentation.

Diagnostic Tests
A. Labs: CBC, urea, creatinine, electrolytes, cardiac troponin, brain natriuretic peptide (BNP), D-dimer, carbon monoxide levels.
B. ECG.
C. Chest x-ray.
D. Pulmonary function tests.
E. Echocardiogram if heart failure is suspected.
F. Anxiety and depression scales as indicated.
G. Stress Test.
H. Assessment for functional exercise capacity (six-minute walk, stair climbing, etc.).

Differential Diagnoses
A. Cardiovascular anomalies, dysfunction, or acute ischaemia.
B. Pulmonary disease, including autoimmune disorders affecting lung tissue.
C. Anxiety.
D. Foreign body or other aspiration syndromes.
E. Anaphylaxis.
F. Airway trauma.
G. Infection of upper or lower airways.
H. Pulmonary hypertension.

Plan

A. General interventions:
  1. The underlying aetiology of the SOB should be considered and treated.
  2. Severe airway compromise should be considered in clients with stridor or change in level of consciousness. Emergency medical services (EMS) should be activated immediately with airway support, including supplemental oxygen.

▶ **B.** Client teaching: *Refer to Client Teaching Guide: Shortness of Breath.*
  1. Discuss the underlying aetiology of SOB with the client and family and establish strategies to prevent further episodes of SOB.

C. Dietary management:
  1. Foods associated with worsening SOB should be avoided.
  2. Swallowing studies should be considered for clients at risk for aspiration.

D. Nonpharmacological and Pharmacological Interventions:
  1. Nonpharmacological interventions and medications should be prescribed according to the underlying aetiology. Interventions specifically for dyspnoea relief in terminal illness in clients under hospice care include positioning, pulmonary rehabilitation (COPD), walking aids, neuromuscular electrical stimulation delivered by a trained provider, chest wall vibrations (clients with COPD or motor neuron disease) if delivered by a trained provider and if client tolerates. Pharmacological interventions include oral or parental opioids, bronchodilators for clients with asthma or COPD, and benzodiazepines for clients who are anxious. There is no evidence of efficacy for the use of benzodiazepines for the treatment of breathlessness but they can be used as second- or third-line management if opioids and nonpharmacological measures fail to relieve breathlessness.

Follow-Up

A. Follow-up should occur frequently until symptoms of SOB have been controlled and the underlying aetiology treated.

Consultation/Referral

A. Activate EMS in acute respiratory distress.
B. Provide supplemental oxygen for all ages until EMS has transported the client.
C. Refer to appropriate specialty care depending on underlying cause of SOB.
D. Consultation to palliative care or hospice services should be considered to relieve dyspnoea based on clients' advance care planning.

Individual Considerations

A. Paediatrics:
  1. Acute respiratory distress should be immediately ruled out in infants and children in an ED setting.

B. Pregnancy:
  1. Dyspnoea occurs in up to two-thirds of clients beginning in the first or second trimester of pregnancy. Underlying pathology during pregnancy should be considered as with all ages.

C. Geriatrics:
  1. Avoid sedating medications that would increase the risk for hypoventilation or aspiration.
  2. Physical changes associated with aging increase the risk for hypoxia.
  3. Elderly clients may report SOB less frequently and assume it is an expectation of aging.

Bibliography

Prescriber's Letter. (2013, May). *Appropriate med use* (Vol. 29). Retrieved from http://prescribersletter.therapeuticresearch.com/pl/ArticleDD.aspx?cs=&s=PRL&pt=6&fpt=31&dd=290501&pb=PRL&searchid=55980185

Schwartzstein, R. M., & Adams, L. (2016). *Murray & Nadel's textbook of respiratory medicine* (6th ed.). Philadelphia, PA: Elsevier-Saunders.

Valentine, N. (2017). Respiratory disorders. In B. Richardson (Ed.), *Pediatric primary care: Practice guidelines for nurses* (3rd ed., pp. 143–158). Burlington, MA: Jones & Bartlett.

Tuberculosis (TB)

Cheryl A. Glass, Melissa A. Hall, and Shelley Ann Walkerley

Definition

A. Tuberculosis (TB) is an infectious disease. TB is a granulomatous disease caused by *Mycobacterium tuberculosis, Mycobacterium bovis,* and other mycobacteria. Humans are the only reservoirs for *M. tuberculosis*. TB may involve multiple organs, including the lungs, liver, spleen, lymph nodes, kidney, brain, eyes, and bone. The WHO estimates that one-third of all people in the world are infected with *M. tuberculosis.*

B. In most immunocompetent individuals, macrophages are successful in containing the bacilli, and the infection is self-limited and often subclinical. As many as 60% of children and 5% of adults with primary TB are asymptomatic. When the pulmonary macrophages are unable to contain the bacilli, this leads to clinically apparent infection-progressive primary TB.

C. Postprimary (reactivation) TB occurs when the initial infection was successfully contained by the pulmonary macrophages, with bacilli remaining viable within the macrophages. Infection results when the host's immune status (T cells) is compromised.

D. Clients with fever of unknown origin, failure to thrive, significant weight loss, or unexplained lymphadenopathy should be evaluated for TB.

E. The lungs are the most common site for the development of TB; 85% of clients present with pulmonary complaints.

Incidence/Prevalence

A. TB is a worldwide infection and is considered a global public health emergency by the World Health Organization (WHO):
  1. The WHO reports more than nine million new cases of TB every year.
  2. TB can affect any age group. More than 60% of cases are aged 25 to 40 years. TB is uncommon in children aged between 5 and 15 years.
  3. Child-to-child transmission is not common because children rarely develop a cough and the sputum is scant.
  4. The incidence of TB in Canada in 2012 was 4.8 new cases per 100,000 population.
  5. Of those new cases 64% were foreign-born individuals, 23% were Canadian-born indigenous people, and 10% were Canadian-born nonindigenous people.

▶ Client Teaching Guides are available at https://connect.springerpub.com/content/reference-book/978-0-8261-9498-5

Ontario has the most cases of TB among the provinces. Ninety percent of these cases were foreign-born occurred in areas with high immigration such as the Greater Toronto Area.

B. Postprimary TB is a significant cause of worldwide morbidity and mortality. Pulmonary morbidity results from a chronic cough, haemoptysis, fibrosis, superinfection, bronchial stenosis, repeated pulmonary infections, or empyema. Morbidity also arises from chronic TB osteomyelitis, chronic renal insufficiency, and central nervous system (CNS) TB.

Pathogenesis

A. Mycobacteria are non-spore-forming, slow-growing bacilli. TB infection occurs by means of inhalation of airborne bacillus droplets from an infected host. The development of an infection depends on prolonged exposure (weeks) to an individual with active pulmonary TB. Bacilli travel through the pulmonary lymphatics or enter the vascular system and are disseminated to the brain, meninges, eyes, bones, joints, lymph nodes, kidneys, intestines, larynx, pericardium, genitourinary system, and skin. The incubation period from infection to positive skin test reaction is two to ten weeks, although disease may not occur for many years or may never occur. The risk of disease is greatest within two years following infection.

Risk Factors for Latent TB Infection

A. Close contact of recently diagnosed infectious case of TB.
B. Immigrants and travellers from countries with high TB incidence.
C. Persons who are homeless or underhoused.
D. Indigenous communities with high rates of latent TB infection (LTBI) or active infection.
E. Persons at risk for occupational exposure: staff and volunteers in hospitals, shelters, correctional facilities, long term care homes.
F. Residents of communal living settings; shelters, correctional facilities, long-term care homes.
G. Injection drug users.

Risk Factors for Development of Active TB Disease Among Those With LTBI

High Risk
A. AIDS.
B. HIV infection.
C. Transplantation (related to immune-suppressing therapy).
D. Silicosis.
E. Chronic renal failure requiring dialysis.
F. Carcinoma of the head and neck.
G. Recent TB infection.
H. Abnormal chest x-ray-fibronodular disease

Increased Risk
A. Treatment with glucocorticoids
B. Tumour necrosis factor-alpha (TNF-alpha) antagonist (used in the treatment of rheumatoid arthritis, psoriasis and other autoimmune diseases)
C. Diabetes (all types)
D. Underweight (<90% ideal body weight; BMI less than or equal to 20).
E. Young age when infected (under four years).
F. Cigarette smoking (one pack per day).
G. Abnormal chest x-ray (granuloma).
H. Alcohol consumption (at least three drinks per day).

Low Risk
A. Infected persons, no known risk factors, normal chest x-ray. (OLA, TB booklet, 2015).

Common Findings
A. Fever (usually low grade at onset but becoming marked with progression of disease).
B. Malaise.
C. Weight loss/difficulty gaining weight.
D. Cough.
E. Night sweats.
F. Chills.
G. Occasional haemoptysis.
H. Fatigue.
I. Paediatric symptoms:
  1. Non-productive cough.
  2. Failure to thrive.
  3. Difficulty gaining weight.
  4. Fever.
  5. Night sweats.
  6. Anorexia.
  7. Wheezing.
  8. Lethargy or irritability.

Other Signs and Symptoms
A. Pulmonary TB: Fatigue, irritability, undernutrition, with or without fever and cough.
B. Glandular TB: Chronic cervical adenitis.
C. Meningeal TB: Fever and meningeal signs, positive cerebrospinal fluid.
D. Failure to thrive.
E. Anorexia.

Subjective Data
A. Determine the onset, duration, and course of illness.
B. Review symptom history: Fever, night sweats, chills, or cough.
C. Review history of weight loss.
D. Review exposure history to someone who has TB.
E. What is the client's living situation (including past history of homelessness)?
F. Review travel history to endemic areas with TB.
G. Review HIV status or need for testing.

Physical Examination
A complete physical examination is mandatory. Physical findings of pulmonary TB are not specific and usually are absent in mild or moderate disease.
A. Record temperature, respirations, pulse, oxygen saturation, blood pressure, and weight.
B. Inspect:
  1. Observe overall appearance.
  2. Check skin for pallor.
  3. Inspect eyes, ears, nose, and throat.
C. Auscultate:
  1. Heart.
  2. Lungs and chest for the following:
     a. Rales in upper posterior chest.
     b. Bronchophony: Voice sounds louder than usual.
     c. Whispered pectoriloquy: Client's whispered sounds are louder than normal.
D. Percuss chest.
E. Palpate.
  1. For lymphadenopathy, usually anterior or posterior cervical and supraclavicular nodes. Less commonly

involved lymph nodes include submandibular, axillary, and inguinal lymph nodes.
   2. To evaluate hepatosplenomegaly.
F. Neurologic examination:
   1. Evaluate the presence of nuchal rigidity.
   2. Assess deep tendon reflexes.

Diagnostic Tests

Diagnosis is based on a combination of tuberculin skin testing, purified protein derivative (PPD) testing, and sputum cultures. Bronchoscopy may be required to obtain specimens. Clients with primary TB may not undergo imaging; however, conventional CXR may be performed, and 15% of clients with primary TB have normal chest radiograph (CXR) findings.

Clients with progressive primary or postprimary TB may need a CT to evaluate parenchymal involvement, satellite lesions, bronchogenic spread, and miliary disease. MRI may be ordered to evaluate complications, such as the extent of thoracic wall involvement with empyema:

A. Tuberculin skin test using the Mantoux test is the recommended method. The dosage of PPD should be injected intradermally into the volar aspect of the forearm using a 27-gauge needle. A wheal should be raised and should measure approximately six to ten mm in diameter. Skilled personnel should read the test in 48 to 72 hours after administration. Measure the amount of induration and note the erythema. Measure transverse to the long axis of the forearm (see Table 9.3).
B. Health Canada has approved two Interferon gamma release assays (IGRAs) for use. Test may not be covered by provincial health plans (OLA, TB booklet, 2015).
C. Annual Mantoux tests are given for those at high risk and have never had a positive skin test. There is no need to repeat PPD once the client has had a documented positive PPD from a reputable source.
D. AP and lateral CXR films: "Snowstorm" appearance indicates miliary TB; segmental consolidation and hilar adenopathy are common; pleural effusion may be present.
E. CBC with differential may be performed.
F. Sputum culture with acid-fast bacilli smears:
   1. Nasopharyngeal secretions and saliva not acceptable.
   2. Gastric aspirate specimens for children younger than six years old. (Young children do not have a cough deep enough for a sputum specimen.)
G. Interferon-gamma release assay (IGRAs) test.
H. HIV testing should be conducted for all clients with a positive TB skin test and no previously documented HIV infection or AIDS.
I. Pregnancy test (if indicated) to guide management.

Differential Diagnoses
A. Bronchiectasis.
B. Asthma.
C. Histoplasmosis.
D. Coccidioidomycosis.
E. Blastomycosis.
F. Malignancies.
G. Other pulmonary infections.
H. Aspiration pneumonia.

Plan
A. General interventions:
   1. Report all positive TB skin tests and confirmed cases of active TB infection to the local public health department (mandatory).
   2. Directly observed therapy (DOT) is available in all Canadian jurisdictions. Generally, it is required for all clients receiving treatment for active TB disease.
B. Client teaching:
   1. Educate clients regarding compliance to therapy, adverse effect of medications, and follow-up care.
C. Pharmacological therapy: For a full discussion of the treatment of TB see the Canadian Tuberculosis Standards, 7th Edition. Public Health Agency of Canada, 2014.
Latent TB Infection:
   1. First-line regime. Isoniazid and vitamin B6.
   2. Second line regime. INH and Rifampin (RMP).
   3. Alternative regime: RMP, orally. Oral RMP for 4 months is now considered a first line treatment for LatentTBI in many Canadian jurisdictions, especially where adherence and completion of the course of medication is an issue. Active TB must be carefully ruled out; an abnormal chest x-ray may warrant specialist referral before starting RMP as treatment for LatentTBI.

TABLE 9.3 Interpretation of Mantoux Tuberculin Skin Test

TB Skin Test Result—Induration Size	Situation Where Reaction Is Considered Positive
0–4 mm	• Generally considered negative; no treatment indicated • Children <5 years old and at high risk for TB
5 mm	• HIV infected • Close contact with a known or suspected tuberculosis within the past two years • Fibronodular disease on CXR • Organ transplantation • TNF-alpha inhibitors • Other immunosuppressive drugs • End-stage renal disease
10 mm	All others, including the following specifics: • TB skin test conversion (within two years) • Diabetes, malnutrition, cigarette smoking, heavy alcohol consumption • Silicosis • Haematological malignancies (leukaemia, lymphoma) and head and neck carcinoma

CXR, chest radiograph; TB, tuberculosis; TNF, tumour necrosis factor.
Source: © All rights reserved. Canadian Tuberculosis Standards, 7th Edition. Public Health Agency of Canada. Adapted and reproduced with permission from the Minister of Health, 2019.

Table 9.4 Treatment for Fully Drug-Sensitive Tuberculosis

Regime	Initial Phase (months)	Continuring Phase (months)	Total (months)
INH/RMP/PZA + EMB	2	4	6
INH/RMP	2	7	9

EMB, ethambutol; INH, isoniazid; PZA, pyrazinamide; RMP, rifampin.
Source: Ontario Lung Association. (2015). Tuberculosis information for health care providers (5th ed., p. 23). *Ontario Lung Association Tuberculosis Committee*. Retrieved from https://www.rcdhu.com/wp-content/uploads/2018/12/TB-Information-for-Health-Care-Providers-5th-edition.pdf

4. Children with LTBI can be treated with INH for nine months. Consultation with a TB specialist is recommended. (OLA, TB booklet, 2015)
D. Active TB disease:
1. Contact public health authorities and TB specialists for up-to-date recommendations on medications. Medication protocols vary and include the following first-line agents: Isoniazid (INH), rifampin (RMP), pyrazinamide (PZA), and ethambutol (EMB; see Table 9.4).
2. Compliance with drug regimen is most important.
3. Cases of drug-resistant TB [multidrug resistant: INH/RMP (MDR-TB) or extensively drug-resistant: INH/RMP + at least two second-line groups of drugs such fluorquinolones (XDR-TB)] should be referred to a TB specialist for management. These clients will be hospitalized for their initial treatment and must be on DOT once discharged. In 2012 eight percent of cases in Canada were INH resistant and 0.6% were MDR-TB. Seven cases of XDR-TB had been diagnosed in Canada as of 2013. (OLA, TB booklet, 2015)
4. The bacilli Calmettend–Guerin (BCG) vaccine is available for the prevention of disseminated TB. BCG is a live vaccine. BCG does not prevent infection with *M. tuberculosis.*

Follow-Up
A. Regular follow-up every four to eight weeks to ensure compliance and to monitor the adverse effects and response of the medications.
B. Repeat CXR may be performed after two to three months of therapy to observe the response to treatment for clients with pulmonary TB.
C. Consider monitoring liver enzymes monthly in the following clients:
1. Severe or disseminated TB.
2. Concurrent or recent hepatic disease or hepatobiliary tract disease from other causes.
3. Those receiving high doses of INH (10 mg/kg/d) in combination with rifampin, pyrazinamide, or both drugs.
4. Women who are pregnant or within the first six weeks postpartum.
5. Clinical evidence of hepatotoxic effects.
6. Liver enzymes should be measured before starting treatment for LTBI or active TB disease.

Consultation/Referral
A. Consult a TB specialist or an Infectious Diseases specialist for the management of all clients with active disease.

Individual Considerations
A. Pregnancy:
1. Clients who are pregnant must be referred to a TB specialist for the management of active TB disease.
2. INH/RMP are considered safe in pregnancy and breastfeeding. There is increased risk of hepatotoxicity during pregnancy and for the first three months postpartum. Defer treatment for LTBI until after this period unless there is a high risk of progression to active disease (HIV, recent TB contact).
3. Chemotherapy:
   a. First-line agents include INH, rifampin, ethambutol and PZA.
   b. Streptomycin and most second-line drugs are contraindicated in pregnancy.
4. All pregnant women on INH therapy should receive pyridoxine.
5. Breastfeeding is safe during treatment.
B. Paediatrics:
1. Most children and adolescents with positive skin tests are asymptomatic.
2. Neonatal symptoms of TB typically develop in the second or third week of life and include poor feeding, poor weight gain, cough, lethargy, and irritability.
3. INH tablets can be crushed and added to food. Isoniazid liquid without sorbitol should be used to avoid osmotic diarrhoea.
4. Rifampin capsules can be opened and the powder added to food.
5. Young children are at high risk of disseminated TB and permanent sequela. Timely treatment is essential.
6. TB is commonly diagnosed clinically and should be considered in children presenting with superficial lymph adenopathy and CNS dysfunction.
C. Geriatrics:
1. The majority of cases of TB in older adults are due to reactivation of previous TB exposure.
2. Most cases of TB in older adults have pulmonary involvement (75%).
3. For long-term care, use a two-step TB PPD test for initial screening of newly admitted residents.
4. Treatment of active TB is the same as in younger adults. Renal and hepatic labs should be monitored according to the manufacturer's recommendations.
5. Adult clients who have recently converted to positive TB status should receive prophylaxis with INH for nine months.

Bibliography
Adams, L. V., & Starke, J. R. (2015, October). Tuberculosis disease in children. *UpToDate*. Retrieved from http://www.uptodate.comcontents/tuberculosis-disease-in-children

Adore, O., Burnell, C., Cuillerier, M., Davis, S., Fawcett, D., & Ontario Lung Association Tuberculosis Committee. (2015). *Tuberculosis: Information for health care providers*. Toronto, ON, Canada: Ontario Lung Association.

American Lung Association. (n. d.). *Tuberculosis*. Retrieved from http://www.lung.org/lung-health-and-diseases/lung-disease-lookup/tuberculosis

Flaherty, E., & Resnick, R (Eds.). (2014). *Geriatric nursing review syllabus: A core curriculum in advanced practice geriatric nursing* (4th ed.). New York, NY: American Geriatrics Society.

Hopewell, P. C., Kato-Maeda, M., & Ernst, J. D. (2016). Tuberculosis. In V. C. Broaddus, R. J. Mason, J. D. Ernst, T. E. King, S. C. Lazarus, J. F. Murray, . . . M. B. Gotway (Eds.), *Nadel's textbook of respiratory medicine* (6th ed., Vol. 1, pp. 593–628). Philadelphia, PA: Elsevier Saunders.

Menzies, D., Adjobimey, M., Ruslami, R., Trajman, A., Sow, O., Kim, H., . . . Benedetti, A. (2018). Four months of rifampin or nine months of isoniazid for latent tuberculosis in adults. *New England Journal of Medicine, 379*(5), 440–453. doi:10.1056/NEJMoa1714283

Pozniak, A. (2016, January 16). Clinical manifestations and complications of pulmonary tuberculosis. *UpToDate.* Retrieved from http://www.uptodate.com/contents/clinical-manifestations-and-complications-of-pulmonary-tuberculosis

Prescriber's Letter. (2013, May). *Appropriate med use* (Vol. 29). Retrieved from http://prescribersletter.therapeuticresearch.com/pl/ArticleDD.aspx?cs=&s=PRL&pt=6&fpt=31&dd=290501&pb=PRL&searchid=55980185

Public Health Agency of Canada. (2014). *Canadian Tuberculosis Standards* (7th ed.). Ottawa, Ontario, Canada https://www.canada.ca/en/public-health/services/infectious-diseases/canadian-tuberculosis-standards-7th-edition.html

Raviblione, M. C. (2015). Tuberculosis. In D. L. Kasper, A. S. Fauci, S. L. Hauser, D. L. Longo, & J. L. Jameson (Eds.), *Harrison's principles of internal medicine* (19th ed.). New York, NY: McGraw-Hill.

Schwartzstein, R. M., & Adams, L. (2016). *Murray & Nadel's textbook of respiratory medicine* (6th ed.). Philadelphia, PA: Elsevier-Saunders.

Sterling, T. R. (2016, January). Treatment of pulmonary tuberculosis in HIV-uninfected adults. *UpToDate.* Retrieved from http://www.uptodate.com/contents/treatment-of-pulmonary-tuberculosis-in-hiv-uninfected-adults

Valentine, N. (2017). Respiratory disorders. In B. Richardson (Ed.), *Pediatric primary care: Practice guidelines for nurses* (3rd ed., pp. 143–158). Burlington, MA: Jones & Bartlett.

10 Cardiovascular Guidelines

Acute Myocardial Infarction

Jill C. Cash, Debbie Gunter, and Krista A. Bradley

Definition
A. Acute myocardial infarction (MI) is a prolonged lack of myocardial oxygenation leading to necrosis of a portion of the heart muscle. It is caused by atherosclerotic coronary artery disease (CAD), which alone or in association with other factors causes complete blockage of one of the coronary arteries. It is important to distinguish between an MI, angina, and nonischaemic pain.

Incidence/Prevalence
A. According to the Report from the Canadian Chronic Disease Surveillance System: Heart Disease in Canada 2018, approximately 578,000 Canadian adults have a history of MI. Of these, 63,000 (2.3 per 1,000) had a first MI. Despite a marked decrease in incidence and mortality during the past three decades, MI continues to be a leading cause of death in this country.

Pathogenesis
A. Abrupt coronary artery occlusion is the primary cause of most MIs. Occlusions can result from atherosclerotic plaque, intracoronary thrombus formation, or arterial spasm.

Predisposing Factors
A. Hypercholesterolaemia: Increased low-density lipoprotein (LDL), decreased high-density lipoprotein (HDL).
B. Hypertriglyceridaemia.
C. Premature familial onset of coronary heart disease (CHD), formerly called CAD, before age 55.
D. Smoking.
E. Hypertension (HTN).
F. Obesity.
G. Sedentary lifestyle.
H. Diabetes mellitus.
I. Aging.
J. Stress.

Common Findings
A. Primary complaint: Pain somewhere in chest, described as worst pain ever experienced.
B. Nausea.
C. Vomiting.
D. Diaphoresis.
E. Indigestion.

Other Signs and Symptoms
A. Pain in abdomen, arm, back, jaw, and neck.
B. Chest heaviness or tightness.
C. Anxiety.
D. Cough.
E. Dyspnoea.
F. HTN or hypotension.
G. Weakness, light-headedness, syncope.
H. Pallor.
I. Orthopnoea.
J. Fatigue.
K. Malaise.

Potential Complications
A. Arrhythmias.
B. Heart failure (HF).
C. Cardiogenic shock.
D. Rupture of left ventricular (LV) papillary muscle.
E. Ventricular septal rupture.
F. Pericarditis or Dressler's syndrome.
G. Ventricular aneurysm.
H. Thromboembolism.
I. Death.

Subjective Data
A. Ask the client what activity brought about or preceded the cardiac symptoms.
B. Ask the client to describe the duration of symptoms and what time of day symptoms began.
C. Ask the client to describe the symptoms; for example, crushing, stabbing, or burning pain, shortness of breath and so on.
D. Ask the client where sensation began and in what direction it radiates.
E. Identify the degree of pain by using a pain scale of 1 to 10, with one being the least painful.
F. Inquire about the duration of the symptoms and whether anything relieves the symptoms.
G. Ask the client to list all medications currently being taken, particularly substances not prescribed and illicit drugs such as cocaine.

Physical Examination
Clients presenting with acute symptoms should be quickly assessed for the need to call emergency services/911 for immediate transport to the hospital.
A. Check pulse, respirations, blood pressure (BP), pulse oxygenation and ECG (if available).

B. Inspect:
　1. General appearance, noting dyspnoea and weakness.
　2. Skin for pallor and diaphoresis.
　3. Legs for oedema.
　4. Chest wall for visible pulsations.
　5. Neck for jugular vein distension.
　6. Nail beds for signs of cyanosis and note capillary filling time.
C. Palpate:
　1. Abdomen for organomegaly.
　2. Peripheral pulses in legs.
　3. Femoral pulses.
D. Auscultate:
　1. Auscultate carotid arteries.
　2. Auscultate abdomen.
　3. Conduct a complete heart examination, checking for dysrhythmias.
　4. Conduct a complete lung examination.
E. Mental status: Assess for confusion and anxiety.

Diagnostic Tests

A. ECG: Shows inverted T waves and ST segment elevation; depending on the timing, Q waves may also be present. One normal ECG initially does not always rule out MI; perform serial ECGs if MI is suspected.
B. Laboratory testing:
　1. Cardiac biomarkers/enzymes.
　2. Troponins: Troponins increase within three to four hours of injury and may remain elevated for one to two weeks.
　3. Creatine kinase (CK): CK-MB levels increase three to 12 hours after the chest pain begins, peak at 24 hours, and return to normal in 48 to 72 hours.
　4. Myoglobin: Urine myoglobin levels rise one to four hours after the chest pain begins (less commonly sent).
　5. Complete blood count (CBC).
　6. Chemistry profile.
　7. Lipid profile.
C. Cardiac imaging: Coronary angiogram.

Differential Diagnoses

A. Unstable angina pectoris.
B. Stable angina.
C. Aortic dissection.
D. Pulmonary embolism (PE).
E. Pericarditis.
F. Oesophageal spasm.
G. Pancreatitis.
H. Biliary tract disease.
I. Anxiety.
J. Chest trauma.
K. Pneumonia.
L. Musculoskeletal pain (nontraumatic).

Plan

A. General interventions:
　1. Educate the client and family regarding the signs and symptoms of an acute MI.
　2. Long-term care and treatment should be reinforced at each client visit.
B. Client teaching:
　1. Educate the client about modifying controllable risk factors, such as keeping diabetes and HTN under control, diet, exercise, and smoking cessation.
　2. If known CHD is present:
　　a. Instruct the client on signs and symptoms of an acute MI.
　　b. Advise the client to have a plan for seeking medical attention or dialing 911 if signs and symptoms occur.
　　c. Advise the client to carry nitroglycerin at all times and to take the nitroglycerin at the first sign of chest pain. If there is no relief after five minutes, 911 should be called. Nitroglycerin may be repeated every five minutes up to a total of three doses.
　　d. Encourage cardiopulmonary resuscitation (CPR) training for family members and close friends.
　　e. Exercise regimen: Encourage routine exercise for the client most days of the week, such as walking, treadmill use, and so on, once released by the cardiologist.
　　f. Advise smoking cessation as indicated. Encourage support groups, classes, and smoking cessation aids as indicated.
C. Dietary management: Counsel the client on nutrition and low-fat, low-cholesterol, low-sodium diet. Recommend the Dietary Approaches to Stop Hypertension (DASH) diet and lifestyle changes. Provide dietary handouts on the DASH diet, a low-fat/low-cholesterol/low-sodium diet. See Appendix B for the DASH diet.
D. Pharmacological therapy:
　1. When MI is suspected: ASA chewed or swallowed as soon as possible. Enteric-coated ASA delays absorption and therefore is not recommended.
　2. Instruct the client on how to take sublingual nitroglycerin tablets and other medications.
　3. Nitrates: Nitroglycerin sublingual tablets or nasal spray every five minutes for ischaemic chest pain in the absence of hypotension up to three doses. Monitor side effects: headache, hypotension.
　4. If pain persists after three doses of nitroglycerin:
　　a. Morphine sulphate IV, repeating every five minutes until pain resolves. Monitor side effects: nausea/vomiting, dizziness, hypotension.
　5. Oxygen therapy.
　6. In-hospital acute management: If there are no contraindications (bradycardia, HF, second- or third-degree heart block, asthma, shock), beta-blockers may be started intravenously (IV) during the acute phase and changed to oral therapy during the course of the treatment.
　7. In-hospital acute management: Fibrinolytic therapy may be used for clients with suspected MI with ST-elevation myocardial infarction (STEMI) or non-ST-elevation myocardial infarction (NSTEMI) with left bundle branch block.
　8. After an MI, if the client is not currently on a statin, a statin should be started.

Follow-Up

A. Follow-up is determined by the client's needs, severity of acute MI, and whether complications are present.

Consultation/Referral

A. If MI is suspected, call 911 and refer the client for immediate hospitalization.
B. According to the 2009 Canadian Cardiovascular Society guidelines, a client who is a candidate for reperfusion who is seen at a percutaneous coronary intervention (PCI)-capable hospital should be sent to the catheterization lab for primary PCI in 90 minutes or less. If the client is at a facility that is non-PCI capable, then a transfer should be made to a PCI

facility as soon as possible in 120 minutes or less. If time lapse will be more than 120 minutes, then it is recommended to administer fibrinolytic therapy within 30 minutes of arrival.
C. Follow up with cardiologist as scheduled when discharged from the hospital.

Individual Considerations
A. Adults:
  1. Women do not always complain of typical chest pain. Suspect MI in clients who complain of shortness of breath, back pain, jaw pain, nausea, just not feeling right.

B. Geriatrics:
  1. Consider MI in clients complaining of atypical chest pain. Symptoms may include dyspnoea, fatigue, dizziness, confusion, altered mental state.
  2. Older adults may not perceive chest pain as being severe and may not consider that symptoms may be related to a heart attack because of an altered pain perception. Educate older adults that pain perception may be diminished as one ages.

Bibliography
Amsterdam, E. A., Wenger, N. K., Brindis, R. G., Casey, D. E., Ganiats, T. G., Holmes, D. R., & Zieman, S. J. (2014). AHA/ACC guideline for the management of patients with non-ST-elevation acute coronary syndromes: A Report of the American College of Cardiology/American Heart Association Task Force on Practice Guidelines and the Heart Rhythm Society. *Circulation, 130*(25), e344–e426. doi:10.1161/CIR.0000000000000133

Drug information. (2016). *Prescribers' digital reference.* Retrieved from www.pdr.net

Eckel, R. H., Jakicic, J. M., Ard, J. D., deJesus, J. M., HoustonMiller, N., Hubbard, V. S., & Yanovsk, S. Z. (2014). 2013 AHA/ACC guideline on lifestyle management to reduce cardiovascular risk: A report of the American College of Cardiology/American Heart Association Task Force on practice guidelines. *Circulation, 129*(25), S76–S99. doi:10.1161/01.cir.0000437740.48606.d1

Goff, D. C., Lloyd-Jones, D. M., Bennett, G., Coady, S., & D'Agostino, B. R., Sr. (2014). 2013 ACC/AHA guideline on the assessment of cardiovascular risk: A report of the American College of Cardiology/American Heart Association Task Force on practice guidelines. *Circulation,* S49–S73. doi:10.1161/01.cir.0000437741.48606.98

O'Gara, P. T., Kushner, F. G., Ascheim, D. D., Casey, D. E., Chung, M. K., deLemos, J. A., & Zhao, D. X. (2013a). 2013 ACCF/AHA guideline for the management of ST-elevation myocardial infarction: A report of the American College of Cardiology Foundation/American Heart Association Task Force on Practice Guidelines. *Circulation, 127*(4), e362–e425. doi:10.1161/CIR.0b013e3182742c84

O'Gara, P. T., Kushner, F. G., Ascheim, D. D., Casey, D. E., Chung, M. K., deLemos, J. A., & Zhao, D. X. (2013b, January). 2013 ACCF/AHA guideline for the management of ST-elevation myocardial infarction: A report of the American College of Cardiology Foundation/American Heart Association Task Force on Practice Guidelines. *Journal of the American College of Cardiology, 61*(4), e78–e140. Retrieved from http://content.onlinejacc.org/article.aspx?articleid=1486115

Public Health Agency of Canada. (2018). *Report from the Canadian chronic disease surveillance system: Heart disease in 2018. Canada.* Retrieved from https://www.canada.ca/content/dam/phac-aspc/documents/services/publications/diseases-conditions/report-heart-disease-canada-2018/pub1-eng.pdf

Welsh, R. C., Travers, A., Huynh, T., Cantor, W. J., & Canadian Cardiovascular Society Working Group. (2009). Providing a perspective on the 2007 focused update of the American College of Cardiology and American Heart Association 2004 guidelines for the management of ST elevation myocardial infarction. *Canadian Journal of Cardiology, 25*(1), 25–32. doi:10.1016/S0828-282X(09)70019-4

Arrhythmias

Jill C. Cash, Debbie Gunter, and Krista A. Bradley

Definition
Arrhythmias are abnormal heart rhythms. Common types are the following:

A. Sinus bradycardia: Heart rate <60 beats per minute (bpm); impulse originates in sinoatrial (SA) node.
B. Sinus tachycardia: Heart rate >100 to 160 bpm; impulse originates in SA node.
C. Supraventricular tachydysrhythmias (SVTs): Heart rate >100 bpm; the origin of impulse is listed as follows:
  1. Atrioventricular (AV) nodal reentrant tachycardia (NRT) is intranodal reentry by means of fast and slow conduction pathways within the AV junction.
  2. Orthodromic atrioventricular reentrant tachycardia (AVRT) is tachycardia across accessory pathways associated with preexcitation.

D. Atrial fibrillation (AF): Chaotic electrical activity caused by rapid discharges from numerous ectopic foci in atria. Atrial rate is difficult to count. There are three types of AF:
  1. Paroxysmal AF occurs in clients who usually have normal sinus rhythm (NSR), but then have an episode of faulty electrical signals and rapid heart rate. This usually starts suddenly and stops on its own. Symptoms can be mild or severe and usually stop in <24 hours, but may last for several days.
  2. Persistent AF is a condition in which the abnormal heart rhythm continues for more than a week. It may stop on its own, or it can be stopped with treatment.
  3. Permanent AF is a condition in which a normal heart rhythm cannot be restored with treatment. Both paroxysmal and persistent AF may become more frequent and, over time, result in permanent AF.

E. Premature ventricular contractions (PVCs) are impulses that form within the Purkinje network.

Incidence/Prevalence
A. SVTs are the most common cardiac arrhythmias presenting to health-care providers.
B. Atrioventricular nodal reentrant tachycardia (AVNRT) accounts for 60% to 70% of all SVTs.
C. AVRTs account for 30% to 40% of all SVTs. Greater than 90% of younger children who present with SVTs are likely to have an AVRT, but once they reach adolescence, AVNRT is the primary cause of SVT in about one-third of these clients.
D. AF is the most common cardiac tachydysrhythmia. According to the Canadian Task Force on Preventative Health Atrial Fibrillation Guidelines (2014), AF affects approximately 4.5% of the general population with a lifetime risk of approximately 25% among clients older than 40 years. The presence of AF is associated with a fivefold increase in the risk of morbidity, a twofold increase in mortality, and an increased incidence of embolic stroke.
E. PVCs are common, and their frequency increases with age.

Pathogenesis
A. Bradycardia: Dominance of the parasympathetic nervous system, with excessive vagal stimulation to the heart, causes a decreased heart rate of sinus node discharge.
B. Tachycardia: Dominant sympathetic nervous system stimulation of the heart or vagal inhibition results in positive chronotropic, dromotropic, and inotropic effects.
C. AVRT: The most classic form of this SVT is Wolff–Parkinson–White (WPW) syndrome. Reentry occurs in a loop using atrial myocardium, AV node–His–Purkinje system, ventricular myocardium, and an accessory AV connection. During sinus rhythm, antegrade conduction through the accessory connection depolarizes the myocardium earlier than would occur by conduction through the AV node–His–Purkinje system, preexcitation is present, and a delta wave

(slurring of initial deflection of the QRS complex) is usually seen on the surface 12-lead ECG.
D. AVNRT: The most common form is antegrade conduction, which occurs through a pathway with a short effective refractory period (ERP) and a longer conduction time. This pathway is often referred to as the *slow pathway*.
E. AF: Multiple, rapid impulses from many foci depolarize the atria in a totally disorganized manner. In the chaos, no P waves, no atrial contraction, no atrial kick, and a totally irregular ventricular response occur. The atria quiver, which leads to formation of mural thrombi and potential embolic events.
F. PVCs: These originate in the ventricles as a result of increased irritability in those cells.

Predisposing Factors
A. Bradycardia:
  1. Increased vagal tone.
  2. Decreased sympathetic drive.
  3. Ischaemia to SA node.
  4. Drugs: Digitalis, sedatives, beta-blockers, diltiazem, verapamil, amiodarone, parasympathomimetics.
  5. Normal variant in athletes.
  6. Atrial enlargement.
  7. Acute myocardial infarction (MI).
  8. Chronic heart failure (CHF).
  9. Rheumatic heart disease.
  10. Hypertensive heart disease.
  11. Hypothyroidism.
  12. Hypothermia.
  13. Electrolyte abnormality.
  14. Acidosis.
  15. Infection.
B. Tachycardia:
  1. Decreased vagal tone.
  2. Increased sympathetic tone.
  3. MI.
  4. Hyperthyroidism.
  5. Caffeine.
  6. Illicit drugs such as cocaine.
C. SVT:
  1. Digitalis toxicity.
  2. Catecholamine surge.
  3. Heart failure.
  4. Thyroid disease.
  5. Chronic lung disease.
  6. Smoking.
  7. Heavy alcohol or caffeine ingestion.
D. AF:
  1. Myocardial ischaemia.
  2. Hypertension.
  3. Heart failure.
  4. Coronary artery disease.
  5. Cardiomyopathy.
  6. Coronary artery bypass surgery.
  7. Myocarditis/pericasrditis.
  8. Pulmonary embolism.
  9. Thyrotoxicosis.
  10. Heavy alcohol use.
E. PVC.
  1. Stress.
  2. Heart failure.
  3. Coronary artery disease.
  4. Hypertension.
  5. Alcohol ingestion.
  6. Caffeine.
  7. Decongestants and antihistamines.
  8. Illicit drugs such as cocaine.

Common Findings
A. Symptoms may not be present; however, client may note irregular heartbeat.
B. Palpitations.
C. Chest discomfort.
D. Shortness of breath (SOB).
E. Dizziness.
F. Diaphoresis.
G. Weakness.
H. Syncope.
I. Nausea.

Subjective Data
A. Obtain an accurate health and medical history.
B. Explore precipitating factors such as emotional stress, alcohol or drug use, or hot tub or bath use.
C. Inquire about the onset and duration of symptoms, also noting the client's age when symptoms began.
D. Explore whether the client has had concomitant weight loss, mood changes, and tremour, which are often associated with hyperthyroidism.
E. Carefully determine the number of previous episodes of palpitations or symptoms and what treatment, if any, was initiated.
F. Review all medications, including prescription, over-the-counter (OTC), and herbal products.

Physical Examination
A. Check pulse, respirations, blood pressure (BP), and weight:
  1. Sinus bradycardia: Pulse rate decreased below 60 bpm.
  2. ECG: Normal.
  3. Sinus tachycardia: Pulse rate increased above 100 bpm:
     a. Pulse regular.
     b. Systolic BP (SBP) constant.
  4. AF:
     a. Pulse irregular.
     b. SBP changing.
  5. AVNRT:
     a. Pulse regular; AV block usual.
     b. Systolic BP (SBP) constant; electrical alternans rare.
  6. AVRT:
     a. Pulse regular; AV block not present.
     b. SBP constant; electrical alternans common, especially at high heart rates.
  7. PVC: Pulse diminished or absent during the PVC.
B. Inspect:
  1. General appearance:
     a. Is the client in respiratory distress? Note SOB, chest pain, dyspnoea.
     b. Does the client look anxious or apathetic? This may be a sign of an anxiety or thyroid problem.
  2. Inspect the skin for flushing or pallor.
  3. Examine the eyes, noting lid lag.
  4. Assess the neck for jugular vein distension or thyromegaly:
     a. With sinus tachycardia, neck vein pulsation is normal.
     b. With AF, neck vein pulsation is irregular; assess for thyromegaly.

c. AVNRT: Assess the neck veins for "frog sign," in which the atria contract against closed AV valves, producing rapid, regular, expansive venous pulsation in the neck, resembling the rhythmic puffing motion of a frog.
d. AVRT: Assess for frog sign.

C. Auscultate the neck for carotid artery bruits and the heart for abnormal heart sounds. Heart rhythm may be regular or irregular, depending on type of dysrhythmia. Have the client perform vagal maneuver (Valsalva's maneuver). If the rapid heart rate responds to the vagal maneuver and the cycle is broken, it is likely the client has AVRT. If it does not respond, it is possible the client has AVNRT:
1. Sinus bradycardia:
   a. Rate less than 60 bpm.
   b. Rhythm regular.
2. Sinus tachycardia:
   a. Rate >100 bpm.
   b. Rhythm regular; gradual onset and cessation.
   c. Constant loudness of first heart sound.
3. AF:
   a. Rate: Atrial rate is nonmeasurable, ventricular rate is variable, usually rapid at onset.
   b. Rhythm: Atrial and ventricular rhythms are irregular.
   c. Loudness of first heart sound changes.
4. AVNRT:
   a. AV block is usually present.
   b. Loudness of first heart sound is constant.
5. AVRT
   a. AV block is not present.
   b. Constant loudness of first heart sound
6. PVC
   a. Rate depends on underlying rhythm.
   b. Rhythm: Prematurity interrupts regularity of rhythm.

Diagnostic Tests
A. ECG.
B. Drug screen:
   1. Digitalis.
   2. Aminophylline.
   3. Illicit drugs.
C. Electrolytes.
D. Arterial blood gases (ABGs) if indicated.

Differential Diagnoses
A. Multifocal atrial tachycardia.
B. Sinus tachycardia with multiple premature atrial contractions.
C. Atrial flutter.
D. Ventricular tachycardia.
E. AV blocks.

Plan
A. General interventions:
   1. Remove as many predisposing factors as possible.
   2. Stop smoking.
   3. Decrease or stop caffeine use.
B. Client teaching:
   1. Teach relaxation techniques.
   2. Teach the client and his or her family signs of haemodynamic compromise, including rapid heart rate, unexplained weight gain or loss, worsening dyspnoea on exertion, and decreased exercise tolerance.
   3. Teach and reassure the client about long-term medication therapy and its side effects.
   4. Educate the client and family regarding safety, dietary restrictions, and complications that may occur (bleeding) with the use of anticoagulant therapy.
   5. Discuss the need for a pacemaker/defibrillator or surgical ablation.
C. Pharmacological therapy:
   1. Selection of treatment modality should be based on underlying pathophysiology.
   2. For reentrant cases (AVNRT, AVRT), agents that block the reentrant circuit are more effective:
      a. Calcium channel blockers (CCBs).
      b. Beta-blockers—long acting.
      c. Digitalis.
   3. Episodes caused by increased automaticity are treated with antiarrhythmic therapy.
   4. Chronic nonvalvular AF is treated with a non–vitamin K antagonist oral anticoagulant (NOAC; Clinical Practice Guideline for the Management of Atrial Fibrillation www. onlinecjc. ca/article/S0828-282X(16)30829-7/pdf).
      a. Start therapy as soon as possible if a history of underlying heart disease is present.
      b. Evaluate prothrombin time/international normalized ratio (PT/INR) on a regular basis to monitor for therapeutic response to warfarin sodium treatment.

Follow-Up
A. Clients who have their first episode of AF should return to the clinic within 24 to 48 hours for reevaluation.
B. Clients on antiarrhythmic agents should have liver enzymes measured during the first four to eight weeks of therapy.
C. Clients with risk factors for developing cardiac complications to therapy, like QT prolongation, should have ECG during the first weeks of therapy and every three to six months thereafter.
D. Monitor clients on digoxin carefully for digitalis toxicity.
E. Clients on digitalis should be carefully monitored for signs of toxicity. Caution the client regarding interactions of medication with digitalis.

Consultation/Referral
A. Clients with haemodynamic instability should be referred to a hospital or 911 immediately.
B. Clients unable to tolerate their dysrhythmia should be hospitalized immediately.
C. Consult a cardiologist if the client has an abnormal ECG pattern, refractory AF, suspicion of WPW syndrome, or sick sinus syndrome, or when questions arise about the difference between a narrow and wide QRS complex.

Individual Considerations
A. Pregnancy: Digitalis is safe during pregnancy.
B. Paediatrics:
   1. Paroxysmal supraventricular tachycardia (PSVT) is probably the most common paediatric arrhythmia.
   2. Instruct young adult clients without underlying heart disease to quit/avoid smoking, avoid sleep deprivation, and limit use of alcohol and stimulants.

Resources
Canadian Task Force on Preventative Health Care Atrial Fibrillation Guidelines: Recommendations for Stroke Prevention and Rate/Rhythm Control: https://canadiantaskforce.ca/portfolios/atrial-fibrillation/

Bibliography

Drug information. (2016). *Prescribers' digital reference*. Retrieved from www.pdr.net

Go, A. S., Mozaffarian, D., Roger, V. L., Benjamin, E. J., Berry, J. D., & Borden, W. B. (2013). Heart disease and stroke statistics—2013 update: A report from the American Heart Association. American Heart Association Statistics Committee and Stroke Statistics Subcommittee. *Circulation*, *127*(1), e6–e245. doi:10.1161/CIR.0b013e31828124ad

Mozaffarian, D., Benjamin, E. J., & Go, A. S. (2015). Heart disease and stroke statistics—2015 update: A report from the American Heart Association. *Circulation*, *131*(4), e29–e322. doi:10.1161/CIR.0000000000000152

Atherosclerosis and Hyperlipidaemia

Jill C. Cash, Debbie Gunter, and Krista A. Bradley

Definition

A. Atherosclerosis is a systemic disease characterized by lipid deposition and smooth muscle cell migration and proliferation in the intima of the larger arteries. Atheromatous changes lead to thrombotic stroke, peripheral vascular disease (PVD), atherosclerotic cardiovascular disease (ASCVD), and myocardial infarction (MI).

B. Hyperlipidaemia is an elevation in serum lipoproteins and a major risk factor in the development of cardiovascular disease (CVD). The two main lipids in blood are cholesterol and triglyceride. Cholesterol is a relatively insoluble lipid that is necessary for cell membrane formation, steroid and bile salt production, and the development of nerve sheaths. Cholesterol is composed of three clinically significant components: high-density lipoprotein cholesterol (HDL-C), low-density lipoprotein cholesterol (LDL-C), and very-low-density lipoprotein (VLDL). Triglyceride is found in VLDL particles, but its role in atherosclerosis is not clear.

C. The atherosclerotic buildup of lipids, cholesterol, calcium, and cellular debris within the intima of the blood vessels causes plaque formation, vascular remodeling, and acute and chronic obstruction of the lumen of the blood vessels, which in turn decreases blood flow causing myocardial ischaemia and decreased oxygen to other vital organs.

D. In 2016, the Canadian Cardiovascular Society (CCS) released updated guidelines for the assessment of cardiovascular risk, lifestyle management, and treatment of cholesterol to reduce ASCVD risks. A downloadable sheet enabling estimation of 10-year and lifetime risk for ASCVD and a web-based calculator are available (see www. ccs. ca/images/Guidelines/Tools_and_Calculators_En/FRS_eng_2017_fnl_grey. pdf). These risk tools are used to drive conversations on client risk factors for ASCVD, potential benefits, negative aspects of risk, and client preferences regarding initiation of relevant therapies. The assessment of ASCVD risk factors is recommended every four to six years in adults 20 to 79 years of age who are free from ASCVD and estimate 10-year ASCVD risk every four to six years in adults aged 40 to 79 years who are free from ASCVD. Long-term and lifetime risk information may be used to motivate therapeutic lifestyle changes (TLCs), and encourage adherence to these changes and pharmacological therapies.

Incidence/Prevalence

A. Atherosclerosis begins in childhood with the development of fatty streaks. The incidence of atherosclerotic diseases increases with age. In Canada, 29% of all death occur as a result of heart disease, with one death from heart disease or stroke occurring every seven minutes. The annual cost to the Canadian economy from CVD is estimated at $20.9 billion.

B. The leading risk factors for CVD are hypertension (HTN), high cholesterol, and smoking:
  1. HTN can increase arterial wall tension, potentially leading to disturbed repair processes and aneurysm formation.
  2. Cigarette smoking is associated with an increase in multiple inflammatory markers, including C-reactive protein (CRP), interleukin-6, and tumour necrosis factor.

Pathogenesis

A. Atherosclerosis is in part attributed to the deposition of cholesterol and lipoproteins in arterial smooth muscle cells. Dietary factors, obesity, drugs, and genetic defects in lipoprotein particle metabolism influence lipid and lipoprotein concentrations in blood.

B. Primary hyperlipoproteinaemias are either caused by single-gene disorders transmitted by simple dominant or recessive mechanisms, or to multifactorial disorders with complicated inheritance patterns.

C. Secondary hyperlipoproteinaemias (such as in thyroid disease and diabetes mellitus) occur as part of a constellation of abnormalities in certain metabolic pathways. The association among atherosclerosis, CVD, and hypercholesterolaemia is well documented. HDL-C comprises about one-fourth of the total serum cholesterol and acts as a scavenger, removing cholesterol from peripheral tissues and returning it to the liver, which produces a favourable cardioprotective effect. Elevated HDL-C levels are desirable. HDL-C levels 1.55 mmol/L are a negative risk factor for CVD; those below 0.91 mmol/L are a major risk factor for CVD.

D. LDL-C constitutes 70% of the total serum cholesterol. It is the most atherogenic cholesterol subgroup. LDL-C particles interact with platelets, damaged arterial endothelium, and smooth muscle cells in the process of plaque formation. LDL-C levels of 4.14 mmol/L or greater are associated with an increased number of cardiac events.

E. VLDL accounts for a small amount of total serum cholesterol and is responsible for carrying triglycerides from the liver. Its role in atherogenesis is uncertain, but an inverse relationship has been observed between VLDL and HDL-C.

Predisposing Factors

A. High-risk factors for cardiovascular disease (CVD) events (CVD risk equivalent):
  1. Clinical CVD.
  2. Symptomatic carotid artery disease.
  3. Peripheral arterial disease (PAD).
  4. Abdominal aortic aneurysm.

B. Presence of major risk factors (other than LDL-C):
  1. **Age is the strongest risk factor for the development of CVD:**
      a. Age greater than 45 years for men and greater than 55 years for women.
      b. Elderly persons experience a higher morbidity and mortality.
  2. Cigarette smoking.
  3. Low HDL-C level, less than 1.04 mmol/L.
  4. Family history of early CVD: MI or sudden cardiac death younger than 55 years in father or other male first-degree relative, or before age 65 years in mother or other female first-degree relative.
  5. HTN (blood pressure [BP] > 140/90 mmHg or on antihypertensive medication).
  6. Sedentary lifestyle.
  7. Obesity.

8. Metabolic syndrome.
9. Diabetes.
10. Chronic inflammation.

HDL-C > 1.55 mmol/L is equal to a "negative" risk factor and removes one risk factor from the total count.

Common Findings
A. There are no complaints or symptoms associated with atherosclerosis and hyperlipidaemia. Most lipid abnormalities are detected by routine laboratory testing or as part of a cardiovascular evaluation.

Subjective Data
A. Ask the client whether there is a history of CVD.
B. Discuss his or her past medical history, including predisposing factors for CVD.
C. Have the client list current medications, including over-the-counter (OTC) and herbal products.
D. Have the client discuss his or her current diet and exercise routine.
E. Explore the client's social habits, including use of alcohol and tobacco.

Physical Examination
A. Check pulse, respirations, BP, height, and weight. Calculate body mass index (BMI) at each subsequent visit. BMI calculators are available online.
B. Inspect:
 1. Funduscopic examination: Examine eyes for premature arcus cornealis, which is a gray opaque line around the cornea caused by lipid degeneration, and for lipaemia retinalis, or a pale retina with white blood vessels caused by excess serum lipids because of VLDL of more than 51.8 mmol/L or alcoholism.
 2. Inspect skin for xanthomas, which appear as red–brown or yellow papules, nodules, or plaque, caused by lipid deposits from high VLDL. Tendinous xanthomas are found on Achilles tendons, patellae, and hands.
 3. Inspect joints for Achilles tendonitis and arthritis.
C. Palpate:
 1. Palpate abdomen for hepatomegaly or splenomegaly.
 2. Palpate neck and thyroid.
D. Auscultate:
 1. Perform a complete heart examination.
 2. Perform a complete vascular examination.

Diagnostic Tests
A. Laboratory testing:
 1. Lipid profile.
 2. Complete blood count (CBC).
 3. Complete metabolic panel (CMP).
 4. Thyroid function studies to exclude disorders of the thyroid.
 5. CRP.
 6. Haemoglobin A1C (if appropriate).
B. Tests/imaging:
 1. Treadmill stress test.
 2. Nuclear stress test.
 3. Multigated Acquisition Scan (MUGA).
 4. CT angiography.
 5. Coronary angioplasty.

Differential Diagnoses
Assess the client for the following secondary causes of ASCVD and hyperlipidaemia:
A. Diabetes mellitus.
B. Hypothyroidism.
C. Nephrotic syndrome.
D. Porphyria.
E. Obesity.
F. Obstructive liver disease.
G. Diuretic use.

Plan
A. General interventions:
 1. TLCs, including exercise, diet, and weight management, are recommended for all clients.
 2. Increased physical activity. The 2016 Canadian Cardiovascular Society's Dyslipidemia Guidelines for Treatment: Health Behavior Interventions outline the physical activity recommendations advising adults to engage. At least 150 minutes of aerobic physical activity in sessions of 10 minutes or more each week. The aerobic exercise should involve moderate to vigorous intensity to reduce BP, LDL-C, and non-HDL-C.
B. Dietary management:
 1. Advise the client that diet modification is the first line of therapy for hyperlipidaemia.
 2. Explain cholesterol-lowering diet, such as the Mediterranean Diet recommended in the 2016 Canadian Cardiovascular Society's Dyslipidemia Guidelines for Treatment: Health Behavior Interventions. Give dietary recommendation sheets. See Appendix B for low-fat/low-cholesterol and DASH dietary approaches to stop HTN.
C. Client teaching:
 1. Weight reduction:
  a. Explain that weight reduction in clients greater than 20% over ideal body weight can lower LDL-C and triglyceride levels.
 2. Other key dietary recommendations include the following:
  a. Reduce intake of saturated fats and trans fats. Aim for 5% to 6% of calories from saturated fat.
  b. Increase intake of poly- and monounsaturated fats.
  c. Increase intake of soluble fiber (psyllium supplement).
  d. Limit intake of alcohol: One drink per day for women and two drinks per day for men.
  e. Increase intake of plant stanols and sterols.
  f. Follow the Dietary Approaches to Stop Hypertension (DASH), Mediterranean, or AHA diet.
  g. Lower sodium intake. Consume no more than 2,400 mg/d of sodium. Further reductions to 1,500 mg/d of sodium are associated with greater reduction in BP.
 3. Discuss smoking cessation *(Refer to Client Teaching Guide: Nicotine Dependence)*.
D. Pharmacological therapy: **Use clinical judgment when deciding potential benefits, possible side effects, and costs of drug treatment:**
 1. First-line treatment: 3 Hydroxy-3 Methyl-Glutaryl Coenzyme A Reductase (HMG-CoA) reductase inhibitors (statins):
  a. Statins suppress the activity of the key enzyme in cholesterol synthesis in the liver; they are highly effective in lowering LDL-C but can cause liver toxicity, myositis, rhabdomyolysis, and low HDL-C.

b. There are four major statin benefit groups:
   i. Individuals with the presence of clinical ASCVD, including acute coronary syndromes, a history of MI, stable or unstable angina, coronary or other arterial revascularization, stroke, transient ischaemic attack (TIA), or PAD.
   ii. Individuals with primary elevations of LDL-C ≥4.92 mmol/L.
   iii. Individuals 40 to 75 years of age with diabetes and LDL-C 1.81 to 4.89 mmol/L and without clinical ASCVD (refer to Chapter 20, Endocrine Guidelines)
   iv. Individuals without clinical ASCVD or diabetes who are 40 to 75 years of age with an LDL-C 1.81 to 4.89 mmol/L and an estimated 10-year ASCVD risk of 7.5% or higher.
c. ASCVD events are reduced by using the maximum tolerated statin intensity in those groups shown to benefit. The expert panel defines intensity of statin therapy on the basis of the average expected LDL-C response to a specific statin and dose. The intensity levels are "high-intensity," "moderate-intensity," and "low-intensity" statin therapy. Full statin treatment recommendations for primary and secondary prevention as well as the high-, moderate-, and low-intensity statin therapy from the 2017 CCS Lipid Guidelines on the treatment of cholesterol are available at www. ccs. ca/images/Guidelines/-Tools_and_Calculators_En/FRS_eng_2017_fnl_grey. pdf.
d. Monitor liver function tests (LFTs) before therapy begins, then four to six weeks after starting drug therapy. Check at six- to 12-month intervals or more frequently, if necessary.
e. Discontinue medications if abnormal laboratory values or adverse symptoms appear.
f. Use caution with the use of statins and other medications. Avoid concomitant drugs such as erythromycin, nicotine, azole antifungals, clofibrate, and gemfibrozil.
2. Statins are harmful or potentially harmful for the fetus and are contraindicated in pregnancy.
3. Nonstatin drug therapy (see Table 10.1 for the nonstatin drugs that affect cholesterol):
   a. Bile acid sequestrants bind bile acids in the gastrointestinal (GI) tract; lower moderately elevated LDL-C by 20%; and may cause constipation, bloating, and poor absorption of other drugs. Bile acid sequestrant therapy is not recommended if triglycerides are >3.39 mmol/L.
   b. Nicotinic acid or niacin: Broad-spectrum lipid-regulating agent. Niacin has been documented to exhibit anti-inflammatory properties (reduction of lipoprotein-associated phospholipase A2 and CRP). Discuss possibilities of flushing. Contraindicated with chronic liver disease and severe gout. The niacin-treated subjects in the Atherothrombosis Intervention in Metabolic Syndrome with Low HDL/High Triglycerides: Impact on Global Health (AIM-HIGH) clinical trial had a trend toward increased stroke incidence.
   c. Fibric acid derivatives: Highly effective in lowering triglycerides; it lowers VLDL-C, causes modest reduction in LDL-C, and raises HDL-C:
      i. The combination of niacin with other lipid-lowering drugs has been shown to reduce progression and promote regression of coronary and carotid atherosclerosis and improve clinical outcomes.
      ii. Fibrates may cause GI distress, rash, pain, blurred vision, anaemia, and gallstones.
      iii. Fibrates may inhibit insulin and oral hypoglycaemic absorption, and potentiates oral anticoagulants.

Nonstatin Drugs Affecting Lipoprotein Metabolism

Drug Class	Agents	Lipid/Lipoprotein Effects	Side Effects	Contraindications
Bile acid sequestrants	Cholestyramine, Colestipol, Colesevelam	LDL-C ↓ 15%–30% HDL-C ↑ 3%–5% TG No change or increase	Gastrointestinal distress Constipation Decreased absorption of other drugs	Absolute: • Dysbeta-lipoproteinaemia • TG >4.52 mmol/L Relative: • TG >2.26 mmol/L
Nicotinic acid	Immediate release (crystalline) nicotinic acid, extended release nicotinic acid, sustained release nicotinic acid	LDL-C ↓ 5%–25% HDL-C ↑ 15%–35% TG ↓ 20%–50%	Flushing Hyperglycaemia Hyperuricaemia (or gout) Upper GI distress Hepatotoxicity	Absolute: • Chronic liver disease • Severe gout Relative: • Diabetes • Hyperuricaemia • Peptic ulcer disease
Fibric acids	Gemfibrozil, Fenofibrate, Clofibrate	LDL-C ↓ 5%–20% (may be increased in clients with high TG) HDL-C ↑ 10%–20% TG ↓ 20%–50%	Dyspepsia Gallstones Myopathy	Absolute: • Severe renal disease • Severe hepatic disease

GI, gastrointestinal; HDL-C, high-density lipoprotein cholesterol; LDL-C, low-density lipoprotein cholesterol; TG, triglyceride.

Follow-Up

A. Measure client's total cholesterol four weeks after initiation of diet and then at three- to four-month intervals.
B. If initiating medication therapy, obtain baseline blood work, including fasting lipid profile with LFTs and a CBC. Recheck tests four to six weeks after starting drug therapy. Then check at six- to 12-month intervals or more frequently, if necessary.

Consultation/Referral

A. Refer to dietitian for dietary modifications.

Individual Considerations

A. Adults:
  1. Clients with high cholesterol who are otherwise at low risk for ASCVD (particularly men older than age 35 years and premenopausal women) are candidates for primary prevention emphasizing diet modification and increased physical activity. It is recommended that drug therapy be used sparingly in these clients.
  2. Lowering serum cholesterol reduces morbidity and mortality in clients with ASCVD, and it also reduces the number of new cardiac events in those without known ASCVD.
  3. Elevated triglycerides increase the risk of pancreatitis and diabetes.

B. Children:
  1. It is uncommon for children to have events secondary to atherosclerosis during childhood; however, the buildup of plaque begins during childhood and progressive changes can lead to heart events during early adulthood. Risk factors for children for this to occur include obesity, high BP, family history of heart disease, depression/bipolar disorder, exposure to cigarette smoking, and underlying chronic conditions.
  2. Educate and lifestyle changes during childhood are imperative to prevent these events in children and early adulthood. Education should include healthy diet, exercise, and avoiding exposures (cigarette smoke) that increase risk factors.
  3. Guidelines for screening children have been developed according to risk factors and can be found in the CCS Dyslipidemia Guidelines in the section "Who to Screen." www. ccs. ca/images/Guidelines/PocketGuides_EN/Lipids_Gui_2016_EN. pdf Page 3.

Resources

Canadian Cardiovascular Society Framingham Risk Score: https://www. ccs. ca/images/Guidelines/Tools_and_Calculators_En/FRS_eng_2017_fnl_grey. pdf

Mediterranean Diet: https://www.nutrition.va.gov/docs/UpdatedPatient-Ed/Mediterraneandiet.pdf

Bibliography

Boudi, F. B. (2016, April 25). Coronary artery atherosclerosis. *Medscape*. Retrieved from emedicine.medscape.com/article/153647-overview

Canadian Cardiovascular Society. (2016). *Dyslipidemia guidelines for treatment: Health behavior interventions*. Retrieved from https://www.ccs.ca/images/Guidelines/Tools_and_Calculators_En/FRS_eng_2017_fnl_grey.pdf

Drug information. (2016). *Prescribers' digital reference*. Retrieved from www.pdr.net

Eckel, R. H., Jakicic, J. M., Ard, J. D., deJesus, J. M., HoustonMiller, N., Hubbard, V. S., & Yanovsk, S. Z. (2014). 2013 AHA/ACC guideline on lifestyle management to reduce cardiovascular risk: A report of the American College of Cardiology/American Heart Association Task Force on practice guidelines. *Circulation*, 129(25), S76–S99. doi:10.1161/01.cir.0000437740.48606.d1. Retrieved from http://circ.ahajournals.org/content/129/25_suppl_2/S76

Go, A. S., Bauman, M. C., King, S. M., Fonarow, G. C., Lawrence, W., Williams, K. A., & Sanchez, E. (2014, April). An effective approach to high blood pressure control: A science advisory from the American Heart Association, the American College of Cardiology, and the Centers for Disease Control and Prevention. *Hypertension*, 63(4), 878–885. doi:10.1161/CIR.0b013e31828124ad. Retrieved from http://hyper.ahajournals.org/content/early/2013/11/14/HYP.0000000000000003.reprint

Goff, D. C., Lloyd-Jones, D. M., Bennett, G., Coady, S., & D'Agostino, B. R., Sr. (2014, June 24). 2013 ACC/AHA guideline on the assessment of cardiovascular risk: A report of the American College of Cardiology/American Heart Association Task Force on practice guidelines. *Circulation*, 129(25 Suppl. 2), S49–S73. doi:10.1161/01.cir.0000437741.48606.98. Retrieved from http://circ.ahajournals.org/content/129/25_suppl_2/S49 Suppl. 2

Lavigne, P. M., & Karas, R. H. (2013). The current state of niacin in cardiovascular disease prevention: A systematic review and meta-regression. *Journal of the American College of Cardiology*, 61(4), 440–446. doi:10.1016/j.jacc.2012.10.030

Mozaffarian, D., Benjamin, E. J., & Go, A. S. (2015). Heart disease and stroke statistics—2015 update: A report from the American Heart Association. *Circulation*, 131(4), e29–e322. doi:10.1161/CIR.0000000000000152

Public Health Agency of Canada. (2018). *Report from the Canadian chronic disease surveillance system: Heart disease in 2018. Canada*. Retrieved from https://www.canada.ca/content/dam/phac-aspc/documents/services/publications/diseases-conditions/report-heart-disease-canada-2018/pub1-eng.pdf

Stone, N. J., Robinson, J., Lichtenstein, A. H., BaireyMerz, C. N., Lloyd-Jones, D. M., Blum, C. B., & Wilson, P. W. (2013, November 7). 2013 ACC/AHA guidelines on the treatment of blood cholesterol to reduce atherosclerotic cardiovascular risk in adults: A report of the American College of Cardiology/American Heart Association Task Force on practice guidelines. *Journal of the American College of Cardiology*, 53(25), 2889–2934.

Summary of the Second Report of the National Cholesterol Education Program Expert Panel on Detection, Evaluation, and Treatment of High Blood Cholesterol in Adults (Adult Treatment Panel II). (1993). *The Journal of the American Medical Association*, 269, 3015–3023. doi:10.1001/jama.269.23.3015

Atrial Fibrillation (AF)

Jill C. Cash, Debbie Gunter, and Krista A. Bradley

Definition

A. Atrial fibrillation (AF) is the irregular and rapid heart rhythm caused by abnormal electrical impulse formation and/or propagation. These impulses make the heart's upper chambers (the atria) beat chaotically and out of sync with the heart's lower chambers (the ventricles), resulting in poor circulation of blood throughout the body.

B. Classification of AF:
  1. Paroxysmal AF:
     a. Also called *intermittent AF*.
     b. Two or more episodes of AF that end spontaneously within seven days or less and usually last <24 hours.
  2. Persistent AF:
     a. AF that does not end spontaneously within seven days.
     b. Usually requires pharmacological interventions and/or cardioversion to restore sinus rhythm.
  3. Permanent AF:
     a. Persistent AF in which rhythm control strategies are no longer effective. (Such strategies are not utilized to restore sinus rhythm.)
  4. "Lone" AF:
     a. The term used to reference clients with paroxysmal, persistent, or permanent AF who do not have structural heart disease.

Incidence/Prevalence

A. According to the Canadian Heart and Stoke Foundation of Canada, 2018, AF is the most common arrhythmia in Canada, affecting approximately 350,000 Canadians.
B. AF is more common in women than in men. Men of any age are more likely than women to develop AF. However, because AF occurs much more often in older adults, and because there are more women than men over age 75, the total number of women and men with AF in this age group is essentially the same.
C. AF is more common in Caucasians.

Pathogenesis

A. Multiple impulses travel throughout the atria, yielding continuous electrical activity and an atrial rate in excess of 300 beats per minute (bpm). The impulses enter the atrioventricular (AV) node in a completely random manner. A small percentage of the impulses are conducted to the ventricle, which results in a lower ventricular rate, usually 100 to 180 bpm, and an irregularly irregular rhythm. This leads to ineffective atrial contractions, a decrease in cardiac output, and an increased risk of thrombus formation.

Predisposing Factors

A. Age, increased occurrence after age 65 years.
B. Coronary artery disease (CAD).
C. Hypertension (HTN).
D. Diabetes.
E. Rheumatic heart disease.
F. Valvular heart disease:
  1. Mitral valve stenosis.
  2. Mitral regurgitation.
  3. Tricuspid regurgitation.
G. Fibrosis or calcification in the vicinity of the AV node.
H. Left ventricular hypertrophy (LVH).
I. Heart failure (HF).
J. Myocardial infarction (MI).
K. Sick sinus syndrome.
L. Hyperthyroidism.
M. Infection.
N. Pericarditis.
O. Obstructive sleep apnoea (OSA).
P. Obesity.
Q. Recent cardiac surgery, including heart transplantation.
R. Pulmonary diseases (related to hypoxia):
  1. Chronic obstructive pulmonary disease (COPD).
  2. Bronchitis, acute or chronic.
  3. Asthma.
  4. Emphysema.
S. Electrolyte imbalances:
  1. Hyperkalaemia and hypokalaemia.
  2. Hypercalcaemia and hypocalcaemia.
  3. Hypermagnesaemia and hypomagnesaemia.
T. Factors that can trigger episodes of AF:
  1. Physical or emotional stress.
  2. Nicotine.
  3. Caffeine.
  4. Alcohol.
  5. Exercise.

Common Findings

A. Palpitations.
B. Angina.
C. Fatigue.
D. Dyspnoea at rest or on exertion.
E. Vertigo or dizziness.
F. Disorientation.
G. Confusion.
H. Syncope.
I. Headache.
J. Urinary frequency or urgency.
K. Anxiety.
L. Asymptomatic presentation, most often seen in the elderly and in clients with permanent AF.

Potential Complications

A. Stroke:
  1. The risk for stroke increases five times during an episode of AF.
B. Pulmonary embolism (PE).
C. Peripheral emboli:
  1. May present as an ischaemic extremity or ischaemic bowel.

Subjective Data

A. Ask the client what activity brought about or preceded the episode.
B. Have the client describe the duration of pain, if any, and what time of day the symptoms began.
C. Ask the client to describe his or her symptoms.
D. Ask the client whether any previous episodes have occurred.
E. Ask the client to list all medications, over-the-counter (OTC), and herbal products currently being taken or recently stopped.
F. Ask the client to quantify his or her smoking history, alcohol history, and caffeine intake.

Physical Examination

A. Clients presenting with an acute cardiovascular episode should be quickly assessed for the need to call emergency services/911 for immediate transport to the hospital.
B. Vital signs: Check blood pressure (BP), pulse, and respirations. Count heart rate for a full minute.
  1. Check orthostatic BP: Sitting, standing, and lying down.
C. Inspect:
  1. Inspect overall physical appearance, noting any distress.
  2. Inspect the neck: Check jugular vein distension and pulsations:
    a. Aborting maneuvers (i.e., carotid massage) should be performed only by a cardiologist.
  3. Inspect extremities: Note oedema, pallor, and cyanosis.
  4. Perform a funduscopic examination: Note haemorrhage, exudates, and papilloedema to determine the presence of malignant HTN.
D. Palpate:
  1. Palpate extremities for peripheral pulses in arm and groin; determine rate and regularity.
  2. Assess capillary refill.
  3. Palpate carotid arteries for thrills and heaves.
E. Auscultate:
  1. Heart: While the client is sitting, standing, and in left lateral recumbent positions, note normal and extra heart sounds (S3 and S4):
    a. S4 is not present during AF.
  2. Neck for carotid bruits.
  3. Lungs: Note the presence of wheezing and crackles.

F. Additional areas for physical examination:
  1. Assess for focal neurologic deficits (orientation, unilateral weakness, dysarthria).

Diagnostic Tests

A. Complete blood count (CBC), basic metabolic panel (BMP; including electrolytes, blood glucose, urea, and creatinine), magnesium, and liver function tests (LFTs).
B. Thyroid profile and lipid profile.
C. Brain natriuretic peptide (BNP).
D. Cardiac profile (including troponin, creatine phosphokinase [CPK] test, creatine kinase, muscle and brain [CK-MB]).
E. Serum drug levels, digoxin, amiodarone, quinidine (if applicable).
F. International normalized ratio (INR), if applicable.
G. Creatinine clearance (CrCl).
H. ECG.
I. 2-D echocardiogram.
J. Chest x-ray.
K. Exercise stress test or thallium stress test, if exercise-induced arrhythmia or CAD is suspected.
L. Holter monitoring.
M. Evaluation of sleep apnoea.

Differential Diagnoses

A. Myocardial infarction (MI).
B. CAD.
C. Heart failure (HF).
D. Mitral stenosis.
E. HTN.
F. Hyperthyroidism.
G. Digitalis intoxication.
H. Acute infections.

Plan

A. General interventions:
  1. The goal of therapy is to improve the client's quality of life by reducing morbidity and prolonging survival.
B. Client teaching:
  1. Encourage weight loss, smoking cessation, and stress management. *Refer to Client Teaching Guide: Atrial Fibrillation.*
  2. Educate clients about the adverse effects of their anticoagulant and antiarrhythmic medications.
  3. Instruct clients taking warfarin to take steps to lessen their risk of falls.
  4. Educate the clients with implanted defibrillators and pacemakers about their susceptibility for external electrical fields and avoidance of exposure.
C. Prevention:
  1. Control other chronic medical conditions, that is, HTN, diabetes, HF, pulmonary diseases, and hyperlipidaemia.
D. Dietary management:
  1. Counsel client on proper nutrition, specifically a low-fat, low-cholesterol, low-sodium diet. Give diet handouts.
  2. Clients taking warfarin should be educated regarding foods that are high in vitamin K. Some foods will interfere with clotting factors. Please see Appendix B, Foods to Avoid While Taking Warfarin, for common foods that interfere with clotting factors.
E. Pharmacological therapy:
  1. Anticoagulant therapy:
    a. Goal of therapy: Prevention of thromboembolism:
      i. Warfarin sodium:
        1) Review all medications that may affect the anticoagulant effects of warfarin.
      ii. Dabigatran etexilate mesylate.
      iii. Rivaroxaban.
      iv. Apixaban.
      v. Edoxaban.
  2. Antiplatelet therapy:
    a. Goal of therapy: Prevention of thromboembolism; modest preventative effect:
      i. ASA.
      ii. Clopidogrel bisulphate.
  3. Combined anticoagulant and antiplatelet therapies:
    a. Prescription of both antiplatelet medications (clopidogrel and ASA) in addition to an anticoagulant is referred to as *triple therapy*. Triple therapy is commonly used to prevent complications when two or more of the following conditions are present:
      i. AF.
      ii. Mechanical valve prosthesis.
      iii. Drug-eluting coronary stent.
    b. Triple therapy is linked with an increase in bleeding complications ranging from mild to life threatening.
  4. Heart rate control therapy:
    a. Goal of therapy: Varies based on client age, but typically involves achieving a ventricular rate between 60 and 80 bpm at rest and 90 and 115 bpm during moderate exercise.
    b. Beta-blockers:
      i. Acebutolol.
      ii. Atenolol.
      iii. Betaxolol.
      iv. Bisoprolol.
      v. Metoprolol.
      vi. Nadolol.
      vii. Propranolol.
      viii. Sotalol.
      ix. Timolol.
    c. Calcium channel blockers (CCBs):
      i. Diltiazem.
      ii. Verapamil.
    d. Fourth-generation CCBs:
      i. Digoxin.
  5. Heart rhythm control therapy: Goal of therapy: The maintenance of a normal rhythm and suppression of AF:
    a. Potassium channel blockers:
      i. Amiodarone.
      ii. Dronedarone.
      iii. Sotalol.
    b. Sodium channel blockers:
      i. Disopyramide.
      ii. Quinidine.
F. Surgical therapies:
  1. Ablation therapy:
    a. Goal of therapy: Prevention of recurrent AF.
    b. Preferred clinical characteristics include the following:
      i. Symptomatic paroxysmal AF.
      ii. Failure of one or more antiarrhythmic medications.
      iii. Normal to mildly dilated atria.

▶ Client Teaching Guides are available at https://connect.springerpub.com/content/reference-book/978-0-8261-9498-5

    iv. Normal to mildly reduced ventricular function.
    v. Absence of severe pulmonary disease.
  c. The long-term efficacy of ablation therapy requires further study, especially with regard to clients with HF and structural heart disease.

Follow-Up
A. AF that is resistant to routine therapy should always be followed by a cardiologist.
B. Laboratory monitoring as indicated by the client's anticoagulant and antiarrhythmic medications:
  1. CrCl for clients taking antiarrhytmics.
  2. INR for clients taking warfarin. Multiple medications affect the anticoagulant property of warfarin.
C. Follow-up is determined by the client's needs, frequency of AF reoccurrence, and the presence of other medical conditions.
D. After defibrillator or pacemaker placement, monitor the client using regular follow-up appointments and ECGs to identify failure of the implanted device, thromboembolism, lead dislodgement, infection, and complicating arrhythmias.

Consultation/Referral
A. If you suspect an acute cardiovascular episode, refer the client for immediate hospitalization in order to initiate thrombolytic therapy, cardioversion, hypertensive management, and additional diagnostic testing.
B. Refer to cardiology as indicated by the client's clinical situation, specifically the frequency of AF reoccurrence and the presence of other complex medical conditions.
C. AF that is resistant to routine therapy should always be followed by a cardiologist.

Individual Considerations
A. Paediatrics: AF is uncommon in the paediatric population; however, when present AF occurs secondary to structural heart disease.

Bibliography
Aschenbrenner, D. (2013). Drug watch: New labeled indications for an anticoagulant. *American Journal of Nursing, 113*(3), 22–23. doi:10.1097/01.NAJ.0000427872.05603.3f

Batra, G., Svennblad, B., Held, C., Jernberg, T., Johanson, P., Wallentin, L., & Oldgren, J. (2016). All types of atrial fibrillation in the setting of myocardial infarction are associated with impaired outcome. *Heart (British Cardiac Society), 102*(12), 926–933. doi:10.1136/heartjnl-2015-308678

Canadian Heart and Stroke Foundation. (2018). *Heart atrial fibrillation*. Retrieved from https://www.heartandstroke.ca/heart/conditions/atrial-fibrillation

Centers for Disease Control and Prevention. (2015, August). *Atrial fibrillation fact sheet*. Retrieved from https://www.cdc.gov/dhdsp/data_statistics/fact_sheets/fs_atrial_fibrillation.htm

Chao, T.-F., Liu, C.-J., Tuan, T.-C., Chen, S.-J., Wang, K.-L., Lin, Y.-J., & Chen, S.-A. (2015). Rate-control treatment and mortality in atrial fibrillation. *Circulation, 132*, 1604–1612. doi:10.1161/CIRCULATIONAHA.114.013709.. Retrieved from http://circ.ahajournals.org/content/early/2015/09/17/CIRCULATIONAHA.114.013709.abstract

Cheng, A., & Kumar, K. (2016, February). Overview of atrial fibrillation. *UpToDate*. Retrieved from www.uptodate.com/contents/overview-of-atrial-fibrillation

Drug information. (2016). *Prescribers' digital reference*. Retrieved from www.pdr.net

Ganz, L. (2015, October). Epidemiology of and risk factors for atrial fibrillation. *UpToDate*. Retrieved from http://www.uptodate.com/contents/epidemiology-of-and-risk-factors-for-atrial-fibrillation

Gonsalves, W. I., Pruthi, R. K., & Patnaik, M. M. The new oral anticoagulants in clinical practice. *Mayo Clinic Proceedings, 88*(5), 495–511. doi:10.1016/j.mayocp.2013.03.006 2013

Heidbuchel, H., Verhamme, P., Alings, M., Antz, M., Hacke, W., Oldgren, J., & Kirchhof, P. (2013). EHRA practical guide on the use of new oral anticoagulants in patients with non-valvular atrial fibrillation: Executive summary. *European Heart Journal, 34*(27), 2094–2106. doi:10.1093/eurheartj/eht134

January, C. T., Wann, L. S., Alpert, J. S., Calkins, H., Cigarroa, J. E., Cleveland, J. C., & Yancy, C. W. (2014). 2014 AHA/ACC/HRS guideline for the management of patients with atrial fibrillation: The Heart Rhythm Society. *A report of the American College of Cardiology/American Heart Association Task Force on Practice Guidelines and, Journal of the American College of Cardiology, 64*(21), e1–e76. doi:10.1161/CIR.0000000000000041

Macle, L., Cairns, J., Leblanc, K., Tsang, T., Skanes, A., & Cox, J. L. (2016). 2016 Focused Update of the Canadian Cardiovascular Society Guidelines for the management of atrial fibrillation. *CCS Atrial Fibrillation Guidelines Committee, Canadian Journal of Cardiology, 32*(10), 1170–1185. doi:10.1016/j.cjca.2016.07.59

Moss, J. D., & Cifu, A. S. (2015). & ACC/AHA Task Force on Practice Guidelines. Management of anticoagulation in patients with atrial fibrillation. *Journal of the American Medical Association, 314*(3), 291–292. doi:10.1001/jama.2015.3088

Palmer, S. (2015). Atrial fibrillation. *British Journal of Cardiac Nursing, 10*(11), 567. doi:10.12968/bjca.2015.10.11.567

Ruff, C. T., Giugliano, R. P., Braunwald, E., Hoffman, E. B., Deenadayalu, N., Ezekowitz, M. D., & Antman, E. M. (2014). Comparison of the efficacy and safety of new oral anticoagulants with warfarin in patients with atrial fibrillation: A meta-analysis of randomised trials. *Lancet, 383*(9921), 955–962. doi:10.1016/S0140-6736(13)62343-0

Verma, A., Cairns, J. A., Mitchell, L. B., Macle, L., Stiell, I. G., Gladstone, D., & Healey, J. S. (2014). 2014 focused update of the Canadian Cardiovascular Society guidelines for the management of atrial fibrillation. *Canadian Journal of Cardiology, 30*(10), 1114–1130. doi:10.1016/j.cjca.2014.08.001

Wigle, P., Hein, B., Bloomfield, H. E., Tubb, M., & Doherty, M. (2013). Updated guidelines on outpatient anticoagulation. *American Family Physician, 87*(8), 556–566.

Yao, S., & Tong, L. (2012). Comparison of anticoagulants used for stroke prevention in patients with atrial fibrillation. *American Journal for Nurse Practitioners, 16*, 29–34.

Chest Pain
Cheryl A. Glass, Debbie Gunter, and Krista A. Bradley

Definition
A. Chest pain is a localized sensation of distress or discomfort that may or may not be associated with actual tissue damage.

Incidence/Prevalence
A. Chest pain is one of the most common complaints of adult clients. Causes can range from minor disorders to life-threatening diseases; every client must be assessed carefully.

Pathogenesis
A. Cardiac aetiology: Ischaemia, atherosclerosis, inflammation, or valvular problems caused by angina, myocardial infarction (MI), pericarditis, endocarditis, dissecting aortic aneurysm, or mitral valve prolapse (MVP; see Table 10.2).
B. Musculoskeletal aetiology: Muscle strain and inflammation caused by costochondritis, chest wall syndrome, cervicodorsal arthritis, or intercostal myositis.
C. Neurologic aetiology: Nerve inflammation and/or compression caused by herpes zoster and nerve root compression.
D. Gastrointestinal (GI) aetiology: Structural defects, inflammation, or infection caused by gastro-oesophageal reflux disease (GORD), hiatal hernia, oesophageal spasm, pancreatitis, cholecystitis, or peptic ulcer disease (PUD).
E. Pleural aetiology: Inflammation, distension, or compression of pleural membranes caused by pneumonia, pulmonary embolus, pulmonary hypertension (HTN), spontaneous pneumothorax, and lung and mediastinal tumours.

TABLE Comparison of Common Chest Pain Aetiologies

Condition	Pain Findings	Associated Symptoms	Precipitating Factors	Relieving Factors	Physical Findings	Diagnostic Tests	Treatment Modalities
Cardiac-stable angina	Substernal, tight, dull pressure, usually lasts longer than 15 minutes		Exertion, cold, emotional stress	Rest, nitroglycerin, Valsalva's maneuver	Sinus tachycardia, bradycardia, xanthomas, signs of HF	Resting ECG, stress ECG, cardiac enzymes, echocardiogram, angiogram	ASA, BB, nitrate, CCB
Prinzmetal's angina (variant)	Substernal, achy, tight, dull pressure		Often occurs at rest; may awaken from sleep	Nitroglycerin	Same as stable angina	Resting ECG, angiogram	ASA, nitrate, CCB
MI	Precordial, substernal, severe, crushing, squeezing, lasts >15 minutes	Dyspnoea, sweating, dizzy, pain radiates to neck/arm/jaw, N&V, cough, fever, unstable VS	Oxygen	Not relieved by nitroglycerin	S3 or S4 murmur, tachycardia, bradycardia, pericardial, friction rub, hyper/hypotension	ECG, serial CK enzymes, echo, radionuclide studies	Analgesia, reperfusion, prevention and treatment complications limit infarcts Thrombolytic therapy for acute MI
MVP	Usually not substernal, often knifelike, may last one to three hours	Palpitations, fatigue, light-headed, arrhythmia, syncope		Recumbent position, BB, nitroglycerin	Midsystolic click and/or murmur, thin body status, SOB	Echo, ECG	Usually none, BB if palpitations or ventricular ectopy becomes disabling
Hypertrophic cardiomegaly	Similar to angina	Dyspnoea with exertion, arrhythmias, light-headed syncope	May be increased by nitroglycerin, exertion	BB, squatting	Systolic murmur, increased upright position, Valsalva's maneuver, more forceful PMI	ECG, CXR, echo, Doppler, cardiac catheterization	BB, CCB, possible pacing and myomectomy, exercise restriction
Pericarditis	Retrosternal, sharp or dull; sudden onset; long duration; radiates to one side of the trapezius	Fever, myalgia, anorexia, anxiety, recent viral infection		Sitting up, leaning forward	Friction rub, SVT1, tachypnoea, crackles, signs of cardiac tamponade	ECG, echo, CBC, ESR	Hospitalize; rule out purulent process Analgesics

(continued)

Comparison of Common Chest Pain Aetiologies (continued)

Condition	Pain Findings	Associated Symptoms	Precipitating Factors	Relieving Factors	Physical Findings	Diagnostic Tests	Treatment Modalities
Endocarditis	Usually dull, retrosternal, may radiate to back	Fever, night sweats, joint pain, back pain, weight loss, headache, murmur			Systolic–diastolic murmur, petechiae, Osler's modes, Roth spots, neck vein distension, pleural or pericardia rub, pain in extremities, splenomegaly, haematuria	CBC, ESR blood cultures, echo	Hospitalize, for antibiotic therapy
GI-oesophageal spasm	May be identical to angina		Alcohol or cold liquids	May be relieved by nitroglycerin		Oesophageal manometry	Nitroglycerin anticholinergics, oesophageal dilation
Oesophagitis	Burning, tightness	Heartburn, water brash	Overeating, alcohol, recumbent position	Antacids	May have slight to moderate epigastric tenderness	Oesophagoscopy	Lifestyle modification, antacid, H2 blocker, PPI, promotility agent
Musculoskeletal costochondr-itis	Sharp, sometimes pleuritic, parasternal costochondral pain		Sneezing, cough on deep inspiration, or twisting motions, reaching overhead		Erythema at sites of tenderness; positive pinpoint tenderness at costochondral junctions	CXR to rule out other causes	NSAIDs, ASA, ibuprofen, naproxen, heat application

BB, beta-blocker; CBC, complete blood count; CCB, calcium channel blockers; CK, creatine kinase; CXR, chest x-ray; ESR, eosinophilic sedimentation rate; HF, heart failure; MI, myocardial infarction; MVP, mitral valve prolapse; NSAIDs, nonsteroidal anti-inflammatory drugs; N&V, nausea and vomiting; PMI, point of maximal impulse; PPI, proton pump inhibitor; SOB, shortness of breath; SVT, supraventricular tachydysrhythmias; VS, vital signs.

F. Psychogenic aetiology: Stress caused by anxiety, depression, or panic disorders.

Predisposing Factors
A. These vary depending on the aetiology of pain.

Common Findings
A. Primary complaint: Pain somewhere in the chest.
B. "Levine's sign": Placing the fist on the center of the chest to demonstrate pain.
C. Fatigue.
D. Cough.
E. Indigestion.
F. Dyspnoea.
G. Syncope.
H. Palpitations.
I. Profound fatigue.

Other Signs and Symptoms
A. Pain may be typical of angina and MI.
B. Musculoskeletal pain may be relieved by position change, aggravated by body movement, reproducible, or caused by injury or trauma.
C. Neurologic pain is associated with skin lesion if herpes zoster is the causative agent.
D. GI pain may be associated with meals, certain positions, belching, or an acid "brash" taste in mouth, or it may be referred to other sites.
E. Pleural pain is accompanied by cough, upper respiratory infection (URI) symptoms, or shortness of breath (SOB).
F. Psychogenic pain or pressure along with SOB and dizziness may be associated with a specific event or time.

Subjective Data
A. How long has the client had chest pain?
B. Has the client ever been treated for chest pain? What treatment, tests, and medications (such as nitroglycerin) were used?
C. What precipitates and relieves the client's chest pain?
  1. Precipitates pain: Exertion, taking a deep breath, eating, cold, stress, and sexual intercourse.
  2. Relieves pain: Resting, eating, taking an antacid, taking nitroglycerin, and positional change.
D. Inquire about character of pain:
  1. Location: Neck, throat, chest, epigastric area, and shoulder.
  2. Radiation: Neck, throat, shoulder, lower jaw, and upper extremity:
     a. **Radiation to both arms is a predictor of acute MI.**
     b. **Chest pain that radiates between the scapulae may be because of thoracic aortic dissection.**
  3. Quality: Squeezing, pressure, strangling, fullness, heavy weight, tightening, constriction, and ripping/tearing (acute aortic dissection).
  4. Intensity: Abrupt onset, gradually getting worse, dull, or insidious.
  5. How long has the pain been occurring? Seconds, minutes, hours, or years?
  6. Frequency: Intermittent, occurs every morning/evening.
E. Are other associated symptoms present?
F. Discuss any risk factors the client may have for cardiac disease: Smoking, hyperlipidaemia, HTN, sedentary lifestyle, diabetes, and family history.
G. Review medical history as noted earlier.
H. Review all medications including prescription (such as sildenafil), over-the-counter (OTC), and herbal products.
I. Review recreational/illicit drug use.
J. Inquire about any new physical labour if musculoskeletal aetiology is suspected.
K. Has the client had any trauma (including domestic violence)?
L. Has the client had a recent infection?

Physical Examination
A. Check temperature (if infection is suspected), pulse, respirations, blood pressure (BP), and pulse oximetry.
B. Inspect:
  1. Inspect general appearance:
     a. Appearance of discomfort/distress.
     b. Any appearance of respiratory distress.
     c. Evaluate jugular venous distension (JVD).
     d. Note client position: Sitting, lying, squatting. Relief of chest pain with recumbency suggests MVP; relief with squatting suggests hypertrophic cardiomyopathy. Noncardiac chest pain may be present along with cardiac chest pain.
  2. Inspect skin for diaphoresis, jaundice, pallor, herpes zoster lesions, rash, or cyanosis.
  3. Inspect chest wall for herpes zoster lesions or signs of trauma.
  4. Inspect eyes by performing funduscopic examination.
  5. Inspect legs for signs of phlebitis: Unilateral swelling, cyanosis, venous stasis, and diminished pulses.
  6. Inspect neck for enlarged thyroid and lymph nodes, midline trachea, and JVD.
C. Palpate:
  1. Palpate chest wall for tenderness and swelling. Chest pain present in only one body position is usually not cardiac in origin.
  2. Palpate abdomen for masses, tenderness, bounding pulses, organomegaly, and ascites.
  3. Palpate femoral and distal pulses.
D. Auscultate:
  1. Auscultate carotid arteries for bruits.
  2. Auscultate lungs for crackles, wheezes, equal breath sounds, and pleural rub.
  3. Auscultate abdomen for bruits and bowel sounds.
  4. Auscultate heart for murmurs, rubs, clicks, irregularities, or extra sounds.
E. Neurologic examination: Perform this examination if neurologic aetiology is suspected.

Diagnostic Tests
A. Testing depends on information collected in the examination. A normal physical examination, ECG, and/or laboratory test results in a client with chest pain does not rule out coronary heart disease (CHD). Typical tests include the following:
  1. ECG.
  2. Chest radiography, whenever diagnosis of chest pain is not clear.
  3. Echocardiogram.
  4. Stress test.
  5. Cardiac catheterization.

6. Barium tests.
7. Endoscopy to rule out GI aetiology.
8. Oesophageal pH, low.
9. Laboratory tests:
   a. Troponin I or T.
   b. Myoglobin.
   c. Creatine kinase (CK).
   d. Creatine kinase-muscle and brain (CK-MB).
   e. C-reactive protein (CRP).
   f. Brain natriuretic peptide (BNP) for clinical findings/risk of heart failure (HF).
   g. D-dimer for suspected venous thrombotic event (deep vein thrombosis [DVT] or pulmonary embolism [PE]).

Differential Diagnoses
A. Cardiac causes:
   1. CHD:
      a. Acute MI: Chest pain lasting more than 15 minutes.
      b. Unstable angina pectoris.
      c. Stable angina pectoris.
      d. Prinzmetal's or variant angina.
   2. Valvular heart disease:
      a. MVP.
      b. Aortic stenosis.
   3. Hypertrophic cardiomyopathy.
   4. Pericarditis.
   5. Endocarditis.
   6. Aortic dissection.
B. Noncardiac causes:
   1. Pulmonary causes:
      a. Pneumonia.
      b. Pleurisy.
      c. PE.
      d. Pulmonary HTN.
      e. Pneumothorax.
      f. Tracheobronchitis.
      g. Lung cancer.
   2. GI causes:
      a. GERD.
      b. Oesophageal spasm.
      c. PUD.
      d. Pancreatitis.
      e. Cholecystitis.
      f. Flatulence.
   3. Rheumatology causes:
      a. Fibromyalgia.
      b. Costochondritis.
      c. Arthritis.
   4. Chest wall causes:
      a. Rib fracture.
      b. Muscle strain.
      c. Cervical or thoracic spine disease.
      d. Metastatic bone disease.
      e. Breast conditions.
   5. Neurologic causes:
      a. Herpes zoster.
      b. Postherpetic pain syndrome.
      c. Nerve root compression.
   6. Psychogenic causes:
      a. Panic disorder.
      b. Generalized anxiety.
      c. Depression.
      d. Somatoform disorders.

Plan
A. General interventions: Direct management toward primary disorder causing the symptom.
B. Client teaching: Teach the client about medications:
   1. Encourage cardiopulmonary resuscitation (CPR) training for the client's family and/or close friends if chest pain is cardiac in origin.
   2. Explain to the client and family when and how to call 911 and the importance of going to the ED immediately so that thrombolytic therapy can be considered. A positive response to nitroglycerin does not confirm the presence of coronary artery disease (CAD).
C. Pharmacological therapy:
   1. Cardiac pain: Nitroglycerin.
   2. GI pain: H2 blocker, proton pump inhibitor (PPI).
   3. Musculoskeletal pain: Nonsteroidal anti-inflammatory drugs (NSAIDs).
   4. Psychogenic pain:
      a. Selective serotonin reuptake inhibitors (SSRIs).
      b. Tricyclic antidepressants (TCAs).
      c. Benzodiazepines.

Follow-Up
A. Follow-up of clients with CAD to be carried out for an indefinite period of time to detect the recurrence or progression of disease.
B. Other follow-up depends on the aetiology of chest pain.

Consultation/Referral
A. Consult a cardiologist when chest pain is cardiac in origin. If a cardiac origin is found in a pregnant client, schedule a cardiology consultation as soon as possible for comanagement.

Individual Considerations
A. Pregnancy:
   1. Evaluate chest pain in the same manner as in nonpregnant clients.
   2. Rule out pregnancy-induced hypertension (PIH) and haemolysis, elevated liver enzymes, low platelets (HELLP) syndrome when a third-trimester client presents with upper epigastric/chest pain.
B. Paediatrics:
   1. Chest pain usually does not represent serious cardiovascular disease (CVD).
   2. Pericarditis is one of the most frequent causes of chest pain associated with a febrile illness.
   3. Exercise-induced chest pain may be indicative of asthma.
   4. A chest wall syndrome, such as costochondritis, is another frequent aetiology.
C. Geriatrics:
   1. Frail elderly clients usually do not present with the "typical" symptom complex of chest pain. Often, the only symptoms of acute MI are lethargy, decreased level of consciousness (LOC), crackles, congestive heart failure (CHF), persistent cough, or hypotension.
   2. Prescribe medications for frail elderly clients in half the usual dosage and then slowly taper upward to the desired effect.

Bibliography
Abid, S., & Shuaib, W. (2015). Chest pain assessment and imaging practices for nurse practitioners in the emergency department. *Advanced Emergency Nursing Journal, 37*, 12–22. doi:10.1097/TME.0000000000000048

Drug information. (2016). *Prescribers' digital reference*. Retrieved from www.pdr.net

Chronic Venous Insufficiency (CVI) and Varicose Veins

Laura A. Petty and Krista A. Bradley

Definition
Peripheral vascular disease (PVD) is a general term that encompasses all occlusive or inflammatory diseases that occur within the peripheral arteries, veins, and lymphatics. These conditions include peripheral arterial disease (PAD), deep vein thrombosis (DVT), superficial thrombophlebitis, lymphoedema, and chronic venous diseases. Chronic venous diseases include chronic venous insufficiency (CVI) and varicose veins.

A. CVI:
1. According to Canada Vein Clinics, CVI is found in 40% of women and 25% of men in Canada.
2. Peak incidence is seen in women older than 50 years.

B. Varicose veins:
1. This is the most common circulatory condition of the lower extremities, affecting up to 20% of the adult population. Varicose veins are usually thought to be more common in females; however, in certain populations the rate is higher in males.

Pathogenesis
A. CVI: Venous insufficiency is caused by incompetent valves that allow valvular reflux and subsequently venous hypertension (HTN). In CVI, venous HTN leads to obstruction of venous flow, which produces local tissue anoxia, inflammation, and at times even tissue necrosis. This process eventually causes subcutaneous fibrosing panniculitis and additional venous and lymphatic outlet obstruction.

B. Varicose veins: Varicose veins are a form of CVI. The same incompetent valves that cause valvular reflux and subsequently venous HTN in CVI also cause varicose veins. This influx of volume and pressure causes the vessels to dilate, twist, and bulge.

Predisposing Factors
A. CVI:
1. Age.
2. Female gender.
3. Prolonged standing or sitting.
4. Prior history of DVT.
5. Stature, more common in tall persons.
6. Obesity.
7. Sedentary lifestyle.

B. Varicose veins:
1. Genetics:
    a. Risk increases to 90% if both parents have varicose veins.
    b. If one parent is affected, the risk increases by 25% for men and 62% for women.
2. Age.
3. Pregnancy.
4. Prolonged standing.
5. Restrictive clothing.
6. Obesity.
7. Ligamentous laxity:
    a. A history of hernia(s) or flat feet.
8. Smoking.

Common Findings
A. CVI:
1. Extremity oedema.
2. Pain worse when standing, usually dull, aching, or cramping.
3. Pain improved with elevation.
4. Itching sensation.
5. Feeling of heaviness in extremity.
6. Hyperpigmentation.
7. Thickening and hardening of the skin.
8. Ulcerations.

B. Varicose veins:
1. Pain, usually burning, aching, or itching.
2. Blue veins that protrude above the surface of the skin.
3. Leg fatigue.
4. Oedema.
5. Symptoms worsen toward the end of the day.
6. Leg heaviness.

Potential Complications
A. CVI:
1. Cellulitis.
2. Peripheral neuropathy.
3. Varicose veins.
4. Abscess.
5. Ulceration.
6. Stasis dermatitis.
7. DVT.

B. Varicose veins:
1. Stasis dermatitis.
2. Stasis ulceration.
3. Petechial haemorrhage.
4. Chronic oedema.
5. Superficial thrombophlebitis.
6. Hyperpigmentation.
7. Eczema.

Subjective Data
A. Ask the client when the symptom(s) were first noticed.
B. Have the client describe the duration of symptoms.
C. Ask the client to describe pain, for example, crushing, stabbing, or burning.
D. Ask the client what makes the symptoms better and what makes them worse.
E. Have the client rate pain on a scale of 1 to 10, with 1 being the least painful.
F. Ask the client to list all medications currently being taken, particularly substances not prescribed and illicit drugs such as cocaine.
G. Review recent history of invasive procedures or surgery.

Physical Examination
A. CVI:
1. Vital signs:
    a. Check blood pressure (BP) and document resting heart rate, respirations, temperature, height, and weight.
2. Inspect:
    a. Inspect extremity for oedema, hyperpigmentation, erythema, and difference in temperature.
    b. Inspect and document any varicosities.
3. Palpate:
    a. Palpate distended veins, noting tenderness.
    b. Perform the cough impulse test to determine turbulent retrograde flow.

c. Perform the tap test to determine if the great saphenous vein is distended with blood.
4. Auscultate:
   a. Heart: Rate rhythm, heart sounds, murmur, and gallops.
   b. Lungs: Assess lung sounds in all fields.
B. Varicose veins:
   1. **Client presenting with any of the following should be quickly assessed for the need to call emergency services/911 for immediate transport to the hospital:**
      a. **A bleeding varicosity with eroded surrounding skin.**
      b. **A varicosity that has bled and is at risk of bleeding again.**
      c. **An ulceration that is worsening and/or painful despite treatment.**
   2. Vital signs:
      a. Check BP and document resting heart rate, respirations, temperature, height, and weight.
   3. Inspect:
      a. Inspect skin for superficial veins that are raised above the skin's surface; client should be standing.
      b. Inspect extremity for oedema, hyperpigmentation, and eczema.
   4. Palpate:
      a. Palpate distended veins, noting tenderness.
   5. Auscultate:
      a. Auscultate heart: Rate rhythm, heart sounds, murmur, and gallops.
      b. Auscultate lungs: Assess lung sounds.

Diagnostic Tests

A. CVI:
   1. Trendelenburg test.
   2. Perthes test.
   3. Doppler ankle/brachial index (ABI).
   4. Duplex ultrasound.
   5. Venography, not utilized often because of expense and risk of phlebitis.
B. Varicose veins:
   1. Trendelenburg test.
   2. Perthes test.
   3. Duplex ultrasound.

Differential Diagnoses

A. CVI:
   1. DVT.
   2. Ulceration.
   3. Infection.
   4. PAD.
   5. Varicose veins with risk of haemorrhage.
B. Varicose veins:
   1. Arthritis.
   2. Peripheral neuritis.
   3. Nerve root compression.
   4. Telangiectasia.
   5. DVT.
   6. Inflammatory liposclerosis.

Plan

A. Prevention: General:
   1. Avoid prolonged standing or sitting.
   2. Exercise on a regular basis.
   3. Encourage smoking cessation, weight loss, and exercise, if applicable.
   4. Encourage strategies to better manage other chronic medical conditions that directly affect the progression of PAD, that is, diabetes, dyslipidaemia, obesity, and HTN.
B. CVI:
   1. Nonpharmacological therapy:
      a. Extremity elevation.
      b. Compression stockings.
      c. Exercise.
      d. Venous ulcerations treated with wound care and compression therapy.
   2. Pharmacological therapy:
      a. Diuretics: Management of oedema, short-term administration:
         i. Hydrochlorothiazide.
         ii. Antiplatelet: May increase the speed of healing to ulcerations:
            1) ASA.
            2) Systemic antibiotics: Management of infection in persons demonstrating an increase in pain, erythema, or size of ulceration.
   3. Surgery:
      a. Venous ablation for clients who continue to be symptomatic after six months of nonpharmacological, therapies. Types of ablation: chemical, thermal, and mechanical.
C. Varicose veins:
   1. Client teaching: *Refer to Client Teaching Guides: Chronic Venous Insufficiency.* and *Varicose Veins*
      a. If prolonged standing is required, shift weight from one leg to the other.
      b. Do not sit with legs dependent.
   2. Nonpharmacological therapy:
      a. Extremity elevation.
      b. Compression stockings.
      c. Exercise.
   3. Surgery:
      a. Radiofrequency ablation.
      b. Endovenous laser therapy.
      c. Phlebectomy.
      d. Foam sclerotherapy.
      e. Vein ligation.

Follow-Up

A. Follow-up is determined by client's needs, frequency and intensity of symptoms, and the presence of other medical conditions.
B. PVD manifesting persistent symptoms should always be followed by a cardiologist.

Consultation/Referral

A. If you suspect acute limb ischaemia, refer client for immediate hospitalization in order to obtain diagnostic testing to determine the presence of a thrombus and restore circulation to the affected extremity.
B. If chronic limb ischaemia has led to ulceration and/or superimposed infection, hospitalization is indicated to initiate a wound care consultation and diagnostic testing to determine the degree of arterial occlusion.
C. Referral to a cardiologist is indicated in the presence of persistent PVD symptoms.

D. Referral to a podiatrist as necessary to trim toenails and assess client for properly fitting shoes.
E. Referral to pain management is indicated if pain is resistant to treatment.

Individual Considerations
A. Nonambulatory clients:
   1. Using rocking chairs is a possible substitute for persons unable to participate in a walking program.
B. Geriatrics:
   1. Be alert to signs and symptoms of depression related to immobility and pain.

Bibliography
Alguire, P. C., & Mathes, B. M. (2015, September). Diagnostic evaluation of chronic venous insufficiency. *UpToDate*. Retrieved from http://www.uptodate.com/contents/diagnostic-evaluation-of-chronic-venous-insufficiency

Alguire, P. C., & Scovell, S. (2015, March). Overview and management of lower extremity chronic venous disease. *UpToDate*. Retrieved from www.uptodate.com/contents/overview-and-management-of-lower-extremity-chronic-venous-disease

AlShammeri, O., AlHamdan, N., Al-Hothaly, B., Midhet, F., Hussain, M., & Al-Mohaimeed, A. (2014). Chronic venous insufficiency: Prevalence and effect of compression stockings. *International Journal of Health Sciences, 8*(3), 231–236. doi:10.12816/0023975

Canada Vein Clinics. (2018). *Vein conditions*. Retrieved from http://www.canadaveinclinics.ca/vein-conditions/

Dooner, J. (n.d.). *Varicose veins. Canadian Society for Vascular Surgery*. Ottawa, ON, Canada. Retrieved from https://canadianvascular.ca/Varicose-Veins

Drug information. (2016). *Prescribers' digital reference*. Retrieved from www.pdr.net

McLafferty, R. B., Lohr, J. M., Caprini, J. A., Passman, M. A., Padberg, F. T., Rooke, T. W., & Wakefield, T. W. (2007). Results of the national pilot screening program for venous disease by the American Venous Forum. *Journal of Vascular Surgery, 45*(1), 142–148. doi:10.1016/j.jvs.2006.08.079

Rooke, T. W., & Felty, C. L. (2014). A different way to look at varicose veins. *Journal of Vascular Surgery. Venous and Lymphatic Disorders, 2*(2), 207–211. doi:10.1016/j.jvsv.2013.08.006

Trayes, K. P., Studdiford, J. S., Pickle, S., & Tully, A. S. (2013). Edema: Diagnosis and management. *American Family Physician, 88*(2), 102–110. doi:10.1097/ACM.0b013e318277d5b2

Vascular Cures. (2016). *Chronic venous insufficiency*. Retrieved from http://www.vascularcures.org/about-vascular-disease/2011-05-05-02-02-59/chronic-venous-insufficiency

Wittens, C., Davies, A. H., Bækgaard, N., Broholm, R., Cavezzi, A., & Chastanet, S. (2015). Editor's choice—Management of chronic venous disease: Clinical Practice Guidelines of the European Society for Vascular Surgery (ESVS). *European Journal of Vascular and Endovascular Surgery: The Official Journal of the European Society for Vascular Surgery, 49*(6), 678–737. doi:10.1016/j.ejvs.2015.02.007

Zhang, S., & Melander, S. (2014). Varicose veins: Diagnosis, management, and treatment. *Journal for Nurse Practitioners, 10*(6), 417–424. doi:10.1016/j.nurpra.2014.03.004

Deep Vein Thrombosis (DVT)

Laura A. Petty and Krista A. Bradley

Definition
A. Peripheral vascular disease (PVD) is a general term that encompasses all occlusive or inflammatory diseases that occur within the peripheral arteries, veins, and lymphatics. PVD includes deep vein thrombosis (DVT). DVT is a condition in which a thrombus forms in one or more veins. DVT greatly increases the risk of pulmonary embolism (PE).

Incidence/Prevalence
A. Thrombosis Canada estimates 45,000 clients in Canada are affected by DVT each year. If untreated, approximately one-third of these may result in a fatal event.

Pathogenesis
A. Changes within the venous system precipitate the formation of a DVT. These changes are formally called Virchow's triad. This triad includes hypercoagulability, venous stasis, and injury to the vessel wall. At least two of the three must be present for a DVT to form. Essentially, an injury to the vessel wall causes inflammation that attracts platelets, especially in a state of altered coagulation. The thrombus that forms spreads in the direction of blood flow and additional layers of platelets are added to the thrombus as time progresses. As it grows, the vessel becomes more occluded and symptoms worsen.

Predisposing Factors
A. Age, 60 years and older.
B. Hip or femur fracture.
C. Recent surgery, especially cardiac or extremity surgery.
D. Prolonged inactivity/immobility.
E. Pregnancy.
F. Medication:
   1. Hormone replacement therapy (HRT).
   2. Oral contraceptives.
   3. Tamoxifen.
G. Smoking.
H. Obesity.
I. Cancer.
J. Inherited hypercoagulable conditions.

Common Findings
Symptoms of a DVT are usually unilateral and have a sudden onset:
A. Extremity oedema.
B. Extremity pain.
C. Increased temperature of extremity.
D. Change in colour or extremity.
E. Asymptomatic, depending on the size and location of the thrombus.

Potential Complications
A. PE.
B. Arterial embolism with atrioventricular (AV) shunting.
C. Myocardial infarction (MI).
D. Chronic venous insufficiency (CVI).
E. Postphlebitic syndrome.
F. Phlegmasia cerulea dolens (painful blue oedema) due to extensive thrombus in a limb that can lead to venous gangrene.

Subjective Data
A. Ask the client when the symptom(s) were first noticed.
B. Have the client describe the duration of the symptoms.
C. Ask the client to describe pain, for example, crushing, stabbing, or burning.
D. Ask the client what makes the symptoms better and what makes them worse.
E. Have the client rate pain on a scale of 1 to 10, with 1 being the least painful.
F. Ask the client to list all medications currently being taken, particularly substances not prescribed and illicit drugs such as cocaine.
G. Review recent history of invasive procedures or surgery.

Physical Examination
Clients presenting with acute shortness of breath (SOB) and/or chest pain should be quickly assessed for the need

to call emergency services/911 for immediate transport to the hospital. Clients presenting with symptoms of DVT that include cyanosis of the distal extremity should be quickly assessed for the need to call emergency services/911 for immediate transport to the hospital.
  A. Vital signs:
    1. Check blood pressure (BP) and document resting heart rate, respirations, height, and weight.
  B. Inspect:
    1. Assess for signs of erythema, increased temperature, and oedema.
    2. Assess for a Homans' sign (i.e., calf pain with forced plantar flexion).
    3. Assess for Moses' or Bancroft's sign (i.e., pain when calf muscle is compressed forward against the tibia).
    4. Assess the Lisker sign (i.e., pain upon tibial percussion).
  C. Palpate:
    1. Pulses distal to affected area, noting symmetry.
    2. Capillary refill.
    3. Extremity for tenderness. Do not perform deep palpation.
  D. Auscultate:
    1. Heart: Rate, rhythm, heart sounds, murmur, and gallops.
    2. Lungs: Assess lung sounds in all fields.

Diagnostic Tests
  A. DVT:
    1. Serum laboratory testing:
      a. D-dimer.
      b. Complete blood count (CBC) with differential.
      c. Coagulation panel (prothrombin time [PT], partial thromboplastin time [PTT], international normalized ratio [INR]).
      d. Testing for idiopathic DVT: Add Factor V Leiden, homocysteine, G20210A prothrombin, Factor VIII, lupus anticoagulant antibody, protein C and protein S levels anticardiolipin antibodies, and antithrombin.
    2. Compression ultrasound.
    3. MRI, if thrombus is suspected in the pelvic veins or vena cava.
    4. Venography, not utilized often because of expense and risk of phlebitis.

Differential Diagnoses
  A. Cellulitis.
  B. Fracture.
  C. Lymphoedema.
  D. Congestive heart failure (CHF).
  E. Vein compression (caused by enlarged lymph nodes or mass).
  F. Filariasis (parasitic disease).
  G. Allergic reaction, localized.
  H. Compartment syndrome.

Plan
▶ A. Client teaching: *Refer to Client Teaching Guide: Deep Vein Thrombosis:*
    1. Clients taking warfarin should be educated regarding foods that are high in vitamin K. Some foods will interfere with clotting factors. Please see Appendix B, Diet Recommendations for common foods that interfere with clotting factors.
    2. Avoid prolonged standing or sitting.
    3. Avoid crossing the legs.
    4. Gradually resume normal activity.
    5. Avoid immobility.
    6. Exercise on a regular basis.
    7. Stop smoking.
    8. Encourage strategies to better manage other chronic medical conditions that directly affect the progression of peripheral arterial disease (PAD), that is, diabetes, dyslipidaemia, obesity, and hypertension (HTN).
  B. Nonpharmacological therapy:
    1. Compression stockings.
  C. Pharmacological therapy:
    1. Thrombolytics: Administered in the inpatient setting.
    2. Anticoagulants:
      a. Heparin, intravenous, administered in the inpatient setting.
      b. Warfarin.
    3. Low-molecular-weight heparin (LMWH):
      a. Enoxaparin sodium.
      b. Dalteparin sodium.
    4. Specific factor Xa inhibitor:
      a. Fondaparinux sodium.
      b. Edoxaban.
      c. Apixaban.
      d. Rivaroxaban.
      e. Dabigatran.
  D. Surgery:
    1. Insertion of vena cava filter to prevent PE.
    2. Venous thrombectomy.

Follow-Up
  A. Follow-up is determined by client's needs, frequency and intensity of symptoms, and presence of other medical conditions.
  B. DVT manifesting persistent symptoms should always be followed by a cardiologist.
  C. Clients taking anticoagulants are best followed by an anticoagulant clinic and/or cardiologist.

Consultation/Referral
  A. If you suspect acute limb ischaemia, refer client for immediate hospitalization in order to obtain diagnostic testing to determine the presence of a thrombus and restore circulation to the affected extremity.
  B. If chronic limb ischaemia has led to ulceration and/or superimposed infection, hospitalization is indicated to initiate a wound care consultation and diagnostic testing to determine the degree of arterial occlusion.
  C. Referral to a cardiologist is indicated in the presence of persistent PVD symptoms.
  D. Refer to pain management if pain is resistant to treatment.
  E. Refer to a registered dietitian as indicated by the client's understanding of dietary modification necessary to improve status of risk factors.

Individual Considerations
  A. Nonambulatory clients:
    1. Using rocking chairs is a possible substitute for persons unable to participate in a walking program.
  B. Geriatrics:
    1. Be alert to signs and symptoms of depression related to immobility and pain.

▶ Client Teaching Guides are available at https://connect.springerpub.com/content/reference-book/978-0-8261-9498-5

Bibliography

Aschenbrenner, D. (2013). Drug watch: New labeled indications for an anticoagulant. *American Journal of Nursing, 113*(3), 22–23. doi:10.1097/01.NAJ.0000427872.05603.3f

Canada Vein Clinics. (2018). *Vein conditions*. Retrieved from http://www.canadaveinclinics.ca/vein-conditions/

Centers for Disease Control and Prevention. (2012, June 8). *Deep vein thrombosis (DVT)/pulmonary embolism (PE)—Blood clot forming in a vein*. Retrieved from www.cdc.gov/ncbddd/dvt/data.html

Centers for Disease Control and Prevention. (2014, March 7). *CDC grand rounds: Preventing hospital-associated venous thromboembolism*. Retrieved from https://www.cdc.gov/mmwr/preview/mmwrhtml/mm6309a3.htm

Centers for Disease Control and Prevention. (2015, June). *Venous thromboembolism (blood clots)*. Retrieved from www.cdc.gov/ncbddd/dvt/data.html

Drug information. (2016). *Prescribers' digital reference*. Retrieved from www.pdr.net

Faiz, A. S., Khan, I., Beckman, M. G., Bockenstedt, P., Heit, J. A., Kulkarni, R., & Philipp, C. S. (2015). Characteristics and risk factors of cancer associated venous thromboembolism. *Thrombosis Research, 136*(3), 535–541. doi:10.1016/j.thromres.2015.06.036

Guyatt, G. H., Akl, E. A., Crowther, M., Gutterman, D. D., & Schüunemann, H. J. (2012). Executive summary: Antithrombotic therapy and prevention of thrombosis, 9th ed: American College of Chest Physicians evidence-based clinical practice guidelines. *Chest, 141*(2 Suppl), 7S–47S. doi:10.1378/chest.1412S3

Kearon, C., Akl, E. A., Ornelas, J., Blaivas, A., Jimenez, D., Bounameaux, H., & Moores, L. (2016). Antithrombotic therapy for VTE disease CHEST guideline and expert panel report. *Chest, 149*(2), 315–352. doi:10.1016/j.chest.2015.11.026

Lip, G., & Hull, R. (2016, May). Overview of the treatment of lower extremity deep vein thrombosis (DVT). *UpToDate*. Retrieved from http://www.uptodate.com/contents/overview-of-the-treatment-of-lower-extremity-deep-vein-thrombosis-dvt

McLafferty, R. B., Lohr, J. M., Caprini, J. A., Passman, M. A., Padberg, F. T., Rooke, T. W., & Wakefield, T. W. (2007). Results of the national pilot screening program for venous disease by the American Venous Forum. *Journal of Vascular Surgery, 45*(1), 142–148. doi:10.1016/j.jvs.2006.08.079

Payne, A. B., Miller, C. H., Hooper, W. C., Lally, C., & Austin, H. D. (2014). High factor VIII, von Willebrand factor, and fibrinogen levels and risk of venous thromboembolism in Blacks and Whites. *Ethnicity & Disease, 24*(2), 169–174.

Thrombosis Canada. (2013). *Deep vein thrombosis treatment*. Retrieved from http://thrombosiscanada.ca/guides/pdfs/DVT_Treatment.pdf

Trayes, K. P., Studdiford, J. S., Pickle, S., & Tully, A. S. (2013). Edema: Diagnosis and management. *American Family Physician, 88*(2), 102–110. doi:10.1097/ACM.0b013e318277d5b2

Heart Failure (HF)

Cheryl A. Glass, Debbie Gunter, and Krista A. Bradley

Definition

Heart failure (HF) is failure of the heart to pump sufficient blood to meet the metabolic demands of the tissues. The Canadian Cardiovascular Society has developed Guidelines for HF which address management of HF.

The Canadian Cardiovascular Society (CCS) Guidelines are available at www.ccs.ca/images/Guidelines/PocketGuides_EN/HF_Gui_2017_PG_EN_web.pdf. These guidelines include the following:

A. HFrEF (HF with reduced ejection fraction):
  1. Ejection fraction (EF) <40% because of weak, inefficient systolic contractions. The left ventricular ejection fraction (LVEF) is a measurement of systolic failure.
  2. An S3 ventricular gallop rhythm commonly occurs.
  3. Systolic failure is often the result of coronary heart disease (CHD) and/or myocardial infarction (MI).
  4. It can result from right- or left-sided failure, or both.

B. HFpEF (HF with preserved EF):
  1. EF is >50%, but with poor compliance of the ventricle, which impedes ventricular diastolic filling (the ventricle is unable to relax).
  2. There are two subgroups:
     a. HFpEF borderline (or intermediate): Clients with an EF of 41% to 49%.
     b. HFpEF with EF >40% who previously had HFrEF (EF <40%) but improvement or recovery was noted in EF.
  3. The client may be asymptomatic for years. HFpEF presents with the same symptoms of systolic failure, pulmonary congestion, and peripheral oedema.
  4. An S4 atrial gallop rhythm commonly occurs.

Incidence/Prevalence

A. HFrEF incidence is higher in older women, chronic hypertension (HTN), obesity, left ventricular hypertrophy (LVH), cardiomyopathy, excessive alcohol use, end-stage chronic obstructive pulmonary disease (COPD), valvular disorders, anaemia, renal failure, atrial fibrillation (AF), coronary artery disease (CAD), or diabetes.

B. Approximately 1% of the Canadian population, or 600,000 people, have HF. By the year 2045, the Canadian Heart Failure Network estimates that rates of HF in Canada will increase by threefold.

Pathogenesis

A. Injuries to the myocardium may cause loss of functioning muscle. Compensatory mechanisms, including cardiac hypertrophy and neurohumoral processes, lead to adverse long-term effects. An inotropic insult results in incomplete emptying (systolic failure), and a compliance abnormality results in incomplete filling (diastolic failure). Most HF has some degree of both abnormalities.

Predisposing Factors

A. Atherosclerotic heart disease.
B. MI.
C. Rheumatic heart disease involving mitral and aortic valves.
D. Cardiomyopathies.
E. Hypertensive heart disease.
F. Aortic stenosis or regurgitation.
G. Thyrotoxicosis.
H. Pregnancy-related disorders such as multiple births with preexisting heart disease.
I. Volume overload.
J. Beta-blockers or other cardiac depressants.
K. Pulmonary embolism (PE).
L. Systemic infection.
M. Arrhythmias.
N. Renal disease.
O. Diabetes.
P. Smoking.

Common Findings

Clients are assigned the New York Heart Association classifications by their tolerance of physical activity and shortness of breath (SOB). This classification may change according to the progression or regression of their cardiovascular disease (CVD; see Table 10.3):

A. Dyspnoea on exertion.
B. Haemoptysis.
C. Fatigue.
D. Cough.
E. Orthopnoea.
F. Oedema/weight gain.
G. Paroxysmal nocturnal dyspnoea.

TABLE 10.3 New York Heart Association Functional Classification for Heart Failure

Functional Class	Activities	Objective Assessment
AHA Class I ACCF Stage A	No limitation. Ordinary activity does not cause undue fatigue, palpitation, dyspnoea, or angina.	No objective evidence of CVD
AHA Class II ACCF Stage B	Slight limitations. Fatigue, palpitation, SOB, angina with ordinary physical activity.	Objective evidence—minimal CVD
AHA Class III ACCF Stage C	Marked limitations. No discomfort at rest. Fatigue, palpitation, SOB, and angina with less than usual activities.	Objective evidence—moderately severe CVD
AHA Class IV ACCF Stage D	Inability to do physical activity without discomfort. Symptoms are present at rest and become worse with activity.	Objective evidence—severe CVD

ACCF, American College of Cardiology Foundation; AHA, American Heart Association; CVD, cardiovascular disease; SOB, shortness of breath.
Source: Modified from the American Heart Association and includes staging by the American College of Cardiology Foundation.

H. Nausea.
I. Right upper abdominal pain or fullness.
J. Chest pain.
K. Palpitations.

Other Signs and Symptoms
A. Haemoptysis.
B. Bibasilar crackles.
C. S3 gallop.
D. Murmurs.
E. Exercise intolerance.
F. Weakness.
G. Cough.
H. Orthopnoea.
I. Nocturnal dyspnoea.
J. Tachycardia.
K. Pallor.
L. Cyanosis.
M. Anorexia.
N. Constipation.
O. Jugular venous distension (JVD).
P. Hepatomegaly.
Q. Hepatojugular reflux (HJR).
R. Murmurs.
S. Exercise intolerance.

Subjective Data
A. Ask the client whether he or she has difficulty breathing.
B. Ask how many pillows he or she sleeps on. Does the client need to sit up in a recliner to sleep?
C. Inquire about how often he or she wakes up at night with SOB.
D. Inquire about how far the client can walk without getting SOB. Have the client describe his or her routine activities of daily living (ADLs) and how well the client tolerates each activity.
E. Discuss the client's history of heart disease, heart attack, HTN, or hyperlipidaemia.
F. Ask the client about current medications: prescription, over-the-counter (OTC), and herbal products.
G. Question the client regarding all symptoms found in section "Common Findings."
H. Discuss drug and alcohol history.
I. Has the client ever been treated for cancer/chemotherapy, and how long ago?
J. What is the client's usual weight; has he or she experienced more symptoms if he or she has pedal oedema?
K. Does the client have a cough? (Consider angiotensin-converting enzyme inhibitors [ACEI] as the cause.)

Physical Examination
A. Check pulse, respirations, blood pressure (BP), height, and weight:
 1. Check BP while client is sitting, standing, and lying down.
 2. Be alert for abnormal vital signs: Hypotension, narrow or wide pulse pressure, tachycardia, bradycardia, and tachypnoea.
 3. Calculate body mass index (BMI).
 4. On all subsequent visits, note weight gain of more than one pound per day over three consecutive days or three pounds in one day.
B. Inspect:
 1. Overall physical appearance. Is the client in distress?
 2. Skin: Note pallor, cyanosis, and temperature.
 3. Neck: Check jugular veins for distension.
 4. Extremities: Note oedema, cyanosis, pallor, and ulcers.
C. Auscultate:
 1. Heart for murmurs; tachycardia; S1, S3, or S4 gallops; and other abnormalities.
 2. Lungs: Note moderate to severe crackles/rales and other abnormal sounds.
 3. Neck and carotid arteries.
D. Palpate:
 1. Abdomen for hepatomegaly and HJR.
 2. Extremities for peripheral pulses.
 3. Chest wall for displaced point of maximal impulse (PMI), lifts, heaves, and thrills.
E. Mental status: Check mental status because confusion may occur, especially in the elderly.

Diagnostic Tests
Initial
A. Chest x-ray.
B. ECG for clients with suspected arrhythmia, ischaemia, or cardiac disease. Identify acute and old ECG changes to rule out pathologic Q wave, ST segment elevation, and left ventricular (LV) hypertrophy.

C. CBC, creatinine, ferritin, thyroid-stimulating hormone (TSH), troponin, glucose.
D. Urinalysis.

If heart failure still suspected:
A. Two-dimensional echocardiography with Doppler to evaluate LVEF.
B. Radionuclide ventriculography may be used to measure LVEF and (LV) volumes.
C. Coronary angiography.
D. Multigated acquisition (MUGA) scan.
E. CT angiography.
F. Natriuretic peptides (brain natriuretic peptide [BNP] or N-terminal pro brain natriuretic peptide [NT-proBNP]) where available.

Differential Diagnoses
A. HFrEF versus HFpEF:
  1. HFpEF borderline clients with an EF of 41% to 49%.
  2. HFpEF clients with an EF >40% who previously had HFrEF (EF, 40%) with improvement noted in EF.
B. Renal disease or nephrotic syndrome.
C. Liver disease.
D. Asthma.
E. COPD: To distinguish between progressing HF and a COPD exacerbation when both conditions are present, the presence of weight gain and an S3 gallop indicates HF, not COPD.

Plan
A. General interventions:
  1. Determine the aetiology of the failure state and treat appropriately.
  2. Treat HF stages:
    a. Stage A: Treat/manage the client's underlying conditions (HTN, AF, hyperlipideamia, diabetes, tobacco cessation, obesity, substance abuse [alcohol, cocaine, etc.]).
    b. Stage B: Begin ACEI with beta-blockers for clients with HFrEF. Add statin therapy if client has a history of MI.
    c. Stage C: HFrEF: Implantable cardioverter defibrillators and consider cardiac resynchronization therapy:
      i. Digoxin may be used to manage symptoms. Hydralazine and isosorbide dinitrate are indicated for African American clients with HFrEF, clients with kidney dysfunction, or clients who cannot take ACEI or angiotensin receptor blocker (ARB) therapy. A diuretic agent is also recommended.
    d. Stage D: Provide advanced treatment such as cardiac transplant, mechanical support, and/or palliative care.
  3. The goals of therapy are to improve the client's quality of life by reducing symptoms, decreasing morbidity, and prolonging survival.
B. Client teaching:
  1. Teach the client to weigh daily at the same time, on the same scale, and in the same clothing. Instruct the client to call if there are gains of more than three pounds in one day or more than one pound a day over a three-day period:
    a. Develop a plan of care for the increase of diuretic dosing for oedema/weight gain in order to decrease dyspnoea and prevent hospitalization.
  2. Encourage weight loss.
  3. Recommend regular, moderate exercise as long as dyspnoea is not induced. Encourage exercise to increase endurance and strengthen muscles even though the client may only tolerate a few minutes of walking.
  4. Encourage smoking cessation.
  5. Encourage medication adherence. Instruct the client about all medications and possible side effects. Do not use OTC medicines without consulting the provider. Non-steroidal anti-inflammatory drugs (NSAIDs) are contraindicated in HF.
  6. Use continuous positive airway pressure (CPAP) or bilevel positive airway pressure (BiPAP) for nighttime sleep and naps for treatment of obstructive sleep apnoea (OSA).
C. Dietary management:
  1. Read food labels for sodium content.
  2. Teach dietary modifications, especially salt restriction of 2,000 to 3,000 mg/d for HFrEF and HFpEF. Less than 2,000 mg sodium per day is recommended in clients with moderate to severe HF symptoms.
  3. Fluid restriction is not recommended unless the client is classified as Stage D or is diagnosed with hyponatraemia with sodium levels <130 mEq/L. Restrict fluid intake to 2,000 mL/d or less for clients with chronic fluid retention despite use of diuretics and sodium restrictions.
  4. Alcohol consumption should be limited to one glass of beer or wine per day. This amount should be counted in the daily fluid restriction.
  5. See Appendix B for the DASH diet (Tables B.3 and B.4).
  6. Other diet changes include low-fat/low-cholesterol foods and the use of the following:
    a. Monounsaturated fats, which decrease cholesterol:
      i. Canola oil.
      ii. Olive oil.
    b. Polyunsaturated fats, which decrease cholesterol but not as well as monounsaturated fats:
      i. Vegetable and fish oils.
      ii. Corn, safflower, peanut, and soybean oils.
    c. Avoid saturated fats:
      i. Animal fats and some plant fats.
      ii. Butter and lard.
      iii. Coconut oil and palm oil.
D. Pharmacological therapy:
  1. Therapy is based on the extent of cardiac impairment and severity of symptoms. Medication regimens include a combination of the following classes: Diuretics, ACEI (ARB if unable to tolerate ACEI), cardioselective beta-blockers, inotropic agents such as digoxin, vasodilators, nitrates, and anticoagulants if there is an increased risk of thrombus formation. In general, calcium channel blockers (CCBs) are not used in HF management.
  2. Drug classifications for antihypertensive and cardiac medication are noted in Table 10.4.
E. Drugs that should be avoided and/or used with caution in HF because they cause exacerbations or are at high risk of adverse reactions include the following:
  1. NSAIDs: Increased renal dysfunction, oedema, impaired response to ACEI.
  2. Cyclooxygenase (COX-2) inhibitors: Increased rate of HF and increased mortality.
  3. ASA: Interaction between ASA and ACEI and interference with benefits of beta-blockers on LVEF.
  4. Metformin: Increased risk of lethal lactic acidosis.

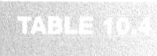

TABLE 10.4 Pharmacologic Treatment for Heart Failure (by Classification)

ACE-Inhibitors (ACE1)	MRA
Enalapril	Sprionolactone
Lisinopril	Eplerenone
Perindopril	**ARNI**
Ramipril	Sacubitril/Valsartan
Trandolapril	**I_f Inhibitor**
ARB	Ivabradine
Candesartan	**Vasodilators**
Valsartan	Isosorbide dinitrate
Beta-blockers	Hydralazine
Carvedilol	
Bisoprolol	
Metoprolol	

ACE, angiotensin converting enzyme; ARB, angiotensin receptor blocker; ARNI, angiotensin receptor-neprilysis inhibitor; MRA, mineralocorticoid receptor antagonists.

5. Thiazolidinediones: Causes fluid retention that may precipitate HF.
6. CCBs: Some data exist on possible effects on systolic dysfunction.
7. Antidepressants (tricyclic antidepressants [TCAs]) and selective serotonin reuptake inhibitors (SSRIs): Major adverse cardiovascular events, including HF, MI, stroke, and cardiovascular death.
8. Phosphodiesterase inhibitors (PDE-3, PDE-4, and PDE-5): Increased mortality.
9. Antiarrhythmic: Negative inotropic activity and further reduction in LV function can impair the elimination and result in toxicity of the antiarrhythmic.
10. Chemotherapy: Many are cardiotoxic.
11. Androgen–testosterone patch: Oedema may increase the rate of HF.
12. Theophylline-serum levels may increase and cause toxicity because of acute decompensation of HF.
13. Sodium bicarbonate contains significant quantities of sodium.
14. Herbal/supplements may also affect HF.

F. Biventricular pacing or an implantable defibrillator may be necessary for advanced HF.
G. Discuss the need for palliative/hospice care when HF does not respond despite maximal therapy.
H. Discuss the client's desire for advanced therapies that might include an evaluation for heart transplant or ventricular assist device.
I. The pneumonia vaccination as well as yearly influenza immunization should be encouraged.

Follow-Up

A. Close follow-up is essential if the client is to be maintained as an outpatient.
B. Appointments every one to two weeks may be necessary, with additional appointments depending on the client's symptoms, such as increasing SOB, inability to lie flat to sleep, nocturnal moist cough, and increase in daily weight.
C. Laboratory monitoring is required for electrolytes, urea, creatinine, proteinuria, and digoxin level.

Consultation/Referral

A. Consult a cardiologist for staging and hospital management.

Individual Considerations

A. Pregnancy:
  1. HF is uncommon in healthy women without coexisting heart disease.
  2. Pregnancy in a client with heart disease is considered high risk.
  3. Refer to a high-risk obstetrician.
B. Paediatrics: HF is usually associated with congenital heart defects.
C. Adults:
  1. The five-year survival rate is 25% for men and 38% for women.
  2. Predictors of poor outcome include an EF of <25%, ischaemic aetiology, ventricular arrhythmias, serum sodium <130 mEq/L, poor functional class, low cardiac index, and high-filling pressures.
D. Geriatrics:
  1. In very frail elderly clients or those in long-term care settings, the only sign may be increased agitation or acute change in level of consciousness (LOC).

Resources

Canadian Cardiovascular Society Heart Failure Guidelines: http://www.ccs.ca/images/Guidelines/PocketGuides_EN/HF_Gui_2017_PG_EN_web.pdf
Canadian Heart Failure Network: www.chfn.ca
Heart and Stroke Canada: www.heartand stroke.ca

Bibliography

Bowers, M. T. (2013, November). Managing patients with heart failure. *Journal for Nurse Practitioners, 9*, 621–628. doi:10.1016/j.nurpra.2013.08.025

Canadian Cardiology Society. (2017). *Guidelines for heart failure*. Retrieved from http://www.ccs.ca/images/Guidelines/PocketGuides_EN/HF_Gui_2017_PG_EN_web.pdf

Centers for Disease Control and Prevention. (2012, October 17). *Heart failure fact sheet*. Retrieved from https://www.cdc.gov/dhdsp/data_statistics/fact_sheets/fs_heart_failure.htm

Drug information. (2016). *Prescribers' digital reference*. Retrieved from www.pdr.net

Dumitru, I. (2013, May 6). Heart failure medication. *Medscape*. Retrieved from emedicine.medscape.com/article/163062-medication

Eckel, R. H., Jakicic, J. M., Ard, J. D., deJesus, J. M., HoustonMiller, N., Hubbard, V. S., & Yanovsk, S. Z. (2014). 2013 AHA/ACC guideline on lifestyle management to reduce cardiovascular risk: A report of the American College of Cardiology/American Heart Association Task Force on practice guidelines. *Circulation, 129*(25), S76–S99. doi:10.1161/01.cir.0000437740.48606.d1. Retrieved from http://circ.ahajournals.org/content/129/25_suppl_2/S76

Go, A. S., Mozaffarian, D., Roger, V. L., Benjamin, E. J., Berry, J. D., & Borden, W. B. (2013). Heart disease and stroke statistics—2013 update: A report from the American Heart Association. American Heart Association Statistics Committee and Stroke Statistics Subcommittee. *Circulation, 127*(1), e6-e245. doi:10.1161/CIR.0b013e31828124ad

Goff, D. C., Lloyd-Jones, D. M., Bennett, G., Coady, S., & D'Agostino, B. R., Sr. (2014). 2013 ACC/AHA guideline on the assessment of cardiovascular risk: A report of the American College of Cardiology/American Heart Association Task Force on practice guidelines. *Circulation, 129*(25 Suppl. 2), S49–S73. doi:10.1161/01.cir.0000437741.48606.98. Retrieved from http://circ.ahajournals.org/content/129/25_suppl_2/S49 Suppl. 2

Jackson, S. M. (2013). Diastolic heart failure. *Advance for NPs & PAs, 4*(2), 23–34.

Mozaffarian, D., Benjamin, E. J., & Go, A. S. (2015). Heart disease and stroke statistics—2015 update: A report from the American Heart Association. *Circulation, 131*(4), e29–e322. doi:10.1161/CIR.0000000000000152

Trayes, K. P., Studdiford, J. S., Pickle, S., & Tully, A. S. (2013). Edema: Diagnosis and management. *American Family Physician, 88*(2), 102–110. doi:10.1097/ACM.0b013e318277d5b2

Yancy, C. W., Jessup, M., Bozkurt, B., Butler, J., Casey, D. E., Drazner, M. H., & Wilkoff, B. L. (2013). 2013 ACCF/AHA guideline for the management of heart failure: A report of the American College of Cardiology Foundation/American Heart Association Task Force on Practice Guidelines. *Journal of the American College of Cardiology, 62*(16), e147–e239. doi:10.1161/CIR.0b013e31829e8776

Yancy, C. W., Jessup, M., Bozkurt, B., Butler, J., Casey, D. E., Drazner, M. H., & Wilkoff, B. L. (2013). 2013 ACCF/AHA guideline for the management of heart failure: A Report of the American College of Cardiology/American Heart Association Task Force on Practice Guidelines and the Heart Rhythm Society. *Circulation, 128*(16), e240–e327. doi:10.1161/CIR.0b013e31829e877

Hypertension (HTN)

Jill C. Cash, Cheryl A. Glass, Debbie Gunter, and Krista A. Bradley

Definition

A. Hypertension (HTN) is considered to be a systolic blood pressure (SBP) of 130 mmHg or more, a diastolic blood pressure (DBP) of 80 mmHg or more, or describes a condition in which a person is taking antihypertensive medications. Hypertension Canada defines HTN in adults as follows (see Table 10.5).
B. Resistant HTN is defined as follows:
  1. BP that is not at target despite a three-drug regimen, with one of the agents being a diuretic appropriate for the client's glomerular filtration rate (GFR).
  2. BP that is controlled while taking four or more medications is also considered resistant HTN.
C. Standing and supine blood pressure (BPs) should be measured before the initiation of combination antihypertensive therapy. Orthostatic (postural) hypotension is diagnosed when, within two to five minutes of quiet standing, one or more of the following is present:
  1. At least a 20 mmHg fall in systolic pressure.
  2. At least a 10 mmHg fall in diastolic pressure.
  3. Symptoms of cerebral hypoperfusion, such as dizziness.
D. The average nocturnal BP is approximately 15% lower than daytime values. Failure of the BP to fall by at least 10% during sleep is called "nondipping" and is a stronger predictor of adverse cardiovascular outcomes than daytime BP.
E. Isolated systolic HTN (ISH) is when the SBP is ≥130 with DBP normal or below normal (<80 mmHg). ISH usually affects the elderly, increasing their risk of stroke or myocardial infarction (MI).
F. Isolated diastolic hypertension (IDH) is defined as a diastolic pressure ≥80 mmHg with a systolic pressure <130 mmHg. IDH is more common in younger men who are overweight/obese and in individuals younger than 40 years.
G. Malignant HTN is marked HTN with retinal haemorrhages, exudates, or papilloedema. Malignant HTN is usually associated with diastolic pressures above 120 mmHg.

Incidence/Prevalence

A. Worldwide, HTN affects about 975 million people.
B. Approximately 7.5 million, or one in five Canadian adults, has HTN.
C. The incidence of resistant HTN is being studied more closely and the current average rate is about 12% of all clients with hypertension.
D. In Canada those at higher risk for HTN include Indigenous peoples, those with South Asian or Black ethnicity, and those with lower socioeconomic status.

Pathogenesis

More than 90% of cases have no identifiable cause, thus constituting the category of primary or essential HTN. The remaining 10% of cases have the following secondary causes:
A. Renal causes:
  1. Glomerulonephritis.
  2. Pyelonephritis.
  3. Polycystic kidney disease.
B. Endocrine causes:
  1. Primary hyperaldosteronism.
  2. Pheochromocytoma.
  3. Hyperthyroidism.
  4. Cushing's syndrome.
C. Vascular causes:
  1. Coarctation of aorta.
  2. Renal artery stenosis.
D. Chemical/medication induced:
  1. Oral contraceptives.
  2. Nonsteroidal anti-inflammatory drugs (NSAIDs).
  3. Decongestants.
  4. Antidepressants.
  5. Sympathomimetics.
  6. Corticosteroids.
  7. Lithium.
  8. Ergotamine alkaloids.
  9. Cyclosporine.
  10. Monoamine oxidase inhibitors (MAOIs), in combination with certain drugs or foods.
  11. Appetite suppressants, in combination with certain drugs or foods.
  12. Cocaine.
  13. Amphetamines.
E. Obstructive sleep apnoea (OSA).

TABLE 10.5 Whelton 2017 High Blood Pressure Clinical Practice Guideline

Blood Pressure Classification	Systolic Blood Pressure (mmHg)	Diastolic Blood Pressure (mmHg)
Normal	<120	and <80
Elevated BP	120–129	>80
Stage 1 HTN	130–139	80–89
Stage 2 HTN	≥140	or ≥90

BP, blood pressure; HTN, hypertension.
Source: Whelton P. K., et al. (2017). High Blood Pressure Clinical Practice Guideline. A guideline for the prevention, detection, evaluation, and management of high blood pressure in adults. Hypertension, DOI: 2017; HYP.0000000000000065.

Predisposing Factors

When making a diagnosis, consider not only the absolute BP reading, but also the presence or absence of other cardiovascular risk factors. Factors include the following:
A. Family history of HTN.
B. Obesity.
C. Alcohol consumption.
D. Stress.
E. Sedentary lifestyle.
F. African American ancestry.
G. Male gender.
H. Age >30 years.
I. Excessive salt intake.
J. Medications.
K. Drug use.

Common Findings
A. HTN is asymptomatic in the majority of clients.

Other Signs and Symptoms
A. Headaches.
B. Advanced disease: Organ-specific complaints with end-organ damage.
C. Retinopathy.

Potential Complications
A. Cerebral vascular accident (CVA).
B. MI.
C. Renal failure.
D. Heart failure (HF).
E. Peripheral arterial disease (PAD).

Subjective Data
A. Ask the client about any family history of HTN or cardiac or renal disease.
B. Ask whether the client has ever been diagnosed with HTN or cardiac or renal disease.
C. Ask whether the client ever had any high BP readings.
D. Ask whether the client has ever been treated for any of the aforementioned problems.
E. Ask the client about other risk factors, such as smoking, drinking, high fat intake, obesity, and/or diabetes.
F. Inquire about the client's lifestyle, exercise regimen, work environment, and stress level.
G. Ask the client about symptoms that suggest secondary aetiology:
  1. Palpitations, headache, diaphoresis (pheochromocytoma).
  2. Anxiety, weight gain, or loss (thyroid abnormality).
  3. Muscle weakness, polyuria (primary hyperaldosteronism).
H. Find out whether the client is taking drugs that elevate BP (noted under "Pathogenesis").
I. Ask whether the client feels nervous when having his or her BP taken in the office ("white coat HTN").
J. Review current medications, including prescription, over-the-counter (OTC), and herbal products.
K. Review current recreational/illicit drug use.

Physical Examination
A. Check pulse, BP, height, weight, waist circumference, and distribution of body fat. Calculate body mass index (BMI):
  1. The diagnosis of HTN is made after averaging two or more properly measured readings at each of the two or more visits after an initial screen.
  2. When the client's SBP and DBP fall into two different categories, use the higher category to classify his or her BP.
  3. For accurate measurement, use the correct size cuff for the client (adult, large adult, or thigh cuff).
B. Inspect:
  1. Observe overall appearance.
  2. Conduct funduscopic examination; look for papilleodema, exudates, atrioventricular (AV) nicking, anterior nicking.
  3. Inspect the neck for jugular vein distension.
  4. Observe for pedal oedema.
C. Auscultate:
  1. Heart; note the point of maximal impulse (PMI).
  2. Lungs; check for bronchospasm and rales.
  3. Neck; assess carotid arteries for bruits.
D. Palpate:
  1. Palpate the neck; check thyroid for enlargement.
  2. Palpate the abdomen for masses or organomegaly.
  3. Palpate the extremities; assess peripheral pulses and note oedema.
  4. Assess deep tendon reflexes (DTRs).

Diagnostic Tests
A. Haematocrit.
B. Liver function tests (LFTs; lactate dehydrogenase [LDH], uric acid).
C. Chemistry profile.
D. Lipid profile (total and HDL cholesterol and triglycerides).
E. Urinalysis for proteinuria.
F. Estimated GFR.
G. ECG.
H. If history, physical examination, or laboratory tests indicate the need, obtain the following:
  1. Intravenous pyelography (IVP).
  2. Renal arteriogram.
  3. Plasma renin.
  4. Catecholamines.
  5. Chest radiography.
  6. Aortogram.
  7. Ultrasonography.
  8. Sleep study.
I. Monitor potassium levels if on angiotensin-converting enzyme inhibitor/angiotensin receptor blocker (ACEI/ARBs) or spironolactone.

Differential Diagnoses
A. Primary HTN.
B. Secondary HTN.
C. Drug-induced HTN.
D. "White coat" syndrome.

Plan
A. General interventions (see Table 10.6):
  1. Advise overweight clients to lose weight. Loss of as little as 10 pounds reduces BP in many clients.
  2. Advise the client to limit or discontinue alcohol intake.
  3. Encourage the client to stop smoking.
  4. Encourage increased physical activity. The Canadian Cardiology Society recommendations 150 minutes of moderate to vigorous activity each week in sessions of 10 minutes or more.
  5. Counsel clients to consider reducing sodium intake to a maximum of 2,000 mg (2 g) of salt per day.
  6. Stress management should be considered where stress might be contributing to high BP.

B. Client teaching:
 1. Stress asymptomatic nature of disease.
 2. Stress importance of ongoing monitoring and treatment under the direction of a health-care provider.
 3. Review risk factors for cardiac, renal, and cerebrovascular disease and possible preventive measures.
 4. Hypertension Canada provides resources for clients that can be downloaded from the website guidelines. hypertension. ca/patient-resources/. Other resources include Smokershelpline.ca, a program that provides support to stop smoking.
C. Dietary management: Review specific dietary measures. Give dietary recommendation sheets. See Appendix B for low-fat/low-cholesterol and DASH dietary approaches to stop HTN:
 1. Diet alone will make only the lowest incremental change in BP; therefore, it should be combined with lifestyle modification and lower sodium intake; smoking cessation, weight loss, and exercise are essential.
 2. It is essential for the client/family to read labels for sodium, fat content, and serving sizes.
 3. Other dietary changes include low-fat/low-cholesterol diets and limiting fats:
  a. Use monounsaturated fats to decrease cholesterol:
   i. Canola oil.
   ii. Olive oil.
  b. Use in limited quantities: Polyunsaturated fats decrease cholesterol, but not as well as monounsaturated:
   i. Vegetable and fish oils.
   ii. Corn, safflower, peanut, and soybean oils.
  c. Limit saturated fats:
   i. Animal fats and some plant fats.
   ii. Butter and lard.
   iii. Coconut oil and palm oil.
D. Pharmacological therapy:
 1. If lifestyle changes alone are not adequate to control HTN, consider drug therapy. Medication doses are dependent on age, ethnicity, and comorbid conditions. Most clients will require two or more medications to control their BP. Consider starting antihypertensives and/or diuretics (see Table 10.5 for drugs and classifications). Hypertension Canada (2018) recommends commencing antihypertensive therapy when average DBP measurements are >100 or average SBP measurements exceed 160 mmHg in the absence of target organ damage or other cardiovascular risk factors.
 2. If there is evidence of target organ damage or in the presence of cardiovascular risk factors, treatment should be initiated when DBP exceeds 90 mmHg or when systolic readings exceed 140 mmHg.
 3. Hypertension Canada (2018) recommends the following approach to managing hypertension:

Initial Monotherapy
A. Thiazide/Thiazide-like diuretic with a preference for a long-acting formulation.
B. Beta-blocker (if age <60 years).
C. An angiotensin converting enzyme (ACE)-inhibitor (not recommended in African American clients).
D. An angiotensin-receptor blocker (ARB).
E. A long-acting calcium channel blocker (CCB).
Recommendations for initial single-pill combined therapy:
A. ACE-inhibitor with CCB.
B. ARB with a CCB.
C. ACE-inhibitor or ARB with a diuretic.
An additional drug chosen from the first-line treatments should be considered if monotherapy is unsuccessful in achieving target BP levels.

Notes: Combining an ACE-inhibitor and an ARB not recommended.
Caution is warranted if combining a nondihydropyridine CCB and a beta-blocker.
Statin therapy should be considered in hypertensive clients with three or more CV risk factors.
Low-dose ASA therapy should be considered in hypertensive clients >50 years.

Management of Isolated Systolic Hypertension
First-line therapies: Single-agent treatment:
A. Thiazide/thiazide-like diuretic.
B. Long-acting dihydropyridine CCB.
C. ARB.

Management of Hypertension in Specific Conditions
Coronary Artery Disease
A. First-line treatment is usually an ACE-inhibitor or an ARB (not used in combination).
B. For clients with stable angina and no history of heart failure, MI or coronary bypass surgery, a beta-blocker or CCB can be used.
Note: Avoid DBP below 60 mmHg as this may contribute to myocardial ischaemia.
C. For clients with a recent MI:
 1. Initial therapy should be a beta-blocker with an ACE-inhibitor.
 2. An ARB can be used if the ACE-inhibitor is not tolerated.
 3. A CCB can be used if a beta-blocker is contraindicated or ineffective.

Ischemic Stroke
A. Antihypertensives should be initiated after the acute phase of a stroke.
B. First-line treatment is with an ACE-inhibitor and a thiazide/thiazide-like diuretic.

Diabetes
A. BP target in clients with diabetes is <130/<80.
B. In the presence of cardiovascular renal disease (microalbuminaemia) or additional cardiovascular risk factors, an ACE-inhibitor or an ARB is the first-line treatment.

TABLE 10.6 Modifiable and Nonmodifiable Risk for Control of HTN

Modifiable	Nonmodifiable
Sedentary lifestyle	Age
Smoking	Gender
Diet	Ethnicity
Lipid control	Diabetes
Sodium intake	Postmenopausal
Alcohol intake	Family history
Obesity	

HTN, hypertension.

C. If combined therapy is needed and an ACE-inhibitor is being considered, then a dihydropyridine CCB is preferred over a thiazide diuretic.
Complete guidelines can be found at Hypertension Canada guidelines. hypertension. ca/.
D. Evaluate the client for secondary causes if severe HTN is resistant to therapy.
E. Resistant HTN; rule out all inadequate responses to the three-drug therapy (ACEI or ARB or CCB + diuretic):
  1. "White coat" HTN: Have the client begin to take and record his or her BP at home and report the values.
  2. Use size-appropriate BP cuffs on obese clients.
  3. Nonadherence to therapy, including side effects, medication regimen too complex, and/or cost/affordability.
  4. Volume overload because of excessive salt intake, progressive renal damage, fluid retention from BP reduction, and inadequate diuretic therapy.
  5. Drug problems: Dose too low, wrong type of diuretic, inappropriate combinations, rapid inactivation, drug actions, and interactions.
  6. Associated conditions: Smoking, obesity, sleep apnoea, insulin resistance, ethanol intake more than 30 mL (1 oz.) per day, panic attacks, chronic pain, and organic brain syndrome.
  7. Adding spironolactones can decrease SBP by 25 mmHg on average and DBP by an average of 12 mmHg in resistant hypertensives.
F. Treat with decongestants very cautiously. Pseudoephedrine HCl has the least cardiovascular effect.
G. Diuretics may worsen gout and diabetes.
H. Beta-blockers are contraindicated in asthma, HF, and heart block.
I. ACEI may cause coughing.
J. Abrupt cessation of therapy with a short-acting beta-blocker, such as propranolol, or the short-acting alpha-2-agonist clonidine, can lead to a potentially fatal withdrawal syndrome. Gradual discontinuation of these agents over a period of weeks should prevent this syndrome.

Follow-Up
A. If drug therapy is initiated, see the client again in two to four weeks for follow-up.
B. Once the client is stable, see him or her every three to six months.
C. Evaluate the client yearly, including uric acid, creatinine, and potassium.
D. Review and discuss drug therapy compliance, effectiveness, and adverse reactions (including effect on sexual activity) at each visit.
E. Home and ambulatory blood pressure monitoring (ABPM) is an adjunctive tool for the management of HTN:
  1. BP tracking apps are available on iTunes for the iPhone, iPod touch, and iPad.
  2. BP tracking apps for Androids are available on Google Play and Amazon Appstore.
  3. Hypertension Canada has BP tracking instructions and a printable BP tracking log located at
  hypertension. ca › Hypertension & You › Managing Hypertension.
F. Consider a sleep study for diagnosis of OSA (see section "Obstructive Sleep Apnoea" in Chapter 9, Respiratory Guidelines,).
G. Clients with pre-HTN without diabetes, chronic kidney disease (CKD), or cardiovascular disease (CVD) should be treated with nonpharmacological therapy (i.e., diet, sodium reduction, weight loss, exercise, smoking cessation) and should be evaluated annually.

Consultation/Referral
A. If the client is pregnant, consult an obstetrician before prescribing medications. Many antihypertensive drugs are harmful to the fetus.
B. Consult a cardiologist if the client is having an acute hypertensive emergency: DBP >130 mmHg.

Individual Considerations
A. Pregnancy: Refer to Chapter 13, Obstetrics Guidelines:
  1. HTN may be either chronic or gestational hypertension.
  2. HTN (BP >140/90) is considered chronic if it is present before pregnancy or diagnosed before the 20th week of gestation.
  3. Gestational hypertension refers to hypertension that develops during pregnancy. When BP readings prior to pregnancy are not known, a reading of 140/90 or higher is considered abnormal.
  4. Maternal as well as fetal mortality and morbidity improve with treatment.
B. Paediatrics:
  1. Evaluate BP at every visit starting at the age of 3 years.
  2. HTN can occur in many acute illnesses, or it may be a chronic problem.
  3. Determine high BP by correlating height indexes with BP readings.
C. Geriatrics:
  1. The optimal BP treatment goal in the elderly has not been determined, as there is not a consensus among various national and international organizations. Earlier Canadian Hypertension Guidelines (The Canadian Hypertension Education Program 2014) proposed that in clients over the age of 80 years with isolated systolic hypertension, goals for initiating drug therapy in the absence of diabetes or target organ damage is >160 mmHg with a BP target of <150. The more recent Hypertension Canada Guidelines (2018) are based on risk factors rather than age.
  2. Elderly persons with HTN are more likely to develop orthostatic and postprandial hypotension, which may result in falls or syncope:
    a. Evaluate side effects, including dizziness and sedation. Beta-blockers may cause depression or confusion in the elderly.
  3. The general approach to drug therapy in the geriatric population is to start low and go slow.
  4. Check the Beers list for harmful drugs in the geriatric population. The 2015 American Geriatrics Society's, Updated Beers Criteria for Potentially Inappropriate Medication Use in Older Adults is available at geriatricscareonline. org/ProductAbstract/american-geriatrics-society-updated-beers-criteria-for-potentially-inappropriate-medication-use-in-older-adults/CL001. A printable pocketcard is available for download at www. americangeriatrics. org/files/documents/beers/Printable-BeersPocketCard. pdf.
  5. To avoid hyperkalaemia in the elderly, potassium-sparing diuretics should not be given with ACEI or ARBs.

Resource
Hypertension Canada has resources for both health care professionals and patients. https://guidelines. hypertension. ca/chep-resources/
The National Kidney Foundation provides online calculators: www. kidney. org/professionals/KDOQI/gfr_calculator

Bibliography

American Diabetes Association. (2013). Executive summary: Standards of medical care in diabetes—2013. *Diabetes Care, 36*(Suppl. 1), S4–S10. doi:10.2337/dc13-S004

American Geriatrics Society. (2015). Updated Beers criteria for potentially inappropriate medication use in older adults. *Journal of the American Geriatrics Society, 63,* 2227–2246. doi:10.1111/jgs.13702

Davis, L. L. (2013, November). Using the latest evidence to manage hypertension. *Journal for Nurse Practitioners, 9,* 621–628. doi:10.1016/j.nurpra.2013.08.013

Drug information. (2016). *Prescribers' digital reference.* Retrieved from www.pdr.net

Go, A. S., Bauman, M., C, King. S. M., Fonarow, G. C., Lawrence, W., Williams, K. A., & Sanchez, E. (2014, April). An effective approach to high blood pressure control: A science advisory from the American Heart Association, the American College of Cardiology, and the Centers for Disease Control and Prevention. *Hypertension, 63*(4), 878—885. doi:10.1161/CIR.0b013e31828124ad. Retrieved from http://hyper.ahajournals.org/content/early/2013/11/14/HYP.0000000000000003.reprint

Go, A. S., Mozaffarian, D., Roger, V. L., Benjamin, E. J., Berry, J. D., & Borden, W. B. (2013). Heart disease and stroke statistics—2013 update: A report from the American Heart Association. American Heart Association Statistics Committee and Stroke Statistics Subcommittee. *Circulation, 127*(1), e6-e245. doi:10.1161/CIR.0b013e31828124ad

Hypertension Canada. (2016). *Hypertension in Canada.* Retrieved from http://www.hypertensiontalk.com/wp-content/uploads/2016/05/HTN-Fact-Sheet-2016_FINAL.pdf

James, P. A., Oparil, S., Carter, B. L., Cushman, W. C., Dennison-Himmelfarb, C., Handler, J., & Ortiz, E. (2014). 2014 evidence-based guideline for the management of high blood pressure in adults: Report from the panel members appointed to the Eighth Joint National Committee (JNC 8). *The Journal of the American Medical Association, 311*(5), 507–520. doi:10.1001/jama.2013.284427

Judd, E., & Calhoun, D. A. (2014). Apparent and true resistant hypertension: Definition, prevalence and outcomes. *Journal of Human Hypertension, 28*(8), 463–468. doi:10.1038/jhh.2013.140

Madhur, M. S. (2013, December 3). Hypertension. *Medscape.* Retrieved from emedicine.medscape.com/article/241381-overview

Mann, J. F. E. (2013, May 25). Choice of therapy in primary (essential) hypertension: Recommendations. *UpToDate.* Retrieved from www.uptodate.com

Mann, J. F. E., & Hilgers, K. F. (2015, January 20). Hypertension: Who should be treated? *UpToDate.* Retrieved from http://www.uptodate.com/contents/hypertension-who-should-betreated?topicKey-NEPH

Mozaffarian, D., Benjamin, E. J., & Go, A. S. (2015). Heart disease and stroke statistics—2015 update: A report from the American Heart Association. *Circulation, 131*(4), e29–e322. doi:10.1161/CIR.0000000000000152

Robert, L. (2013, May 15). *Hypertension meeting has primary care track.* Retrieved from www.consultantlive.com/print/article/10162/2142634

Rutecki, G. W. (2013a, May 16). *Some do's and don'ts for tough-to-treat hypertensives.* Retrieved from http://www.consultantlive.com/print/article/10162/2142822?printable=true

Rutecki, G. W. (2013b, May 22). *Lessons in quality improvement. Reflections on ASH 2013.* Retrieved from www.consultantlive.com/conference-reports/ash2013/content/article/10162/2143452

Spencer, A., Jablonski, R., & Loeb, S. J. (2012). Hypertensive African American women and the DASH diet. *Nurse Practitioner, 37*(2), 41–46. doi:10.1097/01.NPR.0000410278.75362.a2

U.S. Department of Health and Human Services, National Institutes of Health, & National Heart, Lung, and Blood Institute. (2006). *Your guide to lowering your blood pressure with DASH* (NIH Publications No. 06-4082). Bethesda, MD: National Heart, Lung and Blood Institute. Retrieved from http://www.nhlbi.nih.gov/health/public/heart/hbp/dash/new_dash.pdf

U.S. Department of Health and Human Services, National Institutes of Health, National Heart, Lung, and Blood Institute. (2004). *Seventh report of the Joint National Committee on prevention, detection, evaluation, and treatment of high blood pressure.& National High Blood Pressure Education Program & National High Blood Pressure Education Program.* Bethesda, MD: National Heart, Lung and Blood Institute. Retrieved from https://www.nhlbi.nih.gov/files/docs/public/heart/new_dash.pdf

Vongpatanasin, W. (2014). Resistant hypertension: A review of diagnosis and management. *The Journal of the American Medical Association, 311*(21), 2216–2224. doi:10.1001/jama.2014.5180

Wright, B. M., Rutecki, G. W., & Bellone, J. (2013, January). Resistant hypertension: An approach to diagnosis and treatment. *Consultant, 53*(1), 9–16. Retrieved from www.Consultant360.com

Lymphoedema

Jill C. Cash, Debbie Gunter, and Krista A. Bradley

Definition

A. Peripheral vascular disease (PVD) is a general term that encompasses all occlusive or inflammatory diseases that occur within the peripheral arteries, veins, and lymphatic system. Lymphoedema is a chronic condition caused by the accumulation of lymphatic fluid in the interstitial tissue.

Incidence/Prevalence

A. In Canada, 300,000 people have lymphoedema. The incidence worldwide is projected to approach 100 million.

Pathogenesis

A. Lymphoedema occurs when lymph fluid is unable to flow in a normal manner and accumulates in an extremity. The propensity for lymphoedema can be inherited or caused by another condition, such as lymphangitis, malignancy, filariasis, or removal of lymph nodes.

Predisposing Factors

A. Cancer.
B. Radiation therapy.
C. Surgical removal of lymph nodes.
D. Parasitic infection (filariasis).
E. Congenital disorders involving the structure of the lymph system:
  1. Milroy's disease.
  2. Meige's disease.
F. Obesity.
G. Surgical implantation of pacemaker or arteriovenous shunt.
H. Systemic diseases (hyperthyroidism; hypertension; renal or cardiac disease).
I. Vascular disease (chronic venous insufficiency or post-thrombotic syndrome).

Common Findings

A. Severe oedema that is consistent to the distal aspect of the extremity.
B. Hard skin over oedematous area.
C. Loss of range of motion.

Potential Complications

A. Infection, including lymphangitis and cellulitis.
B. Lymphangiosarcoma.

Subjective Data

A. Ask the client when the symptom(s) were first noticed.
B. Have the client describe the duration of symptoms.
C. Review any history of cancer, radiation, and chemotherapy.
D. Review recent history of invasive procedures or surgery.
E. Ask the client to list all medications currently being taken, particularly substances not prescribed and illicit drugs.
F. Ask the client to describe any pain.
G. Ask the client what makes the symptoms better and what makes them worse.
H. Have the client rate discomfort on a scale of 1 to 10, with 1 being the least uncomfortable.

Physical Examination

A. Vital signs:
 1. Check blood pressure (BP) and document resting heart rate, respirations, temperature, height, and weight.

B. Inspect:
 1. Assess for signs of erythema, increased temperature, and oedema.

C. Palpate:
 1. Lymph nodes distal and proximal to the site.
 2. Pulses distal and proximal in all extremities.
 3. Extremity for tenderness.

D. Auscultate:
 1. Heart: Rate, rhythm, heart sounds, murmur, and gallops.
 2. Lungs: Assess lung sounds in all fields.

Diagnostic Tests

A. Serum laboratory tests (complete blood count [CBC] with differential and brain natriuretic peptide [BNP]).
B. CT scan of the affected extremity.
C. Doppler ultrasound of the affected extremity.
D. Testing to assess the extent of the lymphoedema or to rule in/out an aetiology:
 1. CT scan, MRI, and/or Doppler.
E. Lymphoscintigraphy.
F. Additional tests to monitor coexisting systemic and/or vascular disease.

Differential Diagnoses

A. Unilateral limb oedema:
 1. Lymphoedema.
 2. Venous insufficiency.
 3. Deep vein thrombosis or postthrombotic syndrome.
 4. Arthritis.
 5. Baker's cyst.
 6. Presence or reoccurrence of cancer.

B. Symmetrical limb oedema:
 1. Congestive heart failure (CHF).
 2. Chronic venous insufficiency.
 3. Renal dysfunction.
 4. Hepatic dysfunction.
 5. Hypothyroidism (myxoedema).
 6. Medication-induced oedema.
 7. Lipoedema.

Plan

▶ **A.** Client teaching: *Refer to Client Teaching Guide: Lymphoedema:*
 1. Protect the arm or leg while recovering from cancer treatment.
 2. Avoid heavy lifting, if an arm is affected.
 3. Avoid strenuous exercise.
 4. Avoid heat on the arm or leg.
 5. Avoid tight clothing.
 6. Inspect the affected limb daily, noting any cracks or cuts.
 7. Apply lotion daily to protect and prevent dry skin.

B. Nonpharmacological therapy:
 1. Extremity elevation.
 2. Compression stockings or wrapping of affected limb.
 3. Pneumatic compression boot.
 4. Therapeutic massage, specifically manual lymph drainage.
 5. Referral to a lymphoedema therapist.
 6. Referral to physical therapy for home exercise program.

C. Surgery:
 1. Lymphaticovenular bypass.
 2. Lymphovenous bypass.

Follow-Up

A. Follow-up is determined by client's needs, frequency and intensity of symptoms, and presence of other medical conditions.
B. PVD manifesting persistent symptoms should always be followed by a cardiologist.

Consultation/Referral

A. If you suspect acute limb ischaemia, refer the client for immediate hospitalization in order to obtain diagnostic testing to determine the presence of a thrombus and restore circulation to the affected extremity.
B. If chronic limb ischaemia has led to ulceration and/or superimposed infection, hospitalization is indicated to initiate a wound care consultation and for diagnostic testing to determine the degree of arterial occlusion.
C. Referral to a cardiologist is indicated in the presence of persistent PVD symptoms.
D. Referral to a lymphoedema therapist and physical therapist is indicated to best manage chronic lymphoedema.

Bibliography

Alberta Lympheda Network. (n.d.). *Lymphedema*. Retrieved from http://www.lymphaticresearchab.com/lymphedema/
Bernas, M. (2013). Assessment and risk reduction in lymphedema. *Seminars in Oncology Nursing, 29*(1), 12–19. doi:10.1016/j.soncn.2012.11.003
Isl, I. (2013). The diagnosis and treatment of peripheral lymphedema: 2013 consensus document of the International Society of Lymphology. *Lymphology, 46*(1), 1–11.
Piller, N., Partsch, H., Hays, S., & Woodman, R. (2014). What's best for our lymphedema patients? *Journal of Lymphoedema, 9*(2), 6–10.
Trayes, K. P., Studdiford, J. S., Pickle, S., & Tully, A. S. (2013). Edema: Diagnosis and management. *American Family Physician, 88*(2), 102–110. doi:10.1097/ACM.0b013e318277d5b2
Vascular Cures. (2016). *Lymphedema*. Retrieved from http://vasculardisease.org/images/VDF-Diseases-Flyers/lymphedema-flyer%20Vascular%20Cures.pdf

Murmurs

Jill C. Cash, Debbie Gunter, and Krista A. Bradley

Definition

A murmur is turbulent blood flow through the heart as a result of one or more of the following aetiologies:
A. Narrow valve opening, stenosis.
B. Incomplete valve closure, regurgitant or insufficient blood flow.
C. Abnormal opening through chambers, atrial, or ventricular septal defect (VSD).
D. Rapid blood flow through normal valve structures; occurs during pregnancy, with increased physiological demand states, and in children.
E. No abnormality; occurs in clients with thin chest walls and in children.

▶ Client Teaching Guides are available at https://connect.springerpub.com/content/reference-book/978-0-8261-9498-5

Incidence/Prevalence
A. Approximately 80% of children have a physiological murmur at one time or another. Four percent of women studied in the Framingham study had a murmur related to mitral valve prolapse (MVP).

Pathogenesis
A. Pathogenesis depends on specific aetiology, but rheumatic disease, calcific changes, ischaemic insults, congenital abnormalities, and degenerative diseases all contribute to the development of a murmur.

Common Findings
A. Often no symptoms are present, and murmur is found on routine examination.
B. Complaints with advanced valvular disease:
  1. Chest pain.
  2. Dyspnoea.
  3. Palpitations.
  4. Shortness of breath (SOB).
  5. Exercise intolerance.
  6. Postural light-headedness.

Subjective Data
A. Has the client ever been diagnosed with a murmur?
B. Did the client have frequent strep infections as a child?
C. Ask the client about any recent viral infections.
D. Question the client about chest pain; SOB; palpitations; diaphoresis; light-headedness; or syncope, especially with exertion.
E. Ask the client whether any family members had sudden cardiac death before the age of 55 years.

Physical Examination
A. Check temperature, if indicated, pulse, respirations, and blood pressure (BP):
B. Inspect chest for lifts and heaves.
C. Palpate chest for lifts, heaves, and thrills.
D. Auscultate:
  1. Heart for splitting of heart sounds, clicks, rubs, and murmurs; use the bell and diaphragm of the stethoscope to auscultate the client in the left lateral, supine, standing, sitting (and leaning forward), and squatting positions and after having client run in place or do jumping jacks for two to three minutes:
     a. A new, systolic, regurgitant murmur in the setting of an acute myocardial infarction (MI) may indicate a ruptured papillary muscle and possible cardiogenic shock.
     b. When a new murmur is audible, differentiate location, timing, quality, intensity, and duration. Note if radiation to the neck, axilla, or back is present.
     c. Note location of murmur:
        i. Aortic: Second right intercostal space (ICS) next to sternum.
        ii. Pulmonic: Second left ICS next to sternum.
        iii. Tricuspid: Fifth left ICS next to sternum.
        iv. Mitral: Fifth left ICS at midclavicular line.
     d. If murmur is heard, have the client squat, stand, and/or perform the Valsalva maneuver. Squatting will increase the blood to the heart and increase the left ventricle blood volume and stroke volume, which will increase the sound of the murmur. Standing and the Valsalva maneuver will provide the opposite, in which the venous return will drop and decrease the ventricle size and stroke volume and soften the sound of the murmur.
     e. If the sound of the murmur occurs during the opposite action, softer when squatting and louder when standing or during the Valsalva maneuver, consider hypertrophic cardiomyopathy or MVP as the diagnosis.
  2. Assess the neck and axilla for radiation.

Diagnostic Tests
A. ECG.
B. Echocardiogram.
C. Chest radiography.

Differential Diagnoses
Major differentiation should be in the description of murmur, as this aids in identification of the murmur:
A. Timing:
  1. Identify when the murmur occurs in the cardiac cycle.
  2. Systolic murmurs may or may not be normal:
     a. Occurs between the S1 "lub" and the S2 "dub."
  3. Diastolic murmurs are always abnormal and need further evaluation:
     a. Occurs between the S2 "dub" and the S1 "lub."
B. Quality: Is the sound harsh, blowing, musical, rumbling, vibratory, or soft?
C. Intensity: Murmurs are usually graded on a six-point scale:
  1. Grade I. Barely audible.
  2. Grade II. Audible but soft.
  3. Grade III. Easily audible without thrill.
  4. Grade IV. Easily audible, thrill usually palpable.
  5. Grade V. Audible with only the rim of the stethoscope on the chest wall; thrill present.
  6. Grade VI. Audible with the stethoscope barely off the chest wall; thrill present.
D. Duration: Identify location and timing in the specific phase of the cardiac cycle:
  1. Holosystolic: Throughout systole.
  2. Holodiastolic: Throughout diastole.
  3. Midsystolic: Midway between S1 and S3.
  4. Mid-diastolic: Midway between S2 and S1.
  5. Decrescendo: Starts loud at the beginning, then tapers off.
  6. Crescendo: Starts soft at the beginning, then gets louder.
E. Radiation: Murmur can be heard in another place, such as the neck, back, left axilla, or across precordium. Sound usually radiates in the direction of blood flow.
F. Location: Identify location on chest wall where murmur is heard the best. Identify site: Apex, pulmonary area, tricuspid, and aortic areas. Radiation murmur may also include axilla, left fourth ICS, or base of heart.
G. Configuration: The intensity of the murmur over time: Does it plateau, crescendo, decrescendo, or crescendo–decrescendo?
H. Systolic murmurs: Systolic murmurs are benign or pathologic:
  1. Early systolic murmurs:
     a. Mitral regurgitation: Holosystolic, blowing may be loud. Located at fifth ICS and radiates to left axilla/back. Heard best in left lateral position and with sudden squatting; intensity decreases with the Valsalva maneuver and standing.
     b. Tricuspid regurgitation: Holosystolic, heard in left lower sternal border or apex when right ventricle

is enlarged. Intensity increases with inspiration and decreases with expiration. Straight leg raises may increase intensity. May also see hepatojugular reflux (HJR).

c. Physiological: Early to midsystolic, low-pitch normal S1–S2, located at left lower sternal edge at third to fourth ICS. Heard best with bell and supine and disappears when sitting up or holding breath. Commonly seen in children, pregnancy, and infection.

2. Midsystolic to late systolic murmurs:
   a. Aortic stenosis: Loud, hard crescendo–decrescendo at second right ICS that radiates to the neck. Heard best when client is leaning forward, increases with leg raise and lying flat. Decreases with Valsalva and handgrip standing.
   b. Pulmonic stenosis: Prolonged, loud S2 or crescendo–decrescendo, usually >3/6 at second ICS and radiates to neck; increases with inspiration.
   c. Hypertrophic cardiomyopathy (aortic outflow obstruction): Peaks at midsystole; loud, harsh tone at left, lower sternal border that may radiate to neck. Increases with Valsalva maneuver and standing, decreases with sudden squatting. Note brisk carotid upstroke.

3. Late systolic murmurs:
   a. MVP: Midsystolic click heard before late systolic murmur, heard best at fifth left ICS. Heard best with diaphragm; sitting or squatting may increase intensity.
   b. Tricuspid valve prolapse: Heard over the left lower sternal border, delayed onset of murmur with inspiration secondary to an increase in the right ventricular volume.

I. Diastolic murmurs: Murmurs are always pathologic:
1. Early diastolic murmur:
   a. Aortic regurgitation: High-pitch faint, decrescendo may start with S2, at third left ICS and radiate down sternal edge. Heard best when the client is leaning forward, holding breath. Increases with sudden squatting or handgrip. May hear displaced PMI, S3, bounding pulse.
   b. Pulmonary regurgitation: Valvular, dilation of valve annulus, congenital defect (tetralogy of Fallot VSD), pulmonic stenosis. Best heard over left second/third ICS. May sound high pitched with "blowing" sound in clients with hypertension (HTN). May be pansystolic, having decrescendo configuration.

2. Mid-diastolic murmur:
   a. Mitral stenosis: Rumbling extends beyond mid-diastole at fifth ICS, heard best using the bell of the stethoscope. Increases with left lateral position. May hear snap after S2.
   b. Tricuspid stenosis: Increased flow across the tricuspid valve, heard best at the left sternal border. Identified by its increase in intensity of the murmur with inspiration (Carvallo's sign). Commonly seen with mitral stenosis.

Plan

A. General interventions:
1. Major therapeutic goals are to preserve quality of life, increase life expectancy and exercise capacity, and reduce risk of complications.
2. Activity restriction is not necessary in clients with asymptomatic valvular disease.

B. Client teaching:
1. Reassure the client regarding specific diagnosis.
2. Counsel the client regarding his or her specific condition. Teach the client signs and symptoms to report to the health provider, including chest pain, SOB, difficulty breathing, and so forth.

C. Medical and surgical management: Clients who need progressive increases in medications to control symptoms may be candidates for valve replacement surgery.

D. Pharmacological therapy:
1. The 2007 American Heart Association (AHA) guidelines (these remain the most up-to-date) do not recommend endocarditis antimicrobial prophylaxis treatment for common valvular lesions that include bicuspid aortic valve, acquired aortic or mitral valve disease (including MVP with regurgitation), and hypertrophic cardiomyopathy with latent or resting obstruction. The Canadian Dental Association (2014) has endorsed the AHA's Guidelines.
2. The Canadian Paediatric Society (2010/2018) published guidelines for the prevention of infective endocarditis in the paediatric populations. These guidelines are also based on the 2007 American guidelines.

E. Endocarditis prophylaxis treatment: Cardiac conditions:
1. It is recommended for high-risk cardiac condition abnormalities to have prophylactic treatment. Specific cardiac conditions are as follows:
   a. Prosthetic cardiac valve or prosthetic material used for cardiac valve repair.
   b. Previous infective endocarditis.
   c. Certain congenital heart diseases, such as cyanotic congenital heart disease that has not been repaired; a congenital heart disease that has been repaired with an artificial material or device for six months after repair; and repaired congenital heart defects with continued problems, such as leaks or insufficient flow at the prosthetic device or adjacent to the repair endocarditis prophylaxis treatment.
   d. Postcardiac transplant valvulopathy.

2. Procedures for high-risk clients mentioned earlier that require prophylaxis treatment:
   a. All dental procedures with manipulation of gingival tissue or periapical region of teeth or perforation of oral mucosa.
   b. Incision or biopsy of respiratory mucosa or any invasive procedure of the respiratory tract system.
   c. Procedures that include infected skin or musculoskeletal tissue.
   d. Preventative treatment with antibiotics is not recommended for procedures that include the reproductive tract, urinary tract, or gastrointestinal (GI) tract.

3. Antibiotic prophylactic regimens include a single dose 30 to 60 minutes before procedure:
   a. Amoxicillin.
   b. Ampicillin.
   c. Allergy to penicillin (PCN): Cephalexin.
   d. Azithromycin or clarithromycin.
   e. Allergic to aforementioned: Consider cefazolin or ceftriaxone or clindamycin.

4. Other pharmacological treatments depend on the specific valvular abnormality:
   a. Mitral stenosis: The mitral valve has a narrowing that does not allow adequate blood to the left ventricle during diastole, usually because of rheumatic heart disease. Mitral heart disease is the most commonly seen valve effect with rheumatic heart disease.

b. Diuretics, such as furosemide or hydrochlorothiazide, are used to control oedema.
c. Digoxin or beta-blockers are used to control atrial fibrillation (AF) and irregular heart rate.
d. Warfarin and the antiplatelet agent ASA are used to prevent clotting.
e. MVP: The echocardiogram is the recommended test for diagnosis of MVP. Usually no medications are recommended except when symptomatic and required:
  i. Beta-blockers may be used for palpitations.
  ii. Diuretics should be avoided in clients who are volume reserved.
  iii. Oral contraceptives should be avoided in women who exhibit neurologic symptoms.
f. Mitral regurgitation: Diuretics, digitalis, and afterload-reducing agents for congestive heart failure (CHF):
  i. Aortic stenosis.
  ii. Diuretics are used for CHF.
  iii. Avoid vasodilators; they may result in profound, irreversible hypotension.
  iv. Echocardiograms should be performed every six to 12 months to follow the progression of narrowing of the left ventricle across the aortic valve.
g. Aortic regurgitation: Afterload-reducing agents, digitalis, and diuretics are recommended.

Follow-Up
A. Most clients with valvular disease should be evaluated at least once a year.
B. Clients on oral anticoagulation drugs need monthly follow-up or as needed prothrombin time/international normalized ratios (PT/INRs).

Consultation/Referral
A. Consult a cardiologist if the client is diagnosed with a new murmur or exercise-induced symptoms during a sports physical.
B. Refer clients with newly diagnosed murmurs to a cardiologist after obtaining echocardiogram results. Drug therapy should be initiated according to diagnosis and symptoms.
C. Onset of AF with rapid ventricular response is an indication for immediate hospitalization.
D. Refer clients with systemic embolization for emergent anticoagulation therapy and chronic oral anticoagulant therapy. Discuss the possibility of valve replacement with a cardiologist.
E. If a new murmur is diagnosed in a pregnant client with a history of cardiac disease, refer her to a cardiologist immediately.
F. All diastolic murmurs in paediatric clients indicate pathology and need to be evaluated by a cardiologist.

Individual Considerations
A. Pregnancy:
  1. The development of a new, "high-flow" murmur in a healthy woman is not uncommon because of physiological changes occurring during pregnancy.
B. Paediatrics:
  1. Perform a thorough cardiac examination on clients from the time they are newborns through adolescence, so that if a murmur is detected, it can be compared.
C. Geriatrics:
  1. A systolic murmur heard best in the aortic area may indicate aortic sclerosis because of aging of the aortic valve rather than true aortic stenosis.

Resources
American Heart Association Infective Endocarditis prevention: https://www.heart.org/en/health-topics/infective-endocarditis
Canadian Paediatric Society Infective Endocarditis Guidelines: https://www.cps.ca/en/documents/position/infective-endorcarditis-guidelines

Bibliography
American Heart Association. (2013). *Infective endocarditis*. Retrieved from http://www.heart.org/HEARTORG/Conditions/CongenitalHeartDefects/TheImpactofCongenitalHeartDefects/Infective-Endocarditis_UCM_307108_Article.jsp#.WGFOlLnT8rM
Drug information. (2016). *Prescribers' digital reference*. Retrieved from www.pdr.net
National Institute for Health and Care Excellence. (2016, July). *Prophylaxis against infective endocarditis: Clinical guideline 64.1: Methods, evidence and recommendations*. Retrieved from https://www.nice.org.uk/guidance/cg64

Palpitations

Jill C. Cash, Debbie Gunter, and Krista A. Bradley

Definition
A. Palpitations are a feeling or an unpleasant awareness of the heartbeat in the chest. It may be described as feeling a sensation of the heart "flip-flopping" or feeling a "rapid flutter" of the heart.

Incidence/Prevalence
A. The incidence of palpitations may range from 1% to 8% of clients in a general practice setting.

Pathogenesis
Palpitations may be caused by the following:
A. Increase in stroke volume or contractility.
B. Sudden change in heart rate or rhythm.
C. Unusual cardiac movement within thorax.
D. Hyperkinetic states, which cause constant pounding; hyperthyroidism, late-stage pregnancy.
E. Valvular heart disease that produces large stroke volumes.
F. Catecholamine release during anxiety or panic attacks.

Predisposing Factors
A. Cardiac defects.
B. Severe anaemia.
C. Hyperthyroidism.
D. Pregnancy.
E. Fever.
F. Anxiety.
G. Stimulants such as caffeine and certain drugs.
H. Emotions such as fear.
I. Exertion.
J. Diabetes mellitus and insulin reaction.

Common Findings
A. Palpitations are often described as a turning over or flopping sensation in the chest, but symptoms vary enormously.
B. Most clients are free of palpitations at the time of the examination.

Other Signs and Symptoms
A. Fluttering in the chest.
B. Shortness of breath (SOB).
C. Pounding in the chest and neck.
D. Diaphoresis.
E. Light-headedness.
F. Anxiety or fear.

Subjective Data
A. Ask the client when symptoms first presented, including age, and how they have changed.
B. Have the client describe the characteristics of the palpitations, such as rapid, regular, irregular, or slow.
C. Ask the client what precipitates the palpitations. Does anything terminate them, or do they go away on their own?
D. Inquire whether symptoms occur or change with position (standing, bending over, lying down, left lateral decubitus position) and/or exercise.
E. Ask the client about other associated symptoms with the palpitations, such as dizziness or syncope.
F. Ask how often the episodes occur and how long each lasts.
G. Discuss any previous treatments for this condition and the results.
H. Ask the client about risk factors for coronary heart disease (CHD) and prior cardiac history.
I. Question the client's use of over-the-counter (OTC) decongestants and diet pills. Are there any new medications or change in routine medications? Obtain a complete list of medications the client is currently taking.

Physical Examination
A. Check pulse (count the pulse for a full minute), respirations, and blood pressure (BP).
B. Inspect:
  1. Overall appearance.
  2. The skin for diaphoresis and pallor.
  3. The neck for thyromegaly or jugular vein distension.
  4. The legs for oedema.
C. Palpate:
  1. The skin for temperature and dryness.
  2. The lower extremities for oedema and calf tenderness.
  3. The neck for thyroid enlargement.
D. Auscultate:
  1. The heart for abnormal rhythms. Auscultate heart with the client in the sitting, standing, and left lateral decubitus positions. Ask the client to walk quickly down the hallway and back and then auscultate the heart in all positions again.
  2. The lungs.
  3. The neck and carotid arteries for bruits.
E. Mental status: Does the client appear light-headed, anxious, or fearful?

Diagnostic Tests
Diagnostic testing is highly recommended for clients with an arrhythmia, who at risk of an arrhythmia, and clients who are anxious and want to explore causes for their symptoms.
  Testing recommended:
A. Haemoglobin (Hgb) to rule out anaemia, if suggestive on examination.
B. Thyroid-stimulating hormone (TSH) to rule out hyperthyroidism, if suggestive on examination.
C. ECG during episode, if possible.
D. Ambulatory monitoring if symptoms continue, either 24-hour Holter monitor or client-activated transtelephonic monitoring.
E. Treadmill test if palpitations are provoked by exercise.

Differential Diagnoses
A. Palpitations are secondary to the underlying problem, such as anxiety, medications, or cardiac or pulmonary origin.

Plan
A. General interventions:
  1. Provide reassurance if the palpitations result from a neurotic concern.
B. Client teaching:
  1. Caution the client to avoid any factors that trigger episodes. Factors may include stress, exercise, foods, and medications.
  2. Teach the client a vagal maneuver, which is effective in halting palpitations.
C. Medical and surgical management: Correct any underlying problem (e.g., cardiac or pulmonary). Treat medical conditions accordingly. Management of arrhythmias should be monitored by a cardiologist.
D. Pharmacological therapy: Discontinue all nonessential medications that could cause palpitations.

Follow-Up
A. Depending on the aetiology of palpitations and the existence of comorbid conditions, the prognosis in clients with no underlying cardiac disease is generally favourable.

Consultation/Referral
A. If the client has a history of palpitations leading to syncope or near syncope, angina-like chest pain, or dyspnoea, refer to a cardiologist and/or inpatient evaluation. Refer any client with an arrhythmia to a cardiologist.
B. Haemodynamically compromised clients need prompt hospital admission.

Bibliography
Go, A. S., Mozaffarian, D., Roger, V. L., Benjamin, E. J., Berry, J. D., & Borden, W. B. (2013). Heart disease and stroke statistics—2013 update: A report from the American Heart Association. American Heart Association Statistics Committee and Stroke Statistics Subcommittee. *Circulation*, *127*(1), e6-e245. doi:10.1161/CIR.0b013e31828124ad
Mozaffarian, D., Benjamin, E. J., & Go, A. S. (2015). Heart disease and stroke statistics—2015 update: A report from the American Heart Association. *Circulation*, *131*(4), e29–e322. doi:10.1161/CIR.0000000000000152
Trayes, K. P., Studdiford, J. S., Pickle, S., & Tully, A. S. (2013). Edema: Diagnosis and management. *American Family Physician*, *88*(2), 102–110. doi:10.1097/ACM.0b013e318277d5b2

Peripheral Arterial Disease (PAD)

Laura A. Petty and Krista A. Bradley

Definition
A. Peripheral arterial disease (PAD) is a circulatory disorder generally characterized by the buildup of plaque on the interior surface of arteries. These plaques harden and narrow the diameter of the arteries, which reduces the volume of blood circulating to internal organs and extremities. The arteries affected by PAD include all arteries in the body with the exception of the cerebral and coronary arteries. The decreased circulation seen in PAD can also be caused by nonatherosclerotic conditions. Some of these conditions are arteritis, trauma, radiation damage, and fibromuscular dysplasia. Symptoms of PAD can occur in upper or lower extremities.

B. Classification of PAD:
1. Asymptomatic PAD:
a. No symptoms, but the presence of risk factors or a new diagnosis of a common coexisting disease (coronary artery disease [CAD] or cerebrovascular disease) should prompt further evaluation.
2. Intermittent claudication (IC):
a. Discomfort with physical exertion that remits a few minutes after activity ceases.
3. Chronic limb ischaemia.
a. Pain at rest and/or skin ulceration.
4. Acute limb ischaemia:
a. Pain at rest with a pulseless extremity.
C. Other conditions contained within PAD.
1. Buerger's disease (thromboangiitis obliterans): A disease manifested by inflammation, peripheral oedema, and microthrombi leading to gangrene of the hands and feet. Usually caused by tobacco abuse; clients are thought to have a genetic predisposition to develop this condition.
2. Raynaud's disease/phenomenon: A vasospastic disorder manifested by a response in the extremities to cold temperatures or stress during which pallor, cyanosis, numbness, and/or pain are experienced.
3. Leriche syndrome: Involves the triad of claudication, absent or diminished femoral pulses, and erectile dysfunction.

Incidence/Prevalence
A. In Canada, approximately 800,000 people are affected by PAD.
B. PAD is more common in men than in women.
C. PAD is more common in Indigenous Peoples of Canada and people of African and Hispanic descent.

Pathogenesis
A. PAD is most commonly precipitated by atherosclerosis. An atherosclerotic plaque develops in response to turbulent blood flow on the endothelial cells of the vessel wall. The plaque contains inflammatory cells and a thrombogenic lipid core that is covered by a fibrous cap. When the fibrous cap is disturbed, the lipid core can precipitate to the development of a thrombus and lead to occlusion of the vessel.

Predisposing Factors
A. Smoking.
B. Diabetes.
C. Dyslipidaemia.
D. Hypertension (HTN).
E. Obesity.
F. Age, increased occurrence after the age of 60 years.

Common Findings
A. Pain with activity is commonly characterized as cramping and/or aching:
1. Upper extremity pain in the forearm, hand, and digits.
2. Lower extremity pain in the foot, calf, hip, thigh, and/or buttocks:
a. Foot pain is most common in tibial or peroneal artery stenosis.
b. Calf pain is most common with superficial femoral or popliteal artery stenosis.
c. Thigh pain is most common in aortoiliac and common femoral artery stenosis.
d. Hip and buttock pain are most common with aortoiliac arterial stenosis.

B. Pain at rest.
C. Calf weakness or fatigue.
D. Numbness or tingling.
E. Dizziness with upper extremity exertion.
F. Syncope with upper extremity exertion.
G. Extremity ulceration.

Other Signs and Symptoms
A. Decreased peripheral pulses.
B. Blanching of the affected limb with elevation.
C. Ulcerations or infection on distal aspects of extremities.
D. Erectile dysfunction.

Potential Complications
A. Nonhealing lower extremity ulcerations.
B. Infection.
C. Amputation.
D. Common coexisting diseases:
1. CAD; also known as coronary heart disease (CHD).
2. Cerebrovascular disease.

Subjective Data
A. Ask the client what activity brought about or preceded the episode or whether it occurs at rest. If ambulation was the precipitating factor, how far was the client able to walk?
B. Have the client describe the duration of pain and what time of day symptoms began.
C. Ask the client what alleviates his or her pain.
D. Ask the client whether any previous episodes have occurred.
E. Ask the client to list all medications, including over-the-counter (OTC) and herbal products, currently being taken or recently stopped.
F. Ask the client to quantify his or her smoking history.
G. Ask the client whether he or she has a past medical history of an myocardial infarction (MI) or cerebrovascular accident.
H. If the client is male, ask whether he has any history of impotence or erectile dysfunction.

Physical Examination
A. Clients presenting with acute limb ischaemia should be quickly assessed for the need to call emergency services/911 for immediate transport to the hospital:
1. Symptoms of acute limb ischaemia as evidenced by the six Ps—pain, pallor, paresthesia, paralysis, pulselessness, and poikilothermia (the inability to maintain a constant core temperature).
B. Vital signs:
1. Check blood pressure (BP) in both upper extremities:
a. A difference in systolic BP (SBP) of 10 mmHg or greater in the upper extremities is associated with the upper extremity PAD and cerebrovascular disease.
b. A difference in SBP of 15 mmHg or greater in the upper extremities is associated with lower extremity PAD.
2. Check BP in both lower extremities.
3. Document resting heart rate, respirations, height, and weight.
C. Inspect:
1. Perform a funduscopic examination: Check for retinal vascular changes that indicate a retinal vascular occlusion such as macular oedema and neovascularization:
a. Macular oedema is the swelling of the central part of the retina.

b. Neovascularization is the growth of abnormal vessels secondary to decreased perfusion of the retina.
   2. Inspect abdomen for a pulsating abdominal mass.
   3. Inspect extremities. Note oedema, pallor, and cyanosis. Note colour of extremities in dependent and elevated positions.
   4. Inspect distal skin, hair, and nails. Note any temperature discrepancies or trophic changes that are indicative of ischaemia.
   5. Assess lower extremities for any ulcerations or diffuse erythema.
   6. Assess for a Homans' sign (i.e., calf pain with forced dorsiflexion).
   7. Assess whether pain occurs when affected limb is elevated.
D. Palpate:
   1. Palpate pulses, noting symmetry:
      a. Bilateral upper extremities (brachial and radial).
      b. Abdominal (aorta).
      c. Bilateral groin (femoral).
      d. Bilateral lower extremity pulses (popliteal, dorsalis pedis, and posterior tibialis).
   2. Palpate capillary refill.
   3. Perform an Allen test: Occlude the radial and ulnar arteries with the fist closed. Open the hand and then release one of the occluded arteries. Repeat but release the other artery. Each time, prompt capillary refill should occur.
   4. Palpate neck for carotid bruits.
   5. Palpate the abdominal aorta noting any lateral pulsation, indicative of an aortic aneurysm.
E. Auscultate:
   1. Heart: Assess the rate, rhythm, heart sounds, murmur, and gallops.
   2. Carotids, abdomen, and bilateral groin for bruits.
   3. Lungs: Assess lung sounds, noting any sign of heart failure (HF).

Diagnostic Tests

A. Doppler ankle brachial index (ABI):
   1. Interpretation of ABI ratios.
      a. 1.00 to 1.29: Normal.
      b. 0.91 to 0.99: Borderline PAD.
      c. 0.41 to 0.90: Mild to moderate PAD.
      d. 0.00 to 0.40: Severe PAD.
B. Basic metabolic panel (BMP; including urea, creatinine, sodium, and potassium).
C. Lipid profile.
D. C-reactive protein (CRP), homocysteine, D-dimer.
E. ECG (12 lead).
F. Doppler ultrasound.
G. Abdominal ultrasound.
H. Treadmill testing.
I. Computed tomography angiography (CTA).
J. Magnetic resonance angiography (MRA).
K. Arteriography, ordered and performed by surgeon.

Differential Diagnoses

A. Venous stasis.
B. Venous obstruction/claudication.
C. Spinal stenosis.
D. Nerve root compression.
E. Arthritis of the hip.
F. Peripheral neuropathy.
G. Arteritis.

Plan

A. General interventions:
   1. The goal of therapy is to improve the client's quality of life by reducing morbidity and prolonging survival.
B. Client teaching: *Refer to Client Teaching Guide: Peripheral Arterial Disease:*
   1. Encourage smoking cessation, weight loss, and exercise, if applicable.
   2. Encourage strategies to better manage other chronic medical conditions that directly affect the progression of PAD, that is, diabetes, dyslipidaemia, obesity, and HTN.
   3. Proper foot care:
      a. Instruct the client to wear properly fitting shoes that protect the feet.
      b. Inspect inside of shoes before donning.
      c. Encourage the client to inspect feet daily for signs of trauma or infection.
      d. Instruct the client to dry feet well, including between toes, after bathing.
C. Prevention:
   1. Control other chronic medical conditions, that is, diabetes, dyslipidaemia, HTN, and obesity.
D. Dietary management:
   1. To manage dyslipidaemia and HTN: Counsel client on nutrition and low-fat, low-cholesterol, low-sodium diet.
   2. To manage diabetes: Counsel client on diabetic diet and carbohydrate counting.
   3. To manage infection related to PAD: Counsel client on high-calorie, high-protein diet. Consider the addition of vitamins and minerals to promote wound healing, specifically zinc, and vitamins A and C.
   4. Give diet handouts and/or refer to a registered dietitian.
E. Pharmacological therapy:
   1. Goal of therapy: Prevention of thromboembolism:
      a. Pentoxifylline.
      b. Acetylsalicylic acid.
      c. Clopidogrel bisulphate.
   2. Risk factor reduction:
      a. Manage dyslipidaemia:
         i. Low-density lipoprotein (LDL) cholesterol goal: Less than 2.59 mmol/L and <1.81 mmol/L for clients at high risk of CAD.
      b. Manage HTN:
         i. BP goal in clients without diabetes: <140/90 mmHg.
         ii. BP goal in clients with diabetes or chronic kidney disease (CKD): <130/80 mmHg.
      c. Manage diabetes:
         i. Haemoglobin A1C goal: <7.0%.
F. Surgical therapies: Considered in clients with pain at rest, tissue loss, or significant physical limitations that prevent exercise:
   1. Bypass.
   2. Stenting.
   3. Angioplasty/percutaneous transluminal angioplasty.
G. Nonsurgical therapies:
   1. Smoking cessation program.
   2. Daily walking program:
      a. Instruct client to walk to the point of pain, then stop and resume walking when pain remits.
      b. May need to obtain medical clearance for the client to exercise.

▶ Client Teaching Guides are available at https://connect.springerpub.com/content/reference-book/978-0-8261-9498-5

Follow-Up

A. PAD manifesting persistent symptoms should always be followed by a cardiologist visit.
B. Follow-up is determined by the client's needs, frequency and intensity of symptoms, and the presence of other medical conditions.

Consultation/Referral

A. If you suspect acute limb ischaemia, refer the client for immediate hospitalization in order to obtain diagnostic testing to determine the presence of a thrombus and restore circulation to the affected extremity.
B. If chronic limb ischaemia has led to ulceration and/or superimposed infection, hospitalization is indicated to initiate a wound care consultation and diagnostic testing to determine the degree of arterial occlusion.
C. Referral to a cardiologist in the presence of persistent PAD symptoms.
D. Referral to a vascular surgeon for further evaluation of angioplasty, stenting, or bypass surgery.
E. Referral to a podiatrist to trim toenails and assess client for properly fitting shoes.
F. Referral to pain management if pain is resistant to treatment.
G. Referral to a registered dietitian as indicated by the client's understanding of dietary modification necessary to improve status of risk factors.

Individual Considerations

A. Nonambulatory clients:
   1. Using rocking chairs is a possible substitute for persons unable to participate in a walking program.
B. Geriatrics:
   1. Be alert to signs and symptoms of depression related to immobility and pain.

Bibliography

Anderson, J. L., Halperin, J. L., Albert, N. M., Bozkurt, B., Brindis, R. G., Curtis, L. H., & Shen, W. K. (2013). Management of patients with peripheral artery disease (compilation of 2005 and 2011 ACCF/AHA guideline recommendations): A report of the American College of Cardiology Foundation/American Heart Association Task Force on Practice Guidelines. *Circulation, 127*(13), 1425–1443. doi:10.1161/CIR.0b013e31828b82aa

Brazziel, T., Cox, L., Drury, C., & Guerra, M. (2011). Stopping the wave of PAD. *Nurse Practitioner, 36*(11), 28–33; quiz 33–34. doi:10.1097/01.NPR.0000406484.52134.83

Bonneau, C., Caron, N. R., Hussain, M. A., Kayssi, A., Verma, S., & Al-Omran, M. (2017). Periohearal artery disease among Indigenous Canadians: What do we know? *Canadian Journal of Surgery, 61*(5), 305–310.

Drug information. (2016). *Prescribers' digital reference*. Retrieved from www.pdr.net

Goff, D. C., Lloyd-Jones, D. M., Bennett, G., Coady, S., & D'Agostino, B. R., Sr. (2014). 2013 ACC/AHA guideline on the assessment of cardiovascular risk: A report of the American College of Cardiology/American Heart Association Task Force on practice guidelines. *Circulation*, S49–S73. doi:10.1161/01.cir.0000437741.48606.98

Harris, L., & Dryjski, M. (2015, November). Epidemiology, risk factors, and natural history of peripheral artery disease. *UpToDate*. Retrieved from http://www.uptodate.com/contents/epidemiology-risk-factors-and-natural-history-of-peripheral-artery-disease

Mohler III, E. (2014, June). Clinical features and diagnosis of lower extremity peripheral artery disease. *UpToDate*. Retrieved from http://www.uptodate.com/contents/clinical-features-and-diagnosis-of-lower-extremity-peripheral-artery-disease

Mohler III, E. (2015, October). Overview of upper extremity peripheral artery disease. *UpToDate*. Retrieved from http://www.uptodate.com/contents/overview-of-upper-extremity-peripheral-artery-disease

Patel, M. R., Conte, M. S., Cutlip, D. E., Dib, N., Geraghty, P., Gray, W., & Krucoff, M. W. (2015). Evaluation and treatment of patients with lower extremity peripheral artery disease: Consensus definitions from Peripheral Academic Research Consortium (PARC). *Journal of the American College of Cardiology, 65*(9), 931–941. doi:10.1016/j.jacc.2014.12.036. Retrieved from http://content.onlinejacc.org/article.aspx?articleid=2174621#tab1

Then, K., Rankin, J., & Ali, E. (2013). Peripheral arterial disease versus peripheral venous disease: Assessment, diagnosis and treatment. *Canadian Journal of Cardiology, 29*(10), S393. doi:10.1016/j.cjca.2013.07.700

Trayes, K. P., Studdiford, J. S., Pickle, S., & Tully, A. S. (2013). Edema: Diagnosis and management. *American Family Physician, 88*(2), 102–110. doi:10.1097/ACM.0b013e318277d5b2

Superficial Thrombophlebitis

Cheryl A. Glass, Laura A. Petty, and Krista A. Bradley

Definition

A. Superficial thrombophlebitis is the inflammation of a vessel wall accompanied by blood stasis in varicose veins, which may also have clot formation in a vein close to the surface:
   1. Most superficial thrombophlebitis occurs in the lower extremity, but may also occur in the breast and in the penis (Mondor disease).
   2. Superficial thrombophlebitis may also occur in the upper extremities and in the neck after invasive intravenous (IV) catheters are used in medical procedures.
   3. Generally superficial thrombophlebitis is self-limiting, but may persist for a period of time (three to four weeks or longer) before resolution.
B. Superficial phlebitis with an infection is referred to as a *septic thrombophlebitis*.

Incidence/Prevalence

A. Pregnancy carries an increased risk of phlebitis. Eighty percent of thromboembolic events in pregnancy are venous. The incidence of pulmonary embolism (PE) in pregnancy accounts for 1.1 deaths per 100,000 deliveries.
B. The prevalence of superficial thrombophlebitis ranges from 4% to 8% of clients with an indwelling IV catheter.
C. Superficial phlebitis after a vein radiofrequency or laser ablation is common.

Pathogenesis

A. Superficial thrombosis is caused by infection, abuse of IV drugs, chemical irritation from overuse of IV route for diagnostic tests and drugs, and/or trauma. Several episodes can signal an underlying problem, such as carcinoma of the pancreas.
B. A common cause of varicose veins is blood-flow stasis, basically caused by valvular incompetence and/or dilation of the vessel lumen.
C. Thrombi in the upper extremities commonly have iatrogenic causes, such as IV catheters.
D. Thrombophlebitis during pregnancy through the first six weeks postpartum is linked to a reduced fibrinolytic state.

Predisposing Factors

A. Previous thrombophlebitis is the highest risk factor for recurrence.
B. Hypercoagulability such as pregnancy (50% of events) through six weeks postpartum (50% of events).
C. Haemoglobinopathies:
   1. Factor V Leiden mutation.
   2. Protein C deficiency.
   3. Protein S deficiency.
   4. Prothrombin gene mutation.
   5. Antithrombin III deficiency.
   6. Factor XII deficiency.

D. Estrogen therapy:
   1. Oral contraceptives.
   2. High-dose hormone replacement therapy (HRT).
E. Malignancy (especially in the tail of the pancreas).
F. Lupus, positive anticardiolipin antibody.
G. Sepsis.
H. Surgery.
I. Long bone trauma.
J. Recent IV catheter access.
K. Prolonged immobilization.
L. Obesity.
M. Varicose veins.
N. Age older than 60 years.
O. Stroke.
P. Myocardial infarction (MI).
Q. Family history of deep vein thrombosis (DVT).
R. Smoking.
S. Hypertension (HTN).
T. Infection.

Common Findings
A. Warm, tender, inflamed vessel with palpable cord.
B. Redness along the course of the superficial vein.
C. Tenderness or pain localized to the affected vein.

Other Signs and Symptoms
A. Fever/no fever.
B. Localized oedema.

Potential Complications
A. Superficial thrombophlebitis extending into the deep venous system.
B. DVT.
C. Conversion to suppurative thrombophlebitis:
   1. Metastatic abscess formation.
   2. Septicaemia.
   3. Septic emboli.

Subjective Data
A. Query the client regarding the onset, duration, and intensity of symptoms.
B. Ask the client about fever or other related symptoms.
C. Obtain a thorough medical history and account of recent physical activity.
D. Ask the client about any recent experience of any type of injury.
E. Inquire whether the client has ever had similar symptoms or history of previous thrombophlebitis. If so, discuss previous treatment and therapy used and the results.
F. Review current medications: Prescription, over-the-counter (OTC), and herbal products:
   1. Ask specifically about oral contraceptives and hormone therapy.
G. Review the client's occupation for sedentary lifestyle.
H. Review any recent plane travel.
I. Review history for recent invasive procedures.

Physical Examination
A. Check temperature (if indicated with inflammation), pulse, respirations, and blood pressure (BP).
B. Inspect:
   1. Assess overall appearance. Evaluate for the presence of respiratory distress.
   2. Inspect extremities, noting erythema and oedema.
   3. Assess for increased warmth over the affected vein.
C. Auscultate:
   1. Heart, noting rate, rhythm, heart sounds, murmurs, and gallops.
   2. Lungs for lung sounds in all fields.
D. Palpate:
   1. Palpate extremities; check all pulses, including femoral, posttibial, pedal, and radial.
   2. Palpate extremities for tenderness and palpable cord.
   3. Palpate lymph nodes distal and proximal to the site.
   4. Test for Homans' sign in lower extremities bilaterally if DVT is suspected.

Diagnostic Tests
A. Duplex ultrasound identifies the presence, location, and extent of venous thrombosis.
B. Doppler ultrasound.
C. Laboratory tests are ordered dependent on the clinical situation:
   1. Complete blood count (CBC) with differential.
   2. Screening for hypercoagulability should not be considered for one episode of superficial thrombophlebitis.
   3. Screening for hypercoagulability should be considered for recurrent superficial thrombophlebitis.
   4. Blood cultures.

Differential Diagnoses
A. Varicose veins.
B. Cellulitis.
C. Strained muscle.
D. Insect bites.
E. Erythema nodosum.
F. Cutaneous polyarteritis nodosa.
G. Kaposi's sarcoma.
H. Hyperalgesic pseudothrombophlebitis.

Plan
A. General interventions:
   1. Advise all clients to stop smoking.
   2. Advise the client to avoid prolonged sitting or standing and not to cross or massage legs. *Refer to Client Teaching Guides: Superficial Thrombophlebitis* and *Varicose Veins.*
   3. Advise the client to avoid constrictive clothing, such as knee-high hosiery.
   4. Prescribe supportive hose/compression stockings.
   5. Have the client apply heat and elevate extremity for varicose veins or superficial thrombophlebitis.
   6. Prescribe bed rest for superficial thrombophlebitis.
   7. DVT: Hospitalization is required.
   8. Advise clients with thrombophlebitis to discontinue oral contraceptives and hormone replacement.
   9. Alternative forms of birth control recommended by the American College of Obstetricians and Gynecologists (ACOG) include the following:
      a. Intrauterine device, including intrauterine devices (IUDs) that contain progestin.
      b. Progestin-only oral contraceptives.
      c. Progestin-only implants.
      d. Barrier methods.
      e. Surgical procedures: Vasectomy and tubal ligation.

▶ Client Teaching Guides are available at https://connect.springerpub.com/content/reference-book/978-0-8261-9498-5

▶ **B.** Client teaching: *Refer to Client Teaching Guide: Superficial Thrombophlebitis.*
C. Pharmacological therapy for superficial thrombophlebitis:
  1. Nonsteroidal anti-inflammatory drugs (NSAIDs) are used for treatment of pain. No NSAID has been identified as superior for treatment.
  2. The use of anticoagulation therapy for the treatment of lower extremity superficial thrombophlebitis is controversial. Unfractionated heparin and low-molecular-weight heparin (LMWH) are both used for treatment to reduce risk of DVT and/or recurrent phlebitis.
  3. Thrombosis Canada recommends anticoagulation for clients with lower extremity superficial thrombophlebitis at increased risk of thromboembolism. This is defined as a client with:
    a. A concomitant DVT.
    b. An isolated superficial venous thrombosis (SVT), which extends to within 3 cm of the saphenofemoral junction (SFJ).
    c. An isolated SVT >5 cm in length and more than 3 cm from the SFJ.
    d. An isolated SVT <5 cm in length and >3 cm from the SFJ in the presence of severe symptoms or risk factors for extension, such as prior DVTs or PE, cancer, pregnancy, hormonal therapy, or recent surgery or trauma.
    Specific recommendations for anticoagulation for various medical conditions can be found at thrombosiscanada.ca/resourcepage/resources/.
  4. Antibiotics, if infection is suspected.
  5. Oral or topical nonsteroidal anti-inflammatory drugs (NSAIDs) and warm compresses can be used for symptom relief.
D. Surgery:
  1. Biopsy.
  2. Vein ablation, only if symptoms are significant and persistent.
  3. Vein ligation, only if symptoms are significant and persistent.

Follow-Up
A. Schedule a return appointment for clients with superficial thrombophlebitis to return in seven to 10 days or earlier as needed. Repeat physical examination as needed to evaluate resolution or progression of the thrombophlebitis.
B. Periodic follow-up is needed to monitor clients on anticoagulation therapy.
C. After an acute problem is resolved, consider laboratory evaluation for hypercoagulation syndrome (protein C, protein S, and antithrombin III).
D. Monitor bone loss with dual-energy x-ray absorptiometry (DEXA) scan with prolonged use of heparin.
E. Screening all women for thrombophilias before starting oral contraceptives is not recommended by the Society of Obstetricians and Gynaecologists of Canada.
F. Women with a history of thrombosis who have not had a complete evaluation should be tested for both antiphospholipid antibodies and inherited thrombophilias.

Consultation/Referral
A. Hospitalization is required to initiate heparin therapy.
B. Comanage pregnancy with an obstetrician.
C. Consider referral to a haematologist.

Individual Considerations
A. Pregnancy:
  1. Routine anticoagulation therapy for all pregnant women is not recommended. Therapeutic anticoagulation is recommended for women with acute thromboembolism during the current pregnancy or those at high risk of thrombosis, such as women with mechanical heart valves.
  2. Warfarin and NSAIDs are contraindicated.
  3. Heparin is the preferred anticoagulant in pregnancy. Neither unfractionated heparin nor LMWH crosses the placenta.
  4. Warfarin, LMWH, and unfractionated heparin do not accumulate in breast milk and do not induce an anticoagulant effect in the infant and therefore are considered compatible with breastfeeding.
B. Geriatrics:
  1. Prognosis is poor for clients with septic thrombophlebitis.
  2. Using a rocking chair is a possible substitute for persons unable to participate in a walking program.
  3. Be alert to signs and symptoms of depression related to immobility and pain.

Resources
Thrombosis Canada Clinical Practice Guidelines: https://thrombosiscanada.ca/clinicalguides/#

Bibliography
DiNisio, M., & Middeldorp, S. (2014). Treatment of lower extremity superficial thrombophlebitis. *The Journal of the American Medical Association, 311*(7), 729–730. doi:10.1001/jama.2014.520
Drug information. (2016). *Prescribers' digital reference.* Retrieved from www.pdr.net
Fernandez, L., & Scovell, S. (2016, April). Superficial thrombophlebitis of the lower extremity. *UpToDate.* Retrieved from http://www.uptodate.com/contents/superficial-thrombophlebitis-of-the-lower-extremity
Klever, R. G. (2015, June). Superficial thrombophlebitis. *Medscape.* Retrieved from emedicine.medscape.com/article/463256-overview
Nasr, H., & Scriven, J. M. (2015). Superficial thrombophlebitis (superficial venous thrombosis). *The BMJ, 350,* h2039. doi:10.1136/bmj.h2039. Retrieved from http://www.bmj.com/content/350/bmj.h2039
Trayes, K. P., Studdiford, J. S., Pickle, S., & Tully, A. S. (2013). Edema: Diagnosis and management. *American Family Physician, 88*(2), 102–110. doi:10.1097/ACM.0b013e318277d5b2

Syncope
Jill C. Cash, Debbie Gunter, and Krista A. Bradley

Definition
A. Syncope is a brief, sudden loss of consciousness and muscle tone secondary to cerebral ischaemia, or inadequate oxygen or glucose delivery to brain tissue. Recovery is spontaneous.

Incidence/Prevalence
A. Syncope is a common problem in all age groups. An estimated 15% of children experience an episode by adulthood. Between 12% and 48% of healthy young adults have lost consciousness (one-third following trauma), but most do not seek medical attention. Adults older than age 75 years in long-term care facilities have a 6% annual incidence of syncope, and 23% have had previous episodes. Syncopal episodes account for approximately 1% to 6% of hospital admissions and 3% of ED visits.

▶ Client Teaching Guides are available at https://connect.springerpub.com/content/reference-book/978-0-8261-9498-5

Pathogenesis

The most common cause of syncope is inadequate cerebral perfusion caused by one of the following:

A. Vasomotor instability associated with a decrease in systemic vascular resistance and/or venous return. The following may cause syncope:
  1. Vasovagal episodes.
  2. Situational syncope, from coughing, micturition, and defecation.
  3. Medications:
     a. Vasodilators.
     b. Antiarrhythmics.
     c. Diuretics.
     d. Neurologic agents.
     e. Glucose-regulating drugs.
     f. Impotence therapy.

B. Decrease in cardiac output caused by blood flow obstruction within the heart or pulmonary circulation or by arrhythmias. This may be caused by the following:
  1. Aortic, pulmonic, and mitral stenosis.
  2. Idiopathic hypertrophic subaortic stenosis (IHSS).
  3. Pump failure.
  4. Subclavian steal syndrome.
  5. Seizures.

C. Focal or generalized decrease in cerebral perfusion leading to transient ischaemia because of cerebrovascular disease.

D. Metabolic abnormalities:
  1. Hypoglycaemia.
  2. Hypocarbia and hypoxia usually do not result in syncope unless they are profound, although consciousness may be altered.

E. Psychiatric illnesses associated with syncope include the following:
  1. Generalized anxiety.
  2. Panic attacks.
  3. Major depressive disorders.

F. Unexplained cause.

Predisposing Factors

A. Advanced age, caused by altered regulation of cerebral blood flow and/or systemic arterial pressure because of aging process and increased medication use.
B. Other factors, depending on aetiology.
C. Medication use (noted earlier).

Common Findings

A. Dizziness.
B. Light-headedness.
C. Fainting with no memory of events.

Other Signs and Symptoms

A. Neuroautonomic regulations:
  1. Event triggered by changing position, turning head, wearing tight collars.
  2. Nausea, warmth, diaphoresis, weakness one hour after eating.

B. Cardiac causes: Exercise-induced palpitations, chest pain, shortness of breath (SOB) with no warning before episode.

C. Neurologic causes:
  1. Vertigo.
  2. Diplopia.
  3. Facial paresthesias.
  4. Ataxia.
  5. Auditory, visual, or vestibular disturbances.

D. Metabolic or endocrine causes:
  1. Restlessness.
  2. Anxiety.
  3. Confusion.
  4. No recent food intake, low glucose level.

E. Psychiatric: Graceful fainting in presence of an audience.

Subjective Data

A. Inquire whether the client ever experienced similar symptoms or episodes before. If so, when and at what age did it begin?

B. Ask the client or witness of the episode to give a detailed description of the loss of consciousness. Was loss of consciousness complete, and, if so, for how long? What was the posture of the client before, during, and after the event? Did it occur abruptly, or were there symptoms leading up to the event?

C. Question the client regarding events leading up to the episode, noting prodromal symptoms such as headache, aura, nausea/vomiting, light-headedness, diaphoresis, feeling of warmth.

D. Obtain a detailed account of symptoms during and after the episode, noting mental status. Did the client recover on his or her own, or did the client require assistance? Were there any associated symptoms that occurred during the event—SOB, chest pain, loss of bowel or bladder control?

E. If syncope has occurred in the past, are there any events that precipitate an episode? Exertion, exercise, coughing, standing quickly?

F. Obtain a detailed medication history, addressing prescribed and over-the-counter (OTC) drugs, alcohol, and illicit preparations.

G. Review the client's past medical history.

Physical Examination

A. Check temperature, if indicated, pulse, respirations, and blood pressure (BP):
  1. Measure BP and pulse in both arms and legs. Note BP differences between the arms.
  2. Measure BP several times during a two-minute period with the client standing.
  3. Check for orthostatic hypotension, which is defined as a drop of 20 mmHg or more in systolic BP (SBP) on standing.
     a. First, measure BP after the client lies supine for five to 10 minutes.
     b. Then have the client stand, and measure BP several times during a two-minute period.

B. Inspect:
  1. Assess overall appearance of the client, skin colour.
  2. Note the range of motion in the neck.

C. Auscultate:
  1. The heart with position changes. Note murmurs or extra heart sounds to rule out structural disease.
  2. The carotid arteries.
  3. The abdomen for bruits.

D. Palpate the abdomen, noting pulsatile expansion.

E. Neurologic examination:
  1. Perform a complete examination, if indicated, including assessing second to 12th cranial nerves, Babinski's reflex, and gait.

F. Mental status:
  1. Assess mental health, if indicated.

Diagnostic Tests

The following tests are performed depending on history and physical examination results. The 2009 European Society of Cardiology (ESC) guidelines recommend the following testing:

A. Carotid sinus massage in client older than 40 years of age. Avoid if client has a history of transient ischaemic attack (TIA) or stroke in the past three months and in clients with carotid bruits. Recommend cardiology specialist assistance when performing carotid massage. Use caution when performing carotid sinus massage. Please consider contraindications, complications, and protocol for performing procedure.
B. Echocardiogram for clients with a history of heart disease, structural heart disease, or syncope secondary to cardiovascular cause (known heart disease, family history of unexplained sudden death, syncope with exertion or supine, abnormal ECG, sudden onset of palpitation before syncope, or arrhythmia on ECG).
C. ECG for clients with suspected arrhythmia or cardiac disease. Identify acute and old ECG changes to rule out pathologic Q wave, ST segment elevation, and left ventricular hypertrophy (LVH).
D. Orthostatic challenge test if syncope is related to position change or suspect reflex mechanism.
E. Neurologic/serum laboratory testing for other concerns of nonsyncopal loss of consciousness. Laboratory testing includes chemistry profile, thyroid-stimulating hormone (TSH), and free T4. Consider a glucose tolerance test if diabetes is suspected. Brain natriuretic peptide (BNP) may be useful to evaluate cardiac versus noncardiac cause for syncope.
F. Chest radiography, for essential baseline data. Wide mediastinum signals aortic dissection.
G. In-hospital monitoring recommended for unstable, life-threatened clients.
H. Holter monitor for 24 to 48 hours.
I. External event monitor.
J. Exercise testing recommended for clients with syncope that occurs during, or quickly after, cessation of exercise. Echocardiogram is recommended before this testing.
K. Cardiac catheterization.
L. Lung scan.
M. Treadmill test.
N. Electrophysiological studies recommended for clients with unexplained syncope.

Differential Diagnoses

A. Irregular neuroautonomic regulations:
    1. Neurocardiogenic causes.
    2. Situational causes, such as coughing, defecation, diving, micturition, sneezing, swallowing, trumpet playing, vagal stimulation, weight lifting, postprandial state.
    3. Orthostatic causes:
        a. Hyperadrenergic state.
        b. Hypoadrenergic state, primary or secondary autonomic insufficiency.
        c. Carotid sinus syncope.
        d. Cardioinhibitory state.
        e. Vasodepressor stimulation.
        f. Mixed.
B. Cardiac causes:
    1. Mechanical causes such as aortic dissection, aortic stenosis, atrial myxoma, cardiac tamponade, global myocardial ischaemia, hypertrophic cardiomyopathy, mitral stenosis, myocardial infarction (MI), prosthetic valve dysfunction, pulmonary embolism (PE), pulmonary hypertension (HTN), pulmonary stenosis, and Takayasu's arteritis.
    2. Electrical causes, such as atrioventricular (AV) block, long QT syndrome, pacemaker, sick sinus syndrome, supraventricular tachyarrhythmias, and ventricular tachyarrhythmias.
C. Neurologic causes:
    1. Neuralgias: Glossopharyngeal, trigeminal.
    2. Normal pressure hydrocephalus.
    3. Subclavian steal.
    4. Vertebrobasilar artery disease: Compression, migraine, TIA.
D. Metabolic or endocrine causes: Hypoadrenalism, hypoglycaemia, hyponatraemia, hypothyroidism, and hypoxia.
E. Psychiatric causes: Anxiety, hysteria, major depression, panic disorder, somatization, and hyperventilation syndrome.

Plan

A. General interventions:
    1. Management is directed at primary cause for the episode.
B. Client teaching:
    1. If the client has orthostatic hypotension, suggest that he or she wear elastic stockings, change positions slowly, sleep with the head of the bed elevated, and exercise legs before standing.
    2. If syncope is induced by situations, warn the client to avoid or alter his or her approach to such precipitating events.
    3. If the client has prodromal symptoms, such as nausea, light-headedness, pallor, sweating, or palpitations, advise him or her to lie down when they occur.
    4. If the client has hypersensitive carotid sinus reflex, recommend that he or she loosen his or her collar.
    5. Discuss with clients to avoid prolonged standing. If they cannot avoid it, they should contract their calf muscles to increase venous blood flow.
    6. Some driving restrictions exist for clients at risk of recurrent syncope. Driving restrictions are enforced by the state law. Review restrictions with the client and family as indicated by diagnosis.
C. Dietary management: If not contraindicated, instruct clients with orthostatic hypotension to use salt liberally.
D. Pharmacological therapy will depend on the aetiology of the syncope. Therapy for neurocardiogenic syncope includes the following:
    1. Nonpharmacological methods suggested: Avoid volume depletion. Maintain adequate sodium levels by increasing salt intake in the diet. Wear thigh-high elastic support hose with 30- to 40-mmHg pressure. Orthostatic training is also recommended two times a day.
    2. First-line treatment: Beta-blockers.
    3. Fludrocortisone acetate, a corticosteroid, may be used alone or with beta-blockers.
    4. Other drugs include anticholinergic agents and selective serotonin reuptake inhibitors (SSRIs).

Follow-Up

A. Scheduling of return visits depends on aetiology and severity of syncope and whether the client has been placed on medications.

Consultation/Referral

A. Consult with or refer the client to a specialist (cardiologist or neurologist) when cardiac or neurologic involvement is suspected.

Individual Considerations

A. Adults:
   1. In young adult athletes, be aware of symptoms of Marfan syndrome.
   2. In older adults, coronary atherosclerosis may present along with syncope.

B. Geriatrics:
   1. Elderly clients may have multiple comorbid conditions, such as decreased cerebral blood flow and acute viral illness.

Bibliography

Drug information. (2016). *Prescribers' digital reference*. Retrieved from www.pdr.net

Saklani, P., Krahn, A., & Klein, G. (2013). Syncope. *Circulation, 127*(12), 1330–1339. doi:10.1161/CIRCULATIONAHA.112.138396

Walsh, K., Hoffmayer, K., & Hamdan, M. H. (2015). Syncope: Diagnosis and management. *Current Problems in Cardiology, 40*(2), 51–86. doi:10.1016/j.cpcardiol.2014.11.001

11 Gastrointestinal Guidelines

Abdominal Pain

Cheryl A. Glass, Audra C. Malone, and Kristie A. D. Morydz

Definition
A. Abdominal pain is a common nonspecific complaint. The responsibility is for clinicians to determine clients who can be safely observed and treated symptomatically and those who require further investigation or a specialist referral. Pain in the abdomen is secondary to problems relating to abdominal organs, and it is categorized as follows:
   1. Acute pain: Pain of less than a few days that has worsened progressively until presentation.
   2. Chronic pain: Interval of 12 weeks can be used to separate acute from chronic pain, that is, pain has remained unchanged for months or years.
   3. Emergent: Pain that lasts four hours or longer, accompanied by fever or vomiting.
B. Pain may be categorized by description:
   1. Visceral pain is usually dull and aching in character.
   2. Parietal pain is sharp and well localized.
   3. Referred pain is aching and perceived to be near the surface of the body.

Incidence/Prevalence
Abdominal pain is very common. On questioning, abdominal pain is present in 75% of adolescents and in about 50% of all adults. Gastroenteritis and irritable bowel syndrome (IBS) are the most common cause of acute pain, and chronic stool retention is the most common cause of chronic pain. Other causes of abdominal pain include the following:
A. Acute appendicitis: Occurs 10:100,000.
B. Acute cholecystitis: Varies according to age and ethnic origin.
C. Intestinal obstruction, usually small intestines: Accounts for 20% of acute abdominal conditions.
D. Abdominal pain associated with pregnancy: Ectopic pregnancy (1:200 pregnancies), miscarriage, and abruptio placenta.

Pathogenesis
A. Pathogenesis depends on the origin of pain. Pain may result from inflammation, ischaemia, distension, altered motility, obstruction, or ulceration.

Predisposing Factors
A. Abdominal trauma.
B. Motor vehicle accidents.
C. Lactose, gluten, or other food intolerance.
D. Pregnancy.
E. Torsion.
F. Psychogenic pain.
G. Sickle cell disease.
H. Infection.

Common Findings
Clinical presentation of abdominal pain is determined in part by the site of the involvement:
A. Acute or chronic onset of pain.
B. Vomiting.
C. Diarrhoea.

Other Signs and Symptoms
A. Bleeding.
B. Referred shoulder pain.
C. Fever.
D. Nausea and/or projectile vomiting.
E. Rigid abdomen.
F. Changes in vital signs.
G. Abdominal distension.
H. Constipation.
I. Guarding.
J. Rebound tenderness.
K. Biliary pain and right subcostal tenderness.
L. Anorexia.
M. Periumbilical discomfort: Consider appendicitis if within two to 12 hours, pain localizes in right lower quadrant (RLQ) at McBurney's point.
N. Dysuria.
O. Abdominal mass: Do not overlook the possibility of pregnancy as the cause of a mass.
P. Melaena (most common in peptic ulcer disease [PUD]).
Q. Changes in/absence of bowel sounds.

Subjective Data

Evaluate for a "surgical abdomen," defined as a rapidly worsening prognosis in the absence of surgical intervention. Clients should not eat or drink while a diagnosis of a surgical abdomen remains under consideration. Once a surgical abdomen has been excluded, the remainder of the evaluation will be guided by the chronicity of symptoms along with the location of pain.

A. Review the onset, duration, course, and quality of pain:
   1. When did the pain start?
   2. What were you doing when the pain started?
   3. Has this ever occurred before?
   4. What was the primary diagnosis?

5. What was the previous treatment, and was it effective?
6. Is there anyone else in your home having the same symptoms?
7. Review the progression of pain.

B. Determine the pain rating on a 10-point scale, with 0 being no pain and 10 being equivalent to the worst pain the client has ever felt.

C. Qualify the duration of pain in minutes, hours, days, weeks, or months. Does the pain interfere with sleep?

D. Review the pattern of pain:
1. Review aggravating factors.
2. Review alleviating factors.
3. Does the pain radiate?
4. Does the pain have any relationship to food intake?

E. Questions specific to females:
1. Determine the client's last menstrual period (LMP).
2. Has she had a hysterectomy or tubal ligation?
3. Does she have a recent history of dyspareunia or dysmenorrhoea that suggests pelvic pathology?
4. Is there any history of physical abuse?
5. What type of contraception is used? (Specifically evaluate for an intrauterine device [IUD].)

F. Review the client's current medications and drug history, especially antibiotic, laxative, acetaminophen, ASA, and non-steroidal anti-inflammatory drug (NSAID) use. Pain may be significantly masked in clients taking corticosteroids.

G. Rule out abdominal trauma from domestic violence, motor vehicle accidents, falls, or assaults.

H. Review bowel habits and note changes: Constipation, diarrhoea, anorexia, food intolerance, nausea, vomiting, or bloating.

I. Review the client's history for sickle cell disease. Any individual of African American or Mediterranean descent presenting with leg or abdominal pain should be questioned regarding sickle cell disease or trait.

J. Review urinary function. Is there any urinary frequency, urgency, dysuria, flank pain, or back pain? If the client is male, does he have any hesitancy, difficulty starting the urine stream, nocturia, low urinary volume, or any lower abdominal distension indicating urinary retention?

K. Review alcohol intake/history.

L. Has the client had any unexplained weight loss?

M. Evaluate sexual activity to rule out potential sexually transmitted infection (STI):
1. Evaluate whether the client has new partners.
2. Are the partners experiencing any symptoms?

Physical Examination

A. Check temperature, pulse, respirations, and blood pressure (BP); include orthostatic blood pressure.

Tachycardia or hypotension may be the signs of a ruptured aortic aneurysm, septic shock, gastrointestinal (GI) haemorrhage, or volume depletion. Absence of a fever in the elderly or immunosuppressed does not exclude a serious illness.

B. Inspect.
1. Observe general appearance: Facial expressions, walk, skin turgor, refusal to move/writhing; note grimace during examination.
2. Perform eye and mouth examination to rule out iritis and aphthous ulcers of the mouth (extraintestinal manifestations of inflammatory bowel disease [IBD]). Examine eyes for jaundice.
3. Examine the abdomen for the presence of hernia at the umbilicus, groin, or near the site of prior surgical incisions.
4. Examine the abdomen for overt masses or pulsations.
5. Examine skin for jaundice. Observe for any bruising or other signs of domestic violence in the "bathing suit" areas—breasts, abdomen, and the back—that would be easily covered with clothes.

C. Auscultate:
1. Auscultate for bowel sounds in all four quadrants of the abdomen.
2. Evaluate heart and lungs.
3. Check for aortic, iliac, and renal bruits.

D. Percuss the abdomen for tympany and dullness. Percuss liver span. Assess for ascites (fluid wave or shifting dullness).

E. Palpate:
1. Abdomen for masses, rebound tenderness, Murphy's sign, and peritoneal signs:
   a. Before palpating the abdomen, ask the client to bend the knees to help with relaxation of the wall musculature.
   b. Elderly clients may lack classical peritoneal signs of rebound and guarding.
2. Check the abdomen for tender pulsatile mass at midline; it may indicate abdominal aortic aneurysm (AAA).
3. Palpate back; check for costovertebral angle (CVA) tenderness.
4. Perform a bimanual examination in women regardless of whether the client has had a hysterectomy or is post-menopausal:
   a. Evaluate the size and symmetry of the uterus.
   b. Evaluate the adnexal areas for presence of appropriately sized mobile ovaries. A fixed, painful adnexal mass is suggestive of an endometrioma or tubo-ovarian abscess.
   c. Endometriosis is suggested by localized tenderness in the cul-de-sac or uterosacral ligaments, palpable tender nodules, pain with uterine movement, and tenderness fixation of adnexal mass or uterus in a retroverted position.
5. Check for obturator sign, which is abdominal pain in response to passive internal rotation of the right hip from the 90-degree angle knee–hip flexion position; perform this when an inflamed appendix is suspected.
6. Check for iliopsoas sign; perform this when an inflamed appendix is suspected. Positive psoas sign is the presence of lower quadrant pain noted as the supine client raises his or her right leg from the hip while the examiner pushes downward against his or her lower thigh.

F. Perform a rectal examination, including testing of stool for occult blood. **Failure to perform a rectal examination in clients with abdominal pain may be associated with an increased rate of misdiagnosis.**

Diagnostic Tests

Diagnostic testing is ordered based on the following differential diagnoses:

A. **In all women of childbearing age, assume the woman is pregnant until proven otherwise. Vaginal bleeding with or without abdominal pain should prompt a transvaginal ultrasound and a serum human chorionic gonadotropin (HCG) test. HCG should be tested before performing the transvaginal ultrasound.**

B. Complete blood count (CBC) with differential.

C. Electrolytes and calcium.

D. Blood glucose.
E. Urea and creatinine.
F. Amylase.
G. Aminotransferases, alkaline phosphatase (ALP), and bilirubin.
H. Lipase.
I. Urinalysis; save sample for culture.
J. Coproporphyrin, if lead poisoning is suspected.
K. Plain x-ray films of abdomen to rule out obstruction.
L. CT of abdomen with or without contrast.
M. Abdominal ultrasonography.
N. GI series radiography.
O. Consider *Helicobacter pylori* serology or hydrogen breath testing.
P. Sigmoidoscopy.
Q. Barium enema (BE): Avoid with suspected obstruction.
R. Stool guaiac test for occult blood.
S. Consider endoscopic retrograde cholangiopancreatography (ERCP) to visualize the distal common bile duct.
T. ECG to rule out cardiac pain.
U. Consider blood cultures for elderly who present with abdominal pain associated with either fever or hypothermia or when sepsis is suspected.
V. Chest radiography.

Differential Diagnoses

Location and duration of abdominal pain can often significantly help in narrowing the differential diagnosis:

A. Right upper quadrant (RUQ) pain:
  1. Acute cholecystitis and biliary colic:
     a. Biliary tract: Increased serum amylase.
     b. Ascending cholangitis presents with fever and jaundice in a client with RUQ pain.
     c. In acute cholecystitis, the typical pain is maximal in the RUQ or epigastrium, radiating to the scapular region, and is accompanied by nausea, vomiting, and fever without jaundice. Murphy's sign, or inspiratory arrest in response to upper quadrant palpation, may be seen with acute cholecystitis. RUQ tenderness to percussion or pressure of the gallbladder is also a suggestive finding.
     d. Ketoacidosis has been found to present with severe abdominal pain in 8% of instances and may be accompanied by emesis and an elevated white cell count. Acute intra-abdominal events, such as cholecystitis, may be the precipitant of ketoacidosis.
  2. Acute hepatitis.
  3. Hepatic abscess.
  4. Hepatomegaly due to congestive heart failure (CHF).
  5. Perforated duodenal ulcer (DU).

A perforated ulcer is accompanied by an increased serum amylase.

  6. Acute pancreatitis: RUQ and left upper quadrant (LUQ) pain.

Pancreatitis is accompanied by an increased serum amylase.

  7. Herpes zoster.
  8. Myocardial ischaemia.
  9. Pleural or pulmonary pathology (e.g., pneumonia, pulmonary embolism, or empyema).

B. RLQ pain:
  1. Appendicitis often begins with symptoms of dull, steady, periumbilical pain and anorexia before localizing to the RLQ at McBurney's point.
  2. Regional enteritis.
  3. Leaking aneurysm.
  4. Ruptured ectopic pregnancy.
  5. Ovarian cyst.
  6. Ovarian torsion.
  7. Pelvic inflammatory disease (PID).
  8. Ureteral calculi.
  9. Incarcerated, strangulated inguinal hernia.
  10. Endometriosis.
  11. Meckel's diverticulitis.
  12. Abdominal wall haematoma.
C. LUQ pain:
  1. Gastritis.
  2. Acute pancreatitis: Epigastric pain that is relatively sudden, bores in to the back, and is associated with nausea, vomiting, and anorexia.
  3. Splenic enlargement, rupture, infarction, aneurysm.
  4. Myocardial ischaemia.
  5. Left lower lobe pneumonia.
  6. Renal colic: Radiates to the groin.
D. Left lower quadrant (LLQ) pain.
  1. Sigmoid and/or descending diverticulitis.
  2. Regional enteritis.
  3. Leaking aneurysm.

AAA may present with a tender pulsatile mass at the abdominal midline. Vascular disorders such as acute arterial insufficiency due to atherosclerosis or embolus, may present with severe abdominal pain, although mild, constant pain may be the only symptom for several days. Dissection or rupture of an AAA produces severe acute abdominal pain and often radiates to the back or genitalia.

  4. Ruptured ectopic pregnancy.

Rupture of the fallopian tube generally causes sudden, acute, and localized abdominal pain. Internal haemorrhage causes syncope and referred shoulder pain, caused by phrenic nerve irritation. Diagnosis before tubal rupture may be difficult because symptoms and physical findings mimic other conditions such as appendicitis.

  5. Ovarian cyst.
  6. Ovarian torsion.
  7. PID.
  8. Ureteral calculi.
  9. Incarcerated, strangulated inguinal hernia.
E. Generalized abdominal pain:
  1. Trauma:
     a. Any person with a possible blow to the abdomen should have orthostatic blood pressure taken, careful palpation of the abdomen, serial abdominal circumferences measured, and be considered for abdominal imaging. Serial haemoglobin and haematocrit (Hct) measurements should be obtained, if necessary.
     b. In abdominal trauma, the spleen is the most commonly injured organ, especially in blunt abdominal trauma; the onset can be immediate or delayed.

c. Nontraumatic splenic rupture is often associated with acute infectious mononucleosis.

2. Intestinal obstruction: Obstruction that develops slowly over weeks to months may be relatively subtle in presentation.

Acute obstruction presents with severe "colicky" pain or pain that is wavelike in nature; it makes the pain relentless.

3. Peritoneal irritation: Severe pain due to the rich innervation of the parietal peritoneum. Focal injury results in well-localized discomfort that is described as a sharp aching or burning sensation.

4. Metabolic disturbances may mimic intra-abdominal aetiologies.

Porphyria and lead poisoning sometimes simulate bowel obstruction because they can cause cramping, abdominal pain, and hyperperistalsis.

5. Nonspecific dysfunctional abdominal pain and psychogenic abdominal pain are diagnoses of exclusion.

Plan

A. General interventions:
  1. If necessary, prepare the client for emergency transport and hospitalization.
  2. Management and follow-up of other causes of abdominal pain are variable and depend on diagnosis.
B. Client teaching:
  ▶ **1.** *Refer to Client Teaching Guides: Abdominal Pain: Adults* and *Abdominal Pain: Children.*
  2. Counsel the client to keep a pain diary to include activity, foods, and other pain triggers; duration of pain; and what provides relief of symptoms.
C. Pharmacological therapy: Treatment depends on the findings from the history, physical, and testing and clinical diagnosis.

Follow-Up

A. Variable, depending on diagnosis.
B. Review pain diary.

Consultation/Referral

A. Refer to ED for pain related to abdominal trauma.
B. For the obstetric client, consult an obstetrician for any bleeding or abdominal pain.

Individual Considerations

A. Pregnancy: There is no evidence that acute intra-abdominal surgical emergencies are more common during pregnancy if ectopic pregnancy is excluded:
  1. The presence of peritoneal signs, rebound tenderness, and abdominal guarding is never normal in pregnancy.
  2. Bleeding complications include the following:
    a. First trimester: Miscarriage and ectopic pregnancy.
    b. Second and third trimester: Abruptio placenta.
  3. Physiological changes of pregnancy may affect the presentation and evaluation of abdominal pain. The enlargement of the uterus can impede physical examination, affect the normal location of pelvic and abdominal organs, and mask or delay peritoneal signs.
  4. Severe preeclampsia: The clinical manifestations of liver involvement include RUQ or midepigastric pain, elevated transaminases, and, in severe cases, subcapsular haemorrhage or hepatic rupture.
B. Paediatrics:
  1. The caregiver's lap makes the best examining surface; it is much better than having the child lie fixed and supine on a table.
  2. Observe the child's interaction and gait prior to examination. If able to stand, ask the child to hop as an assessment of peritoneal irritation. If the child is unwilling to stand, shaking the examination table or pelvis can also evaluate for peritoneal signs.
  3. An infant's abdomen should be examined during a time of relaxation and quiet, if possible. It is often best to do this at the start of the overall examination, especially before initiating any procedure that may cause distress.
  4. Allowing an infant to suck on a pacifier may help relax him or her.
  5. Tenderness or pain on palpation may be difficult to detect in an infant. However, pain and tenderness are assessed by such behaviours as change in the pitch of crying, facial grimacing, rejection of opportunity to suck, and drawing the knees to the abdomen with palpation.
  6. Urinary tract infections (UTIs) can cause abdominal pain, and often the child with a UTI does not complain of dysuria and frequency as adults typically do.
  7. Young children have inaccurate body perceptions and are inaccurate historians. The practitioner must rely on the caregiver and the examination for data. Consider psychosocial aspects of child care and possible abuse.
  8. Appendicitis is the most common paediatric surgical emergency. The diagnosis can be difficult, because the classic symptoms are often not present.
  9. Intestinal malrotation must be considered when a healthy infant suddenly refuses to eat, vomits, becomes inconsolable, and develops abdominal distension.
  10. Intussusception presents as paroxysmal, colicky pain, and the infant often has currant-jelly stools; a palpable RUQ abdominal mass; and, ultimately, distension.
  11. Young male clients may hesitate to report testicular pain.
C. Adults:
  1. Obesity distorts the abdominal examination, making organ palpation or pelvic examination difficult.
  2. With men older than 40 and women older than 50, suspect cardiac origin when presenting with epigastric pain. Consider obtaining ECG for clients in this age group.

Although myocardial infarction "classically" presents with anterior chest pressure or pain, the client may also have a gastritis or heartburn sensation, coupled with nausea and diaphoresis.

D. Geriatrics:
  1. Elderly clients may have a vague or atypical presentation of pain, varying in location, severity, and presence of a fever or nonspecific findings on examination:
    a. Classic findings of acute peritonitis, rebound tenderness, and local rigidity occur less in the elderly.

▶ Client Teaching Guides are available at https://connect.springerpub.com/content/reference-book/978-0-8261-9498-5

2. Elderly clients have a diminished sensorium, allowing pathology to advance to a dangerous point prior to symptom development:
      a. The level of pain is much less severe at presentation and continues to be at a lower level of pain.
      b. The elderly may present with altered mental status.
   3. In an older client, a similar presentation to IBD with abdominal pain and a change in bowel habits can be the first sign of colon cancer.
   4. AAA is observed almost exclusively in elderly clients. Maintain a high index of suspicion in clients who present with a clinical picture suggestive of renal colic or musculoskeletal back pain:
      a. Approximately 5% of men 65 years and older have AAA.
      b. Maintain a high index of suspicion in clients who present with a clinical picture suggestive of renal colic or musculoskeletal back pain.
   5. Elderly clients with UTI are less likely to have dysuria, frequency, or urgency.
   6. Clients older than 65 years have a 30% to 50% risk of gallstones and may not present with significant pain; less than half have fever, vomiting, or leukocytosis.
   7. Fever and an elevated white blood cell (WBC) count, occur in less than half of the elderly clients with diverticulitis. Only about 25% of the elderly with diverticulitis present with a guaiac positive stool.
   8. The incidence of PUD is more common in the elderly due to the availability and use of NSAIDs. The most common presenting symptom with PUD in the elderly is melena.

Resource
Rome Foundation: http://romecriteria.org/criteria

Bibliography
American College of Gastroenterology. (2011). Pregnancy and gastrointestinal disorders. *Pregnancy monograph*. Retrieved from http://gi.org/wp-content/uploads/2011/07/institute-PregnancyMonograph.pdf
Cartwright, S. L., & Knudson, M. P. (2015). Diagnostic imaging of acute abdominal pain in adults. *American Family Physician*, *91*, 452–460.
Crocket, J. R., Bastian, L. A., & Chireau, M. V. (2013). Does this woman have an ectopic pregnancy? The rational clinical examination systematic review. *Journal of the American Medical Association*, *309*, 1722–1729. doi:10.1001/jama.2013.3914
Fishman, M. B., & Aronson, M. D. (2012, March 5). History and physical examination in adults with abdominal pain. *UpToDate*. Retrieved from http://www.uptodate.com/contents/history-and-physical-examination-in-adults-with-abdominal-pain
National Digestive Diseases Information Clearinghouse. (2012, December). *What I need to know about bowel control*. (NIH Publication No.13-6513). Retrieved from http://digestive.niddk.nih.gov/ddiseases/pubs/bowelcontrol_ez/index.aspx
Nettina, S. (2010). *The Lippincott manual of nursing practice* (9th ed.). Philadelphia, PA: Wolters Kluwer Lippincott Williams & Wilkins.
University of Maryland Medical Center. (2013, June 27). *Gallstones and gallbladder disease*. Retrieved from http://umm.edu/health/medical/reports/articles/gallstones-and-gallbladder-disease
Wehbi, M. (2011, January 12). Acute gastritis. *Medscape*. Retrieved from http://emedicine.medscape.com/article/175909-overview

Appendicitis

Cheryl A. Glass, Audra C. Malone, and Kristie A. D. Morydz

Definition
A. Appendicitis is acute inflammation of the appendix caused by the obstruction of the appendiceal lumen. There is no single sign, symptom, or diagnostic test that accurately confirms the diagnosis of inflammation. Perforation is rare in the first 12 hours, but the rate of possible perforation increases after 72 hours. Prompt, early diagnosis and intervention are the goal of treatment. The differential diagnoses for appendicitis include all abdominal sources of pain.

Incidence/Prevalence
A. Acute appendicitis occurs at a rate of 10:100,000. It is the most common condition in children (1%–8%) and during pregnancy (0.06%–0.1%) that requires emergency abdominal surgery. One in every 2,000 adults older than 65 years will develop appendicitis.

Pathogenesis
A. Foreign bodies, faecal material, tissue hypertrophy, strictures, or a bend or twist in the organ may cause obstruction of the appendix. The obstruction causes colicky pain. Bacterial invasion causes inflammation and leads to gangrene and perforation. The most common bacteria are *Escherichia coli*, pseudomonas, *Bacteroides fragilis*, and *Peptostreptococcus* species.

Predisposing Factors
A. Pregnancy.
B. Torsion.
C. Abdominal trauma.
D. Male gender, age 10 to 30 years.

Common Findings
The classic history of anorexia and periumbilical pain followed by nausea, right lower quadrant (RLQ) pain, and vomiting occurs in only 50% of cases.

A. Adults:
   1. Generalized or localized abdominal pain in the epigastric or periumbilical areas. Within two to 12 hours, pain localizes in RLQ at McBurney's point, and intensity increases.
   2. The location of the appendix is altered in pregnancy and with anatomical variations.
   3. Pain typically develops before vomiting.
   4. Nausea and/or vomiting (may be projectile).
   5. Anorexia signals organic cause of abdominal pain.
   6. Elderly may present with confusion.
B. Paediatrics:
   1. Children younger than two years:
      a. Abdominal distension.
      b. Irritability.
      c. Lethargy.
      d. Fever.
   2. Children older than two years:
      a. Vomiting is often the first symptom.
      b. Abdominal pain in RLQ.
      c. Fever.

Other Signs and Symptoms
A. Rigid abdomen.
B. Changes in pulse (tachycardia), breathing (tachypnoea), or skin temperature.
C. Involuntary guarding.
D. Rebound tenderness.

Subjective Data
Evaluate for a "surgical abdomen," defined as a rapidly worsening prognosis in the absence of surgical intervention.

Clients should not eat or drink while a diagnosis of a surgical abdomen remains under consideration. Once a surgical abdomen has been excluded, the remainder of the evaluation will be guided by the chronicity of symptoms along with the location of pain:

A. Review the onset, duration, course, and quality of pain. Has pain ever occurred before? If so, what was the primary diagnosis? What was the previous treatment, and was it effective?
B. Qualify the duration of pain in minutes, hours, days, weeks, or months. Does it interfere with sleep? Is there a pattern to the pain?
C. Have the client rate the pain on a 10-point pain scale, with 0 being no pain and 10 being the worst pain the client has ever felt.
D. Review the pattern of pain:
   1. Review aggravating factors.
   2. Review alleviating factors.
   3. Does the pain radiate?
   4. Does the pain have any relationship to food?
E. Questions specific to females:
   1. Determine the client's last menstrual period (LMP) to rule out pregnancy.
   2. What type of contraception is used (specifically evaluate for an intrauterine device [IUD])?
   3. Has she had a hysterectomy or tubal ligation?
   4. Does she have a recent history of dysparaeunia or dysmenorrhoea that suggests pelvic pathology?
F. Review current medications and drug history, especially antibiotic and laxative use. Clients taking corticosteroids may have a significant masking of pain.
G. Rule out abdominal trauma, motor vehicle accidents, falls, and assault.
H. Discuss bowel habits, including any changes, such as constipation or diarrhoea, anorexia, food intolerance, nausea and vomiting, and bloating.
I. Ask the client about urinary frequency, urgency, dysuria, flank pain, and back pain. In males, ask about hesitancy, difficulty starting the urine stream, nocturia, low urinary volume, or lower abdominal distension (urinary retention).

Physical Examination

A. Check temperature, pulse, respirations, and blood pressure (BP), including orthostatic BP.
B. Inspect:
   1. Observe general appearance: Facial expressions (grimace during examination), walk, skin colour and turgor, level of consciousness, and acuity level of pain.
   2. Inspect abdomen for surgical scars.
   3. Observe for any bruising or other signs of domestic violence in the "bathing suit" area—breasts, abdomen, or the back—that would be easily covered by clothes.
C. Auscultate:
   1. Abdomen for bowel sounds in all quadrants.
   2. Heart and lungs.
D. Palpate: Note guarding with examination:
   1. Palpate back; note costovertebral angle (CVA) tenderness.
   2. Check for obturator sign, or abdominal pain in response to passive internal rotation of right hip from 90-degree angle hip–knee flexion position. A positive sign indicates pain secondary to irritation of obturator muscle with inflamed appendix.
   3. Assess psoas sign or increased abdominal pain occurring when the client attempts to raise his or her right thigh against the pressure of your hand placed over his or her right knee. Pain is caused by inflammation of the psoas muscle in acute appendicitis.
   4. Check for the Apley rule; the farther the pain from the navel, the more likely it is organic in origin.
   5. Check for Rovsing's sign, or pain in the RLQ on palpation of the left side.
   6. Anatomical variations of the appendix may lead to differences in the location of the pain. For example, the location of the appendix changes with pregnancy (see Figure 11.1), retrocaecal appendix may lead to right loin pain.
E. Percuss abdomen.
F. Perform rectal or pelvic examination if needed. May have right-side pain with subcaecal or pelvic appendix.
G. Palpate abdomen: Palpate at the end of the examination because positive response produces pain and muscle spasm that can interfere with subsequent examination:
   1. Ask the client to bend his or her knees to help relax abdominal wall musculature.
   2. Check for Murphy's sign, which is inspiratory arrest in response to right upper quadrant (RUQ) palpation, seen in acute cholecystitis.
   3. Check for rebound tenderness.
   4. Check for jar tenderness.

Diagnostic Tests

A. Serum human chorionic gonadotropin (HCG): Pregnancy should be excluded in all women of childbearing age. Assume that the woman is pregnant until proven otherwise.
B. Complete blood count (CBC) with differential.
C. C-reactive protein (CRP).
D. Urinalysis, to rule out urinary disorders.
E. Abdominal ultrasonography: Any person with trauma to the abdomen should have an abdominal ultrasound.
F. CT scan with or without contrast.
G. MRI may be used as an alternative diagnostic test in pregnancy to avoid exposure to ionizing radiation.
H. Stool guaiac test for occult blood.

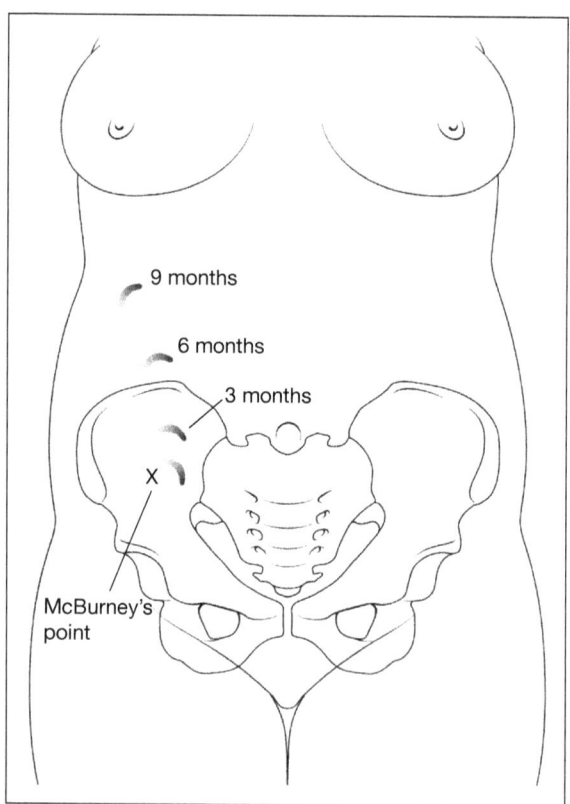

FIGURE 11.1 The position of the appendix alters during pregnancy and so must the site of incision to gain access.

Differential Diagnoses
The appendix has no fixed position. Duration of pain can significantly help in narrowing differential diagnosis. Nonspecific dysfunctional abdominal pain and psychogenic abdominal pain are diagnoses of exclusion:
A. Regional enteritis.
B. Leaking aneurysm.
C. Ruptured ectopic pregnancy.
D. Ovarian cyst.
E. Ovarian torsion.
F. Pelvic inflammatory disease (PID).
G. Mittelschmerz, or ovulatory bleeding or pain.
H. Endometriosis.
I. Ureteral calculi.
J. Incarcerated, strangulated groin hernia.
K. Meckel's diverticulitis.
L. Abdominal wall haematoma.
M. Bowel obstruction.
N. Intestinal malrotation.
O. Intussusception.
P. Testicular torsion.
Q. Inflammatory bowel disease (IBD)/Crohn's disease.
R. Parasites.
S. IUD.
T. Constipation.

Plan
▶ A. Client teaching: *Refer to Client Teaching Guides: Abdominal Pain: Adults* and *Abdominal Pain: Children.*
B. Medical and surgical management: Appendectomy may need to be performed.
C. Pharmacological therapy:
   1. Antibiotics are currently used to treat uncomplicated, nonsurgical appendicitis; however, there is a 5% to 15% rate of complications and a 15% to 30% recurrence rate. More studies are needed to determine the efficacy of antibiotic therapy alone.
   2. Do not give antipyretics to mask fever.
   3. Do not administer cathartics because they may cause rupture.

Follow-Up
A. Postoperative follow-up is with the surgeon.

Consultation/Referral
A. Surgical consultation and possible emergency transport and hospitalization are often required.

Individual Considerations
A. Pregnancy:
   1. Any abdominal pain or bleeding in the first eight weeks after a missed menstrual period must be considered a symptom of possible *ectopic pregnancy.*
   2. The identification of intra-abdominal masses may be compromised by the enlarged uterus, but this problem may be partially obviated by examining the woman in the lateral position.
   3. The intestinal tract is progressively displaced upward, outward, and backward during pregnancy; bowel sounds are best heard lateral or superior to the uterus.

B. Paediatrics:
   1. The caregiver's lap makes the best examining surface; it is much better than having the child lie fixed and supine on a table.
   2. If possible, examine the infant's abdomen during a time of relaxation and quiet. It is often best to do this at the start of the overall examination, especially before initiating any procedure that might cause distress. Allowing the infant to suck on a bottle or pacifier may help relax him or her.
   3. Tenderness or pain on palpation may be difficult to detect in the infant. However, pain and tenderness are assessed by such behaviours as change in the pitch of crying, facial grimacing, rejection of the opportunity to suck, and drawing knees to the abdomen with palpation.
   4. Intestinal malrotation must be considered when a healthy infant suddenly refuses to eat, vomits, becomes inconsolable, and develops abdominal distension.
   5. Young children have inaccurate body perceptions and are inaccurate historians, so rely on caregivers and examination for data, and consider psychosocial aspects such as child care and child abuse.
   6. Intussusception presents as paroxysmal, colicky pain, and the infant often has currant-jelly stools, a palpable RUQ, abdominal mass, and ultimately distension.
C. Adults:
   1. Obesity distorts abdominal examination, making organ palpation or pelvic examination difficult.
   2. Immunocompromised clients are susceptive to infection. They may not exhibit the typical signs and symptoms of appendicitis; only mild tenderness on examination.
   3. CT examination is useful for diagnosis in the immunocompromised.
D. Geriatrics:
   1. The elderly tend to have a diminished inflammatory response, resulting in a less remarkable history and physical examination. Be aware of vague symptoms, such as milder pain, less pronounced fever, and leukocytosis with shift to left on differential.
   2. Confusion is a common presenting symptom.
   3. A redundant sigmoid colon may also cause right-sided pain from sigmoid disease.
   4. Prompt CT scanning is used for diagnosis and differential.

Bibliography
American College of Gastroenterology. (2011). Pregnancy and gastrointestinal disorders. *Pregnancy monograph.* Retrieved from http://gi.org/wp-content/uploads/2011/07/institute-PregnancyMonograph.pdf

Craig, S. (2012, October 26). Appendicitis. *Medscape.* Retrieved from http://emedicine.medscape.com/article/773895

Crocket, J. R., Bastian, L. A., & Chireau, M. V. (2013). Does this woman have an ectopic pregnancy? The rational clinical examination systematic review. *Journal of the American Medical Association, 309,* 1722–1729. doi:10.1001/jama.2013.3914

Ehlers, A. P., Talan, D. A., Moran, G. J., Flum, D. R., & Davidson, G. H. (2016). Evidence for an antibiotics first strategy for uncomplicated appendicitis in adults: A systematic review and gap analysis. *Journal of the American College of Surgeons, 222,* 309–314. doi:10.1016/j.jamcollsurg.2015.11.009

Nettina, S. (2010). *The Lippincott manual of nursing practice* (9th ed.). Philadelphia, PA: Wolters Kluwer Lippincott Williams & Wilkins.

Snyder, J. A., Gurevitz, S. L., Rush, L. S., McKeague, L. C., & Houpt, C. G. (2012, January). Appendicitis review. *Clinician Reviews, 22,* 23–28.

▶ Client Teaching Guides are available at https://connect.springerpub.com/content/reference-book/978-0-8261-9498-5

Celiac Disease

Cheryl A. Glass, Audra C. Malone, and Kristie A. D. Morydz

Definition
A. Celiac disease, previously known as *celiac sprue*, is an autoimmune disorder triggered by a well-defined environmental factor, gluten. Celiac disease is a permanent sensitivity to gluten, specifically; the people are unable to tolerate gliadin, the alcohol-soluble fraction of gluten. Three cereals contain gluten and are considered toxic for clients with celiac disease: wheat, rye, and barley. The disease primarily affects the small intestine. Onset of symptoms depends on the amount of gluten in the diet. Dietary nonadherence is the chief cause of persistent or recurrent symptoms (see Appendix B, Diet Recommendations, Table B.5).
B. Celiac disease is one of the most common causes of chronic malabsorption as a result of injury to the small intestine with loss of absorptive surface area, reduction of digestive enzymes, and consequential impaired absorption of micronutrients such as fat-soluble vitamins, iron, and potentially vitamin B12 and folic acid.
C. Celiac disease is strongly associated with autoimmune conditions, including type 1 diabetes, Addison's disease, and thyroiditis, as well as genetic syndromes including Down syndrome, Williams syndrome, and Turner syndrome. The complications from celiac disease include osteopaenia, osteoporosis, infertility, short stature, delayed puberty, anaemia, gastrointestinal (GI) malignancies, and non-Hodgkin's lymphoma (NHL).
D. After GI symptoms, the second most common manifestation of celiac disease in clients with type 1 diabetes is diminished or impaired bone mineralization.
E. Celiac disease is the most common cause of steatorrhoea in people older than 50 years and the second most common cause in people older than 65 years.
F. A substantial number of clients are misdiagnosed as having irritable bowel syndrome (IBS) for years before the diagnosis of celiac disease.

Incidence/Prevalence
A. Celiac disease can occur at any stage of life. The prevalence of celiac disease in children is unknown. Its prevalence is approximately 1% of the general population in North America. The true incidence is undetermined due to asymptomatic disease and underdiagnosis. It is estimated that 75% of those affected by celiac disease remain underdiagnosed or misdiagnosed.
B. Screening of the general population is not recommended.
C. Newly diagnosed clients with celiac disease should inform their first-degree family members of their increased risk (10%–15% chance) of celiac disease and the recommendations for testing.

Pathogenesis
A. Interactions between gluten and immune and genetic factors result in celiac disease. Gluten is poorly digested. The enzyme tissue transglutaminase (tTG) is the autoantigen against which abnormal immune response is directed. The immune responses promote an inflammatory reaction. Celiac disease primarily affects the mucosal layer of the small intestine. The classic celiac lesion is noted in the proximal small intestine.
B. A hallmark on histology is the presence of villous atrophy. The *Modified Marsh Classification* is used to describe the progressive histologic stages of celiac disease. Marsh 1 and Marsh 2 may be seen in sow and cow's milk allergies:
- Marsh Type 0: Preinfiltrative stage (normal)—celiac disease highly unlikely.
- Marsh Type 1: Increased intraepithelial lymphocytes but no villous atrophy.
- Marsh Type 2: Increased intraepithelial lymphocytes villi normal plus hyperplastic crypts.
- Marsh 3a: Increased intraepithelial lymphocytes, increased crypt hyperplasia and mild atrophy of villi.
- Marsh 3b: Increased intraepithelial lymphocytes, increased crypt hyperplasia and marked atrophy of villi.
- Marsh 3c: Increased intraepithelial lymphocytes, increased crypt hyperplasia and complete atrophy of villi.

Predisposing Factors
A. Female gender.
B. May be precipitated by an infectious diarrhoeal episode or other intestinal disease (e.g., rotavirus).
C. Genetic disorders:
  1. Down syndrome (8%–12%).
  2. Type 1 diabetes (10%).
  3. Turner syndrome (2%–10%).
  4. Williams syndrome (8.2%).
D. Strong hereditary component (10% in first-degree relatives).
E. The introduction of gluten before four months of age is associated with increased disease development.
F. Autoimmune thyroiditis.
G. Selective immunoglobulin A (IgA) deficiency.

Common Findings
A. Asymptomatic.
B. Chronic diarrhoea or explosive watery diarrhoea.
C. Foul-smelling voluminous stools.
D. Anorexia.
E. Abdominal distension.
F. Abdominal pain.
G. Poor weight gain or weight loss.
H. Vomiting.
I. Steatorrhoea (malabsorption of ingested fat).
J. Refusal to eat (children).

Other Signs and Symptoms
A. Behavioural changes, including irritability.
B. Dehydration.
C. Lethargy.
D. Constipation.
E. Failure to thrive (FTT).
F. Short stature and delayed puberty.
G. Dermatitis herpetiformis.
H. Arthritis.
I. Seizures.
J. Weakness and fatigue.
K. Dental enamel hypoplasia of permanent teeth.
L. Iron-deficiency anaemia unresponsive to treatment.
M. Bruising/bleeding tendency.
N. Osteopaenia/osteoporosis.
O. Hair loss.
P. Lactose intolerance.
Q. Aphthous stomatitis.
R. Ataxia.
S. Neuropathy.

Subjective Data
A. Review the onset, duration, course, and type of symptoms.
B. Review the client's weight history.
C. Evaluate family history for celiac disease or members with similar histories.
D. Review current medications and drug history, especially antibiotic, laxative, and herbal products.
E. Review bowel habits and note changes: Constipation, diarrhoea, anorexia, and/or food intolerance.
F. Review the client's tolerance to lactose products.

Physical Examination
A. Check vital signs, including height and weight. Follow serial weights and plot serial height/weight on growth charts.
B. Inspect:
  1. Observe general overall appearance.
  2. Oral examination to evaluate glossitis, dry mucosal membranes (dehydration), and the presence of oral aphthae.
  3. Examine the skin for the presence of dermatitis herpetiformis, a blistering rash involving the scalp, neck, elbows, knees, and buttocks.
  4. Evaluate the abdomen for the presence of bloating and protuberant "potbelly."
  5. Evaluate the client's weight loss, including muscle wasting.
C. Auscultate: Bowel sounds in all four quadrants of the abdomen.
D. Percuss abdomen.
E. Palpate:
  1. Palpate the abdomen for masses, rebound tenderness, and peritoneal signs:
    a. Before palpating the abdomen, ask the client to bend his or her knees to help with relaxation of the wall musculature.
  2. Perform a rectal examination, including testing stool for occult blood.

Diagnostic Tests
The confirmation of a diagnosis of celiac disease is based on the combination of findings from the medical history, physical examination, serology, and upper endoscopy, with histologic analysis of multiple biopsies of the duodenum. **All testing should be performed while clients are following a gluten-rich diet.**
A. Endoscopy for duodenal biopsies is the standard and a critical component for diagnosing celiac disease (Figure 11.2).
B. Screening and monitoring tests for celiac disease (see Table 11.1 for celiac disease tests and possible results):
  1. tTG antibody, IgA class:
    a. Primary test ordered to screen for celiac disease.
    b. Used for monitoring and evaluating the effectiveness of treatment.
    c. Antibody levels should fall when gluten is removed from the diet.
  2. Anti-tTG antibodies, immunoglobulin G (IgG).
  3. Anti-tTG, IgG class.
  4. Deamidated gliadin peptide antibodies (anti-DGP, IgA).
  5. Anti-gliadin antibodies (AGAs) IgG (gliadin is a component of wheat storage protein gluten).
  6. AGA IgA.
  7. IgA endomysial antibody (EMA)—less frequently ordered, measures same as the anti-tTG.
  8. Antireticulin antibody (ARA)—rarely ordered.
  9. Anti-F-actin—is ordered if the disease has been diagnosed; evaluates the severity of intestinal damage. May be used for monitoring.
C. Complete blood count (CBC) and electrolytes.
D. Aspartate transaminase (AST) and alanine transaminase (ALT; liver enzymes normalize on a gluten-free diet).
E. Prothrombin time (PT) may be prolonged with malabsorption of vitamin K.
F. C-reactive protein (CRP).
G. Erythrocyte sedimentation rate (ESR).
H. Total protein.
I. Albumin.
J. Calcium.
K. Iron, transferrin, and ferritin.
L. Vitamin B12 and folate levels.
M. Thyroid screen (autoimmune thyroid disorders and hypothyroidism common in the elderly).
N. Stool culture, ova, and parasites.
O. Faecal fat.
P. Bone density (bone mineral density improves on gluten-free diet).
Q. Human leukocyte antigen (HLA) haplotypes.
R. Colonoscopy if bloody stools or symptoms of colitis.
S. Sweat test to exclude cystic fibrosis (CF).
T. Other testing specific to nutritional deficiencies as needed (vitamin D, B12, folate).
U. Radiograph, including barium swallow study with a small-bowel follow-through, is usually nonspecific and is not indicated.

Differential Diagnoses
A. FTT.
B. Food allergies.
C. Inflammatory bowel disease (IBD):
  1. Crohn's disease (CD).
  2. Ulcerative colitis (UC).
D. Immunodeficiency disorders.
E. Gastroenteritis (viral or bacterial).
F. Parasites.
G. Fungal infection.
H. IBS.
I. Malabsorption.
J. Lymphomas of the small intestine.

Plan
A. Nutrition therapy is the only accepted treatment for celiac disease:
  1. Gluten-free dietary instructions should be given and reinforced.
  2. Reinforce the need to read all food labels.
  3. Stress that wheat-free is not the same as gluten-free.
  4. The gluten-free diet must continue throughout the client's life.
B. The Canadian Association of Gastroenterology recommends a referral to a registered dietitian in order to receive a thorough nutritional assessment and education on a gluten-free diet. A gluten-free diet should be maintained for life. Nutriguides "nutrition guides" apps are available from the iTunes Store for iPhone and iPad and from the Google Store for Android products.
C. Genetic testing does not diagnose celiac disease.
D. Monitor for iron and vitamin deficiencies because substitute flours are not fortified with B vitamins. Supplement with iron, folate, and vitamin B12 as needed.
E. Screen for osteoporosis. Up to 70% of adult and elderly clients with celiac disease have osteopaenia.

ALGORITHM FOR THE EVALUATION OF CELIAC DISEASE

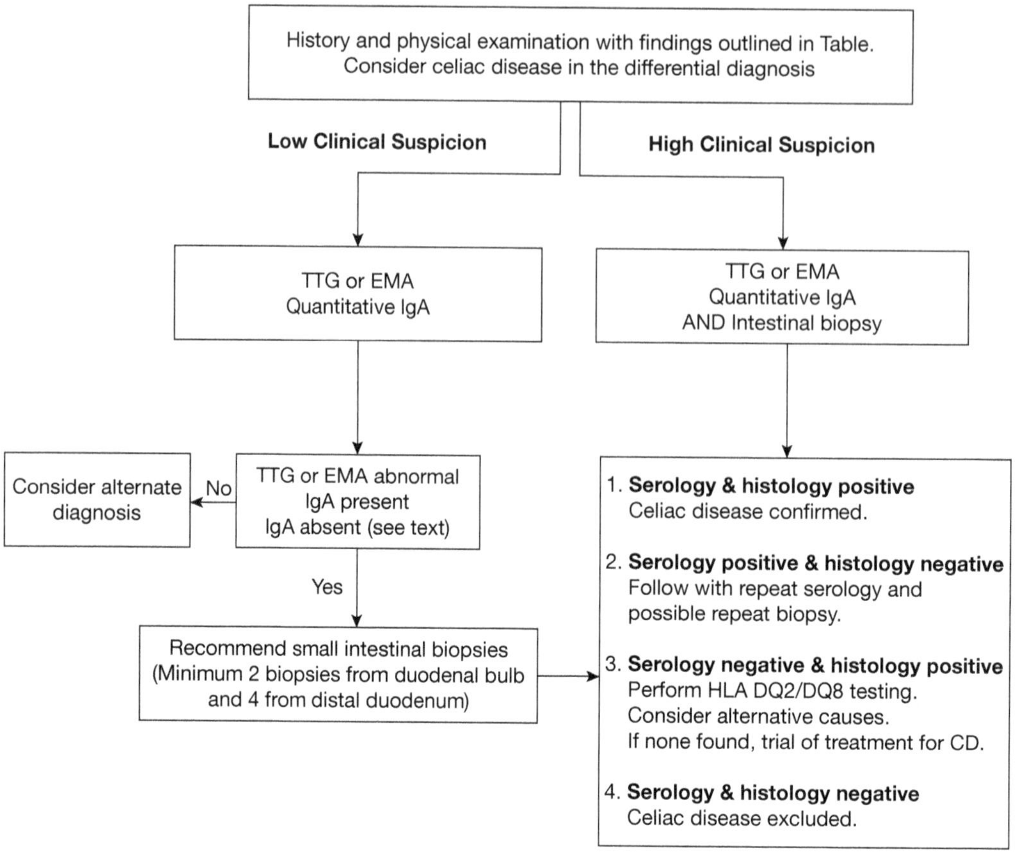

```
History and physical examination with findings outlined in Table.
Consider celiac disease in the differential diagnosis
        │                                    │
Low Clinical Suspicion            High Clinical Suspicion
        ▼                                    ▼
TTG or EMA                        TTG or EMA
Quantitative IgA                  Quantitative IgA
                                  AND Intestinal biopsy
        ▼                                    ▼
Consider alternate ◄── No ── TTG or EMA abnormal
diagnosis                    IgA present
                             IgA absent (see text)
                                  │ Yes
                                  ▼
                        Recommend small intestinal biopsies
                        (Minimum 2 biopsies from duodenal bulb
                        and 4 from distal duodenum)
```

1. **Serology & histology positive**
   Celiac disease confirmed.

2. **Serology positive & histology negative**
   Follow with repeat serology and possible repeat biopsy.

3. **Serology negative & histology positive**
   Perform HLA DQ2/DQ8 testing.
   Consider alternative causes.
   If none found, trial of treatment for CD.

4. **Serology & histology negative**
   Celiac disease excluded.

FIGURE 11.2 Diagnosis of celiac disease.
Source: Butzner, D. (2016). *Screening and diagnosis of celiac disease: A summary from the NASPGHAN, WGO and ACG guidelines.* Canadian Celiac Association.

Some Celiac Disease Tests and Positive Results

Anti-tTG Antibodies, IgA	Total IgA	Anti-tTG Antibodies, IgG	Anti-DGP, IgA	AGAs, IgG	Diagnosis
Positive	Normal	Not performed	Not performed	Not performed	Presumptive celiac disease
Negative	Normal	Negative	Negative	Negative	Symptoms not likely due to celiac disease
Negative	Low	Positive	Negative	Positive	Possible celiac disease (false negative anti-tTG, IgA, and anti-DGP, IgA are due to total IgA deficiency)
Negative	Normal	Negative	Positive	Positive (or not performed)	Possible celiac disease (may be seen in children younger than three years old)

Notes: AGA, anti-gliadin antibodies; DGP, deamidated gliadin peptide; IgA, immunoglobulin A; IgG, immunoglobulin G; tTG, tissue transglutaminase.
Source: American Association for Clinical Chemistry. (2018, October 28). *Celiac disease antibody tests. Lab Tests Online.* Retrieved from https://labtestsonline.org/tests/celiac-disease-antibody-tests. Reprinted with permission from LabTestsOnline.

F. Keep a food/symptom diary in order to eliminate trigger foods. See Appendix B, Diet Recommendations, Table B.5.

G. Gluten has been identified in dietary supplements, over-the-counter (OTC) medications, nonfood items such as lipstick and envelope adhesive, and food items with gluten additives, such as condiments.

H. Gluten rechallenge is not generally recommended unless the diagnosis remains uncertain:
   1. The rechallenge is not mandatory for clients with good improvement of symptoms.
   2. HLA-DQ2/DQ8 gentoyping for genetic risk factors should be used to try to exclude celiac disease prior to a formal gluten challenge.

I. Pharmacology: Corticosteroids may be prescribed for rapid control of symptoms: Prednisone:
   1. Children with celiac disease are rarely given steroids.
   2. Bisphosphonates for osteoporosis.

Follow-Up

A. After the diagnosis of celiac disease and a strict diet has been started, follow up in four to eight weeks or earlier if the client has other comorbidities.

B. Guidelines recommend the measurement of tissue transglutaminase (tTGA) after six months of a gluten-free diet.

C. Newly diagnosed clients with celiac disease should undergo testing and treatment for micronutrient deficiencies.

Deficiency testing should include, but not be limited to, iron, folic acid, vitamin D, and vitamin B12.
D. Refer for dietary consultation with a nutritionist with experience in gluten-free diets.
E. Consider allergy testing.

Consultation/Referral
A. If the gluten-free diet fails or the client experiences new symptoms, a systematic evaluation is required.
B. Endocrine consultation for clients with Hashimoto's thyroiditis and celiac disease.
C. Consultation with a paediatric gastroenterologist.

Individual Considerations
A. Pregnancy: Women with untreated celiac disease are at risk for preterm birth, low-birth-weight babies, recurrent loss, and reduced fertility.
B. Paediatrics:
   1. Children may appear to have a "potbelly" with muscle wasting from malnutrition.
   2. Monitor growth and development. Utilize a growth chart to plot growth rates. As many as 10% of children with idiopathic short stature may have celiac disease.
   3. Breastfeeding has a protective role even if gluten is introduced while breastfeeding.
   4. Biliary sludge and/or gallstones are likely to form in one in five children with haemolytic anaemia before their adolescent years.
C. Geriatrics:
   1. The elderly may present with nonspecific GI symptoms, abdominal discomfort, bloating, constipation, or dyspepsia.
   2. Diarrhoea may be mild or intermittent in the elderly.
   3. Iron-deficiency anaemia may also be a presenting symptom. Anaemia is present in 60% to 80% of elderly clients with celiac disease.
   4. The elderly are at increased risk for falls related to osteopaenia, ataxia, and neuropathy.
   5. Autoimmune thyroid disorders are common with elderly celiac clients. The majority present with hypothyroidism.
   6. The risk for NHL is increased in people with celiac disease aged 50 years and older.

Resources
http://www.celiac.com/categories/Gluten-Free–Recipes-c-3400.html
www.glutenfreedrugs.com
www.celiac.ca

Bibliography
Academy of Nutrition and Dietetics. (n.d.). *Celiac disease evidence-based nutrition practice guideline.* Retrieved from http://www.adaevidencelibrary.com/topic.cfm?cat=3677

American Association for Clinical Chemistry. (2015, February 24). Celiac disease antibody tests. *Lab Tests Online.* Retrieved from labtestsonline.org/understanding/analytes/celiac-disease/tab/test

American College of Gastroenterology. (2011). Pregnancy and gastrointestinal disorders. *Pregnancy monograph.* Retrieved from http://gi.org/wp-content/uploads/2011/07/institute-PregnancyMonograph.pdf

Butzner, D. (2016). *Screening and diagnosis of celiac disease: A summary from the NASPGHAN, WGO and ACG guidelines.* Canadian Celiac Association.

Ciclitira, P. J. (2009, May 1). Management of celiac disease in adults. *UpToDate.* Retrieved from http://www.uptodate.com/online/content/topic.do?topicKey=mal_synd/5722&view=print

Freeman, H. J. (2008). Adult celiac disease in the elderly. *World Journal of Gastroenterology, 14*, 6911–6914. doi:10.3748/wjg.14.6911

Gainer, C. L. (2011, September). Helping patients live gluten-free. *Nurse Practitioner, 36,* 14–20. doi:10.1097/01.NPR.0000393969.13812.2e

Goebel, S. U. (2013, 2014, July 14). Celiac spruce. *Medscape.* Retrieved from http://emedicine.medscape.com/article/171805-overview

Green, P. H. R., & Cellier, C. (2007). Celiac disease medical progress. *New England Journal of Medicine, 357*(17), 1731–1744. doi:10.1056/NEJMra071600

Hill, I. D. (2009, May 1). Management of celiac disease in children. *UpToDate.* Retrieved from http://www.uptodate.com/online/content/topic.do?topicKey=pedigast/9506&view=print

Kagnoff, M. F. (2006). American Gastroenterological Association Institute medical position statement on the diagnosis and management of celiac disease. *Gastroenterology, 131,* 1977–1980. doi:10.1053/j.gastro.2006.10.003

Kelly, C. P. (2013, January 16). Diagnosis of celiac disease. *UpToDate.* Retrieved from http://www.uptodate.com/contents/diagnosis-of-celiac-disease

Nettina, S. (2010). *The Lippincott manual of nursing practice* (9th ed.). Philadelphia, PA: Wolters Kluwer Lippincott Williams & Wilkins.

North American Society for Pediatric Gastroenterology, Hepatology and Nutrition. (2005). Guideline for the diagnosis and treatment of celiac disease in children: Recommendation of the North American Society for Pediatric Gastroenterology, Hepatology and Nutrition. *Journal of Pediatric Gastroenterology and Nutrition, 40*(1), 1–19. doi:10.1097/00005176-200501000-00001

Rubio-Tapia, A., Hill, I. D., Kelly, C. P., Calderwood, A. H., & Murray, J. A. (2013, May). ACG clinical guidelines: Diagnosis and management of celiac disease. *American Journal of Gastroenterology, 108,* 656–676. doi:10.1038/ajg.2013.79

Sadowski, D. C., & van Zanten, S. V. (2015). Dyspepsia. *CMAJ, 187*(4), 276–276. doi:10.1503/cmaj.141606

Sharma, G. D. (2013, June 17). Cystic fibrosis. *Medscape.* Retrieved from http://emedicine.medscape.com/article/1001602-overview

University of Chicago Celiac Disease Center. (n.d.). *Gluten free diet.* Retrieved from http://www.celiacdisease.net/glutenfree-diet

University of Maryland Medical Center. (2013, June 27). *Gallstones and gallbladder disease.* Retrieved from http://umm.edu/health/medical/reports/articles/gallstones-and-gallbladder-disease

Zhu, J., Mulder, C. J. J., & Dieleman, L. A. (2018). Celiac disease: Against the grain in gastroenterology. *Journal of the Canadian Association of Gastroenterology,* 1–9. doi:10.1093/jcag/gwy042

Cholecystitis

Cheryl A. Glass, Audra C. Malone, and Kristie A. D. Morydz

Definition
A. Cholecystitis is the acute or chronic inflammation of the gallbladder. Acute cholecystitis has associated stone formation (cholelithiasis) in 90% of all cases, causing obstruction and inflammation. Biliary sludge is a feature of chronic cholecystitis.

Incidence/Prevalence
A. Gallbladder disease afflicts 16% to 18% of Canadians. The incidence in children is not known. Most clients with an acute attack of cholecystitis have complete remission in one to five days; however, approximately 20% require surgical intervention. Mortality related to acute cholecystitis is 5% to 10%, with the highest risk for clients older than 60 years. The most common complication is the development of gallbladder gangrene with the potential for subsequent perforation (2%). Gangrenous cholecystitis is most common in older clients, diabetics, or clients who delay treatment.
B. Cholecystectomy for recurrent biliary colic or acute cholecystitis is the most common major surgical procedure performed by general surgeons.

Pathogenesis
A. Cholecystitis occurs subsequent to bile stasis, bacterial infection, ischaemia, or obstruction by a gallstone. Acute cholecystitis is related to the impaction of a calculus in the

neck of the gallbladder in approximately 90% of cases. Spontaneous resolution may occur after the reestablishment of cystic duct patency.
B. *Escherichia coli* is the primary microorganism in 80% of cholecystitis infections.
C. Oestrogen-induced alteration in bile salts may favour stone formation. Stones occur when cholesterol supersaturates the bile in the gallbladder and precipitates out of the bile. Cholesterol stones are the most common type of gallstones in the United States.
D. Pigment stones occur when free bilirubin combines with calcium. Pigment stones are found in clients with cirrhosis, haemolysis, and infections in the biliary tree.
E. Acalculous cholecystitis is associated with infection and local inflammation. Formation of gallstones is not necessary for the obstruction of the bile duct.

Predisposing Factors
A. Female gender.
B. Sudden starvation/prolonged fasting.
C. Medications:
  1. Cholesterol-lowering drugs: Stone formation increases in users of cholesterol-lowering drugs, which are known to increase biliary cholesterol saturation.
  2. Oestrogen usage (oral contraceptive pills [OCPs] and hormone replacement therapy [HRT]). Stone formation increases in users of contraceptives and oestrogens, which are known to increase biliary cholesterol saturation.
  3. Furosemide.
  4. Ceftriaxone.
  5. Cyclosporine.
  6. Opiate narcotic analgesics.
D. Bile acid malabsorption.
E. Genetic predisposition: Indigenous, Chinese, or Japanese clients have a high incidence.
F. Total parenteral nutrition (TPN).
G. Obesity.
H. Status post bariatric surgery.
I. Pregnancy secondary to elevated progesterone.
J. Increasing age.
K. Haemolytic anaemia.
L. Diabetes.
M. High serum triglyceride and low high-density lipoprotein (HDL) levels.
N. High-caloric and refined carbohydrate diet.
O. Cirrhosis, Crohn's disease, and gallbladder stasis.

Common Findings
A. Abrupt, severe abdominal pain lasting 24 hours.
B. Constant aching pain in the right upper quadrant (RUQ), right subcostal region, with radiation to the back and right shoulder.
C. Nausea and vomiting.
D. Acalculous cholecystitis may present with fever and sepsis alone.

Other Signs and Symptoms
A. Anorexia.
B. Heartburn.
C. Upper abdominal fullness.
D. Biliary colic: Sudden onset of severe pain in the epigastrium or right hypochondrium that subsides relatively slowly. Tenderness may remain for days.
E. Fat intolerance.
F. Fever (low grade).
G. Mild jaundice (20%).
H. Complicated disease such as an abscess or perforation; symptoms include more severe localized persistent pain, tenderness, fever, chills, and leukocytosis.
I. Chronic diarrhoea (four to 10 bowel movements every day for at least 3 months).

Subjective Data
A. Review the onset, location, duration, course, and quality of pain.
B. Use a pain-rating scale, such as a 10-point pain scale, with 0 being no pain and 10 being equivalent to the worst pain the client has ever felt. Determine the progression of the pain as well.
C. Review any alleviating factors, such as antacids, and any worsening factors, such as deep inspiration.
D. Review any pain radiating to the jaw, neck, shoulder, or arm.
E. Review the onset of pain in relation to last meal and foods ingested.
F. Ask the client about recurrent history of epigastric pain.
G. Obtain history and demographic data that may indicate the risk factors for biliary disease.
H. Review the date of the client's last menstrual period (LMP), and, if she is pregnant, establish gestational age.

Physical Examination
The absence of physical findings does not rule out the diagnosis of cholecystitis:
A. Check temperature, pulse (tachycardia), respirations, and blood pressure (BP).
B. Inspect: Observe general appearance, facial expressions, walk, skin colour (15% have jaundice) and turgor, and grimace during examination. Overall appearance is generally unremarkable between attacks; ill appearance occurs during acute attack.
C. Auscultate:
  1. Heart.
  2. Lung fields.
  3. Abdomen for bowel sounds in all four quadrants.
D. Percuss the abdomen.
E. Palpate:
  1. Palpate the abdomen; check for tenderness in the RUQ, especially with inspiration; assess for guarding and rebound tenderness.
  2. Check Murphy's sign. Positive Murphy's sign is inspiratory arrest secondary to extreme tenderness when the subhepatic area is palpated during deep inspiration.
F. Perform rectal examination, if indicated.

Diagnostic Tests
A. Laboratory tests:
  1. Amylase (will be normal in classic cholecystitis).
  2. Complete blood count (CBC) with differential (leukocytosis).
  3. Alkaline phosphate (normal in classic cholecystitis).
  4. Bilirubin (normal to mildly elevated in classic cholecystitis).
  5. Aspartate transaminase (AST; slightly elevated to normal).
  6. Alanine transaminase (ALT; slightly elevated to normal).
  7. Urinalysis to rule out pyelonephritis and renal calculi.
  8. Pregnancy test if childbearing age.
  9. Stool guaiac test for occult blood to rule out bleeding.

B. Radiography:
1. **Ultrasonography: Can often establish the diagnosis. Positive findings include presence of stones, gallbladder wall thickening, or enlargement and fluid.**
2. Cholescintigraphy (hepatobiliary iminodiacetic acid [HIDA]) scan is indicated if the diagnosis is uncertain after an ultrasound.
3. MR cholangiography.
4. CT scan (can identify extrabiliary disorders and complications of acute cholecystitis).
5. Chest radiography to rule out pneumonia.
C. ECG to rule out myocardial infarction (MI).

Differential Diagnoses
A. Biliary colic.
B. Acute pancreatitis.
C. Appendicitis.
D. Peptic ulcer disease (PUD)/perforation.
E. Acute hepatitis.
F. Pneumonia or pleurisy.
G. MI.
H. Renal calculi.
I. Gastro-oesophageal reflux disease (GORD).
J. Pregnancy: Urolithiasis, pyelonephritis.

Plan
A. General interventions: Clients with a single episode of biliary colic are reasonable candidates for expectant management, as long as they continue to be free of recurrent pain.
B. Client teaching:
1. No activity restriction is required.
2. Treatment depends on acuteness of attack. Heat may be used as needed for pain. If pain continues to worsen, have the client contact his or her health-care provider. Hospitalization and/or surgery may be required depending on the severity of the attack.
C. Dietary management:
1. Counsel the client to avoid fatty foods.
2. Encourage the client to avoid fasting and starvation diets, which make the bile even more lithogenic.
D. Surgical management:
1. Cholecystectomy may be recommended for symptomatic clients. **The standard of care is the laparoscopic cholecystectomy.** Conversion from a laparoscopic procedure to an open surgical procedure is approximately 5%.
E. Pharmacological therapy:
1. Acetaminophen may be used as needed for pain.
2. Anticholinergics are not helpful.
3. Oral bile acid therapy decreases the amount of cholesterol produced by the liver and absorbed by the intestines:
   a. Ursodiol.
4. Antibiotics, such as ampicillin or cefazolin, may be used for mild attacks.
5. Antiemetics for nausea and vomiting.
6. Drug dissolution therapy with ursodeoxycholic acid and extracorporeal shock wave lithotripsy have lower cure rates.

Follow-Up
A. See the client at next pain attack to reevaluate.
B. Surgical follow-up in two weeks or as indicated.

Consultation/Referral
A. For acute attack, surgical consultation referral.
B. Refer to surgeon for elective cholecystectomy when client has documented gallstones and recurrent biliary colic or a history of complication of gallstone disease such as pancreatitis.
C. Refer to a gastroenterologist for consideration of endoscopic retrograde cholangiopancreatography (ERCP).

Individual Considerations
A. Pregnancy:
1. RUQ pain in pregnancy differential includes preeclampsia, pancreatitis, and appendicitis.
2. In the absence of pancreatitis, maternal mortality should be rare, and foetal loss is generally estimated to be no more than 5%. However, if secondary pancreatitis is present, maternal mortality is 15%, and foetal loss is reported as high as 60%.
B. Paediatrics:
1. Clients with sickle cell disease are at higher risk for developing cholecystitis.
2. Infants with cholecystitis may present with irritability, jaundice, and acholic (pale white) stools.
3. The most common complication of gallstones in children is pancreatitis.
C. Geriatrics:
1. Signs and symptoms may be nonspecific and vague.
2. Localized tenderness may be the only presenting sign.
3. The response of Murphy's sign may be diminished in the elderly.
4. Early cholecystectomy is advocated for elderly clients with gallstone disease. The most important risk factor for postoperative morbidity and mortality is advanced age.
5. Biliary sludge and/or gallstones are likely to form in one in five children with haemolytic anaemia before their adolescent years.

Bibliography
American College of Gastroenterology. (2011). Pregnancy and gastrointestinal disorders. *Pregnancy monograph*. Retrieved from http://gi.org/wp-content/uploads/2011/07/institute-PregnancyMonograph.pdf
American College of Obstetricians and Gynecologists. (2009, June). ACOG practice bulletin bariatric surgery and pregnancy. *Obstetrics & Gynecology, 113*, 1405–1413. doi:10.1097/AOG.0b013e3181ac0544
Bloom, A. A. (2016, April 15). Cholecystitis. *Medscape*. Retrieved from http://emedicine.medscape.com/article/171886-overview
Heuman, D. M. (2014, April 2). Cholelithiasis. *Medscape*. Retrieved from http://emedicine.medscape.com/article/175667-overview
Nettina, S. (2010). *The Lippincott manual of nursing practice* (9th ed.). Philadelphia, PA: Wolters Kluwer Lippincott Williams & Wilkins.
Schwarz, S. M. (2011, March 29). Pediatric cholecystitis. *Medscape*. Retrieved from http://emedicine.medscape.com/article927340-overview
University of Maryland Medical Center. (2013, June 27). *Gallstones and gallbladder disease*. Retrieved from http://umm.edu/health/medical/reports/articles/gallstones-and-gallbladder-disease
Zakko, S. F., & Afdhal, N. H. (2015, August 15). Acute cholecystitis: Pathogenesis, clinical features and diagnosis. *UpToDate*. Retrieved from http://www.uptodate.com/contents/acute-cholecystitis-pathogenesis-clinical-features-and-diagnosis

Colic

Cheryl A. Glass and Kristie A. D. Morydz

Definition
A. Colic is a benign disorder characterized by abdominal spasms and rigidity that results in abdominal pain. Infants with colic exhibit persistent, unexplained, and inconsolable crying lasting more than three hours a day, occurring more than three days in a week for three weeks in an otherwise healthy infant aged two weeks to four months. The infant

is in good health, eats well, and gains weight appropriately, despite the daily crying episodes. Colic is self-limited. No disease process found on examination.

Incidence/Prevalence
A. Between 8% and 30% of all infants exhibit colic, regardless of ethnicity, gender, gestational age, breast- versus bottlefed, or socioeconomic status.

Pathogenesis
A. Research has never conclusively identified a cause for colic, and many interventions are based on hypothesized causes, such as immature gastrointestinal (GI) function, milk allergy to casein or whey, and maternal anxiety. Exposure to cigarette smoke may be linked to colic. There has been a causal relationship between colic and family stress.

Predisposing Factors
A. Age: 2 weeks to 4 months; usually resolves by 6 months of age.
B. Male gender: Occurs more in males than females.
C. First in birth order.
D. Fruit juice intolerance (sorbitol-containing fruit juices).

Common Findings
Crying characteristics:
A. Intense crying: Louder, higher, and more variable in pitch.
B. The cry may sound like the baby is in pain or is screaming rather than crying.
C. Inconsolable.

Other Signs and Symptoms
A. Hands clenched.
B. Abdominal distension.
C. Legs flexed over abdomen.
D. Short sleep cycles.
E. Flatus.
F. Fussiness.
G. Red flags include distended abdomen, fever, and lethargy.

Subjective Data
A. Review when the crying occurs and how long it lasts. What techniques help?
B. Review basic infant needs with caregivers, such as determining whether the infant is hungry or wet, has air bubbles, or is in an uncomfortable position.
C. Review feeding methods, technique, and burping. Crying that occurs directly after feeding may be associated with swallowing too much air or gastro-oesophageal reflux.
D. If the infant is breastfed, review maternal diet for offending foods, including chocolate, pizza, spicy foods, cabbage, and so forth.
E. If the infant is breastfed, review prescribed maternal drugs and any over-the-counter (OTC) medications that she is taking, such as laxatives.
F. If the infant is bottlefed, review preparation of formula and type of formula.
G. Review intake of fruit juices for possible carbohydrate intolerance to sorbitol.
H. Rule out the early introduction of solid foods.
I. Review any history of fever and high-pitched or shrill cry.
J. Have caregiver describe colour, frequency, and softness of stools.
K. Review secondhand smoke exposure: There is an association between maternal smoking and colic.
L. Have caregiver describe nature, colour, and frequency of any emesis.

Physical Examination
A. Check temperature, pulse, respirations, blood pressure (BP), and weight.
B. Plot growth parameters: Length, head circumference, and weight. **Note signs of failure to thrive (FTT). Failure to gain approximately one ounce per day may indicate FTT.**
C. Inspect:
   1. Evaluate the skin for signs of abuse.
   2. Check fontanelles.
   3. Conduct ear, nose, and throat examination.
   4. Evaluate the skin and mucosa for signs of dehydration.
D. Auscultate abdomen, heart, and lungs.
E. Percuss the abdomen.
F. Palpate:
   1. Palpate the abdomen for tenderness, masses, and distension.
   2. Feel anterior and posterior fontanelles.
   3. Perform testicular examination to evaluate torsion.

Diagnostic Tests
A. Colic is a diagnosis of exclusion and must be differentiated from identifiable causes of prolonged crying.
B. Laboratory tests and radiographic examination are not required if the infant is gaining weight and has a normal physical examination.
C. Consider urinalysis.
D. Check stool for occult blood to rule out cow's milk allergy.

Differential Diagnoses
A. Infection.
B. Obstruction.
C. Injury.
D. Abuse.
E. FTT.
F. Gastro-oesophageal reflux disease (GORD).
G. Intussusception.
H. Meningitis.
I. Otitis media.
J. Protein intolerance.
K. Testicular torsion.
L. Strangulated inguinal hernia.
M. Pyloric stenosis (depending on age at presentation).

Plan
A. Client teaching:
   1. Encourage parents and caregivers to keep a diary of crying and fussing spells for review.
   2. Review feeding and burping techniques, making sure the baby is not over- or underfed.
   3. Reassure the family that the baby has no evidence of infant developmental problems and the problem is not related to poor parenting skills.
   4. Reassure families that colic does resolve over time.
   5. Encourage parents to take time away from the infant to rest and recoup the energy needed to deal with the demands of a crying baby.
   6. Empathize with parental frustration and provide coping techniques.

Physical abuse of the infant with colic may occur when crying is prolonged and parents have inadequate resources to cope.

7. Consider a hypoallergenic diet (e.g., protein hydrolysate formula). The literature does not support the use of fiber-enriched formulas.
8. *Refer to Client Teaching Guide: Colic: Ways to Soothe a Fussy Baby.*
9. Teach caregivers to assess the child for signs of emergent abdominal problems such as fever, pallor, sweating, vomiting, diarrhoea, a rigid and tender abdomen.

B. Dietary management:
1. Dietary changes such as eliminating cow's milk proteins is indicated only in cases of suspected intolerance to protein (e.g., positive family history, eczema, onset after the first month, association with other GI symptoms such as vomiting or diarrhoea).
2. Use of soy-based formula is not recommended because many infants allergic to cow's milk protein may also develop an intolerance to soy protein.
3. For breastfeeding mothers, suggest a period of elimination of allergic foods (e.g., dairy, nuts, soy, and citrus) in order to evaluate the baby's response.
4. For formula-fed infants, consider hydrolyzed formula.
5. Educate caregivers to avoid the use of homegrown mint teas for fussy babies. Fatalities have been reported secondary to ingestion of the pennyroyal form of mint, which produces toxic oil.

C. Pharmacological therapy:
1. Simethicone has little therapeutic benefit versus a placebo for treating colic by randomized controlled trials.
2. Antispasmodics have adverse effects, including apnoea, seizures, and coma. Dicyclomine is contraindicated in infants younger than six months of age and is not considered for the indication of colic by the manufacturer.
3. Lactase is not a therapeutic option for colic.
4. For breastfed infants, consider *Lactobacillus reuteri*. Evidence does not support other forms of probiotics or prebiotics.
5. Sedatives should not be used for the treatment of colic.
6. Herbal remedies are common in many cultures, but few herbal products have been evaluated for colic.

Follow-Up
A. Reevaluate the child periodically to provide support and assess for other problems.
B. Review signs of emergent abdominal problems such as fever, pallor, sweating, vomiting, diarrhoea, and rigid and tender abdomen.

Consultation/Referral
A. Consider a home-based nursing consultation.
B. Refer the breastfeeding mother to a lactation specialist or breastfeeding clinic.

Bibliography
Barclay, L. (2010, December 2). American Academy of Pediatrics reviews use of probiotics, prebiotics. *Medscape.* Retrieved from http://www.medscape.com/viewarticle/733463

Deshpande, P. G. (2015, September 3). Colic. *Medscape.* Retrieved from http://emedicine.medscape.com/article/927760

Kheir, A. E. M. (2012). Infantile colic, facts and fiction. *Journal of Pediatrics, 38,* 34–37. doi:10.1186/1824-7288-38-34

Nettina, S. (2010). *The Lippincott manual of nursing practice* (9th ed.). Philadelphia, PA: Wolters Kluwer Lippincott Williams & Wilkins.

Turner, T. L., & Palamountain, S. (2009a, May 1). Clinical features and etiology of colic. *UpToDate.* Retrieved from http://www.uptodate.com/online/content/topic.do?topicKey=behavior/2155&view=print

Turner, T. L., & Palamountain, S. (2009b, May 1). Evaluation and management of colic. *UpToDate.* Retrieved from http://www.uptodate.com/online/content/topic.do?topicKey=behavior/4542&view=print

Colorectal Cancer Screening

Cheryl A. Glass and Kristie A. D. Morydz

Definition
Screening for colorectal cancer has increased early detection and the ability for early intervention of premalignant localized cancer. The Canadian Task Force on Preventative Health recommends:

Faecal occult blood test (FOBT) or faecal immunochemical test (FIT) testing every two years or flex sigmoidoscopy every 10 years for those ages 50 to 74. This does not include those at high risk.

Incidence/Prevalence
A. In Canada, colorectal cancer is the third leading cause of cancer-related death for women and second leading cause of death for men.
B. This disease affects both men and women with 1/13 and 1/16, respectively, being diagnosed.
C. Colorectal cancer is rare before age 40. Colorectal cancer is most frequently diagnosed among adults aged 65 to 74 years. You would consider screening in older clients if symptoms are present and life expectancy is >10 years.
D. 94% of the cases of colorectal cancer occur after 50 years of age.
E. 12.4% of colorectal cancer in men and 8.7% in women in Canada is associated with smoking.
F. Obesity is associated with colon cancer but not an increase in rectal cancer. Abdominal obesity is a stronger risk factor than truncal obesity or body mass index (BMI).

Pathogenesis
A. The usual pathogenesis is an adenomatous polyp that grows slowly, followed by dysplasia and, finally, cancerous cells.

Predisposing Factors
A. Age: 50 years and older.
B. Easter European Jewish and African Canadian descent.
C. Inflammatory bowel diseases (IBDs; Crohn's disease [CD], and ulcerative colitis [UC]).
D. Family history/genetic:
1. Familial adenomatous polyposis (FAP).
2. Nonpolyposis colorectal cancer (Lynch syndrome).
E. Smoking.
F. Obesity.
G. Diet high in red meat and fats.

Common Findings
A. Asymptomatic screening.

Subjective Data
A. Review the client's age and risk factors to discuss screening for colorectal cancer.

B. Review family history of colorectal cancer.
C. Review smoking history.
D. Review the client's diet evaluating red meat; processed meats; and lack of grains, fruits, and vegetables.
E. Review all medications currently being taken, including over-the-counter (OTC) medications and herbal products.

Physical Examination
A. Examinations are not required for discussion on colorectal screening testing.
B. A physical examination and vital signs should be taken as indicated for other presenting complaints.

Diagnostic Tests
A. Stool-based testing:
  1. Guaiac-based faecal occult blood test (gFOBT) or FIT every two years.
  or
  2. Flexible sigmoidoscopy every 10 years.
  There is a lack of evidence of the efficacy of colonoscopy compared with other screening tests. If clients do press for colonoscopy for screening, it should not be done any sooner than every 10 years. Clinical trials do not demonstrate a mortality benefit with the use of computed tomographic colonography, faecal DNA tests, barium enema, digital rectal exam, or serologic tests, and there are no recommendations made for these tests in the setting of general screening.

Differential Diagnosis
A. None related to screening.

Plan
A. Client teaching:
  1. Educate the client about modifying controllable risk factors with diet, exercise, and smoking cessation.
  2. Discuss the procedures and the preparation needed for each test.
B. Pharmacological therapy:
  1. Bowel prep depends on the test, client's age, and other comorbidities.

Follow-Up
A. Follow-up and consultations are determined by client's needs, severity, and whether complications are present.
B. Clients with classic FAP (>100 adenomas) should be advised to have genetic counselling.
C. Nonsteroidal anti-inflammatory drugs (NSAIDs) have been associated with a decrease in the risk of developing colorectal cancer. There is insufficient evidence to recommend the use of NSAIDs as a prevention strategy.
D. The United States Preventive Services Task Force (USP-STF) has made a recommendation on ASA use for primary prevention of cardiovascular disease and colorectal cancer in average-risk adults (www.uspreventiveservicestaskforce.org).

Consultation/Referral
A. Referral to a gastroenterologist and/or surgeon as indicated.

Individual Considerations
A. Geriatrics:
  1. The benefit of early detection of and intervention for colorectal cancer declines after age 75 years. Screening for adults aged 76 to 85 years should be made on an individual basis, taking into account the client's overall health and prior screening history.

Resources
Canadian Cancer Society: http://www.cancer.ca/en/cancer-information/cancer-type/colorectal/colorectal-cancer/?region=on
Canadian Task Force on Preventative Health Care: Colorectal cancer (2016): https://canadiantaskforce.ca/guidelines/published-guidelines/colorectal-cancer/
The Canadian Partnership against Cancer: https://www.cancerview.ca/preventionandscreening/colorectalcancerscreeningpage/
National Cancer Institutes at the National Institutes of Health Tests to Detect Colorectal Cancer and Polyps: www.cancer.gov/cancertopics/factsheet/detection/colorectal-screening

Bibliography
Canadian Task Force on Preventative Health Care. (2016). Recommendation on screening for colorectal cancer in primary care. *CMAJ*, *188*(5), 340–348. doi:10.1503/cmaj.151125
Centers for Disease Control and Prevention. (n.d.). *Screening tests at-a-glance*. Retrieved from https://www.cdc.gov/cancer/colorectal/pdf/SFL_inserts_screening.pdf
Medicare.gov. (n.d.). *Your medicare coverage, colorectal cancer screening*. Retrieved from www.medicare.gov/coverage/colorectal-cancer-screenings.html
Nettina, S. (2010). *The Lippincott manual of nursing practice* (9th ed.). Philadelphia, PA: Wolters Kluwer Lippincott Williams & Wilkins.
Qaseem, A., Denberg, T. D., Hopkins, R. H., Humphrey, L. L., Levine, J., Sweet, D. E., & Shekelle, P. (2012). Screening for colorectal cancer: A guidance statement from the American College of Physicians. *Annals of Internal Medicine*, *156*, 378–386. doi:10.7326/0003-4819-156-5-201203060-00010
Rex, D. K., Johnson, D. A., Adnerson, J. C., Schoenfeld, P. S., Burke, C. A., & Inadomi, J. M. (2009). American College of Gastroenterology guidelines for colorectal cancer screening 2008. *American Journal of Gastroenterology*. doi:10.1038/ajg.2009.104. Retrieved from www.amjgasro.com
Statistics Canada, Canadian Cancer Registry. (2017). *Canadian cancer statistics, CANSIM Table 103-0554*.
U.S. Preventive Services Task Force. (2016, June 21). Screening for colorectal cancer. U.S. Preventive Task Force recommendation statement. *Journal of the American Medical Association*, *315*, 2564–2575.

Constipation

Cheryl A. Glass, Audra C. Malone, and Kristie A. D. Morydz

Definition
Constipation is infrequent and difficult defecation of hard stools and a sensation of incomplete evacuation or straining. Constipation may also refer to a decrease in the volume or weight of stool and the need for enemas, suppositories, or laxatives to maintain bowel regularity. Constipation is a symptom, not a disease. The lower limit of normal stool frequency is three bowel movements (BMs) a week. The Rome Consensus criterion defines constipation as two or fewer stools weekly, lumpy/hard stools, straining, sensation of incomplete evacuation/obstruction or blockage, and/or the need for digital removal of stool.

Classification of constipation includes the following:
A. Normal-transit constipation (most common).
B. Functional constipation (slow transit).
C. Irritable bowel syndrome (IBS; constipation dominant).
D. Outlet obstruction (sudden onset).

Incidence/Prevalence
A. The incidence of constipation is unknown due to frequent self-treatment. Constipation is commonly self-reported. Constipation occurs in more than 50% of clients with colorectal cancers; it may be an early symptom of rectal cancer or a symptom of advanced disease in colon cancer.

TABLE 11.2 Drugs/Drug Classifications That Cause and Increase Constipation

• Analgesics	• Chemotherapy agents
• Anticholinergics (atropine, antidepressants, neuroleptics, antiparkinsonian drugs)	• Opiates
	• Antacids (aluminum hydroxide and calcium carbonate)
• Anticonvulsants	• Antispasmodics
• Antidiarrhoeal agents	• Iron supplements
• Antiemetics	• NSAIDs
• Antihistamines	• Cholestyramine (binds bile salts)
• Antihypertensives (calcium channel blockers, clonidine, hydralazine, MAOI, methyldopa)	• Ganglionic blockers, analgesics, antidiarrhoeals, antiemetics, antispasmotics, chemotherapy
• Antipsychotics	
• Diuretics	

MAOI, monoamine oxidase inhibitor; NSAIDs, nonsteroidal anti-inflammatory drugs.

Pathogenesis
A. Constipation can be caused by an alteration of the filling of the rectum by colonic transportation and/or reflex defecation of stool.
B. Lack of exercise decreases propulsion of bowel contents.
C. During pregnancy, progesterone has a relaxing effect on the muscles of the gastrointestinal (GI) tract and causes a decrease in peristalsis. The compression of the intestines by the enlarging uterus causes constipation during pregnancy.
D. Habitual use of laxatives is associated with impaired motor activity and has the potential of producing hypokalaemia.
E. Hypokalaemia can produce a generalized ileus and is most often seen in clients who take diuretics.
F. Psychiatric disease and psychosocial distress have important roles. The exact mechanisms by which emotional difficulties lead to constipation remain unclear, but their contribution is widely recognized.
G. Drugs (see Table 11.2).

Predisposing Factors
A. Insufficient nutrition:
  1. Low-fiber diet.
  2. Low fluid intake.
B. Neurologic causes:
  1. Spinal cord injury.
  2. Parkinson's disease.
  3. Multiple sclerosis.
  4. Aganglionosis (Hirschsprung's disease [HD]).
  5. Sacral nerve trauma/tumour.
C. Sedentary lifestyle.
D. Laxative misuse.
E. Travel.
F. Ignoring urge to defecate.
G. Drug use (individual medications and polypharmacy).
H. Pregnancy, especially third trimester.
I. Psychosocial problems:
  1. Depression.
  2. Sexual abuse.
  3. Unusual attitudes to food and bowel function.
J. Extremes of ages: infants and geriatrics.
K. Hypothyroidism.
L. Colorectal cancer.
M. IBS.
N. Pelvic floor disorders:
  1. Impaired function of the pelvic floor and/or external sphincter.
  2. Pelvic floor obstruction.
  3. Rectal prolapse.
  4. Enterocele and/or rectocele.
  5. Rectal intussusception.

Common Findings
A. Hard, infrequent stools.
B. Straining.
C. Inability to defecate when desired.
D. Need for digital manipulation to facilitate evacuation.

Other Signs and Symptoms
A. Hard, pebbly, rocklike stools.
B. Painful defecation.
C. Abdominal pain.
D. Weight loss.
E. Blood in stools.

Potential Complications
A. A rectal prolapse of the mucosa is pink and looks like a doughnut or rosette. Complete prolapse involving the muscular wall is larger and red, and it has circular folds.

Subjective Data
A. Review the onset, duration, and course of symptoms:
  1. Is constipation a chronic or acute problem?
  2. If there has been a change in bowel habits, was it gradual or sudden?
  3. What feature does the client rate most distressing?
B. Review bowel habits:
  1. Does the client have a regular time for defecation?
  2. Review size, colour, consistency, and frequency of stools. Has there been a change in the calibre of stools?
  3. Is there any blood?
  4. Are there any periods of diarrhoea?
  5. How often are laxatives being used, and at what doses?
  6. Are suppositories and enemas also required?
  7. Does the client have the urge to defecate?

8. Does the client have a sensation of incomplete evacuation?
9. Does the client need to digitally remove stool?
10. Does the client have faecal incontinence?

C. Review the client's daily diet and fluid intake. Has there been any dietary change?
D. Review the client's medication history: Prescription and over-the-counter (OTC; refer to Table 11.2).
E. Review the client's daily physical activity.
F. Review the client's psychosocial history of stress, depression, anxiety, and coping mechanisms.
G. Review the client's other health problems, such as diabetes, depression, hypothyroidism, and hypercalcaemia.
H. Review family history of constipation and colorectal cancer.
I. Review surgical history.

Physical Examination

A. Check pulse, respirations, blood pressure (BP), and weight. Check temperature if indicated.
B. Inspect:
1. General overall assessment of nutritional status.
2. Examine the skin, especially the rectum, for pallor and signs of dehydration and hypothyroidism.
3. Evaluate for the presence of hernias.
4. Inspect the anus, including the position, anal wink, prolapse, presence of excoriation, presence of perianal erythema, haemorrhoids, fissures, and skin tags.
5. Examine the lower back to rule out spinal lesions—hairy or hyperpigmented patches, gluteal fold asymmetry, cutaneous dimples, sinus tracts, and lipomas.

C. Auscultate all four abdominal quadrants for bowel sounds. Bowel sounds may be high pitched or absent.
D. Percuss the abdomen.
E. Palpate:
1. The abdomen for masses, tenderness, distension, and faecal mass.
2. The liver and spleen.

F. Digital rectal examination:
1. Examine the rectum for an anorectal mass, stricture, haemorrhoids, fissures, fistula, prolapse, inflammation, and anal warts.
2. Evaluate for impaction, hard stool in ampulla.
3. Perform an anal reflex test by a light pinprick or scratch.
4. Evaluate sphincter tone:
   a. Disordered innervation of the anus is indicated by finding that the anal canal opens wide when the puborectalis muscle is pulled posteriorly.
   b. Evaluate the resting tone of the sphincter and squeezing effort.
   c. Instruct the client to "expel the examination finger" to evaluate the force of expulsion.
   d. Have the client do a Valsalva maneuver to diagnose a rectocele, prolapse, pelvic floor descent, or puborectalis dysfunction.

G. Perform a neurologic examination for tone, strength, and reflexes to search for focal deficits and the delayed relaxation phase of the ankle jerks, suggestive of hypothyroidism.
H. Perform pelvic examination to evaluate a prolapse or rectocele. Evaluate when the client is at rest and with straining.
I. Perform mental state examination for signs of depression and somatization.

Diagnostic Tests

A. No tests are required for *common* constipation.
B. Tests to rule out differential diagnoses:
1. Complete blood count (CBC) with differential.
2. Thyroid studies.
3. Potassium and calcium: Clients taking diuretics should have serum potassium checked. Hypokalaemia may reduce bowel contractility and produce an ileus.
4. Urinalysis.
5. Serum glucose to rule out diabetes.
6. Barium enema (BE) to evaluate megacolon and redundant sigmoid colon.
7. Flexible sigmoid or colonoscopy is recommended if the client meets the guidelines for general screening or weight loss >10 pounds, anaemia, or blood in the stool.
8. Stool for occult blood.
9. Anorectal function tests:
   a. Manometry.
   b. Electromyography.

Differential Diagnoses

A. Intestinal obstruction: Acute onset of constipation requires ruling out an ileus, especially when accompanied by abdominal discomfort.
B. Hypothyroidism.
C. Psychosocial dysfunction.
D. Faecal impaction.
E. Neurologic disorders.
F. Multiple sclerosis.
G. Spinal cord injury.
H. Cancer.
I. Drug use.
J. Crohn's disease (CD): Constipation is often the presenting complaint in CD.
K. Diabetes (chronic dysmotility).

Plan

A. Client teaching:
1. *Refer to Client Teaching Guide: Constipation Relief.*
2. Encourage the client to exercise. Both exercise and dietary fiber stimulate the natural wavelike contraction of the colon that triggers the urge to defecate.
3. Reassure the client that recommended dietary changes and exercise help with constipation.
4. Warn chronic laxative users that it may take four to six weeks before spontaneous BMs return.
5. Teach the client about potential complications of long-term constipation.
6. Ask the client to keep a stool diary to bring to the next appointment.

B. Dietary management: See Appendix B, Diet Recommendations.
C. Surgical and medical management:
1. Treatment of constipation is symptomatic and should begin with lifestyle and dietary changes.
2. Evaluate and stop medications, if possible, that cause constipation.
3. Glycerin suppositories may be needed for rectal disimpaction in infants. Enemas are to be avoided.
4. Faecal impaction may require enemas or manual removal to relieve the situation. Enemas should not be given routinely to treat constipation because they disrupt

▶ Client Teaching Guides are available at https://connect.springerpub.com/content/reference-book/978-0-8261-9498-5

normal defecation reflexes and the client becomes dependent. Disimpaction by enema treatments includes three enemas per day:
  a. The first enema of the day includes the use of a phosphate-based enema plus saline solution.
  b. The second and third enema of the day includes only the saline solution and no phosphate-based enema.
  c. **Clients should never receive more than one phosphate enema per day because of the risk of phosphate intoxication, hypoglycaemia, and hyponatraemia.**
  d. **Soap suds, tap water, and magnesium enemas in children are not recommended because of potential toxicity.**
  5. Pelvic floor physiotherapy may be offered.
  6. Biofeedback has been effective for short-term treatment of intractable constipation.
  7. Manual removal of faecal impaction can stimulate the vagus nerve and cause syncope and tachycardia. It is contraindicated in the following conditions:
  a. Pregnancy.
  b. After genitourinary, rectal, perineal, abdominal, or gynaecologic surgery.
  c. Myocardial infarction, coronary insufficiency, pulmonary embolus, congestive heart failure (CHF), or heart block.
  d. GI or vaginal bleeding.
  e. Blood dyscrasias or bleeding disorders.
  f. Haemorrhoids, fissures, and rectal polyps.
D. Pharmacological therapy:
  1. Bulk-forming agents decrease abdominal pain and improve stool consistency. They should be used if an increase in dietary fiber does not work. They act by causing retention of fluid and increasing faecal mass. They must be taken with plenty of fluids to prevent formation of an obstructing bolus. Flatulence and abdominal distension may occur, but long-term use is safe.
  2. Stimulant laxatives act by directly stimulating the colonic nerves. Suppositories are faster (20–60 minutes) versus oral laxatives (8–12 hours).
  3. Osmotic laxatives act by retaining fluid in the bowel by osmosis, changing the water distribution in the faeces. Good hydration is important. (Table 11.3).
  4. Lubiprostone is approved for treatment of chronic idiopathic constipation in adults, opioid-induced constipation in adults with chronic noncancer pain, and IBS–constipation predominant in women 18 years or older.
  5. Methylnaltrexone bromide is currently approved for treatment of opioid-induced constipation in adult clients with chronic noncancer pain.
  6. When severe depression requires the use of antidepressants, the least constipating agent should be selected (i.e., one with minimal anticholinergic activity).
  7. Treat other identified causes, for example, hypothyroidism.

Follow-Up
A. Repeat assessment in four to six weeks. Ask the client to keep a stool diary and bring it for subsequent appointments.
B. If there is no evidence of obstruction, anaemia, or occult blood loss, follow the client expectantly for a few weeks on a conservative program that includes increased dietary fiber and increased exercise, and follow stool guaiac.
C. Failure to improve may indicate a serious underlying cause and need for referral.

TABLE 11.3 Laxatives

Bulk laxatives	Psyllium Polycarbophil Inulin
Lubricating agents	Mineral oil[a]
Stimulant laxatives	Docusate (would be considered softener) Bile acids Bisacodyl[b] Castor oil Senna[a] Aloes Rhubarb
Osmotic agents	Magnesium and phosphate salts Lactulose Sorbitol[a] Polyethylene glycol Glycerin suppositories[a]
Selective 5-HT$_4$ receptor agonists	Prucalopride
Activator	Lubiprostone

[a]Considered safe and effective in children.
[b]After a thorough evaluation, use in low doses for selected children when constipation is hard to manage.

Consultation/Referral
A. Consider consultations with a gastroenterologist (adult or paediatric), paediatrician, gynaecologist, surgeon, or psychologist/psychiatrist as indicated.

Individual Considerations
A. Pregnancy:
  1. Constipation is very common in pregnancy secondary to progesterone and the enlarging uterus (see section "Pathogenesis").
  2. Constipation that results from iron supplementation can be avoided by increasing the intake of fluid and high-fiber foods, and increasing physical activity such as walking.
  3. Bulking agents and lactulose will not enter breast milk. Senna, in large doses, will enter breast milk and may cause diarrhoea and colic in infants.
B. Paediatrics:
  1. In infancy and childhood, most constipation is functional. Constipation can be associated with coercive toilet training, sexual abuse, excessive parental interventions, and toilet phobia.
  2. An empty contracted anal canal in a constipated child may suggest HD:
  a. Bloody mucoid diarrhoea in an infant with a history of constipation could be an indication of enterocolitis complicating HD.
  b. If HD is suspected, the client should be evaluated by a paediatric gastroenterologist and a paediatric surgeon.
  3. Reinforce the idea that each infant has individual stool patterns. Formula-fed infants generally pass at least one stool each day, whereas breastfed infants may pass a stool after every feeding or, occasionally, only one every two to three days.
  4. Educate the parent that constipation really is dry, hard, and marblelike stools.

5. Infants may get red in the face and appear to be straining when having a BM, but it is normal behaviour and does not indicate constipation.
6. Rectal prolapse in children has been associated with cystic fibrosis (CF).
7. Use a high-fiber diet and fluids first before other therapies. Prune, pear, and apple juices may decrease constipation.
8. Common times when constipation is likely to occur in the paediatric population are the following:
   a. Upon introduction of solid foods or cow's milk:
      i. Recommended fiber intake is 20 g/d.
      ii. Minimum fluid intake depends on the child's age.
      iii. Consumption of cow's whole milk should be limited to 24 oz./d.
   b. During toilet training: A potty seat that provides appropriate foot support and leverage for elimination should be used.
   c. On school entry.

C. Adults:
1. The most common cause of chronic constipation in adults is failure to initiate defecation.
2. Diabetics should avoid stimulant laxatives, such as lactulose and sorbitol. Their metabolites may influence blood glucose levels.

D. Geriatrics:
1. Constipation in old people is not a result of aging; it is usually related to an increase in constipating factors such as chronic illnesses, immobility, dietary factors, medications, neurologic factors, and psychiatric conditions. **Acute onset of constipation is considered a red flag in the geriatric population.**
2. An important diagnostic concern in the elderly is the possibility of constipation due to a colonic neoplasm. More than 25% of clients with colorectal carcinomas present with constipation.
3. Check for a faecal impaction, especially in elderly clients with a history of chronic constipation. Faecal impaction ranks as one of the major sources of anorectal discomfort among the elderly and bedridden. Chronic, incomplete evacuation leads to formation of an obstructing bolus of desiccated hard stool in the rectum. Faecal incontinence may be a sign of faecal impaction.
4. Diarrhoea, rather than constipation, is sometimes the only complaint because of the collection of liquid stool distending the proximal colon and passing around the obstructing bolus.
5. Dietary fiber supplementation has been shown to allow discontinuation of laxatives in 59% to 80% of elderly clients with chronic idiopathic constipation.

Resource

The Rome Foundation: https://theromefoundation.org/
Update of Rome IV Criteria: https://www.ncbi.nlm.nih.gov/pmc/articles/PMC5378729/pdf/11894_2017_Article_554.pdf

Bibliography

American College of Gastroenterology. (2011). Pregnancy and gastrointestinal disorders. *Pregnancy monograph*. Retrieved from http://gi.org/wp-content/uploads/2011/07/institute-PregnancyMonograph.pdf
Basson, M. D. (2013, May 6). Constipation. *Medscape*. Retrieved from http://emedicine.medscape.com/article/184704
Chatoor, D., & Emmnauel, A. (2009). Constipation and evacuation disorders. *Best Practice & Research Clinical Gastroenterology*, 23, 517–530. doi:10.1016/j.bpg.2009.05.001
Dinning, P. G., & Di Lorenzo, C. (2011). Colonic dysmotility in constipation. *Best Practice & Research Clinical Gastroenterology*, 25, 89–101. doi:10.1016/j.bpg.2010.12.006
Greenberger, N. J. (2013, November). Constipation. *The Merck manual for health care professionals*. Retrieved from http://www.merckmanuals.com/professional/gastrointestinal_disorders/symptoms_of_gi_disorders/constipation.html
Levitt, M. A. (2011, August 11). Management of severe pediatric constipation. *Medscape*. Retrieved from http://emedicine.medscape.com/937030-overview
Levitt, M. A. (2015, August 28). Management of severe pediatric constipation. *Medscape*. Retrieved from http://emedicine.medscape.com/article/937030-overview
Mason, D., Tobias, N., Lutkenhoff, M., Stoops, M., & Ferguson, D. (2004). The APN's guide to pediatric constipation management. *Nurse Practitioner*, 29(7), 13–21. doi:10.1097/00006205-200407000-00003
Moses, S. (2014, May 17). *Chronic constipation*. Retrieved from http://www.fpnotebook.com/GI/Constipation/ChrncCnstptn.htm
Nettina, S. (2010). *The Lippincott manual of nursing practice* (9th ed.). Philadelphia, PA: Wolters Kluwer Lippincott Williams & Wilkins.
NHS Choices. (n.d.). *Constipation*. Retrieved from http://www.nhs.uk/Conditions/constipation/Pages/Introduction.aspx
North American Society for Pediatric Gastroenterology Hepatology and Nutrition. (2006). Clinical practice guideline. Evaluation and treatment of constipation in infants and children: Recommendations of the North American Society for Pediatric Gastroenterology, Hepatology and Nutrition. *Journal of Pediatric Gastroenterology and Nutrition*, 43, e1–e13. doi:10.1097/01.mpg.0000233159.97667.c3
Paquette, I. M., Varma, M., Ternent, C., Melton-Meaux, G., Rafferty, J. F., Feingold, D., & Steele, S. R. (2016). The American Society of Colon and Rectal Surgeons' clinical practice guidelines for the evaluation and management of constipation. *Diseases of the Colon & Rectum*, 59, 479–492. doi:10.1097/DCR.0000000000000599
Sharma, G. D. (2013, June 17). Cystic fibrosis. *Medscape*. Retrieved from http://emedicine.medscape.com/article/1001602-overview
Tack, J., Müller-Lissner, S., Stanghellini, V., Boeckxstaens, G., Kamm, M. A., Simren, M., & Fried, M. (2011). Diagnosis and treatment of chronic constipation—A European perspective. *Neurogastroenterology and Motility*, 23, 697–710. doi:10.1111/j.1365-2982.2011.01709.x
Vargas, H. D. (n.d.). *Constipation expanded version*. Retrieved from https://www.fascrs.org/patients/disease-condition/constipation-expanded-version

Crohn's Disease

Cheryl A. Glass, Audra C. Malone, and Kristie A. D. Morydz

Definition

A. Crohn's disease (CD) is a chronic inflammatory bowel disease (IBD) of the gastrointestinal (GI) tract that produces ulceration, fibrosis, and malabsorption. CD can involve any segment of the GI tract from the mouth to the anus; the terminal ileum and colon are the most common sites. Paediatric clients are more likely to present with the disease limited to the small intestine.
1. In 2003, CD was subclassified based on age, location (ileal, colonic, ileocolonic, or upper GI), and clinical presentation (nonstricturing/nonpenetrating to penetrating) using the Montreal classification.
2. Elderly clients with IBD can be subdivided into two groups:
   a. Elderly clients with onset of IBD at a late age (late-onset IBD).
   b. Elderly clients with long-standing IBD; first diagnosed as having IBD at a younger age (long-standing IBD).

B. The disease is chronic, relapsing, and incurable. CD is characterized by episodes of remission and exacerbation. The most frequent cause of death in persons with IBD is the primary disease, followed by malignancy and thromboembolic disease. In most cases, symptoms do correspond well with the degree of inflammation present. The diagnosis is usually established with endoscopic finding in a client with a compatible clinical history. Objective evidence for disease activity should be sought before administering medication with significant adverse effects.

C. More than 70% of clients with CD undergo surgery within 20 years of the diagnosis. Indications for surgery include stricture, intractable or fulminant disease, anorectal disease, and intra-abdominal abscess. Approximately 30% of clients who have surgery for CD have a recurrence within three years, and up to 60% will have a recurrence within 10 years.
D. The lifetime risk of fistulae development is 20% to 40%.
E. The incidence of small bowel and colorectal adenocarcinoma in CD is higher than in the general population. Lymphoma is also increased, especially for clients with IBD treated with azathioprine (AZA; 6-mercaptopurine [6-MP]).

Incidence/Prevalence
A. IBS affects 13% to 20% of Canadians.
B. The peak incidence of CD is most common in late adolescence to the third decade of life: Children younger than five years and elderly persons aged 70 to 80 years. CD may involve the entire GI tract; note the incidence according to the location:
  1. About 80% have small-bowel involvement, usually in the distal ileum. In severe cases of ileitis, complications may include fistulas or an abscess in the right lower quadrant (RLQ) of the abdomen.
  2. About 50% have ileocolitis (involving both the ileum and colon). This type is associated with significant weight loss.
  3. About 20% have disease limited to the colon, with roughly one-half having sparing of the rectum.
  4. A small percentage has predominant involvement of the mouth (aphthous ulcers) or gastroduodenal area; fewer have involvement of the oesophagus (odynophagia and dysphagia) and proximal small bowel.
  5. One-third have perianal disease (perianal pain, drainage from large skin tags, anal fissures, perirectal abscesses, and anorectal fistulae).
  6. 15% to 20% have arthralgias. Arthritis is the most common complication.

Pathogenesis
Pathogenesis is unknown. The common end pathway is inflammation of the mucosal lining of the intestinal tract, causing ulceration, oedema, bleeding, and fluid and electrolyte loss. Speculation for the pathogenesis includes the following:
A. Pathogenic organism (remains unidentified).
B. Immunologic response.
C. Autoimmune process.
D. Potential genes linked to IBD:
  1. Chromosome 16 (*IBD1* gene).
  2. *CARD15* gene, which is noted to be a susceptibility gene for CD.
  3. Susceptibility genes on chromosomes 5 (5q31) and 6 (6p21 and 19p).

Predisposing Factors
A. Age between 15 and 35 years.
B. Genetic predisposition/family history of CD:
  1. First-degree relatives five- to 20-fold increased risk.
  2. Children of a parent with IBD have 5% risk.
  3. About 70% incidence in identical twins versus 5% to 10% in nonidentical twins.
  4. Jewish populations.
C. Smoking (increased risk for CD, but reduces risk in ulcerative colitis [UC]).

Common Findings
The following cardinal symptoms occur in about 80% of clients:
A. Chronic or nocturnal diarrhoea.
B. Abdominal pain, the classic location being in the RLQ (appendicitis like).
C. Fatigue, commonly related to pain, inflammation, and anaemia.

Other Signs and Symptoms
Symptoms vary, depending on the location of the intestinal tract and extent of disease:
A. Constipation: Early sign.
B. Weight loss.
C. Abdominal mass.
D. Cramping with bowel movement (BM).
E. Urgent need to move bowels.
F. Rectal bleeding or blood in stools.
G. Perianal discomfort or soft or semiliquid irritating rectal discharge.
H. Vomiting.
I. Low-grade fever.
J. Folate deficiency.
K. Anorexia.
L. Fissures and fistulas, abscesses sometimes extending to skin.
M. Weight loss, diarrhoea, and growth restriction may be presenting signs in children.
N. Extraintestinal symptoms:
  1. Erythema nodosum (correlates well with the activity of disease).
  2. Inflammation of the eyes.
  3. Inflammation of the skin.
O. Paediatric:
  1. Failure to grow.
  2. Delayed development of secondary sex characteristics.
P. Loss of normal menstrual cycle.

Subjective Data
A. Ask about the onset, duration, and course of symptoms. Have any of the presenting symptoms occurred at any time in the past (flares of CD may have gone undiagnosed in the past)?
B. Review the client's history and extent of diarrhoea, including frequency, consistency, colour, quantity, and odour of stools. Evaluate if there is blood, mucus, pus, or food particles in the stools.
C. Inquire about recent travel to foreign countries.
D. Ask the client if diarrhoea represents a change in bowel habits. Is there nocturnal diarrhoea?
E. Ask the client what makes the diarrhoea worse or better.
F. Inquire about previous GI surgery.
G. Review the client's usual weight and any history of weight loss. If weight loss has occurred, how many pounds? How is client's appetite?
H. Review family history of CD, colon cancer, UC, and malabsorption syndrome.
I. How has the duration of current complaints affected the client's work or usual social activities?
J. Review for duration and extraintestinal symptoms, including the following:
  1. Urinary complications: Renal calculi.
  2. Sclerosing cholangitis: Fatigue and jaundice.

3. Skin diseases:
     a. Erythema nodosum: Painful, tender, raised, purple lesion on the tibia.
     b. Pyoderma gangrenosum: Inflamed patch of skin that has progressed to ulceration.
     c. Herpetic lesions related to immune suppression.
  4. Arthritic symptoms.
  5. Ocular inflammation.
  6. Hypercoagulabilty.
K. Review medications, especially antibiotics and nonsteroidal anti-inflammatory drugs (NSAIDs).
L. Review the client's current tobacco/cigarette use.

Physical Examination
A. Check temperature, pulse, respirations, blood pressure (BP), and weight. Paediatrics: Plot height/weight on growth curves to follow growth failure.
B. Inspect:
  1. Observe general appearance, noting pallor, wasting, apathetic appearance, ecchymosis, skin ulcerations, jaundice, and signs of Kaposi's sarcoma.
  2. Inspect the head and neck for aphthous ulcers, glossitis, stomatitis, and poor dentition.
  3. Inspect the abdomen for surgical scars.
  4. Order eye examination for uveitis.
  5. Inspect joints for warmth and redness.
C. Auscultate the abdomen in all quadrants for altered bowel sounds (obstruction).
D. Palpate:
  1. Palpate the neck for goiter and lymphadenopathy.
  2. Palpate the abdomen for distension, ascites, tenderness rebound, guarding, and masses.
  3. Palpate for hepatomegaly in RLQ.
  4. Palpate the joints for tenderness.
E. Rectal examination:
  1. Check anal sphincter for tags, control, and discharge.
  2. Palpate for masses, fissures, fistulas, tags, and inflammation.
  3. Perform digital rectal examination to assess for anal strictures and rectal mass.
F. Neurologic examination: Assess for signs of vitamin B12 deficiency including tingling sensation and numbness in the hands or feet.

Diagnostic Tests
A. Laboratory tests:
  1. Complete blood count (CBC) with differential.
  2. Electrolytes and albumin.
  3. Erythrocyte sedimentation rate (ESR).
  4. Serum cobalamin (vitamin B12).
  5. Serum iron studies.
  6. Folate.
  7. Liver enzymes and functioning tests (international normalized ratio [INR]) and bilirubin.
  8. HIV.
  9. Celiac antibody testing should be considered..
  10. Thiopurine methyltransferase (TPMT) activity should be assessed before AZA or MP.
B. Stool studies:
  1. Guaiac.
  2. Stool culture.
  3. *Clostridium difficile* toxin assay.
  4. Ova and parasites.
C. Imaging:
  1. Abdominal flat plate.
  2. Barium enema (BE):
     a. Classic "string sign": Narrow band of barium flowing through an inflamed or scarred area in terminal ileum; differentiates CD from UC.
     b. "Rectal sparing": Suggests CD in the presence of inflammatory changes in other parts of the colon.
     c. "Thumbprinting": Indicates mucosal inflammation (may be seen on flat plate of abdomen).
     d. "Skip lesions": Areas of inflammation with normal-appearing areas.
  3. Small-bowel follow-through GI series.
  4. Fistulogram: Used to guide the surgical correction.
  5. CT scan of the abdomen and pelvis (limited use in IBD but may detect fistulae).
D. Procedures with/without biopsy.
  1. Colonoscopy: Mucosa has a characteristic cobblestone appearance.
  2. Flexible sigmoidoscopy with biopsy: Reveals "skip areas" in colon, significant small-bowel involvement, fistulas, and granulomas.
  3. Upper endoscopy: Aphthous ulcerations occur in the stomach and duodenum in 5% to 10%.
  4. Capsule enteroscopy: The major risk is the potential for the camera to become lodged at the point of stricture and require operative intervention.
  5. Skin biopsy.
E. Tuberculin purified protein derivative (PPD) skin test.

Differential Diagnoses
A. UC.
B. Other forms of colitis (ischaemic, medication induced).
C. Appendicitis.
D. Colon cancer.
E. Irritable bowel syndrome (IBS).
F. Anorexia nervosa.
G. Perianal abscess.
H. Intestinal protozoan and bacterial aetiologies.
I. Food poisoning.
J. Cytomegalovirus (CMV).
K. Intestinal tuberculosis (TB).

Plan
A. **CD should be managed jointly with a gastroenterologist, colorectal surgeon, and specialists such as a rheumatologist and a nutritionist.**
B. Client teaching: *Refer to Client Teaching Guide: Crohn's Disease.*
C. Dietary management:
  1. Adequate nutrition is critical to promote healing. Sufficient protein and calories limit the stress on an inflamed and often strictured bowel.
  2. Clients with cramps and diarrhoea should alter the fiber content of their diets. Diet should include high fiber, low fat (see Appendix B, Diet Recommendations).
  3. Those with steatorrhoea benefit from decrease in fat intake to <80 g/d. Give the client a copy of the low-fat/low-cholesterol diet (see Appendix B, Diet Recommendations).
  4. An empiric trial of restricting milk products may terminate diarrhoea due to lactase deficiency.
  5. Clients with severe diarrhoea may require partial bowel rest, which removes the stimulus that food has on bowel motility and secretion.

6. Elemental diet preparations have been found to induce remission, improve symptoms, and decrease disease activity in clients with acute disease.

7. Total parenteral nutrition (TPN) is used when the client's oral intake is not adequate or when surgery is indicated.

8. Pretreatment screening for TB, using Mantoux (a PPD) skin testing, is needed prior to initiation of immunomodulators and thiopurines.

9. Immunization status:
   a. Immunizations with inactivated vaccines should be brought up-to-date and rigorously maintained during treatment, including influenza, meningococcus, and pneumococcus.
   b. Check varicella titres prior to treatment with immunomodulators and reimmunize if titres are low.
   c. The risk of administering live vaccines (polio, rubella, and yellow fever) to clients on immunomodulators has not been established; however, most experts avoid live vaccines during treatment.

D. Medical and surgical management:
   1. Consider hospitalization for fulminate disease, cachexia, fever, vomiting, and evidence of obstruction and/or abscess:
   a. Surgery does not cure the client and is reserved for intractable disease, perforation, obstruction, or severe bleeding.
   b. The objective of surgery is to remove grossly involved bowel and to spare as much normal-appearing bowel as possible.
   c. Postoperative recurrence rates are estimated at 30% to 50% per decade and are inversely related to preoperative disease duration.

E. Pharmacological therapy: The medical management of CD can be divided into treatment of an acute exacerbation and maintenance of remission. In acute exacerbation, triggers, such as underlying infection, fistula, perforation, and other pathology, must be ruled out prior to the intravenous (IV) administration of glucocorticoids. The goal of chronic therapy is the remission of bowel inflammation. Therapies include the following:

   1. Vitamin, mineral, and folic acid supplements are necessary for proper healing and avoidance of secondary complications, such as bone disease and anaemia:
   a. Client should take a multiple vitamin supplement containing about five times the normal daily vitamin requirements.
   b. Folic acid supplementation is required for clients on sulphasalazine because it impairs folic acid absorption.
   c. Vitamin B12 replacement is required for clients who have ileal surgery.
   d. Vitamin D, 4,000 international units (IU) is required for clients with steatorrhoea.

   2. Opiates provide symptomatic relief of diarrhoea during acute phases of illness and chronic active colitis. Diphenoxylate and atropine, codeine, tincture of opium, and loperamide all limit the number of BMs. Tincture of belladonna and other anticholinergics help control cramping.

   3. Stepwise medication approach (see Table 11.4 for adult dosing):
   a. 5-Aminosalicylates (5-ASA) are a mainstay of therapy because of their anti-inflammatory activities and rapid absorption throughout the small intestines. Several formulations are available for targeting a specific region of the bowel. The 5-ASA drugs are not specifically approved by the Food and Drug Administration (FDA) for use in CD.
      i. Sulphasalazine is primarily released in the colon:
         1) Reduced absorption of folic acid and digoxin have been reported when administered with sulphasalazine.
      ii. Mesalamine can be released in the duodenum to the distal colon.
      iii. Mesalazine is targeted for release in the distal ileum and colon.
      iv. Multi-Matrix System (MMX) releases mesalamine in the colon. *Not recommended for children younger than 18 years.*
      v. Mesalamine is specific for the rectum and distal colon.
   b. Corticosteroids are used if IBD fails to respond to 5-ASA. Corticosteroids should be tapered as rapidly as possible and do not have a role in maintaining remission:
      i. Budesonide is designed to be effective only in the treatment of disease involving the ileum and ascending colon. Budesonide is effective in the maintenance of short-term (three months) but not long-term (one year) remission.
      ii. Prednisone or prednisolone:
         1) Paediatrics: Prednisone or prednisolone brings rapid improvement but should serve as a short-term induction therapy due to long-term side effects, including growth failure, osteopaenia, hirsutism, diabetes, psychosis, cataracts, and altered body shape and image. As soon as the acute disease subsides, taper steroid for two weeks to minimum necessary to control symptoms.
   c. Immunomodulatory agents may be initiated for IBD refractory to corticosteroids or frequent flares that require steroids. These agents require monitoring of blood counts due to haematologic toxicity. A 3% incidence of pancreatitis, allergic reactions, infections, and marrow toxicity is associated with their use. The main drawback to the use of AZA and 6-MP is their slow onset. The effect of therapy is noted after three to six months of treatment. The FDA recommends that individuals should have TPMT genotype or phenotype assessment before initiation of therapy with AZA or 6-MP to detect individuals who have low-enzyme activity or who are homozygous deficient in TPMT:
      i. 6-MP:
         1) Clients with inherited little or no TPMT activity are at increased risk for severe Purinethol toxicity and generally require substantial dose reduction.
      ii. AZA:
         1) Monitoring includes CBC, including platelet counts weekly during the first month, twice monthly for the second and third months of therapy, then monthly or more frequently if dosage alteration is necessary.
         2) TPMT testing: Testing is recommended for consideration to either genotype or phenotype clients for TPMT.
         3) Doses for adults and paediatrics must be lowered for reduced TPMT activity.

TABLE 11.4 Medications for Crohn's Disease and Ulcerative Colitis

\multicolumn{2}{l}{**5-ASA anti-inflammatory activities and rapid absorption throughout the GI tract.**}
Sulphasalazine	Treatment of mild to moderate UC and as adjunctive therapy in severe UC. Converted to mesalamine in the colon
Olsalazine	Release is delayed in the colon. Converted to mesalamine in the colon
Mesalazine	Targeted for release in the distal ileum and colon
Mesalamine	Mild to moderate disease. Released in the duodenum to the distal colon
Mesalamine suppository	Specific to the rectum and distal colon
Mesalamine retention enema	Specific to the rectum and distal colon
Corticosteroids nonspecifically suppress the immune system. They are the mainstay of treatment for active flares.	
Budesonide	Treatment of mild to moderate CD involving the ileum and/or ascending colon; released in the distal small intestine and right colon **Rectal 5-ASA is the first-line therapy in distal UC**
Prednisone (most common oral steroid used) Methylprednisolone (IV)	Used in acute treatment but is not preventative IV steroids are used in clients in severe disease who require hospitalization
Hydrocortisone enemas	Colonic disease—proctitis requiring topical/rectal formulations
Hydrocortisone acetate foam and steroid suppositories Betamethasone enema	
Immunomodulatory agents: Thiopurines—The 2013 AGA recommends against using thiopurine monotherapy to induce remission with clients with moderately severe CD. Because of the delay in the onset of action of 6-thiopurines, concomitant therapy with systemic corticosteroids or an anti-TNF-alpha drug is required for rapid system relief with moderately severe CD. AGA suggests against using MTX to induce remission in clients with moderately severe CD. AGA suggests using MTX over no immunomodulator therapy to maintain corticosteroid-induced remission in clients with CD.	
6-Mercaptopurine	Slow onset—The onset of therapy is noted after three to six months
Azathioprine	Converts to its active form 6-MP. Slow acting, can take up to three months to work
MTX folic acid antagonist	Improvement generally in three to six weeks; full benefit may not be seen for 12 weeks
Biologics—TNF-alpha blocker. The AGA recommends using anti-TNF-alpha monotherapy to induce remission in clients with moderately severe CD. The AGA recommends using anti-TNF-alpha with thiopurines over thiopurines monotherapy to induce remission in clients with moderately severe CD. The AGA recommends using anti-TNF-alpha over no anti-TNF-alpha to maintain corticosteroid or anti-TNF-alpha-induced remission in clients with CD.	
Infliximab IV infusion	Moderate to severe CD with fistulizing CD or resistance to steroids and conventional therapy
Infliximab-dyyb	Approved for adult and paediatric clients with moderate to severe Crohn's disease
Certolizumab pegol Subcutaneous (subq) in the abdomen or thigh	Moderate to severe CD resistance to steroids and conventional therapy
Adalimumab Subcutaneous in the abdomen or thigh	Moderate to severe CD resistance to steroids and conventional therapy
Golimumab	Moderate to severe UC resistance to steroids and conventional therapy
Vedolizumab Ustekinumab	Moderate to severe CD and UC resistance to steroids and conventional therapy; moderate to severe CD
Antiadhesion molecule	
Natalizumab	Moderate to severe CD for adults who failed anti-TNF therapy
Antibiotics—Used for treatment of bacterial infections that cause abscesses and can be helpful with treatment of fistulas	
Ciprofloxacin	
Metronidazole	

AGA, American Gastroenterology Association; CD, Crohn's disease; 5-ASA, 5-aminosalicylates; GI, gastrointestinal; IV, intravenous; MTX, methotrexate; TNF, tumour necrosis factor; UC, ulcerative colitis.

[a]Natalizumab users carry an increased risk of a severe brain condition called progressive multifocal leukoencephalopathy (PML), resulting from infection with the John Cunningham (JC) virus. It is important to be tested for JC virus prior to starting natalizumab; clients who are negative for JC virus have a much lower risk of developing PML.

Source: Adapted from the American College of Gastroenterology Guidelines (2013). Retrieved from gastro.org/guidelines.

iii. Methotrexate ([MTX] folic acid antagonist) has adverse effects, including leukopaenia, GI upset, and hypersensitivity pneumonitis:
    1) Subcutaneous dosing for children is recommended to ensure absorption until the client enters remission; then switch to oral MTX.
    2) Folic acid supplement may reduce the likelihood of oral ulcers.
d. Tumour necrosis factor (TNF)-alpha blocker:
  i. Infliximab is a chimeric monoclonal antibody to TNF-alpha. Infliximab is effective for moderate to severe CD and for clients with fistulizing CD or who are resistant to steroids and conventional therapy. Infliximab can close perianal fistulas refractory to therapy with antibiotics and 6-MP. Infliximab has a half-life of approximately 10 days:
    1) Paediatrics: Recommended for people ages six to 17 years with severe active CD whose disease has not responded to conventional therapy including corticosteroids, immunomodulators, and conventional therapy.
  ii. Certolizumab is given subcutaneously in the abdomen or thigh:
    1) *Paediatrics: Not recommended.*
  iii. Adalimumab is an antibody directed against TNF. It is also administered subcutaneously in the abdomen or thigh:
    1) *Paediatrics: Not recommended for those younger than 18 years.*
e. Natalizumab, a monoclonal antibody, is an effective induction agent for CD in adults. It is given in a certified TYSABRI Outreach: Unified Commitment to Health (TOUCH) centre. IV infusion is given over one hour and requires a one-hour observation period post infusion.
f. *Paediatrics: Not recommended for those younger than 18 years.*
g. Antibiotics are utilized in adults for perianal disease or inflammatory mass. Paediatric doses have not been established in either metronidazole or ciprofloxacin for CD.

Follow-Up

A. Have the client record his or her weight daily to monitor changes.
B. Assess frequency and consistency of stools to evaluate volume losses and effectiveness of therapy.
C. Instruct clients on self-medication to call the health provider's office if fever develops, diarrhoea worsens, bleeding occurs, or abdominal pain becomes marked.
D. Monitoring clients on 5-ASA should include a CBC at least twice a year and urinalysis at least annually.
E. Monitoring clients on 6-MP requires frequent monitoring, including CBC and aminotransferase levels (alanine transaminase [ALT] and aspartate transaminase [AST]) before treatment, and again at two, three, eight and 12 weeks after initiating therapy. When stable, monitor every three months thereafter, and two to three weeks after a change in dosage.
F. Monitoring clients on MTX includes a CBC and aminotransferases as with 6-MP/thiopurine therapies.
G. Periodic bone mineral density assessment is recommended for clients on long-term corticosteroid therapy (longer than three months). Osteopaenia should be treated aggressively. The primary intervention includes dietary counselling and supplementation to ensure adequate intake of vitamin D and calcium.
H. Annual ophthalmologic examinations are recommended for clients on long-term corticosteroids.
I. Clients who are using corticosteroids should be monitored for glucose intolerance and other metabolic abnormalities.

Consultation/Referral

A. Refer the client to a gastroenterologist initially for evaluation. Treatment requires multidisciplinary management with the gastroenterologist and other subspecialists, including a nutritionist, surgeon, rheumatologist, ophthalmologist, and social workers.
B. Promptly hospitalize for parenteral management clients who are toxic, bleeding heavily, in severe pain, or too sick to obtain adequate nutrition orally.
C. Consider a referral for genetic testing.

Individual Considerations

A. Pregnancy:
  1. Active disease at the time of conception is associated with increased incidence of miscarriage and postpartum exacerbation. It may also predispose the client to other maternal and prenatal risks such as premature labour, small-for-gestational-age babies, and stillbirth.
  2. Oral and topical mesalamine, oral balsalazide, sulphasalazine, corticosteroids, and ciprofloxacin (after the first trimester) are safe and effective during nursing or pregnancy.
  3. Women on prednisone should receive supplementary steroids during labour and delivery as well as during other highly stressful times.
  4. Counsel women to attempt pregnancy only when the disease has been quiescent for several months.
  5. Withholding sulphasalazine for two to three days before delivery may be advisable to minimize neonatal jaundice due to bilirubin displacement.
  6. MTX is a FDA category X drug.
B. Paediatrics:
  1. Approximately 30% of children with CD are refractory to or dependent on steroids despite concomitant use of 6-MP. These clients may require conversion from thiopurine to MTX maintenance therapy, or treatment with a biologic agent.
  2. Sulphasalazine and olsalazine can be compounded into a suspension for young children to drink. It is recommended that other 5-ASA be swallowed whole; however, mesalazine may be opened and administered by sprinkling the granules on soft food.
  3. Psychological counselling may be required in children secondary to the chronic relapsing nature of the illness and effects on body appearance and image, such as short stature and pubertal delay.
  4. Children with CD should undergo colonoscopy for cancer screening beginning eight to 10 years after the diagnosis of CD. The frequency of screening should be determined by the findings on the initial colonoscopy (around every one to three years).
  5. The National Institute for Health and Clinical Excellence (NICE) clinical guideline recommendations include consideration of monitoring for changes in bone mineral density in children and young people with risk factors, such as low body mass index (BMI), low-trauma fracture, or continued or repeated glucocorticosteroid use.

C. Geriatrics:
   1. **Unexplained diarrhoea, weight loss, and perianal disease in the elderly should arouse suspicions regarding CD. Elderly clients have worse outcomes because of delayed presentation and comorbid conditions.**
   2. Elderly clients tend to have CD confined to the distal colon, with only 40% having proctitis.
   3. With an increase in cancers in elderly clients with CD, it is imperative to evaluate and exclude cancer before beginning immunosuppressant or biologic therapies.
   4. Review CD therapies, with comorbid conditions in mind, due to side effects, interactions, need for increased laboratory monitoring (e.g., INR, as well as digoxin levels and phenytoin levels), and risk of infection.
   5. Anti-TNF-alpha agents are contraindicated in clients with New York Heart Association (NYHA) class III and IV heart failure (HF).

Resource
Crohn's and Colitis Foundation of Canada: http://crohnsandcolitis.ca/

Bibliography
American College of Gastroenterology Guidelines (2013). Retrieved from gastro.org/guidelines

Beth Israel Deaconess Medical Center. (2013). *What are the treatments for Crohn's disease?* Retrieved from http://www.bidmc.org/CentersandDepartments/Departments/DigestiveDiseaseCenter/InflammatoryBowelDiseaseProgram/CrohnsDisease/WhatarethetreatmentsforCrohnsdisease.aspx

Bousvaros, A., & Leichtner, A. (2012, September 17). Overview of the management of Crohn's disease in children and adolescents. *UpToDate*. Retrieved from http://www.uptodate.com/contents/overview-of-the-management-of-crohns-disease-in-children-and-adolescents

Crohn's and Colitis Foundation of America. (2014, February 6). *Biologic therapies*. Retrieved from http://www.ccfa.org/resources/biologic-therapies.html

Crohn's and Colitis Foundation of America. (n.d.-a). *Crohn's disease medication options*. Retrieved from http://www.ccfa.org/what-are-crohns-and-colitis/what-is-crohns-disease/crohns-medication.html

Crohn's and Colitis Foundation of America. (n.d.-b). *Crohn's treatment options*. Retrieved from http://www.ccfa.org/what-are-crohns-and-colitis/what-is-crohns-disease/crohns-treatment-options.html

Crohn's and Colitis Foundation of America. (n.d.-c). *Types of Crohn's disease and associated symptoms*. Retrieved from http://www.ccfa.org/what-are-crohns-and-colitis/what-is-crohns-disease/types-of-crohns-disease.html

Global, R. P. H. (2016, March 10). *TNF inhibitors—Biological response modifiers (BRMs)*. Retrieved from http://www.globalrph.com/TNFinhibitors.htm

Hvas, A. M., & Nexo, E. (2006). Diagnosis and treatment of vitamin B12 deficiency. An update. *Haematologica/The Hematology Journal, 91*, 1506–1512.

Lichtenstein, G. R., Hanauer, S. B., Sandborn, W. J., & The Practice Parameters Committee of the American College of Gastroenterology. (2009). Management of Crohn's disease in adults. *American Journal of Gastroenterology, 104*(2) 465–483. doi:10.1038/ajg.2008.168. Retrieved from http://s3.gi.org/physicians/guidelines/CrohnsDiseaseinAdults2009.pdf

National Institute for Health and Clinical Excellence. (2012, October). Crohn's disease, management in adults, children, and young people. *NICE Clinical Guideline, 152*. Retrieved from http://guidance.nice.org.uk/cg152

Nettina, S. (2010). *The Lippincott manual of nursing practice* (9th ed.). Philadelphia, PA: Wolters Kluwer Lippincott Williams & Wilkins.

Rao, S. S. C., & Meduri, K. (2011). What is necessary to diagnose constipation? *Best Practice & Research Clinical Gastroenterology, 25*, 127–140. doi:10.1016/j.bpg.2010.11.001

Surawicz, C. M., Brandt, L. J., Binion, D. G., Ananthakrishnan, A. N., Curry, S. R., Gilligan, P. H., & Zuckerbraun, B. S. (2013). Guidelines for diagnosis, treatment, and prevention of *Clostridium difficile* infections. *American Journal of Gastroenterology, 108*, 478–498. doi:10.1038/ajg.2013.4

Terdiman, J. P., Gruss, C. B., Heidelbaugh, J. J., Sultan, S., & Falck-Ytter, V. T. (2013). American Gastroenterological Association Institiute Guideline on the use of thiopurines, methotrexate, and anti-TNF-α biologic drugs for the induction and maintenance of remission in inflammatory Crohn's disease. *Gastroenterology, 145*, 459–1463. doi:10.1053/j.gastro.2013.10.047

Cyclosporiasis

Cheryl A. Glass, Audra C. Malone, and Kristie A. D. Morydz

Definition
A. Cyclosporiasis is a one-cell parasite that infects the upper small intestines. Causes of cyclosporiasis include ingesting infected water or produce (fresh fruits, especially raspberries, and vegetables) or exposure to the organism during travel to countries where it is endemic.
B. Cyclosporiasis manifests as protracted and relapsing gastroenteritis. The clinical syndrome consists of explosive watery diarrhoea, nausea, anorexia, weight loss, fatigue, and abdominal cramps that may persist for seven days to several weeks, with a waxing and waning course.
C. In an immunocompromised host, onset is insidious; the condition becomes chronic with symptoms, and the shedding of oocysts continues indefinitely.
D. The oocysts are resistant to most disinfectants used in food and water processing and can remain viable for prolonged periods.

Incidence/Prevalence
A. The incidence of infection is unknown, although it is common around the world.
B. Most outbreaks in the United States and Canada have been associated with consumption of imported fresh produce, including raspberries, basil, snow peas, and mesclun lettuce.

Pathogenesis
A. Infection is caused by an 8- to 10-mcg, spore-forming coccidian protozoan called *Cyclospora cayetanensis*. Transmission of oocysts is by the oral–faecal route. The incubation period ranges from two days to two weeks after excretion, depending on temperature and humidity.

Predisposing Factors
A. Incompetent or compromised immune system (e.g., infection with AIDS).
B. Travel to underdeveloped or tropical countries.
C. Ingestion of contaminated food or water.
D. Contact with animals that carry the parasite.

Common Findings
A. Abrupt, profuse, malodourous, watery diarrhoea.
B. Nausea.
C. Vomiting.
D. Anorexia.
E. Substantial weight loss.
F. Flu-like symptoms.
G. Abdominal cramps and bloating.

Other Signs and Symptoms
A. Asymptomatic.
B. Low-grade fever.
C. Nausea and vomiting.
D. Profound fatigue.
E. Yellow- to khaki-green stools.
F. Flatus.
G. Dehydration.

Subjective Data
A. Review the onset, duration, and course of symptoms. Is diarrhoea acute or chronic?

B. Question the client about travel to areas known for cyclospora, such as Haiti, Puerto Rico, Pakistan, India, Mexico, Nepal, New Guinea, and Peru. It has also been seen in Chicago, Los Angeles, New York, Florida, and Massachusetts.
C. Review the client's intake of medications and other substances that can cause diarrhoea, especially antibiotics, laxatives, quinidine, magnesium-containing antacids, digitalis, loop diuretics, antihypertensives, alcohol, caffeine, herbal teas, and sorbitol-containing (sugar-free) gum and mints.
D. Ask about the nature of the client's bowel movements (BMs), including frequency; consistency; volume; and presence of blood, pus, or mucus.
E. Review associated symptoms that need evaluation: Fever, abdominal pain, and anorexia.
F. Ask the client if other family members or sexual contacts are also ill.
G. Establish the client's normal weight and any recent weight loss. How much weight was lost and over what period of time?

Physical Examination
A. Check temperature, pulse, respirations, blood pressure (BP), and weight (vital signs are normal in most cases).
B. Inspect:
  1. General appearance for signs of illness and dehydration:
    a. Inspect mucous membranes.
    b. Inspect infants' fontanelles.
    c. Note for decreased skin turgor.
C. Auscultate the abdomen for bowel sounds in all quadrants.
D. Palpate:
  1. The abdomen for masses, rebound tenderness, and guarding; may exhibit right upper quadrant (RUQ) pain (biliary disease)
  2. Lymph nodes for enlargement.
E. Perform rectal examination.

Diagnostic Tests
Identification may be made by microscopic examination of stool under ultraviolet light, by modified acid-fast staining, or by review of wet mounts of stool by experienced microscopists. Finding large numbers of white cells suggests an inflammatory or invasive diarrhoea. The following tests are done:
A. Acid-fast Ziehl–Neelsen stained slide of stool.
B. Stool culture for ova and parasites: Parasites are passed intermittently, so three or more stools on alternating days should be examined.
C. Endoscopy with small-bowel biopsy.

Differential Diagnoses
A. Inflammatory bowel disease (IBD; Crohn's disease [CD] or ulcerative colitis [UC]).
B. Giardiasis.
C. Malabsorption.
D. *Escherichia coli* infection: *E. coli* causes diarrhoea within hours of ingesting contaminated food. Confirm by checking if others were affected.
E. Irritable bowel syndrome (IBS): Leukocyte-free mucus is the hallmark of IBS.
F. Viral diarrhoea.
G. Lactose intolerance.
H. Other bacterial infections, for example, *Shigella*, *Salmonella*, and *Campylobacter*.
I. Cholera.

Plan
A. General interventions:
  1. Avoid food and water that is contaminated with faeces.
  2. Fresh produce should always be washed thoroughly before it is eaten.
B. Client teaching: *Refer to Client Teaching Guide: Diarrhoea:*
  1. Teach contact precautions to those caring for diapered and/or incontinent children.
C. Dietary management:
  1. Encourage the client to increase fluids. Fluid replacement is the basic approach to prevent dehydration from diarrhoea.
  2. Advise the client to restrict milk products to rule out lactose intolerance.
  3. Give the client a copy of a diet plan to control nausea and vomiting (children and adults).
D. Pharmacological therapy:
  1. First-line treatments are trimethoprim with sulphamethoxazole (TMP/SMZ). They can reduce shedding, and stop diarrhoea within two days.
  2. Ciprofloxacin is the alternative treatment for clients with allergies to sulphamethoxazole.

Follow-Up
A. See the client in one week to verify continuing clinical improvement.
B. If diarrhoea persists two weeks or longer, a second evaluation is indicated.
C. Retest stools for blood and leukocytes; do a stool culture for ova and parasites.
D. Report cases of cyclosporiasis to the health department.

Consultation/Referral
A. Consult an infectious disease specialist and/or gastroenterologist if the client has no symptom relief after completing therapies or has a prolonged or severe case.

Individual Considerations
Pregnancy:
A. TMP/SMZ is a pregnancy category C drug. Use during pregnancy if the potential benefits outweigh the risk to the foetus.
B. TMP/SMZ should be avoided near term because of the potential for hyperbilirubinaemia and kernicterus in the newborn.

Resource
Government of Canada: https://www.canada.ca/en/public-health/services/diseases/cyclosporiasis-cyclospora/health-professionals-cyclosporiasis-cyclospora.html

Bibliography
American Academy of Pediatrics. (2012). Cyclosporiasis. In L. K. Pickering (Ed.), *Red book: 2012 report of the Committee on Infectious Diseases* (29th ed., pp. 299–300). Elk Grove Village, IL: Author. Retrieved from https://redbook.solutions.aap.org/DocumentLibrary/RB12_interior.pdf

▶ Client Teaching Guides are available at https://connect.springerpub.com/content/reference-book/978-0-8261-9498-5

Centers for Disease Control and Prevention. (2015, February 28). *Parasites—Cyclosporiasis (Cyclospora infection)*. Retrieved from www.cdc.gov/parasites/cyclosporiasis

Nettina, S. (2010). *The Lippincott manual of nursing practice* (9th ed.). Philadelphia, PA: Wolters Kluwer Lippincott Williams & Wilkins.

Shoff, W. H. (2012, November 16). Cyclospora. *Medscape*. Retrieved from http://emedicine.medscape.com/article/236105-overview

Diarrhoea

Cheryl A. Glass, Audra C. Malone, and Kristie A. D. Morydz

Definition

A. Diarrhoea is an abnormally high fluid content in the stool. Generally, diarrhoea also involves an increase in the frequency of bowel movements (BMs), which can range from fourfiveto 5 to more than 20 times a day. Diarrhoea may be an acute onset or chronic/persistent diarrhoea.
B. Acute diarrhoea is usually self-limited; the most common complication of diarrhoea is dehydration.
C. Chronic diarrhoea is defined as lasting longer than 14 days.

Incidence/Prevalence

A. The incidence of diarrhoea is unknown; however, it is responsible for 20% of paediatric referrals in children younger than 2 years and for 10% in children younger than 3 years. Morbidity has decreased because of the use of oral rehydration solutions; however, the global rate of mortality from acute diarrhoea is 18% of children younger than 5 years.
B. The incidence of *Clostridium difficile* infection is approximately 7%, and 28% of clients who were hospitalized have positive cultures for the organism. *C. difficile*–associated diarrhoea has a mortality rate as high as 25% in the frail elderly.
C. 20% to 27% of cases of *C. difficile* are community acquired.

Pathogenesis

A. The increased water content in diarrhoea stools is due to an imbalance in the physiology of the small and large intestinal processes. A bacterial infection is usually the cause of acute diarrhoea in children. Other causes of diarrhoea in children include malabsorption syndrome (see Table 11.5).

TABLE **Organisms That Cause Diarrhoea**

Viral organisms	Rotavirus Norovirus Adenovirus Calicivirus Astrovirus
Invasive bacteria	*Escherichia coli* *Klebsiella* *Clostridium difficile* *C. perfringens* *Shigella* *Salmonella* *Campylobacter* *Cholera* *Yersinia* *Plesiomonas* *Aeromonas*
Parasites	*Giardia* *Entamoeba* organisms *Cryptosporidium* *Giardia lamblia*

Predisposing Factors

A. Enteric infections.
B. Females have a higher incidence of *Campylobacter* species infections.
C. Young children.
D. Institutional: Day care and skilled nursing facilities.
E. Food: Raw or contaminated food.
F. Contaminated water or inadequate chlorinated water supply.
G. Travel.
H. Chemotherapy or radiation induced.
I. Vitamin deficiencies (niacin and folate).
J. Vitamin toxicity (C, niacin, and vitamin B3).
K. Ingestion of heavy metals (copper, tin, or zinc) or toxins.
L. Ingestion of plants, mistletoe, or mushrooms.
M. Antibiotics.
N. Antacids containing magnesium.

Common Findings

A. Frequent watery stool.
B. Foul-smelling stools (fat malabsorption).
C. Flatulence.
D. Abdominal cramping.

Other Signs and Symptoms

A. Lethargy.
B. Fever.
C. Nausea and vomiting.
D. Currant jelly stool (blood and mucus).
E. Anorexia.
F. Dehydration in adults:
 1. Thirst.
 2. Less frequent urination.
 3. Dark urine.
 4. Dry skin.
 5. Fatigue.
 6. Dizziness.
 7. Light-headedness.
G. Dehydration in infants and young children:
 1. Dry mouth and tongue.
 2. No tears when crying.
 3. No wet diapers for three hours or more.
 4. Sunken eyes, cheeks, or fontanelles.
 5. High fever.
 6. Listlessness or irritability.

Subjective Data

A. Review the onset of diarrhoeal stools. What is the normal stool pattern?
B. Review the consistency, colour, volume, and frequency of the stools.
C. Review dietary intake of raw foods, contaminated food, and nonabsorbable sugars including lactulose or lactose in lactose malabsorbers.
D. Review any contact with others who may have the same symptoms.
E. Have any of the stools contained blood? Bloody stool may be an indication of bacterial infection.
F. Review travel history, including camping vacations.
G. Review any exposure to turtles or young dogs or cats.
H. Review medication history, including antibiotics, vitamins, herbal production, laxatives, antacids that contain magnesium, opiate withdrawal, and methylxanthines (caffeine, theobromine, and theophylline).
I. Review any food allergies and history of lactose intolerance.

J. Evaluate the presence of other symptoms, such as fever, nausea, vomiting and abdominal pain, or tenesmus.
K. Evaluate for symptoms of dehydration, including thirst, dizziness, mental status changes, and decreased urine output.

Physical Examination

A. Check temperature, pulse, respirations, blood pressure (BP; standing and sitting), and weight.
B. Inspect:
  1. Observe the client's general overall appearance, the presence of lethargy or depressed consciousness, or grimace during examination.
  2. Evaluate muscle tone, skin turgor, reduced muscle, and fat mass.
  3. Examine mouth, lips, and mucous membranes for signs, symptoms, and severity of dehydration.
  4. Perianal examination for skin breakdown, erythema, and fissures.
C. Auscultate:
  1. Assess heart and lungs.
  2. Auscultate the abdomen in all four quadrants.
  3. Assess the presence of borborygmi (significant increase in peristaltic action that may be audible and/or palpable).
D. Percuss abdomen.
E. Palpate:
  1. Palpate the abdomen for masses, guarding, rebound tenderness, and peritoneal signs.
  2. For a newborn, palpate fontanelles.
  3. Palpate for lymphadenopathy.
  4. Perform a rectal examination, including testing of stool for occult blood.

Diagnostic Tests

A. Stool specimens for the evaluation of the following:
  1. *C. difficile*.
  2. Faecal leukocytes.
  3. Blood.
  4. Culture.
  5. Ova and parasites.
  6. Faecal alpha-1 antitrypsin levels.
  7. Viral antigen testing.
B. Specific enzyme immunoassay (EIA) and direct florescence antibody (DFA) assays are becoming the standard for the diagnosis of giardiasis.
C. Complete blood count (CBC): White blood cell (WBC) may be elevated.
D. Albumin.
E. Electrolytes.
F. A colonoscopy for intestinal biopsy for chronic or protracted diarrhoea or clients with AIDS should be done. A sigmoidoscopy alone may not reveal any abnormality.
G. Abdominal ultrasound to identify intussusception.
H. Abdominal CT.

Differential Diagnoses

A. Diarrhoea: Infectious aetiology.
B. Inflammatory bowel disease (IBD):
  1. Crohn's disease (CD).
  2. Ulcerative colitis (UC).
C. Cystic fibrosis (CF).
D. Giardiasis.
E. Protozoan.
F. Malabsorption syndromes.
G. Intussusception.
H. Stool impaction.
I. Irritable bowel syndrome (IBS).
J. Meckel's diverticulum.
K. Intolerance to lactose, carbohydrates, and protein.
L. Medication induced:.
  1. Antibiotic-associated diarrhoea.
  2. Antacids containing magnesium.
  3. Cancer drugs.
M. Pseudomembranous colitis.
N. Toxic megacolon.
O. Appendicitis.

Plan

A. Client teaching: *Refer to Client Teaching Guide: Diarrhoea:*
B. Examination of stools for ova and parasites should be done every other day or every three days.
C. Rehydrate with oral fluids for each diarrhoeal stool. Administer small amounts at frequent intervals.
D. Hold foods until hydration is completed. No evidence shows that bananas, rice, applesauce, and toast (BRAT) are useful; these are not currently recommended.
E. Use antibiotics (or the discontinuation of antibiotics in the case of *C. difficile*) or use antiparasitic agents, depending on the aetiology.
F. The use of probiotics, *Lactobacillus GG* (I, A) and *Saccharomyces boulardii* (II, B), has been found to be effective and may reduce the spread of rotavirus.
G. Encourage proper hygiene and food preparation to prevent spread and future infections.
H. Water should be boiled for at least one minute if contamination is suspected.

Follow-Up

A. Follow-up depends on the severity of diarrhoea and the age of the client. Neonates require strict follow-up within a few days of illness.
B. Monitor children who require labour-intensive oral hydration. Hospitalization for intravenous (IV) hydration may be required.
C. Rotavirus vaccine is available for the prevention of rotavirus gastroenteritis.

Consultation/Referral

A. Evaluate the need for a surgical consultation (fulminant colitis, peritonitis, and toxic megacolon) or one with an infectious disease specialist or a gastroenterologist.

Individual Considerations

A. Paediatrics:
  1. Stool patterns vary widely. Breastfed children may have up to five to six stools per day. Breastfed infants with acute diarrhoea should continue on breast milk.
  2. The younger the child, the higher the risk for severe, life-threatening dehydration and nutrient malabsorption.
B. Geriatrics:
  1. Review any hospitalizations within the last 72 hours as a cause of diarrhoea.
  2. Advanced age is a risk factor for *C. difficile* infection.
  3. Diarrhoea may be related to fecal impaction.
  4. Dehydration is more common in the elderly.
  5. Because of polypharmacy risk in the elderly, review all medications for drug-to-drug interactions.

▶ Client Teaching Guides are available at https://connect.springerpub.com/content/reference-book/978-0-8261-9498-5

Resources

Drugs.com Drug Interaction Checker: https://www.drugs.com/drug_interactions.html

Medscape Drug Interaction Checker: http://reference.medscape.com/drug-interactionchecker

RxList Drug Interaction Checker: http://www.rxlist.com/drug-interaction-checker.htm

Bibliography

American Academy of Pediatrics. (2012). Shigella infections. In L. K. Pickering (Ed.), *Red book: 2012 report of the Committee on Infectious Diseases* (29th ed., pp. 645–647). Elk Grove Village, IL: Author. Retrieved from https://redbook.solutions.aap.org/DocumentLibrary/RB12_interior.pdf

American College of Gastroenterology. (2011). Pregnancy and gastrointestinal disorders. *Pregnancy monograph*. Retrieved from http://gi.org/wp-content/uploads/2011/07/institute-PregnancyMonograph.pdf

Barclay, L. (2010, December 2). American Academy of Pediatrics reviews use of probiotics, prebiotics. *Medscape*. Retrieved from http://www.medscape.com/viewarticle/733463

Centers for Disease Control and Prevention. (2011, April 11). *Rotavirus*. Retrieved from www.cdc.gov/rotavirus/index.html

Centers for Disease Control and Prevention Vaccines & Immunizations. (2012, November 30). *Vaccines and preventable diseases: Rotavirus vaccination*. Retrieved from www.cdc.gov/vaccines/vpd-vac/rotavirus/default.htm#ed

National Digestive Diseases Information Clearinghouse. (2011, January). *Diarrhea*. (NIH Publication No. 11-2749). Retrieved from http://digestive.niddk.nih.gov/ddiseases/pubs/diarrhea/Diarrhea_208.pdf

Nettina, S. (2010). *The Lippincott manual of nursing practice* (9th ed.). Philadelphia, PA: Wolters Kluwer Lippincott Williams & Wilkins.

Sharma, G. D. (2013, June 17). Cystic fibrosis. *Medscape*. Retrieved from http://emedicine.medscape.com/article/1001602-overview

Surawicz, C. M., Brandt, L. J., Binion, D. G., Ananthakrishnan, A. N., Curry, S. R., Gilligan, P. H., & Zuckerbraun, B. S. (2013). Guidelines for diagnosis, treatment, and prevention of *Clostridium difficile* infections. *American Journal of Gastroenterology, 108,* 478–498. doi:10.1038/ajg.2013.4

Diverticulosis and Diverticulitis

Cheryl A. Glass, Audra C. Malone, and Kristie A. D. Morydz

Definition

A. Diverticula are saclike protrusions of mucosa through the muscular colonic wall. Protrusions can occur in weakened areas of the bowel wall and blood vessels. Diverticulosis is the presence of diverticula, but it does not imply a pathologic condition. Diverticulitis occurs when the diverticula become plugged and inflamed. Surgery is often the first-line treatment for young symptomatic clients. Diverticular disease is one of the most common causes of lower gastrointestinal (GI) haemorrhage and a leading consideration in clients who present with brisk rectal bleeding.

B. There is no evidence of a relationship between the development of diverticula and smoking, caffeine, and alcohol consumption. However, an increased risk of developing diverticular disease is associated with a diet that is high in red meat and total fat content. This risk can be reduced by a diet high in fiber content, especially with fruits and vegetables (cellulose); see Appendix B, Diet Recommendations, Table B.6).

C. Diverticulosis is often diagnosed as an incidental finding on a barium enema (BE) or sigmoid/colonoscopy.

D. Recurrent attacks of diverticulitis can result in the formation of scar tissue, leading to narrowing and obstruction of the colonic lumen.

E. Complicated diverticulitis includes those episodes associated with free perforation, abscess, fistula, obstruction, or stricture.

Incidence/Prevalence

Diverticulosis is very common and increases with age.

A. Prevalence by age:
  1. Age 40 years: 5%.
  2. Age 60 years: 30%.
  3. Age 80 years: 65% to 80%.

B. No significant difference in prevalence by gender: Diverticulosis is symptomatic in 70% of cases. It leads to diverticulitis in 5% to 25%; and is associated with bleeding in 5% to 15%. The sigmoid colon is commonly affected. There are two types of diverticular disease and diverticulitis:
  1. Simple, with no complications; responds to treatment such as dietary changes without the need for surgery.
  2. Complicated, with abscesses, fistula, obstruction, perforation, and peritonitis leading to sepsis; usually requires surgery.

Pathogenesis

A. The exact aetiology of diverticular disease is not known.

B. The present theory that fiber is a protective agent against the development of diverticula and subsequent diverticulitis holds that insoluble fiber causes the formation of bulkier stool, which leads to decreased effectiveness in colonic segmentation. The overall result is that intracolonic pressure remains close to the normal range during colonic peristalsis. Diverticular sac can become inflamed when undigested food residues and bacteria get trapped in the thin-walled sacs. If this occurs, blood supply is mechanically compromised and bacterial invasion ensues.

Predisposing Factors

A. Advanced age.
B. Obesity (84%–96%).
C. Low-residue diet.
D. Complicated diverticular disease is exacerbated by the following:
  1. Smoking.
  2. Nonsteroidal anti-inflammatory drugs (NSAIDs).
  3. Acetaminophen use (especially paracetamol).
  4. Opioids.
  5. Steroids.
E. Indication that genetics is a predisposing factor:
  1. Left-sided diverticula is most common.
  2. Right-sided (caecal) diverticula is predominant in Asia.

Common Findings

A. Diverticulosis is usually asymptomatic.
B. Painless rectal bleeding is the hallmark of diverticular bleeding, with intermittent passage of maroon or bright red blood.
C. Common diverticulitis symptoms:
  1. Left lower quadrant (LLQ) pain.
  2. Constipation.

Other Signs and Symptoms

A. Back pain.
B. Flatulence.
C. Periodic abdominal distension.
D. Borborygmi, or loud, prolonged gurgles caused by hyperactive intestinal peristalsis.
E. Diarrhoea.
F. Nausea or vomiting.
G. Dysuria.

H. Tenderness on palpation, possible guarding.
I. Fever, low-grade.

Subjective Data
A. Review the onset, duration, and course of symptoms, including size, colour, consistency, and frequency of stools.
B. Ask the client whether constipation is a chronic or acute problem, and whether it alternates with diarrhoea. Has the client ever had a bowel obstruction?
C. Review the client's daily diet and fluid intake.
D. Ask the client about medication use, including iron supplements, NSAIDs, and acetaminophen.
E. Inquire about the colour, amount, and frequency of rectal bleeding. Does the client strain when having a bowel movement (BM)?
F. Review the client's history of pain with defecation.
G. Review the client's history of kidney stones, as it can mimic diverticulitis.

Physical Examination
The constellation of LLQ tenderness with or without peritoneal findings, fever, and leukocytosis is suggestive of sigmoid diverticulitis:
A. Check temperature, pulse, respirations, blood pressure (BP), and weight.
B. The physical examination may be relatively unremarkable, but most commonly reveals abdominal tenderness or a mass.
C. Inspect:
   1. Observe the general overall appearance for signs of pain.
   2. Inspect the abdomen in detail, assessing for distension and guarding.
D. Auscultate all four quadrants of the abdomen. Bowel sounds may be decreased or normal in early diverticulitis.
E. Percuss the abdomen.
F. Palpate:
   1. Palpate the abdomen for rebound tenderness or masses signaling possible abscess and tenderness.
   2. Palpate beneath the right costal arch, checking for Murphy's sign or pain on deep inspiration.
   3. Consider a pelvic examination to rule out gynaecologic sources of the abdominal pain.
G. Rectal examination: Evaluate for haemorrhoids, masses, fissures, fistulas, inflammation, and stool in the ampulla.

Diagnostic Tests
The diagnosis of acute diverticulitis can often be made following a focused history and examination, especially in clients with recurrent diverticulitis whose diagnosis has been previously confirmed:
A. The diagnosis of diverticular colitis is made endoscopically and histologically.
B. CT scan of the abdomen and pelvis is the optimal method of investigation for suspected acute diverticulitis.
C. Complete blood count (CBC) with differential: White blood cell (WBC) may show leukocytosis with a shift to the left; haemoglobin and haematocrit (Hct) may be low with chronic or acute bleeding.
D. C-reactive protein (CRP; >50 in the client with LLQ pain and no vomiting is highly suggestive of diverticulitis).
E. Radiography: Flat plate and upright films of abdomen to evaluate ileus or obstruction, free air, and perforation.
F. Abdominal ultrasonography to evaluate masses or abscess.
G. Proctosigmoidoscopy.
H. BE after infection subsides. Caution: A BE during the acute phase may increase intraluminal pressure and cause bowel perforation.
I. Haemoccult: Stool.
J. Pregnancy test if there is a possibility of pregnancy.
K. Urinalysis (excludes urinary tract infections [UTIs]).

Differential Diagnoses
A. Hernia.
B. Renal colic.
C. Acute appendicitis.
D. Bowel obstruction.
E. Ischaemic colitis.
F. Colon cancer.
G. Haemorrhoids.
H. Constipation or impaction.
I. Inflammatory bowel disease (IBD).
J. Urologic disorder: Pyelonephritis.
K. Tubo-ovarian abscess/pelvic inflammatory disease (PID).
L. Torsion (testicular or ovarian).
M. Ectopic pregnancy.
N. Cholecystitis.
O. UTI.

Plan
A. Stress the importance of strict adherence to diet.
B. Dietary management:
   1. Nothing by mouth (NPO) status for acute treatment.
   2. Full-liquid diet or low-fiber diet if not on bowel rest.
   3. Long-term dietary management:
      a. High-fiber diet including bran, beans, fruits, and vegetables.
      b. Bulk agents if unable to tolerate bran.
      c. Note foods to avoid, such as nuts.
C. Medical and surgical management: Acute treatment has not been well defined in diverticular disease:
   1. Acute treatment may include the following:
      a. Nasogastric (NG) tube placement.
      b. Intravenous (IV) fluids.
   2. Surgical intervention is required for abscess, peritonitis, obstruction, fistula, or failure to improve after several days of medical management, or recurrence after successful medical management.
D. Pharmacological therapy: Optimal treatment has not been defined:
   1. Conservative management of diverticulosis: Psyllium.
   2. Diverticulitis initial attack: Ciprofloxacin and metronidazole. Amoxicillin/clavulanic acid or sulfamethoxazole-trimethoprim may also be used with metronidazole.
   3. 5-Aminosalicylates (5-ASA) may be added if there is a lack of response.
   4. Relapse: May repeat with the same antibiotic regimen for one month.
   5. Chronic disease: Use long-term ciprofloxacin but not metronidazole.
   6. Avoid laxatives, enemas, and opiates.
   7. NSAIDs should be avoided due to a moderately increased risk of occurrence of diverticulitis.

Follow-Up
A. Follow up in two to three days. Continue conservative management if the client has no signs of complications.
B. A colonoscopy should be performed from six to eight weeks after recovery to evaluate the extent of the diverticulosis/rule out other manifestations.

Consultation/Referral

A. Arrange for prompt hospitalization and surgical consultation if the client's temperature rises above 38.3°C, his or her pain worsens, peritoneal signs develop, or WBC continues to rise. Surgery consultation is required for abscess, peritonitis, obstruction, fistula, or failure to improve after several days of medical management.

Individual Considerations

A. Immunocompromised and elderly clients may have a normal WBC without a left shift and still have a severe infection.

Bibliography

Feingold, D., Steele, S. R., Lee, S., Kaiser, A., Boushey, R., Buie, W. D., & Frederick Rafferty, J. (2014). Practice parameters for the treatment of sigmoid diverticulitis. *Diseases of the Colon & Rectum, 57*, 284–294. doi:10.1097/DCR.0000000000000075

Natesan, A., & Bury, C. (2015, April). *Diverticulitis: Evaluation and management*. Retrieved from http://www.ahcmedia.com/articles/135320-diverticulitis-evaluation-and-management

Nettina, S. (2010). *The Lippincott manual of nursing practice* (9th ed.). Philadelphia, PA: Wolters Kluwer Lippincott Williams & Wilkins.

Nguyen, M. C. T. (2011, September 22). Diverticulitis. *Medscape*. Retrieved from http://emedicine.medscape.com/article/173388-overview

World Gastroenterology Organisation Practice Guidelines. (2007). *Diverticular disease*. Retrieved from http://www.worldgastroenterology.org/assets/downloads/en/pdf/guidelines/07_diverticular_disease.pdf

Young-Fadok, T., & Pemberton, J. H. (2012, November 15). Treatment of acute diverticulitis. *UpToDate*. Retrieved from http://www.uptodate.com/contents/treatment-of-acute-diverticulitis

Elevated Liver Enzymes

Cheryl A. Glass, Audra C. Malone, and Kristie A. D. Morydz

Definition

Liver function tests (LFTs) used to determine the health of the liver are not direct measures of its function. The liver has excretory, metabolic, protective, detoxification, haematologic, and circulatory functions. LFTs may be abnormal even in clients with a healthy liver. Normal laboratory chemistry values may vary according to age, gender, ethnicity, blood group, and postprandial state, as well as other factors, such as exercise and pregnancy. Common rationales for ordering liver chemistry tests (see Table 11.6) include the following:

A. Making differential diagnosis of the different types of jaundice.
B. Assessing the severity of hepatocellular injury.
C. Following the trend of the disease.
D. Diagnosing the presence of latent liver disease (i.e., differential diagnosis of ascites or haematemesis).
E. Screening the suspected case during outbreaks of infective hepatitis.
F. Screening the persons exposed to hepatotoxic drugs.
G. Evaluating cholestatic problems.

Incidence/Prevalence

A. The incidence of elevated liver enzymes is undetermined. Abnormal elevations of serum liver chemistries may occur in 1% to 4% of the asymptomatic population.

Pathogenesis

A. Pathogenesis varies by diagnosis.

Predisposing Factors

A. Predisposing factors are dependent on the suspected or known medical diagnosis.

Common Findings

A. Asymptomatic.
B. Pruritus.
C. Jaundice.
D. Ascites.
E. Fatigue.
F. Weight loss.
G. Change in the colour of urine (dark) or stools (clay coloured).
H. Loss of appetite.

Subjective Data

A complete medical history is the single most important part of the evaluation of the client with elevated LFTs.

A. Review medications, including prescription medications, statins, and over-the-counter (OTC) medications, as well as herbal therapies.
B. Determine the duration of LFT abnormalities (if known).
C. Review the presence of accompanying symptoms, including arthralgias, myalgias, rash, abdominal pain, fever, pruritus, and changes in the colour of urine or stool.
D. Has the client experienced any anorexia or weight loss? Over what period did weight loss occur?
E. Review parenteral exposures, including transfusions, intravenous (IV) and intranasal drug use, tattoos, and sexual history.
F. Review the client's recent travel history and possible exposure to contaminated foods.
G. Review the client's exposure to people with jaundice.
H. Review the client's occupational history and exposure to hepatotoxins.
I. Review the client's history of alcohol consumption, including when started, amount, type of alcohol (beer, liquor, and moonshine), and frequency.
J. Evaluate the gestational age of pregnancy. Haemolysis, elevated liver enzymes, and low platelets (HELLP) syndrome is generally present in the third trimester of pregnancy.

Physical Examination

A. Temperature (if indicated), pulse, respirations, and blood pressure (BP).
B. Observation:
  1. Observe for temporal and proximal muscle wasting.
  2. Perform eye and mouth (mucous membranes) examination for icterus.
  3. Perform dermal examination for icterus, spider nevi, palmar erythema, and presence of caput medusae (the presence of dilated veins seen on the abdomen; noted with cirrhosis of the liver and portal hypertension).
  4. Evaluate the presence of gynaecomastia.
  5. Observe for the presence of jugular venous distension (JVD), a sign of right-sided heart failure (HF) that suggests hepatic congestion.
C. Auscultate heart and lungs.
D. Percuss the abdomen.
E. Palpate:
  1. Abdominal examination:
    a. Evaluate the presence of hepatomegaly; focus on the size and consistency of the liver.
    b. Evaluate the presence of splenomegaly; focus on the size of the spleen. An enlarged spleen is most easily appreciated with the client in the right lateral decubitus position.

TABLE 11.6 Liver Chemistry Tests and Implications

Liver Chemistry Test	Clinical Implication of Abnormality
ALT	Hepatocellular damage
AST	Hepatocellular damage
ALP	Cholestasis, infiltrative disease, or biliary obstruction
Albumin	Synthetic function
Alpha-fetoprotein	Cancer marker when elevated
Bile acids: urine bile salts, bile pigments, and urobilinogen	Cholestasis or biliary obstruction, impaired hepatic update or secretion, or portal-systemic shunting
Bilirubin: serum total, direct, and indirect bilirubin	Cholestasis, impaired conjugation, or biliary obstruction
Cholesterol, serum triglycerides	Lipoprotein production and metabolism, chronic cholestasis
Fibrinogen	Liver damage/cirrhosis, acute liver insufficiency, poisoning
GGT	Cholestasis or biliary obstruction, malignant involvement in hepatocellular disease, more sensitive than other enzymes in alcoholism
Hepatitis surface antigen, IgM, antibody, RNA, genotype, viral load	Differentiation of type of hepatitis
LDH	Hepatocellular damage not specific for hepatic disease
Total proteins, albumin globulin (A/C ratio)	Hepatitis, advanced liver disease
PT	Synthesis function in hepatocellular disease, fulminate hepatitis
Plasma ammonia	Central nervous system dysfunction/toxicity or end-stage liver disease
5NT	Cholestasis or biliary obstruction
Urea	End-stage liver disease

ALP, alkaline phosphatase; ALT, alanine transaminase; AST, aspartate transaminase; CNS, central nervous system; 5NT, 5'-nucleotidase; GGT, gamma-glutamyl transpeptidase; IgM, immunoglobulin M; LDH, lactate dehydrogenase; PT, prothrombin time; RNA, ribonucleic acid.

    c. Assess for ascites: Note presence of a fluid wave or shifting dullness.
    d. Assess for an abdominal mass.
  2. Lymph nodes: Evaluate lymphadenopathy.
  3. Conduct testicular examination for testicular atrophy (increased oestrogen/reduced testosterone).

Diagnostic Tests
A. The particular LFT tests ordered are related to the suspected or identified medical diagnosis. Table 11.7 shows common serologic tests for viral hepatitis.

Differential Diagnoses
A. Table 11.8 shows differential diagnoses with elevated liver enzymes.

Plan
A. The clinical significance of any liver chemistry test abnormality must be interpreted in the context of the clinical situation. The plan of care is dependent on the suspected or identified medical diagnosis. Lifestyle modifications, including discontinuance of medications and alcohol, weight loss, and dietary changes, can be recommended as appropriate.
B. Clients with marked abnormalities of liver tests, or with signs and symptoms of chronic liver disease or hepatic decompensation (i.e., ascites, encephalopathy, coagulopathy, or portal hypertension), should be evaluated and treated in a more expeditious manner than asymptomatic clients.

Follow-Up
A. Follow-up testing for elevated LFTs, including abdominal/liver ultrasonography, CT, MRI, and liver biopsy, is dependent on the risk factors for disease, symptoms and history, and physical finding of the suspected or identified medical diagnosis. A liver chemistry test that is normal does not ensure that the client is free of liver disease. If a laboratory error is suspected, the laboratory test should be repeated.

Consultation/Referral
A. Consider a consultation or referral to a hepatologist, gastroenterologist, or infectious disease specialist.

Individual Considerations
Pregnancy: HELLP syndrome is a severe form of pregnancy-induced hypertension (PIH or preeclampsia). It may occur anywhere from the mid-second trimester to immediately postpartum. The HELLP syndrome occurs in 0.1% to 0.8% of pregnancies. The aetiology is unknown. The presence of laboratory abnormalities confirms the diagnosis. Treatment of the HELLP syndrome will not be covered. However, the laboratory abnormalities that are noted include the following:
A. Haemolytic anaemia.
B. Proteinuria.
C. Serum aspartate transaminase (AST) level (>70 IU/L).
D. Low platelet count ($<100 \times 10^9$ /L).
E. Serum lactate dehydrogenase (LDH) level (>600 IU/L or 10 μkat/L).
F. Total bilirubin level (>20.52 mmol/L).

TABLE 11.7 Serologic Tests for Viral Hepatitis

Virologic Test	Usual Clinical Implication of a Positive Test
Hepatitis A-IgM	Positive in acute hepatitis A
Hepatitis A-IgG	Positive in response to previous hepatitis A infection or vaccination
HBsAg	Positive during active hepatitis B infection Positive in response to previous hepatitis B infection or vaccination
Hepatitis B core antibody-IgM	Positive during active hepatitis B infection
Hepatitis B core antibody-IgG	Positive in response to current or prior hepatitis B infection
HBV-DNA	Positive during active hepatitis B infection
Hepatitis B e antigen	Positive test indicates replicative state of wild-type hepatitis B infection
Hepatitis B e antibody	Positive after replicative state of wild-type hepatitis B infection
HBV viral load	Assess hepatitis B virology
HCV antibody ELISA	Positive during or after hepatitis C infection
HCV-immunoblot assay (RIBA)	Positive during or after hepatitis C infection
HCV-RNA	Positive during hepatitis C infection
HCV viral load	Assess hepatitis C virology
HCV genotype	Genotyping is used for evaluation of the length of therapy

ELISA, enzyme-linked immunosorbent assay; HBV, hepatitis B virus; HCV, hepatitis C virus; HBsAg, hepatitis B surface antigen; IgG, immunoglobulin G; IgM, immunoglobulin M; RIBA, Recombinant ImmunoBlot Assay; RNA, ribonucleic acid.

TABLE 11.8 Differential Diagnosis With Elevated Liver Enzymes

Infiltrating Diseases of the Liver	
• Sarcoidosis • TB • Fungal infection • Amyloidosis	• Lymphoma • Metastatic malignancy • Hepatocellular carcinoma

Acute viral hepatitis (A–E, EBV, CMV, herpes)	Wilson's disease (genetic disorder of biliary copper excretion)
Cholestasis disease	Acute bile duct obstruction
Chronic hepatitis B, C	Haemolysis
Steatosis/nonalcoholic steatohepatitis	Myopathy
Hereditary haemochromatosis	Thyroid disorders
Medication/herbal induced	Strenuous exercise–induced changes
Alpha-1-antitrypsin deficiency	Pregnancy—HELLP syndrome
Cirrhosis	Toxin(s) exposure
Celiac disease	Acute Budd–Chiari syndrome
Alcohol-related liver injury	Anorexia nervosa

CMV, cytomegalovirus; EBV, Epstein–Barr virus; HELLP, haemolysis, elevated liver enzymes, and low platelets; TB, tuberculosis.

Bibliography

Green, R. M., & Flamm, S. (2002). AGA technical review on the evaluation of liver chemistry tests. *Gastroenterology, 123,* 1367–1384. doi:10.1053/gast.2002.36061

Nettina, S. (2010). *The Lippincott manual of nursing practice* (9th ed.). Philadelphia, PA: Wolters Kluwer Lippincott Williams & Wilkins.

Utah Library of Medicine. (n.d.). *Hepatitic pathology: Caput medusae.* Retrieved from http://library.med.utah.edu/WebPath/LIVEHTML/LIVER061.html

Gastroenteritis, Bacterial and Viral

Cheryl A. Glass, Audra C. Malone, and Kristie A. D. Morydz

Definition

A. Bacterial and viral gastroenteritis is an acute inflammation of the gastrointestinal (GI) mucosa of the middle or lower intestine. It is primarily an acute, self-limiting illness.

Table 11.9 Infectious Agents Causing Gastroenteritis

Causative Agent	Incubation Period
Noroviruses	12 hours–2 days
Escherichia coli	24–72 hours
Campylobacter	2–5 days
Staphylococcus	1–6 hours
Shigella	8–24 hours
Botulism	12–36 hours
Giardia lamblia	7–21 days
Salmonella	6–72 hours
Rotaviruses	1–3 days
Astrovirus	1–5 days
Adenoviruses	5–8 days
C. perfringens	10–12 hours
Clostridium difficile	Variable
Listeria species	20 hours

Immunocompromised clients can develop unremitting or fatal symptoms from gastroenteritis.

Incidence/Prevalence

A. Gastroenteritis is very common, occurring in all age groups. Epidemic outbreaks of bacterial gastroenteritis occur in groups who have ingested contaminated food. Viral excretion can begin before symptoms. Gastroenteritis is responsible for an estimated eight million health-care visits and 250,000 hospitalizations a year.
B. Rotavirus is most common in young children, with peak incidence at three to 15 months of age.
C. Norovirus most commonly infects older children and adults.
D. Astrovirus usually infects infants and young children; however, it can infect people of all ages.
E. Adenoviruses primarily affect children younger than two years.

Pathogenesis

A. Gastroenteritis is commonly caused by infectious agents—viruses, bacteria, and parasites (see Table 11.9). There are four viral agents: rotavirus, norovirus, enteric adenovirus, and astrovirus (Lee et al., 2013). Rotavirus is the most common cause of severe diarrhoea in children. Exotoxins produced by some organisms induce hypersecretion or increased peristalsis resulting in diarrhoea or vomiting. Bacteria, such as *Escherichia coli* and *Salmonella*, penetrate and invade the gastric mucosa and lead to diarrhoea accompanied by fever and faecal leukocytes. Viruses destroy enterocytes of the upper jejunal villi, often producing secondary lactose intolerance.

Predisposing Factors

A. Travel to areas where cholera or *Giardia* is epidemic:
  1. Ingestion of raw or undercooked seafood or drinks containing cholera-contaminated ice or water.
  2. Ingestion of *Giardia*-contaminated water supplies.
B. Ingestion of food contaminated with *Salmonella* or *Shigella*. Foods that are often implicated are domestic fowl and eggs, custard-filled pastries, processed meats, foods warmed on steam tables, poultry, red meat, raw seafood, raw milk, rice, and bean sprouts, due to the following:
  1. Inadequate cooking time and temperatures.
  2. Poor hygiene, lack of handwashing.
  3. Improper storage of food.
  4. Ingestion of fruits and vegetables contaminated by an infected person or by animal products.
C. Infection by person-to-person spread:
  1. Day-care centres: Rotavirus can be found on toys and hard surfaces.
  2. Overcrowded environments, inadequate health care or education.
  3. Schools/dormitories.
  4. Nursing homes.
  5. Banquet halls, cruise ships.
D. Contact with *Salmonella*-infected turtles, iguanas, and other reptiles.
E. Seasonal outbreaks:
  1. Rotavirus and astrovirus occur from October to April.
  2. Adenovirus occurs throughout the year.
  3. Norovirus occurs throughout the year but tends to increase in cooler months (November to April).
  4. Astrovirus is most common in the winter.

Common Findings

A. Abrupt onset of nausea and vomiting.
B. Abrupt onset of diarrhoea (with or without blood and mucus).
C. Fever, sometimes.

Other Signs and Symptoms

A. Explosive flatulence.
B. Cramping abdominal pain.
C. Abdominal tenderness.
D. Frequent watery diarrhoea.
E. Mucoid stools with or without blood.
F. Tenesmus.
G. Myalgia.
H. Headache.
I. Weakness.
J. Malaise.
K. Potential for seizures in children with high fever or electrolyte abnormalities.

Subjective Data

A. Review the onset, duration, and course of symptoms, including presence of abdominal pain and frequency of bowel movements (BMs). Ask the client if anyone else in the family has the same symptoms.
B. Ask the client about travel history, including travel by cruise ships or travel to foreign countries and camping with ingestion of water from streams, springs, or untreated wells.
C. Ask the client about crowded or unsanitary living conditions, use of day-care centres, and institutional living.
D. Take a 24-hour diet history, including ingestion of prunes or beans.
E. Review diarrhoea history:
  1. How many stools?
  2. How frequent are the diarrhoeal stools?
  3. What colour is the stool?
  4. Does the stool contain mucus?
  5. Has there been blood in the stool?
  6. Does the client have tenesmus (constant feeling of the need to pass stool)?

F. Inquire about other symptoms, such as fever or respiratory problems.
G. If the client is an infant, ask the caregiver about activity level, irritability, sleep pattern, fluid intake, and number of wet diapers.
H. If the client is a child, ask about activity level and dietary and fluid intake.
I. Review drug history intake, including laxatives, antacids, antibiotics, quinine, or anticancer medications.
J. Has the client been vaccinated with the rotavirus vaccine?

Physical Examination

A. Check temperature, pulse, respirations, blood pressure (BP), and weight:
   1. Bacterial infections: Temperatures between 38.3°C and 38.9°C.
   2. Viral infections: Temperatures of 39.4°C and above.
   3. Note hypotension and tachycardia.
B. Inspect:
   1. Inspect general appearance; note whether the client is very ill.
   2. Assess hydration status. Signs of dehydration:
      a. Mild: Slightly dry buccal mucous membranes, increased thirst, decreased urine output.
      b. Moderate: Sunken eyes, sunken fontanelle in infants, loss of skin turgor, dry buccal mucous membranes, decreased urine output.
      c. Severe: Signs of moderate dehydration and one or more of the following: rapid thready pulse, tachypnoea, lethargy, and postural hypotension.
   3. Assess activity level and behaviour in infant or child.
C. Auscultate the abdomen in all quadrants for bowel sounds; note hyperactive bowel sounds, absent or hypoactive bowel sounds (common with botulism), and borborygmi.
D. Palpate the abdomen for diffuse tenderness, slight distension, masses, rebound tenderness, and spasm. Observe for muscle guarding during the examination.
E. Rectal examination: Check for masses, fissures, inflammation, perianal erythema, or stool in ampulla.
F. Neurologic examination:
   1. Check for dizziness, difficulty swallowing, and other neurologic signs.
   2. Neurologic signs and symptoms indicate botulism and require emergency intervention.

Diagnostic Tests

A. No immediate laboratory tests are required if dehydration is absent or mild and the client feels well except for frequent diarrhoea.
B. Complete blood count (CBC) with differential: Serologic studies can detect viral pathogens.
C. Sedimentation rate: Elevated with infections or inflammation.
D. Electrolytes, sodium, chlorides, potassium, calcium and urea, and creatinine,
E. Blood gases to assess acid–base balance, if indicated,
F. Blood cultures, if indicated,
G. Stool for guaiac, leukocytes, ova, and parasites; test specimens three times, every other day. Stool guaiac is usually negative in viral infections, positive in invasive bacterial infections. Large numbers of white cells in stool suggest inflammatory or invasive diarrhea, such as occurs with *Shigella, Salmonella, Campylobacter*, invasive *E. coli*, or *Entamoeba*. Mononuclear cells in stool are characteristic of salmonellosis.
H. Stool culture if blood or mucus, fever more than 24 hours, or leukocytes are present.
I. Special cultures for *Campylobacter* and cholera are required.
J. Urinalysis: Excludes urinary tract infection (UTI) as cause of nonspecific diarrhoea; urine specific gravity to assess dehydration.
K. Sigmoidoscopy: Skip bowel prep with gross blood, large numbers of leukocytes in stool, or severe illness.
L. Culture food from suspected foci for *Salmonella*.
M. Real-time reverse transcriptase-polymerase chain reaction (RT-qPCR) is the most widely used assay for detecting norovirus in stool, vomitus, and environmental specimens. The best detection is in stool specimens.

Differential Diagnoses

A. Acute viral hepatitis.
B. Acute appendicitis.
C. Cholecystitis.
D. Inflammatory bowel disease (IBD).
E. Pelvic inflammatory disease (PID).
F. Intussusception.
G. Bowel obstruction for other causes.

Plan

A. General interventions:
   1. Meticulous handwashing is the single most important measure to decrease transmission. Hand sanitizers are an option when access to soap or clean water is limited.
   2. Advise the client to begin bed rest with progression to regular activities.
   3. If the client is diapered and/or incontinent, discuss strict contact precautions with the client or caregiver. Alcohol-based handwashing may decrease the spread.
   4. Diaper-changing areas should be separate from food preparation areas.
   5. Chlorine-based disinfectants inactivate rotavirus and may prevent disease transmission from contact with environmental surfaces.
B. Client teaching: *Refer to Client Teaching Guide: Diarrhoea.*
C. Dietary management:
   1. Clients should comply with nothing by mouth (NPO) and then slowly add clear liquids to maintain hydration.
   2. Hydration is one of the most important factors in the prevention of complications.
   3. Rehydrate with oral fluids for each diarrhoeal stool.
   4. Administer small amounts at frequent intervals.
   5. Hold foods until hydration is completed. No evidence shows that bananas, rice, applesauce, and toast (BRAT) are useful; these are not currently recommended. See section "Nausea and Vomiting Diet Suggestions (Children and Adults)" in Appendix B, Diet Recommendations.
D. Pharmacological therapy:
   1. The primary treatment for viral gastroenteritis is fluid replacement. There are no specific antiviral pharmacological therapies. Intravenous (IV) rehydration of fluids and electrolytes may be required in severe dehydration.
   2. Antibiotics may or may not be prescribed according to the bacterial source. Antimicrobial therapy is not indicated for uncomplicated (noninvasive) gastroenteritis because therapy does not shorten duration of the

▶ Client Teaching Guides are available at https://connect.springerpub.com/content/reference-book/978-0-8261-9498-5

disease and can prolong duration of excretion of *Salmonella* organisms.

3. Antidiarrhoeal therapy delays transit time and can reduce the severity and duration of abdominal cramping; however, it may prolong the course of some bacterial diarrhoea such as *Shigella* and *E. coli*. Bismuth subsalicylate is not recommended for young children with gastroenteritis due to the potential toxicity from salicylate absorption.

4. Stop other medications that may be triggering diarrhoea.

5. Vaccinate children with rotavirus live vaccine. Both available vaccinations are oral:

   a. The rotavirus vaccine can be administered together with diphtheria, tetanus, and pertussis (DTaP) vaccine, *Haemophilus influenzae* type b (Hib) vaccine, inactivated polio vaccine (IPV), hepatitis B vaccine, and the pneumococcal conjugate vaccine.

   b. In March 2010, the Centers for Disease Control and Prevention (CDC) learned that a virus (or parts of a virus), *Porcine circovirus* (PCV), is present in both rotavirus vaccines. There is no evidence that PCV is a safety risk or causes illness in humans. Information related to PCV and rotavirus vaccines is available on the CDC and Health Canada website: www.canada.ca/en/health-canada/services/drugs-health-products/biologics-radiopharmaceuticals-genetic-therapies/activities/fact-sheets/questions-answers-porcine-circovirus-rotavirus-vaccines.html

   c. Some postmarketing studies from outside the United States have detected a low-level increased risk of intussusception following rotavirus vaccination, particularly shortly after the first dose. The CDC continues to recommend both ROTARIX and RotaTeq to prevent severe rotavirus disease in infants and children. The CDC continues to monitor data on intussusception.

Follow-Up

A. Advise the client to return if the condition worsens or if signs and symptoms have not abated in 48 to 72 hours. However, diarrhoea due to *Salmonella* may be expected to persist for up to two weeks.

B. Renal function tests and CBC should be done in approximately one week after the start of symptoms in clients with *E. coli* O157:H7 to detect early-onset haemolytic-uremic syndrome.

C. If diarrhoea persists for two weeks or more, the client should present for a secondary evaluation.

D. Reporting surveillance systems:

   1. The Public Health Agency of Canada (www.canada.ca/en/public-health/services/food-safety.html) works with health-care providers to monitor and track outbreaks of foodborne illness.

Consultation/Referral

A. Refer clients to a hospital immediately if they have dehydration, rebound tenderness, severe abdominal pain, neurologic symptoms, and intussusception.

B. Immediately refer infants under age two years with paroxysmal, severe abdominal pain and vomiting followed by currant-jelly stool; they need immediate evaluation for intussusception.

C. Refer any client with diarrhoea longer than seven days who has had no response to usual treatment.

D. Refer an immunocompromised client.

Individual Considerations

A. Paediatrics:

   1. Very young children are at a higher risk of mortality.
   2. Affected children may exhibit chronic diarrhoea, or more than five watery or loose stools a day, but they develop normally and show no signs of malnutrition.
   3. Rotavirus is the most common cause of nosocomial diarrhoea in children and an important cause of acute gastroenteritis in day-care centres. Children whose stool cannot be contained by diapers or toilet use should be excluded from day care until diarrhoea stops.
   4. Breastfeeding can continue during diarrhoea.
   5. Children should not attend day-care facilities until 24 hours or more after diarrhoea ceases.
   6. In cases of *Shigella,* the health department may not permit return to day-care facilities until there are one or more stool cultures negative for *Shigella*.
   7. Children should not go to water parks/swimming pools for one week after symptoms resolve.

B. Adults: Those with concomitant chronic debilitating disease are at a higher risk of mortality.

C. Geriatrics:

   1. Elderly are at a higher risk of mortality secondary to dehydration. Signs of dehydration include the following:
      a. Confusion.
      b. Muscle weakness.
      c. Fever.
      d. Dizziness.
      e. Poor skin turgor.
      f. Hypotension.
      g. Tachycardia.
   2. Diminished thirst mechanism and decreased body water exacerbate dehydration.
   3. New residents to nursing/group homes should be isolated from ill clients.

Resource

Public Health Agency of Canada: https://www.canada.ca/en/public-health/services/food-safety.html

Bibliography

Alexandraki, I., & Smetana, G. W. (2016, October). Acute viral gastroenteritis in adults. *UpToDate*. Retrieved from http://www.uptodate.com/contents/acute-viral-gastroenteritis-in-adults

American Academy of Pediatrics. (2012). Shigella infections. In L. K. Pickering (Ed.), *Red book: 2012 report of the Committee on Infectious Diseases* (29th ed., pp. 239–240). Elk Grove Village, IL: Author. Retrieved from https://redbook.solutions.aap.org/DocumentLibrary/RB12_interior.pdf

Bonheur, J. L. (2015, October 13). Bacterial gastroenteritis. *Medscape*. Retrieved from http://emedicine.medscape.com/article/176400-overview

Boyce, T. G. (2014, July). Overview of gastroenteritis. *Merck manual*. Retrieved from http://www.merckmanuals.com/professional/gastrointestinal-disorders/gastroenteritis/overview-of-gastroenteritis

Centers for Disease Control and Prevention. (2011, April 11). *Rotavirus*. Retrieved from www.cdc.gov/rotavirus/index.html

Centers for Disease Control and Prevention Vaccines & Immunizations. (2012, November 30). *Vaccines and preventable diseases: Rotavirus vaccination*. Retrieved from www.cdc.gov/vaccines/vpd-vac/rotavirus/default.htm#ed

Lee, R. M., Lessler, J., Lee, R. A., Rudolph, K. E., Reich, N. G., Perl, T. M., & Cummings, D. A. (2013). Incubation periods of viral gastroenteritis: A systematic review. *BMC Infectious Diseases, 13*, 446. doi:10.1186/1471-2334-13-446

Nettina, S. (2010). *The Lippincott manual of nursing practice* (9th ed.). Philadelphia, PA: Wolters Kluwer Lippincott Williams & Wilkins.

RotaTeq (Rotavirus Vaccine, Live, Oral, Pentavalent). (2013). *Highlights of prescribing information*. Retrieved from http://www.fda.gov/downloads/BiologicsBloodVaccines/Vaccines/ApprovedProducts/UCM142288.pdf

Surawicz, C. M., Brandt, L. J., Binion, D. G., Ananthakrishnan, A. N., Curry, S. R., Gilligan, P. H., & Zuckerbraun, B. S. (2013). Guidelines for diagnosis, treatment, and prevention of *Clostridium difficile* infections. *American Journal of Gastroenterology, 108*, 478–498. doi:10.1038/ajg.2013.4

World Health Organization. (2010, September 22). *Statement on Rotarix and Rotateq vaccines and intussusception.* Retrieved from http://www.who.int/immunization/sage/3_Rotarix_statement.pdf

Gastro-esophageal Reflux Disease

Cheryl A. Glass, Audra C. Malone, and Kristie A. D. Morydz

Definition
A. Gastro-esophageal reflux disease (GERD) is symptoms or complications resulting from the reflux of gastric contents into the oesophagus or beyond, into the oral cavity (including larynx) or lung.
B. GER is considered a normal physiological process in healthy infants, children, and adults. Most episodes last <3 minutes, and most often occur 30 to 60 minutes after meals and with reclining positions. GORD is present when the symptoms occur more than twice a week.
C. Complications of GERD include erosive oesophagitis, oesophageal strictures, and Barrett's oesophagus.
D. A very large population of clients will present after self-medicating with antacids, bicarbonate soda, and over-the-counter (OTC) medications. Management of GERD should be tailored to the frequency, severity, and duration of symptoms.

Incidence/Prevalence
A. GERD is very common. Daily heartburn typically occurring postprandially has been estimated to affect 17% to 65% of the normal adult population. Reflux oesophagitis affects 30% to 80% of women at some time during pregnancy. It is estimated that 30% to 90% of asthmatics have GERD. Barrett's oesophagus, which affects fewer than 1% of adults, is commonly associated with GERD.

Pathogenesis
A. GERD is relaxation or incompetence of the lower oesophagus persisting beyond the newborn period. Relaxation of the lower oesophageal sphincter (LOS) allows reflux of gastric acid and pepsin into the distal oesophagus. Heartburn occurs when reverse peristaltic waves cause regurgitation of acidic stomach contents into the oesophagus. Anatomical abnormalities, such as a hiatal hernia, predispose persons to GERD. Improper diet and nervous tension are also precipitating factors.
B. GERD has been identified as a trigger for asthma, possibly by the activation of vagal reflexes and/or microaspiration. Asthma may promote GERD, and GERD may provoke asthma. Some asthma medications may reduce LOS tone, further complicating the picture. Conversely, a client with GERD may experience pulmonary disease as a response to the oesophageal acid exposure.

Predisposing Factors
A. Obesity.
B. Consuming large meals.
C. Pregnancy.
D. Immature, weak sphincter in newborns.
E. Emotional stress.
F. Increased abdominal pressure from tight clothes, straining to lift or defecate, or swallowing air.
G. Ingesting drugs and foods that promote LOS relaxation:
  1. Nonsteroidal anti-inflammatory drugs (NSAIDs).
  2. Benzodiazepines.
  3. Calcium channel blockers.
  4. Theophylline.
  5. Nitrates.
  6. Anticholinergics.
  7. Alcohol.
  8. Chocolate and peppermint.
H. Smoking: Increases stomach acid and LOS pressure.
I. Ingestion of caustic agents such as lye.
J. Infection by agents, such as *Candida*, herpes simplex, or cytomegalovirus (CMV), that directly attack the oesophageal mucosa.
K. Compromised immunity, from AIDS, diabetes, or chemotherapy.
L. Asthma.

Common Findings
A. Heartburn.
B. Regurgitation of fluid or food.
C. Chest pain.

Alarm Symptoms
A. Dysphagia (difficulty swallowing).
B. Unintentional weight loss.
C. Predominant upper abdominal pain.
D. Haematemesis (vomiting blood).
E. Melaena (black faeces/blood stool).
F. Odynophagia (painful swallowing).
G. Severe symptoms.

Other Signs and Symptoms
A. Retrosternal aching or burning.
B. Nocturnal aspiration, water or "acid" brash.
C. Harsh taste in the mouth upon awakening.
D. Chronic cough, especially at bedtime.
E. Hoarseness.
F. Globus sensation.
G. Nausea.
H. Dental erosion.
I. Infants: Failure to thrive (FTT), vomiting.

Subjective Data
A. Review the onset, duration, and course of heartburn or other symptoms.
B. Review medication history, including OTC medication and herbals.
  1. Has the client been taking OTC antacids, H_2 blockers, or OTC proton pump inhibitors (PPIs)?
  2. How long has the client been using these OTCs?
  3. Is the client taking drugs that induce oesophagitis, such as the following?
    a. Antibiotics.
    b. Alendronate.
    c. NSAIDs.
    d. Ascorbic acid.
    e. Potassium chloride.
    f. Quinidine.
    g. Iron.
C. Ask the client about alleviating and aggravating factors.
D. Review the client's habits, including smoking and alcohol intake.
E. Inquire about other symptoms, such as weight loss, dysphagia, blood loss, regurgitation, and diarrhoea.

F. Establish the client's usual weight to determine the extent of the problem.
G. Ask the client about any history of asthma and Crohn's disease (CD).
H. Rule out ingestion of caustic agents, especially in the paediatric population.
I. Review the client's dietary history for bulimia.

Physical Examination
A. Check pulse, respirations, blood pressure (BP), and weight.
B. General observation of respiratory distress, including stridor.
C. Inspect:
  1. Examine throat and evaluate mouth for dental erosion.
  2. Assess swallowing ability.
D. Auscultate:
  1. Evaluate the presence of wheezing in the lungs.
  2. Auscultate the heart.
  3. Evaluate the abdomen in all four quadrants.
E. Palpate:
  1. Palpate the abdomen for the presence of hepatosplenomegaly and masses.
  2. Assess the abdomen for tenderness or distension.
F. Perform rectal examination (if indicated for any history of haematemesis).

Diagnostic Tests
A. Clinical examination and history alone usually confirm the diagnosis in the vast majority of reflux sufferers.
B. Rule out cardiac/noncardiac chest pain before institution of therapy (see section "Chest Pain" in Chapter 10, Cardiovascular Guidelines).
C. Endoscopy is not required for the presence of typical GORD symptoms but is recommended for the presence of alarm symptoms or for screening clients at high risk for complications.
D. Endoscopy with biopsy is usually the first diagnostic tool in cases of caustic ingestion or suspected infectious aetiology. The American College of Gastroenterology (ACG) does not recommend an endoscopy to establish the diagnosis of GORD-related asthma, chronic cough, or laryngitis.
E. Ambulatory 24-hour pH monitoring: Prolonged monitoring is the best clinical tool for diagnosing GORD in asthmatics. However, it is very expensive and not universally available.
F. Upper gastrointestinal (GI) series or barium contrast radiography is not used to diagnose GORD, but rules out anatomic abnormalities of the upper digestive tract.
G. Oesophageal manometry is not used for the diagnosis of GORD. It is used to evaluate clients who have failed to respond to an empiric trial of PPIs.
H. Guaiac test for occult blood: Bleeding may accompany reflux oesophagitis and be slow and chronic, resulting in iron-deficiency anaemia, or brisk, resulting in haematemesis. GORD may not be obvious to the clinician when obtaining a client history, especially in an asthmatic client with confounding respiratory symptoms.
I. Consider *Helicobacter pylori* testing.

Differential Diagnoses
A. Cancer—gastric or oesophageal.
B. Myocardial infarction (MI)/angina.
C. Oesophageal spasm.
D. Gallbladder disease.
E. Pyloric stenosis.
F. Infections: CMV, herpes simplex virus, and *Candida*.
G. Peptic ulcer.
H. Ingestion of caustic substance.
I. Self-induced vomiting/bulimia.
J. Food allergy.
K. Eosinophilic oesophagitis.
L. Autoimmune skin disorders affecting the oesophagus.

Plan
A. General interventions: Management depends on the cause and severity of symptoms.
B. Client teaching: *Refer to Client Teaching Guide: Gastroesophageal Reflux Disease.*
C. Dietary management:
  1. Weight loss is advised for overweight or obese clients with GERD symptoms.
  2. At present, there is no supporting data for special dietary precautions; however, a dietary elimination of foods helps to identify triggers.
D. Medical and surgical management:
  1. The Nissen fundoplication is a surgical procedure used to treat GERD in asthmatics. It improves the antireflux barrier and provides a lasting solution. Because it is not always successful, it is reserved for severe cases. The Nissen operation is often performed as a laparoscopic procedure. Achalasia or severe hypomotility (scleroderma-like oesophagus) are conditions that would be contraindications to Nissen fundoplication.
  2. Surgical therapy is not recommended for clients who do not respond to PPI therapy.
  3. The ACG guidelines note that surgical therapy is as effective as medical therapy for carefully selected clients with chronic GERD when performed by an experienced surgeon.
  4. Clients on NSAIDs who experience upper gastric pain, including reflux, need to be referred for endoscopy as soon as possible.
E. Pharmacological therapy:
  1. The potentially adverse effects of acid suppression include the increased risk of community-acquired pneumonia and GI infections, including, *Clostridium difficile*–associated diarrhoea.
  2. Long-term use of acid suppression therapy without a diagnosis is not advised.
  3. The target of pharmacological therapy is improvement in quality of life through the reduction/relief of symptoms and healing of EO.
  4. On-demand or self-directed therapy has been shown to be effective; however, client's use and response should be evaluated.
  5. Histamine-2 receptor antagonists (H_2 blockers) are effective in managing milder, infrequent GI symptoms. Tolerance occurs with chronic use of H_2 blockers. Several H_2 blockers are currently available by prescription or OTC: famotidine, cimetidine, and ranitidine.
  6. PPIs are used for both GERD and EO and are considered the "gold standard" of treatment:
    a. Initiation of a PPI should be prescribed once a day, before the first meal of the day. For maximal pH

control, the traditional delayed-release PPI should be administered 30 to 60 minutes before a meal.
    b. Avoid the concomitant use of clopidogrel with omeprazole or esomeprazole because of the significant reduction of the antiplatelet activity of copidogrel. This is a Food and Drug Administration (FDA) safety labelling change.
    c. Dosages are age- and weight-based.
    d. Long-term therapy should be titrated down to the lowest effective dose based on symptom control.
    e. Clients may experience a relapse in their GERD symptoms after discontinuance, and therefore may need to be tapered off or use a stepdown approach with an antacid or an H_2 blocker.
    f. No PPI is approved for use in infants younger than one year.
    g. PPIs are currently available by prescription and OTC (see Table 11.10).
    h. Clients with known osteoporosis can remain on PPI therapy except for long-term use in clients with other risks for hip fracture.
    i. PPI therapy can be a risk factor for *C. difficile* infection, and should be used with care for clients at risk.

Follow-Up
A. Noncardiac chest pain due to GERD should have a diagnostic evaluation before institution of therapy.
B. Empiric treatment with a PPI may be attempted for a short period except for clients presenting with any alarm symptoms. Schedule a return visit in one to two weeks to evaluate the relief of symptoms.
C. Clients have been having frequent relapses; failure to adequately respond or long-term OTC H_2 blockers and PPI use should have an endoscopic evaluation.
D. The need for prescribed long-term PPI treatment or the presence of alarm symptoms requires a gastroenterology consultation.
E. Consider bone density studies for clients with long-term PPI use.

Consultation/Referral
A. GERD diagnosis should not be made without a full evaluation in infants with vomiting or poor weight gain; refer to a paediatric gastroenterologist for evaluation.
B. Referral is necessary if the client fails to improve after trying two different medications, or if the client has dysphagia, recent weight loss, or blood loss.
C. PPI nonresponders need to be referred for evaluation.

Individual Considerations
A. Pregnancy:
    1. The diagnosis of heartburn during pregnancy is usually made by taking a thorough history. Underlying causes of GERD in pregnancy are diminished gastric motility and displacement of stomach by enlarging uterus.
    2. Sodium bicarbonate–containing antacids should be avoided as they may lead to metabolic alkalosis and fluid overload in both the foetus and mother.
    3. To rule out pregnancy-induced hypertension (PIH), evaluate the client immediately for signs and symptoms of sudden-onset discomfort with no relief from antacids (PIH or haemolysis, elevated liver enzymes, and low platelets [HELLP] syndrome).
B. Paediatrics:
    1. Some regurgitation is normal in neonates because the cardiac sphincter is immature and weak. However, vomiting is an abnormal sign associated with overfeeding, sepsis, metabolic disorders such as galactosaemia, increased intracranial pressure (ICP), and intestinal atresia and stenosis. Regurgitation and vomiting must be differentiated:
      a. Regurgitation most frequently occurs within the first hour after feeding in conjunction with burping or spontaneous eructation of air.
      b. Infants may exhibit refusal to eat, irritability, or arching of their back during or immediately after feeding.
      c. Vomiting, often projectile in nature, can occur at any time and results in the loss of significant amounts of body fluids and electrolytes.
    2. Milk protein sensitivity should be ruled out.
    3. There is no evidence to eliminate specific foods in children and adolescents to manage GERD.
    4. The major agents used in children are gastric acid buffering agents, mucosal surface barriers, and gastric antisecretory agents.
C. Geriatrics:
    1. GERD prevalence increases with age and may be asso-associated with a hiatal hernia.
    2. Prolonged reflux results in oesophagitis and may lead to stricture development. Chronic recurrence may develop into Barrett's syndrome.
    3. Treatment of GERD is the same as for general adults; however, do diagnostic testing in short-time sequence secondary to stricture and cancer in the elderly.

Resources
Canadian Society on Intestinal Research: https://www.badgut.org/
The Rome Foundation: https://theromefoundation.org/
The 2013 guidelines for the diagnosis and management of gastroesophageal reflux disease: http://gi.org/wp-contents/uploads/2013/03/ACG_Guideline_GERD_March_2013.pdf
https://www.cag-acg.org/images/publications/GERD_Enhanced_Primary_Care_Pathway_July_2016.pdf

Bibliography
American College of Gastroenterology. (2011). Pregnancy and gastrointestinal disorders. *Pregnancy monograph*. Retrieved from http://gi.org/wp-content/uploads/2011/07/institute-PregnancyMonograph.pdf
Fallone, C. A., Chiba, N., van Zanten, S. V., Fischbach, L., Gisbert, J. P., Hunt, R. H., & Marshall, J. K. (2016). The Toronto consensus for the treatment of Helicobacter pylori infection in adults. *Gastroenterology*, 151(1), 51–69. doi:10.1053/j.gastro.2016.04.006
Kahrilas, P. J., Shaheen, N. J., & Vaezi, M. F. (2008, October). American Gastroenterological Association Medical position statement on the management of gastroesophageal reflux disease. *Gastroenterology*, 135, 1383–1391. doi:10.1053/j.gastro.2008.08.045. Retrieved from http://www.gastrojournal.org/issues?_key-S0016-5085(08)X0010-1
Katz, P. O., Gerson, L. B., & Vela, M. F. (2013, February). Guidelines for the diagnosis and management of gastroesophageal reflux disease. *American Journal of Gastroenterology*, 108, 308–328. doi:10.1038/ajg.2012.444
Nettina, S. (2010). *The Lippincott manual of nursing practice* (9th ed.). Philadelphia, PA: Wolters Kluwer Lippincott Williams & Wilkins.
Poh, C. H., Navarro-Rodriguez, T., & Fass, R. (2010). Review: Treatment of gastroesophageal reflux disease in the elderly. *American Journal of Medicine*, 123, 496–501. doi:10.1016/j.amjmed.2009.07.036

TABLE 11.10 Proton Pump Inhibitors

Omeprazole
Lansoprazole
Rabeprazole
Pantoprazole
Esomeprazole
Dexlansoprazole

Saad, R. J., & Chey, W. D. First-line treatment strategies for *Helicobacter pylori* infection. *Gastroenterology & Endoscopy News,* June 23, 2015, 1–8. Retrieved from http://www.gastroendonews.com/Review-Articles/Article/06-15/First-Line-Treatment-Strategies-for-Helicobacter-nbsp-pylori-Infection/32678/ses=ogst

Surawicz, C. M., Brandt, L. J., Binion, D. G., Ananthakrishnan, A. N., Curry, S. R., Gilligan, P. H., & Zuckerbraun, B. S. (2013). Guidelines for diagnosis, treatment, and prevention of *Clostridium difficile* infections. *American Journal of Gastroenterology, 108,* 478–498. doi:10.1038/ajg.2013.4

Giardiasis

Cheryl A. Glass, Audra C. Malone, and Kristie A. D. Morydz

Definition
A. *Giardia intestinalis* (formerly *Giardia lamblia*) is the leading parasitic cause of diarrhoea. Infestation can lead to malabsorption by coating large areas of the small bowel, particularly the lower duodenum and upper jejunum. Most people infected with *G. intestinalis* remain asymptomatic, and most infections are self-limited.

Incidence/Prevalence
A. Giardiasis has a worldwide distribution. It is common in areas where water supplies are contaminated by human sewage. The age-specific prevalence of giardiasis is highest in children one to nine years and adults 35 to 44 years of age. The peak onset occurs annually during early summer through early fall.

Pathogenesis
A. *G. intestinalis* is a flagellated protozoan. The infective form is the cyst. Humans are the principal reservoir of infection, but *Giardia* can infect dogs, cats, beavers, and other animals that can contaminate water with faeces containing cysts.
B. People become infected either directly, by hand-to-mouth transfer of cysts from faeces of an infected person (e.g., child care), or indirectly, by ingestion of faeces-contaminated water or food. Most community-wide epidemics result from contaminated water supplies.
C. Incubation period is one to 3 weeks, with an average of seven to 10 days. Infection is limited to the small intestine and the biliary tract. Disease is communicable for as long as the infected person excretes cysts.

Predisposing Factors
A. About 50% to 75% of outbreaks occur in child care settings.
B. Travel to endemic areas.
C. Subjection to unsanitary food handling.
D. Exposure to contaminated water supplies.
E. Anal intercourse.
F. Cystic fibrosis (CF).
G. Immunocompromised individuals are at high risk.

Common Findings
Acute complaints:
A. Explosive, foul-smelling diarrhoea.
B. Mucus in stools, bulky stools.
C. Upper abdominal pain or discomfort.
D. Flatulence.
E. Nausea.
F. Anorexia.
G. Weight loss.

Other Signs and Symptoms
Chronic complaints:
A. Intermittent loose stools (but not diarrhoea).
B. Steatorrhoea.
C. Increased flatulence or distension.
D. Vague abdominal discomfort.
E. Fatigue related to anaemia.
F. Profound weight loss (10%–20% of body weight).
G. Malabsorption.
H. Urticaria.
I. Dehydration.

Subjective Data
A. Review the onset, duration, and course of symptoms. Is diarrhoea acute or chronic?
B. Ask the client about travel to areas known for giardiasis.
C. Review the client's intake of medications and other substances that can cause diarrhoea, especially antibiotics, laxatives, quinidine, magnesium-containing antacids, excess alcohol, caffeine, herbal teas, digitalis, loop diuretics, antihypertensive agents, and sorbitol-containing (sugar-free) gums and mints.
D. Review the nature of the client's bowel movements (BMs), including frequency; consistency; volume; and presence of blood, pus, or mucus.
E. Does diarrhoea have any relationship to meals? Onset of diarrhoea within hours of ingesting a potentially contaminated food is suggestive of bacterial infection such as *Escherichia coli*; this is confirmed by checking whether others were similarly affected.
F. Ask the client about associated symptoms that need evaluation, such as fever, abdominal pain, or rash.
G. Ask the client if other family members or sexual contacts are also ill.
H. Establish the client's normal weight, and, if any weight has recently been lost, review amount and over what period of time.

Physical Examination
The physical examination may reveal no specific finding:
A. Check temperature, pulse, respirations, blood pressure (BP), and weight.
B. Inspect general appearance for signs of dehydration; include evaluation of mucous membranes and infants' fontanelles.
C. Auscultate abdomen for bowel sounds in all quadrants.
D. Palpate:
 1. Palpate the abdomen for masses, tenderness, guarding, and rebound. Clients with periumbilical or right lower quadrant (RLQ) pain and copious volumes of watery stool are likely to have a small-bowel aetiology.
 2. Palpate lymph nodes for enlargement.
E. Perform rectal examination.

Diagnostic Tests
A. Enzyme immunoassay (EIA) and are becoming the standard for diagnosis of giardiasis in the United States.
B. Stool bacteria culture and sensitivity.
C. Mucous stool for leukocytes: Mucus free of leukocytes is the hallmark of irritable bowel syndrome (IBS); a large number of white cells suggests inflammatory or invasive diarrhoea.
D. Stool for ova and parasites; test three times on alternate days. Parasites are passed intermittently, so examine stools on alternating days.
E. Stool for occult blood.

F. Endoscopy to identify cyst in duodenal fluid or small-bowel tissue.

Differential Diagnoses
A. Crohn's disease (CD).
B. Malabsorption.
C. *E. coli* infection.
D. IBS.
E. Viral diarrhoea.
F. Lactose intolerance.
G. Other bacterial infections, such as *Shigella, Salmonella,* and *Campylobacter.*
H. Celiac disease.

Plan
A. General interventions:
   1. Advise children and adult workers with diarrhoea to stay away from day-care centres until they become asymptomatic.
   2. Advise the client's household and sexual contacts to seek medical examination and treatment.
B. Client teaching:
   1. *Refer to Client Teaching Guide: Diarrhoea.*
   2. Discuss safe sexual practices. Avoiding oral–anal and oral–genital sex can decrease venereal transmission.
   3. Recommend contact precautions for duration of illness for diapered and/or incontinent children.
   4. People with diarrhoea caused by *Giardia* should not use recreational water venues, including swimming pools and water slides, for two weeks after symptoms resolve.
C. Dietary management:
   1. Encourage the client or caregiver to prevent dehydration from diarrhoea by increasing fluids.
   2. Advise restricting milk products to rule out lactose intolerance. Postgiardia lactose intolerance occurs in 20% to 40% of clients.
   3. Advise backpackers, campers, and people likely to be exposed to contaminated water to avoid drinking directly from streams. To make water for safe drinking, boil water, or use chemical disinfection or filtration. Boiling water is the most reliable method to make water safe for drinking.
D. Pharmacological therapy:
   1. Treatment of asymptomatic carriers is not generally recommended.
   2. **Fluid and electrolyte management is critical in clients with large-volume diarrhoeal losses.**
   3. Treat children with acute or chronic diarrhoea who manifest failure to thrive (FTT), malabsorption, or other gastrointestinal (GI) tract symptoms when giardia has been identified.
   4. Metronidazole, tinidazole, and nitazoxanide are first-line treatment:
      a. Metronidazole is the principal agent used to treat giardiasis.
      b. Tinidazole as a one-time dose for children three years of age and older; it has fewer side effects than metronidazole.
      c. Nitazoxanide oral suspension has similar efficacy to metronidazole and has the advantage of treating other intestinal parasites; it has been approved for children one year of age and older.
   5. Paromomycin, a nonabsorbable aminoglycoside, is recommended for treatment of symptomatic infection in pregnant women in the second and third trimesters.

Follow-Up
A. Relapses after treatment are common, especially in immunocompromised clients.
B. Schedule follow-ups at six weeks and six months after treatment, as indicated.
C. If diarrhoea persists for two weeks or more, secondary evaluation is indicated. Stools should be examined again for blood, leukocytes, and parasites.
D. Clients who remain undiagnosed after an extensive evaluation and trial of metronidazole often turn out to have IBS or surreptitious laxative misuse.

Consultation/Referral
A. Severely dehydrated or malnourished clients should be admitted to hospital for further care.
B. Consultations with a paediatric infectious disease specialist and paediatric gastroenterologist are recommended.

Individual Considerations
A. Pregnancy:
   1. Treatment of clients during pregnancy is recommended. Giardiasis in pregnancy is associated with dehydration, malabsorption, or severe symptoms.
   2. Malabsorptive symptoms may persist as regeneration of functioning intestinal mucosa requires time.
   3. Breastfeeding appears to protect infants from *G. intestinalis*.
B. Paediatrics:
   1. **When an outbreak is suspected in a child-care setting, the local health department should be notified to investigate.**
   2. Children who are carriers do not have to be excluded from childcare; however, personal hygiene/universal precautions should be followed.

Resources
Ontario Ministry of Health and Long-Term Care Giardisis Fact Sheet: http://www.health.gov.on.ca/en/public/publications/disease/giardiasis.aspx
Public Health Agency of Canada Giardia Fact Sheet: https://www.canada.ca/en/public-health/services/laboratory-biosafety-biosecurity/pathogen-safety-data-sheets-risk-assessment/giardia-lamblia.html

Bibliography
American Academy of Pediatrics. (2012). Giardia intestinalis infections. In L. K. Pickering (Ed.), *Red book: 2012 report of the Committee on Infectious Diseases* (29th ed., pp. 333–335). Elk Grove Village, IL: Author. Retrieved from https://redbook.solutions.aap.org/DocumentLibrary/RB12_interior.pdf
Gardner, T. B., & Hill, D. R. (2001). Treatment of giardiasis. *Clinical Microbiology Reviews, 14*(1), 114–128. doi:10.1128/CMR.14.1.114-128.2001
Leder, K., & Weller, P. F. (2009, May 1). Epidemiology, clinical manifestations, and diagnosis of giardiasis. *UpToDate*. Retrieved from http://www.uptodate.com/online/content/topic.do?topicKey=parasite/7013&view=print
Nazer, H. (2016, February 15). Giardiasis. *Medscape*. Retrieved from http://emedicine.medscape.com/article/176718-overview
Nettina, S. (2010). *The Lippincott manual of nursing practice* (9th ed.). Philadelphia, PA: Wolters Kluwer Lippincott Williams & Wilkins.
Sharma, G. D. (2013, June 17). Cystic fibrosis. *Medscape*. Retrieved from http://emedicine.medscape.com/article/1001602-overview
Weller, P. F., & Kaplan, S. L. (2015, June 16). Treatment and prevention of giardiasis. *UpToDate*. Retrieved from http://www.uptodate.com/contents/treatment-and-prevention-of-giardiasis

▶ Client Teaching Guides are available at https://connect.springerpub.com/content/reference-book/978-0-8261-9498-5

Haemorrhoids

Cheryl A. Glass, Audra C. Malone, and Kristie A. D. Morydz

Definition
A. Haemorrhoids are clusters of vascular tissues, smooth muscle, and connective tissue of the anal canal. Internal haemorrhoids are above the anorectal line, covered by rectal mucosa, and can be found at any position in the rectum. Internal haemorrhoids are graded by severity (see Table 11.11).
B. External haemorrhoids are below the anorectal line, covered by anal skin, and appear as painless, flaccid skin tags (see Figure 11.3).
C. When blood within the haemorrhoid becomes clotted due to obstruction, the haemorrhoids are referred to as thrombosed and appear as blue, shiny masses.
D. Although rectal bleeding is commonly associated with haemorrhoids, it may be a symptom of other disease processes, such as colorectal cancer, inflammatory bowel disease (IBD), other colitides, diverticular disease, and angiodysplasia.

Incidence/Prevalence
A. The incidence of haemorrhoids is unknown. Clients tend to present after utilization and failure of over-the-counter (OTC) treatments. Haemorrhoids are common in people over 20 years of age. They are uncommon in people under age 20 years except secondary to pregnancy.

Pathogenesis
A. Mechanism is unknown. Prolapse may be initiated by shearing force from passage of large firm stool, by increased venous pressure from heart failure (HF) or pregnancy, or by straining that occurs with lifting or defecation.

Predisposing Factors
A. Increased abdominal pressure (constipation, pelvic congestion, pregnancy, portal hypertension, cirrhosis).
B. Altered bowel function (constipation, diarrhoea).
C. Poor muscle tone.
D. Low-fiber diet.
E. Sedentary jobs, such as driving trucks, piloting planes.
F. Loss of muscle tone due to advanced age.
G. Anal intercourse.
H. Obesity.
I. Colon malignancy.
J. Rectal surgery.
K. IBD.

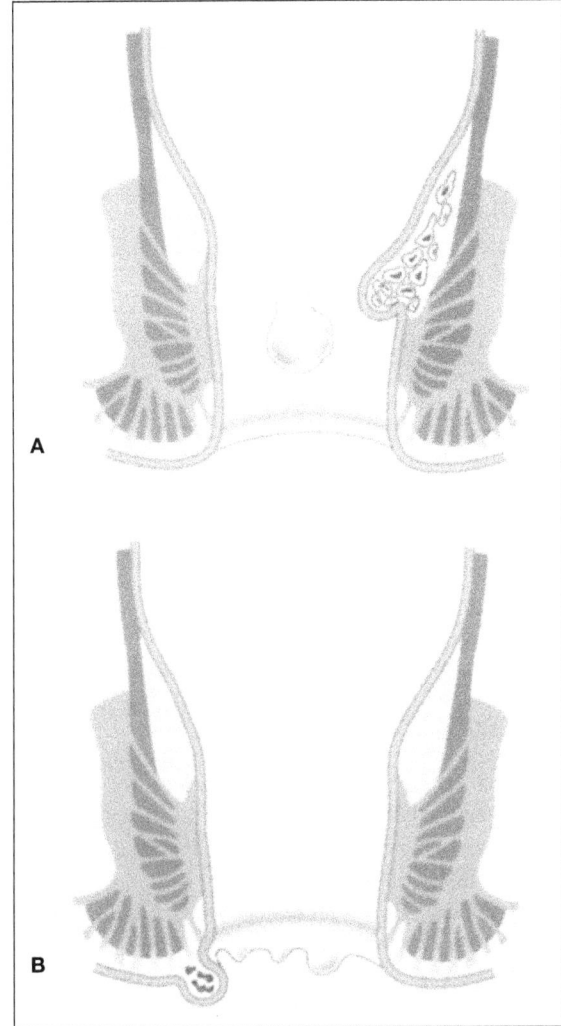

FIGURE 11.3 Internal and external haemorrhoids. (A) Internal haemorrhoid: Covered by a thin sheet of tissue called mucous membrane, an internal haemorrhoid bulges into the rectal opening and may sink a bit during bowel movements. (B) External haemorrhoid: Covered by skin, an external haemorrhoid protrudes from the rectum.

Common Findings
A. Cardinal features:
  1. Bleeding: Painless, bright red bleeding with defecation (internal).
  2. Anal pruritus.
  3. Prolapse.
  4. Pain related to thrombosis.

Other Signs and Symptoms
A. Visible prolapsed mass.
B. Incomplete defecation.
C. Leakage of faeces (internal haemorrhoids).
D. Excessive moisture.
E. Weakness or fatigue, with anaemia.
F. External haemorrhoid: Covered by skin, an external haemorrhoid protrudes from the rectum.

Subjective Data
A. Review the onset and duration of symptoms, especially the history of rectal bleeding, prolapse, and issues of hygiene and pain.
B. Review the client's history of haemorrhoids and treatments, including surgery.

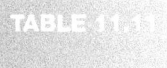 **Severity of Haemorrhoids to Guide Treatment Options**

Grade	Severity
I	The haemorrhoids bleed but do not prolapse.
II	The haemorrhoids prolapse upon defecation but reduce spontaneously.
III	The haemorrhoids prolapse upon defecation and must be reduced manually.
IV	The haemorrhoids are prolapsed and cannot be reduced manually.

C. Ask the client about recent pregnancy, liver disease, and constipation.
D. Inquire about the client's job and level of daily activity.
E. Review the client's sexual practices for anal intercourse.
F. Review the client's dietary history for fluid intake and sources/amount of fiber.
G. Ask about bowel habits, including frequency, consistency, and ease of evacuation.
H. Review a detailed family history, with emphasis on intestinal disease.

Physical Examination
A. Check temperature (if indicated), pulse, respirations, blood pressure (BP), and weight.
B. Inspect:
  1. Observe rectal area for skin tags, prolapse, irritation, fissures, and condyloma:
     a. Internal haemorrhoids are usually not visible unless prolapsed.
     b. External haemorrhoids protrude with straining or standing.
  2. Using anoscopy: Visualize internal rectum for haemorrhoids, fissures, or masses.
C. Palpate:
  1. Palpate abdomen for masses.
  2. Internal haemorrhoids are usually not palpable unless thrombosed.
  3. Perform digital rectal examination.

Diagnostic Tests
A. Haematocrit (Hct) and haemoglobin, if bleeding present.
B. Anoscopy: Reveals internal haemorrhoids as bright red to purplish bulges. Digital rectal examination alone can neither diagnose nor exclude internal haemorrhoids; anoscopy is required.
C. Sigmoidoscopy or colonoscopy (geriatric population).
D. Stool for guaiac testing.
E. Air-contrast barium enema (BE) for atypical bleeding.

Differential Diagnoses
A. Condyloma acuminata.
B. Rectal prolapse.
C. Rectal bleeding due to one of the following:
  1. Colorectal cancer.
  2. Polyps.
  3. Anal fissure.
  4. Fistula.
  5. Perianal abscess.
  6. IBD, including ulcerative colitis (UC) and Crohn's disease (CD).
  7. Diverticulitis.
  8. Pelvic tumour.

Plan
A. General interventions: No treatment is necessary if the client is asymptomatic except for maintaining regular bowel habits and performing comfort measures.
▶ B. Client teaching: *Refer to Client Teaching Guide: Haemorrhoids.*
C. Dietary management: High-fiber diet and an adequate fluid intake should be continued indefinitely in order to maintain a soft bulky stool that can be passed without straining (see Appendix B, Diet Recommendations, Table B.6).
D. Medical and surgical management:
  1. Use warm sitz baths up to three times a day for irritation and pruritus.
  2. Conservative treatment for thrombosed haemorrhoid includes lying prone and applying ice pack to the area.
  3. Incision and evacuation of thrombosis or clot may be performed under local anesthaesia. Other treatments for thrombosed haemorrhoids noted in clinical trials have included the following:
     a. Topical nitroglycerin 0.2% topical ointment for temporary analgesia. The most common side effect is headache.
     b. Topical nifedipine.
     c. In a small study, one intrasphincter injection of botulinum toxin relieved pain within 24 hours.
  4. Symptomatic Grade I, Grade II, and some Grade III haemorrhoids may be treated by the following:
     a. Rubber band ligation is the first-line treatment for Grades I and II internal haemorrhoids. Rubber band ligation is the most widely used and is associated with fewer complications than surgery.
     b. Bipolar, infrared, and laser coagulation (may require more than one treatment).
     c. Sclerotherapy.
     d. Stapled haemorrhoidopexy can be performed in clients with Grade III haemorrhoids.
  5. External haemorrhoids usually do not require surgical therapy except in cases of thrombosis. For selective Grade III and Grade IV internal and strangulated haemorrhoids that fail medical and nonoperative therapies, surgical treatment is required. Stapled haemorrhoidopexy has a faster recovery but has a higher recurrence rate. Haemorrhoidectomy is the treatment of last choice because it requires hospitalization and an extended recovery period, and it risks compromising competence of the anal sphincter. Haemorrhoidectomy complications include the following:
     a. Urinary retention.
     b. Urinary tract infection (UTI).
     c. Faecal impaction.
     d. Pain.
     e. Haemorrhage.
     f. Stricture formation (1%) or sphincter damage (rare).
     g. Nonhealing wound.
     h. Fistula formation.
     i. Anal leakage.
E. Pharmacological therapy:
  1. First-line treatment: Bulk-forming agents such as psyllium seed, methylcellulose, or calcium polycarbophil.
  2. Stool softener: Docusate sodium or docusate calcium.
  3. For irritation and pruritus, topical creams and anesthetics are found in OTC products such as pramoxine HCl and topical hydrocortisone preparations.
  4. Nonsteroidal anti-inflammatory drugs (NSAIDs) supplemented with narcotics. An oral analgesic such as codeine may be prescribed for thrombosed haemorrhoids. However, codeine causes constipation.

Follow-Up
A. None is necessary if resolution occurs and the client is asymptomatic.
B. Reevaluate the client in two weeks for further treatment if symptoms persist.
C. Evaluate the client with an intervention in seven to 10 days.

▶ Client Teaching Guides are available at https://connect.springerpub.com/content/reference-book/978-0-8261-9498-5

Consultation/Referral

A. The onset of urinary retention and fever immediately after an office-based procedure may be the initial sign of perianal sepsis and mandates emergent client evaluation.

B. Refer the client to a surgeon if haemorrhoids bleed repeatedly, prolapse, produce intractable pain, or are thrombosed, and if three to five consecutive days of treatment do not provide relief.

Individual Considerations

A. Pregnancy:
  1. Labour, which results in pressure on the pelvic floor by the presenting part of the foetus and the expulsive efforts of the woman, may aggravate haemorrhoids, causing protrusion and inflammation during the puerperium. Haemorrhoids may be pushed back after delivery to prevent them from becoming swollen and painful.
  2. Surgical treatment is contraindicated in pregnancy because of the risk of inducing labour.
  3. Conservative treatment is recommended with excision of thrombosed external haemorrhoids if necessary.

B. Paediatrics: Rectal prolapse in children is associated with cystic fibrosis (CF).

Prolapse looks like a pink doughnut or rosette; complete prolapse involving the muscular wall is larger and red, and it has circular folds.

C. Geriatrics:
  1. Prolapse of rectal mucosa is more common in the elderly.
  2. Colonoscopy is recommended in the geriatric population to exclude malignancy or other underlying disease.

Bibliography

American College of Gastroenterology. (2011). Pregnancy and gastrointestinal disorders. *Pregnancy monograph*. Retrieved from http://gi.org/wp-content/uploads/2011/07/institute-PregnancyMonograph.pdf

Bleday, R. (2009, May 1). Patient information: Hemorrhoids. *UptoDate*. Retrieved from http://www.uptodate.com/online/content/topic.do?topicKey=digestiv/8271&view=print

Bleday, R., & Breen, E. (2009, May 1). Treatment of hemorrhoids. *UpToDate*. Retrieved from http://www.uptodate.com/online/content/topic.do?topicKey=colosurg/6160&view=print

Clinical Practice Committee. (2004). American Gastroenterological Association Institute medical position statement: Diagnosis and treatment of hemorrhoids. *Gastroenterology, 126*, 1461–1462.

Fargo, M. V., & Latimer, K. M. (2012). Evaluation and management of common anorectal conditions. *American Family Physician, 85*, 624–630.

Madoff, R. D., & Fleshman, J. W. (2004). American Gastroenterological Association technical review on the diagnosis and treatment of hemorrhoids. *Gastroenterology, 126*(5), 1463–1473. doi:10.1053/j.gastro.2004.03.008

Mounsey, A. L., Halladay, J., & Sadiq, T. S. (2011). Hemorrhoids. *American Family Physician, 84*(2), 204–210.

Nettina, S. (2010). *The Lippincott manual of nursing practice* (9th ed.). Philadelphia, PA: Wolters Kluwer Lippincott Williams & Wilkins.

Rivadeneira, D. E., Steele, S. R., Ternent, C., Chalasani, S., Buie, W. D., & Rafferty, J. L. (2011). Practice parameters for the management of hemorrhoids (revised 2010). *Diseases of the Colon & Rectum, 54*, 1059–1064. doi:10.1097/DCR.0b013e318225513d

Sharma, G. D. (2013, June 17). Cystic fibrosis. *Medscape*. Retrieved from http://emedicine.medscape.com/article/1001602-overview

Thornton, S. C. (2012, September 12). Hemorrhoids. *Medscape*. Retrieved from http://emedicine.medscape.com/article/775407-overview

Hepatitis A

Cheryl A. Glass, Audra C. Malone, and Kristie A. D. Morydz

Definition

A. Hepatitis A is an acute self-limited illness with inflammation of the liver caused by a viral infection. Hepatitis A virus (HAV) is spread by viral shedding. All cases of hepatitis A are reportable to the public health department.

B. The highest titres of HAV in the stool of infected clients occur one to two weeks before the onset of illness (jaundice or elevation of liver enzymes), during which time clients are most likely to transmit infection. Risk subsequently diminishes and is minimal in the week after the onset of jaundice. Few children younger than six years have concomitant jaundice, whereas up to 70% of older children and adults will have jaundice. Fulminant hepatitis is rare, and chronic infectious and carrier states do not occur.

C. Duration of HAV infection is typically eight weeks, but prolonged disease, as long as six months, can occur in 10% to 15% of symptomatic clients, especially in neonates and young children.

D. The major methods of prevention include improved sanitation of water sources, improved hygiene practice prior to food preparation and diaper changes, immunization with the hepatitis A vaccine, and administration of immune globulin (IG).

Incidence/Prevalence

A. Outbreak in custodial institutions accounts for about 10% to 15% of reported HAV in the United States. No appreciable seasonal variation in incidence has been noted.

B. The incidence of mortality from HAV is 0% to 1%. The single most important determinant of illness severity is age; a direct correlation between increasing age and the likelihood of adverse events is present.

Pathogenesis

A. HAV is a small, RNA enterovirus classified as a member of the picornavirus group. Viral replication depends on hepatocyte uptake and synthesis, and assembly occurs exclusively in liver cells. Transmission of HAV is person-to-person primarily by the faecal–oral route and parenterally. The incubation period is 15 to 50 days, with an average of 25 to 30 days. It does not cause chronic infection.

B. Common-source and food- and waterborne epidemics have occurred, including several caused by shellfish contaminated with human sewage. Nosocomial outbreaks have occurred as a result of shedding of HAV from infected, asymptomatic neonates, children, or adults.

Predisposing Factors

A. Ingestion of infected water, food, and shellfish:
  1. Undercooked HAV-contaminated foods are a source of outbreaks.
  2. Cooked foods also can transmit HAV if the temperature during food preparation is inadequate to kill the virus.
  3. Food contaminated after cooking is associated with infected food handlers.

B. Close personal contact with an HAV-infected person:
  1. Contact with a child who attends a child-care centre (especially with children in diapers).
  2. Anal intercourse.
  3. Vertical transmission from mother to foetus (limited).
  4. Personal contact with a newly arriving international adoptee.
C. Poor sanitation or personal hygiene.
D. Crowded living conditions.
E. International travel.
F. Intravenous (IV) drug misuse.
G. Persons with clotting factor disorders.
H. Persons working with nonhuman primates.

Common Findings
A. Asymptomatic, particularly in young children.
B. Malaise.
C. Anorexia.
D. Nausea with/without vomiting.
E. Low-grade fever.
F. Jaundice—icteric phase (70% of older children and adults):
  1. Tea-coloured urine.
  2. Clay-coloured stool.
  3. Abdominal pain.
  4. Pruritus.
  5. Enlarged liver.

Other Signs and Symptoms
A. Infants and children: Mild, nonspecific, flu-like symptoms without jaundice.
B. Adults: Severe, prolonged course with fatigue, headache, vomiting, and symptoms noted earlier.
C. Relapsing hepatitis A is more common in the elderly. There generally has been a protracted course of symptoms, then a relapse of symptoms following an apparent resolution.

Subjective Data
A. Review the duration, onset, and severity of symptoms, including specifics about urine or stool colour changes.
B. Ask the client about family members and sexual contacts with similar symptoms.
C. Review the client's history of blood transfusions, IV drug use, and alcohol misuse.
D. Inquire about occupational exposure.
E. Ask the client about recent international travel or exposure to newly arrived international adoptees.
F. Review immunization status.
G. Review medications for a possible acetaminophen overdose or Ecstasy use as a cause for acute drug-induced liver injury.

Physical Examination
A. Check temperature (acute illness), pulse, respirations, blood pressure (BP), and weight.
B. Inspect:
  1. Note general appearance.
  2. Inspect the skin for slight jaundice or rash.
  3. Inspect mucous membranes and nail beds.
  4. Inspect eyes for yellow sclera.
C. Auscultate lung fields, all quadrants of the abdomen, and the heart.
D. Percuss the abdomen.
E. Palpate: All quadrants of the abdomen for masses, liver tenderness, and hepatosplenomegaly (about 10% of cases).

Diagnostic Tests
A. Viral serology for typing HAV, immunoglobulin G (IgG), and immunoglobulin M (IgM). Serum IgM presents at the onset of illness and disappears within four months, generally indicating current or recent infection. However, it may persist for six months or longer. Presence of IgG anti-HAV antibodies without virus-specific IgM indicates past infection and lifelong immunity.
B. Liver function studies including alanine transaminase (ALT), aspartate transaminase (AST), lactate dehydrogenase (LDH), and alkaline phosphatase (ALP).
C. Bilirubin, direct and indirect.
D. Complete blood count (CBC).
E. Prothrombin time (PT).
F. Urinalysis: Reveals proteinuria and bilirubinuria.
G. Imaging studies are usually not indicated for hepatitis A infection. An ultrasound may be used to exclude other pathology.

Differential Diagnoses
A. Exclusion of other hepatitis types.
B. Mononucleosis.
C. Cancer.
D. Obstructive jaundice.
E. Alcoholic hepatitis or cirrhosis.
F. Hepatotoxic drug use:
  1. Drug-induced liver injury (e.g., acetaminophen, Ecstasy).
  2. Drug-induced hypersensitivity reaction (e.g., sulphasalazine hypersensitivity).
G. Food poisoning.
H. Cytomegalovirus (CMV).
I. Acute HIV infection.

Plan
A. General interventions:
  1. Contact precautions are recommended for diapered and/or incontinent clients for one week after the onset of symptoms.
  2. Children and adults with acute HAV infection should be excluded from school, work, and child-care centres for one week after the onset of illness.
  3. Hepatitis is self-limiting and does not require therapy. Treatment is supportive:
    a. Limit activities secondary to malaise.
    b. Oral contraceptive pills (OCPs) and hormone replacement therapy (HRT) should be stopped to avoid cholestasis.
    c. Alcohol consumption is not advised.
    d. Adults who work as food handlers should not work for one week after the onset of the illness.
  4. Encourage strict handwashing.
B. Client teaching:
  1. *Refer to Client Teaching Guide: Jaundice and Hepatitis.* ◀
  2. Teach the client that major methods for prevention are improved sanitation (e.g., of water sources and in food preparation) and personal hygiene.
  3. Food and travel precautions include the following:
    a. Avoid uncontrolled water resources: Use bottled water, boil water, or add iodine to inactivate the virus.

      b. Avoid raw shellfish.
      c. Avoid uncooked foods.
      d. All fruit should be washed and peeled.
C. Dietary management: Encourage optimum nutrition.
D. Pharmacological therapy:
  1. HAV vaccine preexposure is preferred in all populations unless contraindicated.
  2. Postexposure IG administration given intramuscularly (IM) within two weeks of HAV exposure is 80% to 90% effective in preventing symptomatic infection:
      a. Time of exposure: two weeks or less.
      b. Postexposure prophylaxis with IG is recommended for the following:
         i. Household and sexual contacts of infected persons.
         ii. Newborn infants of HAV-infected mothers.
         iii. Child-care centre staff, children, and their household contacts.
         iv. Students when transmission within school is documented.
         v. Staff in institutions and hospitals.
         vi. People who ingested HAV-contaminated food or water, within two weeks of last exposure.
  3. Vaccines:
      a. Three inactivated HAV vaccines (adult and paediatric formulations) are available in Canada.
      b. A combination of hepatitis A and hepatitis B vaccine is also available for use in both paediatric and adult populations in Canada (see Table 11.12).
  4. Hepatitis A vaccine is recommended for the following:
      a. People 6 months of age or older who are at high risk of infection or those who wish to decrease their risk of infection.
      b. Clients with chronic liver disease.
      c. Homosexual and bisexual men (both adolescents and adults).
      d. Users of illegal injected and noninjected drugs.
      e. Those with occupational risk of exposure, such as handlers of nonhuman primates and persons working with HAV in a laboratory setting.
      f. Travelers who need preexposure immunoprophylaxis. The first dose of hepatitis A vaccine should be administered as soon as travel is considered.
      g. Clients with clotting factor disorders, such as haemophilia.
      h. Routine HAV vaccination is *not* indicated for the following groups:
         i. Child-care centre staff and children.
         ii. Clients and staff in custodial care institutions.
         iii. Hospital personnel; if a client with hepatitis A is admitted to the hospital, routine infection-control precautions will prevent transmission to hospital staff.
         iv. Food service workers.
         v. Clients with haemophilia.
         vi. Sewage workers.
  5. HAV vaccine may be administered simultaneously with other vaccines, including hepatitis B, diphtheria, poliovirus (oral and inactivated), tetanus, oral and IM typhoid, cholera, Japanese encephalitis, rabies, and yellow fever. The HAV vaccine should be given in a separate syringe and at a separate site.
  6. The need for an additional hepatitis A booster beyond the two-dose primary immunization has not been established; however, the CDC reports that extra doses of HAV vaccine are not harmful.
  7. Immune response in immunocompromised clients, such as those with HIV or on haemodialysis, may be suboptimal. The vaccine is inactivated; therefore, no special precautions are needed when vaccinating immunocompromised clients.
  8. Vaccine side effects are generally mild and may include the following:
      a. Local pain at the immunization site.
      b. Localized induration at the injection site.
  9. Acetaminophen may be administered for fever and arthralgia, but maximum dose should be respected.

Follow-Up
A. Dehydration may require hospital admission.
B. Follow up in two weeks for reevaluation.

TABLE 11.12   Dosages and Schedules for Hepatitis A-Containing Vaccines

Vaccine	Antigen(s)	Dose	Schedule (Months: First dose = month 0)	Age
AVAXIM®	160 antigen units HA	0.5 mL	0, 6–36	12 years and older
AVAXIM® Paediatric	80 antigen units HA	0.5 mL	0, 6–36	6 months to less than 16 years
HAVRIX® 1440	1440 ELISA units HA	1.0 mL	0, 6–12	19 years and older
HAVRIX® 720 Junior	720 ELISA units HA	0.5 mL	0, 6–12	6 months to less than 19 years
VAQTA®	50 units HA	1.0 mL	0, 6–18	18 years and older
VAQTA® Paediatric	25 units HA	0.5 mL	0, 6–18	6 months to less than 18 years
ViVAXIM®	160 antigen units HA, *Salmonella typhi*	1.0 mL	0, booster dose of HA vaccine at month 6–36 or HA-Typh-I vaccine at month 36	16 years and older

ELISA, enzyme-linked immunosorbent assay; HA, hepatitis A; HB, hepatitis B.
Source: Canadian Immunization Guideline. (2018). *Part4-Active vaccines*. Retrieved from https://www.canada.ca/en/public-health/services/publications/healthy-living/canadian-immunization-guide-part-4-active-vaccines/page-6-hepatitis-a-vaccine.html.

C. Check for hepatitis B immunity and vaccinate.
D. Hepatitis A is reportable to the public health department.

Consultation/Referral
A. Only if necessary.

Individual Considerations
A. Pregnancy:
   1. Pregnant women recently exposed to HAV should receive prophylactic gamma globulin.
   2. HAV is an inactivated vaccine and is considered safe during pregnancy.
   3. HAV infection during pregnancy is associated with increased risk of premature labour and delivery.
B. Paediatrics:
   1. Children who have received HAV vaccine rarely have detectable anti-HAV IgM titres.
   2. Risk of outbreak in child-care centres increases with the number of children under age two years who wear diapers.
   3. Immunization is recommended routinely for children 12 through 23 months of age (follow the childhood immunization schedule).
   4. The hepatitis A vaccine is not currently licensed for children younger than 12 months.
C. Geriatrics:
   1. The elderly have greater numbers of HAV antibodies, resulting in fewer cases.
   2. Symptoms are usually vague. Fatigue; pruritus; and the classic symptoms of jaundice, hepatomegaly, and liver tenderness are commonly absent in the elderly.
   3. Diagnostic test results in the elderly include elevated bilirubin, lower or normal transaminase and ALP, and normal ultrasonography.
   4. Treatment is supportive. Corticosteroids may relieve symptoms but prolong the disease state due to prolonged viral replication.
D. Special populations:
   1. People with chronic liver disease are at risk of fulminant hepatitis and should be immunized.
   2. People who are awaiting or have received liver transplants should be immunized.

Bibliography

American Academy of Pediatrics. (2012). Hepatitis A. In L. K. Pickering (Ed.), *Red book: 2012 report of the Committee on Infectious Diseases* (29th ed., pp. 361–369). Elk Grove Village, IL: Author. Retrieved from https://redbook.solutions.aap.org/DocumentLibrary/RB12_interior.pdf

Canadian Immunization Guideline. (2018). *Part4-Active vaccines*. Retrieved from https://www.canada.ca/en/public-health/services/publications/healthy-living/canadian-immunization-guide-part-4-active-vaccines/page-6-hepatitis-a-vaccine.html

Centers for Disease Control and Prevention. (2016, July 13). *Viral hepatitis—Hepatitis A information*. Retrieved from https://www.cdc.gov/hepatitis/HAV/index.htm

Division of Viral Hepatitis, CDC. (2014). *Viral hepatitis surveillance United States, 2014*. Retrieved from https://www.cdc.gov/hepatitis/statistics/2014surveillance/pdfs/2014hepsurveillancerpt.pdf

Nettina, S. (2010). *The Lippincott manual of nursing practice* (9th ed.). Philadelphia, PA: Wolters Kluwer Lippincott Williams & Wilkins.

Hepatitis B

Cheryl A. Glass, Audra C. Malone, and Kristie A. D. Morydz

Definition
A. Hepatitis B is inflammation of the liver caused by hepatitis B virus (HBV). Acute HBV infection cannot be distinguished from other forms of acute viral hepatitis on the basis of clinical signs and symptoms or nonspecific laboratory findings. Acutely infected clients may be asymptomatic or symptomatic. The likelihood of developing symptoms of acute hepatitis is age dependent.
B. Chronic HBV infection is defined as the presence of hepatitis B surface antigen (HBsAg) in serum for at least six months or by the presence of HBsAg in a person who tests negative for antibody of the immunoglobulin M (IgM) subclass to hepatitis B core antigen (IgM anti-hepatitis B core antigen).
C. HBV is the main cause of cirrhosis and hepatocellular carcinoma (HCC) worldwide. For selected candidates, liver transplantation currently seems to be the only viable treatment for the latest stages of hepatitis B.
D. Antiviral treatment may be effective in approximately one-third of the clients who receive it. Eight genotypes (A through H) have been identified. The progression of the disease seems to be more accelerated, and the response to treatment with antiviral agents is less favourable for clients infected by genotype C compared with those infected by genotype B. Genotypes A or B have a better response to interferon (IFN) treatment compared with clients infected by genotype C or D.
E. Acute HBV is undistinguishable from other forms of hepatitis in the acute viral stage on the basis of clinical symptoms.
F. Testing is recommended for the following:
   1. All pregnant women.
   2. Persons born in regions with intermediate or high rates of hepatitis B (HBsAg prevalence ≥2%).
   3. Canadian-born persons not vaccinated as infants whose parents were born in regions with high rates of hepatitis B (HBsAg prevalence of ≥8%).
   4. Infants born to HBsAg-positive mothers.
   5. Household, needle-sharing, or sex contacts of HBsAg-positive persons.
   6. Men who have sex with men (MSM).
   7. Injection drug users.
   8. Clients with elevated liver enzymes (alanine transaminase [ALT]/aspartate transaminase [AST]) of unknown aetiology.
   9. Haemodialysis clients.
   10. Persons needing immunosuppressive or cytotoxic therapy.
   11. HIV-infected persons.
   12. Donors of blood, plasma, organs, tissues, or semen.
   13. Adults with diabetes mellitus are at an increased risk of acquiring HBV infection if they share diabetes care equipment such as blood glucose metres, fingerstick devices, syringes, and/or insulin pens. Adults with diabetes age <60 years are, therefore, recommended to receive hepatitis B vaccination and those aged >60 years are to be considered for vaccination.

Incidence/Prevalence
A. An estimated one-third of the global population has been infected with HBV. Approximately 350 million people are lifelong carriers, and only 2% spontaneously seroconvert annually. Of chronically infected clients, 15% to 40% will develop cirrhosis, progressing to liver failure and/or HCC.
B. In 2014, rates were highest for persons age 30 to 39 years; the lowest rates were among children and adolescents age <19 years.
C. Acute hepatitis B occurs in one to two out of every 1,000 pregnancies, and chronic infection occurs in five to 15 out of every 1,000 pregnancies. The course of maternal HBV infections does not seem to be affected by coexistent pregnancy. However, premature labour and delivery is increased.

D. Chronic HBV infections with persistence of HBsAg occur in as many as 90% of infants infected by perinatal transmission; in 30% of children 1 to 5 years old infected after birth; and in 5% to 10% of older children, adolescents, and adults with HBV infection.

Pathogenesis

A. HBV is a hepadnavirus. HBV-related liver injury is largely caused by immune-mediated mechanisms mediated via cytotoxic T-lymphocyte lysis of infected hepatocytes. The virus is transmitted through blood or body fluids, such as wound exudates, semen, cervical secretions, and saliva, that are HBsAg positive. It is not transmitted by the faecal–oral route or by water. Blood and serum contain the highest concentration of virus; saliva contains the lowest.
B. The incubation period is 45 to 160 days (two to five months), with an average of 120 days. An infected person can infect others four to six weeks before symptoms appear and for an unpredictable time thereafter.
C. The production of antibodies against HBsAg confers protective immunity and can be detected in clients who have recovered from HBV or in those clients who have been vaccinated. The IgM subtype indicates an acute infection or reactivation. Immunoglobulin G (IgG) subtype indicates chronic infection.

Predisposing Factors

A. Higher prevalence in:
  1. Indigenous populations.
  2. Asian origin.
  3. Incarcerated individuals.
B. Sexual contact is the major mode of transmission:
  1. High number of sexual partners.
  2. An early age of first intercourse.
  3. Homosexuality/bisexuality.
C. Intravenous (IV) drug use, sharing needles.
D. Occupational exposure.
E. Household exposure.
F. Perinatal exposure, by vertical infection.
G. Receiving blood transfusions or blood products for haemophilia and haemodialysis.
H. Breastfeeding, by transmission in breast milk.
I. Staffing or residing in institutions.
J. International travel.
K. Incarceration in long-term correctional facilities.
L. Percutaneous contact with inanimate objects contaminated with HBV; virus can survive one week or longer.
M. Diabetics.
N. Recipient of dialysis or kidney transplant.

Common Findings

A. The following symptoms occur in the acute phase of HBV:
  1. Anicteric hepatitis: Asymptomatic (majority of clients).
  2. Icteric hepatitis: Associated with a prodromal period:
     a. Anorexia.
     b. Nausea and vomiting.
     c. Low-grade fever.
     d. Headache.
     e. Diarrhoea.
     f. Myalgia.
     g. Fatigue.
     h. Aversion to food and cigarettes.
     i. Intermittent, mild to moderate right upper quadrant (RUQ) and epigastric pain.
  3. Hyperacute, acute, and subacute hepatitis symptoms:
     a. Hepatic encephalopathy.
     b. Somnolence.
     c. Disturbances in sleep pattern.
     d. Mental confusion.
     e. Coma.
B. The following symptoms occur in the chronic phase of HBV:
  1. Asymptomatic: May be healthy carriers without any evidence of active disease.
  2. During the replicative state common symptoms are the following:
     a. Fatigue.
     b. Anorexia.
     c. Nausea.
     d. Mild upper quadrant pain or discomfort.
     e. Hepatic decompensation.

Other Signs and Symptoms

A. In young children:
  1. Jaundice and other symptoms may not be present.
  2. Symptoms may be prolonged and insidious compared with hepatitis A virus (HAV).
B. Icteric phase (10 days after the appearance of constitutional symptoms and lasts for one to three months):
  1. Jaundice of sclera and skin.
  2. Tea-coloured urine.
  3. Clay-coloured stools, often precede jaundice.
  4. RUQ tenderness.
  5. Enlarged liver.

Subjective Data

A. Review the onset, duration, course, and severity of symptoms. Ask the client for specifics about urine and stool colour:
  1. Ask whether the client has ever been treated for any type of hepatitis.
B. How long ago was he or she treated?
  1. Did the client complete the therapy? If not, why?
  2. What was the client's response to therapy (i.e., nonresponder)?
C. Review vaccination status.
D. Review family history for HCC.
E. Ask the client about other family members and sexual contacts with similar symptoms.
F. Discuss the client's history of blood transfusions, intravenous (IV) drug use, and alcohol misuse.
G. Review the client's occupational exposure.
H. Inquire about recent international travel.
I. Review for a history of variceal bleeding.
J. Is the client coinfected with hepatitis C virus (HCV) or HIV?

Physical Examination

A. Check temperature (if indicated), pulse, respirations, blood pressure (BP), and weight. Establish the client's usual weight; note amount of any weight lost and over what length of time.
B. Inspect:
  1. Observe general appearance, muscle wasting, ascites, and peripheral oedema.
  2. Inspect the skin for jaundice, palmar erythema, rash, spider nevi, spider angioma, and dehydration.
  3. Inspect the eyes for yellow sclera.

Table 11.13 Diagnostic Tests for HBV Antigens and Antibodies

Factors to be Tested	HBV Antigen or Antibody	Indication
HBsAg	HBsAg	Detects acutely or chronically infected; antigen used in hepatitis B vaccine
Anti-HBs	Antibody to HBsAg	Identifies resolved HBV infections; determines immunity after immunization
HBeAg	HBeAg	Identifies at risk of transmitting HBV
Anti-HBe	Antibody to HBeAg	Identifies lower risk of transmitting HBV
Anti-HBc	Antibody to hepatitis B core antigen; IgM (HBcAg)	Identifies acute, resolved, or chronic HBV infection. Anti-HBc is not present after immunization
IgM anti-HBc Anti-HAV	IgM antibody to HBcAg	Identifies acute or recent HBV infections (includes HBsAg-negative during the window phase of infection); determines need for vaccination

HAV, hepatitis A virus; HB, hepatitis B: HBcAg, hepatitis B core antigen; HBeAg, hepatitis B envelope antigen; HBsAg, hepatitis B surface antigen; HBV, hepatitis B virus; IgM, immunoglobulin M.

4. Inspect the mucous membranes and nail beds.
5. Evaluate for the presence of gynaecomastia.
C. Auscultate:
  1. Lung fields and the heart.
  2. All quadrants of the abdomen.
D. Percuss the abdomen.
E. Palpate:
  1. All quadrants of the abdomen for masses, liver enlargement or tenderness, hepatomegaly, and splenomegaly.
  2. The lymph nodes for lymphadenopathy.
  3. For testicular atrophy.

Diagnostic Tests

A. Diagnostic tests for HBV antigens and antibodies (see Table 11.13).
B. Complete blood count (CBC) with differential.
C. Complete liver panel:
  1. AST/ALT.
  2. Total bilirubin.
  3. International normalized ratio (INR).
  4. Albumin.
  5. Alkaline phosphatase.
D. Other viral infection markers: HCV and hepatitis delta virus (HDV).
E. Alkaline phosphatase (ALP).
F. Serum iron levels.
G. Gamma-glutamyl transpeptidase (GGT; rule out other causes of chronic liver disease).
H. Alpha-fetoprotein (AFP; rule out other causes of liver disease).
I. HBV genotype.
J. HBV DNA viral load quantitation.
K. Serum fibrosis panel:
  1. APRI = aspartate aminotransferase (AST)-to-platelet ratio index used for estimating hepatic fibrosis. Online calculator can be found at www.hepatitisc.uw.edu/page/clinical-calculators/apri.
  2. Fibrosis-4 (FIB-4) is an index for estimating hepatic fibrosis based on a calculation derived from AST, ALT, platelet concentrations, and age. Online calculator can be found at www.hepatitisc.uw.edu/page/clinical-calculators/fib-4.
  3. FibroTest (FibroSure)—commercial biomarker test that uses the results of six blood markers to estimate hepatic fibrosis.
L. Imaging:
  1. Abdominal ultrasound.
  2. FibroScan—Transient shear wave elastography measures liver stiffness as a surrogate for fibrosis.
  3. CT or MRI to help exclude biliary obstruction.
M. Liver biopsy to assess the severity of disease.
N. Pregnancy testing before antiviral therapy.
O. Before oral antiviral therapy is introduced, all clients should be screened for HIV.
P. HCV and HIV testing to rule out coinfection.

Differential Diagnoses

A. Exclusion of other types of hepatitis (A, C, D, E, viral, or autoimmune hepatitis).
B. Infectious mononucleosis.
C. Hepatotoxic drug ingestion, for example, chloramphenicol, acetaminophen, or methyldopa.
D. Metastatic cancer to the liver.
E. Alcoholic cirrhosis.
F. Haemochromatosis.
G. Wilson's disease.

Plan

A. General interventions:
  1. No specific therapy for acute HBV infection is available.
  2. Before any form of HBV therapy is started, and optimally at the first presentation, the client needs to be provided with information about the natural history of chronic hepatitis B infection and the fact that most infections remain entirely without symptoms even in those with severe disease, so that there is a need for regular lifelong monitoring.
  3. Hepatitis B immune globulin (HBIG) and corticosteroids are not effective treatment.
B. Client teaching.
  1. *Refer to Client Teaching Guide: Jaundice and Hepatitis.* ◀
  2. Advise the client to avoid sexual activity until he or she is free of HBsAg.

▶ Client Teaching Guides are available at https://connect.springerpub.com/content/reference-book/978-0-8261-9498-5

3. History of anaphylactic reaction to common baker's yeast is a contraindication to HBV vaccination.
4. There are no dietary restrictions with acute and chronic hepatitis (without cirrhosis). Decompensated cirrhosis, portal hypertension, or encephalopathy are prescribed:
   a. Low-sodium diet (1.5 g/d).
   b. High-protein diet (white-meat protein, e.g., pork, turkey, and fish).
   c. Fluid restriction of 1.5 L/d in the presence of hyponatraemia.

C. Pharmacological therapy: The goal of treatment is to prevent progression to cirrhosis, hepatic failure, and HCC:
   1. Primary prevention includes vaccination of high-risk individuals, including teens. Vaccination is up to 95% effective.
   2. HBV vaccine is the recommended preexposure for the following groups:
      a. Prevention of perinatal HBV infection through routine screening of all pregnant women for HBV infection and provision of hepatitis B vaccine and immunoprophylaxis to infants born to HBsAg-positive mothers
      b. All infants: All major authorities recommend that all children receive a complete series of HBV immunizations during the first 18 months of life. **Recommended vaccination schedules vary by province. Consult your provincial health department for guidance.**
      c. Routine vaccination of previously unvaccinated children and adolescents.
      d. Children at risk of acquiring HBV by person-to-person (horizontal) transmission.
      e. All adolescents.
      f. IV drug users.
      g. Sexually active individuals with more than one sex partner in the previous six months or those who have a sexually transmitted infection (STI), MSM, and persons who inject drugs (PWID).
      h. Health-care workers and others at occupational risk.
      i. Residents and staff of institutions for developmentally disabled persons.
      j. Staff of nonresidential childcare centres.
      k. Clients undergoing haemodialysis.
      l. Clients with bleeding disorders who receive clotting factor concentrates.
      m. Household contacts and sexual partners of HBV carriers.
      n. Members of households with adoptees who are HBsAg positive.
      o. International travelers to areas of high or intermediate endemicity.
      p. Inmates of long-term correctional facilities.
   3. Hepatitis B vaccine can be given concurrently with other vaccines.
   4. Early prophylaxis is paramount after an HBsAg needle stick. HBIG should be administered immediately, no later than 48 hours, after exposure. Postexposure prophylaxis HBV vaccine is recommended.
   5. The length of therapy is dependent on the genotype and previous treatment:
      a. Treatment: Naïve—not previously treated for HCV.
      b. Relapser: Reappearance of HCV occurs after therapy is discontinued.
      c. Partial responder: HCV declines at week 12 of therapy but is still positive at week 24 after completion of treatment.
   6. Management of side effects with therapeutic agents is targeted to the symptoms.
   7. There are multiple drug–drug interactions; consult with a pharmacological reference before instituting drug therapy.
   8. Dose adjustment is required in the presence of renal impairment and dialysis, and is used with caution in clients with a history of pancreatitis.
   9. Orthotopic liver transplantation (OLT) is the first-line treatment for clients with fulminant hepatic failure who do not recover and for clients with end-stage liver disease.
   10. The guidelines for treatment are rapidly changing. The most current guideline recommendations are available at the Canadian Liver Foundation, at www.liver.ca/wp-content/uploads/2017/09/HBV-QR-EN-_FINAL_Web.pdf, as well as the Canadian Association for the Study of the Liver: www.cmaj.ca/content/cmaj/suppl/2018/05/29/190.22.E677.DC1/170453-guide-1-at.pdl. Guidelines include the following:
      a. Acute liver failure, management.
      b. Ascites due to cirrhosis, management.
      c. Gastro-oesophageal varices and variceal haemorrhage in cirrhosis, management.
      d. Hepatic encephalopathy.
      e. Hepatitis B, guidance.
      f. Hepatitis C, guidance.
      g. HCC, management.
      h. Liver biopsy.
   11. The current World Health Organization (WHO) *Guidelines for the Prevention, Care, and Treatment of Persons With Chronic Hepatitis B Infection* is at www.who.int/hiv/pub/hepatitis/hepatitis-b-guidelines/en.

Follow-Up

A. Laboratory monitoring:
   1. Monitor liver function (ALT) every three to six months for active disease.
   2. Monitor hepatitis B envelope antigen (HBeAg) every three to six months, depending on ALT levels.
   3. Monitor CBC and creatinine every month (one to two days before treatment).
   4. Monitor HBV DNA every three to six months when the client is on treatment in the reactivation phase.

B. Risk of exposure to HBsAg ceases when antigen disappears from the bloodstream, usually within six to eight weeks of infection. Repeated serum determinations of HBsAg can help define when precautions may be relaxed.

C. Laboratory, physical examination, and psychosocial evaluation are required for antiviral therapy.

D. The Canadian Association for the Study of Hepatocellular Carcinoma recognizes the populations at risk as defined by the American Association for the Study of Liver Disease (AASLD). It is recommended HCC surveillance using ultrasound in the following types of clients with chronic HBV:
   1. Asian men older than 40 years and Asian women older than 50 years.
   2. All clients with cirrhosis, regardless of age.
   3. Clients with a family history of HCC; any age.
   4. Africans older than 20 years and any carriers older than 40 years with persistent or intermittent ALT evaluation and/or HBV DNA level >2,000 IU/mL should be screened with an ultrasound every six to 12 months.
   5. Any individual with HBV/HIV coinfection.

E. Routine booster doses of hepatitis B vaccine are not recommended for children or adults with normal immune status.

Consultation/Referral
A. Clients with persistently elevated serum transaminase concentrations (exceeding twice the upper limits of normal), as well as those with elevated serum AFP concentrations or abnormal ultrasounds, should be referred to a gastroenterologist for further management.

Individual Considerations
A. Pregnancy:
1. No adverse effect on the developing foetus has been observed when pregnant women are vaccinated against HBV.
2. There are insufficient data to recommend delivery by cesarean section.
3. The Public Health Agency of Canada suggests antiviral therapy to reduce the risk of perinatal transmission of hepatitis B in HBsAg-positive pregnant women with an HBV DNA level >200,000 IU/mL.
4. The only antivirals studied in pregnant women are lamivudine, telbivudine, and tenofovir.
5. Antiviral therapy was started at 28 to 32 weeks of gestation and discontinued at birth to three months postpartum in most studies.
6. Pregnancy and lactation are not a contraindication to vaccination.
7. Prenatal HBsAg testing of all pregnant women is recommended to identify newborns who require immediate postexposure prophylaxis.
8. Breastfeeding by an HBsAg-positive mother poses no additional risk for acquisition of HBV infection by infant.

B. Paediatrics:
1. Infants born to HBsAg-positive mothers need no special precautions for spread of infectious disease other than removal of maternal blood by a gloved attendant and standard universal precautions.
2. Infants of all HBsAg-positive women should receive immunoprophylaxis (HBV vaccination ± hepatitis B immunoglobulin) per WHO and Canadian Public Health recommendations.
3. All infants, including those who are premature, born to HBsAg-positive mothers need HBIG within 12 hours of birth.
4. More than 90% of infants infected perinatally will develop chronic HBV infection.
5. Adoptees from countries where HBV infection is endemic should be screened for HBsAg. If a child is HBsAg positive, previously unimmunized family members and other household contacts should be vaccinated, preferably before adoption.
6. Persons infected as infants or young children are at higher risk of death due to liver disease than those infected as adults. Children with chronic HBV should be screened periodically for hepatic complication using serum liver transaminase tests, AFP concentration, and abdominal ultrasound.
7. All children 11 to 12 years should have their immunization records reviewed and should complete the vaccine series if they have not received the vaccine or did not complete the immunization series.
8. Children who stop antiviral therapy should be monitored every three months for at least one year for recurrent viraemia, ALT flares, and clinical decompensation.

C. Adults:
1. Most HBV infections are acquired in adolescence or adulthood, largely as a result of IV drug use, sexual contact, or occupational or household exposure. HBV infection is associated with other sexually transmitted diseases (STDs), including syphilis.
2. Clients who have received a blood transfusion should refrain from blood donation for six months, the incubation period for HBV. Blood should never be donated if the client is a hepatitis B carrier or was infected with hepatitis C.

D. Geriatrics:
1. The elderly have fewer cases of HBV due to diminished immune response; however, they tend to be asymptomatic HBV carriers.
2. The disease has a greater tendency to deteriorate into chronic liver failure or chronic hepatitis.

Resources
Canadian Association for the study of the Liver: https://hepatology.ca/Centers for Disease Control and Prevention: www.cdc.gov//hepatitis
Canadian Liver Foundation: www.liver.ca
Hepatitis and HIV: www.hivandhepatitis.com
Hepatitis B Foundation: www.hepb.org
Hepatitis Foundation International: www.hepfi.org
Public Health Agency of Canada Hepatitis B Facts: https://www.canada.ca/en/public-health/services/surveillance/blood-safety-contribution-program/bloodborne-pathogens-section/hepatitis/hepatitis-b-facts.html
World Health Organization: who.int

Bibliography
American Academy of Pediatrics. (2012). Hepatitis B. In L. K. Pickering (Ed.), *Red book: 2012 report of the Committee on Infectious Diseases* (29th ed., pp. 369–390). Elk Grove Village, IL: Author. Retrieved from https://redbook.solutions.aap.org/DocumentLibrary/RB12_interior.pdf
Burak, K. W., & Sherman, M. (2015). Hepatocellular carcinoma: Consensus, controversies and future directions: A report from the Canadian Association for the Study of the Liver Hepatocellular Carcinoma Meeting. *Canadian Journal of Gastroenterology and Hepatology, 29*(4), 178–184. doi:10.1155/2015/824263
Division of Viral Hepatitis, CDC. (2014). *Viral hepatitis surveillance United States, 2014*. Retrieved from https://www.cdc.gov/hepatitis/statistics/2014surveillance/pdfs/2014hepsurveillancerpt.pdf
Hepatitis B, Foundation. (2012, February 3). *Approved drugs for adults*. Retrieved from http://www.hepb.org/patients/hepatitis_b_treatment.htm
Loc, A. S. F., & McMahon, B. J. (2009). *AASLD practice guideline update: Chronic hepatitis B: Update 2009*. Retrieved from http://www.aasld.org/sites/default/files/guideline_documents/ChronicHepatitisB2009.pdf
Nettina, S. (2010). *The Lippincott manual of nursing practice* (9th ed.). Philadelphia, PA: Wolters Kluwer Lippincott Williams & Wilkins.
World Health Organization. (2015, March). *Guidelines for the prevention, care and treatment of persons with chronic hepatitis B*. Geneva, Switzerland: Author.

Hepatitis C

Cheryl A. Glass and Kristie A. D. Morydz

Definition
A. Hepatitis C is an inflammation of the liver caused by the hepatitis C virus (HCV). HCV has signs and symptoms often undistinguishable from those of hepatitis A virus (HAV) or hepatitis B virus (HBV). The disease tends to be asymptomatic to mild and has an insidious onset. Acute fulminate infection is rare. The major feature of HCV is its propensity to become chronic. Persistent infection occurs in at least 75% to 85% of clients, even in the absence of biochemical evidence of liver disease. Approximately 60% to 70% of clients develop chronic hepatitis, and 5% to 20% develop cirrhosis.

B. Multiple (six) HCV genotypes and subtypes exist. The genotype is a major factor in the effectiveness of the client's response to therapy. Approximately 50% of clients infected with genotype 1 and approximately 80% of clients with genotypes 2 and 3 achieve a sustained virologic response (SVR). SVR is defined as undetectable HCV RNA 12 months or more after treatment cessation.
C. The development of chronic hepatitis and its complications increase with several factors, including older age at acquisition, HIV infection, excessive alcohol consumption, and male gender. Among children, liver disease progression appears to be accelerated with comorbid conditions, including cancer, iron overload, thalassaemia, or coinfection with HIV.
D. HCV is the leading cause of nonalcoholic hepatic failure and cirrhosis, and the cause of 90% of posttransfusion hepatitis. Primary hepatic cellular carcinoma (HCC) also occurs in these clients.

Incidence/Prevalence
A. Worldwide, more than 170 million individuals are chronically infected with HCV.
B. The "emerging epidemic" of acute HCV resulted from people who have transitioned from oral prescription opioid misuse to injection of these opioids and heroin.
C. Seroprevalence rates among individuals vary according to their associated risk factors. The highest rates occur in persons with large or repeated direct percutaneous exposure to blood or blood products, such as intravenous (IV) drug users and clients with haemophilia who have received multiple blood transfusions.
D. Seroprevalence among pregnant women has been estimated at 1% to 2%. Maternal–foetal (vertical) transmission is only 5% from women who are HCV RNA positive at the time of delivery. Maternal coinfection with HIV has been associated with increased risk of perinatal transmission of HCV RNA.
E. Serum anti-HCV antibody and HCV RNA have been detected in colostrum. However, although only a limited number of clients have been studied, the rate of transmission among breastfed infants is the same as among bottlefed infants.
F. More than 20% of adults with chronic infection progress to cirrhosis an average of 20 years after their initial infection. Clients with cirrhosis have a secondary risk of portal hypertension, liver failure, and other complications. HCV is the leading indication for liver transplantation among adults in the United States.
G. HCC is diagnosed an average of 30 years after initial HCV infection in 1% to 5% of clients, most of whom have underlying cirrhosis.

Pathogenesis
A. HCV is a small, single-stranded RNA virus with a lipid envelope and is a member of the Flavivirus family. Infection is spread primarily by parenteral exposure to blood and blood products from HCV-infected persons. In the United States, the current risk of HCV infection following blood transfusion is estimated at 0.1% or less because of exclusion of high-risk individuals from the pool of blood donors and screening for HCV. Sexual transmission of HCV is uncommon except with high-risk behaviour.
B. The incubation period averages six to seven weeks, with a range of two weeks to six months. The time from exposure to the development of viraemia generally is one to two weeks.

Predisposing Factors
All people with HCV RNA in their blood are considered to be infectious. The following groups are at high risk of HCV infection and should be tested:
A. IV drug users who have shared needles.
B. Intranasal cocaine users, presumably resulting from epistaxis and shared equipment.
C. Haemophiliacs, haemodialysis clients, and those who received blood transfusions before 1992.
D. Recipients of solid organ transplants before 1992.
E. Health-care workers with percutaneous exposures.
F. Individuals with multiple sexual partners.
G. Transmission among contacts living with infected persons may occur with percutaneous or mucosal exposure to blood.
H. Infants of infected mothers, by vertical transmission.
I. More common in males than females.
J. Tattooing, body piercing, and acupuncture with unsterile equipment.
K. HIV.

Common Findings
A. Chronic HCV is asymptomatic unless there is progressive inflammation and complications from cirrhosis.
B. Malaise.
C. Anorexia.
D. Nausea.
E. Myalgia.
F. Fever.
G. Abdominal pain.

Other Signs and Symptoms
A. Jaundice (occurs in <20% of clients).
B. Hepatomegaly is present in one-third of clients with an acute infection.
C. Ascites.
D. Spider nevi.
E. Dark urine.

Subjective Data
A. Review the onset, duration, course, and severity of symptoms. Ask the client for specifics about urine and stool colour.
B. Ask the client about other family members and sexual contacts with similar symptoms.
C. Review the client's history of blood transfusions, tattoos, incarceration, IV drug use, and alcohol misuse.
D. Ask the client about occupational exposure.
E. Ask about high-risk sexual practices.
F. Review family history of HCC.
G. When was HCV diagnosed?
H. Has the client had a liver biopsy? When?
I. Ask if the client has ever been treated for any type of hepatitis:
   1. How long ago the client treated?
   2. Did the client complete therapy? If not, why?
   3. What was the client's response to therapy (i.e., nonresponder, relapser)?
J. Review for a history of variceal bleeding.

Physical Examination
A. Check temperature (acute infection), pulse, respirations, blood pressure (BP), and weight.
B. Inspect:
   1. Observe general appearance, muscle wasting, oedema, and demeanour. **Administer a depression self-assessment tool at each visit when on HCV therapy.**

2. Inspect the skin for jaundice, rash, dehydration, palmar erythema, excoriations, spider nevi, and tattoos/piercings.
3. Inspect the eyes for yellow sclera.
4. Inspect mucous membranes and nail beds for clubbing and cyanosis.
5. Inspect for gynaecomastia and small testes.
C. Auscultate:
1. Lung fields and heart.
2. All quadrants of the abdomen and evaluate for abdominal bruit.
D. Percuss the abdomen.
E. Palpate:
1. All quadrants of the abdomen for masses; liver enlargement or tenderness; characteristics of cirrhosis; and hepatosplenomegaly, which occurs in about 10% of cases.
2. The lymph nodes for lymphadenopathy and enlarged parotid.

Diagnostic Tests

A. Laboratory tests:
1. Immunoglobulin G (IgG) antibody enzyme immunoassays (EIAs) for HCV and nucleic acid amplification (NAA) tests to detect HCV RNA.
2. HCV genotyping.
3. HCV viral load: Quantitative assay used as a prognostic indicator for clients undergoing antiviral therapy.
4. Alanine transaminase (ALT) and aspartate transaminase (AST).
5. Hepatitis A immunoglobulin (IgM) and IgG.
6. Hepatitis B surface antigen (HBsAg) and antibody, core antibody.
7. Cytomegalovirus (CMV)IgM and IgG (and/or CMV in urine culture).
8. Epstein–Barr virus IgM and IgG.
9. HIV IgG enzyme-linked immunoassay (ELISA).
10. Alpha-fetoprotein.
B. Ultrasonography is used for monitoring HCV-related complications. FibroScan—transient shear wave elastography—measures liver stiffness as a surrogate for fibrosis.
C. Serum fibrosis panel:
1. APRI = AST-to-platelet ratio index used for estimating hepatic fibrosis. Online calculator can be found at hepcbc.ca/tests/non-invasive-tests/apri/.
2. Fibrosis-4 (FIB-4) is an index for estimating hepatic fibrosis based on a calculation derived from AST, ALT, platelet concentrations, and age. Online calculator can be found at www2.gov.bc.ca/assets/gov/health/practitioner-pro/special-authority/fibrosis-info-sheet.pdf.
3. FibroTest: Commercial biomarker test that uses the results of six blood markers to estimate hepatic fibrosis.
D. Liver biopsy is the most accurate method of evaluating the extent of HCV-related liver disease. Liver biopsy is the gold standard for determining the histologic grade and stage of fibrosis/cirrhosis. The *absolute* requirement for a liver biopsy prior to the institution of medication therapy is currently under discussion. For clients with genotypes 2 and 3, the likelihood of response to therapy is so high that the benefits of treatment may outweigh the risk of biopsy and histologic considerations.
E. Prior to the institution/during antiviral therapy, perform the following tests:

1. Complete blood count (CBC) with platelets.
2. Viral load.
3. Liver function (alanine aminotransferase [ALT]/aspartate aminotransferase [AST]).
4. Pregnancy test.
5. Thyroid profile.
6. Blood glucose/haemoglobin A1C.
7. Consider a dilated retinal examination.
8. Consider a stress test.
9. Screen for alcohol misuse, drug misuse, and/or depression.

Differential Diagnoses

A. Hepatitis A.
B. Hepatitis B.
C. Alcoholic liver disease.
D. Drug toxicities.
E. Opportunistic infections associated with HIV infection.

Plan

A. Client teaching:
1. *Refer to Client Teaching Guide: Jaundice and Hepatitis.* ◀
2. Warn the client of the possibility of transmission to others, and advise the client to refrain from donating blood, organs, tissues, or semen and from sharing toothbrushes and razors.
3. All clients with chronic HCV should be immunized against hepatitis A and hepatitis B.
4. Counsel the client to avoid hepatotoxic medications and alcohol.
5. Immunoprophylaxis for postexposure prophylaxis with immune globulin (IG) is not recommended.
6. The Canadian Association for the Study of the Liver (hepatology.ca/) recommends anyone born between 1945 and 1975 be tested for HCV.
B. Clients and their spouses should be counselled to not become pregnant while on therapy and for six months after the completion of treatment. Pregnancy tests should be done prior to institution of HCV therapy and monthly thereafter.
C. Pharmacological therapy is aimed at inhibiting HCV replication, eradicating infection, progression of fibrosis, and prevention of HCC:
1. The length of therapy is dependent on the genotype and previous treatment:
   a. Treatment: Naïve—not previously treated for HCV.
   b. Relapser: Reappearance of HCV after therapy is discontinued.
   c. Partial responder: HCV declines at week 12 of therapy but is still positive at week 24 after completion of treatment:
      i. Manage side effects with therapeutic agents related to symptoms.
      ii. If there are multiple drug–drug interactions, consult with a pharmacological reference before instituting of drug therapy.
      iii. The guidelines for treatment are rapidly changing. The most current guideline recommendations are available from the American Association for the Study of Liver Diseases (AASLD), the Canadian Association for the Study of the Liver, and the Infectious Diseases Society of America

▶ Client Teaching Guides are available at https://connect.springerpub.com/content/reference-book/978-0-8261-9498-5

(IDSA) at www.aasld.org/publications/practice-guidelines-0. Guidelines break down therapy in detail by genotype, length of therapy, and medications. The Canadian guidelines also include the following:
1) Acute liver failure, management.
2) Ascites due to cirrhosis, management.
3) Gastro-oesophageal varices and variceal haemorrhage in cirrhosis management.
4) Hepatic encephalopathy.
5) Hepatitis B guidance.
6) Hepatitis C guidance.
7) HCC management.
8) Liver biopsy.

2. The World Health Organization (WHO) *Guidelines for the Screening, Care, and Treatment of Persons With Hepatitis C Infection* is available at apps.who.int/iris/bitstream/10665/111747/1/9789241548755_eng.pdf?ua=1&ua=1

Follow-Up
A. Test the client within five to six weeks after the onset of hepatitis; 80% of clients are positive for serum anti-HCV antibody.
B. Persons with chronic HCV infections should be vaccinated against hepatitis A and B, unless they have previously been demonstrated to be nonsusceptible.
C. Children with chronic infection should be screened periodically for chronic hepatitis with serum liver function tests (LFTs) because of their potential long-term risk for chronic liver disease. Definitive recommendations on frequency have not been established.
D. Monitor for mental dysfunction related to interferon (IFN), including depression, psychosis, aggressive behaviour, hallucinations, violent behaviour, suicidal ideation, suicide attempt, and homicidal ideation (rare), even without previous history of psychiatric illness.

Consultation/Referral
A. Referrals include gastroenterologist, psychiatrist, endocrinologist, neurologist, haematologist, dietitian, and social workers.
B. Clients who are coinfected with HBV or HIV or have end-stage renal disease should be referred for treatment.
C. Children with severe disease or histologically advanced pathology (bridging necrosis or active cirrhosis) should be referred to a specialist in the management of chronic HCV infection.
D. Children with persistently elevated serum transaminase concentrations, or those exceeding twice the upper limits of normal, should be referred to a gastroenterologist for further management.

Individual Considerations
A. Pregnancy:
1. No data currently exist to support counselling a woman against pregnancy (unless under active treatment).
2. Routine serologic testing of pregnant women for HCV infection is not recommended. Women with significant risk factors for HCV should be offered antibody screening.
3. According to current guidelines of the U.S. Public Health Service and the American Academy of Pediatrics, maternal HCV infection is not a contraindication to breastfeeding. HCV-positive mothers should consider abstaining from breastfeeding if their nipples are cracked or bleeding.
4. Ribivarin (RBV) is a pregnancy category X drug with abortifacients potential.
5. IFN is a pregnancy category C drug and should be used only if the benefits outweigh the risk to the foetus. **IFN is a pregnancy category X drug when combined with RBV.**
6. The method of delivery has not been shown to increase the risk of vertical transmission of HCV. Cesarean delivery is reserved for obstetric indications.
B. Paediatrics:
1. Serologic testing for anti-HCV antibodies in children born to women previously identified to be HCV infected is recommended because approximately 5% acquire the infection. Duration of passive maternal antibody in infants is unknown. Testing for anti-HCV antibodies should not be performed until after 12 months of age.
2. Exclusion of children with HCV infections from out-of-home childcare centres is not indicated.
3. The need for testing for alpha-fetoprotein concentration and for abdominal ultrasonography in children has not been determined.
4. Routine serologic testing of adoptees, either domestic or international, is not recommended.
C. Adults:
1. In 2017, the Canadian Task Force on Preventative Health Care recommended against screening for hepatitis C in asymptomatic adults unless risk factors are identified.
2. Infected persons with steady partners do not need to change their sexual practices. However, they should be informed of the possible risk of transmission and of what precautions to use to prevent transmission.
3. Persons with multiple partners should be advised to reduce the number of partners and to use condoms to prevent transmission.
4. The best means of limiting transfusion-associated HCV is to rely exclusively on volunteer rather than commercial blood donors and to screen donors for anti-HCV antibodies.
D. Geriatrics: There are fewer cases of HCV in the elderly than in other age groups. However, they tend to develop chronic hepatitis or hepatic failure.

Resources
American Association for the Study of Liver Diseases: www.aasld.org
American Liver Foundation: www.liverfoundation.org
Canadian Association for the study of the Liver
Canadian Liver Foundation www.liver.ca
Centers for Disease Control and Prevention: www.cdc.gov/hepatitis
Hepatitis and HIV: www.hivandhepatitis.com
Hepatitis Foundation International: www.hepfi.org
Public Health Agency of Canada Hepatities C information for Health Professionals: https://www.canada.ca/en/public-health/services/diseases/hepatitis-c/health-professionals-hepatitis-c.html
World Health Organization: www.who.int/en

Bibliography
American Academy of Pediatrics. (2012). Hepatitis C. In L. K. Pickering (Ed.), *Red book: 2012 report of the Committee on Infectious Diseases* (29th ed., pp. 391–395). Elk Grove Village, IL: Author. Retrieved from https://redbook.solutions.aap.org/DocumentLibrary/RB12_interior.pdf
Centers for Disease Control and Prevention. (2012a, August 17). Recommendations for the identification of chronic hepatitis C virus infection among persons born during 1945–1965. *Morbidity and Mortality Weekly Report, 61*(4), 1–32. Retrieved from https://www.cdc.gov/mmwr/preview/mmwrhtml/rr6104a1.htm?s_cid=rr6104a1_w

Centers for Disease Control and Prevention. (2012b, October 22). *Hepatitis C FAQS for the public.* Retrieved from https://www.cdc.gov/hepatitis/c/cfaq.htm#cFAQ21

Chou, R., & Wasson, N. (2013, June 4). Blood tests to diagnose fibrosis or cirrhosis in patients with chronic hepatitis C infection. *Annals of Internal Medicine, 158,* 807–820 and W-328–W330. doi:10.7326/0003-4819-158-11-201306040-00005

Dhawan, V. K. (2013, June 17). Hepatitis C. *Medscape.* Retrieved from http://emedicine.medscape.com/article/177792-overview

Dienstag, J. L., & McHutchison, J. G. (2006). American Gastroenterological Association medical position statement on the management of hepatitis C. *Gastroenterology, 130,* 225–230. doi:10.1053/j.gastro.2005.11.011

Division of Viral Hepatitis, CDC. (2014). *Viral hepatitis surveillance United States, 2014.* Retrieved from https://www.cdc.gov/hepatitis/statistics/2014surveillance/pdfs/2014hepsurveillancerpt.pdf

Ghany, M. G., Nelson, D. R., Strader, D. B., Thomas, D. L., & Seeff, L. B. (2011). An update on treatment of genotype 1 chronic hepatitis C virus infection: 2011 practice guideline by the American Association for the Study of Liver Diseases. *Hepatology, 54,* 1433–1444. doi:10.1002/hep.24641

HepCnet. (2003, March 7). *Drugs & liver damage.* Retrieved from http://www.hepcnet.net/drugsandliverdamage.html

Hofmann, W. P., & Zeuzem, S. (2011, May). A new standard of care for the treatment of chronic HCV infection. *Nature Reviews Gastroenterology & Hepatology, 8,* 257–264. doi:10.1038/nrgastro.2011.49

Nettina, S. (2010). *The Lippincott manual of nursing practice* (9th ed.). Philadelphia, PA: Wolters Kluwer Lippincott Williams & Wilkins.

Page, J. (2012). Recent developments in the treatment of chronic hepatitis C. *Journal for Nurse Practitioners, 8,* 225–230. doi:10.1016/j.nurpra.2011.09.022

Shah, H., Bilodeau, M., Burak, K. W., Cooper, C., Klein, M., Ramji, A., & Feld, J. J. (2018). The management of chronic hepatitis C: 2018 guideline update from the Canadian Association for the Study of the Liver. *CMAJ, 190*(22), E677–E687. doi:10.1503/cmaj.170453

Hernias, Abdominal

Cheryl A. Glass and Kristie A. D. Morydz

Definition
A hernia is the protrusion of a peritoneum-lined sac through a defect in the abdominal wall. Abdominal-wall hernias are the most common of surgical procedures. Hernias are a leading cause of disability and work loss. Abdominal hernias can be congenital or acquired. Types include the following:
A. Umbilical hernia: Occurs when the intestinal muscles fail to close around the umbilicus, allowing the omentum and/or intestines to protrude into the weaker area.
B. Incisional hernia: Caused by a defect in the abdominal musculature that develops after a surgical incision.
C. Epigastric hernia: Protrusion of fat or omentum through the linea alba between the umbilicus and the xiphoid. Epigastric hernias are generally <2 cm in diameter.
D. Diastasis recti: Acquired hernia most often due to pregnancy and obesity. The right and left rectus muscles separate, but there is no fascial defect.
E. Obturator hernia: Follows the path of the obturator nerves and muscles.

Incidence/Prevalence
A. Umbilical hernias are more common in premature infants and infants of African American descent, women, and the elderly. This type of hernia has a higher risk of incarceration and strangulation and, therefore, a greater mortality because the large bowel is frequently entrapped.
B. Epigastric hernias are most common in men 20 to 50 years old.
C. Incisional hernias typically are noted in the early postoperative period; however, there is an increase in incisional hernias during pregnancy. These iatrogenic hernias occur in 2% to 10% of abdominal operations. In addition to hernias, separation of the recti abdominis muscles (diastasis recti) is often caused by pregnancy or obesity.
D. Obturator hernias occur more commonly in females. Females have a larger canal diameter, which is noted predominantly in thin elderly women.

Pathogenesis
A. Incisional hernias are due to failure of fascial tissues to heal and close.
B. Epigastric hernias are defects in the abdominal midline between the umbilicus and the xiphoid process. They are usually related to a congenital weakness, increased intra-abdominal pressure, surrounding muscle weakness, or chronic abdominal-wall strain.
C. An umbilical hernia is caused by failure of the umbilical ring to obliterate after birth. In the infant, the umbilical ring often closes spontaneously within the first one to two years of life. Increased abdominal pressure or congenital defects cause abdominal hernias that allow abdominal contents to protrude through the opening defect. In adults with an umbilical hernia, obesity increases the danger of incarceration.
D. Parastomal hernia is caused by the bowel intrusion into the defect in the abdominal wall when the ileostomy or colostomy was created.

Predisposing Factors
A. Congenital predisposition.
B. Gender.
C. Obesity.
D. Multiparity.
E. Cirrhosis and ascites.
F. Trauma or straining.
G. African American ancestry and infancy.
H. Chronic cough; can precipitate or worsen herniation.
I. Previous abdominal surgery.
J. Straining, coughing, and sneezing in infancy.
K. Straining with chronic constipation.
L. Incisional hernia factors:
   1. Smoking.
   2. Connective tissue disorder.
   3. Infection.
   4. Malnutrition.
   5. Immunosuppressive medications.
M. Age: Obturator hernias occur predominately in the elderly.
N. Maternal smoking is associated with an increased prevalence of omphalocele and gastroschisis.

Common Findings
A. Bulge of abdomen or of a previous scar.
B. Symptoms aggravated by cough and straining.
C. Small hernias may be asymptomatic, or, as the hernia progresses, varying degrees of discomfort and pain occur.
D. The only sign of a hernia may be increased irritability.

Other Signs and Symptoms
A. Incisional: Bulge through incision wall (may be intermittent).
B. Epigastric: Small, usually painless subcutaneous mass.
C. Umbilical:
   1. Adult: Vague, intermittent pain; palpable mass.
   2. Infant: Vomiting and irritability.
D. Reducible or irreducible: Signs and symptoms are related to the degree of pressure of their contents rather than to size. Most clients are asymptomatic or complain of only mild pain.

E. Strangulated: Colicky abdominal pain, nausea, vomiting, abdominal distension, hyperperistalsis.

Subjective Data
A. Review the onset, duration, and course of symptoms.
B. Ask the client about previous abdominal surgeries, wound infection, and pregnancies.
C. Review the history of straining, trauma, or physical labour.
D. Determine whether the client has signs and symptoms of strangulation of entrapped bowel: Pain, nausea, vomiting, distension, and fever.
E. Determine whether the client can reduce the hernia.
F. Ask the client whether the hernia is enlarging and uncomfortable.
G. Review the client's bowel history, specifically constipation.
H. Review the client's history for chronic obstructive pulmonary disease (COPD)/chronic cough.
I. Review the client's history for symptoms of obstructive uropathy.
J. Review how the hernia affects the client's activities of daily living (ADL).

Physical Examination
Examination is the same for all types of abdominal hernias. Perform examination while the client is standing and supine. History and physical examination are the best means of diagnosing hernias:
A. Check temperature (if indicated), pulse, respirations, and blood pressure (BP).
B. Inspect:
   1. Inspect contour and symmetry of the abdomen for bulges or masses. The bulge may be asymmetric.
   2. Inspect irreducible hernias for discolouration, oedema, and ascites.
   3. Assess:
      a. Have the client perform Valsalva's maneuver while standing.
      b. Have the client lie supine, lift head from examination table, and then bear down to tense abdomen.
C. Auscultate all quadrants of the abdomen for bowel sounds.
D. Percuss liver, spleen, and abdomen.
E. Palpate:
   1. The entire abdomen for masses, hepatomegaly, and ascites. Umbilical hernias may be obscured by subcutaneous fat.
   2. The groin.
   3. The hernia; to try to gently reduce it.

Diagnostic Tests
A. None is required if the hernia is easily reducible (depending on the type of hernia).
B. Complete blood count (CBC): White blood cell (WBC) increased, haematocrit (Hct) increased.
C. Electrolytes: Na+ increased or decreased.
D. Abdominal radiography: Reveals abnormally high levels of gas in bowel.
E. Ultrasonography, if strangulation is suspected.
F. CT scan of the abdomen and pelvis may be indicated. In obese clients, the CT of the abdomen is the best imaging study.

Differential Diagnoses
A. Diastasis recti.
B. Ascites.
C. Abdominal wall tumour or cyst.
D. Bowel obstruction.

Plan
A. Client teaching:
   1. Discuss the hernia and available options for treatment.
   2. Teach the client signs and symptoms of strangulation.
   3. Instruct the client to refrain from heavy lifting.
   4. Advise the client to wear a support garment.
B. Medical and surgical management:

Reduction should not be attempted if there are signs of inflammation or obstruction.

   1. Try to reduce the hernia unless strangulated:
      a. Easily reducible: Abdominal contents can be easily returned to their original compartment. Allows symptomatic relief.
      b. Incarcerated: Cannot be returned to its original compartment. The incarcerated tissue may be bowel, omentum, or other abdominal contents.
      c. Strangulated: Surgical emergency—blood supply to the herniated tissue is compromised.
   2. Do not try to reduce strangulated hernias because reduction can cause gangrenous bowel to enter the peritoneal cavity.
   3. A truss fits snugly over a hernia to prevent abdominal contents from entering the hernial sac. It does not cure a hernia and is used only when the client is not a surgical candidate.
   4. Umbilical hernia repair is best performed under general anaesthesia in children.
   5. Surgery may be done laparoscopically or through an open procedure and by sutured or mesh repair, depending on the age of the person, type and size of the hernia, and the presence of strangulation.

Follow-Up
A. Instruct the client to call the office if fever or severe pain occurs. Otherwise, no follow-up is required unless for postoperative repair. Postoperative follow-up is with the physician who performed the surgery.

Consultation/Referral
Consult a gastroenterologist if the client has abdominal tenderness, discolouration, or oedema at the site; fever; or signs of bowel obstruction.
A. Pregnancy:
   1. Incisional hernias are more common during pregnancy because of increased intra-abdominal pressure.
   2. Bowel obstruction secondary to previous scarring may also be seen and is most common when the uterus emerges from the pelvis early in the second trimester, when the uterus is maximally distended at term, and in immediate puerperium when the uterus promptly decreases in size.
B. Paediatrics:
   1. Infants with umbilical hernias require no special treatment because the majority of these hernias close by the fifth year.

2. The infant's abdomen should be soft. Masses may be due to enlargement of tumours or liver. The liver is normally felt 1 to 3 cm below the right costal margin.
3. Discuss with caregivers that the umbilicus normally everts when a baby cries. However, they should report if the lump becomes large or irreducible, particularly if the baby is vomiting. These signs indicate strangulation and the need for urgent surgery.
4. Genetic testing should be considered in infants with an omphalocele. An omphalocele is associated with chromosomal abnormalities, including trisomy 13, trisomy 18, trisomy 21, or Klinefelter syndrome.
C. Geriatrics:
1. Because of the anatomic position of the obturator hernia, the presentation is more common as a bowel obstruction than as a protrusion of bowel contents:
    a. The geriatric population is more prone to develop electrolyte and acid–base imbalances from obstruction.
2. The geriatric population has a higher rate of ventral hernias attributed to the loss of muscle strength in the anterior abdominal wall and the prevalence of comorbidities that lead to an increased intra-abdominal pressure.

Bibliography

Brooks, D. C. (2014, October 4). Overview of abdominal wall hernias in adults. *UpToDate*. Retrieved from http://www.uptodate.com/contents/overview-of-abdominal-wall-hernias-in-adults

Nettina, S. (2010). *The Lippincott manual of nursing practice* (9th ed.). Philadelphia, PA: Wolters Kluwer Lippincott Williams & Wilkins.

Rather, A. A. (2015, December 1). Abdominal hernias. *Medscape*. Retrieved from http://emedicine.medscape.com/article/189563-overview

Hernias, Pelvic

Cheryl A. Glass and Kristie A. D. Morydz

Definition

A hernia is the protrusion of a peritoneum-lined sac through some defect from one anatomical space to another. As shown in Figure 11.4, there are three types of pelvic (inguinal) hernias distinguished by presentation:
A. Indirect: Protrudes through internal inguinal ring; can remain in canal, exit external ring, or pass into scrotum; unilateral or bilateral.
B. Direct: Protrudes through external inguinal ring; is located in region of Hesselbach's triangle; rarely enters scrotum.
C. Femoral: Protrudes through femoral ring, femoral canal, and fossa ovalis.

Incidence/Prevalence

A. Indirect inguinal hernias are the most common type of hernia. They affect both sexes, but most often are seen in children and young males (7:1 male-to-female ratio). Incidence increases with age.
B. Direct inguinal hernias are less common than indirect inguinal hernias. They occur more often in males and are more common in those older than 40. Primary inguinal hernias occur in 1% to 5% of infants and in 9% to 10% of those born prematurely.
C. Femoral hernias are the least common type of hernias. They are rarely seen in children and occur more often in females (1.8:1 female-to-male ratio). Right-side presentation is more common than left.
D. Among inguinal hernias, a sliding component is found in 3%; they are overwhelmingly on the left side (left-to-right ratio, 4.5:1). Sliding hernias are much more common in men than in women, and the predominance increases with age. Female infants have a high incidence of sliding tube, ovary, or broad ligament hernias.
E. Primary perineal hernias occur most often in elderly multiparous women.

Pathogenesis

Pelvic hernias occur because there is a potential space for protrusion—commonly of the bowel, but occasionally of the omentum:
A. Indirect and direct hernias arise along the course that the testicle travels as it exits the abdomen and enters the scrotum during intrauterine life. Indirect hernias may be due to a congenital defect in which the processus vaginalis remains patent.
B. Femoral hernias occur at the fossa ovalis, where the femoral artery exits the abdomen.

Predisposing Factors

A. Pregnancy.
B. Straining.
C. Age.
D. Obesity.
E. Gender.
F. Repetitive stress/hard physical labour.
G. Congenital defect.
H. Premature birth.
I. Chronic cough.
J. Chronic constipation.
K. Family history of hernia.
L. History of an abdominal aortic aneurysm (AAA).

Common Findings

A. Bulging or swelling localized in the groin or scrotum.
B. Dull ache in lower abdomen or groin.
C. Swelling of labia majora in women.
D. Children with inguinal hernias have minimal symptoms and may present with a history of an intermittent mass noted when straining or crying.
E. Bowel obstruction.

Other Signs and Symptoms

A. Ability to reduce hernia.
B. Exacerbation on standing, straining, or coughing.
C. Strangulation:
    1. Colicky abdominal pain.
    2. Nausea or vomiting.
    3. Hyperperistalsis.
    4. Fever.
    5. Oedema.
    6. Discolouration.
    7. Tenderness.
D. Infants:
    1. Distress.
    2. Vomiting.
    3. Poor feeding.
    4. Irritable and crying.

Subjective Data

A. Review the time of onset, duration, and course of hernia, and swelling.

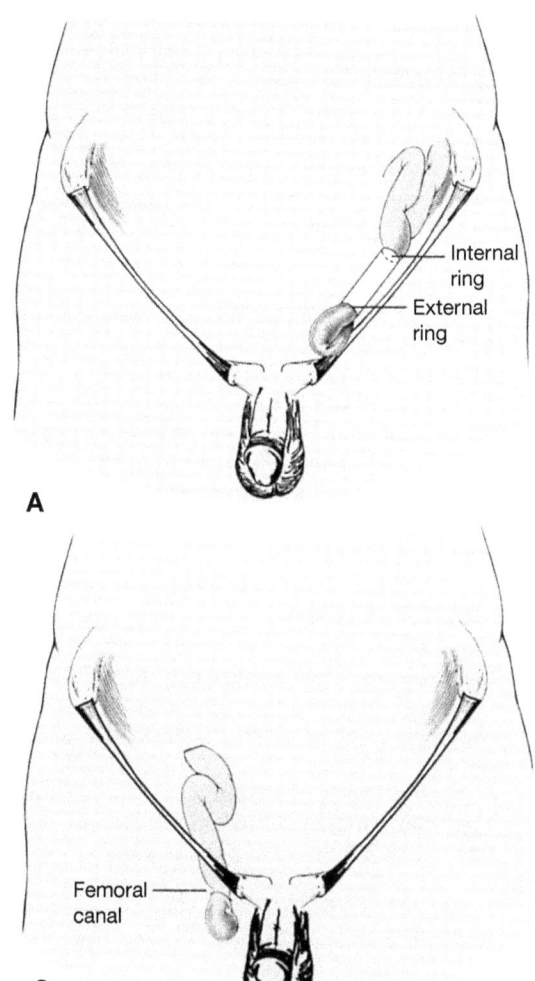
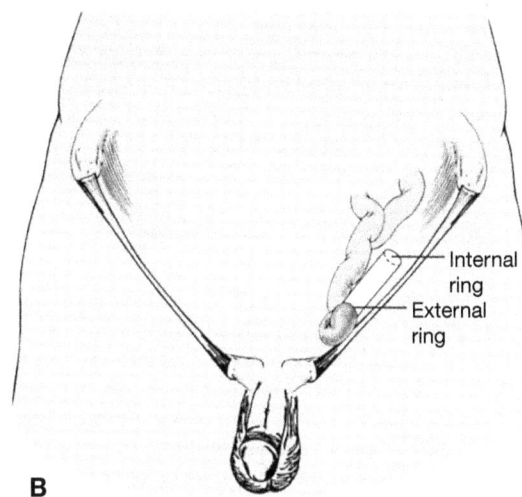

FIGURE 11.4 Pelvic hernias. (A) Indirect hernia comes down the canal and touches the fingertip on examination. (B) Direct hernia bulges anteriorly and pushes against the side of the finger on examination. (C) Femoral hernia protrudes through the femoral ring, femoral canal, and fossa ovalis, so the inguinal canal is empty on examination.

B. Review any symptoms and quality of pain. Outright pain with hernias is unusual, and its presence should raise the possibility of incarceration or strangulation.
C. Ask the client about history of straining, trauma, physical labour, and pregnancy.
D. Inquire about symptoms of obstruction or strangulation of entrapped bowel: Pain, nausea, and vomiting. Groin pain and tenderness are generally absent in strangulated femoral hernias.
E. Determine whether the client can reduce the hernia.
F. Review irritating (e.g., exercise, straining, and cough) and alleviating factors.
G. Review bowel habits, particularly constipation.
H. Evaluate history of chronic obstructive pulmonary disease (COPD) and cough.

Physical Examination

Physical examination is the same for all types of hernias and is directed at determining the type of hernia and whether it is reducible, incarcerated, or strangulated. Perform the examination while the client is standing or supine. Palpation is best done with the client standing:
A. Check temperature (if indicated), pulse, respirations, and blood pressure (BP).
B. Inspect:
  1. Inspect for discolouration and oedema of the herniated area.
  2. Inspect for visible hernia. Instruct the client to perform Valsalva's maneuver to increase intra-abdominal pressure.
  3. Transillumination of the scrotum is performed to evaluate any bowel contents.
  4. Inspect for the presence of ascites.
C. Auscultate abdomen for bowel sounds.
D. Palpate:
  1. Palpate the groin for lymphadenopathy, masses, and tenderness. *The right side is more commonly affected in both genders:*
    a. Males: Using the second or third finger, invaginate the scrotal skin, with and without cough and strain. There will be some degree of pressure with this maneuver, but a true hernia can typically be felt as a "silky" impulse tapping against the finger. Palpate the scrotum: Scrotal lump is either soft or unusually firm.
    b. Females: Visually examine for a bulge, and then place two or three fingers across the inguinal canal and ask the client to bear down or cough to elicit the characteristic bulge or impulse. Palpate the labia for swelling: Either soft or unusually firm.

Diagnostic Tests

A. History and physical examination remain the best means of diagnosing hernias.
B. Ultrasonography for abdominal masses and strangulation.

C. MRI appears to be able to differentiate inguinal and femoral hernias with a high sensitivity.
D. Sigmoidoscopy is not recommended as a screening test.
E. Plain abdominal x-rays are of limited value in the evaluation of an incarcerated hernia.
F. Karyotyping should be considered when a testicle is palpable in the inguinal canal or found at herniorrhaphy in phenotypic females.
G. Routine laboratory work is not recommended.

Differential Diagnoses
A. Acute conditions:
   1. Testicular torsion causes sudden, excruciating pain in or around the testicle, which may spread to the lower abdomen; the pain may get worse with standing. Other signs and symptoms include swelling, rising of the affected testicle, nausea, vomiting, fever, and fainting or light-headedness.
   2. Epididymitis.
B. Nonacute conditions:
   1. Testicular tumour.
   2. Muscle strain.
   3. Hip arthritis.
   4. Undescended testicle.
   5. Hydrocele.
   6. Varicocele.
   7. Spermatocele.
C. Bowel obstruction.

Plan
A. Client teaching:
   1. Advise the client to call the office right away if he finds a lump or swelling in the scrotum, even if it is small or painless. Testicular tumours are usually painless.
   2. Discuss the condition and treatment options with the client:
      a. Surgery is the only effective treatment. Open hernia repair and laparoscopic repair are the two types of haerniorrhaphy.
      b. Watchful waiting rather than surgical repair is an option if the client is asymptomatic as long as he or she is aware of the risk and understands the need for prompt attention should symptoms of complication occur.
      c. Nonsurgical therapy for groin hernias is the use of a truss. There are insufficient data to determine the efficacy of trusses in controlling symptoms. A truss has the potential risk of bowel constriction; prolonged use of a truss can lead to atrophy of the spermatic cord or fusion to the hernial sac.
   3. Teach the client signs of strangulation.
   4. Instruct the client to avoid heavy lifting.
B. Medical and surgical management: Gently reduce a groin hernia while the client lies supine with hips slightly flexed to relax the abdominal muscles.

Follow-Up
A. Advise the client to return to the office if fever, severe pain, or strangulation occurs.
B. Postoperative evaluation for hernia recurrences as needed:
   1. Immediately from repair.
   2. Greater than six months and up to five years from repair.
   3. Late recurrences beyond five years from the repair.

Consultation/Referral
A. Refer clients with femoral hernias to a surgeon. These hernias need to be repaired as soon as possible because of increased risk of incarceration and strangulation.
B. Contemporary practice triages surgical repair versus watchful waiting according to the severity of symptoms, type of hernia, and gender:
   1. Females should undergo inguinal herniorrhaphy once a diagnosis is established instead of watchful waiting.
   2. Surgical repair is indicated for males with moderate to severe symptoms from an inguinal hernia.
   3. Surgical repair is indicated in men with scrotal or recurrent hernias, even though they are asymptomatic or may only have minimal symptoms.
   4. Strangulated hernias are nonreducible, and blood supply to protruded tissue is compromised. Refer clients for immediate surgical intervention.

Individual Considerations
A. Pregnancy:
   1. Preexisting groin hernias may become more symptomatic during the first trimester of pregnancy. The symptoms must be differentiated from round ligament pain.
   2. Surgical repair of a groin hernia during a pregnancy is generally contraindicated. Generally, elective repair is deferred until four weeks' postpartum.
B. Paediatrics:
   1. A high incidence (16%–25%) of inguinal hernias occurs in premature infants. The incidence is inversely related to weight.
   2. In infants, the only symptom of a hernia may be increased irritability.
C. Geriatrics:
   1. Groin hernias are one of the most frequently encountered pathologies occurring in old age, secondary to the presence of constipation, coughing, abdominal fat deposits, and loss of strength of the abdominal wall.
   2. Signs and symptoms of prostatism are frequently present in men with hernias and may require relief before herniorrhaphy.
   3. Excessive waiting time for elective repair increases the risk of strangulation, bowel resection, and mortality, especially with older clients.

Bibliography
Brooks, D. C. (2016, May 3). Overview of treatment for inguinal and femoral hernia in adults. *UpToDate*. Retrieved from http://www.uptodate.com/contents/overview-of-treatment-for-inguinal-and-femoral-hernia-in-adults

Brooks, D. C., Obeid, A., & Hawn, M. (2013, January 25). Classification, clinical features and diagnosis of inguinal and femoral hernias in adults. *UpToDate*. Retrieved from www.uptodate.com/contents/classification-clinical-features-and-diagnosis-of-inguinal-and-femoral-hernias-in-adults?topicKey=SURG%2F3686

National Institute of Diabetes and Digestive and Kidney Diseases. (2014, June). *Inguinal hernia*. Retrieved from www.niddk.nih.gov/health-information/health-topics/digestive-diseases/inguinal-hernia/Pages/facts.aspx

Nettina, S. (2010). *The Lippincott manual of nursing practice* (9th ed.). Philadelphia, PA: Wolters Kluwer Lippincott Williams & Wilkins.

Nicks, B. A. (2012, June 6). Hernias. *Medscape*. Retrieved from http://www.emedicine.medscape.com/article/775630-overview

Ramsook, C., & Endom, E. E. (2012, September 12). Overview of inguinal hernia in children. *UpToDate*. Retrieved from www.uptodate.com/contents/overview-of-inguinal-hernia-in-children

Hirschsprung's Disease or Congenital Aganglionic Megacolon

Cheryl A. Glass and Kristie A. D. Morydz

Definition
A. Hirschsprung's disease (HD) is the major cause of intestinal obstruction in newborns. HD is congenital or present at birth. HD is a motor disorder of the gut. The aganglionic segment is aperistaltic and remains in a state of contraction, causing a functional obstruction. The majority of HD clients are diagnosed in the neonatal period. Although infants appear normal at birth, more than half do not pass meconium for more than 48 hours. Absence of peristalsis causes faeces to accumulate proximal to the defect and leads to intestinal obstruction. Bacterial enterocolitis is the most severe complication of untreated HD, and mortality from the complications may be as great as 25% to 30%.

Incidence/Prevalence
A. HD occurs in approximately one in every 5,000 live births. It is uncommon in premature infants.
B. Occurrence is more common in males; however, long-segment disease increases in females.
C. About 10% to 50% of cases have familial incidence. Around eight genetic mutations have been identified. One in 100 children with Down syndrome also have HD.
D. HD is associated with other chromosomal abnormalities and syndromes:
    1. Trisomy 21 (Down syndrome).
    2. Cardiac disease (septal defects).
    3. Bardet–Biedl syndrome (BBS).
    4. Congenital central hypoventilation syndrome (CCHS).
    5. Waardenburg syndrome.
    6. Smith–Lemli–Opitz syndrome.
    7. Multiple endocrine neoplasia type 2.
    8. Shprintzen–Goldberg syndrome.
    9. Piebaldism.
    10. Yemenite deaf–blind syndrome.
    11. Neurocristopathy syndromes.
E. Approximately 80% of affected clients have the disorder limited to the rectum or rectosigmoid region.
F. From 3% to 5% of affected clients have aganglionosis of the entire colon.
G. The disease is three times more common in people of European ancestry.
H. Around 25% of HD clients have associated congenital anomalies of the kidney and urinary tract (hydronephrosis and renal hypoplasia).

Pathogenesis
A. The disorder is due to congenital absence of ganglion cells in both Meissner's (submucosal) and Auerbach's (myenteric) plexus. It occurs secondary to the failure of migration of ganglia from the neural crest, which normally occurs before the 12th week of gestation. The disorder starts in the distal rectum and extends proximally to involve a varying amount of the bowel.

Predisposing Factors
A. Full-term infant of normal weight.
B. European ancestry.
C. Male gender.
D. Family history of disorder.
E. Down syndrome.

Common Findings
A. Newborns: Failure to pass meconium for more than 48 hours.
B. Blast sign: Explosive expulsion of gas and stool after a digital rectal examination.
C. Children: Failure to grow.
D. Constipation.
E. Abdominal distension.

Other Signs and Symptoms
A. Newborns:
    1. Overflow-type diarrhoea.
    2. Bile- or faeces-stained vomitus.
    3. Failure to thrive (FTT).
    4. Anorexia due to early satiety, abdominal discomfort, and distension.
    5. Temporary relief with enema.
B. Older infants and children (nearly all children with HD are diagnosed during the first two years of life):
    1. Constipation since birth; may have a history of requiring a daily enema.
    2. Older presentation is more common in breastfed infants; constipation will typically develop around the time of weaning.
    3. Intestinal obstruction.
    4. Progressive abdominal distension with visible peristaltic activity.
    5. Temporary relief with enema.
    6. Ribbonlike, fluidlike, or pellet stools.
    7. FTT.
    8. Anaemia.

Subjective Data
A. In newborns, review the onset, duration, and course of symptoms, including number of bowel movements (BMs), passage of first stool, and expulsion of flatus.
B. Ask the client or caregiver about family history of HD.
C. Review the infant's weight and growth parameters.
D. Inquire about other symptoms of bowel obstruction, such as vomiting and diarrhoea.
E. Ask about other complications such as blood in stool.
F. Review the history of BMs and feeding habits, including onset of constipation, character of stools (ribbonlike or fluid filled), frequency of BMs, and use of enemas.

Physical Examination
A. Check temperature (if indicated), pulse, respirations, blood pressure (BP), weight, and growth parameters including length and head circumference.
B. Inspect:
    1. Note general appearance, level of activity, abdominal distension, and signs of malnutrition.
    2. Inspect fontanelles for signs of dehydration.
    3. Inspect the lower back for evidence of spinal cord involvement, such as a hairy or hyperpigmented patch, gluteal fold asymmetry, cutaneous dimples, sinus tracts, and lipomas.
C. Auscultate the abdomen for bowel sounds in all quadrants.
D. Percuss the abdomen for organomegaly.
E. Palpate the abdomen for distension and masses. Specifically examine the left quadrant for the presence of stool.

F. Neurologic examination to evaluate other systemic disease related to constipation.
G. Rectal examination:
  1. Check for "tight" anal sphincter and absence of stool in rectal ampulla.
  2. Many infants have relief of symptoms and pass large amounts of stool and flatus after examination (Blast sign).
  3. Test the perineal sensation and the anocutaneous "wink" reflex by stroking the skin around the anus using a cotton-tipped swab.

Diagnostic Tests
A. Full-thickness rectal biopsy is considered the gold standard for diagnosis of HD. The biopsy is obtained by mucosal suction.
B. Contrast barium enema (BE): 25% of cases appear normal.
C. Anorectal manometry.
D. Ultrasonography.
E. Plain abdominal x-ray (distended bowel loops and air in the rectum).
F. Chemistry panel to evaluate fluid and electrolyte management.

Differential Diagnoses
A. Constipation.
B. Meconium peritonitis.
C. Meconium plug syndrome.
D. Meconium ileus.
E. Intestinal obstruction.
F. Enterocolitis.
G. Megacolon (acute, chronic, or toxic).
H. Hypothyroidism.
I. Irritable bowel syndrome (IBS).

Plan
A. Client teaching:
  1. Prepare caregivers or the client for referral or consultation.
  2. Teach caregivers or the client about HD and treatment therapy.
B. Medical and surgical management:
  1. Treatment consists of colostomy performed proximal to aganglionic segment with biopsies taken at the time of surgery to identify level of involvement. Definitive repair can then be performed when the infant is six to 12 months old.
    a. There are two types of surgical procedures:
      i. Pull-through procedure involves removal of the affected part of the large intestine and anastomose to the healthy part of the anus.
      ii. Ostomy surgery reroutes the intestine through the abdominal wall, forming a stoma.
  2. The mainstay of treatment is surgery; however, in older children when symptoms are chronic but not severe, treatment may consist of isotonic enemas, stool softeners, and low-residue diet.

Follow-Up
A. Paediatric surgeons and gastroenterologists should generally care for children with HD.

Consultation/Referral
A. Consult or refer the client to a paediatrician if HD is suspected in an infant:
  1. Bloody mucoid diarrhoea in an infant with a history of constipation could be an indication of enterocolitis complicating HD.
  2. An empty contracted anal canal in a constipated child may suggest HD.
B. Consider genetic testing.

Individual Considerations
A. Paediatrics:
  1. Recurrence risk is proportional to the length of aganglionic segment of the colon.
  2. Infants who have symptom relief after rectal examination and pass large amounts of stool and gas (Blast sign) can have recurrence of symptoms, often fail to grow normally, can have constipation or diarrhoea, and may have protein loss in their stool.

Bibliography
National Institute of Diabetes and Digestive and Kidney Diseases. (2015, September). *Hirschsprung disease*. Retrieved from https://www.niddk.nih.gov/health-information/health-topics/digestive-diseases/hirschsprung-disease/Pages/ez.aspx

Nettina, S. (2010). *The Lippincott manual of nursing practice* (9th ed.). Philadelphia, PA: Wolters Kluwer Lippincott Williams & Wilkins.

Neville, H. L. (2012, May 8). Pediatric Hirschsprung disease. *Medscape*. Retrieved from http://emedicine.medscape.com/article/929733-overview

Wagner, J. P. (2015, August 18). Hirschsprung disease. *Medscape*. Retrieved from http://emedicine.medscape.com/article/178493-overview

Wesson, D. E. (2012, December 13). Congenital aganglionic megacolon (Hirschsprung disease). *UpToDate*. Retrieved from http://www.uptodate.com/contents/congenital-aganglionic-megacolon-hirschsprung-disease

Hookworm

Cheryl A. Glass and Kristie A. D. Morydz

Definition
A. Hookworm is a chronic, debilitating parasitic disease with vague symptoms that vary in proportion to the degree of iron-deficiency anaemia and hypoproteinaemia of the host. The adult hookworm attaches to the small intestinal wall and ingests the host's blood and nutrients. Chronic infection in children may lead to physical growth delay, cognitive deficits, and developmental delay. Anaemia and hypoproteinaemia are produced by the blood-clotting activity of adult nematodes in the intestines.

Incidence/Prevalence
A. Incidence in Canada is unknown. Globally, about 740 million are infected with hookworms.

Pathogenesis
A. Disease is caused by infection with *Ancylostoma duodenale, Ancylostoma ceylonicum*, and *Necator americanus* (soil-transmitted helminthes) intestinal parasites. Mixed infections are common. Humans are the major reservoir. *A. duodenale* may be ingested. Eggs of the nematode hatch into larvae that penetrate the soles of feet and palms of hands from contact with contaminated soil. Contact for five to 10 minutes results in skin penetration. Larvae are carried by circulation to lungs and eventually to their final habitat, the small intestines. Eggs are passed in stools of infected persons. Although hookworms are not transmitted from person to person, infected persons can contaminate soil by defecation as long as they are untreated.

B. Incubation period, or the time from exposure to eggs excreted in stool to the development of noncutaneous symptoms, is four to 12 weeks. The appearance of parasites in the blood is four to six weeks. Adult worms or larvae are rarely seen.

Predisposing Factors
A. Living in or travelling to rural, tropic, or subtropic areas where soil contamination with human faeces is common.
B. Exposure to loose, sandy, moist, shady, well-aerated, warm soil where larvae and eggs thrive.
C. Agricultural workers.
D. Tourists with bare feet or open footwear that exposes skin to contaminated soil.
E. Military troops in endemic areas.
F. Children.

Common Findings
A. Intense stinging or burning at penetration site, followed by pruritus and papulovesicular rash that persists for one to two weeks.
B. Fatigue.
C. Weight loss.
D. Vague abdominal discomfort.
E. Loss of appetite.

Other Signs and Symptoms
A. **Anaemia is the principal manifestation of hookworm infestation; it occurs secondary to blood loss.** *Severe anaemia affects children and pregnant women disproportionately due to their preexisting iron stores.* **Severe anaemia symptoms include the following:**
  1. Fatigue.
  2. Syncope.
  3. Exertional dyspnoea.
  4. Tachycardia.
  5. Pallor.
B. Pharyngeal itching after oral ingestion.
C. Hoarseness.
D. Nausea or vomiting.
E. Cough or wheeze from pulmonary infiltration due to heavy infestation.
F. Colicky abdominal pain or diarrhoea: late sign, occurring with marked eosinophilia 29 to 38 days after exposure.
G. Oedema.
H. Mild diarrhoea.

Subjective Data
A. Review the onset, duration, and course of symptoms including recent episodes of intense itching of feet, palms of hands, or buttocks.
B. Establish client's normal weight and amount of any weight lost, over what length of time.
C. Inquire about abdominal symptoms, including onset and intensity.
D. Review other gastrointestinal (GI) symptoms such as diarrhoea.
E. Review any transitory chest symptoms, such as cough or wheezing. Is there a history of asthma?
F. Ask the client if any other family members are exhibiting the same symptoms.

Physical Examination
A. Check temperature (if indicated), pulse, respirations, blood pressure (BP), and weight.
B. Inspect skin on the entire body, especially the soles of both feet. Erythematous, papular vesicular lesions may be excoriated from scratching. Rash persists for one to two weeks.
C. Palpate the abdomen for masses and tenderness.
D. Auscultate the abdomen and lungs.

Diagnostic Tests
A. Identification of hookworm eggs in faeces is diagnostic. Faecal egg excretion does not become detectable until around two months after dermal exposure. Repeated stool samples may be needed for diagnosis.
B. Haemoglobin (Hgb) and haematocrit (Hct) for anaemia.
C. Complete blood count (CBC) with differential: May have mild eosinophilia.
D. Beaver direct smear, Stoll egg-counting, or Kato–Katz techniques quantify infection.
E. Endoscopic examination may reveal the adult worms.

Differential Diagnoses
A. Growth failure/failure to thrive (FTT).
B. Acute or chronic anaemia.
C. Asthma.
D. Poor nutrition.
E. Giardiasis.
F. Amoebiasis.
G. Ascariasis.
H. Gastroenteritis.

Plan
A. Client teaching:
  1. Discuss with the client the dangers of going barefoot outdoors.
  2. Explain that good handwashing is critical, especially after defecation.
  3. There is no direct person-to-person transmission.
  4. Use good sanitary practices to prevent soil contamination.
B. Dietary management: Teach the client how to correct anaemia through good nutrition.
C. Pharmacological therapy:
The dosage is the same for children as adults:
  1. Mebendazole is first-line treatment.
  2. Pyrantel pamoate.
  3. Iron replacement therapy and nutritional supplements (proteins and vitamins including folate) may be needed to correct anaemia.
  4. At the present time, there is no hookworm vaccine.

Follow-Up
A. Stool should be examined again two weeks after therapy is completed. If results are positive, repeat therapy is indicated.
B. Reinfection is common.
C. Iron supplement should be continued even after Hgb values return to normal.

Consultation/Referral
A. Refer pregnant clients to an obstetrician.
B. Refer children if Hgb is <60 g/L. Cardiac decompensation occasionally develops in children with Hgb concentrations of <60 g/L.

Individual Considerations
A. Pregnancy:

1. Anthelmintics are in pregnancy category C; however, the potential risks to the foetus versus benefits should be considered.
2. The World Health Organization (WHO) has determined that the benefit of pharmacological treatment outweighs its risk:
   a. The WHO allows the use of albendazole in the second and third trimesters of pregnancy.
   b. The WHO allows the use of pyrantel pamoate in the second and third trimesters of pregnancy.
3. Adequate protein and iron nutrition should be maintained throughout pregnancy.
4. Consider delaying treatment until after delivery if necessary.

B. Paediatrics:
1. All medications are advised for children:
   a. The WHO guidelines for mass prevention campaigns indicate albendazole can be used in children as young as 1 year old.
   b. Mebendazole and pyrantel pamoate are on the WHO Model List of Essential Medicines for Children, intended for the use in children up to 12 years of age.
2. Severely affected children may require a blood transfusion.
3. Pysical and cognitive growth can be affected.

Bibliography

American Academy of Pediatrics. (2012). Hookworm infections (*Ancylostoma duodenale* and *Necator americanus*). In L. K. Pickering (Ed.), *Red book: 2012 report of the Committee on Infectious Diseases* (29th ed., pp. 411–413). Elk Grove Village, IL: Author. Retrieved from https://redbook.solutions.aap.org/DocumentLibrary/RB12_interior.pdf

Centers for Disease Control and Prevention. (2013, January 10). *Parasites—Hookworms*. Retrieved from https://www.cdc.gov/parasites/hookworm/health_professionals/index.html#tx

Haburchak, D. R. (2016, February 24). Hookworm disease treatment & management. *Medscape reference.* Retrieved from http://emedicine.medscape.com/article/218805

Nettina, S. (2010). *The Lippincott manual of nursing practice* (9th ed.). Philadelphia, PA: Wolters Kluwer Lippincott Williams & Wilkins.

Weller, P. F., & Leder, K. (2016, July 1). Hookworm infection. *UpToDate.* Retrieved from http://www.uptodate.com/contents/hookworm-infection

Irritable Bowel Syndrome (IBS)

Cheryl A. Glass and Kristie A. D. Morydz

Definition

Irritable bowel syndrome (IBS) is the most common of the gastrointestinal (GI) motility disorders. IBS is responsible for significant direct and indirect health-care costs. It is a relapsing functional disturbance of intestinal motility marked by a common symptom complex that includes bloating and abdominal pain or discomfort associated with defecation. Bladder dysfunction has been identified in 50% of clients with IBS. Clients commonly transition between subgroups.

IBS is defined by symptom-based diagnostic criteria, in the absence of detectable organic causes. Rome III criteria for IBS are related to stool characteristics:

A. IBS with diarrhoea predominant (IBS-D): Loose stools (small volume, pasty/mushy or watery) more than 25% of the time and hard stools <25% of the time.
B. IBS with constipation (small, hard, pellet-like stools) predominant (IBS-C): Hard stools >25% of the time and loose stools<25% of the time.
C. IBS with alternating bouts of constipation and diarrhoea, mixed or cyclic pattern (IBS-M): Both hard and soft stools >25% of the time.
D. On clinical grounds, other subclassifications are used:
1. Based on symptoms:
   a. IBS with predominant bowel dysfunction.
   b. IBS with predominant pain.
   c. IBS with predominant bloating.
2. Based on precipitating factors:
   a. Postinfectious irritable bowel syndrome (PI-IBS).
   b. Food induced (meal induced).
   c. Stress related.

Incidence/Prevalence

A. IBS is common, accounting for about 40% of GI complaints seen by health-care professionals, and is a major cause of morbidity in Canada. Studies suggest nearly 20% of all adults suffer from some form of the condition; however, only a fraction seek medical help. IBS is recognized in children; symptoms consistent with IBS are reported in 16% of students aged 11 to 17 years. IBS is not described in preschool-aged children.
B. IBS-D is more common in men.
C. IBS-C is more common in women.

Pathogenesis

A. IBS has an absence of detectable pathology, and laboratory tests are unrevealing. The understanding of IBS has evolved from a disturbance in bowel motor activity to a more integrated understanding of visceral hypersensitivity and brain–gut interaction. It is thought to be both a normal response to severe stress and a learned visceral response to stress:
1. Nonpropulsive colonic contractions lead to IBS-C predominant.
2. Increased contraction in the small bowel and proximal colon with diminished activity in the distal colon lead to IBS-D predominant.

B. Most clients with functional disorders appear to have inappropriate perception of physiological events and altered reflex responses in different gut regions.
C. The brain–gut transmitters act at different sites in the brain and gut and lead to varied effects on GI motility, pain control, emotional behaviour, and immunity. Serotonin plays a critical role in the regulation of GI motility, secretion, and sensation. Studies have shown that IBS may be related to an imbalance in mucosal serotonin and 5-hydroxytryptamine (5-HT) availability caused by defects in 5-HT production, serotonin receptors, or serotonin transport.

Predisposing Factors

A. Age:
1. IBS mainly occurs between the ages of 15 and 65 years:
   a. About 50% of IBS occurs before age 35 years.
   b. About 40% of IBS occurs between ages 35 and 50 years.
B. Gender:
1. Women are two to three times more likely to have IBS.
2. In paediatrics, both sexes are equally affected.
C. Emotional factors and situational stress.
D. Prior GI infection–induced IBS.
E. Genetics.
F. Carbohydrate intolerance may produce significant symptoms.

Common Findings
A. Chronic relapsing stool pattern:
   1. Diarrhoea, over three loose stools per day.
   2. Alternation of diarrhoea with constipation. Diarrhoea is typically small in volume, has visible mucus, and may follow a hard movement by a few hours.
   3. Constipation: Less than three bowel movements (BMs) per week.
B. Feeling of incomplete evacuation.
C. Abdominal distension and bloating.
D. Straining with BMs.
E. Aching or cramps in periumbilical or lower abdominal region.
F. Pain relief with BM.

Other Signs and Symptoms
A. Change in bowel function.
B. Clear mucous stool.
C. Pain may be precipitated by meals.
D. Pain radiates to the left chest or arm, from gas in splenic flexure. Nocturnal pain is unusual and is considered a warning sign.
E. Flatulence.
F. Nausea.
G. Anxiety.
H. Depression.
I. Preoccupation with bowel symptoms.
J. Extraintestinal symptoms:
   1. Dysmenorrhoea.
   2. Urinary frequency, urgency, and incomplete bladder emptying.
   3. Impaired sexual function and dyspareunia.
   4. Fibromyalgia.
K. Menses may exacerbate IBS symptoms.
L. Red-flag symptoms and differential diagnoses for IBS (see Table 11.14).

Subjective Data
A. Review pattern of main symptoms, including the onset, duration, and usual course.
B. Ask the client what are the predominant symptoms—abdominal pain, diarrhoea, or constipation.
C. Review the client's history for stress factors, and ask whether recurrent symptoms occur in relation to them.
D. Ask what other symptoms occur with the pain, diarrhoea, or constipation, such as bloating, blood in stool, or nighttime BMs. **Bleeding, weight loss, and nocturnal diarrhoea are not characteristic of IBS. IBS symptoms disappear during sleep.**
E. Establish client's normal weight history, and determine amount of weight loss, if any, over what time period.
F. Review the client's diet, including the following:
   1. Response to milk or lactose products.
   2. Artificial sweeteners.
   3. Alcohol intake.
   4. Irregular or inadequate meals.
   5. Insufficient fluid intake.
   6. Excessive fiber intake.
   7. Obsession with dietary hygiene.
   8. Response to gluten (wheat, barley, rye) ingestion.
G. Inquire about the client's prescription, herbal, and over-the-counter (OTC) medications. Ask specifically about the use of laxatives.
H. Review travel and food history for dominant history of diarrhoea.
I. Ask the client if there is a family history of colon cancer, ulcerative colitis (UC), Crohn's disease (CD), or malabsorption.
J. Is there any fever accompanying lower abdominal pain?
K. What is the relation of symptoms to menstruation?

Physical Examination
A. Check temperature (if indicated), pulse, respirations, blood pressure (BP), and weight.
B. Inspect:
   1. Observe general appearance. Does the client appear anxious or depressed?
   2. Inspect abdominal contour for masses and bulges.
C. Auscultate all quadrants of the abdomen for bowel sounds; note whether they are normal or mildly hyperactive.
D. Percuss the abdomen for tympany or dullness.
E. Palpate the abdomen:
   1. Evaluate the abdomen for mild tenderness, rigidity, guarding, and masses.

TABLE 11.14 Common and Red-Flag Differential Diagnoses for IBS

Disorder	Signs and Symptoms	Diagnostic Tests
Ulcerative colitis	Peaks ages 15–35 years Bloody diarrhoea with mucus, fever, abdominal pain, tenesmus, weight loss	Sigmoidoscopy, colonoscopy, BE
Crohn's disease	Onset ages 15–35 or 70–80 year: Fever, abdominal pain, diarrhoea, fatigue, weight loss, anorectal fissures, fistulae, abscesses	Sigmoidoscopy, colonoscopy, BE
Infectious diarrhoea	Chronic diarrhoea with cramps with or without blood and mucus	Microscopy, stool studies, sigmoidoscopy
Diverticulitis	Lower left abdominal pain, fever, altered bowel habits	CBC, CT, BE
Colorectal malignancy	Age 50 years or older: Rectal bleeding, altered bowel habits, abdominal or back pain, anaemia, occult blood in stool, weight loss	Colonoscopy
Medication side effects	Antacids, laxatives, SSRIs, thyroid hormones, metformin, narcotics, calcium channel blockers, anticholinergics	History of concordance of symptoms with medication initiation, trial of drug holiday or reducing dosage, rechallenge

BE, barium enema; CBC, complete blood count; IBS, irritable bowel syndrome; SSRIs, selective serotonin reuptake inhibitors.

2. Evaluate for hepatosplenomegaly.
3. Evaluate for lymphadenopathy.
F. Rectal examination:
   1. Check for masses and tenderness.
   2. Obtain stool for diagnostic tests.
   3. Rectal examination is normal with IBS.

Diagnostic Tests

A. The Canadian Association of Gastroenterology recommends that clients younger than 50 years who do not have alarm features need not undergo routine colonic imaging. Clients with IBS symptoms who have alarm features, such as anaemia or weight loss, or those who are older than 60 years, should undergo colonic imaging to exclude organic disease.
B. Diagnosis of IBS is usually suspected on the basis of the client's history and physical examination without additional tests (see Table 11.15).
C. Diagnostic tests are performed to exclude organic disease that may masquerade as IBS:
   1. Complete blood count (CBC).
   2. Sedimentation rate or C-reactive protein (CRP).
   3. Serum potassium, if the client is on diuretics; hypokalaemia may reduce bowel contractility and produce an ileus.
   4. Blood glucose, if diarrhoea predominates; rule out diabetes mellitus, which may present as diarrhoea resulting from diabetic gastroenteropathy.
   5. Thyroid function study.
   6. Stool specimen: Culture for leukocytes and fat, ova and parasites, and occult blood; leukocyte-free mucus is a hallmark of IBS.
   7. Stool cultures for *Clostridium difficile* toxin assay, if clinically indicated.
   8. Barium enema (BE) and/or proctosigmoidoscopy for severe signs and symptoms, after consultation or referral.
   9. Celiac serology, if appropriate,
   10. A mucosal biopsy is appropriate if a colonoscopy or sigmoidoscopy is performed.
   11. Oesophagogastroduodenoscopy (EGD) and distal duodenal biopsy in clients with diarrhoea should be considered to rule out celiac disease, tropical sprue, giardiasis, and for clients in whom abdominal pain and discomfort is located more in the upper abdomen.
   12. Hydrogen breath test to evaluate lactose intolerance and small-intestinal bowel overgrowth (SIBO).

TABLE 11. **Rome IV Diagnostic Criteria for IBS**

Onset of symptoms at least six months before diagnosis
Recurrent abdominal pain or discomfort on average, at least one day per week during the past three months
At least two of the following features: **A.** Related to defecation **B.** Association with a change in frequency of stool **C.** Association with a change in stool form

IBS, irritable bowel syndrome.

Differential Diagnoses

A. Inflammatory bowel disease (IBD; CD/UC).
B. Viral or bacterial gastroenteritis.
C. GI neoplasm.
D. Acute diarrhoea caused by protozoa or bacteria.
E. Lactose insufficiency/deficiency.
F. Laxative misuse.
G. Drug side effect.
H. Diabetes.
I. Celiac spruce/gluten aetiology.
J. Diverticulitis.
K. Failure to thrive (FTT) in children.
L. Endometriosis/pelvic inflammatory disease (PID).
M. Zollinger–Ellison syndrome.

Plan

A. General interventions:
   1. Advise the client to keep a diary of events of BMs and precipitating factors.
   2. Encourage the client to quit smoking because nicotine may aggravate symptoms.
   3. Recommend daily exercise to reduce stress.
   4. Stress management should be encouraged, including counselling, tapes, meditation, and yoga.
B. Client teaching: *Refer to Client Teaching Guide: Irritable Bowel Syndrome.*
C. Dietary management:
   1. Prescribe a high-fiber diet.
   2. Encourage the client to avoid foods that aggravate the bowel, including gas-producing foods such as broccoli, beans, onions, garlic, and so forth. When diarrhoea predominates, dietary review is essential for clues of intolerance to lactose or sorbitol.
D. Pharmacological therapy:
   1. Advise the client to stop all nonessential medications that may affect bowel function, especially irritant laxatives. Avoid narcotics, depressants, and other long-term drug use if possible.
   2. Recommend eliminating sorbitol-containing candy and restricting lactose-containing milk products.
   3. First-line treatment: Psyllium hydrophilic mucilloid. This treats both diarrhoea and constipation.
   4. Pain relief:
      a. Opiates should be avoided due to the risk of dependence and addiction in chronic conditions.
      b. Nonsteroidal anti-inflammatory drugs (NSAIDs) have an undesirable side effect on the GI tract.
      c. Antispasmodics and anticholinergic agents (IBS-D predominant):
         i. Hyoscyamine.
         ii. Dicyclomine.
      d. Tricyclic antidepressants for IBS-D predominant. Tricyclics should be avoided for constipated clients:
         i. Amitriptyline.
         ii. Nortriptyline.
         iii. Desipramine.
         iv. Imipramine.
   5. Antidiarrhoeals:
      a. Opiate-derived medications are reserved for very severe cases, secondary to the potential for misuse.
      b. Loperamide.

▶ Client Teaching Guides are available at https://connect.springerpub.com/content/reference-book/978-0-8261-9498-5

c. Alosetron, a 5-HT$_3$ receptor antagonist, is indicated only for women with severe IBS-D predominant.
  6. Laxatives and stool softeners (IBS-C predominant) along with dietary measures and fiber supplements:
   a. Mineral oil.
   b. Stimulant laxatives may be necessary intermittently for short periods, but prolonged use of stimulant laxatives should be avoided.
   c. Lactulose is a colonic acidifier that promotes laxation. Transit time through the colon may be slow; 24 to 48 hours may be required to produce a BM. Lactulose contains galactose and lactose, and should be used with caution for clients with diabetes. Safety in paediatric clients has not been established.
  7. Lubiprostone, a selective C-2 chloride-channel activator, is indicated for women 18 years and over with IBS-C predominant.
  8. Probiotics.
  9. Linaclotide, guanylate cyclase-C (GC-C) agonist is used for both IBS-C and chronic idiopathic constipation (CIC).
  10. Eluxadoline, a mu-opioid receptor agonist, is indicated for IBS-D predominant. There are two recommended dosings:
   a. Alternative dosing is needed for clients with the following conditions:
    i. Do not have a gallbladder.
    ii. Unable to tolerate 100 mg BID.
    iii. Are receiving concomitant OATP1B1 inhibitor, such as the lipid-lowering drug gemfibrozil and its metabolite gemfibrozil 1 O beta.
    iv. Have mild or moderate hepatic impairment.
   b. If a dose is missed, clients should not compensate by taking two doses at once.

Follow-Up
A. Reevaluate the effectiveness of treatment in two weeks. Treatment may be challenging for symptom management and numerous tests that are inconclusive but rule out pathology.
B. If symptoms persist without relief, have the client return as needed.
C. Return if diarrhoea/constipation lasts more than two weeks on medication therapy.

Consultation/Referral
A. Refer to a gastroenterologist for red-flag symptoms.
B. Refer to a paediatric gastroenterologist if findings from the client's history, physical examination, or screening laboratory tests are suggestive of organic disease.
C. Consider a psychiatric consultation, if indicated, for anxiety, depression, somatization, and symptom-related fears.

Individual Considerations
A. Paediatrics:
  1. IBS is recognized in children, and many clients trace the onset of symptoms to childhood.
  2. Children who have a history of recurrent abdominal pain are at increased risk of IBS during adolescence and young adulthood.
  3. The recommended daily intake of fiber (in grams) for children is estimated by adding four to their age in years.

B. Adults:
  1. Annual rectal examination and sigmoidoscopy are recommended after age 50 years.
  2. When constipation predominates, rule out malignancy, particularly in clients older than 40 years who have weight loss or a family history of colon cancer.

Resource
Health Canada Canadian Drug Database
Rome Foundation: https://theromefoundation.org/

Bibliography
American College of Gastroenterology. (2011). Pregnancy and gastrointestinal disorders. *Pregnancy monograph*. Retrieved from http://gi.org/wp-content/uploads/2011/07/institute-PregnancyMonograph.pdf

Andersen, S. (2012, August). Beware the irritable bowel deciphering the overlap of symptoms. *ADVANCE for NPs & PAs, 3*(21–24), 32.

Attara, G. P., Gray, J., & Aumais, G. (2018). A269 Irritable bowel syndrome patient experience in Canada. *Journal of the Canadian Association of Gastroenterology, 1*(Suppl. 1), 467–468. doi:10.1093/jcag/gwy008.270

Beltrán, B. (2011, June 14). Old-age inflammatory bowel disease onset: A different problem? *World Journal of Gastroenterology, 17*, 2734–2739. doi:10.3748/wjg.v17.i22.2734

Burger, D., & Travis, S. (2011). Conventional medical management of inflammatory bowel disease. *Gastroenterology, 140*, 1827–1837. doi:10.1053/j.gastro.2011.02.045

Carter, M. J., Lobo, A. J., & Travis, S. P. L. (2004). Guidelines for the management of inflammatory bowel disease in adults. *Gut, 53*(Suppl. 5), V1–V16. doi:10.1136/gut.2004.043372. Retrieved from http://gut.bmj.com/content/53/suppl_5/vl.extract

Ford, A. C., Moayyedi, P., Lacy, B. E., Lembo, A. J., Saito, Y. A., Schiller, L. R., & Task Force on the Management of Functional Bowel Disorders. (2014). American College of Gastroenterology monograph on management of irritable bowel syndrome and chronic idiopathic constipation. *American Journal of Gastrenterology, 109*, S2–S26. doi:10.1038/ajg.2014.187

Gisbert, J. P., & Chaparro, M. (2014). Inflammatory bowel disease in the elderly. *Medscape*. Retrieved from http://www.medscape.com/viewarticle/820753

Lehrer, J. K. (2015, June 16). Irritable bowel syndrome treatment & management. *Medscape*. Retrieved from http://emedicine.medscape.com/article/180389-treatment

Lichtenstein, G. R., Abreu, M. T., Cohen, R., & Tremaine, W. (2006). American Gastroenterological Association Institute medical position statement on corticosteroids, immunomodulators, and infliximab in inflammatory bowel disease. *Gastroenterology, 130*, 935–939. doi:10.1053/j.gastro.2006.01.047

Medical Letter®. (March, 2012). Treatment guidelines from the medical letter, drugs for inflammatory bowel disease. *Medical Letter, 10*(15), 19–30.

Nettina, S. (2010). *The Lippincott manual of nursing practice* (9th ed.). Philadelphia, PA: Wolters Kluwer Lippincott Williams & Wilkins.

Rowe, W. A. (2013, June 18). Inflammatory bowel disease. *Medscape*. Retrieved from http://emedicine.medscape.com/article/179037-overview

Sartor, R. B. (2015, July 6). Antibiotics for treatment of inflammatory bowel diseases. *UpToDate*. Retrieved from http://www.uptodate.com/contents/antibiotics-for-treatment-of-inflammatory-bowel-diseases

Satsangi, J., Silverberg, M. S., Vermeire, S., & Colombel, J.-F. (2006). The Montreal classification of inflammatory bowel disease: Controversies, consensus, and implications. *Gut, 55*, 749–753. doi:10.1136/gut.2005.082909

Surawicz, C. M., Brandt, L. J., Binion, D. G., Ananthakrishnan, A. N., Curry, S. R., Gilligan, P. H., & Zuckerbraun, B. S. (2013). Guidelines for diagnosis, treatment, and prevention of *Clostridium difficile* infections. *American Journal of Gastroenterology, 108*, 478–498. doi:10.1038/ajg.2013.4

World Gastroenterology Organisation Global Guidelines. (2009, June). *Inflammatory bowel disease: A global perspective*. Retrieved from http://www.worldgastroenterology.org/assets/downloads/en/pdf/guidelines/21_inflammatory_bowel_disease.pdf

World Gastroenterology Organisation Global Guidelines. (2015, September). *Irritable bowel syndrome: A global perspective*. Retrieved from http://www.worldgastroenterology.org/guidelines/global-guidelines/irritable-bowel-syndrome-ibs/irritable-bowel-syndrome-ibs-english

Jaundice

Cheryl A. Glass and Kristie A. D. Morydz

Definition
A. Jaundice is a yellow tinge to the skin or mucous membranes. It is a symptom, not a disease. The diagnostic approach begins with gathering a comprehensive history, physical examination, and screening laboratory tests. The differential diagnosis is formulated, and further testing may be warranted. The onset of jaundice usually prompts the client or family to seek medical attention. Jaundice can reflect a medical emergency secondary to massive haemolysis, ascending cholangitis, unconjugated hyperbilirubinaemia in the neonatal period, and fulminant liver failure.

Incidence/Prevalence
A. Incidence is variable according to pathogenesis, age, and population.

Pathogenesis
The mechanism responsible for jaundice includes excess bilirubin production, decreased hepatic uptake, impaired conjugation, intrahepatic cholestasis, extrahepatic obstruction, and hepatocellular injury (see Table 11.16). However, it is important to recognize that more than one mechanism can be operating in a given case (i.e., sickle cell anaemia and HIV):
A. Excess bilirubin production results from accelerated red cell destruction. The excessive amounts of haemoglobin and resultant bilirubin released into the bloodstream overwhelm the liver's normal capacity for uptake, and an unconjugated hyperbilirubinaemia ensues.
B. With decreased uptake and conjugation, there is often a concurrent, acquired illness such as infection, cardiac disease, or cancer. Hereditary conditions, such as Gilbert and Crigler–Najjar syndromes, are responsible.
C. Intrahepatic cholestasis may occur at a number of levels: Intracellularly (e.g., hepatitis), at the canalicular level (when oestrogen is induced), at the ductule (phenothiazine exposure), at the septal ducts (primary biliary cirrhosis), and at the intralobular ducts (cholangiocarcinoma).
D. Extrahepatic obstruction occurs when a stone, stricture, or tumour blocks the flow of bile within the extrahepatic biliary tree. A history of gallstones, biliary tract surgery, or malignancy may be elicited.

Predisposing Factors
A. Previous blood transfusion.
B. Travel to an area endemic for hepatitis.
C. Raw shellfish consumption.
D. Intravenous (IV) drug misuse.
E. High-risk sexual practices.
F. Family history of episodic jaundice.
G. History of gallstones.
H. Biliary obstruction/previous biliary tract surgery.
I. Alcoholism.
J. Chemical exposure.
K. Working in the health-care profession.
L. Sickle cell disease.
M. Pregnancy (intrahepatic cholestasis).
N. Cancer.

Common Findings
A. Pruritus.
B. Dark, tea-coloured urine, from conjugated bilirubinuria.
C. Light, clay-coloured stools, from absence of bile.
D. Fatigue.
E. Right upper quadrant (RUQ) pain.

Other Signs and Symptoms
A. Enlarged liver.
B. Splenomegaly.
C. Fever.
D. Chills.
E. Gastrointestinal (GI): Appetite loss, weight loss, abdominal pain, nausea, or vomiting.
F. Ascites.
G. Shortness of breath.
H. Palpitations.
I. Ecchymosis.
J. Steatorrhoea, severe.
K. Asterixis (tremor).
L. Myalgias.
M. Malaise.

Subjective Data
A. Review the onset, duration, and course of symptoms.
B. Review medication history for drugs/herbals that may induce jaundice (see Table 11.17).
C. Inquire about recent blood transfusions. Are there any known blood disorders in the client's family history?
D. Ask about contact with a person who has an infection such as infectious hepatitis.
E. Ask about unprotected sexual activity/HIV status.
F. Review ingestion of potentially contaminated food or water, including *Amanita* mushrooms, milk, or shellfish.
G. Ask about the client's exposure to any toxic chemicals such as carbon tetrachloride, chloroform, phosphorus, arsenic, ethanol, or halothane (Fluothane).
H. Review the client's history of nonsterile needle punctures.
I. Review the client's medical/surgical history for gallstones, hepatitis, tumour, pancreatitis, Wilson's disease, Budd–Chiari syndrome, liver surgery, or transplantation. Is there a family history of gallstones?
J. Ask how much alcohol the client has ingested over the years.
K. Ask about dark urine or white- or clay-coloured stool.
L. Inquire about dyspepsia, anorexia, nausea, vomiting, RUQ or epigastric pain, or pain radiating to back or shoulder blade. Ask about the relationship of pain to eating.
M. Inquire about fever, fatigue, malaise, loss of vigour and strength, easy bruising, and weight loss.
N. Review travel history.

Classification of Jaundice According to Bile Pigment and by Mechanism

Unconjugated Hyperbilirubinaemia	Conjugated Hyperbilirubinaemia
Increased/overproduction of bilirubin	Hepatocellular injury/disease
Impaired/decreased hepatic uptake of bilirubin	Intrahepatic cholestasis
Impaired/decreased conjugation	Extrahepatic cholestasis (biliary obstruction)

TABLE 11.17 Drugs and Herbals Associated With Jaundice

- ACE inhibitors
- Acetaminophen
- Alkylated steroids
- Aminobenzoic acid
- Antibiotics
- Antidiabetic drugs
- Arsenic
- Chloramphenicol
- Chlorpromazine
- Ethinyl estradiol/oral contraceptives/hormone replacement
- Herbal medications (e.g., Jamaican bush tea)
- Isoniazid
- Mercaptopurine
- Methyldopa
- Monoamine oxidase inhibitors
- Nitrofurantoin
- Perphenazine
- Phenothiazine derivatives
- Probenecid
- Propylthiouracil
- Rifampin
- Sulphonamides
- Tamoxifen
- TPN

ACE, angiotensin-converting enzyme; TPN, total parenteral nutrition.

Physical Examination

A. Check temperature (if indicated), pulse, respirations, blood pressure (BP), and weight. Marked weight loss accompanied by jaundice suggests carcinoma of the head of the pancreas or metastatic disease obstructing the common duct. Note breath odour for fetor hepaticus (breath of the dead).
B. Inspect:
  1. Skin, mouth, palms, and sclera for yellow tinge. Severe jaundice may cause greenish tinge from oxidation of bilirubin to biliverdin:
      a. In fair-skinned people, discolouration is most evident on the face, trunk, and sclera (sclera icterus).
      b. In dark-skinned people, discolouration is most evident in sclera and roof of mouth.
      c. In newborns, jaundice first appears over the face or upper body, then progresses over larger areas; it can also be seen in conjunctivae of the eyes.
      d. Jaundice is most noticeable in natural sunlight. In artificial or poor light, it may be hard to detect.
  2. The skin for spider angiomata, rashes or scratches from severe itching due to pruritus, and for bruising or petechiae.
  3. The palms for erythema or overt bleeding.
  4. The chest for gynaecomastia.
C. Palpate the abdomen for tenderness, masses, liver enlargement in RUQ, and ascites:
  1. Extrahepatic obstruction and intrahepatic cholestasis may be identical in presentation.
  2. Tenderness is minimal unless cholangitis or rapid distension occur.
  3. Splenomegaly is unlikely except in primary biliary cirrhosis.
  4. Gallbladder may be palpable (Courvoisier sign). Sudden onset of pain results from passage of stone that becomes wedged into a common duct; fever and sepsis shortly thereafter indicates cholangitis.
  5. Malignancy usually presents as a rock-hard mass.
  6. Absence of abdominal pain does not rule out obstruction, especially when it develops slowly from tumour growth or primary biliary cirrhosis.
  7. Advanced hepatocellular disease is indicated by a small liver, signs of portal hypertension (ascites, splenomegaly, and prominent abdominal venous pattern), asterixis, peripheral oedema (from hypoalbuminaemia), spider angiomata, gynaecomastia, palmar erythema, and testicular atrophy.
D. Percuss the abdomen.
E. Auscultate the heart, lungs, and abdomen for bowel sounds.
F. Neurologic examination:
  1. Note level of consciousness.
  2. Asterixis test can be used to test for peripheral neuritis caused by impaired liver function. Screen for a flapping tremor occurring with wrist dorsiflexed.
G. Rectal examination: Check for masses and occult blood.

Diagnostic Tests

The diagnostic approach begins with a careful history, physical examination, and screening laboratory studies. A differential is formulated and appropriate further testing is performed to narrow the diagnosis.
A. Initial laboratory tests:
  1. Serum bilirubin: Direct, indirect (unconjugated), and total; clinically, jaundice becomes noticeable when levels reach 34 to 42 umol/L:
      a. Intrahepatic cholestasis and extrahepatic obstruction: Elevated conjugated bilirubin, elevated serum alkaline phosphatase (ALP), mild to moderate rise in transaminase.
      b. Gilbert syndrome is the most common cause of decreased uptake and unconjugated hyperbilirubinaemia. It is a benign disorder that produces recurrent self-limited episodes of mild jaundice. Typically, the unconjugated fraction rises to no more than 25 to 50 umol/L. In Gilbert syndrome, fasting and minor illness can precipitate jaundice.
  2. ALP.
  3. Aspartate transaminase (AST)/alanine transaminase (ALT).
      a. Elevation of ALT and AST may indicate liver cell damage or may be caused by opiates and ASA.
      b. ASA may also decrease AST and ALT.
  4. Prothrombin time (PT):
      a. PT may be prolonged due to malabsorption, but it is reversible by vitamin K injection.
      b. Prolonged PT unresponsive to parenteral vitamin K strongly suggests hepatocellular failure.
      c. Cholestasis and obstruction may also produce prolongation of PT but can be reversed by vitamin K.
      d. Phenazopyridine (pyridium) may cause a false-positive bilirubin result.
B. Other laboratory testing as needed:
  1. Total serum protein.
  2. Serum albumin and globulin:
      a. Albumin decreases with cirrhosis and chronic hepatitis.

b. Globulin increases with cirrhosis, chronic obstructive jaundice, and viral hepatitis.
   c. To interpret albumin level, consider dietary intake and sources of possible protein loss.
   3. Cholesterol.
   4. Lactate dehydrogenase (LDH).
   5. Gamma-glutamyl transpeptidase (GGT).
   6. Serum ammonia.
   7. Bile acid radioimmunoassay: Elevated levels indicate hepatic disease.
   8. Serologic tests for viral hepatitis.
   9. Serum iron, transferrin, and ferritin to evaluate haemochromatosis.
   10. Serum ceruloplasmin levels to evaluate Wilson's disease.
   11. Alpha-1 antitrypsin activity to evaluate alpha-1 antitrypsin deficiency.
   12. Urine for bilirubin—bilirubinuria may be an early sign of liver disease:
      a. Collect specimens over a two-hour period after lunch.
      b. Place specimen in a dark brown container and send to the laboratory immediately to prevent decomposition.
C. Abdominal ultrasound is considered the screening procedure of choice. More selective imaging procedures are ordered based on clinical evaluation.
D. Other imaging procedures:
   1. Endoscopic ultrasound.
   2. HIDA scan: Uses radioactive isotopes.
   3. Oral cholecystography.
   4. Endoscopic retrograde cholangiopancreatography (ERCP).
   5. Percutaneous transhepatic cholangiography (PTC).
   6. Helical CT.
   7. Magnetic resonance cholangiopancreatography (MRCP) is an alternative to ERCP.
   8. Liver biopsy may be indicated for definitive diagnosis.

Differential Diagnoses
A. Cirrhosis.
B. Cancer of pancreas.
C. Obstruction of biliary tract.
D. Icteric phase of hepatitis.
E. Right-sided heart failure (HF).
F. Chronic haemolysis from prosthetic heart valve.

Plan
A. Management depends on primary diagnosis. Most clients can be managed on an ambulatory basis, unless they are unable to maintain hydration or begin to show evidence of severe hepatocellular failure.
B. Cholestyramine may be used to help relieve itching. Cholestyramine is ineffective with complete biliary obstruction.

Follow-Up
A. See the client two to four weeks after initial diagnosis and referral.
B. Subsequent routine evaluations are related to primary diagnosis.

Consultation/Referral
A. Consult with a gastroenterologist familiar with liver disease and needle biopsy techniques when hepatocellular disease is suspected; when there is evidence of hepatic failure, portal hypertension, or encephalopathy; or when jaundice persists longer than three months.
B. Consultation with a gastroenterologist, surgeon, or radiologist experienced in evaluation of jaundice can be very useful when there is clinical suspicion of extrahepatic obstruction.
C. Admission is mandatory when jaundice is complicated by a fever and peritoneal signs indicative of cholangitis. IV antibiotics and prompt surgical consultation are required.

Individual Considerations
A. Pregnancy:
   1. Viral hepatitis is the most frequent cause of jaundice in pregnancy.
   2. Intrahepatic cholestasis in pregnancy is associated with modest maternal risks, including increased risk of peripartum bleeding and increased likelihood of subsequent cholelithiasis.
   3. Cholestyramine resin has been reported to afford some relief of pruritus in 50% of affected women, presumably by removing a portion of the bile acids by irreversible binding in the gut.
   4. Pregnant women who take cholestyramine are at increased risk for depletion of vitamin K–dependent coagulation factors and should be followed with serial PT times. Such women should also receive prophylactic vitamin K supplementation. If PT becomes prolonged, medication should be discontinued.
   5. Liver dysfunction and jaundice are common in clients with hyperemesis gravidarum.
B. Paediatrics:
   1. Hepatitis predominates as a cause of jaundice.
   2. Neonatal jaundice is more common when the mother is an insulin-dependent diabetic, probably resulting from a higher haematocrit (Hct) developed in utero, especially if oxygen availability is decreased. Newborn jaundice due to liver immaturity is common. It begins on day two, peaks at one week, and disappears in two to three weeks. About half of all full-term newborns and 90% of premature newborns have some degree of jaundice. Jaundice is usually mild and can be treated with hydration and ultraviolet lamp exposure.
   3. Intense, persistent jaundice suggests liver disease or severe, overwhelming infection.
   4. In Rh isoimmunization infants without appropriate treatment (exchange transfusion), progressive jaundice leads to brain damage (kernicterus), death, or severe handicap (deafness, spasticity, and choreoathetosis).
   5. Acute jaundice in young, healthy individuals suggests acute viral hepatitis.
   6. An overdose of acetaminophen is a common cause of jaundice in the young adult.
C. Geriatrics:
   1. The most frequent cause of jaundice in clients older than 65 years is cholelithiasis.
   2. The second most frequent cause of jaundice for clients 65 years and older is cancer, especially of the gallbladder.
   3. Painless jaundice in the elderly with weight loss and a mass, but with minimal pruritus, suggests biliary obstruction caused by cancer.

Bibliography
Chowdhury, N. R., & Chowdhury, J. R. (2009, May 1). Diagnostic approach to the patient with jaundice or asymptomatic

hyperbilirubinemia. *UpToDate*. Retrieved from http://www.uptodate.com/online/content/topic.do?topicKey=hep_dis/8241&view=print

Herrine, S. K. (2016, May). Jaundice. *Merck manual professional version*. Retrieved from http://www.merckmanuals.com/professional/hepatic-and-biliary-disorders/approach-to-the-patient-with-liver-disease/jaundice

Nettina, S. (2010). *The Lippincott manual of nursing practice* (9th ed.). Philadelphia, PA: Wolters Kluwer Lippincott Williams & Wilkins.

Sadowski, D. C., & van Zanten, S. V. (2015). Dyspepsia. *CMAJ, 187*(4), 276–276. doi:10.1503/cmaj.141606

University of Maryland Medical Center. (2013, June 27). *Gallstones and gallbladder disease*. Retrieved from http://umm.edu/health/medical/reports/articles/gallstones-and-gallbladder-disease

Malabsorption

Cheryl A. Glass and Kristie A. D. Morydz

Definition
A. Malabsorption syndrome is a group of signs and symptoms that occur as a result of digestive problems and problems with absorption of nutrients. There may be a resultant decrease in absorption of fat-soluble vitamins A, D, E, and K. Poor absorption of carbohydrates, minerals, and proteins may also occur.
B. The presentation of malabsorption varies from severe overt symptoms with weight loss to discrete oligosymptomatic changes in haematologic/laboratory tests that are found incidentally. Malabsorption can result from congenital defects or from acquired defects, such as bariatric surgery, and may be either global or partial. The degree of nutrient malabsorption from bariatric surgery is dependent on the type of bariatric procedure.

Incidence/Prevalence
A. Incidence is unknown.

Pathogenesis
A. Deficiency of intestinal enzymes: Lactase deficiency.
B. Inadequate digestion caused by diseases of the pancreas, liver (such as cystic fibrosis [CF]), or gallbladder.
C. Change in bacteria that normally live in the intestinal tract.
D. Disease of intestinal walls, such as helminths (worms) or parasites, tropical sprue, and celiac disease.
E. Surgery that reduces the intestinal tract, decreasing the area for absorption (such as bariatric surgery).
F. Intolerance to gluten or celiac sprue.
G. Atrophic gastritis results in hypochlorhydria and achlorhydria. The body does not produce enough pepsin and hydrochloric acid to release the food-bound vitamin B12 from protein.

Predisposing Factors
A. Lactose deficiency:
   1. Incidence is increased in African Canadians, Indigenous groups, and Asians.
   2. People of Jewish ethnicity typically have onset in adulthood.
B. Family history of malabsorption or CF.
C. Use of drugs such as mineral oil or other laxatives.
D. Excess alcohol consumption.
E. Travel to foreign countries.
F. Intestinal surgery:
   1. Partial or total gastrectomy.
   2. Small-bowel resections (jejunum, ileum, or ileocaecal).
   3. Partial or total resection of the pancreas.
G. Chronic pancreatitis.
H. Advanced age (increased risk for malabsorption and malnutrition).
I. Long-term adherence to a strict vegetarian or vegan diet (exclusion of all forms of animal protein, including eggs and dairy products).
J. HIV infection.

Common Findings
A. Diarrhoea stools that are pale, greasy, and copious.
B. Foul-smelling stools, frequently with mucus.
C. Weight loss despite adequate food intake.
D. Gas or vague abdominal discomfort.
E. Anorexia.

Other Signs and Symptoms
A. Early malabsorption:
   1. Minimal weight loss.
   2. Softer, more frequent stools.
   3. Steatorrhoea; stools "float" because of increased trapped gas.
   4. Abdominal discomfort.
   5. Bloating.
B. Later signs: Aforementioned symptoms plus the following:
   1. Marked weight loss.
   2. Foul-smelling, bulky, greasy stools.
C. Malabsorption of fats and carbohydrates: Previous symptoms plus the following:
   1. Foul-smelling, bulky, greasy, "sticky" stools that may be difficult to flush down the toilet.
   2. Ecchymosis.
   3. Bone pain.
   4. Glossitis.
   5. Muscle tenderness.
   6. Cramping in lower abdomen after bowel movement (BM).
D. Malabsorption of lactose:
   1. Nausea and bloating.
   2. Cramps.
   3. Diarrhoea after ingesting more than customary intake of milk products.
   4. Absent or mild weight loss and steatorrhoea.
   5. Good appetite.
E. Oedema: With severe protein depletion.
F. Ecchymosis and bleeding disorders secondary to vitamin K malabsorption.
G. Vitamin malabsorption:
   1. Generalized motor weakness (pantothenic acid, vitamin D).
   2. Peripheral neuropathy (thiamine).
   3. Sense of loss for vibration and position (cobalamin).
   4. Night blindness (vitamin A).
   5. Seizures (biotin).

Subjective Data
A. Review the onset, duration, and course of symptoms. Are there any other family members with the same history/symptoms?
B. Ask the client about dietary intake history.
C. Review any changes in BMs and stool characteristics.
D. Inquire about recent travel to areas known for giardiasis or other parasites.
E. Document weight loss, how much, and over what period of time.

F. Review previous gastrointestinal (GI) surgery, including the bariatric procedures and reversals, small-bowel resections, and partial or total resection of the pancreas.
G. Ask the client about signs and symptoms of inflammatory bowel disease (IBD), such as easy bruising, paraesthesia, and sore tongue.
H. Ask about any irradiation treatment.

Physical Examination

A. Check temperature, pulse, respirations, blood pressure (BP; may have orthostatic hypotension), and weight. Follow serial weight loss and plot on growth charts.
B. Inspect:
  1. Observe general appearance, noting wasting and apathetic appearance.
  2. If the client experiences a BM after the examination, observe the stool for volume, appearance, presence of blood, mucus, and gross worms/parasites.
  3. Inspect the skin for ecchymosis, jaundice, pallor, surgical scars, stigmata of hyperthyroidism or hepatocellular failure, or signs of Kaposi's sarcoma. Alopaecia or seborrhoeic dermatitis may be present.
  4. Inspect the ears, nose, and throat for glossitis, stomatitis, aphthous ulcers, poor dentition, and goiter.
C. Auscultate:
  1. The heart for tachycardia.
  2. The abdomen in all four quadrants for bowel sounds, noting borborygmi.
D. Percuss the abdomen.
E. Palpate:
  1. All lymph nodes; look for lymphadenopathy.
  2. The abdomen for organomegaly, focal tenderness, masses, distension, and ascites.
F. Neurologic examination: Assess for signs of vitamin B12 deficiency, including motor weakness, peripheral neuropathy, or ataxia.
G. Rectal examination: Note tenderness, discharge, blood, and stool.

Diagnostic Tests

A. Assessment of stool fat: Qualitative assessment on a single specimen.
B. Quantitative assessment of a 72-hour stool collection while the client is following a 100 g fat per-day diet.
C. Increased faecal fat: Test for celiac disease.
D. Abdominal ultrasound.
E. Colonoscopy to evaluate and obtain biopsies.
F. Endoscopy to evaluate and obtain biopsies.
G. Barium studies.
H. Consider CT of the abdomen.
I. Endoscopic retrograde cholangiopancreatography (ERCP) helps to document malabsorption due to pancreatic or biliary-related disorders.
J. Breath tests for carbohydrate malabsorption.
K. Complete blood count (CBC) and electrolytes.
L. Serum iron, vitamin B12, and folate concentrations.
M. Prothrombin time (PT): May be prolonged due to vitamin K deficiency.
N. Vitamin levels: Vitamins A, D, E, and K may be decreased.
O. Total protein: May be decreased.
P. Albumin: May be decreased.
Q. Serum amylase.
R. Stool for ova and parasites; obtain on alternate days for three or more specimens because parasites are passed intermittently.
S. Serum IgA—used to rule out IgA deficiency.
T. Three-stage Schilling test (vitamin B12 deficiency).

Differential Diagnoses

A. Worms or parasites.
B. AIDS.
C. Alcoholism.
D. Milk or protein allergy.
E. CF.
F. Failure to thrive (FTT).
G. Crohn's disease (CD).
H. Tropical sprue.
I. Side effect from bariatric surgery.
J. Disaccharidase deficiencies (lactase).
K. Fructose intolerance.
L. Whipple disease.
M. Zollinger–Ellison syndrome.
N. Chronic pancreatitis.
O. Cirrhosis.

Plan

A. General interventions: Treatment depends on underlying cause.
B. Client teaching: *Refer to Client Teaching Guide: Lactose Intolerance and Malabsorption.*
C. Dietary management: In most clients, diet modification, such as gluten-free diet for celiac disease, or dietary supplements restore health.
D. Pharmacological therapy:
  1. Vitamin supplements: Fat-soluble vitamins A, D, and K are most likely to be depleted. Supplements help prevent malnutrition, even though caloric intake may be replenished:
    a. Vitamin A.
    b. Vitamin D.
    c. Vitamin K.
    d. Vitamin B12.
  2. Enzyme replacements: These replace endogenous exocrine pancreatic enzymes and aid in digestion of starches, fat, and proteins:
    a. Pancrelipase: This must be given with each meal or snack.
  3. Antispasmodics:
    a. Anticholinergic agents are used to reduce the cholinergic stimulation of colonic activity that occurs in response to a meal.
    b. First-line treatment: Dicyclomine hydrochloride.
  4. Iron and folic acid supplementation are usually required for celiac disease.
  5. Calcium and magnesium supplementation are required after extensive small intestine resection.
  6. Antibiotic therapy for bacterial overgrowth.
  7. Corticosteroids and anti-inflammatory agents to treat regional enteritis.

Follow-Up

A. If examination is normal, observe the client for one month and have the client keep a diary of food intake and weight.

▶ Client Teaching Guides are available at https://connect.springerpub.com/content/reference-book/978-0-8261-9498-5

B. For persistent malabsorption, monitor for osteoporosis/bone mass with a dual-energy x-ray absorptiometry (DEXA) scan.

Consultation/Referral
A. Any client with weight loss of 15 kg is likely to have a life-threatening condition and requires prompt consultation and hospitalization.
B. Consult a gastroenterologist when malabsorption is documented by 72-hour stool fat assessment.
C. Consider a dietary consultation.
D. Refer back to the bariatric surgeon/centre, depending on surgical complications from bariatric surgery.
E. Consider a referral for allergy testing for milk and proteins.

Individual Considerations
A. Geriatrics:
  1. To identify impediments to adequate food intake, question the client about social isolation, depression, bereavement, physical impairment, poor dentition/edenulous, inability to fix meals, and poverty.
  2. Loss of taste is sometimes responsible for poor intake and should be checked.

Bibliography
American College of Obstetricians and Gynecologists. (2009, June). ACOG practice bulletin bariatric surgery and pregnancy. *Obstetrics & Gynecology, 113*, 1405–1413. doi:10.1097/AOG.0b013e3181ac0544

Goebel, S. U. (2014, December 16). Malabsorption. *Medscape*. Retrieved from http://emedicine.medscape.com/article/180785-overview

Hvas, A. M., & Nexo, E. (2006). Diagnosis and treatment of vitamin B12 deficiency. An update. *Haematologica/The Hematology Journal, 91*, 1506–1512.

Kushner, R. F., & Cummings, S. (2012, July 5). Medical management of patients after bariatric surgery. *UpToDate*. Retrieved from www.uptodate.com/contents/medical-management-of-patients-after-bariatric-surgery

Mason, J. B., & Milovic, V. (2009, May 1). Overview of the treatment of malabsorption. *UpToDate*. Retrieved from http://www.uptodate.com/online/content/topic.do?topicKey=mal_synd/7320&view=print

Milovic, V., & Mason, J. B. (2009, May 1). Clinical features and diagnosis of malabsorption. *UpToDate*. Retrieved from http://www.uptodate.com/online/content/topic.do?topicKey=mal_synd/6513&view=print

Nettina, S. (2010). *The Lippincott manual of nursing practice* (9th ed.). Philadelphia, PA: Wolters Kluwer Lippincott Williams & Wilkins.

Ren, C. J., & Fielding, G. A. (2003). Laparoscopic adjustable gastric banding: Surgical technique. *Journal of Laparoendoscopic & Advanced Surgical Techniques, 13*, 257–263. doi:10.1089/109264203322333584

Ruiz, A. R. (2014, May). Overview of malabsorption. *The Merck manual for health care professionals*. Retrieved from http://www.merckmanuals.com/professional/gastrointestinal_disorders/malabsorption_syndromes/overview_of_malabsorption.html

Sharma, G. D. (2013, June 17). Cystic fibrosis. *Medscape*. Retrieved from http://emedicine.medscape.com/article/1001602-overview

Tyler-Evans, M. E., & Meyer, B. (2009). Post-bariatric surgery: Management considerations for NPs. *American Journal for Nurse Practitioners, 13*, 29–33.

Nausea and Vomiting

Cheryl A. Glass and Kristie A. D. Morydz

Definition
Nausea and vomiting are common symptoms for many conditions and diseases and include several terms to describe the symptoms (see Table 11.18).
A. Hyperemesis gravidarum is a condition of persistent, uncontrollable vomiting that begins in the first weeks of pregnancy and improves by the end of the first trimester; however, it may persist throughout pregnancy.
B. Chronic nausea and vomiting is defined as lasting at least one month in duration.
C. Complications of nausea and vomiting include fluid depletion, hypokalaemia, and metabolic alkalosis.
D. Vomiting is also considered a protective mechanism to remove harmful ingested substances.

Incidence/Prevalence
A. Nausea and vomiting are very common, and the aetiology is dependent on the disease/condition.
B. During pregnancy, 50% to 90% of women experience nausea and/or vomiting; 50% have both nausea and vomiting. Onset after the initial nine weeks of pregnancy should direct especially careful evaluation for another cause within the differential diagnoses of nausea and vomiting in nonpregnant clients.
C. Hyperemesis gravidarum occurs in 0.3% to 2% of pregnancies.
D. Severe hyperemesis requires hospitalization in 0.3% to 2% of pregnancies.

TABLE 11.18   Definitions of Terms Used to Describe Nausea and Vomiting

Term	Definition
Vomiting	Forceful oral expulsion of gastric contents associated with contraction of the abdominal and chest wall musculature
Nausea	The unpleasant sensation of the imminent need to vomit, usually referred to the throat or epigastrium; a sensation that may or may not ultimately lead to vomiting
Regurgitation	The act by which food is brought back into the mouth without the abdominal and diaphragmatic muscular activity that characterizes vomiting
Anorexia	Loss of desire to eat; a true loss of appetite
Sitophobia	Fear of eating because of subsequent or associated discomfort
Early satiety	Fear of feeling full after eating an unusually small quantity of food
Retching	Spasmodic respiratory movements against a closed glottis with contraction of the abdominal musculature without expulsion of any gastric contents, referred to as "dry heaves"
Rumination	Chewing and swallowing of regurgitated food that has come back into the mouth through voluntary increase in abdominal pressure within minutes of eating or during eating; rumination may be accompanied by weight loss and bulimia

E. Approximately one-third of surgical clients have nausea and/or vomiting after general anaesthesia.
F. The incidence of nausea and/or vomiting subsequent to cancer treatment is high.

Pathogenesis
A. Protective mechanisms are activated by numerous gastrointestinal (GI) and non-GI causes. Normal function of the upper GI tract involves an interaction between the gut and the central nervous system (CNS).
B. Nausea and vomiting in pregnancy are related to increased hormones, including human chorionic gonadotropin (HCG), oestrogen, and progesterone, as well as decreased gastric motility and relative hypoglycaemia that results from a night-long fast.

Predisposing Factors
A. Acute nausea and vomiting:
  1. Medications: Digitalis toxicity, opiate use, chemotherapy agents, drug withdrawal, nicotine/nicotine patches, antibiotics, hormones, and antivirals.
  2. Ketoacidosis.
  3. Pregnancy or hormones.
  4. Binge drinking.
  5. Hepatitis.
B. Recurrent or chronic nausea and vomiting:
  1. Psychogenic vomiting.
  2. Metabolic disturbances.
  3. Gastric retention.
  4. Bile reflux.
  5. Pregnancy.
  6. Radiation.
  7. Gastroparesis.
C. Nausea and vomiting with abdominal pain:
  1. Viral gastroenteritis.
  2. Acute gastritis.
  3. Food poisoning.
  4. Peptic ulcer disease (PUD).
  5. Acute pancreatitis.
  6. Small-bowel obstruction.
  7. Acute appendicitis.
  8. Acute cholecystitis.
  9. Acute cholangitis.
  10. Acute pyelonephritis.
  11. Inferior myocardial infarction (MI).
D. Nausea and vomiting with neurologic symptoms:
  1. Increased intracranial pressure (ICP).
  2. Midline cerebellar haemorrhage.
  3. Vestibular disturbances.
  4. Migraine headaches.
  5. Autonomic dysfunction.
  6. Head trauma.
  7. Multiple sclerosis.

Common Findings
A. Food aversion.
B. Inability to retain food or liquids.
C. "Queasy" sensation.

Other Signs and Symptoms
A. Increased salivation.
B. Bitter taste, "acid brash": Indicates ulcer or small-bowel obstruction.
C. Weight loss.
D. Dehydration.
E. Sweating.
F. Fast pulse.
G. Pale skin.
H. Rapid breathing.
I. Light-headedness.

Subjective Data
A. Review the onset, duration (acute or chronic problem?), and course of symptoms, including the quality (projectile?) and quantity of emesis. What was the colour, taste, and consistency of the emesis? Was blood present?
  1. Vomiting bright red blood indicates a haemorrhage—*peptic ulcer.*
  2. Dark red blood indicates a haemorrhage—*oesophageal or gastric varices.*
  3. Coffee-ground material is indicative of digested blood from a slowly bleeding gastric or duodenal ulcer (DU).
  4. Vomiting faecal material is a sign of distal *small-bowel obstruction* and blind-loop syndrome.
B. Ask the client about other symptoms, including pain, fever, diarrhoea, and headache.
C. Inquire if other family members are also ill and what are their symptoms.
D. Review the timing of vomiting in relation to meals, time of day, odours, and activity. Does vomiting occur before or after food intake?
E. Ask the client about medication intake, such as antibiotics, chemotherapy, herbals, digitalis, opiates, and birth control pills.
F. Ask about self-image, binge eating, and self-induced emesis.
G. Review any exposure to hepatitis or travel to places with poor sanitation and outbreaks of cholera.
H. Review the client's medical history for vertigo, head injury, jaundice, diabetes, hypertension, and pregnancy.
I. Inquire about first day of last period and birth control method used.
J. Establish usual weight. Has there been any recent weight change, how many pounds, and over what period of time?
K. Ask about the client's history of diabetes, gallbladder disease, ulcer disease, or cancer.

Physical Examination
A. Check temperature; blood pressure (BP) and pulse, which should be evaluated both standing and lying down; respirations; and weight.
B. Inspect:
  1. Observe general overall appearance of skin for pallor and signs of dehydration. Tenting of skin when it is rolled between your thumb and index finger may indicate dehydration.
  2. Inspect for signs of autonomic insufficiency. Postural hypotension, lack of sweat, or blunted pulse and BP responses to Valsalva's maneuver suggest autonomic dysfunction and a bowel motility problem as the underlying aetiology of nausea and vomiting. Postural hypotension indicates marked volume depletion or circulatory collapse.
  3. Oral examination: Inspect mouth, teeth, and gums.
  4. Inspect fontanelles in infants.
C. Palpate:
  1. The abdomen for masses, distension, tenderness, signs of peritonitis, and organomegaly.
  2. The back; note costovertebral angle tenderness.
D. Percuss the abdomen.

E. Auscultate:
  1. The abdomen for bowel sounds in all quadrants.
  2. The heart and lungs.
F. Perform rectal examination (if indicated).
G. Perform a neurologic examination (if indicated).

Diagnostic Tests
The cause of an acute episode of nausea and vomiting is typically determined through a detailed history and physical examination. Only if the cause is unclear should further testing be performed.
A. Urine: Urinalysis, pregnancy test, culture and sensitivity, if indicated.
B. Urinalysis for ketones and specific gravity.
C. Serum labs: Multiple chemistry profile, including amylase, electrolytes, urea, creatinine, glucose, bilirubin, and transaminase.
D. Hepatitis panel.
E. Drug screen.
F. Upper GI.
G. Ultrasonography:
  1. Obstetric ultrasound to rule out multiple gestations or molar pregnancy if persistent nausea and vomiting, especially after 16 weeks' gestation
  2. Upper abdominal ultrasound, if clinically indicated, to evaluate the pancreas and/or biliary tree.
H. Stool for occult blood.
I. Endoscopy.
J. CT scan:
  1. Head CT scan, if indicated.
  2. Abdominal CT, if appendicitis is suspected.
K. Gastric scintigraphy, to rule out gastroparesis if indicated.
L. ECG, if chest pain/myocardial infarction (MI) is suspected.

Differential Diagnoses
A. See section "Predisposing Factors."

Plan
A. General interventions: Assess hydration status. Proceed to intravenous (IV) hydration and antiemetics until ketones clear.
B. Dietary management: See section "Nausea and Vomiting Diet Suggestions (Children and Adults)" in Appendix B, Diet Recommendations.
C. Pharmacological therapy (not an exhaustive list).

Antiemetics should not be used in vomiting of unknown aetiology in children and adolescents.

  1. Anticholinergics: Scopolamine.
  2. Antihistamines: Dimenhydrate, diphenhydramine (motion sickness), doxylaminesuccinate/pyridoxine.
  3. Benzamides: Domperidone, metoclopramide.
  4. Cannabinoids: Nabilone.
  5. Phenothiazidines: Prochlorperazine.
  6. Seratonin antagonists: Granisetron, Ondansetron.
  7. Steroids: Dexamethasone.
D. Outpatient IV hydration in pregnancy: Lactated Ringer's solution to correct dehydration and restore electrolyte balance. Check urine ketones after first litre to determine if additional litre is necessary to clear ketones.

Follow-Up
A. Advise the client to call or visit the office in 24 hours to check response and nutritional intake.
B. Advise parents who are giving simple treatment at home to call the office promptly if projectile or prolonged vomiting occurs.

Consultation/Referral
A. *If overdose is suspected Contact the provincial or regional poison control or the ED immediately.*
B. Hyperemesis gravidarum is the most severe form of nausea and vomiting in pregnancy. Hyperemesis gravidarum may require hospitalization to correct fluid and electrolyte imbalance, and nutritional deficiencies.
C. Hospitalize the client promptly if there is evidence of bowel obstruction; increased ICP; or another GI, neurologic, or metabolic emergency. **First priority is to rule out acute surgical aetiology such as bowel obstruction and peritonitis.**
D. Call for a paediatric consultation immediately for vomiting lasting more than 24 hours, projectile vomiting, vomiting after a fall or head injury, or prolonged vomiting coupled with diarrhoea.
E. Call for a psychiatric consultation for suspected psychogenic nausea and vomiting.
F. If postural hypotension occurs, especially in elderly clients, hospital admission for parenteral fluid and electrolyte replacement is indicated.
G. Endocrinologist, gastroenterologist, and surgical consultations for treatment, consideration, and placement of a gastric stimulator for diabetes gastroparesis.

Individual Considerations
A. Pregnancy:
  1. Determine whether the woman is ingesting nonfood substances, such as starch, clay, or toothpaste, which would indicate pica.
  2. Intractable nausea and vomiting require ultrasonography to rule out hydatidiform mole.
  3. First-line treatment for nausea and vomiting in pregnancy is pyridoxine monotherapy or doxylamine/pyridoxine. H_1 receptor antagonists should be considered in chronic or acute nausea episodes in pregnancy. Metoclopramide can be used as adjunct therapy, as can phenothiazines. When others have failed, ondansetron can be used as an adjunct therapy. Corticosteroids can be considered after the first trimester.
  4. Uncorrected hyperemesis gravidarum can result in severe electrolyte imbalance and possible hepatic and renal damage. The major concern for foetal well-being is uncorrected ketosis, which may result in foetal abnormalities or death in early pregnancy.
  5. Encourage the client to eat toast or a dry cracker; to eat small, frequent meals and snacks; to drink fluids separately from meals; and to avoid fatty, fried, greasy, or spicy foods and foods with strong odours.
B. Paediatrics:
  1. The differential diagnosis of vomiting is age dependent.
  2. For neonates and young infants, the most frequent diagnostic considerations are the following:
    a. Gastro-oesophageal reflux disease (GORD).
    b. Excessive feeding volume.
    c. Increased ICP/meningitis.
    d. Food allergy.

e. Intestinal obstruction:
      i. Malrotation without volvulus.
      ii. Hirschsprung's disease (HD).
      iii. Intussusception.
      iv. Intestinal atresia.
      v. Pyloric stenosis.
   3. Older infants and children differential diagnoses include the following:
      a. Gastroenteritis.
      b. GORD.
      c. Gastroparesis.
      d. Mechanical obstruction.
      e. Munchausen syndrome by proxy.
   4. Adolescent disorders include the disorders affecting children as well as the following:
      a. Appendicitis.
      b. Inflammatory bowel disease (IBD).
      c. Pregnancy.
      d. Bulimia or psychogenic vomiting.
   5. Question caregivers regarding the infant's feeding, activity level, irritability, lethargy, and number of wet diapers.
   6. Otitis media, pharyngitis, and urinary tract infections (UTIs) may present with nausea and/or vomiting in the paediatric population.
   7. Rumination syndrome is a behavioural disorder that is most commonly identified among mentally disadvantaged children and adolescents with cognitive disabilities. The behaviour consists of daily, effortless regurgitation of undigested food within minutes of starting or completing ingestion of a meal.
C. Geriatrics:
   1. Use of the lower dose ranges of an antiemetic is sufficient for most elderly clients due to their susceptibility to hypotension and neuromuscular reactions.
   2. Dosages should be increased more gradually in the elderly.

There should be a low threshold for hospitalization of the elderly to treat dehydration and correction of fluid and electrolyte imbalance.

Resources
Canadian Cancer Society: http://www.cancer.ca
Rome Foundation: https://theromefoundation.org/

Bibliography
American College of Gastroenterology. (2011). Pregnancy and gastrointestinal disorders. *Pregnancy monograph*. Retrieved from http://gi.org/wp-content/uploads/2011/07/institute-PregnancyMonograph.pdf
American Gastroenterological Association. (2001). American Gastroenterological Association medical position statement: Nausea and vomiting. *Gastroenterology, 120*, 261–262. doi:10.1053/gast.2001.20515
Campbell, K., Rowe, H., Azzam, H., & Lane, C. A. (2016). The management of nausea and vomiting of pregnancy. *Journal of Obstetrics and Gynaecology Canada, 38*(12), 1127–1137. doi:10.1016/j.jogc.2016.08.009
Emetrol. (2015). *Nausea relief for you and your family*. Retrieved from http://emetrol.com/otc-nausea-medication/
Longstreth, G. F. (2013, April 5). Approach to the adult with nausea and vomiting. *UpToDate*. Retrieved from http://www.uptodate.com/contents/approach-to-the-adult-with-nausea-and-vomiting
Nettina, S. (2010). *The Lippincott manual of nursing practice* (9th ed.). Philadelphia, PA: Wolters Kluwer Lippincott Williams & Wilkins.
Ogunyemi, D. A. (2015, November 14). Hyperemesis gravidarum. *Medscape*. Retrieved from http://emedicine.medscape.com/article/254751-overview#a4
Wehbi, M. (2011, January 12). Acute gastritis. *Medscape*. Retrieved from http://emedicine.medscape.com/article/175909-overview

Peptic Ulcer Disease (PUD)

Cheryl A. Glass and Kristie A. D. Morydz

Definition
A. Peptic ulcer disease (PUD) is circumscribed ulceration of the gastrointestinal (GI) mucosa occurring in areas exposed to acid and pepsin. The client's prior ulcer history tends to predict future behaviour and risk of future complications. Complications include bleeding ulcer, perforation, and obstruction.
B. The stomach is divided on the basis of its physiological functions into two main portions. The proximal two-thirds, the fundic gland area, acts as a receptable for ingested food and secretes acid and pepsin. The distal third, the pyloric gland area, mixes and propels food into the duodenum and produces the hormone gastrin. "Peptic" lesions may occur in the oesophagus (oesophagitis), stomach (gastritis), or duodenum (duodenitis).
C. There is often no correlation between the presence of an active ulcer, noted by endoscopy, and symptoms. The disappearance of symptoms does not guarantee ulcer healing.

Incidence/Prevalence
A. The annual incidence of peptic ulcer is estimated to range from 0.1% to 1.8%. The ulcer incidence in *Helicobacter pylori*–infected individuals is about 1% per year. The recurrence rate is 50% to 80% during the six to 12 months following the initial ulcer healing, although relapses are not always symptomatic. Some peptic ulcers heal spontaneously, and 2% to 20% of clients have multiple simultaneous ulcers.
B. From 16% to 31% of ulcers are caused by nonsteroidal anti-inflammatory drugs (NSAIDs). Epidemiologic studies show that risks of peptic ulcer and death are three to six times higher among people who take NSAIDs.
C. Cigarette smokers are twice as likely to develop ulcers as nonsmokers.

Pathogenesis
A. Although the precise mechanisms of ulcer formation remain incompletely understood, the process appears to involve the interplay of acid production, pepsin secretion, *H. pylori* bacterial infection, and mucosal defense mechanisms. Excess acid production is the hallmark of duodenal ulcer (DU) disease. Pepsin secretion is also elevated in DU disease.
B. The relation of ASA and other NSAIDs to ulcer disease is due largely to the drugs' potent inhibition of gastric mucosal prostaglandin synthesis. In addition to prostaglandin inhibition, many NSAID preparations produce acute diffuse mucosal injury by means of a direct erosive effect.

Predisposing Factors
A. *H. pylori* infection is the most common cause of ulceration.
B. Use of NSAIDs, especially ASA, ibuprofen, and naproxen, is associated with acute erosive gastritis.
C. Smoking.
D. Genetic factors: Family history of ulcer disease.
E. Age:
   1. DU occurs between ages 25 and 75 years.
   2. Gastric ulcer (GU) occurs between ages 55 and 65 years.
F. Gender:
   1. The ratio of males to females for gastritis is 1:1.
   2. The ratio of males to females for peptic ulcers is 2:1.

G. Excessive alcohol consumption, which stimulates acid secretion.
H. Medications:
1. Corticosteroids potentiate ulcer risk in clients who use NSAIDs concurrently.
2. Anticoagulants.
3. Bisphosphonates.
4. Spironolactone.
5. Selective serotonin reuptake inhibitors (SSRIs).
I. Improper diet, irregular meals, and skipped meals.
J. Severe physiological stress:
1. Burns.
2. Central nervous system (CNS) trauma.
3. Surgery.
4. Severe medical illness:
   a. Cirrhosis.
   b. Chronic obstructive pulmonary disease (COPD).
   c. Renal failure.
   d. Organ transplantation.
   e. Celiac disease.
   f. Crohn's disease (CD).
K. Other causes.
1. Radiation-induced ulcer.
2. Chemotherapy-induced ulcer.
3. Vascular insufficiency.
4. Duodenal obstruction.
L. Zollinger–Ellison syndrome.
M. Bile reflux.
N. Illicit drugs: Crack cocaine.

Common Findings
A. Pain described as aching, boring, gnawing, or burning feeling.
B. Epigastric pain in right upper quadrant (RUQ) and left upper quadrant (LUQ) of the abdomen or occasionally below breast.
C. Pain that awakens the client at night or in early morning.
D. Perforated peptic ulcer presents with a sudden onset of severe sharp abdominal pain.

Other Signs and Symptoms
A. Asymptomatic.
B. GI distress one to three hours after a meal, on an empty stomach.
C. Pain relieved by food, antacids, or vomiting.
D. Nausea and vomiting.
E. Haematemesis.
F. Chest discomfort.
G. Blood in stools, "grape jelly-" or maroon-coloured stools.
H. Loss of appetite or weight.
I. Weight gain; those with DU may eat more to ease pain.
J. Anaemia.

Signs and Symptoms of Bleeding
A. Massive bleeding:
1. Acute, bright red haematemesis or large amount of melaena with clots in the stool, or "grape jelly" stool.
2. Rapid pulse, drop in, hypovolaemia, and shock.
B. Subacute bleeding:
1. Intermittent melaena or coffee-ground emesis.
2. Hypotension.
3. Weakness and dizziness.
C. Chronic bleeding:
1. Intermittent appearance of blood.
2. Increased weakness, paleness, or shortness of breath.
3. Occult blood.

Subjective Data
A. Ask the client to describe the onset, duration, type, and location of pain. Does it occur at any special time, for example, before meals, after meals, or during the night?
B. Has the client had a previous ulcer? What was the treatment; if oral treatment was prescribed, did the client complete the therapy?
C. Have the client describe what alleviates pain, such as taking antacids, and what worsens pain, such as use of ASA, oral steroids, or NSAIDs.
D. Review associated symptoms, such as nausea, vomiting, and heartburn.
E. Ask the client whether any first-degree relatives have ulcers.
F. Inquire whether the client is a smoker. If so, how much and for how long?
G. Ask the client about alcohol consumption: How much and for how long?
H. Inquire whether any blood has ever been vomited or passed in stool. If so, have the client describe it.
I. Take the client's dietary history, including time of meals, frequency of skipped meals, weight loss, and so forth.
J. Review all medications, including a review of over-the-counter (OTC) and herbal products such as ginkgo biloba.
K. Obtain past medical history of associated diseases such as cirrhosis, pancreatitis, arthritis, chronic obstructive pulmonary disease (COPD), and hyperparathyroidism.
L. If the client suspects blood in stool, ask whether there has been a change in bowel pattern, presence of abdominal pain or tenderness, and whether the client recently ingested food such as red beets.

Physical Examination
A. Check temperature (if indicated), pulse, respirations, BP, and weight.
B. Palpate the abdomen for tenderness, guarding, rigidity, masses, and liver or spleen enlargement.
C. Percuss the abdomen for hepatosplenomegaly.
D. Auscultate the abdomen for bowel sounds in all quadrants.
E. Rectal examination:
1. Check for tenderness and masses.
2. Take stool specimen.

Diagnostic Tests
A. Complete blood count (CBC).
B. Stool for occult blood.
C. Coagulation studies.
D. Testing for *H. pylori*:
1. **Endoscopy with biopsy is the most accurate test.**
2. **Rapid urease test is the diagnostic test of choice.**
3. Urea breath test (UBT) is preferred.
4. Serum test for *H. pylori* antibodies.
5. Stool *H. pylori* antigen testing—more accurate than antibody testing and less expensive.
E. Radiography with barium meal.
F. Mucosal biopsy, after GI consultation, to rule out cancer.
G. Fasting gastrin level (screen for Zollinger–Ellison syndrome).

Differential Diagnoses
A. Gastro-oesophageal reflux disease (GORD).
B. Zollinger–Ellison syndrome: Fasting serum gastrin level 500 pg/mL in the presence of acid hypersecretion is diagnostic.

C. Cancer:
   1. Gastric lymphoma.
   2. Gastric cancer.
   3. Pancreatic cancer.
D. Pancreatitis (acute or chronic).
E. Myocardial ischaemia.
F. Abdominal aneurysm.
G. Diverticulitis.
H. Drug-induced dyspepsia:
   1. Theophylline.
   2. Digitalis.
I. CD involving the stomach or duodenum.
J. Gastric infections.
K. Cholelithiasis.

Plan

A. General interventions: Goals are to alleviate pain, promote healing, limit complications, and prevent recurrences while minimizing costs and side effects of treatment:
   1. Encourage the client to stop taking NSAIDs, unless medically indicated:
      a. If NSAID use is unavoidable, the lowest possible dose and duration and cotherapy with a proton pump inhibitor (PPI) based on triple therapy is recommended.
   2. Smoking cessation should be highly encouraged at each visit.
▶ B. Client teaching: *Refer to Client Teaching Guide: Ulcer Management.*
C. Dietary management: Advise the client to avoid alcohol, coffee (including decaffeinated), and other caffeine-containing beverages, because they stimulate acid secretion. (See Appendix B, Diet Recommendations, Table B.8.)
D. Medical and surgical management:
   1. Diagnostic evaluation of the ulcer is by means of endoscopy.
   2. Test for *H. pylori*:
      a. A single negative *H. pylori* test should be interpreted cautiously, especially in the face of active bleeding. Blood in the stomach can alter the pH indicator in the rapid urease test. False negatives are likely, and additional testing for *H. pylori* is essential.
      b. Concurrent use of a PPI, antibiotics, or bismuth will cause a false-negative test.
   3. Surgery remains an option for treatment of refractory disease and complications. The most serious indications for surgery include brisk bleeding of 6 to 8 units of blood in 24 hours, recurrent bleeding episodes, perforation, gastric outlet obstruction refractory to medical therapy, and failure of a benign GU to heal after 15 weeks. Emergency intervention may be required, such as withholding food and oral fluids, starting an IV, placing a nasogastric (NG) tube, oxygen therapy, or blood transfusion. If life-threatening bleeding occurs, treat shock.
E. Pharmacological therapy:
   1. The treatment of peptic ulcer begins with the eradication of *H. pylori* in infected individuals. Empiric therapy for the infection is reasonable for uncomplicated cases in the absence of NSAID use. Documenting infection, even in clients with known ulcers, is an essential step prior to initiating antimicrobial therapy:
      a. Quadruple therapy anti–*H. pylori* regimen for 14 days: PPI + bismuth + metronidazole + tetracycline OR PPI + bismuth + metronidazole + clarithyromicin. Consider resistance patterns when selecting antibiotic agents:
         i. PPI-based regimen (choose one):
            1) Rabeprazole.
            2) Esomeprazole.
            3) Lansoprazole.
            4) Omeprazole.
   2. Antisecretory therapy is the mainstay of therapy in uninfected clients and is used for maintenance therapy in selected cases. Full doses of an H_2 receptor antagonist provide effective initial therapy; however, PPIs are more effective.
   3. Clients with uncomplicated, small (<1 cm) DU or GU who have received adequate treatment for *H. pylori* probably are asymptomatic and do not need any further therapy directed at ulcer healing. Maintenance acid suppression with a PPI for one year following *H. pyloric* eradication is recommended for clients with a complicated DU. If the ulcer is giant (>2 cm), showing densely fibrosed ulcer beds, or if the client is a high-risk client with a protracted prior history, then the client should be kept on a PPI until a follow-up endoscopy is performed:
      a. H_2 receptor antagonists: Split-dose, evening, and nighttime therapy are all effective in GU management:
         i. Cimetidine.
         ii. Ranitidine.
         iii. Famotidine.
         iv. Metiamide—classified in Canada as experimental.
      b. PPIs are effective in inducing ulcer healing. The PPIs are the most potent inhibitors of gastric acid secretion. Once-daily dosing is generally sufficient for acid inhibition; however, a second dose may be necessary and should be given before the evening meal. Once-daily PPI dosing inhibits acid output by 66% after five days. Optimal dosing is immediately before breakfast:
         i. Omeprazole.
         ii. Esomeprazole.
         iii. Lansoprazole.
         iv. Pantoprazole.
         v. Rabeprazole.
         vi. Dexlansoprazole.
      c. PPIs should not be given concomitantly with prostaglandins, or other antisecretory agents, because of the marked reduction in their effects. An H_2 antagonist can be used with a PPI if given after a sufficient interval between their administrations; the minimal times have not been established. The H_2 antagonist could be given at bedtime for breakthrough symptoms after a morning dose of a PPI.
   4. Sucralfate. Sucralfate is not recommended for *H. pylori* or NSAID ulcers.
   5. Misoprostol is effective for peptic ulcers caused by NSAID use; peptic ulcers respond well.

Follow-Up

A. Therapeutic trial of lifestyle changes combined with an H_2 receptor antagonist, sucralfate, or omeprazole for one to two weeks should provide relief. Reevaluate the client after two weeks, and if symptoms are improved, prescribe a full course of six to eight weeks.

B. Reevaluate the client again at eight weeks, after the full course of therapy is completed.
C. Consider repeating breath test to confirm eradication of *H. pylori*.
D. Some authorities advocate routine endoscopic or radiologic documentation of healing. However, no studies show this to be cost-effective in uncomplicated cases in which symptoms resolve within four to six weeks and do not recur.
E. For refractory GU—that is, persistent pain after eight weeks despite a full medical regimen or unresponsive to treatment for *H. pylori*—endoscopic examination and biopsy are needed, especially in clients older than 40 who are at increased risk of gastric cancer. Barium study is not sufficient, because even malignant ulcers may shrink in size in response to therapy.
F. Evaluate refractory cases for Zollinger–Ellison syndrome, especially when there are multiple ulcers, occurrences in unusual places, marked abdominal pain, or a secretory diarrhoea.
G. There is an increased risk of osteoporotic fracture from the long-term use of PPIs.
H. Clients beginning long-term NSAID therapy should first be tested for *H. pylori*.

Consultation/Referral
A. Consult both a surgeon and a gastroenterologist and admit the client in a hospital when symptoms of haemorrhage, penetration, perforation, or gastric outlet obstruction are present.
B. Refer clients with recurrences or refractory disease for evaluation for *H. pylori* infection by endoscopy or breath test. If present, eradicate with a two-week course of triple therapy.

Individual Considerations
A. Pregnancy: The drugs misoprostol and ranitidine are abortifacients. They cross the placental barrier and are excreted in breast milk and are contraindicated in pregnancy or suspected pregnancy. Use in sexually active women of childbearing age should be done with proper warning and detailed client education.
B. Adults:
  1. DUs are more common in people between ages 45 and 54 years; GUs, between 55 and 64 years.
  2. Clients older than 40 years are at greater risk of gastric cancer and should undergo either an upper GI series or endoscopy to document the nature and location of lesions when there is strong clinical suspicion of ulcer disease.
  3. Gastritis not associated with reflux is present in 75% of people older than 50 years.
C. Geriatrics:
  1. Silent disease is particularly common among the elderly and those using NSAIDs.
  2. Lethargy, confusion, slurred speech, agitation, and visual hallucinations have been reported with cimetidine, particularly in the elderly.
  3. In the elderly, DU symptoms remain classic with early morning awakening to pain, then quick relief by food or antacids. GU symptoms are less obvious, with burning or gnawing pain experienced in <50% of elderly clients.
  4. Anaemia may be the only symptom of gastric cancer. Cancer must always be considered and confirmed by endoscopy with biopsy.
  5. When prescribing an NSAID to the elderly, use the lowest dose, for the shortest period of time, and avoid prescribing a long-acting NSAID such as indomethacin and piroxicam.
  6. Due to other medications taken for comorbid health conditions, the elderly are especially at risk with the combination of NSAIDs and the following:
   a. ASA.
   b. Clopidogrel.
   c. Dabigatran.
   d. Dipyridamole.
   e. Prasugrel.
   f. Ticlopidine.
   g. Warfarin.

Bibliography
American College of Gastroenterology. (2011). Pregnancy and gastrointestinal disorders. *Pregnancy monograph*. Retrieved from http://gi.org/wp-content/uploads/2011/07/institute-PregnancyMonograph.pdf
American Gastroenterological Association. (2016, July). *Peptic ulcer disease*. Retrieved from https://www.gastro.org/patient-care/conditions-diseases/peptic-ulcer-disease
Anand, B. S. (2015, January 9). Peptic ulcer disease. *Medscape*. Retrieved from http://emedicine.medscape.com/article/181753-overview
Fallone, C. A., Chiba, N., van Zanten, S. V., Fischbach, L., Gisbert, J. P., Hunt, R. H., & Marshall, J. K. (2016). The Toronto consensus for the treatment of Helicobacter pylori infection in adults. *Gastroenterology*, *151*(1), 51–69. doi:10.1053/j.gastro.2016.04.006
Lanza, F. L., Francis, K. L., Chan, M. D., Eammonn, M. M., Quigley, M. D., & The Practice Parameters Committee of the American College of Gastroenterology. (2009, March). Guidelines for prevention of NSAID-related ulcer complications. *American Journal of Gastroenterology*, *104*, 728–738. doi:10.1038/ajg.2009.115
Nettina, S. (2010). *The Lippincott manual of nursing practice* (9th ed.). Philadelphia, PA: Wolters Kluwer Lippincott Williams & Wilkins.
Saad, R. J., & Chey, W. D. (2015, June 23). First-line treatment strategies for *Helicobacter pylori* infection. *Gastroenterology & Endoscopy News*, 1–8. Retrieved from http://www.gastroendonews.com/Review-Articles/Article/06-15/First-Line-Treatment-Strategies-for-Helicobacter-nbsp-pylori-Infection/32678/ses=ogst
Sadowski, D. C., & van Zanten, S. V. (2015). Dyspepsia. *CMAJ*, *187*(4), 276–276. doi:10.1503/cmaj.141606
Wehbi, M. (2011, January 12). Acute gastritis. *Medscape*. Retrieved from http://emedicine.medscape.com/article/175909-overview

Pinworm

Cheryl A. Glass, Audra C. Malone, and Kristie A. D. Morydz

Definition
A. Pinworm, *Enterobius vermicularis*, is the most common helminth infection. It is characterized by a white, threadlike worm infestation.

Incidence/Prevalence
A. Pinworm is very common. *E. vermicularis* occurs worldwide and commonly occurs in family clusters. It has a high incidence of reinfection. Exact data are not available because helminth infestations are not reportable.

Pathogenesis
A. The *E. vermicularis* adult nematode, or roundworm, lives in the human rectum or colon and emerges onto the perianal skin to lay eggs. It is transmissible by direct transfer of infective eggs to mouth, or indirectly through clothing, bedding, food, or other articles contaminated with eggs of the parasite. The period of communicability is as long as female nematodes are discharging eggs on perianal skin. Eggs remain infective in an indoor environment, usually two to three weeks. Humans are the only known hosts; dogs and cats do not harbour *E. vermicularis*.
B. The incubation period is one to two months or longer, from ingestion of an egg until an adult gravid female migrates to the perianal region.

Predisposing Factors
A. Preschool and school age.
B. Member of a family of an infected person.
C. Institutional residence.
D. Overcrowded living conditions.

Common Findings
A. Intense nighttime anal pruritus.
B. Irritability in infants and children.

Other Signs and Symptoms
A. Disturbed sleep or insomnia.
B. Pruritus vulvae.
C. Urethritis.
D. Vaginitis.
E. Local irritation.
F. Secondary infections from scratching.
G. Loss of appetite or weight loss.
H. Grinding teeth at night.

Subjective Data
A. Review the onset, duration, course, and time of symptoms, especially anal itching.
B. Ask the client about symptoms in other family members.
C. Inquire about genital irritation symptoms in female children.

Physical Examination
A. Check temperature (if indicated), pulse, respirations, blood pressure (BP), and weight.
B. Inspect anus and female genitals for irritation and skin abrasions.

Diagnostic Tests
A. Press sticky side of transparent (not translucent) cellulose tape against perianal folds, and then press tape on glass slide. Eggs will be visible under a microscope:
   1. The "tape method" should be conducted on three consecutive mornings.
   2. Eggs are most likely to be present on awakening and before the person bathes or uses the toilet.
B. Pinworm eggs may be obtained from a scraping sample from under the fingernails.
C. Order urinalysis to rule out urinary tract infection (UTI).
D. Obtain stool specimen for ova and parasite; adult worms in faeces are diagnostic.
E. Serologic tests are not available for diagnosing pinworm infections.

Differential Diagnoses
A. UTI.
B. Poor hygiene.
C. Chemical irritants, soaps, and bubble baths.

Plan
A. Client teaching:
   1. Refer to *Client Teaching Guide: Roundworms and Pinworms.*
   2. Teach the caregiver how to obtain a specimen from a child.
   3. Infected people should bathe or shower in the morning to remove eggs:
      a. Showering is better than taking a bath. Showering avoids potentially contaminating the bath water with pinworm eggs.
      b. Infected people should not bathe with others during their time of infection.
   4. Use good handwashing habits after using the toilet and before eating or preparing food.
   5. Keep fingernails short and avoid nail biting.
   6. All household members should be treated as a group when there are multiple instances of infection.
   7. Thoroughly launder bedding and clothing to destroy any eggs.
B. Pharmacological therapy:
   1. Mebendazole is the most common drug for the treatment of pinworms.
   2. Pyrantel pamoate.
   3. Piperazine and pyrvinium are second-line nonprescription drugs that may be used to treat pinworms.
   4. It is recommended that all household members be treated at the same time.

Follow-Up
A. If single-dose therapy is not effective, a second course of medication is advised in two weeks.
B. Reinfection is common.

Consultation/Referral
A. Consult an obstetrician if the client is pregnant.

Individual Considerations
A. Pregnancy:
   1. Anthelmintics are in pregnancy category C; however, the potential risks to the foetus versus benefits should be considered.
   2. Breastfeeding should not be withheld during mebendazole therapy.
   3. World Health Organization (WHO) has determined the benefit of pharmacological treatment outweighs the risk:
      a. WHO allows the use of albendazole in the second and third trimesters of pregnancy.
      b. WHO allows the use of pyrantel pamoate in the second and third trimesters of pregnancy.
B. Paediatrics:
   1. All medications are advised for children:
      a. In the WHO guidelines for mass prevention campaigns, albendazole can be used in children as young as 1 year.
      b. Mebendazole and pyrantel pamoate are on the WHO Model List of Essential Medicines for Children, intended for use in children up to 12 years of age.
   2. Pinworms may predispose children to developing UTIs.
   3. No unusual cleansing other than basic hygiene measures should be undertaken. Excessive zeal in this regard can induce guilt and is counterproductive.
   4. The best time to examine a child is two to three hours after he or she falls asleep.
C. Adults have the lowest incidence of pinworms.

Bibliography
American Academy of Pediatrics. (2012). Pinworm infections (*Enterobius vermicularis*). In L. K. Pickering (Ed.), *Red book: 2012 report of the Committee on Infectious Diseases* (29th ed., pp. 566–567). Elk Grove

Village, IL: Author. Retrieved from https://redbook.solutions.aap.org/DocumentLibrary/RB12_interior.pdf

Centers for Disease Control and Prevention. (2016, February 3). *Parasites—Enterobiasis (also known as pinworm infection)*. Retrieved from https://www.cdc.gov/parasites/pinworm/health_professionals/index.html

Nettina, S. (2010). *The Lippincott manual of nursing practice* (9th ed.). Philadelphia, PA: Wolters Kluwer Lippincott Williams & Wilkins.

Weller, P. F. (2009, May 1). Anthelminthic therapies. *UpToDate*. Retrieved from http://www.uptodate.com/online/content/topic.do?topicKey=antibiot/7691&view=print

Roundworm

Cheryl A. Glass, Audra C. Malone, and Krisite A. D. Morydz

Definition

A. Roundworm, *Ascaris lumbricoides*, is a helminthic parasitic infection of the lumen of the small intestines and sometimes the lungs. Most infections with *A. lumbricoides* are asymptomatic. Roundworms are brownish, are the size and shape of earthworms, and can be seen easily without a microscope. The majority of worms are noted in the jejunum but can be noted from the oesophagus to the rectum. Ova can survive for prolonged periods, up to 10 years. The eggs are resistant to normal water purification but can be removed by boiling and water filtration.

Incidence/Prevalence

A. *A. lumbricoides* are very common. Approximately 25% to 33% of the world's population, more than 1.4 billion people, are infected with these human intestinal nematodes. It is the third most frequent helminth infection; only the hookworm and whipworm exceed it. It occurs worldwide, especially in tropical and warm climates. It affects people of all ages but is most common in young children between 3 and 8 years of age.

B. Individuals can be asymptomatic and continue to shed eggs for years. The parasitic eggs are extremely durable in various environments, and each roundworm produces a large number of eggs. Complications secondary to *A. lumbricoides* range from 11% to 67% in infected individuals, with intestinal and biliary tract obstruction the most common serious sequelae. Bowel obstruction or perforation is the highest in children.

C. Many individuals infected with *A. lumbricoides* are also coinfected with other intestinal parasites, including trichuriasis (*Trichuris trichiura*) and hookworm (*Necator americanus* and *Ancylostoma duodenale*).

Pathogenesis

A. *A. lumbricoides* is a large roundworm that infects humans. The nematode measures 15 to 35 cm in length in adulthood. It is contracted by ingesting eggs in contaminated soil through eating the soil (pica), children playing in contaminated soil, eating unwashed fruits and raw vegetables, drinking water contaminated with faeces, or touching food with soil-contaminated hands. Occasionally, transplacental migration of larvae has been reported.

B. The life cycle of *A. lumbricoides* is four to eight weeks, and faeces contain eggs about two months after ingestion of embryonated eggs. Female roundworms produce 200,000 eggs per day, which are excreted in stool and must incubate in soil for two to three weeks for the embryo to form and become infectious (second-stage larvae). The interval between ingestion of egg and development of egg-laying adults is approximately eight weeks. If infection is untreated, adult worms can live six to 24 months, resulting in daily excretion of large numbers of ova.

C. The ingested ova hatch in the small intestine (jejunum or ileum) and release larvae. They then may migrate via blood or via the lymphatic system to the heart, lungs, the biliary tree, and occasionally the kidney or brain. It takes approximately four days for the larvae to reach the lungs. After maturation, they are passed through the bronchi and the trachea and are subsequently swallowed.

D. Eggs are not shed in the stool until roughly 40 days after the development of pulmonary symptoms.

Predisposing Factors

A. Crowded or unsanitary living conditions.
B. Tropical or warm climates, including the southern United States.
C. Preschool or early school age (2–10 years).
D. Tend to cluster in families.
E. Residence in areas where human faeces are used as fertilizer.
F. Travelers to endemic areas (Asia, Africa, and South America).
G. Recent immigrants (especially from Latin America and Asia).
H. International adoptees.

Common Findings

A. Asymptomatic.
B. Restlessness at night.
C. Colicky abdominal pain.
D. Frequent fatigue.
E. Worms found in bowel movements (BMs) or in bed.

Other Signs and Symptoms

A. Transient respiratory symptoms during migration.
B. Nausea and vomiting.
C. Anorexia and erratic or poor appetite.
D. Fever.
E. Irritability.
F. Diarrhoea or constipation.
G. Weight loss or gain.
H. Dry cough or wheezing, from larvae in lungs.
I. Parasites regurgitated or passed through nares of febrile clients.
J. Acute transient pneumonitis.
K. Acute obstructive jaundice.
L. Appendicitis.
M. Urticaria.
N. Impaired absorption of protein, lactose, and vitamin A.
O. Burning chest pain.

Subjective Data

A. Review the onset, duration, and course of symptoms.
B. Ask about any problems with pica.
C. Inquire about worms in stool or emesis.
D. Review history of pets treated for worms.
E. Establish normal weight for evaluation.

Physical Examination

A. Check temperature (as indicated), pulse, respirations, blood pressure (BP), and weight. Plot the child's height and weight on a growth curve.
B. Inspect the skin to rule out jaundice and evaluate urticaria.
C. Auscultate:
   1. Auscultate the lungs to evaluate the presence of rales, wheezes, diminished breath sounds, and tachypnoea.

2. Auscultate the heart.
3. Auscultate the abdomen.

D. Palpate the abdomen for distension, tenderness, and masses (worm bolus). Upper right quadrant, lower right quadrant, or hypogastrium tenderness may suggest complications of ascariasis.

E. Percuss the abdomen: Dullness may be noted.

Diagnostic Tests

A. None, if the worm is visualized; they are occasionally passed from the rectum and nose, and are seen in vomitus.
B. Stool for occult blood, ova, and parasites, and culture.
C. Complete blood count (CBC): Eosinophilia may be noted particularly during the migration of larvae through the lungs.
D. Plain abdominal radiograph.
E. Ultrasound/CT to diagnose hepatobiliary or pancreatic ascariasis. Endoscopic retrograde cholangiopancreatography (ERCP) is used for diagnosis and removal.
F. Chest radiography is rarely needed.
G. Microscopic wet prep of sputum may be helpful with respiratory symptoms.

Differential Diagnoses

A. Impaired growth/failure to thrive (FTT).
B. Asthma.
C. Pneumonia.
D. Poor nutrition.
E. Giardiasis.
F. Pancreatitis from other causes.
G. Iron-deficiency anaemia.
H. Appendicitis.
I. Bowel obstruction (large or small).
J. Intussusception.

Plan

A. Client teaching:
  1. *Refer to Client Teaching Guide: Roundworms and Pinworms.*
  2. Stress the importance of maintaining a clean play area for children.
  3. Stress sanitary disposal of faeces.
  4. Explain that household bleach is ineffective in killing eggs *or* worms.
  5. All family members must be treated with medication.
  6. There is no direct person-to-person transmission.

B. Pharmacological therapy:
  1. Treatment of symptomatic and asymptomatic infections may be achieved by a single dose of the following agents:
    a. Pyrantel pamoate.
    b. Mebendazole.
    c. Anthelmintic therapy is not usually given at the time of pulmonary symptoms. Dying larvae may increase complications with migrating larvae.
  2. Administer the drug to all family members to decrease risk of spreading infection.
  3. Consider vitamin A supplement if growth is retarded.
  4. Inhaled beta-agonists may be indicated for respiratory symptoms.

Follow-Up

A. Reexamine a stool specimen in two weeks to determine if the therapy was successful in eliminating the worms. If the client is not cured, give a second course of medication.
B. Therapy is effective for adult worms only. Reevaluate in two to three months for detectable eggs.
C. Endoscopy or laparoscopic extraction of worms may be required with hepatobiliary infestations.

Consultation/Referral

A. Consult with an obstetrician if the client is pregnant.
B. Bowel or hepatobiliary obstruction may require surgical or gastroenterologic consultation.

Individual Considerations

A. Pregnancy:
  1. Anthelmintics are pregnancy category C; however, the potential risks to the foetus versus benefits should be considered.
  2. The World Health Organization (WHO) has determined that the benefit of pharmacological treatment outweighs the risk:
    a. The WHO allows the use of albendazole in the second and third trimesters of pregnancy.
    b. The WHO allows the use of pyrantel pamoate in the second and third trimesters of pregnancy.

B. Paediatrics:
  1. All medications are advised for children:
    a. The WHO guidelines for mass prevention campaigns: Albendazole can be used in children as young as 1 year old.
    b. Mebendazole and pyrantel pamoate are on the WHO Model List of Essential Medicines for Children, intended for use in children up to 12 years of age.
  2. Children are more prone to acute intestinal obstruction because they have smaller diameters of the intestinal lumen and often have large numbers of worms.

C. Adults: Acute intestinal obstruction may develop with heavy infestation.

Bibliography

American Academy of Pediatrics. (2012). Ascaris lumbricoides infections. In L. K. Pickering (Ed.), *Red book: 2012 report of the Committee on Infectious Diseases* (29th ed., pp. 239–240). Elk Grove Village, IL: Author. Retrieved from https://redbook.solutions.aap.org/DocumentLibrary/RB12_interior.pdf

Dora-Laskey, A. (2016, May 18). Ascaris lumbricoides. *Medscape.* Retrieved from http://emedicine.medscape.com/article/788398-overview

Leder, K., & Weller, P. F. (2016, June 16). Ascariasis. *UpToDate.* Retrieved from http://www.uptodate.com/contents/ascariasis

Nettina, S. (2010). *The Lippincott manual of nursing practice* (9th ed.). Philadelphia, PA: Wolters Kluwer Lippincott Williams & Wilkins.

Shoff, W. H. (2012, November 16). Pediatric ascariasis. *Medscape.* Retrieved from http://emedicine.medscape.com/article/996482-overview

Weller, P. F. (2009, May 1). Anthelminthic therapies. *UpToDate.* Retrieved from http://www.uptodate.com/online/content/topic.do?topicKey=antibiot/7691&view=print

Ulcerative Colitis

Cheryl A. Glass and Kristie A. D. Morydz

Definition

A. Ulcerative colitis (UC) is one of the two inflammatory bowel diseases (IBDs), along with Crohn's disease (CD).

UC is limited to the colon; it extends proximally from the anal verge in an uninterrupted pattern to a part of or the entire colon. Extracolonic manifestations also include uveitis, pyoderma gangrenosum, pluritis, erythema nodosum, ankylosing spondylitis, and spondyloarthropathies (Table 11.19).
B. Neither UC nor CD should be confused with IBS, which affects the motility of the colon. Smoking is negatively associated with UC; the relationship is reversed in CD. The general course of UC is intermittent exacerbations and remissions. In severe cases, surgery may result in a cure. The choice of treatment depends on disease activity and extent of pathology, client acceptability, and mode of drug delivery.
C. Histologically, most of the pathology of UC is limited to the mucosa and submucosa. The extent of UC is defined by the following:
   1. Pan-ulcerative (total colitis): Extensive disease with evidence of UC proximal to the splenic flexure. Massive dilation of the colon (toxic megacolon) may lead to bowel perforation.
   2. Left-sided disease: Continuous UC that is present from the rectum and the descending colon up to, but not proximal to, the splenic flexure.
   3. Proctosigmoiditis: Disease limited to the rectum and sigmoid colon involvement.
   4. Ulcerative proctitis: Disease limited to the rectum—usually less than the full rectum.
D. In 2015, the Toronto Consensus Clinical Practice Guidelines for the Management of Nonhospitalized UC published 34 recommendations, including statements on 5-aminosalicylates (5-ASA), corticosteroids, immunosuppressants, anti-tumour necrosis factor (TNF) therapy, and other agents, including probiotics. The guidelines are available at www.gastrojournal.org/article/S0016-5085(15)00303-0/abstract.
E. The 2015 Toronto Consensus guidelines defined remission and response with UC as follows:
   1. Complete remission: Both symptomatic remission and endoscopic healing defined as follows:
      a. Endoscopic healing: Normal mucosa, vascular blurring, or chronic changes (e.g., inflammatory polyps, scarring) without friability.
      b. Symptomatic remission: Normal stool frequency (less than or equal to three per day) and no blood in the stool.
   2. Symptomatic response: Meaningful improvement in symptoms as judged by both the client and provider in the absence of remission; response should not be considered a desirable final outcome but is useful to assess early response to treatment.

Definition of Severity of UC

Mild UC	• Four or fewer stools per day with or without blood
	• No systemic toxicity
	• Normal ESR
	• Mild abdominal pain or cramping
Moderate UC	• More than four bloody stools per day
	• No signs of systemic toxicity
	• Pulse <90 beats per minute
	• Temperature <37.5°C (99.5°F)
	• Haemoglobin >105 g/L
	• ESR <30 mm/hr
	• Moderate abdominal pain
	• Six or more bloody stools per day or observable massive and significant blood BM
Acute severe UC[a]	• One or more symptoms of systemic toxicity
	• Tachycardia >90 beats per minute
	• Temperature >37.8°C (100.4°F)
	• Haemoglobin <105 g/L
	• Increased ESR (>30 mm/hr)
	• >10 stools per day
	• Continuous rectal bleeding
	• Systemic toxicity
	• Tachycardia >90 beats per minute
Fulminant UC	• Fever >37.8°C (100.4°F)
	• Anaemia requiring blood transfusions
	• Abdominal tenderness and distension
	• Colonic dilation on radiography
	• May lead to toxic megacolon or colonic perforation

BM, bowel movement; ESR, erythrocyte sedimentation rate; UC, ulcerative colitis.
[a]Acute severe colitis is defined by Truelove and Witt's Criteria (1955).

Incidence/Prevalence
A. The annual incidence of UC is 10.4 to 12 per 100,000, depending on the country.
B. UC is three times more common than CD.
C. The most common cause of death in clients with UC is toxic megacolon.
D. Adenocarcinoma of the colon develops in 3% to 5% of clients with UC; the risk increases with the duration of the disease.
E. Approximately 6.2% of clients with IBD have a major extraintestinal manifestation:
   1. Uveitis is the most common—3.8%.
   2. Primary sclerosing cholangitis—3%.
   3. Ankylosing spondylitis—2.7%.
   4. Erythema nodosum—1.9%.
   5. Pyoderma gangrenosum—1.2%.

Pathogenesis
A. The exact aetiology is unknown.
B. UC may be considered an autoimmune disease. Persons with UC often have p-antineutrophil cytoplasmic antibodies (p-ANCAs). Abnormalities of humoral and cell-mediated immunity and/or generalized enhanced reactivity against intestinal bacterial antigen may also be causes of UC.

Predisposing Factors
A. Caucasian.
B. Jewish descent.
C. 30% more females than males.
D. Genetic susceptibility (chromosomes 12 and 16).

Common Findings
A. Frequent small-volume diarrhoea.
B. Bloody diarrhoea with or without mucos.

C. Severe bowel urgency.
D. Abdominal cramps and pain with bowel movement (BM).
E. Constipation.
F. Anorexia.
G. Anaemia.
H. Nocturnal BMs.

Other Signs and Symptoms
A. Tenesmus (rectal urgency/constant feeling of need to pass stool).
B. Abdominal tenderness.
C. Arthralgias.
D. Fatigue secondary to anaemia.
E. Failure to thrive (FTT) in children.
F. Severe UC:
   1. Fever.
   2. Tachycardia.
   3. Significant abdominal tenderness.
   4. Signs of volume depletion.

Subjective Data
A. Review the onset, duration, signs, and symptoms (number of stools, presence/absence of blood in the stool, fever, and abdominal pain).
B. Review the client's recent travel history or camping trips for the presence of intestinal infection.
C. Review the client's medication history, including antibiotics and nonsteroidal anti-inflammatory drugs (NSAIDs; one-third of clients with exacerbation of UC report recent NSAID use).
D. Review family history for IBD, celiac disease, and colorectal cancer.
E. Review the client's smoking status.
F. Review the client's history or contact related to tuberculosis (TB; testing required before biologic therapy).
G. Evaluate if the client has symptoms of uveitis, including light sensitivity, floaters, blurry vision, or pain/tenderness to touch.

Physical Examination
A. Check temperature (if indicated), pulse, blood pressure (BP), and weight. Follow serial weights.
B. Inspect:
   1. Observe the general overall appearance for nutritional status, cachexia, and pallor.
   2. Observe the perianal region for the presence of tags, fissures, fistulas, and abscess.
   3. Observe the abdomen for distension and presence of surgical scars.
   4. Examine the eyes for redness, irritation, and ocular complications (episcleritis, scleritis, and uvetis).
   5. Evaluate for the presence of dermatological findings, including erythema nodosum and pyoderma gangrenosum.
C. Auscultate:
   1. The heart and lungs.
   2. All four quadrants of the abdomen.
D. Palpate:
   1. Palpate all four quadrants of the abdomen, observing for tenderness, rebound, and guarding.
   2. Evaluate the presence of hepatomegaly.
   3. Perform digital rectal examination to assess for anal strictures and rectal masses.
   4. Palpate the joints for warmth, tenderness, and range of motion.

Diagnostic Tests
A. **Diagnosis is best made with endoscopy and biopsy.**
B. Laboratory tests:
   1. Complete blood count (CBC) with electrolytes.
   2. Platelet count.
   3. Sedimentation rate.
   4. C-reactive protein (CRP).
   5. Cytomegalovirus (CMV; chronic immunosuppressive steroids).
   6. HIV.
C. Stool testing:
   1. Evaluate bacterial, viral, or parasitic causes of diarrhoea.
   2. Occult blood.
   3. Faecal leukocytes.
D. Plain abdominal radiograph.
E. CT scan.
F. MRI.
G. Ultrasound.
H. Double-contrast barium enema.
I. Celiac antibody testing should be considered.
J. Intestinal TB testing should be considered.

Differential Diagnoses
A. Ischaemic colitis (especially in the elderly).
B. Toxic megacolon.
C. Colon cancer.
D. Adenocarcinoma.
E. Rectal cancer.
F. Radiation colitis.
G. Intestinal infections.
H. Intestinal lymphoma.
I. Chronic diverticulitis.
J. Amoebiasis.

Plan
A. General interventions:
   1. See Table 11.19 for the definition of severity of UC.
   2. Severe UC should be managed jointly by a gastroenterologist in conjunction with a colorectal surgeon (Table 11.20).
   3. Stress reduction and stress management may improve symptoms.
   4. Pretreatment screening for TB, using Mantoux (a purified protein derivative [PPD]) skin testing, is needed before initiation of immunomodulators and thiopurines.
   5. Immunization status:
      a. Immunizations with inactivated vaccine should be brought up-to-date and rigorously maintained during treatment, including influenza, meningococcus, and pneumococcus.
      b. Check varicella titres prior to treatment with immunomodulators and reimmunize if titres are low.
      c. The risk of administering live vaccines (polio, rubella, and yellow fever) to clients on immunomodulators has not been established; however, most experts avoid live vaccines during treatment.
B. Client teaching: *Refer to Client Teaching Guide: Crohn's Disease.*
C. Dietary management:

TABLE 11-20 Management of Mild to Moderate Distal Ulcerative Colitis With Topical Agents

Topical agent	Proximal extent/distribution of agent
Suppository	10 cm
Hydrocortisone foam	15–20 cm
Enema	As far as the splenic flexure

Source: Adapted from the AGA Ulcerative Colitis in Adult Practice Guidelines (2010).

1. Adequate nutrition is critical to promotion of healing. Sufficient protein and calories limit the stress on an inflamed bowel.
2. Many clients with UC have concurrent lactose intolerance. (See Appendix B, Diet Recommendations, for lactose-intolerance dietary recommendations.)
3. Decrease dietary fiber during increased disease activity.
4. Low-residue diet may decrease the frequency of BMs.
5. High-residue diet may be helpful in ulcerative proctitis when constipation is the dominant symptom (see Appendix B, Diet Recommendations, Table B.6).

D. Pharmacological therapy: Refer to the Canadian Clinical Practice Guidelines for Ulcerative Colitis, at static1.squarespace.com/static/52f8f139e4b0bae912c96d0d/t/559fddcce4b03b0e8a104ce7/1436540364414/UC+guidelines.pdf

1. The choice of topical agents is guided by the proximal distribution of UC into the bowel, as well as client preference.
2. Stepwise medication approach:

5-ASA class of anti-inflammatory drugs is the most common treatment for clients with mild (fewer than four bloody stools per day) or moderate active disease (more than four bloody stools a day without systemic toxicity). Left-sided colitis is treated with rectal or oral + rectal 5-ASA. More extensive diseases are treated with oral 5-ASA with or without rectal therapy. (Figure 11.5)

3. Corticosteroids suppress the immune system and are used for moderate to severe UC (Figure 11.6).
4. If symptom control is achieved after 14 days of corticosteroid therapy, maintenance therapy should be initiated with oral 5-ASA, thiopurine therapy, anti-TNF therapy, or vedolizumab.

E. Indications for the consideration of a total colectomy:
1. Failed medical therapy: Refractory UC.
2. Severe haemorrhage.
3. Fulminate colitis not responsive to treatment.
4. Toxic megacolon.
5. Obstruction or stricture.
6. FTT in children.

F. Indications for consideration for elective surgery:
1. Long-term steroid dependence.
2. Dysplasia or adenocarcinoma found on screening biopsy.
3. Disease present seven to 10 years.

Follow-Up

A. Screening colonoscopy is recommended for all clients with UC for eight to 10 years after the onset of symptoms due to the increase in colonic neoplasia.
B. Clients with extensive UC or left-sided colitis with negative findings on the screening colonoscopy should begin surveillance colonoscopy in one to two years.
C. Steroids should not be used as maintenance therapy. Clients who require long-term steroids are at increased risk of osteoporosis.
D. Subsequent laboratory monitoring tests are dependent on the prescribed therapy.

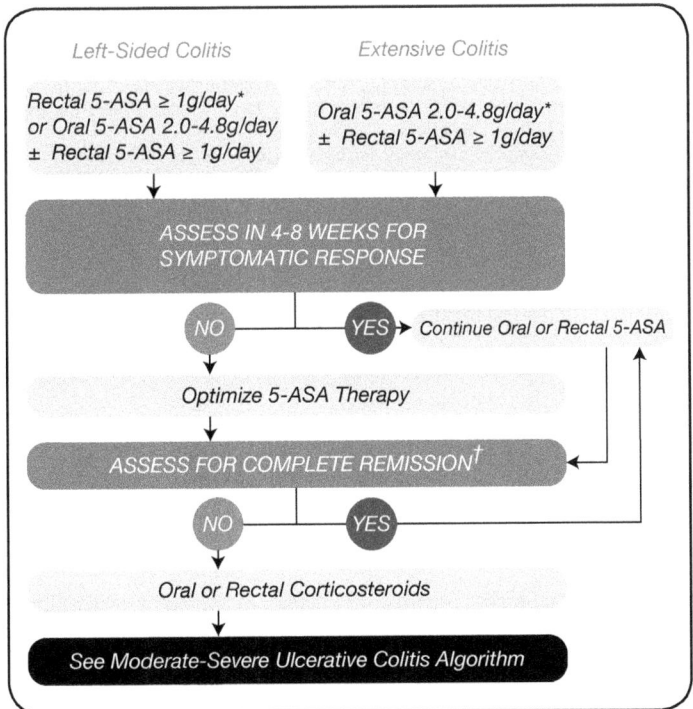

FIGURE 11.5 Stepwise management of ulcerative colitis.
Source: From CARE Canadian Clinical Practice Guidelines for Ulcerative Colitis. Retrieved from https://static1.squarespace.com/static/52f8f139e4b0bae912c96d0d/t/559fddcce4b03b0e8a104ce7/1436540364414/UC+guidelines.pdf.

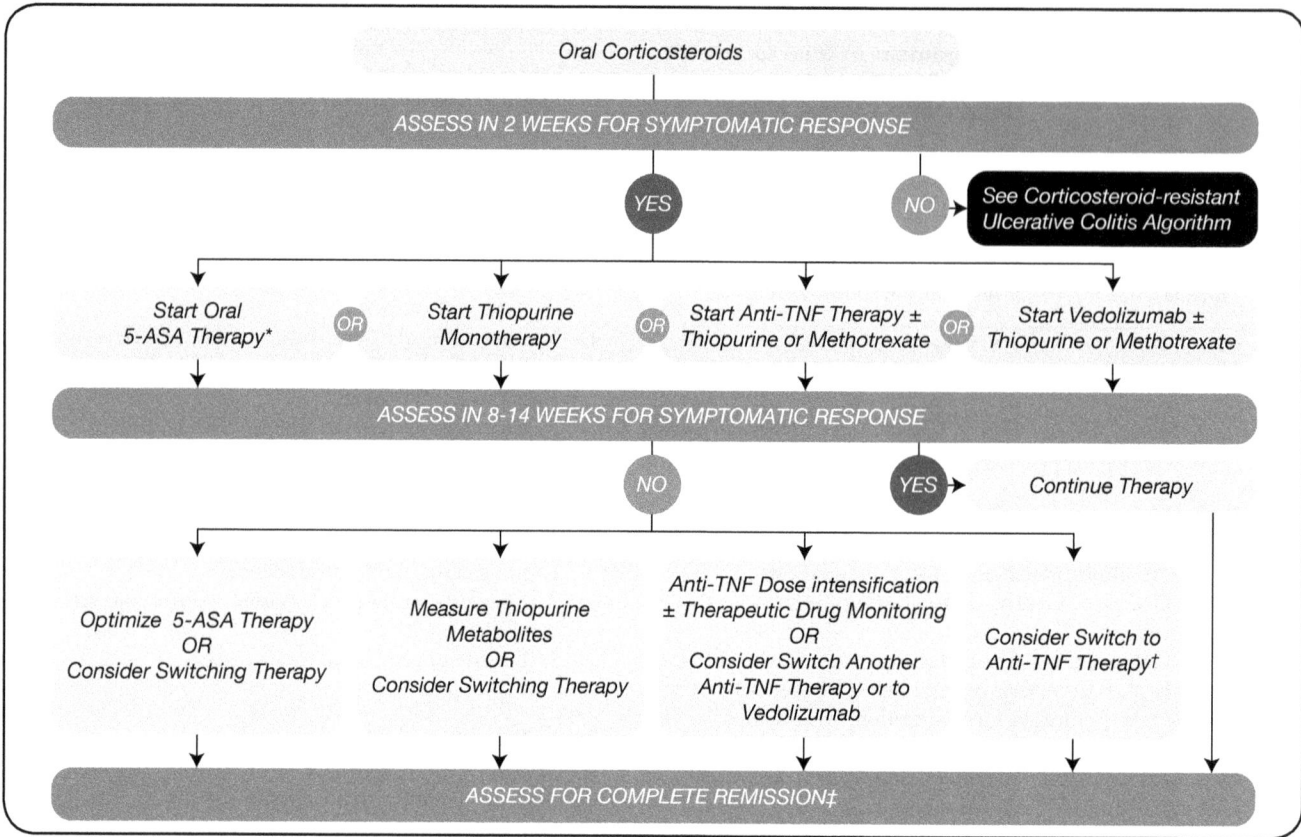

FIGURE 11.6 Moderate to severe active UC treatment algorithm.
UC, ulcerative colitis.
Source: From CARE Canadian Clinical Practice Guidelines for Ulcerative Colitis. Retrieved from
https://static1.squarespace.com/static/52f8f139e4b0bae912c96d0d/t/559fddcce4b03b0e8a104ce7/1436540364414/UC+guidelines.pdf

E. Anxiety and depression are higher in clients with IBD. Screen for depression at each visit.

Consultation/Referral

A. Gastroenterologist for confirmatory diagnosis with a colonoscopy.
B. Surgeon for severe or fulminant colitis. Toxic megacolon is a life-threatening complication and requires urgent surgical intervention.
C. Clients with ocular complications require an urgent consultation.
D. Clients who have had UC for eight to 10 years are at risk of colon cancer; therefore, colonoscopy for surveillance is recommended.

Individual Considerations

A. Live vaccinations should not be administered to immunocompromised clients. If required, vaccines should be administered at the time of UC diagnosis:
  1. The flu and pneumonia vaccines should be routinely administered.
  2. Consider administering the human papilloma virus vaccine.
B. Women with IBD have reported to have a high incidence of abnormal Pap smears. Adherence to Pap smear guidelines are recommended by the American College of Gastroenterology (ACG).
C. Abnormal sperm counts, motility, and morphology are seen with sulphasalazine.
D. Paediatrics:
  1. UC is uncommon in persons younger than 10 years.
  2. Fulminant disease occurs more in children than adults.
  3. Children may present with systemic complaints, including fatigue, arthritis, failure to gain weight, and delayed puberty.

Resources

American College of Gastroenterology: http://gi.org
CARE Ulcerative Colitis Guidelines Overview: https://static1.squarespace.com/static/52f8f139e4b0bae912c96d0d/t/559fddcce4b03b0e8a104ce7/1436540364414/UC+guidelines.pdf
Crohn's and Colitis Canada: http://crohnsandcolitis.ca

Bibliography

Basson, M. D. (2015, November 18). Ulcerative colitis. *Medscape.* Retrieved from http://emedicine.medscape.com/article/183084-overview
Bressler, B., Marshall, J. K., Berstein, C. N., Bitton, A., Jones, J., Leontiadis, G. I., & Fegan, B. (2015). Clinical practice guidelines for the medical management of nonhospitalized ulcerative colitis: The Toronto consensus. *Gastroenterology, 148,* 1035–1058. doi:10.1053/j.gastro.2015.03.001
Crohn's and Colitis Foundation of America. (n.d.). *Types of ulcerative colitis.* Retrieved from http://www.ccfa.org/what-are-crohns-and-colitis/what-is-ulcerative-colitis/types-of-ulcerative-colitis.html
Kornbluth, A., & Sachar, D. B. (2010). Ulcerative colitis practice guidelines in adults: American College of Gastroenterology, Practice Parameters Committee. *American Journal of Gastroenterology, 105,* 501–523. doi:10.1038/ajg.2009.727
National Digestive Disease Information Clearinghouse. (2014, March 5). *Ulcerative colitis.* Retrieved from http://digestive.niddk.nih.gov/DDISEASES/PUBS/colitis/index.aspx
Nettina, S. (2010). *The Lippincott manual of nursing practice* (9th ed.). Philadelphia, PA: Wolters Kluwer Lippincott Williams & Wilkins.
Truelove, S. C., & Witts, L. J. (1955). Cortisone in ulcerative colitis final report on a therapeutic trial. *British Medical Journal, 2,* 1041–1048. doi:10.1136/bmj.2.4947.1041

12 Genitourinary Guidelines

Benign Prostatic Hypertrophy

Cheryl A. Glass, Debbie Gunter, and Kristie A. D. Morydz

Definition
A. Benign prostatic hypertrophy (BPH) is enlargement of the prostate gland that constricts the urethra, causing urinary symptoms. BPH is not believed to be a risk factor for prostate cancer. BPH occurs primarily in the central or transitional zone of the prostate, whereas prostate cancer originates primarily in the peripheral part of the prostate.
B. The voiding dysfunction that results from prostate enlargement and bladder outlet obstruction (BOO) is termed lower urinary tract symptoms (LUTS).

Incidence/Prevalence
A. BPH prevalence increases progressively with age. The prevalence of prostatic hypertrophy increases from 8% in men aged 31 to 40 years to 40%, to 50% in men aged 51 to 60 years, and to more than 90% in men older than 80 years.

Pathogenesis
A. The exact cause is unknown; BPH may be a response to the androgen hormone. The process of aging and the presence of circulating androgens lead to the development of BPH. Hyperplasia, in which the normally thin and fibrous outer capsule of the prostate becomes spongy and thick, and the contraction of muscle fibers cause pressure on the urethra. This requires the bladder musculature to work harder to empty urine.

Predisposing Factors
A. Advancing age.
B. Genetic predisposition: Increases with a positive family history of BPH having moderate to severe LUTS.
C. Obesity.
D. Diabetes.
E. High levels of alcohol consumption.
F. Physical inactivity.

Common Findings
A. The clinical manifestations of BPH are LUTS that typically appear slowly and progress gradually over a period of years:
  1. Difficulty starting urine flow.
  2. Dribbling.
  3. Bladder does not feel like it completely empties.
  4. Frequency of urination.

Other Signs and Symptoms
A. Obstructive symptoms:
  1. Hesitancy.
  2. Diminution in size and force of urinary stream.
  3. Stream interruption (double voiding).
  4. Urinary retention.
  5. Straining/Valsalva maneuver to fully empty the bladder.
B. Irritative voiding symptoms:
  1. Urgency.
  2. Frequency.
  3. Nocturia.
  4. Painless haematuria: An early symptom; may also indicate malignancy.
C. Severe late symptoms with untreated BPH:
  1. Acute urinary retention.
  2. Recurrent urinary tract infections (UTIs).
  3. Hydronephrosis.
  4. Loss of renal concentrating ability.
  5. Systemic acidosis and renal failure.

Subjective Data
A. Have the client complete the International Prostate Symptom Score (IPSS) assessment tool at each visit to track and assess the severity of symptoms of BPH (www.urospec.com/uro/Forms/ipss.pdf).
B. Review the onset, duration, and course of symptoms. The I-PSS assessment tool can be used to quantitatively assess BPH symptoms over time.
C. Does the client have signs of a UTI?
D. Is there any blood in the urine or pain in the bladder region? (Evaluate bladder tumour or calculi.)
E. Does the client have new symptoms such as bone or back pain, loss of appetite, or weight loss (rule out cancer)?
F. Review the client's history for medical illness, including diabetes and neurologic problems.
G. Review previous urinary problems, surgeries, infections, treatments, success of treatments, and testing.
H. Review the client's history of sexual dysfunction and any new sexual partners (sexually transmitted infections [STIs]).
I. Review the client's history of urethral trauma, urethritis, cor urethral instrumentation that could have led to urethral stricture.
J. Review medications, both prescription and over-the-counter (OTC) drugs, including sinus or cold products, anticholinergic drugs (impair bladder function), and sympathomimetic drugs (increase outflow resistance).
K. Review family history of BPH and prostate cancer.
L. Review fluid intake, especially caffeinated/carbonated drinks.

M. Evaluate how bothersome the symptoms are to the client's quality of life:
1. How often does he have interrupted sleep to get up to go to the bathroom?
2. How often does he urinate?
3. Does he have to wear an absorptive underwear pad?

Physical Examination
A. Check temperature (if indicated), blood pressure (BP), and weight (if indicated).
B. Inspect:
1. Inspect general appearance for discomfort or acute discomfort with urinary retention.
2. Consider having the client void: Normal urination for a man is the ability to empty the bladder of 300 mL of urine in 12 to 15 seconds.
3. Examine the urethral meatus for discharge.
4. Retract foreskin (if present) and assess for hygiene and smegma.
5. Check the shaft of the penis, glans, and prepuce for lesions.
6. Check inguinal and femoral areas for bulges or hernias; have the client bear down and cough, and reexamine him.
7. Perform a neurologic examination (evaluate sensory and motor deficits).

C. Palpate:
1. Palpate the abdomen for masses or bladder distension.
2. Palpate lymph nodes in the groin for enlargement.
3. Check costovertebral angle (CVA) tenderness.
4. Palpate the testes and epididymides for inflammation, tenderness, and masses.
5. Palpate the scrotum for hydrocele or varicocele.

D. Digital rectal examination (DRE): Use the index finger of the dominant hand for the DRE:
1. Note sphincter tone, nodules or masses, and tenderness. Decreased anal sphincter tone or the lack of muscle reflex may indicate an underlying neurologic disorder.
2. Palpate the two lateral lobes of the prostate gland and its median sulcus for irregularities, nodules, induration, swelling, or tenderness just above the prostate anteriorly; determine whether the rectum lies adjacent to the peritoneal cavity. If possible, palpate this region for peritoneal masses and tenderness.

Diagnostic Tests
A. Urinalysis: Evaluate for infection and haematuria.
B. Urine culture if indicated (clients with BPH are more susceptible to UTIs).
C. Prostate-specific antigen (PSA): Recommended in men with at least a 10-year life expectancy and if prostate cancer knowledge changes management. PSA is recommended at age 50 for most men, at age 45 for those at high risk; and should be discontinued at age 70 for most men or consider discontinuing at age 60 for those with a PSA <1 ng/mL.
D. Optional studies:
1. Serum creatinine.
2. Urine cytology.
3. Uroflowmetry.
4. Postvoid residual.

E. Not routinely recommended:
1. Cytology.
2. Cystoscopy.
3. Urodynamics.
4. Radiological evaluation.
5. Prostate ultrasound.
6. Prostate biopsy.

Differential Diagnoses
A. Classifications of BPH from the score of the I_PSS symptom assessment tool:
1. Mild = total score 0 to 7.
2. Moderate = total score 8 to 19.
3. Severe = total score 20 to 35.

B. Other obstructive causes: prostate cancer, urethral obstruction, urethral stricture, and vesical neck obstruction.
C. Neurogenic bladder.
D. Cystitis.
E. Prostatitis.
F. Bladder calculi.

Plan
A. General interventions:
1. Have the client complete a 24-hour voiding chart with assessment of frequency and volume.
2. Any client with other than mild symptoms needs referral to a urologist to discuss treatment options (surgery or drugs).
3. Monitor the client with mild symptoms every three to six months to determine the progression of symptoms. Imaging studies are not routinely necessary in typical cases of BPH unless there is haematuria, an elevated creatinine, or another indication.
4. Treat concurrent UTI and STIs.

B. Client teaching: *Refer to Client Teaching Guide: Prostatic Hypertrophy/Benign.*
1. Clients should be instructed about the hypotensive effect, asthaenia, nasal congestion, and effect on ejaculation of the long-acting alpha-1 antagonists. The hypotensive effects can be potentiated by concomitant use of phosphodiesterase-5 (PDE-5) inhibitors sildenafil, tadalafil, or vardenafil.
2. Alpha-1 antagonists have been associated with intraoperative floppy iris syndrome. Clients need to discuss using these medicines with their ophthalmologist before eye surgery (i. e., cataract).

C. Pharmacological therapy:
1. Five long-acting alpha-1 antagonists are recommended for the treatment of LUTS secondary to BHP by the Canadian Urological Association (CUA):
   a. Terazosin requires dose titration to minimize side effects.
   b. Doxazosin increases hypotensive effect with PDE-5 inhibitor. Doxazosin requires dose titration to minimize side effects.
   c. Tamsulosin decreases ejaculate volume.
   d. Alfuzosin generally does not cause ejaculation problems.
   e. Silodosin may produce retrograde ejaculation.
2. Prazosin, a short-acting alpha-1 antagonist, approved for the treatment of hypertension (HTN) improves urine flow rates and may be considered for a client with HTN and urinary symptoms.
3. Two 5-alpha-reductase inhibitors are approved for BPH with an enlarged prostate. The major side effects of

these drugs are decreased libido and ejaculatory or erectile dysfunction (ED):
    a. Providers should be aware of safety information related to the use of the 5-alpha-reductase inhibitors because of an increased risk of a more serious form of prostate cancer (high-grade prostate cancer).
    b. Women who are, or may become, pregnant should not handle the 5-alpha-reductase inhibitors. They are pregnancy category X, known to cause birth defects.
    c. Finasteride.
    d. Dutasteride.
    e. Dutasteride–tamsulosin.
  4. Dual-drug combination.
  5. Phosphodiesterase inhibitors for those with male lower urinary tract symptoms (MLUTS) and erectile dysfunction:
    a. Tadalafil.
  6. There is no recommendation for phytotherapeutic agents.

Follow-Up
A. See the client in two to three weeks to monitor symptoms after specialty referral.
B. PSA testing: Baseline testing should begin at age 50 years (45 years for those at increased risk of prostate cancer) in men who have a life expectancy of 10 years or greater.
C. Age to discontinue screening determinant on PSA level and life expectancy:
  1. Those 60 years old with PSA <1 ng/mL—consider discontinuing PSA screening.
  2. Discontinue screening at 70 years old.
  3. Discontinue screening with those who have a life expectancy of <10 years.
D. PSA testing intervals—CUA recommendations:
  1. PSA <1 ng/mL—repeat every four years.
  2. PSA 1 to 3 ng/mL—repeat PSA every two years.
  3. PSA >3 ng/mL—repeat more frequently or add additional testing methods.

Consultation/Referral
A. Refer to a urologist for any complicated LUTS, including the following:
  1. History of prostate cancer.
  2. Elevated PSA.
  3. Urethral stricture.
  4. Spinal cord injury.
  5. Stroke.
  6. Recurrent/persistent UTI.
B. The presence of microscopic haematuria requires an evaluation of the complete urinary system and needs a referral to a urologist.
C. Refer for procedures after failed medication therapy:
  1. Minimally invasive therapy:
    a. Transurethral microwave therapy (TUMT).
    b. Transurethral incision of the prostate (TUIP).
  2. Surgical therapies:
    a. **Transurethral resection of the prostate (TURP) is considered the gold standard of surgical treatment of BPH.** Sexual dysfunction may occur after a TURP, including decreased libido, impotence, and ejaculatory difficulties. Balloon dilation may be used to reduce symptoms; however, relapse is common.
    b. Open prostatectomy.
    c. Laser procedures:
      i. Laser vaporization of the prostate.
      ii. Laser enucleation of the prostate.
    d. Transurethral needle ablation (TUNA).
    e. Photoselective vaporization of the prostate (PVP).

Individual Consideration
A. Geriatrics: Elderly men require special attention because their symptoms may be poorly expressed or confusing.

Bibliography
American Urological Association. (2010, revised 2014). *American urological association guideline: Management of benign prostatic hyperplasia (BPH)*. Retrieved from https://www.auanet.org/education/guidelines/benign-prostatic-hyperplasia.cfm

American Urological Association. (2016a, July). *Education and research Inc. American urologic association symptom score*. Retrieved from https://www.auanet.org

Associates in Urology. (n.d.[a]). *Patient questionnaire: AUA symptom score (AUASS)*. Retrieved from www.njurology.com/_forms/auass.pdf

Bechis, S. K., Otsetov, A. G., Ge, R., & Olumi, A. F. (2014). Personalized medicine for the management of benign prostatic hyperplasia. *Journal of Urology*, 192(1), 16–23. doi:10.1016/j.juro.2014.01.114

Canadian Urological Association guideline on male lower urinary tract symptoms/benign prostatic hyperplasia (MLUTS/BPH): 2018 update. *Canadian Urological Association Journal*, 12(10), 303–312. doi:10.5489/cuaj.5616

Deters, L. A. (2015 October 12). Benign prostatic hypertrophy. *Medscape*. Retrieved from http://emedicine.medscape.com/article/437359-overview

Patel, N. D., & Parsons, J. K. (2014). Epidemiology and etiology of benign prostatic hyperplasia and bladder outlet obstruction. *Indian Journal of Urology*, 30(2), 170–176. doi:10.4103/0970-1591.126900

Chronic Kidney Disease (CKD) in Adults

Angelito Tacderas, Debbie Gunter, and Kristie A. D. Morydz

Definition
Chronic kidney disease (CKD) is a disorder that leads to progressive kidney damage from a variety of causes, including diabetes, hypertension (HTN), cardiovascular (CV) disease, urinary obstructions, prolonged use of nephrotoxic medications, and inherited diseases such as polycystic kidney disease. Associated comorbidities of CKD include renal osteodystrophy, anaemia, metabolic acidosis, and malnutrition. Early recognition of CKD as well as treatment of complications can improve long-term outcomes.

CKD is specifically defined as follows:
A. The persistent and usually progressive reduction in glomerular filtration rate (GFR) <60 mL/min/1.73 m^2
B. Albuminuria: More than 30 mg of urinary albumin per gram of urinary creatinine.

Stages of CKD
A. Stage 1 disease is defined by a normal GFR (>90 mL/min/1.73 m^2) and persistent albuminuria.
B. Stage 2 disease is a GFR between 60 and 89 mL/min/1.73 m^2 and persistent albuminuria.
C. Stage 3 disease is a GFR between 30 and 59 mL/min/1.73 m^2.
D. Stage 4 disease is a GFR between 15 and 29 mL/min/1.73 m^2.
E. Stage 5 disease is a GFR of <15 mL/min/1.73 m^2 or end-stage renal disease (ESRD).

Incidence/Prevalence
A. Approximately two million Canadians are affected by chronic kidney disease. CV disease and diabetes often coincide with chronic kidney disease. Management of CV risk factors are critical as many clients will succumb to CV events before ESRD development.

B. By age group, CKD is more prevalent among persons older than 60 years than among persons aged 40 to 59 years or persons aged 20 to 39 years. CKD prevalence is greater among persons with diabetes than among those without diabetes and among persons with CV disease than among those without CV disease. CKD prevalence is higher among persons with HTN than among those without HTN.

Pathogenesis

Blood from the renal arteries and their subdivisions is delivered to the glomeruli. The glomeruli form an ultrafiltrate, nearly free of protein and blood elements, which subsequently flows into the renal tubules. The tubules reabsorb and secrete solute and/or water from the ultrafiltrate. The final tubular fluid, the urine, leaves the kidney, draining sequentially into the renal pelvis, ureter, and bladder, from which it is excreted through the urethra. The causes of CKD are traditionally classified by which portion of the renal anatomy is most affected by the disorder.

A. Vascular disease: Vascular disorders of the kidneys may involve partial or complete occlusion of large, medium, or small renal vessels. Examples of macrovascular or large renal vessel disease are renal artery stenosis and atherosclerotic disease. Benign hypertensive arteriolar nephrosclerosis results when chronic HTN damages small blood vessels, glomeruli, renal tubules, and interstitial tissues. Glomerulosclerosis is a severe microvascular or small vessel kidney disease caused by diabetes and uncontrolled HTN in which glomerular function of blood filtration is lost as fibrous scar tissue replaces the glomeruli. Loss of glomerular function leads to proteinuria, haematuria, HTN, and nephrosis, with variable progression to ESRD. Proteinuria occurs because of changes to capillary endothelial cells, the glomerular basement membrane (GBM), or podocytes that normally filter serum protein selectively by size and charge.

B. Tubular and interstitial disease: As with vascular disease, chronic tubulointerstitial nephritis (CTIN) can be primary or secondary to glomerular damage and renovascular disease. CTIN arises when chronic tubular insults cause gradual interstitial infiltration and fibrosis, tubular atrophy and dysfunction, and a gradual deterioration of renal function, usually over years. Causes of CTIN are immune disorders, infections, reflux or obstructive nephropathy, and drugs. Analgesic abuse nephropathy (AAN) is a type of CTIN caused by cumulative lifetime use of large amounts of certain analgesics such as nonsteroidal anti-inflammatory drugs (NSAIDs).

Predisposing Factors

A. Diabetes.
B. HTN.
C. CV disease.
D. Chronic use of analgesics such as NSAIDs.
E. Autoimmune disorder.
F. Polycystic kidney disease.
G. Urinary tract obstructions such as benign prostatic hypertrophy (BPH) or kidney stones.
H. Recurrent urinary tract infections (UTIs).
I. Older than 60 years.
J. African Canadian or Indigenous heritage.
K. Smoking.
L. Exposure to toxins.
M. Family history of kidney disease.

Common Findings

A. For CKD Stages 1 and 2, there are usually no presenting complaints; however, HTN is usually present. CKD is usually identified through routine screening of kidney function and urine tests for microalbumin.

Other Signs and Symptoms

A. In CKD Stage 3, the person will develop CKD complications but will still not usually have identifiable signs/symptoms:
  1. HTN.
  2. Decreased dietary calcium absorption.
  3. Reduced renal phosphate excretion.
  4. Elevation of parathyroid hormone.
  5. Altered lipoprotein metabolism.
  6. Reduced spontaneous protein intake.
  7. Anaemia.
  8. Left ventricular hypertrophy.
  9. Salt and water retention.
  10. Decreased renal potassium excretion.

B. These complications gradually worsen as the person moves to CKD Stage 4. The person will begin to display signs and symptoms of complications:
  1. Changes in bone density.
  2. Fatigue and pallor related to anaemia.
  3. Oedema.
  4. Decrease in muscle mass.

C. As the CKD progresses to Stage 5, in addition to gradual worsening of the signs/symptoms noted in Stages 3 and 4, the person will experience symptoms indicating chronic uraemia:
  1. Impaired sleep.
  2. Nocturia.
  3. Fatigue.
  4. Anorexia, nausea, vomiting, and weight change.
  5. Decreased mental acuity.
  6. Pruritus.
  7. Oedema.
  8. Respiratory symptoms, including orthopnea and dyspnoea.
  9. Muscle cramps, twitching, and restless legs.
  10. Peripheral neuropathy.

Subjective Data

A. Review the client's medical history to identify risk factors for CKD (previously noted in section "Predisposing Factors").
B. Elicit information about how well risk factors such as diabetes mellitus (DM) and HTN are controlled.
C. Review the onset and duration of signs/symptoms of CKD complications and uraemia.
D. Review all medications—including all over-the-counter (OTC) medications, especially NSAIDs, and supplements. Obtain specific information about dosing and length of time the drug was used.
E. Elicit smoking history.

Physical Examination

A. Observe general demeanor, attentiveness, and signs of fatigue.
B. Measure:
  1. Height, weight, and body mass index (BMI).
  2. Vital signs, including orthostatic blood pressure (BP) and pulse.
C. Inspect:
  1. Skin for colour, moisture, turgor, and signs of scratching because of chronic pruritus.
  2. Neck for jugular venous distension.
  3. Abdomen for distension.

4. Extremities for oedema, muscle mass, and signs of pain disorders such as arthritis.
D. Auscultate:
   1. Lungs for crackles.
   2. Heart for cardiac heave, gallop, or rub.
   3. Abdominal or femoral bruit.
E. Palpate:
   1. Abdomen for masses, distension.
   2. Bladder, and assess for flank tenderness.
F. Neurologic examination:
   1. Assess for sensation and vibratory sense on both feet.

Diagnostic Tests

Laboratory testing is critical in ascertaining the stage, course, chronicity, and complications (and associated comorbid conditions) of CKD.
A. Routine kidney function tests:
   1. Serum creatinine.
   2. Urea.
   3. Urinalysis.
   4. Measuring GFR: The severity of CKD should be classified based on the level of the estimated glomerular filtration rate (eGFR). Serum creatinine alone should *not* be used as a measure of kidney function. Kidney function in clients with CKD should be assessed by formula-based eGFR, preferably using the four-variable Modification of Diet in Renal Disease (MDRD) equation. Clinicians who do not have access to an automated tool may use a web-based tool, which is available at www.nkdep.nih.gov/professionals/gfr_calculators/index.htm. Calculate eGFRs using the actual MDRD equation, $eGFR = 186 \times (SCr) - 1.154 \times (age) - 0.203 \times (0.742$ if female$) \times (1.210$ if African Canadian$)$
   where SCr is serum creatinine concentration.
B. Assessing proteinuria:
   1. When screening adults at increased risk for CKD, albumin in the urine should be measured in a spot urine sample using:
      a. Albumin-specific dipstick.
      b. Albumin-to-creatinine ratio:
         i. It is usually not necessary to obtain a timed urine collection (overnight or 24 hours).
         ii. First-morning specimens are preferred, but random specimens are acceptable if first-morning specimens are not available.
         iii. In most cases, screening with urine dipsticks is acceptable for detecting proteinuria.
         iv. Standard urine dipsticks are acceptable for detecting increased total urine protein.
         v. Albumin-specific dipsticks are acceptable for detecting albuminuria.
   2. Clients with a positive dipstick test (1 or greater) should undergo confirmation of proteinuria by a quantitative measurement (protein-to-creatinine ratio or albumin-to-creatinine ratio) within three months.
   3. Clients with two or more positive quantitative tests spaced apart by one to two weeks should be diagnosed as having persistent proteinuria and undergo further evaluation and management for CKD.

Other Tests to Determine CKD Complications

A. Complete blood count (CBC).
B. Haemoglobin (Hgb): If Hgb level is <120 g/L in females and <130 g/L in adult males, also do blood cell indices, absolute reticulocyte count, serum iron, total iron-binding capacity, percent transferrin saturation, serum ferritin, white blood cell (WBC) count and differential, platelet count, and testing for blood in stool.
C. Lipid profile and triglycerides.
D. Comprehensive metabolic profile (serum total protein, serum albumin, glucose, calcium, sodium, potassium, chloride, bicarbonate, urea, creatinine, alkaline phosphatase, alanine aminotransferase [ALT], aspartate aminotransferase [AST], bilirubin).
E. Prealbumin.
F. Phosphorus.
G. Parathyroid hormone.
H. Urine immunofixation study.
I. Antinuclear antibody (ANA), anti-neutrophil cytoplasmic autoantibody (ANCA), complement 3 and complement 4 (C3 and C4):
   1. Test is done to rule out autoimmune disorder, lupus, vasculitis, and cancer.
   2. No fasting is needed.
J. Hepatitis B surface antigen (HBsAg) and hepatitis C antibody.
K. Anti-GBM antibody.
L. Renal ultrasound to rule out postobstructive uropathy.
M. Renal Doppler to rule out renal artery stenosis.

Differential Diagnoses

Evaluation is meant to determine whether kidney disease is acute or chronic and to determine prerenal, intrarenal, or postrenal causation.

Plan

The treatment plan will focus on clients in earlier stages of CKD—Stages 1, 2, and 3. Persons with CKD Stage 4 and 5 need specialized interventions provided by nephrologists and should be referred immediately.
A. General interventions:
   1. Provide support to the client.
   2. Initiate appropriate referrals for a nephrologist, client education, and social and financial support as soon as possible.
   3. For CKD Stage 4 or 5, access devices for hemodialysis, such as a primary arteriovenous fistula or graft, require months to mature and should be in place for six months before the start of dialysis.
B. Client teaching: *Refer to Client Teaching Guide: Kidney Disease: Chronic.* ◀
   1. Instruct the client in how kidneys work and how his or her body is affected by the CKD.
   2. Emphasize the importance of following instructions to prevent further kidney damage:
      a. Follow medication management instructions as carefully as possible.
      b. No OTC medications should be taken that are not approved by the provider.
      c. Keeping diabetes and HTN under control is crucial to maintaining kidney function.
      d. Preventing CV complications by lowering cholesterol and BP is more important for clients with CKD.
      e. Smoking cessation is an important way to prevent worsening kidney function.
      f. Routine follow-ups with provider are necessary to monitor kidney function. Clients should be encouraged to keep all appointments.

▶ Client Teaching Guides are available at https://connect.springerpub.com/content/reference-book/978-0-8261-9498-5

g. Follow dietary instructions regarding protein, fats, sodium, and minerals.
h. Dietary intake of protein is usually restricted to 0.8 to 1.0 g/kg/d of high biologic value protein.
i. Dietary sodium should be restricted to no more than 2 g daily.
j. Potassium should be restricted to 40 to 70 meq/d.
k. Calories should be restricted to 35 kcal/kg/d; if the body weight is >120% of normal or the client is older than 60 years, a lower amount may be prescribed.
l. Fat intake should be about 30% to 40% of total daily caloric intake.
m. Phosphorus should be restricted to 600 to 800 mg/d.
n. Calcium should be restricted to 1,400 to 1,600 mg/d.
o. Magnesium should be restricted to 200 to 300 mg/d.

3. Instruct when to notify the provider with urgent signs/symptoms or changes in kidney function:
a. Changes in urine volume.
b. Anorexia, nausea, and vomiting.
c. Increased oedema.
d. Shortness of breath (SOB).
e. Increased fatigue.
f. Difficulty concentrating.
g. Muscle weakness, cramping, or twitching.
h. Fever.
i. Chest pain.

C. Pharmacological therapy:
General principles of medications used to prevent progression of CKD and to manage symptoms of complications of CKD:

1. Always prescribe the smallest effective dose of any medication.
2. Start with a low dose and gradually increase. Dosage intervals may need to be extended.
3. Monitor the effect of any new medication on kidney function with appropriate laboratory follow-up.
4. Discuss with the client signs/symptoms to report to the provider immediately regarding drug therapy.
5. Avoid use of nephrotoxic drugs such as radiographic contrast materials, aminoglycoside antibiotics, and NSAIDs to prevent nephrogenic systemic fibrosis. If radiocontrast material use cannot be avoided because the benefit outweighs the risks, protect the kidney with acetylcysteine on the day of intravenous (IV) contrast.
6. Immunizations: Some vaccines in usual doses provide protection, while other vaccines require more frequent dosing or larger doses to achieve and maintain protective antibodies. Protective antibody titres may fall and booster doses should be given if appropriate. In general, the recommendations are the following:
a. Annual influenza vaccination.
b. Pneumococcal vaccine with a single booster dose five years after the initial dose.
c. Hepatitis B vaccine series for clients before starting dialysis.
7. HTN control and kidney protection: It is recommended that HTN therapy achieve a goal of BP of 130/80 mmHg or less. Use of an angiotensin-converting enzyme (ACE) inhibitor or angiotensin II receptor blocker (ARB) therapy in early stages of CKD with persons who have proteinuria can preserve kidney function. The clinician should monitor serum potassium on initiation of the therapy. It is common for the serum potassium to initially rise and then return to normal levels in two to three months. Follow-up serum potassium levels are recommended. In the early stages of CKD, with no proteinuria, the ACE inhibitors and ARBs have not been shown to be effective in protecting kidney function. HTN control can still be achieved with the ACE/ARB drugs, but other antihypertensive drugs can also be used.
8. Fluid overload: Occurs when sodium intake exceeds sodium excretion. The combination of sodium restrictions and a loop diuretic, such as furosemide, can lower intraglomerular pressure and provide some kidney protection.
9. Hyperkalaemia: Hyperkalaemia is managed with a low-potassium diet in combination with prescribing a loop diuretic such as furosemide. If a client is on an ACE or ARB, the addition of the loop diuretic will compensate for the elevation of serum potassium related to the ACE/ARB treatment.
10. Metabolic acidosis: Buildup of hydrogen ions causes bicarbonate levels to fall below acceptable levels. Sodium bicarbonate in a daily dose is often given. This prevents the symptoms of metabolic acidosis, which can increase muscle mass loss and worsen bone disease.
11. Renal osteodystrophy: The development of renal osteodystrophy is caused by hyperphosphataemia and hypocalcaemia that are secondary to decreased kidney function. In order to compensate, the client will develop secondary hyperparathyroidism. Dietary restriction of phosphate to 800 mg/d is recommended. In CKD Stage 3, the client will usually require an oral phosphate binder such as calcium carbonate or calcium acetate to prevent hyperphosphataemia. Oral phosphate binders must be taken with meals to be effective. It is imperative to avoid phosphate binders that contain aluminum or magnesium. To suppress parathyroid hormone secretion, the client is given calcitriol, a vitamin D analog.
12. Anaemia: Use of elemental iron, such as ferrous sulfate, is recommended to maintain the percent transferrin saturation >20% and the serum ferritin level >100 ng/mL.
Although primarily used in clients with ESRD, erythropoietic (EPO) agents, such as epoetin alfa and darbepoetin alfa, are also used to correct anaemia in those with CKD who do not yet require dialysis. Dosages of the EPO agents should be prescribed in order to maintain Hgb levels in the range of 110 to 120 g/L in predialysis clients with CKD.
13. Dyslipidaemia: Management of dyslipidaemia has been shown to slow the progression of CKD. Statins and fibrates are commonly prescribed to lower total cholesterol and low-density lipoprotein (LDL) and triglycerides. The incidence of untoward side effects with statins and fibrates is increased in persons with CKD; therefore, lower dosages and careful monitoring are required.

Follow-Up

A. Regular, consistent follow-up appointments to monitor progression of CKD, management of complications of CKD, and management of comorbidities such as DM and HTN are recommended.

Consultation/Referral

A. Early referral to a nephrologist is recommended for anyone who has CKD. Referral to a nephrologist must be done as quickly as possible for symptomatic clients with CKD Stage 4 or 5. Consultation with an endocrinologist or HTN specialist may be helpful in cases in which DM and HTN continue to be poorly controlled.

B. After the client is evaluated as a candidate for kidney transplantation, counseling on renal transplantation should be completed by a nephrologist about types of transplant available and how the transplant process works.

C. Referral to a dietitian for nutritional counseling and education to assist the client to understand and follow complex dietary instructions is recommended.

D. Clients with CKD Stage 4 or 5 may benefit from counseling regarding the psychosocial and financial impact of progressive renal disease. Referral to a renal social worker or case manager can help the client understand his or her health insurance benefits, and to help the client deal with concerns about work or family life.

E. Clients should be referred to educational and support organizations for further education regarding CKD.

F. Websites:
   1. The Kidney Foundation of Canada: www.kidney.ca.
   2. National Kidney Foundation: www.kidney.org.
   3. National Kidney Disease Education Program: www.nkdep.nih.gov.

Individual Consideration

A. Although renal replacement therapy is widely available, some clients, especially the more debilitated elderly or those who have a terminal illness, may request end-of-life counseling, including advance directives.

Bibliography

Aora, P. (2015, April 7). Chronic kidney disease. *Medscape*. Retrieved from http://emedicine.medscape.com/article/238798-overview

Borrelli, S., De Nicola, L., Stanzione, G., Conte, G., & Minutolo, R. (2013). Resistant hypertension in nondialysis chronic kidney disease. *International Journal of Hypertension, 2013*, 929183. doi:10.1155/2013/929183

Carrero, J. J., Burrowes, J., & Wanner, C. (2016). A long road to travel: Adherence to dietary recommendations and adequate dietary phosphorus control. *Journal of Renal Nutrition, 26*(3), 133–135. doi:10.1053/j.jrn.2016.03.004

Inker, L. A., Astor, B. C., Fox, C. H., Isakova, T., Lash, J. P., Peralta, C. A., & Feldman, H. I. (2014). KDOQI U. S. commentary on the 2012 KDIGO clinical practice guideline for the evaluation and management of CKD. *American Journal of Kidney Disease, 63*(5), 713–735. doi:10.1053/j.ajkd.2014.01.416

Kidney Disease Improving Global Outcomes. (2012). *KDOQI 2012 clinical practice guideline for the evaluation and management of chronic kidney disease*. Retrieved from http://kdigo.org/home/guidelines/ckd-evaluation-management

Levin, A, Hemmelgarn, B, Culleton, B., Tobe, S., McFarlane, P., Ruzicka, M., Burns, K., Manns, B., White, C, Madore, F., Moist, L., Klarenbach, S., Barret, B., Foley, R., Jindal, K., Senior, P., Pannu, N., Shurraw, S., Akbari, A., Cohn, A., Reslerova, M., Deved, V., Mendelssohn, D., Nesrallah, G., Kappel, J., Tonelli, M., and the Canadian Society of Nephrology (2008) CMAJ< 179(11), 1154-62.

National Kidney and Urologic Diseases Information Clearinghouse, National Institutes of Health. (n.d.). *Kidney disease*. Retrieved from https://www.niddk.nih.gov/health-information/kidney-disease

National Kidney Disease Education Program. (n.d.[a]). *Glomerular filtration rate (GFR) calculators*. Retrieved from https://www.niddk.nih.gov/healthinformation/healthcommunicationprograms/nkdep/lab-evaluation/gfr-calculators/Pages/gfrcalculators.aspx

National Kidney Disease Education Program. (n.d.[b]). *Manage patients with CKD*. Retrieved from https://www.niddk.nih.gov/health-information/health-communication-programs/nkdep/identify-manage/manage-patients/Pages/manage-patients.aspx

National Kidney Foundation. (2012). *KDOQI clinical practice guidelines for chronic kidney disease: Evaluation, classification, and stratification*. Retrieved from https://www.kidney.org/professionals/guidelines/guidelines_commentaries/chronic-kidney-disease-classification

Steiber, A. L. (2014). Chronic kidney disease: Considerations for nutrition interventions. *Journal of Parenteral and Enteral Nutrition, 38*(4), 418–426. doi:10.1177/0148607114527315

The Clinical Advisor. *Kidney guide features albuminuria testing*. Retrieved from www.clinicaladvisor.com/kidney-guide-features-albuminuria-testing/article/279307

Epididymitis

Cheryl A. Glass, Debbie Gunter, and Kristie A. D. Morydz

Definition

Epididymitis is acute infection of the epididymis, the coiled segment of the spermatic duct that connects the efferent duct from the posterior aspect of the testicle to the vas deferens. Epididymitis is commonly found to develop during strenuous exertion in conjunction with a full bladder. **Testicular torsion should be considered in all cases—this is a surgical emergency.**

A. Acute epididymitis: Duration of symptoms lasts less than six weeks.
   1. Acute epididymitis often involves the testis (epididymo-orchitis).
B. Chronic epididymitis: Duration of symptoms lasts more than six weeks.
   1. Inflammation chronic epididymitis.
   2. Obstructive chronic epididymitis.
   3. Chronic epididymalgia.

Incidence/Prevalence

A. Epididymitis is the fifth most common urologic diagnosis in men aged 18 to 50 years. Sexually transmitted infection (STI) accounts for two-thirds of epididymitis (47% *Chlamydia trachomatis* and 20% *Neisseria gonorrhoeae*) in men under 35 years. About 75% of cases can be attributed to coliforms or pseudomonas in those over 35.

Chronic epididymitis may account for up to 80% of scrotal pain noted in the outpatient setting. The mumps, measles, and rubella (MMR) vaccine has markedly reduced the incidence of mumps orchitis.

Pathogenesis

A. The exact pathophysiology is unclear. The cause may be the retrograde passage of infected urine from the prostatic urethra to the epididymis from the ejaculatory ducts and vas deferens. Reflux may be induced by having the client perform the Valsalva maneuver or by strenuous exertion. Pathogens include *Chlamydia trachomatis, Neisseria gonorrhoeae, Escherichia coli, Proteus* species, *Klebsiella* species, *Pseudomonas, Mycoplasma* species, and *Treponema pallidum*.

Predisposing Factors

A. Age:
   1. Age <35 years is generally associated with urethritis with the following organisms:
      a. *C. trachomatis* (chlamydia).
      b. *N. gonorrhoeae* (gonorrhea).
   2. Benign prostatic hyperplasia (BPH) is more common for men older than 35 years and common organisms include the following:
      a. *E. coli*.
      b. *Pseudomonas* species.
      c. *Proteus* species.
      d. *Klebsiella* species.
   3. The older populations of men usually have nonsexual epididymitis related to urinary tract instrumentation, surgery, and immunosuppression.

B. Men who have sex with men (MSM) who are the insertive partner during anal intercourse may have epididymitis with the following organisms:
  1. *E. coli*.
  2. *Pseudomonas*.
  3. Coliform bacteria.
C. Urinary tract infections (UTIs).
D. Tuberculosis (TB; should be considered if there is a history of or recent exposure to TB).
E. Vasectomy.
F. Indwelling urethral catheter.
G. Urethral stricture.
H. Amiodarone—high drug concentrations (dose-dependent).
I. Prolonged sitting (sedentary job, travel).
J. Mumps.

Common Findings
A. Swelling and tenderness of the scrotum (usually located on one side).
B. Fever.
C. Chronic epididymitis:
  1. Epididymal pain and inflammation that last more than six weeks.
  2. May be accompanied by scrotal induration.

Other Signs and Symptoms
A. Gradual onset of localized, unilateral testicular pain. The client may get relief with elevation of the scrotum, which is a positive **Prehn's sign**.
B. Urethral discharge.
C. Dysuria, frequency, urgency.
D. Haematuria.
E. Fever and chills (in only 25% of adults with acute epididymitis but in up to 71% of children with the condition).

Subjective Data
A. Elicit the onset, duration, and course of the client's symptoms.
B. Review the client's history for vasectomy or trauma to the groin.
C. Are there any other symptoms, including fever, dysuria, or discharge?
D. What makes the pain better? Ask about elevating the scrotum.
E. Does the client's sexual partner(s) have any symptoms or discharge?
F. Has there been any recent instrumentation or catheterization?
G. Is the pain unilateral or bilateral?
H. Review medication history for amiodarone.
I. Does the client have a recent TB exposure?

Physical Examination
A. Check temperature, blood pressure (BP), and pulse.
B. Inspect:
  1. Examine the client generally for discomfort before and during examination.
  2. Check the urethral meatus for discharge. Retract foreskin (if present) and assess for hygiene and smegma. Check the shaft of the penis, glans, and prepuce for lesions.
  3. Check the inguinal and femoral areas for bulges and hernias; have the client bear down and cough, and reexamine him.
C. Palpate:
  1. Palpate testes and epididymides for inflammation, tenderness, and masses. In chronic cases, the epididymis feels firm and lumpy. Vas deferens may be beaded.
  2. Check Prehn's sign by elevating the affected hemiscrotum. This action relieves the pain of epididymitis but exacerbates the pain of torsion.
  3. Elicit a cremasteric reflex. Stroking the inner thigh should result in rise of the testicle and scrotum on the affected side. A normal cremasteric reflex indicates that testicular torsion is less likely.
  4. Palpate the scrotum for hydrocele or varicocele.
  5. Check for costovertebral angle (CVA) tenderness.
  6. Examine the abdomen for masses, urinary distension, tenderness, and organomegaly.
  7. Palpate lymph nodes in the groin.
  8. Evaluate for an inguinal hernia.
D. Rectal examination: Check for symmetry, swelling, tenderness, and enlarged prostate.

Diagnostic Tests
A. Urethral swab for Gram stain.
B. Specimens for identification of *N. gonorrhoeae* and *C. trachomatis* (intraurethral exudate or urine):
  1. Samples for *N. gonorrhoeae* for both culture and nucleic acid amplification test (NAAT) should be considered based on clinical situation; strongly recommended in symptomatic MSM or where there is increased probability of treatment failure.
C. Microscopy and culture of mid-stream urine.
D. Doppler ultrasound—useful to help differentiate epididymitis from testicular torsion, if done without delay.
E. No role for epididymal aspiration in routine clinical practice. Recurrent infection that fails to respond to therapy or in clients with suspected abscess formation may require aspiration.
F. Not routinely recommended:
  1. Intravenous pyelography (IVP).
  2. Doppler ultrasonography.
  3. Scrotal ultrasonography.
  4. Radionuclide scrotal imaging.

Differential Diagnoses
A. Epididymitis:
  1. Bacterial.
  2. Viral epididymo-orchitis (mumps and *Haemophilus influenzae*).
B. Testicular torsion (surgical emergency).
C. Testicular tumour.
D. Prostatitis.
E. Incarcerated inguinal hernia.
F. Orchitis (occurs with parotitis).
G. Trauma.
H. Vasectomy side effect.
I. Folliculitis.
J. Herpes outbreak.

Plan
A. General interventions:
  1. Encourage and stress the importance of adequate fluid intake.
  2. Stress the importance of taking all antibiotics as directed.

B. Client teaching: *Refer to Client Teaching Guide: Epididymitis*.
   1. Offer supportive therapy.
C. Pharmacological therapy:
   1. Antibiotic therapy (both partners must be treated for STI). Treat empirically until laboratory test results are available.
   2. Acute epididymitis should be treated for 10 to 14 days.
   3. Chronic epididymitis should be treated for four to six weeks for bacterial pathogens, especially chlamydia.
   4. Nonsteroidal anti-inflammatory drugs (NSAIDs) for pain management.
   5. Antitubercular triple therapy consists of rifampin, isoniazid, and pyrazinamide for six months.
   6. Amiodarone epididymitis usually responds to a dosage reduction or discontinuation.

For Canadian guidelines for the treatment of STIs, see www.canada.ca/en/public-health/services/infectious-diseases/sexual-health-sexually-transmitted-infections/canadian-guidelines/sexually-transmitted-infections/canadian-guidelines-sexually-transmitted-infections-20.html

Follow-Up

A. See the client in two to seven days depending on severity of infection:
   1. Pain typically improves within one to three days, but may take up to two to four weeks.
   2. Inadequate treatment can result in abscess formation and decreased fertility.
B. Culture urine at the end of treatment (test of cure).
C. Failure to recognize and treat both partners for STIs has potential legal ramifications; test for all STIs and do not just focus on chlamydia and gonorrhea.
D. Consider testing for HIV.
E. Tuberculous epididymitis should be suspected if clinical signs worsen despite appropriate antibiotic therapy.
F. Men older than 50 years should be evaluated for urethral obstruction secondary to prostatic enlargement.

Consultation/Referral

A. Obtain an immediate consultation with a urologist if testicular torsion, scrotal abscess, or failed medical treatment is suspected.
B. Refer pediatric clients for evaluation of an underlying congenital anomaly.

Individual Considerations

A. Partner: Treat sexual partners for STI. Consider testing for HIV. Confirmed gonococcal epididymitis must be reported to local public health authority.
B. Pediatric: Epididymitis is rare prepubertally, and testicular torsion is more common in this age group.
C. Geriatrics:
   1. Epididymitis in the elderly is often caused by an enlarged prostate gland.
   2. Trouble voiding can be an early finding.

Bibliography

Centers for Disease Control and Prevention. (2015, June 15). *2015 sexually transmitted diseases treatment guidelines: Epididymitis*. Retrieved from https://www.cdc.gov/std/tg2015/epididymitis.htm

Ching, C. B. (2015, December 20). Epididymitis treatment and management. *Medscape*. Retrieved from http://emedicine.medscape.com/article/436154-treatemt

ClinicalKey. (n.d.). *Epididymitis*. Retrieved from https://www.cdc.gov/std/tg2015/epididymitis.htm

National Kidney Foundation. (2015). KDOQI clinical practice guideline for hemodialysis adequacy 2015 update. *American Journal of Kidney Disease, 66*(5), 884–930. doi:10.1053/j.ajkd.2015.07.015. Retrieved from www.kidney.org/professionals/guidelines/hemodialysis2015

Erectile Dysfunction (ED)

Nancy Pesta Walsh and Kristie A. D. Morydz

Definition

Erectile dysfunction (ED), also known as impotence, is the persistent inability to achieve or maintain penile erection sufficient for satisfactory sexual performance. ED occurs with reduced blood flow to the penis or nerve damage as well as psychological triggers. Low self-esteem, performance anxiety, depression, stress, and effects to quality of life occur secondary to ED. ED is noted to be a precursor to symptomatic coronary artery disease (CAD).

Age-associated changes in sexual function in men include delay in erection, diminished intensity and duration of orgasm, and decreased force of seminal emission. ED lasting three months or longer should have further evaluation and consideration of treatment.

The Sexual Health Inventory for Men (SHIM) questionnaire can be accessed at www.pcf.org/c/the-sexual-health-inventory-for-men-shim-questionnaire/ in which male sexual dysfunction questionnaires are available.

Incidence/Prevalence

A. ED can occur at any age; however, it is more common in men older than 60 years.
B. The Canadian Study of Erectile Dysfunction found 49.4% of men over age 40 are affected by ED and 5% to 20% with moderate to severe ED.
C. By 2025, it is estimated that 322 million men worldwide will have ED.
D. Men with ED have a 65% to 85% increased risk of subsequent CAD.
E. Reduced libido is estimated as affecting 5% to 15% of men.

Pathogenesis

A. Normal pathology: The dorsal nerve of the penis provides innervation, the dorsal somatic nerve provides sensation, and the autonomic nervous system, via the cavernosal nerves, regulates blood flow to the penis, allowing for erection to occur. The ability to maintain an erection relies on the dorsal nerve, the peripheral nerves, penile vasculature, and biochemical releases within the corpora.
B. Multiple factors may contribute to ED:
   1. Vascular (most common):
      a. This system is responsible for delivering and trapping the blood in the corporal sinusoids. Usually, the blood flowing in is not the problem; rather, the ED is the result of venous leaking from the corporal sinusoids.
      b. Arterial insufficiency contributes to decreased blood flow to the cavernosal sinuses. The cavernosal dysfunction causes difficulty with retaining blood in the penis thus making it difficult to sustain an erection:
         i. Chronic diseases such as cardiovascular (CV) disease, hypertension (HTN), dyslipidaemia, and obesity.

    ii. Certain medications can contribute to this physiological effect.
    iii. Smoking is also a contributing factor, especially in the presence of existing CV disease, because of the vasoconstrictive effects it causes.
  2. Psychological.
    a. Direct inhibition of the spinal erection center and/or excessive sympathetic nervous system biochemical release occurs, which increases the smooth muscle tone of the penis, preventing erection:
      i. Age-related decline.
      ii. Lack of sexual response.
      iii. Personal intimacy-related issues.
      iv. Partner-specific intimacy issues.
      v. Performance anxiety.
      vi. Depression or life stress related.
  3. Neurologic:
    a. Any disease affecting the brain, spinal cord, and cavernous and penile nerves can impair the ability to achieve erection such as spinal cord injury, stroke, or diabetes.
    b. Surgery in the pelvic region, including prostatectomy, perineal resection, and sphincterotomy.
  4. Endocrine:
    a. Decreased testosterone level.
    b. Increased prolactin level.
    c. Hyperthyroidism.
    d. Hypothyroidism.

Predisposing Factors
A. CV disease.
B. Diabetes (neurologic and vascular problems).
C. HTN.
D. Hyperlipidaemia.
E. Advanced age (>60 years).
F. Peripheral neuropathy.
G. Obesity.
H. Neurologic disorders:
  1. Spinal cord injuries.
  2. Brain injuries.
  3. Multiple sclerosis.
  4. Parkinson's disease.
I. Alcohol/tobacco abuse.
J. Drug abuse:
  1. Heroin.
  2. Cocaine.
  3. Marijuana.
K. Side effect of medication (e.g., serotonin reuptake inhibitors, antihypertensives, antihistamines, diuretics, nonsteroidal anti-inflammatories, muscle relaxants).
L. Surgical/radiation therapy for cancers of the pelvis or pelvic trauma.
M. Hypogonadism.
N. Psychological and psychiatric disorders.
O. Peyronie's disease (deformity of the penis).
P. Obstructive sleep apnea.
Q. Physical inactivity.

Common Findings
A. Inability to achieve or sustain an erection.
B. Erection is not firm enough for penetration.
C. Absent or delayed ejaculation.
D. Inability to control the timing of ejaculation.
E. Lack of interest or desire (most common).
F. Pain with intercourse.

Other Signs and Symptoms
A. Diminished self-esteem.
B. Depression.
C. Anxiety.
D. Reduced libido.
E. Relationship difficulties.
F. Premature ejaculation (PE).

Subjective Data

History taking for ED includes sexual, medical, surgical, emotional, and medication evaluations.
ED, erectile dysfunction.

A. Sexual history:
  1. Did the onset of ED coincide with a specific event?
  2. How long has the client had trouble attaining or maintaining an erection?
  3. Is he able to obtain an erection in order to penetrate? On a scale of 0 to 10, how hard is the erection?
  4. Is the ED getting worse?
  5. Is he about to achieve orgasm and ejaculate?
  6. How long is the client able to have intercourse before ejaculation?
  7. Is there pain or discomfort with ejaculation?
  8. Does the client have nocturnal or morning erections?
  9. How frequently does the client have sexual activity?
    a. Is the activity planned or does it occur spontaneously?
    b. How much foreplay occurs?
    c. Do the client and partner agree on the frequency of intercourse?
    d. Is the client's partner satisfied?
  10. Has the client tried any treatment(s) for ED?
    a. What treatments have been tried?
    b. Inquire about his desire to try any particular therapy. Is he opposed to try any particular therapy?
B. Medical history:
  1. Does the client have HTN? When was HTN diagnosed? What is his usual blood pressure (BP)?
  2. Does the client have diabetes?
    a. Is he insulin dependent?
    b. Does he have any peripheral neuropathy?
  3. Does the client have heart disease? When was his heart disease diagnosed?
  4. Has the client ever had cancer, including any surgery, chemotherapy, and radiation?
  5. Does the client have dyslipidaemia? What were the results of his last laboratory tests?
  6. Does the client smoke? How much, including the number of pack years?
  7. Does the client drink? How much, how often?
  8. Does the client have penile curvature (Peyronie's disease)?
  9. Does the client have any neurologic disorders?
C. Surgical history:
  1. Has the client had any prior surgeries, including pelvic, prostate, or trauma?
  2. Has the client had any invasive cardiac procedures or surgery?
D. Emotional history:
  1. Has the client ever had a traumatic sexual experience?
  2. Has the client had a loss of libido?
  3. Does the client have a history of depression or mood disorders?

4. Is the client experiencing any problems related to work and/or family?
5. Does the client have any intrapartner problems such as separation or divorce?

E. Medication history: Ask the client to list all medications currently being taken, particularly substances not prescribed, including herbal products and illicit drugs. Multiple drug classifications have medications that contribute to ED. Review medications from these drug classes:
  1. Nitrates.
  2. Antihypertensives (particularly alpha blockers).
  3. Anti-ulcer medications.
  4. Lipid-lowering medications.
  5. 5-alpha reductase inhibitors (e.g., finasteride or dutasteride).
  6. Antidepressants.
  7. Herbal products.
  8. Illicit drugs.
  9. Caffeine.

Physical Examination

A. **Vital signs:** Check BP, height, and weight. Calculate body mass index (BMI).
B. Inspect:
  1. Inspect general appearance, noting dyspnea and weakness.
  2. Inspect skin for jaundice, pallor, and diaphoresis.
  3. Inspect legs for oedema, cyanosis, and venous stasis.
  4. Perform a *funduscopic* examination.
  5. Evaluate visual field defects (present in hypogonadal men with pituitary tumours).
  6. Inspect for penile plaques (indicates Peyronie's disease).
  7. Inspect the testicles:
     a. Check for presence of atrophy.
     b. Assess asymmetry.
     c. Evaluate the cremasteric reflex by stroking the inner thighs and observe ipsilateral contraction of the scrotum.
C. Palpate:
  1. Palpate abdomen for masses, tenderness, bounding pulses, and organomegaly.
  2. Palpate peripheral pulses in legs.
  3. Palpate femoral pulses.
  4. Examine breast to detect gynecomastia.
  5. Palpate the testicles for masses.
  6. Perform a rectal examination to evaluate the prostate.
D. Auscultate:
  1. Carotid arteries for bruits.
  2. Abdomen for bruits and bowel sounds.
  3. Heart for murmurs, rubs, clicks, irregularities, or extra sounds.
  4. Femoral bruits (possible pelvic blood occlusion).
  5. All lung fields.
E. Observe ipsilateral contraction of the scrotum.
F. Mental status: Assess for depression.
G. Perform a neurologic examination if neurologic etiology is suspected.

Diagnostic Tests

Hormonal testing and treatment of ED should be individualized based on clinical presentation, including libido, premature ejaculation, fatigue, testicular atrophy, and muscle atrophy that suggests a hormonal abnormality.
A. Serum laboratory tests:
  1. Glucose or haemoglobin A1C.
  2. Lipid profile.
  3. Triglycerides (optional).
  4. Testosterone and other hormone levels, such as prolactin level, if high index of suspicion for prolactinoma, including visual disturbances or headache are optional.
  5. Thyroid-stimulating hormone (TSH), luteinizing hormone, follicle-stimulating hormone, prolactin, complete blood count, and urinalysis for protein and glucose are optional.
B. Duplex ultrasound of the cavernous arteries and other vascular testing as indicated. Penile perfusion ultrasound may be done to evaluate arterial perfusion of the penis. (Rarely used.).
C. Nocturnal penile tumescence (NPT) as indicated. This determines the quality and number of nighttime erections. This test is not routinely used and is typically used in younger, more complicated clients. Has limited availability in Canada, cost is not covered in all provinces.
D. Other tests as indicated for abnormal findings on physical examination.

Differential Diagnoses

A. Testosterone deficiency.
B. Decreased libido.
C. Anorgasmia.
D. Peyronie's disease.

Plan

A. General interventions:
  1. A prolonged erection (priapism) lasting more than four hours is a medical emergency often requiring immediate urologic attention.
  2. Lifestyle modifications to include weight loss, increased physical activity, limited alcohol consumption, and smoking cessation.
  3. Control of comorbidities, including CV disease, diabetes, and HTN, is desired.
B. Client teaching:
  1. Educate client about modifying controllable risk factors such as keeping diabetes and HTN under control, diet, exercise, and smoking cessation.
     a. Failure to respond to phosphodiesterase-5 (PDE-5) inhibitor treatment may result from improper instructions or an inadequate dosage of medication.
  2. The initial administration of an alprostadil intraurethral suppository should be done in the office in order to demonstrate correct administration.
  3. The initial intrapenile administration of alprostadil should be done in the office in order to demonstrate correct administration.
  4. Stepwise therapy for ED includes pharmacologicals and surgery.
C. Pharmacological therapy:
  1. **First-line therapy**: Treatment with PDE-5 inhibitors is the first-line therapy for the treatment of ED. PDE-5 inhibitors are not initiators of erection and require sexual stimulation for an erection to occur. The evidence shows that PDE-5 inhibitors improve erections and successful intercourse, with approximately 80% success rate. The use of PDE-5 inhibitors has been extensively studied; however, they are not without side effects.
     a. Contraindications to PDE-5 inhibitors include high-risk conditions and the concomitant use of nitrites. If the client develops angina while using a PDE-5 inhibitor, other antianginal agents should be used instead of nitroglycerin.

b. High-risk clients/conditions are defined as:
   i. Unstable or refractory angina.
   ii. Refractory angina.
   iii. Uncontrolled HTN.
   iv. Congestive heart failure (CHF; Canadian Cardiovascular Society (CCS) classes III and IV).
   v. Myocardial infarction (MI) or a CV accident within the previous two weeks.
   vi. High-risk arrhythmias.
   vii. Hypertrophic obstructive and other cardiomyopathies.
c. Before proceeding to other ED therapies, clients reporting failure of PDE-5 inhibitors should be evaluated to determine whether the medication trial was adequate; evaluate:
   i. Food/drug interactions.
   ii. Timing and frequency of dosing.
   iii. Lack of adequate sexual stimulation.
   iv. Heavy alcohol use.
   v. Relationship issues.
   vi. Using a licensed PDE-5 inhibitor medication.
d. After evaluation and reeducation and counseling on the medications and partner–partner expectations, titrate to the maximum dosing or prescribe different PDE-5 inhibitor.
e. Discuss other options for ED if the client has a contraindication to, or an unsuccessful trial of, PDE-5 inhibitors.

2. **Testosterone therapy—for those with hypogonadism**.
3. **Second-line therapy:** Pharmacological therapy with intracavernous injection is the second-line therapy for the treatment of ED. Penile injection therapy involves injection of alprostadil, a vasoactive drug, into the corpora cavernosa of the penis to expand the blood vessels and increase the blood flow to produce an erection. The most common side effect of alprostadil is burning and a prolonged erection lasting over four hours. Hypotension is also a potential side effect. Prolonged erections require medical intervention to reverse the erection:
   a. Alprostadil intercavernal injections are titrated according to client erection response, within the health-care clinic setting. Very specific dosing requirements exist, based upon brand name; create a high potential for priapism.
   b. Alprostadil urethral pellet.

D. Surgical alternatives:
1. Penile implant is the third-line therapy for the treatment of ED. Penile prostheses (implants) are surgically implanted items, semirigid rods or a hydraulic device to ensure a rigid erection. The prosthesis does not usually affect urination, sex drive, orgasm, or ejaculation. Pain and/or reduced sensation, infection, or mechanical failure may occur from the prosthesis.
2. Vacuum erection devices are external cylinders used to pump the penis into the cylinder and produce an erection by drawing blood into the penis. An occluding band is then placed at the base of the penis in order to prevent the blood from leaving, with subsequent loss of the erection. **Only vacuum constrictor devices containing a vacuum limiter should be used. The occluding band to maintain the erection should be limited to 30 minutes.**
3. Penile arterial revascularization is indicated for young men (younger than 45 years) with no known risk factors for atherosclerosis. The goal of the surgery is to correct injury by rerouting the blood vessel around a blockage or injured blood vessel. Men with insulin-dependent diabetes or widespread atherosclerosis are not candidates for this surgery.
4. Venous ligation surgery is rarely used. Men with insulin-dependent diabetes or widespread atherosclerosis are also not candidates for venous surgery.

Follow-Up
A. Follow up in one to three weeks after treatments are initiated to monitor client satisfaction and the quality of erections.
B. At the time of prescription renewal, clients prescribed PDE-5 inhibitors should have a review of the effectiveness, side effects, and any significant change in health status, including all medications.

Consultation/Referral
A. Client should be directed to go to the emergency department if an erection lasts for more than four hours.
B. Clients whose CV risk is indeterminant for PDE-5 inhibitors should undergo further evaluation by a cardiologist before receiving therapies for sexual dysfunction.
C. Surgical consultation: Men with penile deformities may require surgical correction.
D. Urologist consultation should be considered for surgical therapies, including implantation of penile prosthesis.
E. Endocrinology consultation for complex endocrine disorders.
F. Psychosexual counseling may be considered for the client and/or couple.
G. Psychotherapy is recommended when ED is related to anxiety and/or depression.

Individual Considerations
A. Adults:
1. A mild prolongation of the QT interval has been observed with vardenafil. The product labeling for vardenafil recommends that caution be used in clients with known history of QT prolongation or in clients who are on current medications that prolong the QT interval.
2. Testosterone therapy is not indicated in the treatment of ED if the client has a normal serum testosterone level.
3. Men who present with sleep disorders should also be questioned about the presence of ED.
4. In clients with diabetes, PDE-5 inhibitors may fail.
5. PDE-5 inhibitors are contraindicated in clients with high CV risk and for clients on nitrates.
6. Men with ED are associated with a higher incidence of CV events.

B. Geriatrics:
1. Dose medications on the lower end for elderly clients:
   a. Sildenafil: Renal and hepatic dosing required.
   b. Vardenafil: Renal and hepatic dosing required.
   c. Tadalafil: Renal and hepatic dosing required.

Resource
Canadian Urological Association Guidelines: https://www.cua.org/en/guidelines

Bibliography
Akre, C., Berchtold, A., Gmel, G., & Suris, J. (2014). The evolution of sexual dysfunction in young men aged 18–25 years. *Journal of Adolescent Health, 55*(6), 736–743. doi:10.1016/j.jadohealth.2014.05.014

Annam, K., Voznesensky, M., & Kreder, K. J. (2016). Understanding and managing erectile dysfunction in patients treated for cancer. *Journal of Oncology Practice, 12*(4), 297–305. doi:10.1200/JOP.2016.010678

Associates in Urology. (n.d.[b]). *Sexual health inventory for men (SHIM)*. Retrieved from http://www.njurology.com/_forms/shim.pdf

Chung, E., Gilbert, B., Perera, M., & Roberts, M. J. (2015). Premature ejaculation: A clinical review for the general physician. *Australian Family Physician*, *44*(10), 737–743.

Cunningham, G. R., & Rosen, R. C. (2013, May 31). Overview of male sexual dysfunction. *UpToDate*. Retrieved from http://www.uptodate.com/contents/overview-of-male-sexual-dysfunction

Dean, R. C. & Lue, T. F. (2005). Physiology of penile erection and pathophysiology of erectile dysfunction. *Urologic Clinics of North America*, *32*(4), 379–395, v. doi:10.1016/j.ucl.2005.08.007

Hilz, M. (2015). Assessment and treatment of male and female sexual dysfunction. *Journal of the Neurological Sciences*, *357*(1), 498–499. doi:10.1016/j.jns.2015.09.295

International Society for Sexual Medicine. (2014). *ISSM client information sheet on premature ejaculation*. Retrieved from http://www.issm.info/images/uploads/ISSM_Client_Information_Sheet_on_PE_-_website.pdf

Kim, E. D. (2013, February 4). History taking in the erectile dysfunction patient. *Medscape*. Retrieved from http://emedicine.medscape.com/article/1980342-overview

Kim, E. D. (2015, October 12). Erectile dysfunction treatment & management. *Medscape*. Retrieved from http://emedicine.medscape.com/article/444220-treatment

McCabe, M. P., & Connaughton, C. (2014). Psychosocial factors associated with male sexual difficulties. *Journal of Sex Research*, *51*(1), 31–42. doi:10.1080/00224499.2013.789820

Paco, J. S., & Pereira, B. J. (2016). New therapeutic perspectives in premature ejaculation. *Urology*, *88*, 87–92.

Rajfer, J., Valeriano, J., & Sinow, R. (2013). Early onset erectile dysfunction is usually not associated with abnormal cavernosal arterial inflow. *International Journal of Impotence Research*, *25*(6), 217–220. doi:10.1038/ijir.2013.17

Urological Association. (2011, June). *The management of erectile dysfunction: An update*. Retrieved from https://www.auanet.org/education/guidelines/erectile-dysfunction.cfm

Urology Care Foundation. (2016a). *ED: Non-surgical management (erectile dysfunction)*. Retrieved from http://www.urologyhealth.org/urology/index.cfm?article=60

Urology Care Foundation. (2016b). *ED: Surgical management (erectile dysfunction)*. Retrieved from http://www.urologyhealth.org/urology/index.cfm?article=28

Walsh, T. J., Hotaling, J. M., Smith, A., Saigal, C., & Wessells, H. (2014). Men with diabetes may require more aggressive treatment for erectile dysfunction. *International Journal of Impotence Research*, *26*(3), 112–115. doi:10.1038/ijir.2013.46

Weinberg, A. E., Eisenberg, M., Patel, C. J., Chertow, G. M., & Leppert, J. T. (2013). Diabetes severity, metabolic syndrome, and the risk of erectile dysfunction. *Journal of Sexual Medicine*, *10*(12), 3102–3109. doi:10.1111/jsm.12318

Haematuria

Cheryl A. Glass, Debbie Gunter, and Kristie A. D. Morydz

Definition

A. Haematuria is blood in the urine. Haematuria is a symptom of an underlying disease/condition; however, routine screening is not recommended. Microscopic haematuria is defined as three or more red blood cells (RBCs) per high-power microscope field (HPF) in urinary sediment from two of three properly collected, clean-catch midstream urine specimens.

B. Asymptomatic microscopic haematuria can range from minor findings that do not require treatment to highly significant, life-threatening lesions. Microscopic haematuria is an incidental finding. The Canadian Urological Association (CUA) recommends an appropriate renal or urologic evaluation with asymptomatic microscopic haematuria for clients who are at risk of urologic disease or primary renal disease.

C. If the excretion rate exceeds one million RBCs, macroscopic or gross haematuria is noted. Gross haematuria (macroscopic haematuria) is suspected when red or brown urine is present. Glomerulonephritis is associated with brown urine, while bleeding from the lower urinary tract is suggested by pink or red urine. Gross haematuria with passage of clots almost always indicates a lower urinary tract source.

Incidence/Prevalence

A. The prevalence of asymptomatic haematuria is from 1% to 20% of the general population. Less than 3% excrete 10 RBC/HPF. Every disease of the genitourinary (GU) tract can produce haematuria.

Pathogenesis

A. Prerenal pathology:
   1. Coagulopathy: Haemophilia or idiopathic thrombocytopaenia purpura (ITP).
   2. Drugs: Anticoagulants, ASA.
   3. Sickle cell disease or trait.
   4. Collagen vascular disease; lupus.
   5. Wilms' tumour.
B. Renal pathology:
   1. Nonglomerular pathology:
      a. Pyelonephritis.
      b. Polycystic kidney disease.
      c. Granulomatous disease; tuberculosis (TB).
      d. Malignant neoplasm.
      e. Congenital and vascular anomalies.
   2. Glomerular pathology:
      a. Glomerulonephritis.
      b. Berger's disease.
      c. Lupus nephritis.
      d. Benign familial haematuria.
      e. Vascular abnormalities; vasculitis.
      f. Alport's syndrome; familial nephritis.
C. Postrenal pathology:
   1. Renal calculi.
   2. Ureteritis.
   3. Cystitis.
   4. Prostatitis.
   5. Benign prostatic hypertrophy (BPH).
   6. Epididymitis.
   7. Urethritis.
   8. Malignant neoplasm.
D. False haematuria:
   1. Vaginal bleeding.
   2. Recent circumcision.
   3. Pigmentation:
      a. Food: Beets, blackberries.
      b. Medications: Quinine sulphate, phenazopyridine, and rifampin.
E. Other causes:
   1. Trauma.
   2. Strenuous exercise (marathons).
   3. Fever.

Predisposing Factors

A. See section "Pathogenesis."
B. Risk factors for malignancy:
   1. Age >35 years.
   2. Smoking (current use or past history).
   3. Chemical exposure (cyclophosphamide, benzenes, or aromatic amines).
   4. History of pelvic irradiation.
   5. Prior urologic disease or treatment.
   6. Chronic urinary tract infections (UTIs).

Common Findings

A. Pink or red urine (clots may be present) or brown, cola-coloured urine on toilet tissue is the common complaint.

Other Signs and Symptoms

A. Pain may or may not be present. Colicky flank pain radiating to the groin suggests a kidney stone. Significant flank pain of renal colic is usually secondary to renal calculi, but may occasionally be associated with passage of clots.
B. Frequency, dysuria, urgency, and suprapubic pain occur with cystitis and inflammatory lesions of the lower urinary tract.
C. Dull flank pain with fever and chills may accompany pyelonephritis.
D. Hesitancy and dribbling of urine suggest BPH.

Subjective Data

A. Elicit the onset, duration, and occurrence (beginning, ending, or during voiding) of haematuria. Describe the colour and amount: Is it "pink on tissue" or bright red in the toilet and tissue?
B. Question the client regarding past medical history of renal disease, systemic disease such as lupus, or sickle cell disease.
C. Review all medications including over-the-counter (OTC) and herbal products. Evaluate specifically for the use of ASA, ibuprofen, warfarin, and laxatives containing phenolphthalein. Rifampin and phenazopyridine HCl can change the colour of urine to orange or red.
D. Review other symptoms, such as dysuria, fever, chills, pain, and hesitancy with voiding.
E. Female clients:
  1. Establish whether the blood was urinary or vaginal (after intercourse or during menstruation).
  2. Is the client postpartum?
  3. Is there a history of endometriosis?
F. Does the client bruise easily? Does the client have bleeding when flossing or brushing teeth?
G. Has the client had a recent bout of pharyngitis with a rash, haematuria, oedema, or hypertension (HTN [glomerulonephritis])?
H. Has he or she had any recent trauma, car accident, or strenuous exercise (i. e., running a marathon)?
I. Does the client know if there was any exposure to TB?
J. Is there any family history of kidney disease, stones, and familial nephritis?
K. Does the client have any current outbreaks of herpes or other sexually transmitted infections (STIs)?
L. Review the client's smoking history.
M. Review occupational exposure to chemicals or dyes (benzenes or aromatic amines).
N. Review intake of foods such as beets and blackberries.
O. Does the male client have any hesitancy and dribbling (signs of prostatic obstruction)?
P. Evaluate if there is rectal bleeding from hemorrhoids from straining with a bowel movement (BM).

Physical Examination

A. Check temperature, blood pressure (BP), and weight in the presence of recent weight gain or oedema.
B. Male and female clients:
  1. Inspect:
    a. Inspect mouth: Check tonsils for enlargement and gums for petechiae.
    b. Examine skin for signs of bleeding or bruises and pallor.
    c. Examine for oedema.
  2. Palpate:
    a. Check the back and abdomen for costovertebral angle (CVA) tenderness.
    b. Check the abdomen for masses, urinary distension, tenderness, and organomegaly.
    c. Palpate groin lymph nodes for enlargement.
  3. Auscultate:
    a. The heart and lungs.
    b. For abdominal bruits.
C. Female clients:
  1. Inspect:
    a. Direct visualization of the external genitalia for inflammation, ulcerations, nodules, lesions, and haemorrhoids.
    b. Ask the client to bear down to check for cystocele and rectocele.
    c. Speculum examination: Observe for atrophic vaginitis, torn tissue, discharge, and friable cervix.
  2. Palpate:
    a. Milk urethra for discharge.
    b. Bimanual examination: Check for cervical motion tenderness (CMT) and adnexal masses.
    c. Rectal examination: Check for the presence of haemorrhoids.
D. Male clients:
  1. Inspect:
    a. Direct visualization of the genitals; check the urethral meatus for discharge.
    b. Retract the foreskin (if present) and assess for hygiene and smegma. Check the shaft of the penis, glans, and prepuce for lesions or urethral meatal erosion.
  2. Palpate:
    a. Palpate the testes and epididymides for inflammation, tenderness, and masses; palpate the scrotum for hydrocele or varicocele.
    b. Check the inguinal and femoral areas for bulges and hernias; have the client bear down and cough, and reexamine him.
    c. Rectal examination:
      i. Check for swollen or tender prostate.
      ii. Check for the presence of haemorrhoids.

Diagnostic Tests

A. Urinalysis:
  1. Centrifuge the urine specimen to see if the red or brown colour is in the urine sediment or supernatant.
  2. If the supernatant is red to brown, test for heme (hemoglobin [Hgb] or myoglobin) with a urine dipstick. Semen is in urine after ejaculation and may cause a positive heme reaction on the dipstick.
  3. A positive dipstick must always be confirmed with a microscopic examination.
  4. Urine culture and sensitivity.
  5. Urine cytology.
  6. Complete blood count (CBC) with differential.
  7. Urea/creatinine.
  8. Prothrombin time (PT), partial thromboplastin time (PTT), platelet count, and bleeding time (if indicated).
  9. Sickle cell testing (if indicated).
  10. CT urography (CTU) is considered the preferred initial imaging in most clients for any unexplained persistent haematuria. CT is considered the best imaging modality for the evaluation of urinary stones, renal and perirenal infections, and associated complications. Intravenous pyelography (IVP) and ultrasound are not as sensitive in the evaluation.
  11. Cystoscopy (the combination of a CTU and cystoscopy) provides a complete evaluation.

12. A CT scan of the abdomen or pelvis should be considered with a history of trauma to determine the source of blood.

B. Based on history, consider the following tests:
1. Strep testing to detect poststreptococcal glomerulonephritis.
2. Antinuclear antibody to detect lupus nephritis.

C. Urologic referral testing includes the following:
1. CTU and cystoscopy.
2. MRI if a mass is suspected.
3. Renal biopsy.

Differential Diagnoses
A. See the section "Pathogenesis" for differential diagnoses.

Plan
A. General interventions:
1. Investigate and diagnose cause(s). Only a limited workup (electrolytes, CBC) is needed in clients younger than 35 years with normal physical examination.
2. Clients older than 35 years need detailed investigation and referral.
3. Microhaematuria in clients on an anticoagulant requires a urologic/nephrology workup regardless of the type or level of anticoagulation.
4. Repeat urinalysis in two weeks.

B. Client teaching:
1. There is no one specific treatment for all cases of haematuria.
2. Treatment is aimed at the specific underlying cause, if a cause can be identified.

C. Pharmacological therapy: None is recommended for haematuria unless an infection is diagnosed.

Follow-Up
A. For clients at risk of malignancy who have a negative workup:
1. Urinalysis, urine cytology, and BP check at 6, 12, 24, and 36 months.
2. If gross haematuria occurs after the initial negative urinalysis, repeat a full evaluation.

B. For clients with HTN, proteinuria and/or an increase in creatinine needs to be reevaluated for renal disease.

C. For persistent asymptomatic microhaematuria—after a negative workup by the urologist, a yearly urinalysis is needed.

D. For persistent or recurrent asymptomatic microhaematuria after the initial negative workup, consider repeating the evaluation within three to five years.

E. Culture urine for acid-fast bacillus if sterile pyuria and haematuria persist.

Consultation/Referral
A. If all benign causes for haematuria have been ruled out, found conditions treated, and it persists, referral to a urologist or a nephrologist should be made.

B. The presence of significant proteinuria (excretion of more than 1000 mg per 24 hours), red cell cast or renal insufficiency, or a predominance of dysmorphic RBCs in the urine should prompt an evaluation for renal parenchymal disease by a nephrologist. Red cell casts are considered virtually pathognomonic for glomerular bleeding.

C. New gross haematuria should be promptly reevaluated.

Individual Considerations
A. Women:
1. Nonpregnant: Rule out menstruation and sexual activity.
2. Pregnant: Rule out vaginal bleeding such as threatened abortion, abruptio placentae, or placenta previa.
3. Ultrasound can be used to evaluate the pregnant woman. CTU should not be used secondary to the radiation exposure.

B. Paediatrics:
1. UTI is the most common cause for haematuria in children. Irritation or ulceration of the perineum or urethral meatus is the next most common cause, followed by trauma.
2. The majority of children who present with gross haematuria have an easily recognizable and apparent cause. The underlying etiology is generally easy to establish by a complete history, physical examination, and urinalysis.
3. Renal ultrasound is the preferred modality for evaluation in children.
4. Cystoscopy is rarely indicated for haematuria in children. It is usually reserved for the child with a bladder mass noted on ultrasound and the child with urethral abnormalities because of trauma.

C. Geriatrics: The risk of malignancy increases among older individuals with a significant history of smoking or analgesic abuse.

Bibliography
American Urological Association. (2012). *Diagnosis, evaluation and follow-up of asymptomatic microhematuria (AMH) in adults: AUA guideline*. Retrieved from https://www.auanet.org/education/guidelines/asymptomatic-microhematuria.cfm

Canadian guidelines for the management of asymptomatic microscopic hematuria in adults https://www.cua.org/themes/web/assets/files/guidelines/en/amh_2008_e.pdf

Feldman, A. (2015, March 18). Etiology and evaluation of hematuria in adults. *UpToDate*. Retrieved from http://www.uptodate.com/contents/etiology-and-evaluation-of-hematuria-in-adults

Gulati, S. (2016, February 7). Hematuria. *Medscape*. Retrieved from http://emedicine.medscape.com/article/981898-overview

Sharp, V. J., Barnes, K. T., & Erickson, B. A. (2013). Assessment of asymptomatic microscopic hematuria in adults. *American Family Physician*, 88(11), 747–754.

Hydrocele

Cheryl A. Glass, Debbie Gunter, and Kristie A. D. Morydz

Definition
A. Hydrocele is the collection of fluid between layers of the processus vaginalis producing swelling in the scrotum or inguinal area. Cystic masses containing fluid or sperm often develop spontaneously. Inguinal hernia and hydrocele share a similar etiology and pathophysiology and may coexist.

Incidence/Prevalence
A. Incidence/prevalence is unknown; hydrocele occurs in 6% of the male pediatric population at birth or in the neonatal period. It occurs infrequently in adulthood.

B. A parasitic infection, filariasis, caused by *Wuchereria bancrofti*, is the cause in more than 120 million people worldwide.

Pathogenesis
A. Congenital: Patent processus vaginalis (PPV).
B. Reactive: Inflammatory condition in the scrotum (e.g., trauma, torsion, infection).
C. Idiopathic: Arises over a long period (most common).
D. Hydroceles are believed to arise from an imbalance of secretion and reabsorption of fluid from the tunica vaginalis.

Predisposing Factors
A. Males; most commonly seen in childhood.
B. *W. bancrofti* parasite.
C. Viral illness.
D. Chronic increased intra-abdominal pressure.
E. Increased abdominal fluid production.

Common Findings
A. Swollen scrotum is the common indication.

Other Signs and Symptoms
A. Painless swollen scrotum; pain increases with the size of the mass.
B. Rarely does a hydrocele become infected and cause pain.

Subjective Data
A. Elicit the onset, duration, and course of swelling: Is scrotal sac full all day, or does the client have a flat scrotum in the morning and a gradual increase in fluid during the day?
B. Was the hydrocele noted in the neonatal period?
C. How old is the client? Has this ever occurred before? If so, what happened, and how was it treated?
D. Review the client's history for injury to the scrotum.
E. Is there any pain or other symptoms related to hernia with the swelling?
F. Review other symptoms such as discharge, dysuria, fever, or backaches.
G. Review birth control method (vasectomy).

Physical Examination
A. Check temperature (if indicated) and blood pressure (BP).
B. Inspect: Careful examination is necessary to rule out masses and tumour:
  1. Examine in the supine and standing positions.
  2. Genital examination: Note amount of swelling, symmetry, lesions, discharge, hernias, varices, and colour of scrotum.
  3. Transilluminate the scrotum to determine if the lesion is cystic, solid, or a varicocele. In a dark room, transillumination light appears as a red glow with serous fluid. If normal, blood and tissue do not transilluminate; however, the bowel may transilluminate.
C. Auscultate:
  1. Scrotum for bowel sounds to rule out hernia.
D. Palpate:
  1. Check warmth, tenderness, swelling, and any nodularity; if mass is present, check if it has a solid versus cystic feel.
  2. Palpate lymph nodes: Supraclavicular, chest, abdomen, and groin.
  3. Check for inguinal hernia.
  4. Palpate the abdomen for masses, rebound, and tenderness.

Diagnostic Tests
A. Laboratory evaluation is not required for the evaluation of hydroceles.
B. Scrotal ultrasonography.

Differential Diagnoses
A. Hydrocele: Nontender, smooth, firm; palpation should reveal confinement to the scrotum unless hydrocele has been present for a long time. A hydrocele will transilluminate.
B. Varicocele: Feels like a "bag of worms."
C. Hernia: Herniated bowel makes gurgling sounds upon auscultation of the scrotum.
D. Testicular tumours tend to occur in young men and are the most common tumours in males from ages 15 to 30 years. Consider a tumour if the onset is acute. Tumours feel firm, nontender, and fixed, and do not transilluminate. Inguinal lymphadenopathy may also be seen. The client may complain of heaviness with a tumour.
E. Testicular torsion.
F. Orchitis: Rare except with mumps. Orchitis is usually unilateral and is associated with fever, swelling, pain, and tenderness. On occasion, parotitis is absent.
G. Epididymitis: Inflammation is often concurrent with a urinary tract infection (UTI). Epididymis is very tender; scrotal elevation may relieve the pain.
H. Spermatocele: Cystic swelling of the epididymis. It is not as large as a hydrocele, but it also transilluminates.

Plan
A. General interventions:
  1. Monitor children every three months until resolution or until a decision is made to refer to a specialist for evaluation.
  2. Factors that indicate surgical repair:
    a. Failure to resolve by 2 years of age.
    b. Continued discomfort.
    c. Enlargement or waxing and waning in volume.
    d. Unsightly appearance.
    e. Secondary infection.
B. Client teaching:
  1. Most hydroceles are painless.
  2. In adults, if there are no symptoms, it can be left alone and monitored.
C. Pharmacological therapy: None is recommended.

Follow-Up
A. Monitor every three months.

Consultation/Referral
A. Refer to a urologist for evaluation, as needed.
B. A persistent hydrocele or the association of discomfort may indicate the need for a surgical referral.

Individual Considerations
A. Pediatrics: An infant testicle usually measures 1 cm. The parent may notice a hydrocele that fluctuates slightly in size and usually resolves on its own by 6 months of age.
B. Adults: If an adult experiences a hydrocele, he should be instructed to return for evaluation if the hydrocele becomes larger or uncomfortable, or if it interferes with sexual intercourse.

Bibliography
Lee, S. L. (2015, December 8). Hydrocele. *Medscape*. Retrieved from http://emedicine.medscape.com/article/438724-overview

Interstitial Cystitis (IC)

Cheryl A. Glass, Debbie Gunter, and Kristie A. D. Morydz

Definition
A. Interstitial cystitis (IC) is a chronic condition that results in recurring discomfort or suprapubic pain, pressure in the bladder and surrounding pelvic region, related to bladder filling. IC is also commonly known as painful bladder syndrome (PBS). IC/PBS includes all cases of urinary pain with persistent urge to void or urinary frequency that cannot be attributed to other causes (i.e., infection, stones, or other pathology).
B. The persistent urge to void helps to distinguish the symptoms of IC/PBS from those of overactive bladder (OAB). IC/PBS affects the quality of life related to social activities, lost work productivity, sleep deprivation because of urinary frequency, fatigue, and even depression.
C. The Canadian Urology Association states that the symptoms should last more than six weeks in order for therapy to begin.
D. IC/PBS clients void to avoid or relieve pain, whereas clients with OAB void to avoid incontinence.

Incidence/Prevalence
A. Actual prevalence is unknown because of the variability of diagnostic criteria. It is not uncommon for clients to experience a lag time of five to seven years before diagnosis. The majority of the affected persons are women (10:1 rated over males). The symptom complex is the same for males. IC also occurs in children.

Pathogenesis
A. The pathophysiology of IC/PBS remains unclear. It is not established whether IC/PBS is a localized condition just involving the bladder or whether it is a systemic disease that affects the bladder.

Predisposing Factors
A. In both genders with a higher prevalence in females.
B. Mean age of diagnosis is 42 to 45 years.
C. Urinary tract infection (UTI).
D. Prostatitis.
E. Chronic yeast infections.
F. Posthysterectomy or other pelvic surgery.
G. Medications:
  1. Calcium channel blockers.
  2. Cardiac glycosides.
H. Other hypersensitivity conditions that coexist with IC:
  1. Fibromyalgia.
  2. Irritable bowel syndrome (IBS).
  3. Chronic headaches.
  4. Vulvodynia.
  5. Sjögren's syndrome.

Common Findings
A. Mild discomfort to intense pain with bladder filling and/or emptying is the hallmark symptom. The pain is not limited to the bladder/suprapubic area but includes symptoms throughout the pelvic area, lower abdomen, and back.
B. Persistent urge to void/frequency.
C. Frequency.
D. Urgency.
E. Nocturia.

Other Signs and Symptoms
A. Combination of urgency and frequency.
B. Pressure.
C. Increase in symptoms during menstruation.
D. Pain during vaginal intercourse.
E. Low back pain with bladder filling.

Subjective Data
A. Review the onset, frequency, duration, and severity of symptoms.
B. Evaluate if the pain of bladder filling is partially or completely relieved by voiding.
C. Does the client void frequently in order to maintain a low bladder volume and avoid discomfort versus voiding frequently to avoid urge incontinence (OAB)?
D. Are there any OAB triggers (e.g., citrus, beer, coffee) that exacerbate symptoms?
E. Are symptoms increased after stress, exercise, intercourse, being seated for a long period, or during the menstrual cycle?
F. How much do the symptoms affect the client's quality of life (e.g., sleep disturbance, loss of work, avoiding activities)?
G. Does the client have any other chronic pain syndromes such as IBS, chronic fatigue, dyspareunia, or fibromyalgia?
H. Review the client's surgical history and history of genitourinary (GU) cancers.
I. Any GU trauma or falls onto the coccyx?
J. Review the client's history of UTIs, urinary retention, and urinary tract stones.
K. Review all medications including over-the-counter (OTC) and herbal products.
L. Administer a pain/symptom evaluation tool at each visit.
  1. The Pelvic Pain and Urgency/Frequency (PUF) Patient Symptom Scale is available at defeatic.com/wp-content/themes/bones/library/patient/assets/files/PUF-questionnaire.pdf.
  2. The Interstitial Cystitis Symptom Index (ICSI) is available at www.essic.eu/pdf/ICSIandICPI.pdf

Physical Examination
A. Temperature (if indicated to rule out infection; fever is not associated with IC) and blood pressure (BP).
B. Inspect:
  1. Note the general appearance for signs of depression and discomfort before and during examination.
  2. Inspect the male external genitalia for redness, oedema, lesions, and discharge.
  3. Inspect female genitalia for discharge, lesions, fissures; inspect cervix for cervicitis.
C. Auscultate:
  1. Heart and lungs.
  2. Bowel sounds in all four quadrants.
D. Palpate:
  1. Palpate back; note costovertebral angle (CVA) tenderness.
  2. Palpate the abdomen for suprapubic tenderness, rebound masses, or pain.
  3. Perform bimanual examination to rule out other infections and pelvic inflammatory disease (PID; tenderness of the cervix, uterus, and adnexa should be absent). During the pelvic examination, evaluate locations of tenderness and trigger points.
  4. Males: Complete palpation of external genitalia, prostate, and rectal examination.
E. Percuss:
  1. Bladder.
  2. Back for CVA tenderness.

F. Neurologic:
  1. Perform a limited neurologic examination to rule out an occult problem.

Diagnostic Tests
A. Urinalysis with microscopy to exclude haematuria.
B. Urine culture and sensitivity may be ordered even with a negative urinalysis to evaluate low levels of bacteria.
C. Postvoid residual (PVR) volume by straight catheter or ultrasound.
D. Urodynamic testing is not currently considered to have a role in the diagnosis of IC/PBS.
E. Ultrasound is optional for select clients.
F. Cystoscopy is optional.
G. Hydrodistension is not required for diagnosis or treatment, considered optional in select clients.
H. Bladder biopsy is not required for diagnosis; however, it is used for exclusion of other disorders.
I. The potassium sensitivity test is not recommended for routine use as results are nonspecific for IC/PBS.

Differential Diagnoses
A. UTI.
B. IBS.
C. Females:
  1. Endometriosis.
  2. Vulvodynia.
D. Males:
  1. Chronic prostatitis.
  2. Benign prostatic hypertrophy (BPH).

Plan
A. General interventions:
  1. Behaviour modifications are recommended. Restrict fluids to 64 ounces per day, divided into 16 ounces per meal, and 8 ounces between meals.
  2. Progressively timed voiding on a two- to three-hour schedule. If the client is unable to hold urine for this interval, progressively increase urine storage time between void by 15 minutes per week until the goal of a two- to three-hour interval is reached.
  3. Kegel exercises should be avoided with IC.
  4. Psychosocial support is an integral part of chronic pain disorders.
B. Client teaching.
  1. Several foods have been identified as bladder irritants, including foods rich in potassium. Clients may try to eliminate foods/drinks and reintroduce them one at a time to identify any items that make their symptoms worse. Examples:
    a. Alcohol.
    b. Tomatoes.
    c. Spices/spicy foods.
    d. Chocolate.
    e. Caffeinated beverages.
    f. Coffee.
    g. Artificial sweeteners.
    h. Citrus: Lemons, limes, and oranges (including citrus-flavored beverages).
    i. Cranberries/cranberry juice.
C. Physical Therapies:
    a. Pelvic floor physiotherapy.
    b. Physiotherapy and massage.
    c. Acupuncture.
    d. Trigger point injections.
D. Pharmacological therapies:
  1. Pentosan polysulfate sodium.
  2. Amitriptyline is used in the treatment of other pain syndromes, including IC.
  3. Cimetidine—used after conservative measures have failed.
  Canadian pharmacological guidelines are available at www.canada.ca/en/public-health/services/infectious-diseases/sexual-health-sexually-transmitted-infections/canadian-guidelines/sexually-transmitted-infections/canadian-guidelines-sexually-transmitted-infections-20.html
  4. Bladder instillation:
    a. Intravesical dimethyl sulfoxide (DMSO) is the only drug approved by the Food and Drug Administration (FDA) for bladder instillation.
    b. Heparin instillation.
    c. Lidocaine instillation.
    d. "Bladder cocktail" combination of sodium bicarbonate, heparin, lidocaine, and/or triamcinolone. There are various formulas/combinations.
  5. Medications may be instituted for treating any comorbid depression.
  6. Medications for treating any comorbid infections (e.g., UTIs, sexually transmitted infections [STIs]), inflammatory bowel disease, or endometriosis.
  7. Other medications that have been used for symptomatic relief:
    a. Hydroxyzine hydrochloride.
    b. Gabapentin requires careful dose titration because of sedation.
    c. Nonsteroidal anti-inflammatory drugs (NSAIDs).
  8. Cyclosporine A has been used when other treatments have not provided relief or control of symptoms for clients with inflammation.
E. Intradetrusor botulinum toxin A (BTX-A)—this therapy may require posttreatment intermittent self-catheterization.
F. Laser or electrocautery if Hunner's ulcers are present.
G. Surgical options are available if all other therapies have failed.
H. Therapies that are not recommended/should not be offered include the following:
  1. Long-term antibiotics.
  2. High-pressure, long-duration hydrodistention.
  3. Systemic steroids.
  4. Intravesical resiniferatoxin (ultrapotent capsaicin analog).
  5. Intravesical Bacillus Calmette–Guérin (BCG).
  6. Potassium sensitivity test—not recommended for routine use. It is nonspecific and is a painful test.

Follow-Up
A. Allodynia, the perception of nonnoxious stimuli, such as touch being noxious or painful, may be present; therefore, an adequate pelvic examination may not be possible. Consider empiric treatment and have the client return for a pelvic examination to finish evaluation.
B. Have the client keep a one-day bladder diary before visits to evaluate a pattern of low urine volume frequency characteristic of IC/PBS.
C. As with all medications, start at the lowest dose and titrate/increase doses if there is an improvement in symptoms.

Consultation/Referral
A. Refer to a urologist for more thorough workup and testing.
B. Refer to a pain management specialist if indicated.

Individual Considerations
A. Pediatrics:
  1. The evaluation for interstitial cystitis is essentially the same in children as it is for the adult.
  2. Treatment options are similar to those discussed, including dietary modifications and self-help strategies.

Resources
CUA guideline: Diagnosis and treatment of interstitial cystitis/ bladder pain syndrome Canadian Urological Association: www.cua.org
International Painful Bladder Foundation: www.painful-bladder.org
Interstitial Cystitis Association (ICA): www.ichelp.org
Interstitial Cystitis Network: www.ic-network.com
Pelvic Pain and Urgency/Frequency Patient Symptom Scale: defeatic.com/wp-content/themes/bones/library/patient/assets/files/PUF-questionnaire.pdf

Bibliography
American Urological Association. (2014b, September). *Diagnosis and treatment of interstitial cystitis/bladder pain syndrome*. Retrieved from https://www.auanet.org/education/guidelines/ic-bladder-pain-syndrome.cfm
Clemens, J. Q. (2015, July 24). Pathogenesis, clinical features, and diagnosis of interstitial cystitis/bladder pain syndrome. *UpToDate*. Retrieved from www.uptodate.com/contents/pathogenesis-clinical-features-and-diagnosis-of-interstitial-cystitis-bladder-pain-syndrome
Cox, A., Golda, N., Nadeau, G., Nickel Curtis, J., Carr, L., Corcos, J., & Teichman, J. (2016). CUA guideline: Diagnosis and treatment of interstitial cystitis/bladder pain syndrome. *Canadian Urological Association Journal*, *10*(5-6), E136–E155. doi:10.5489/cuaj.3786. Retrieved from https://www.cua.org/themes/web/assets/files/3786v3.pdf
Patolia, S. (2015, January 9). Cystitis empiric therapy. *Medscape*. Retrieved from http://emedicine.medscape.com/article/1976451-overview#a1
Rovner, E. S. (2015, December 9). Interstitial cystitis. *Medscape*. Retrieved from http://emedicine.medscape.com/article/2055505-overview

Premature Ejaculation (PE)
Cheryl A. Glass, Debbie Gunter, and Kristie A. D. Morydz

Definition
A. Premature ejaculation (PE) is defined as the inability to control or delay ejaculation, which causes personal distress for the male. Two subtypes exist, based on intravaginal ejaculation latency time (IELT):
  1. Lifelong PE is an IELT of less than one minute. Onset is typically from the first sexual encounter. Males have no ability to control the ejaculation.
  2. Acquired PE is an IELT of less than three minutes. Onset is at any point in sexual history. The ability to delay ejaculation is decreased or absent.
  Two subtypes exist based on personal experience; neither is a true sexual dysfunction.
  3. Variable PE is irregular and not the result of psychogenic cause. Onset is at any point in sexual history. The ability to delay ejaculation is decreased or absent.
  4. Subjective PE is self-reported rapid ejaculation despite normal ejaculation time. Onset is at any point in sexual history. The ability to delay ejaculation is decreased or absent.

Incidence/Prevalence
A. PE is reported in approximately 21% to 31% of males. It is the most common type of sexual dysfunction. Erectile dysfunction (ED) commonly coexists.
B. Approximately 31% of men report problems with sexual function.

Pathogenesis
A. The exact cause is unknown.
B. Organic: Chronic prostatitis, hyperthyroidism, genetic disorders.
C. Psychogenic: Relationship problems, psychological preoccupation with performance:
  1. Iatrogenic: Nerve damage from surgery or trauma.

Predisposing Factors
A. Depression.
B. Consumption of alcohol.
C. Obesity.
D. High blood pressure (BP).
E. High cholesterol.
F. Diabetes.
G. Obesity.
H. Smoking.
I. Depression and anxiety medication use.

Common Findings
A. Men.
  1. Inability to achieve or sustain erection.
  2. Absent or delayed ejaculation.
  3. Inability to control the timing of ejaculation.
B. Both sexes.
  1. Lack of interest or desire (most common).
  2. Inability to become aroused.
  3. Pain with intercourse.

Other Signs and Symptoms
A. Diminished self-esteem.
B. Depression.
C. Anxiety.
D. ED.
E. Reduced libido.
F. Relationship difficulties.

Subjective Data
A. Include full medical history, sexual history, and psychological, social, and drug history using open-ended questions.
B. Ask:
  1. Partner(s)' sexual history.
  2. Perceived ejaculatory control.
  3. Estimated IELT.
  4. Previous interventions used to correct the issue.
  5. Impact on personal life and relationships.
  6. If the issue has been lifelong or acquired.
  7. If a loss of erection occurs before ejaculation, to distinguish ED from PE.
C. Screening tools:
  1. PE Diagnostic Tool available at www.sexhealthmatters.org/resources/premature-ejaculation-diagnostic-tool.

Physical Examination
A. Vital signs: Check BP, pulse, and respiration.
B. Inspect:
  1. Thyroid for nodules.
  2. Abdomen for surgical scars.
  3. Neurologic examination for deficiencies.
  4. Lower extremities for hair distribution pattern, lesions, or trauma.

5. Genitalia for abnormalities.
6. Any additional examination should be based on history and previous examination findings.
C. Palpate:
1. Thyroid for nodules.
2. Abdomen for masses or tenderness.
3. Lower extremities for pain and pulses.
4. Neurologic examination of lower extremities.
5. Genitalia for lesions, masses, or pain.

Diagnostic Tests
A. Should be based on individual history and physical findings.

Differential Diagnoses
A. ED.
B. Testosterone deficiency.

Plan
A. General interventions:
1. The treatment plan should include the client and the sexual partner.
2. The client and partner should be educated about the possible interventions outlined as follows:
   a. Both should be educated in treatment options.
   b. Client and partner satisfaction is the desired outcome.
B. Client teaching:
1. Consider the impact of the severity of the issue on the client, any treatable causes, and client wishes.
2. Effectiveness of psychotherapy may diminish over time.
3. Behavioural therapy: "Stop-and-start" method of ceasing genital stimulation until arousal sensation diminishes, or the "squeeze" method of squeezing the glans prepuce at heightened arousal.
C. Psychotherapy: Recommended for lifelong, acquired, or variable, and is the first-line treatment for subjective PE.
D. Pharmacological therapy: Off-label medications include selective serotonin reuptake inhibitors (SSRIs) and eutectic mixture of local anesthetics (EMLA):
1. Paroxetine.
2. Fluoxetine or other SSRIs can be considered such as citalopram, escitalopram, and sertraline.
3. Lidocaine.

Follow-Up
A. The client should be seen in two to four weeks if medication was started to assess for efficacy. SSRIs typically achieve maximum effect after one to two weeks.

Consultation/Referral
A. May refer to urologist or sexual health specialist/counselor.
B. Psychotherapy: Recommended for lifelong, acquired, or variable, and is the first-line treatment for subjective PE. Referral to a practitioner who specializes in sexual therapy is recommended.

Individual Considerations
A. Adults:
1. Off-label SSRIs should be used with caution for the increased risk of serotonin syndrome.
2. Off-label EMLA cream used without a condom may result in vaginal wall numbness in the sexual partner.
3. Prolonged application of lidocaine may result in loss of erection if used for 30 to 45 minutes.
B. Geriatrics:
1. Renal and hepatic dosing of paroxetine is required.
2. Hepatic dosing of fluoxetine and sertraline is required.
3. Taper to discontinue any SSRIs is required.

Bibliography
American Urological Association. (n.d.). *Guideline on the pharmacologic management of premature ejaculation*. Retrieved from https://www.auanet.org/education/guidelines/premature-ejaculation.cfm

Chung, E., Gilbert, B., Perera, M., & Roberts, M. J. (2015). Premature ejaculation: A clinical review for the general physician. *Australian Family Physician*, 44(10), 737–743.

International Society for Sexual Medicine. (2015, January). *ISSM patient information sheet on premature ejaculation*. Retrieved from http://www.issm.info/images/uploads/ISSM_Patient_Information_Sheet_on_PE_-_website_JAN_2015.pdf

Ogunyemi, O. (2015, December 11). Testicular torsion. *Medscape*. Retrieved from http://emedicine.medscape.com/article/2036003-overview

Paco, J. S., & Pereira, B. J. (2016). New therapeutic perspectives in premature ejaculation. *Urology*, 88, 87–92. doi:10.1016/j.urology.2015.11.003

Prostatitis

Cheryl A. Glass, Debbie Gunter, and Kristie A. D. Morydz

Definition
Prostatitis is acute or chronic infection of the prostate gland. Prostatitis is the most important cause of urinary infection in men. There are four types of prostatitis:
A. Acute bacterial prostatitis (least common).
B. Chronic bacterial prostatitis.
C. Chronic prostatitis/chronic pelvic pain syndrome (common in men of any age):
1. Inflammatory (presence of white blood cells in the semen, expressed prostatic secretions [EPSs], or voided bladder urine postprostatic massage).
2. Noninflammatory (absence of white cells).
D. Asymptomatic inflammatory prostatitis.

Incidence/Prevalence
A. Prostatitis symptoms occur in approximately 9% of Canadian men each year.
B. Acute and chronic bacterial prostatitis occurs in about 1 in 10 men.
C. Nonbacterial prostatitis occurs in about 6 in 10 men.
D. Prostatodynia occurs in about 3 in 10 men.

Pathogenesis
A. Nonbacterial prostatitis is an inflammatory condition with an unknown etiology. Infection results in prostatitis in four ways:
1. Ascending infection of urethra.
2. Reflux of infected urine into the prostate through ejaculatory and prostatic ducts that empty into the prostatic urethra.
3. Haematogenous spread, causing bacterial prostatitis.
4. Invasion by rectal bacteria by direct extension or lymph system spread.
B. Causative organisms: *Escherichia coli, Klebsiella, Pseudomonas, Enterococcus, Ureaplasma, Gardnerella vaginalis, Trichomonas vaginalis, Chlamydia trachomatis, Chlamydia, Mycoplasma,* or *Neisseria gonorrhoeae*; cytomegalovirus

(CMV); *Mycobacterium tuberculosis*; and fungi have been associated with prostatitis in HIV-infected clients.
C. Incubation period depends on pathogen.

Predisposing Factors
A. More common in younger and middle-aged men.
B. Sexual transmission of bacteria.
C. Neuromuscular dysfunction.
D. Structural voiding dysfunction.
E. Benign prostatic hypertrophy (BPH).
F. History of allergies and asthma (increase in nonbacterial prostatitis).

Common Findings
A. Dysuria.
B. Perineal, rectal, or suprapubic pain (chronic pain syndrome).
C. Less urine flow.
D. Spiking fever.
E. Back pain.
F. Sexual dysfunction.

Other Signs and Symptoms
A. Acute bacterial prostatitis:
   1. Fever and chills, malaise.
   2. Acute onset of dysuria.
   3. Hesitancy.
   4. Urinary frequency and low back pain.
   5. Pain with intercourse and with defecation.
   6. Initial or terminal haematuria and oedema with acute urinary retention.
   7. Arthralgia or myalgia.
   8. Nocturia.
B. Chronic bacterial prostatitis:
   1. Usually presents with recurrent urinary tract infection (UTI).
   2. May be asymptomatic between acute episodes; some men have large fluctuation in symptom severity.
   3. Perineal, inguinal, or suprapubic pain, or irritative symptoms on voiding such as frequency and urgency.
   4. Haematuria, haematospermia, or painful ejaculations.
   5. Prostatic calculi.
C. Nonbacterial prostatitis (most common):
   1. Vague discomfort or increasing pain: Prostatic, lower back, perineum, groin, scrotum, or suprapubic pain; ejaculatory pain.
   2. Dysuria, urinary frequency, urgency, hesitancy, and decreased urine flow.
   3. Penile discharge, especially noted during the first bowel movement (BM) of the day.
   4. Sexual difficulty.
   5. Low sperm count.
   6. Blood or urine in ejaculate.
D. Asymptomatic inflammatory prostatitis is found when looking for causes of infertility and testing for prostate cancer.
E. Prostatodynia (cause is unknown):
   1. Prostate irritation.
   2. Pain and discomfort in the prostate, testicles, penis, and urethra.
   3. Difficulty urinating.

Subjective Data
A. Ask the client to complete the National Institutes of Health Chronic Prostatitis Symptom Index (NIH-CPSI) self-evaluation form. The assessment tool evaluates pain, urinary symptoms, and the impact on quality of life. An online NIH symptom index that self-scores is available at www.prostatitis.org/symptomindex.html:
   1. Mild = 0 to 14 total score.
   2. Moderate = 15 to 29 total score.
   3. Severe = 30 to 43 total score.
B. Review the onset, duration, and course of symptoms.
C. Are there any other symptoms such as discharge, pain, haematuria, hesitancy, back pain, or weight loss?
D. Has the client ever had the same symptoms? If so, how were they treated?
E. Does any sexual partner(s) have any symptoms, lesions, or known sexually transmitted infections (STIs)?
F. Does the client engage in anal intercourse?
G. Has the client noted any impaired urinary flow?
H. Has the client required any recent urethral catheterization or instrumentation?

Physical Examination
A. Check temperature and blood pressure (BP).
B. Inspect:
   1. Examine the client generally for discomfort before and during examination.
   2. Check the urethral meatus for discharge.
   3. Retract foreskin (if present) and assess for hygiene and smegma.
   4. Check the shaft of the penis, glans, and prepuce for lesions.
C. Palpate:
   1. Palpate testes and epididymides for inflammation, tenderness, and masses; palpate scrotum for hydrocele or varicocele.
   2. Check back for costovertebral angle (CVA) tenderness.
   3. Evaluate for an enlarged tender bladder because of urinary retention.
   4. Palpate the abdomen for masses, urinary distension, suprapubic tenderness, and organomegaly.
   5. Palpate inguinal lymph nodes; check the inguinal and femoral areas for bulges and hernias; have the client bear down and cough, and reexamine him.
   6. Rectal examination:
      a. Before the rectal examination, have the client obtain a clean-catch urine specimen for culture. Check for symmetry, swelling, tenderness, and enlarged prostate.
      b. In acute prostatitis, rectal examination reveals the prostate gland to be exquisitely tender and boggy.
      c. A fluctuant prostatic mass suggests an abscess that may require surgical intervention.
      d. Perform prostate massage for postmassage urine sample (see Section II: Procedure: Prostatic Massage Technique: 2-Glass Test).

Diagnostic Tests
A. Acute infection.
   1. Complete blood count (CBC) with differential.
   2. Urinalysis and urine culture.
   3. Culture for STIs.
   4. Gram stain, culture of EPS:
      a. Avoid vigorous massage when obtaining specimen because of the risk of inducing bacteraemia.
      b. Gram stain of EPS demonstrates infectious organisms or white blood cells (WBCs) typical of an immune response (>10 WBC/high-power

microscope field [HPF] is abnormal). Clients with abnormal WBC but no bacterial growth may have chlamydial or *Ureaplasma* infection and need to be tested or treated empirically.
B. Chronic infection:
 1. Urea.
 2. CBC with differential.
 3. Creatinine.
C. Chronic bacterial prostatitis:
 1. If recurrent infections are confirmed, evaluate for structural or functional abnormality with CT scan.
 2. Measure residual urine after voiding.
 3. If no urologic abnormalities are found and repeated cultures indicate the same bacterial strain, chronic bacterial prostatitis is likely.
D. Other tests, such as ultrasound, MRI, and biopsies, are used as required to rule out other pathology.

Differential Diagnoses
A. Prostatitis:
 1. Acute: Readily evident by clinical presentation and examination.
 2. Chronic: More difficult to diagnose. The hallmark symptom is recurrent UTI. It often resembles prostatic hypertrophy, strictures, and prostatic carcinoma.
 3. Chronic pelvic pain syndrome.
B. Pyelonephritis.
C. Epididymitis.
D. Anal fistulas and fissures.
E. BPH causes urinary retention due to obstruction.
F. Urethral stricture or stone.
G. Chronic pain syndromes/back pain.

Plan
A. General interventions:
 1. Clients with acute prostatitis may need hospitalization and intravenous (IV) therapy for severe infection (high fever, increased WBC, and dehydration). Less toxic clients may be treated on an outpatient basis.
 2. Older men without evidence of infection with lower tract symptoms should have urine cytology to rule out malignancy.
▶ B. Client teaching: *Refer to Client Teaching Guide: Prostatitis.*
 1. Client teaching.
 2. Having the client self-massage to reduce symptoms is questionable; the massage of an acutely infected gland is contraindicated because of the risk of bacteraemia.
 3. Recommend sitz baths two to three times daily.
C. Dietary management. Increase fluid intake:
 1. Decrease caffeine and alcohol, which can irritate the urethra.
D. Pharmacological therapy:
 1. Analgesics (nonsteroidal anti-inflammatory drugs [NSAIDs]) and stool softeners may be needed.
 2. Discontinue or reduce the dosage (if possible) of the client's anticholinergics, sedatives, and antidepressants because they may impair bladder function.
 3. Inpatient: Broad-spectrum penicillin, third-generation cephalosporins with or without aminoglycosides, or fluoroquinolones.

 4. Acute outpatient therapy: The usual course of treatment is 14 to 28 days of therapy. Chronic bacterial prostatitis and chronic pain may require four to six weeks of antibiotic therapy, including fluoroquinolones, trimethoprim, tetracyclines, or macrolides.
 5. Low-dose suppressive therapy with an agent that has been shown to be effective may be considered.
 6. There are no formal guidelines for the management of chronic bacterial prostatitis or chronic pelvic pain syndrome. Strategies are currently focused on symptomatic relief.
 7. Alpha blockers may be used to control symptoms by reducing bladder outlet obstruction (BOO).

Follow-Up
A. See the client in 2 to 10 days depending on the client's symptoms and course.
B. Culture urine at completion of drug therapy. Test of cure for antibiotics requires elimination of bacteria from prostatic fluid to prevent chronic flares. Some clients may not achieve cure even after 6 to 12 weeks of therapy.
C. Clients who achieve a partial response may be given a second course of antibiotics. Those failing to demonstrate an organism may benefit from a course of doxycycline or erythromycin for *Chlamydia* and/or *Ureaplasma* coverage.
D. Notify public health for reportable STIs.

Consultation/Referral
A. Obtain a referral to a urologist for recurrent acute bacterial prostatic infections or infections that persist.
B. Cystoscopy may be required to rule out interstitial cystitis (IC).
C. Urinary retention concomitant with acute prostatitis may require hospitalization.

Individual Considerations
A. Adults:
 1. Prostatitis is the most common prostate infection in men younger than 50 years.

Resources
Canadian Urological Association (AUA): http://www.cua.org/themes/web/assets/files/guidelines/en/1121__1_pdf
The Prostatitis Foundation: www.prostatitis.org

Bibliography
American Urological Association. (2013, April). *Early detection of prostate cancer: AUA guideline*. Retrieved from https://www.auanet.org/education/guidelines/prostate-cancer-detection.cfm
Associates in Urology. (n.d.[c]). *Quality of life questionnaire*. Retrieved from http://www.njurology.com/_forms/qualityoflife.php
Deem, S. (2015, December 9). Acute bacterial prostatitis. *Medscape*. Retrieved from http://emedicine.medscape.com/article/2002872-overview
Nickel, J. C. (2011). Prostatitis. *Canadian Urological Association Journal*, 5(5), 306–315.
Rendon, R., Mason, R., Marzouk, K., Finelli, A., Saad, F., So, A., & Violette, P. (2017). Canadian Urological Association recommendations on prostate cancer screening and early diagnosis. *Canadian Urological Association Journal*, 11(10), 298–309. doi:10.5489/cuaj.4888
Turek, P. J. (2016, February 11). Prostatitis. *Medscape*. Retrieved from http://emedicine.medscape.com/article/785418-overview

▶ Client Teaching Guides are available at https://connect.springerpub.com/content/reference-book/978-0-8261-9498-5

Proteinuria

Cheryl A. Glass, Debbie Gunter, and Kristie A. D. Morydz

Definition

Proteinuria is excess protein (albumin) in urine. Proteinuria may be an incidental finding and have no symptoms. Use of a urine dipstick for screening is acceptable for first detecting proteinuria (see Table 12.1); however, the dipstick should not be used to quantify the amount of urinary protein. Protein concentration is a function of urine volume as well as the quantity of protein present.

The measurement of protein excretion is used to establish the diagnosis and to follow the course of glomerular disease. The normal rate of albumin excretion is <20 mg/d; the rate is about 4 to 7 mg/d in healthy young adults and increases with age and an increase in body weight. Persistent albumin excretion between 30 and 300 mg/d is called microalbuminuria. Values of 300 mg/d of protein are considered overt proteinuria or macroalbuminuria.

When proteinuria coexists with haematuria, the likelihood of clinically significant renal disease is high. In clients with diabetes, microalbuminuria usually indicates incipient diabetic nephropathy. In nondiabetics, the presence of microalbuminuria is associated with cardiovascular (CV) disease. Protein is also the cardinal sign of pregnancy-induced hypertension (PIH).

Functional/transient proteinuria is associated with fever, exercise, dehydration, cold exposure, and stress, and is not associated with underlying renal disease. Orthostatic proteinuria, a transient proteinuria condition, is related to postural changes that affect the glomerular hemodynamics. Orthostatic proteinuria rarely exceeds 1 g/d. Significant renal disease is not usually found upon further testing and workup.

Persistent proteinuria is defined as >4 mg/m^2/hr of protein in a 24-hour urine collection or >0.02 mg/mg of protein-to-creatinine ratio (PCR) on a spot urine. Persistent proteinuria requires further evaluation to rule out underlying renal pathology.

There are three types of mechanisms of persistent proteinuria:

A. Glomerular proteinuria (albuminuria): Caused by increased filtration of macromolecules across the glomerular capillary wall. The standard urine dipstick is able to detect glomerular proteinuria. Some causes of glomerular proteinuria include diabetes; hypertension (HTN); nephrotic syndrome; infections including hepatitis, HIV, cytomegalovirus (CMV), malaria, syphilis, and streptococcal infections; chemotherapeutic agents; Alport syndrome,;and hemolytic uremic syndrome.

B. Tubular proteinuria: Related to interference with proximal tubular reabsorption. A urinary dipstick is unable to detect tubular proteinuria. Some causes of tubular proteinuria include toxins, pyelonephritis, nonsteroidal anti-inflammatory drugs (NSAIDs), antibiotics, and inherited causes such as Lowe syndrome and Wilson disease.

C. Secretory (overflow) proteinuria: Increased excretion from the tubules secondary to an overproduction of a particular protein, most commonly noted in interstitial nephritis. A urinary dipstick is unable to detect overflow protein.

It is currently recommended that a diagnosis of kidney damage can only be made if at least two measurements are elevated.

Incidence/Prevalence

A. Approximately 6% of males and 7% of females have proteinuria detected by a single routine dipstick test.
B. The incidence of proteinuria found on a urine dipstick in school-age children is approximately 10%. When repeat testing is done, the incidence decreases to 0.1% of school-age children.
C. The prevalence of orthostatic proteinuria is 2% to 5%and is noted more commonly in older children and adolescents.
D. The prevalence of proteinuria is higher in the elderly and in clients with comorbidities.

Pathogenesis

A. Pathogenesis depends on the underlying etiology. An alteration in glomerular filtration that increases excretion (filtration) of plasma proteins occurs. Increased glomerular permeability, increased production of abnormal proteins (Bence Jones protein), decreased tubular reabsorption, surgical traumas, and infections may increase urinary protein. Urinary protein may also be affected by dietary protein intake.

Predisposing Factors

A. Fever.
B. Increased exercise.
C. Urinary tract infection (UTI)/pyelonephritis.
D. Medications:
  1. Penicillamine.
  2. NSAIDs.
  3. Angiotensin-converting enzyme (ACE) inhibitors.
  4. Aminoglycosides.
  5. Cisplatin.
  6. Bevacizumab.
  7. Amphotericin B.
  8. Quinolones.
  9. Sulfonamides.
  10. Cimetidine.
  11. Allopurinol.
  12. Antiretroviral drugs can be nephrotoxic.
E. Heavy metal exposure:
  1. Gold.
  2. Cadmium.
  3. Mercury.
  4. Lead.
  5. Copper.
F. Collagen vascular disease or vasculitis.

TABLE 12.1 Dipstick Analysis—Detecting and Quantifying Proteinuria

Dipstick Grade	Quantity of Protein (mg/dL)
Negative	<10
Trace	10–20
1+	30
2+	100
3+	300
4+	1,000

Source: Cox, A., Golda, N., Nadeau, G., Curtis Nickel, J., Carr, L., Corcos, J., & Teichman, J. (2016). CUA guideline: Diagnosis and treatment of interstitial cystitis/bladder pain syndrome. *Canadian Urological Association Journal, 10*(5–6), E136–E155. doi:10.5489/cuaj.3786. Retrieved from https://www.cua.org/themes/web/assets/files/3786v3.pdf

G. Family history of proteinuria or pyelonephritis.
H. HTN.
I. Renal disease.
J. Congestive heart failure (CHF) or endocarditis.
K. Diabetes.
L. Lupus.
M. Infections:
   1. HIV.
   2. Syphilis.
   3. Hepatitis B and C.
   4. Group A beta-hemolytic *Streptococcus*.
   5. Viral infection (e.g., mononucleosis).
   6. Malaria.
N. Malignancy:
   1. Lymphoma.
   2. Hodgkin's disease.
   3. Breast tumour.
   4. Lung tumour.
   5. Colon tumour.
O. Heroin use.
P. PIH.
Q. Radiocontrast media.

Common Findings
A. Asymptomatic.
B. Increased weight.
C. Decreased urine output.
D. Pediatrics:
   1. Growth failure.
   2. Deafness or visual impairment suggests hereditary nephritis.

Other Signs and Symptoms
A. Oedema: Periorbital, presacral, genital, or ankle.
B. Nephrotic syndrome: Hypercholesterolaemia and hypertriglyceridaemia.
C. Protein malnutrition: Anorexia and vomiting.
D. "Frothy" urine.

Subjective Data
A. Review the onset, course, and duration of presenting complaints.
B. Question the client concerning urinary output, thirst or fluid intake, oedema, and increase in weight. Establish usual weight history.
C. If a woman, establish the first day of the client's last period. Is she pregnant? If so, what is the fetus's gestational age? Is there oedema, HTN, headache, visual changes (scotoma), hyperreflexia, and/or right upper quadrant pain?
D. Review the client's past medical history for renal disease, diabetes, CHF, systemic disorders such as lupus, and substance abuse.
E. Does the client have signs or symptoms of a UTI or pyelonephritis?
F. Review the client's recent history for exertion, emotional stress, surgical trauma, fever, and any acute illness.
G. When was the client's last evaluation for cholesterol? Is he or she on any special diet?
H. Review medication list, including prescribed and over-the-counter (OTC) medications and herbal products.
I. Review the client's occupational exposure, smoking history, and risk factors for infectious diseases.

Physical Examination
The client's physical examination may have few abnormalities unless there are features of multisystem disease.

A. Check temperature (if indicated), blood pressure (BP), pulse, respiration, and weight.
B. Inspect:
   1. Inspect overall general appearance for oedema (pedal, hand, facial, or periorbital oedema), butterfly rash (lupus), or ascites.
   2. Evaluate for protein wasting.
   3. Evaluate for jugular vein distension.
   4. *Funduscopic* examination: Evaluate for retinopathy.
   5. Inspect for pharyngitis.
C. Auscultate:
   1. The heart and lungs.
D. Palpate:
   1. Examine the abdomen; evaluate bladder distension, suprapubic tenderness, masses or ascites, and abdominal tenderness.
   2. Palpate for costovertebral angle (CVA) tenderness.
   3. Check deep tendon reflexes, especially in pregnant women.

Diagnostic Tests
A. Urine dipstick is a good screening tool in the outpatient setting.
B. Single-void "spot" urine testing:
   1. The first urine specimen of the morning is optimal and is guideline recommended. Evaluation of the first morning specimen excludes any postural effect on the protein component.
   2. The gold standard for measurement of protein excretion is a 24-hour urine collection, but is now being replaced by the easier-to-obtain and less-complicated spot test. The 24-hour urine is considered impractical for generalized testing, especially in the pediatric population.
C. PCR test or albumin-to-creatinine ratio (ACR) test on a first-morning or a random spot specimen. The PCR or ACR is useful in following trends in the client's proteinuria.
D. Complete blood count (CBC) and serum electrolytes.
E. Serum creatinine (if renal disease is suspected).
F. Lipid profile.
G. Urea: Serves as an index of renal excretory capacity. Urea is the nitrogenous end product of protein metabolism.
H. Urinalysis, urine culture, and sensitivity (if indicated).
I. Ultrasound of the full urinary tract.
J. Screen for diabetes and other testing related to physical findings.
K. Renal biopsy is required to establish the diagnosis in most cases.

Differential Diagnoses
A. See the section "Predisposing Factors."

Plan
A. General interventions:
   1. Current guidelines for screening for evaluation of albuminuria/proteinuria vary by country, but recommendations include at-risk individuals with diabetes, HTN, obesity, smokers, indigenous populations, family history of chronic kidney disease (CKD), age >50 years, structural renal tract disease, renal calculi, prostatic hypertrophy, vascular disease, and autoimmune disease.
   2. Management for nephrotic syndrome includes diet with sodium and protein restriction, loop and distal-acting diuretics, control of cholesterol (low-saturated-fat, low-cholesterol diet), lipid-lowering agents, pneumococcal and influenza vaccines to prevent infections, and use of steroids and immunosuppressive agents as necessary.

3. Clients with haematuria and proteinuria need a 24-hour urine collection for protein and creatinine clearance.
B. Client teaching:
   1. Encourage low-fat/low-cholesterol diet if hyperlipidaemia is present.
   2. Encourage sodium- and protein-restricted diet for nephrotic syndrome.
C. Pharmacological therapy: There is no specific drug therapy for excess protein. Use drug therapy appropriate to the underlying medical disease-causing proteinuria. In clients with CKD, the administration of ACE inhibitors and/or angiotensin II receptor blockers (ARBs) is aimed at reducing the degree of proteinuria.

Follow-Up
A. If proteinuria is found on a dipstick and the first-morning test results are trace or negative for protein, repeat a first-morning test in one year.
B. There is no consensus on how often to screen for proteinuria. Guidelines include annual screening, every five years for clients older than 50 years or smokers, and every three years for clients who have HTN, obesity, indigenous, or a family history of kidney disease. Monitoring should always include BP, quantitative testing by PCR or ACR, and a serum creatinine.
C. Client should be assessed at routine examination appointments for vasculitic skin changes, rashes, retinopathy, lymphadenopathy, signs of heart failure, abdominal masses, organomegaly, guaiac stools, prostatic enlargement, and joint inflammation.

Consultation/Referral
A. Consider client referral if kidney damage is progressing from medical disease (systemic lupus erythematosus, HTN, diabetes).
B. Refer the client as necessary; HTN is a poor prognostic sign for significant renal impairment.
C. Consultation for diagnostic tests to be considered: kidney, ureter, and bladder (KUB), intravenous pyelography (IVP), renal ultrasonography, renal biopsy.
D. Referral to a nephrologist should be considered if a definitive diagnosis is required or a renal biopsy is considered.

Individual Considerations
A. Pregnancy:
   1. Protein excretion is considered abnormal in pregnancy when it exceeds 300 mg/24 hr or >0.3 g of protein per gram of creatinine in a random urine specimen. A urine specimen with 1+ protein is considered the cutoff for proteinuria.
   2. The gestational age at which proteinuria is first documented is important in establishing the likelihood of PIH versus other renal diseases. Proteinuria before or early in pregnancy suggests preexisting renal disease.
   3. Monitor urine protein and BP at each prenatal visit and refer the client if urinary protein remains elevated.
   4. Monitor for intrauterine growth restriction (IUGR).
   5. Proteinuria (or HTN) that persists longer than three months after delivery should be followed closely.
B. Pediatrics:
   1. The Canadian Paediatrics Society does not recommend routine screening for children.
   2. Although there are no set guidelines for children, a child with persistent proteinuria should be initially worked up with a physical examination, BP, urinalysis, serum creatinine, and urea every 6 to 12 months.
   3. When the child is stable, the follow-up should be done annually.
   4. There are no dietary or physical activity limitations.
C. Geriatrics: Renal function deteriorates in the elderly who may also have coexisting medical conditions (HTN, diabetes) that may cause nephropathy.

Bibliography
American College of Obstetricians and Gynecologists. (2013). *Hypertension in pregnancy*. Retrieved from http://www.acog.org/Resources-And-Publications/Task-Force-and-Work-Group-Reports/Hypertension-in-Pregnancy

Amin, S. V., Illipilla, S., Hebbar, S., Rai, L., Kumar, P., & Pai, M. V. (2014). Quantifying proteinuria in hypertensive disorders of pregnancy. *International Journal of Hypertension, 2014*, 941408. doi:10.1155/2014/941408

Gagnadoux, M. (2016, May). 31). Evaluation of proteinuria in children. *UpToDate*. Retrieved from www.uptodate.com/contents/evaluation-of-proteinuria-in-children

Lane, J. (2016, May 16). Pediatric nephrotic syndrome. *Medscape*. Retrieved from http://emedicine.medscape.com/article/982920-overview

Lerma, E. V. (2015, December 10). Proteinuria. *Medscape*. Retrieved from http://emedicine.medscape.com/article/238158-overview

Rovin, B. (2014, September 14). Assessment of urinary protein excretion and evaluation of isolated non-nephrotic proteinuria in adults. *UpToDate*. Retrieved from www.uptodate.com/contents/assessment-of-urinary-protein-excretion-and-evaluation-of-isolated-non-nephrotic-proteinuria-in-adults

Thadhani, R. (2015, November 30). Proteinuria in pregnancy: Evaluation and management. *UpToDate*. Retrieved from www.uptodate.com/contents/proteinuria-in-pregnancy-evaluation-and-management

The Clinical Advisor. *Kidney guide features albuminuria testing*. Retrieved from www.clinicaladvisor.com/kidney-guide-features-albuminuria-testing/article/279307

Pyelonephritis

Cheryl A. Glass, Debbie Gunter, and Kristie A. D. Morydz

Definition
A. Pyelonephritis is an acute infection and inflammatory disease of the upper urinary tract (renal pelvis, tubules, and interstitial tissue) of one or both kidneys. Acute pyelonephritis is an ascending urinary tract infection (UTI) that has progressed from the lower urinary tract.
B. Fever has been strongly correlated with the diagnosis of acute pyelonephritis; therefore, clients with clinical symptoms of pyelonephritis in the absence of fever should be evaluated for alternative diagnoses.
C. Acute pyelonephritis characteristically causes some scarring to the kidney and may lead to significant damage, kidney failure, abscess formation, and sepsis. Antibiotic therapy is essential to prevent the progression of pyelonephritis.

Incidence/Prevalence
A. Thirty percent of the female population have at least one UTI in their lifetime.
B. Annual rates of pyelonephritis in women are 15 to 17 cases per 10,000 and 3 to 4 cases per 10,000 for men.
C. The incidence of pyelonephritis in pregnancy is 2%. Most cases develop as a consequence of undiagnosed or inadequately treated lower UTI.
D. Upper UTIs are less common and more serious than lower UTIs. After puberty, the prevalence of UTIs increases slightly in females, but remains low in males.
E. After age 65 years, UTIs are more common with an equal incidence in both sexes.

Pathogenesis

A. Pyelonephritis is caused by ascending infection from the bladder, usually caused by *Escherichia coli* (75%–90%) and other gram-negative bacteria including *Proteus mirabilis* (5%), *Klebsiella pneumoniae* (5%), *Enterobacter* (3%), and Group B *Streptococcus* (GBS: 1%). Gram-positive causative agents are less common; 10% to 15% of cases are caused by *Staphylococcus saprophyticus*.
B. Bacteria can also reach the kidneys through the bloodstream from intravenous (IV) drug abuse and endocarditis.
C. In women, the short urethra in close proximity to the perirectal area makes colonization possible. In pregnancy, the increased glycosuria, increase in urinary amino acids, urinary stasis, and the presence of vesicoureteral reflux facilitate bacterial growth.
D. In children, vesicoureteric reflux is the most common pathology.
E. In men, benign prostatic hypertrophy (BPH) causing bladder obstruction is a common pathology.
F. Indwelling catheters increase ascending infections and pyelonephritis.

Predisposing Factors

A. Previous UTI, cystitis, and pyelonephritis.
B. Sickle cell disease.
C. Diabetes.
D. Urinary catheterization.
E. Obstruction: Calculi, tumours, and urethral strictures.
F. Neurogenic bladder disease: Strokes, multiple sclerosis, and spinal cord injuries.
G. Urinary reflux.
H. HIV.
I. Trauma.
J. Chronic constipation (children).
K. Incomplete bladder emptying related to medications (e.g., anticholinergics).
L. Gender:
  1. Females:
     a. Increased sexual activity, failure to void after intercourse, diaphragms, and spermicides.
     b. Pregnancy.
     c. Atrophic vaginal mucosa predisposes to the colonization of pathogens and UTIs.
  2. Males:
     a. Homosexuality.
     b. Sexual partner with colonization.
     c. Obstruction: Prostatic hypertrophy.
     d. Age 50 years or older.
     e. Acute or chronic bacterial prostatitis.

Common Findings

A. Shaking, chills, and fever.
B. Flank pain or tenderness.
C. Urinary frequency or urgency.
D. Costovertebral angle (CVA) tenderness.
E. Guarding.
F. Urinary frequency, nocturia, haematuria, and dysuria (not always present in upper tract infections).
G. Blood in urine secondary to haemorrhagic cystitis (unusual in males with pyelonephritis).

Other Signs and Symptoms

A. Adults (particularly the elderly): May be asymptomatic with cystitis.
B. Abdominal pain and suprapubic heaviness.
C. Pregnancy: Uterine contractions.
D. Shortness of breath (SOB).
E. Anorexia.
F. Children:
  1. Fever may be a child's only presenting symptom.
  2. Nausea and vomiting.
  3. Irritability.
  4. Diarrhea.
  5. Abdominal pain/tenderness.
  6. Feeding difficulty.
  7. Failure to thrive.
G. Elderly:
  1. Mental status change.
  2. Generalized deterioration.

Subjective Data

A. Review the onset, course, and duration of symptoms.
B. Are there any problems with voiding such as frequency, urgency, and dysuria?
C. Review the client's history of fever and any treatment.
D. Are there any other symptoms, odour, and nausea?
E. Have the client point to the area of the backache. Is it unilateral or bilateral? What makes the backache better?
F. In women, rule out pregnancy; review first day of last menses.
G. Rule out sickle cell disease, diabetes, and multiple sclerosis.
H. Review the client's previous history of genitourinary (GU) tract problems, stones, UTIs, previous pyelonephritis, any previous testing, and any previous anomalies.
I. Review the strength and character of the urinary stream, especially in older men. Ask if the client has ever been diagnosed with BPH.
J. Review the client's history for active herpes lesion. Does urine flow hurt when urine stream begins? Or is the pain noted when urine passes over the lesion?
K. Review drug allergies.
L. Review all medications, including over-the-counter (OTC) and herbal products. Review medications for a recent history of an incomplete course of antibiotics and current use of anticholinergics.

Physical Examination

A. Check temperature, pulse, and blood pressure (BP); note orthostatic hypotension. Tachycardia may or may not be present, depending on associated fever, dehydration, and sepsis.
B. Inspect:
  1. Note general appearance for respiratory distress and dehydration.
  2. Inspect the male external genitalia for redness, oedema, lesions, and discharge.
  3. Inspect the female genitalia for discharge, lesions, and fissures; inspect cervix for cervicitis.
C. Palpate:
  1. Palpate the back; check CVA tenderness (usually unilateral over the involved kidney).
  2. Palpate the abdomen for suprapubic tenderness, rebound masses, or pain.
  3. Perform a pelvic examination to rule out other infections and pelvic inflammatory disease (PID; tenderness of the cervix, uterus, and adnexa should be absent).
D. Auscultate:
  1. The lungs and heart.

E. Pregnancy:
  1. Check fetal heart rate; fetal tachycardia may be present with fever.
  2. Palpate for uterine tenderness and contractions.
  3. Pelvic examination for cervical dilation, if indicated for increased risk of preterm labour.
F. Males: Complete palpation of external genitalia, prostate, and rectal examination.

Diagnostic Tests

A. Urine culture and sensitivity should always be performed before initial empiric treatment with antibiotics.
B. Urinalysis for evaluation of pyuria. Pyuria is present in almost all women with acute cystitis and pyelonephritis; its absence strongly suggests an alternative diagnosis:
  1. Leukocyte esterase on dipstick detects pyuria or white blood cells (WBCs).
  2. Significant pyuria is greater than two to five leukocytes per high-power microscope field (HPF).
  3. Urine may need to be obtained from straight in-and-out catheterization if the client is incontinent or has dementia.
C. Complete blood count (CBC) with differential or WBC, especially with systemic symptoms.
D. Blood culture, if indicated.
E. Arterial blood gases (ABGs), if indicated.
F. Consider sedimentation rate, especially with severe illness and in the elderly.
G. Culture for gonorrhea and chlamydia, if symptoms are associated with sexually transmitted infections (STIs).
H. Wet prep, if symptoms are associated with STI.
I. Imaging studies are not routinely required for the diagnosis of acute pyelonephritis but can be helpful:
  1. CT scan to identify altered parenchymal perfusion, hemorrhage, nonrenal disease, inflammatory masses, and obstruction. CT with contrast medium is considered the imaging modality of choice for nonpregnant women.
  2. MRI to rule out masses or obstruction.
  3. Renal ultrasonography.
  4. Scintigraphy to detect focal renal abnormalities.
  5. Voiding cystourethrogram.
  6. Intravenous pyelography (IVP), if indicated.

Differential Diagnoses

A. Appendicitis/acute abdomen.
B. Cholecystitis.
C. Pancreatitis.
D. Diverticulitis.
E. Pneumonia.
F. Prostatitis.
G. Epididymitis.
H. PID.
I. Nephrolithiasis.

Plan

A. General interventions:
  1. Optimal therapy for acute uncomplicated pyelonephritis depends on the severity of the illness at presentation.
  2. Many severe infections (increased WBC, dehydration or vomiting, high fever) may need hospital admission for IV therapy. Risk factors include older adult, coexisting illness, pregnancy, and uncontrolled vomiting.
B. Client teaching:
  1. Give instruction on early recognition of UTIs.
  2. Client teaching.
C. Dietary management:
  1. Increase fluids; have the client drink at least one large glass of water every hour while awake.
  2. Encourage the client to drink cranberry juice to help fight and prevent UTIs. If the taste is objectionable, he or she may mix cranberry juice 1:1 with another juice such as grape juice.
  3. There are no dietary restrictions with pyelonephritis.
D. Pharmacological therapy:
  1. Acetaminophen for fever.
  2. Urinary analgesic as needed to relieve dysuria. Dysuria is usually diminished fairly quickly after the start of antibiotics.
  3. Antiemetics as needed; however, if the client is not able to tolerate oral fluids, he or she should be hospitalized.
  4. Antibiotics: Empiric antibiotic selection should be guided by local antibiotic resistance patterns, allergies, and culture results. Clients with delayed response to therapy should also receive a longer course of antibiotics of 14 to 21 days:
     a. Adults:
        i. First-line therapy:
        ii. Ciprofloxacin
        iii. Trimethoprim/sulfamethoxazole (TMP/SMX). Because of the high rate of resistance of *E. coli*, the empirical use of TMP/SMX should be avoided in clients who require hospitalization.
        iv. Levofloxacin
     b. Children younger than 2 years are usually treated for 7 to 14 days. Children older than 2 years who are afebrile and without abnormalities of the urinary tract or have previous episodes of UTIs are usually treated for five days:
        i. Amoxicillin-clavulanate.
        ii. Sulfonamide–TMP/SMX.
        iii. Cephalosporin-cefuroxime.
     c. Antibiotics that should not be used for pyelonephritis:
        i. Nitrofurantoin and fosfomycin should not be used to treat pyelonephritis in adults or children; it is excreted in the urine but does not achieve therapeutic serum levels.
        ii. Fluoroquinolones are not used in children because of potential concerns about sustained injury to developing joints.
        iii. Tetracyclines should not be used in children because of tooth staining.
        iv. Fluoroquinolones are not used in pregnancy because of the risk of auditory and vestibular toxicity in the fetus.
        v. Aminoglycosides are contraindicated in pregnancy because of the risk of permanent ototoxicity to the fetus.

Follow-Up

A. Follow up with the client in 24 to 48 hours depending on the evaluation of the initial severity of symptoms:
  1. Clients with persistent fever or clinical symptoms after 48 to 72 hours of appropriate antibiotic therapy should undergo initiation of another class of antibiotics and consider radiologic evaluation.

2. If the client feels that he or she is not progressing well or is getting worse, evaluate the client emergently and consider hospital admission and IV antibiotics.

B. Follow-up urine cultures are not needed for clients with acute cystitis or pyelonephritis if symptoms resolved on antibiotics; however, repeat cultures for clients with recurrent symptoms or any complicated course of illness.

C. Women with recurrence of pyelonephritis need further urologic investigation.

Consultation/Referral

A. Consider hospitalization for infants with both lower and upper infections, children with pyelonephritis, and children with recurrent infections.

B. Consult or refer the client to a specialist if he or she requires IVP, cystoscopy, or renal biopsy.

C. IV therapy and hospitalization are needed in all cases suggestive of bacteraemia in children who are vomiting, children younger than 2 years, and children with documented parenchymal damage.

D. Males with persistent bladder infections need a urologic consultation.

E. Pyelonephritis in men suggests structural problems and requires hospitalization and further evaluation (IVP).

F. Consult an infectious disease specialist for clients with unusual or resistant pathogens.

G. For pregnancy, consultation with an obstetrician is required.

Individual Considerations

A. Pregnancy:
 1. Pyelonephritis is the most common urinary tract complication in pregnancy.
 2. Untreated asymptomatic bacteriuria (ASB) is a risk factor for acute cystitis and pyelonephritis in pregnancy.
 3. Based on the higher risk of complications in pregnancy, pyelonephritis has traditionally been treated with hospitalization and IV antibiotics until the woman is afebrile for 48 hours and symptoms improve.
 4. Once the pregnant client is discharged from the hospital, oral antibiotics should continue for 10 to 14 days of treatment.
 5. A urine culture should be obtained one to two weeks after completion of therapy and monthly thereafter to monitor for recurrent infection.
 6. Aminoglycosides should be avoided because of the potential risk of ototoxicity following prolonged fetal exposure.
 7. Fluoroquinolones are contraindicated during pregnancy because of the risk of auditory and vestibular toxicity in the fetus.

B. Pediatrics:
 1. Always order a urine culture and sensitivity on children suspected of UTI.
 2. Suprapubic aspiration of the bladder should be considered in young infants.
 3. A voiding cystogram should be considered in all children younger than 16 years with a documented UTI.
 4. Indications for hospitalization:
  a. Age less than 2 months.
  b. Clinical urosepsis or potential bacteraemia.
  c. Immunocompromised client.
  d. Vomiting or inability to tolerate oral medication.
  e. Lack of adequate outpatient follow-up (e.g., no phone, lives far from hospital).
  f. Failure to respond to outpatient therapy.
 5. Vesicoureteric reflux is responsible for up to 50% of pyelonephritis in children younger than 6 years.
 6. Assess the child for chronic constipation as a potential cause for urinary obstruction.

C. Males:
 1. Consider ordering renal function tests (urea and creatinine).
 2. Men older than 50 years: Consider urologic consultation and IVP.

D. Geriatrics:
 1. Clients may need hospitalization for IV antibiotics and hydration.
 2. Bladder or kidney infections may be common in clients with long-term urinary catheters and can lead to septicaemia if untreated or unrecognized.
 3. Fluoroquinolone use in the elderly has the potential to cause neuropsychiatric symptoms, including seizures to worsening dementia.

Bibliography

Fulop, T. (2015, August 11). Acute pyelonephritis. *Medscape*. Retrieved from http://emedicine.medscape.com/article/245559-overview

Hooton, T. M. (2016a, January 5). Acute uncomplicated cystitis and pyelonephritis in men. *UpToDate*. Retrieved from http://www.uptodate.com/contents/acute-uncomplicated-cystitis-and-pyelonephritis-in-men

Hooton, T. M. (2016b, February 9). Acute complicated cystitis and pyelonephritis. *UpToDate*. Retrieved from http://www.uptodate.com/contents/acute-complicated-cystitis-and-pyelonephritis

Hooton, T. M., & Gupta, K. (2016, May 26). Acute uncomplicated cystitis and pyelonephritis in women. *UpToDate*. Retrieved from www.uptodate.com/contents/acute-uncomplicated-cystitis-and-pyelonephritis-in-women?topicKey=ID%2F8063

Renal Calculi or Kidney Stones (Nephrolithiasis)

Cheryl A. Glass, Debbie Gunter, and Kristie A. D. Morydz

Definition

A. Renal calculi, or kidney stones, are caused by the formation of crystals in the urinary system from the kidneys to the bladder. *Nephrolithiasis* refers to renal stone disease; *urolithiasis* refers to the presence of stones in the urinary system. The majority of stones (80%) consist of calcium, usually as calcium oxalate, but they can contain uric acid, struvite (magnesium, ammonium, and phosphate), oxalic acid, phosphate salts, or the amino acid cysteine. Spontaneous passage of a stone is related to the stone size and location. Approximately one half of symptomatic clients require intervention for stone removal. An untreated staghorn (branch-shaped) with persistent renal obstruction can destroy renal tissue with potential for life-threatening sepsis.

Incidence/Prevalence

A. Renal calculi are very common, with a higher incidence noted in males. The overall incidence is rising. At least 12% of men and 7% of women have one symptomatic stone by age 70 years. Initial cases typically occur between ages 30 and 40 years, and the prevalence increases with age. Idiopathic nephrolithiasis is common in males, whereas primary hyperparathyroidism is more common in females.

B. Most kidney stones pass spontaneously; however, 10% to 30% do not pass and can cause continuing pain, infection, or obstruction.

C. Nephrolithiasis is uncommon in children.

D. Stones because of infection (struvite) are more common in women.
E. The incidence of stones in pregnancy is 1 in every 1500 to 3000 pregnancies.
F. The recurrence rate for calculi is 50% within five years.

Pathogenesis
A. The formation of uric acid stones requires continued and excessive oversaturation of urine with stone-forming constituents, uric acid, calcium, and oxalate. Dehydration, hyperuricosuria, and significantly acidic urine contribute to uric acid supersaturation and stone formation. Struvite stones form only when the urinary tract is infected with urea-splitting organisms such as *Proteus* species.
B. Hydroureteronephrosis is the most significant renal alteration in pregnancy. Dilatation is greater on the right side than the left because of pressure because of physiological engorgement of the right ovarian vein and dextrorotation of the uterus.

Predisposing Factors
A. Male.
B. Dehydration (poor intake and immobility).
C. Chronic obstruction with stasis of urine.
D. Hypercalcaemia caused by hyperparathyroidism; renal tubular acidosis; multiple myeloma; or excessive intake of vitamin D, milk, and alkali.
E. Diet high in purines and abnormal purine metabolism (gout).
F. Pregnancy.
G. Chronic infections.
H. Foreign bodies.
I. Excessive oxalate absorption in inflammatory bowel disease, bowel resection, or ileostomy.
J. Previous stone formation.
K. Family history of nephrolithiasis.
L. Medications:
  1. Vitamins A, C, and D.
  2. Loop diuretics.
  3. Acetazolamide.
  4. Ammonium chloride.
  5. Calcium-containing medications, including alkali and antacids.
  6. Indinavir.
  7. Sulfadiazine.
  8. Atazanavir.
  9. Guaifenesin.
  10. Sulfa drugs.
  11. Topiramate.
  12. Acyclovir.
M. Obesity.
N. Gastric bypass/bariatric surgical procedures.
O. Diabetes.

Common Findings
A. Severe flank and groin pain.
B. Blood in urine.
C. Asymptomatic (dependent on the size of the stone).

Other Signs and Symptoms
A. Unilateral flank pain that radiates to the groin.
B. Sudden onset of colicky pain.
C. Haematuria.

The timing and appearance of haematuria are important. Haematuria seen at the beginning of the urine stream may indicate bleeding in the urethra. Terminal haematuria, or blood in the end of the urine stream, denotes bladder neck or the prostate as the source. Finally, blood throughout the entire urine stream suggests a lesion.

D. Nausea and vomiting.
E. Restlessness.
F. Symptoms common with cystitis or inflammatory lesions of the lower tract are usually absent: frequency, dysuria, urgency, and suprapubic pain.

Subjective Data
A. Review the onset, duration, and course of symptoms.
B. Review other signs and symptoms of urinary tract infection (UTI) or pyelonephritis: frequency, dysuria, and fever.
C. Have the client describe pain (colicky); note intensity (use a 1- to 10-point scale, 10 being the worst pain) and the characteristics of pain (constant or intermittent).
D. Has the client ever had a stone before? How was it treated? What tests were performed? Has the client ever seen a urologist?
E. Review dietary intake of high animal protein in the diet, milk, and other calcium-containing products for excessive intake.
F. Review the client's medication history including excessive vitamin C or D supplements, antacids that contain calcium, and other medications noted in the predisposing factors.
G. Ask the client to describe any haematuria or blood clots passed.
H. Ask about recent trauma to the back or abdomen.
I. Is there a family history of stone formation?
J. Is the client pregnant?

Physical Examination
A. Check temperature, blood pressure (BP), and pulse (may have tachycardia). Children: Growth measurements to evaluate poor weight gain and/or failure to thrive (congenital and chronic conditions).
B. Inspect:
  1. Inspect general appearance for discomfort before and during examination. Clients with renal colic are extremely restless and exhibit active movement on presentation.
  2. During the examination, evaluate voluntary guarding of the abdominal musculature.
  3. Inspect external genitalia (male or female) for lesions, discharge, inflammation, and ulcerations.
  4. Assess for peripheral oedema.
C. Auscultate:
  1. The abdomen, noting bruits if present.
  2. Bowel sounds.
D. Palpate:
  1. "Milk" the urethra for discharge.
  2. Palpate the abdomen for masses and tenderness, organomegaly, and suprapubic tenderness.
  3. Palpate the groin; check lymph nodes.
  4. Palpate the back and abdomen.
  5. Check for the presence of costovertebral angle (CVA) tenderness.
E. Perform pelvic or bimanual examination, if indicated, to rule out pelvic inflammatory disease (PID).

Diagnostic Tests
The diagnosis of nephrolithiasis can be made on the basis of clinical symptoms alone, but diagnostic testing is needed to confirm.
A. Laboratory tests:
 1. Urea.
 2. Creatinine.
 3. Calcium.
 4. Uric acid.
 5. Serum electrolytes; consider fasting serum calcium and phosphorus and parathyroid hormone.
 6. Pregnancy test (if indicated) to rule out an ectopic pregnancy.
B. Stone for analysis.
C. Urinalysis:
 1. Urine dipstick for a gross screen.
 2. pH determination (pH >7.5 is compatible with infection lithiasis, and a pH <5.5 favors uric acid lithiasis).
 3. Red cell casts strongly suggest glomerulonephritis.
 4. Evaluate urine sediment for crystalluria.
D. Urine culture, if indicated.
E. 24-hour urine for creatinine, calcium, uric acid, oxalate, pH, sodium, potassium, citrate, and cystine measurement:
 1. Client should be on his or her usual diet before taking 24-hour specimen.
 2. Collection should be months after any interventions, including shock-wave lithotripsy, ureteroscopy, or percutaneous stone removal.
F. Noncontrast helical CT scan is the imaging standard to assess the urinary tract in acute renal colic.
G. Renal ultrasound is the procedure of choice for pregnancy.
H. x-Ray of the kidney, ureter, and bladder (KUB) is often ordered with the pelvic CT or ultrasound.
I. Intravenous pyelography (IVP).
J. Nuclear renal scan.

Differential Diagnoses
A. Kidney stone(s): Associated with colicky flank pain radiating to the groin. Significant flank pain of renal colic is usually secondary to renal calculi, but may occasionally be associated with passage of clots.
B. UTI: Passage of large, bulky blood clots implicates the bladder as the source, whereas long, shoestring-shaped specks or thin, stringy clots suggest an upper urinary tract or ureteral origin.
C. Acute abdomen/appendicitis.
D. Cholecystitis.
E. Pyelonephritis: Associated with dull flank pain with fever and chills. In evaluating urine sediment, the presence of white blood cells (WBCs) and bacteria favors a diagnosis of pyelonephritis or interstitial nephritis.
F. PID.
G. Inflammatory bowel disease.
H. Urinary tract obstruction.
I. Constipation.
J. Ectopic pregnancy.

Plan
A. General interventions.
 1. Increase fluids to allow passage of stone. Strain all urine to recover stone for analysis.
 2. Reduce possibility of recurrence with dietary modifications.
 3. The client is usually referred for imaging after evaluation of creatinine.
 4. Clients can be managed on an outpatient basis with close follow-up if stones are small (<6 mm).
B. Client teaching/dietary management
 1. Force fluids to maintain a daily output of 2 to 3 L of urine. Fluid intake that increases urinary production of at least 2 L of urine per day increases the flow rate and lowers the urine solute concentration.
 2. Dietary consultation may be needed secondary to stone analysis.
C. Pharmacological therapy:
 1. Pain medication (narcotic and nonnarcotic) is a priority:
  a. Nonsteroidal anti-inflammatory drugs (NSAIDs) should be discontinued three days before shock-wave lithotripsy to decrease the risk of bleeding.
 2. Antibiotics should be given for infection.
 3. Antiemetics if needed.
 4. Other medical/pharmacological management depends on the etiology of the stone.
D. Surgical options are dependent on stone size and location:
 1. Percutaneous nephrolithotomy is the first treatment option for most clients and is considered the first-line treatment for clients with staghorn calculi.
 2. Extracorporeal shock-wave lithotripsy is the least invasive of the surgical methods.
 3. Percutaneous nephrostomy should be the last procedure for most clients.
 4. Open nephrostomy may also be used.

Follow-Up
A. Reevaluate the client in 24 hours by phone or in the clinic.
B. Evaluate sooner if pain increases, because of the potential to progress to complete obstruction.
C. Recurrent stone formation is a manifestation of a systemic disease; evaluate for the management of the metabolic abnormality.

Consultation/Referral
A. Clients with severe pain, nausea, and vomiting need hospitalization for intravenous (IV) hydration and pain control.
B. Clients with severe symptoms and persistent obstruction beyond three to four days should be referred for urologic evaluation.
C. Refer to urology for surgical interventions: Lithotripsy, urethroscope interventions, extracorporeal shock-wave lithotripsy, and percutaneous ultrasonic lithotripsy may be indicated. Treatment varies based on the location and size of the stone. Laparoscopy may be indicated for the removal of large or severely impacted ureteral calculi.

Individual Considerations
A. Pregnancy:
 1. Urolithiasis is the most common cause of nonobstetrical abdominal pain that requires hospitalization in pregnancy.
 2. Approximately 80% to 90% are diagnosed in the first trimester.
 3. Renal ultrasound is the first-line screening test for pregnant clients. A transvaginal ultrasound may also be performed.
 4. Low-dose CT is reserved for complex cases in the second and third trimesters.
 5. Conservative treatment is used: Bed rest, hydration, and analgesia.

6. Invasive measures include stent placement, ureteroscopy, and percutaneous nephrostomy.
7. Upon presentation, rule out:
    a. Ectopic pregnancy.
    b. Abruptio placentae.
    c. Preterm labour.

B. Pediatrics:
1. Young children generally do not present with the classic acute onset of flank pain; instead, they may present with abdominal pain. Stone may be detected when abdominal imaging is performed.
2. Haematuria can present as the sole symptom or in conjunction with abdominal pain.
3. Ten percent of children present with symptoms of dysuria and urgency.
4. Shock-wave lithotripsy and percutaneous-based therapy may be considered in children.

Bibliography

American Urological Association. (2016, April). *Surgical management of stones: American Urological Association/Endourological Society guideline*. Retrieved from www.auanet.org/education/guidelines/surgical-management-of-stones.cfm

Curhan, G. C., Aronson, M. D., & Preminger, G. M. (2015, November 11). Diagnosis and acute management of suspected nephrolithiasis in adults. *UpToDate*. Retrieved from www.uptodate.com/contents/diagnosis-and-acute-management-of-suspected-nephrolithiasis-in-adults?topicKey=NEPH%2F7366

Preminger, G. M., & Curhan, G. C. (2015, October 21). Nephrolithiasis during pregnancy. *UpToDate*. Retrieved from www.uptodate.com/contents/nephrolithiasis-during-pregnancy?topicKey=NEPH%2F7370

Smith, J., & Stapleton, F. B. (2015, June 9). Clinical features and diagnosis of nephrolithiasis in children. *UpToDate*. Retrieved from www.uptodate.com/contents/clinical-features-and-diagnosis-of-nephrolithiasis-in-children?topicKey=PEDS%2F6123

Wayment, R. O. (2015, April 17). Pregnancy and urolithiasis. *Medscape*. Retrieved from http://emedicine.medscape.com/article/455830-overview

Wolfe, J. S. (2013a, February 11). Nephrolithiasis. *Medscape*. Retrieved from http://emedicine.medscape.com/article/437096-overview

Wolfe, J. S. (2013b, February 11). Nephrolithiasis treatment & management. *Medscape*. Retrieved from http://emedicine.medscape.com/article/437096-treatment

Testicular Torsion

Cheryl A. Glass, Debbie Gunter, and Kristie A. D. Morydz

Definition

A. Testicular torsion is twisting of the testicle around the vas deferens, with compromise in the blood supply and possible necrosis to the testicles. Testicular torsion is a urologic emergency and is the most frequent cause of testicle loss in the adolescent male population. Approximately 40% of all cases of acute scrotal pain and swelling are diagnosed with testicular torsion. There is often a history of recurrent episodes of testicular pain before torsion.

B. Testicular torsion is most commonly misdiagnosed as epididymitis:
1. Epididymitis usually presents with gradual onset of pain that is localized posterior to the testes that gradually radiates to the lower abdomen.
2. These symptoms are rare with torsion.

Incidence/Prevalence

A. Incidence in males younger than 25 years is approximately 1 in 4000. Although torsion can occur at any age, the largest number of cases occur during adolescence.

B. The bell clapper congenital anomaly is present in approximately 12% of males, and 40% have the abnormality in the contralateral testicle.

Pathogenesis

A. Testicular torsion and torsion of the spermatic cord occur because of abnormal fixation of the testicle to the scrotum, allowing free rotation. The bell clapper deformity allows the testicle to twist spontaneously on the spermatic cord. Venous occlusion and engorgement cause arterial ischaemia and infarction of the testicle.

Predisposing Factors

A. Age: More common in adolescence.
B. Trauma to testicle.
C. Spontaneous occurrence.
D. Congenital bell clapper anomaly.
E. Exercise.
F. Undescended testicle.
G. Active cremasteric reflex.

Common Findings

A. Sudden onset of severe unilateral scrotal pain (<24 hours).
B. Swelling of scrotal sac.
C. High position of the testicle.
D. Abnormal cremasteric reflex.

Other Signs and Symptoms

A. Sudden onset of testicular pain, may radiate to groin.
B. Possible oedema.
C. Abdominal pain (22%–30%).
D. Nausea and vomiting (50% of cases).
E. Fever (16%).
F. Urinary frequency (4%).

Subjective Data

A. Review the onset, duration, and course of symptoms.
B. Review for a history of prior episodes of intermittent testicular pain that resolved spontaneously.
C. Review abdominal symptoms such as pain, nausea and vomiting, and fever.
D. Review urethral discharge (possible sexually transmitted infection [STI]) and dysuria.
E. Review the client's history for trauma to the scrotum or testicle.

Physical Examination

A. Check temperature, blood pressure (BP), pulse, and respiration.
B. Inspect:
1. Observe the client generally for pain before and during examination.
2. Visualize the scrotal sac for oedema, symmetry, lesions, discharge, colour (especially for blue dot superior to the affected testicle). Testis is located high in the scrotum as a result of shortening of the cord by twisting.
3. Check the inguinal and femoral areas for bulges and hernias.
C. Auscultate:
1. Auscultate all four quadrants of the abdomen; note bowel sounds.
2. Assess the scrotum for bowel noise.

D. Palpate:
1. Palpate the abdomen for masses, rebound, and tenderness or guarding.
2. Palpate the groin; check the lymph nodes.
3. Examine for an inguinal hernia.
4. Genital examination:
   a. Check warmth, tenderness, swelling, and any nodularity; if a mass is present, check if it is solid or cystic. The testes should be sensitive to gentle compression, but not tender. They should feel smooth, rubbery, and free of nodules.
   b. Elicit a cremasteric reflex by stroking the inner thigh with a blunt object (reflex hammer or ink pen). The testicle and scrotum should rise on the stroked side. Cremasteric reflex is usually absent in testicular torsion.
   c. Elevate the scrotum; there is usually no relief in pain with torsion. Elevation of the scrotum may improve the pain of epididymitis (Prehn's sign).

Diagnostic Tests
A. Urinalysis: Normal in 90% of cases of testicular torsion.
B. Doppler ultrasonography for blood flow and scrotal ultrasonography.

Differential Diagnoses
A. Testicular torsion: Firm, tender mass of acute onset in an afebrile young man with a history of prior episodes must be considered to represent torsion until proven otherwise.
B. Epididymitis.
C. Orchitis.
D. Hydrocele.
E. Testicular tumour: Usually a hard, enlarged, painless testicle.
F. Acute appendicitis.
G. Scrotal/testicular trauma.
H. Varicocele.

Plan
A. General interventions:
1. Testicular torsion is a urologic emergency requiring surgery.
2. Immediately refer the client to a urologist and/or emergency department.
3. Symptoms for more than six hours can indicate testicular necrosis.
4. The opposite testicle is usually stabilized during the same surgery.
B. Pharmacological therapy:
1. None.

Follow-Up
A. Client should follow up with the urologist as directed.

Consultation/Referral
A. All clients with suspected testicular torsion need to be immediately referred to a urologist.

Individual Considerations
A. Pediatrics: Neonatal testicular torsion is rare. The exact mechanism is unknown. The torsion may occur prenatal (at or within 24 hours of delivery) or postnatal (within first 30 days of delivery). On physical examination, a hardened, fixed nontender scrotal mass with a discoloured scrotum is noted. Management is controversial because of the lack of data on whether the testis can be salvaged and the risk for concomitant or subsequent torsion of the contralateral side.
B. Geriatrics: In older males, rule out epididymitis, especially with new sexual partners or with symptoms of dysuria and urethral discharge.

Undescended Testes or Cryptorchidism

Cheryl A. Glass, Debbie Gunter, and Kristie A. D. Morydz

Definition
A. Undescended testicle(s) or cryptorchidism is a testicle that is not within the scrotum and cannot be manipulated from the inguinal canal into the scrotum or is absent. Spontaneous descent of testes usually happens at the end of the first year. Bilaterally absent testicles is anorchia.

Incidence/Prevalence
A. Approximately 10% of males have bilateral cryptorchidism.
B. In unilateral cases, left-side predominance is noted.
C. Between 2% and 5% of full-term and 30% of premature male infants are born with an undescended testicle.
D. 20% to 30% of boys have at least one nonpalpable testis.

Pathogenesis
A. An absent testicle may occur because of agenesis or an intrauterine vascular problem such as torsion. It may also be related to the lack of gonadotropic and androgenic hormones during fetal development. Most undescended testes are a result of a mechanical factor, a hernia sac, or a shortened spermatic artery that impedes the testes' descent into the scrotum.

Predisposing Factors
A. Prematurity; the testes descend into the scrotum at approximately 36 weeks' gestation. Most testicles will complete their descent within the first few months of life.
B. Birth weight is the principal determining factor for undescended testes from birth to 1 year of age.
C. Twinning.
D. Maternal exposure to oestrogen during the first trimester of pregnancy.
E. Family history.
F. Congenital disorder of testosterone secretion or testosterone action:
1. Kallmann syndrome.
2. Abdominal wall defects.
3. Neural tube defects.
4. Cerebral palsy.
5. Genetic syndromes:
   a. Trisomy 18.
   b. Trisomy 13.
   c. Noonan syndrome.
   d. Prader–Willi syndrome.
G. Exposure to dibutyl phthalate (endocrine-disrupting chemical).

Common Findings
A. Empty scrotum.
B. Small, flat, undeveloped scrotum.
C. Inguinal hernia.

Other Signs and Symptoms
A. Absence of testicle noted on newborn examination or by parents during a bath or diaper change.

Subjective Data
A. Review the course, duration, and symptoms. Have the testes ever been noticed in the scrotum during a bath or while the baby has been relaxed?
B. Note gestational age and birth weight at delivery (term vs. preterm).
C. Has any health-care provider ever noted that the testis was not descended or was absent on examination?
D. Review the maternal history for evidence of an endocrine disturbance during pregnancy.
E. Review family history of congenital abnormalities, genital anomalies, and abnormal pubertal development.
F. Review whether the client has undergone prior inguinal surgery.

Physical Examination
A. Temperature, blood pressure (BP), pulse, and respiration.
B. Inspect:
   1. Check the scrotum for size, shape, rugae, and any anomaly, particularly hypospadias.
   2. Look for a bulge in the inguinal area.
   3. Transilluminate the scrotum to look for testes and note fluid (if present).
     a. To locate the testis, darken the room and shine a bright light from behind the scrotum. In a normal male, the testis stands out as the darker area.
C. Palpate:
   1. Before you palpate the scrotum, place the thumb and index finger of one hand over the inguinal canals at the upper part of the scrotal sac. This maneuver helps prevent retraction of the testes into the inguinal canal or abdomen.
   2. Check each side of the scrotum to detect the presence of the testes and other masses. If either of the testicles is not palpable, place a finger over the upper inguinal ring and gently push toward the scrotum. You may feel a soft mass in the inguinal canal. Try to push it toward the scrotum and palpate it with your thumb and index finger. The testicle of a newborn is approximately 1 cm in diameter.
   3. When any mass other than the testicle or spermatic cord is palpated in the scrotum, determine whether it is filled with fluid, gas, or solid material. It is most likely to be a hernia or hydrocele. If it is reducible, then transilluminate to differentiate a hydrocele from a hernia.
   4. Check the cremasteric reflex: Scrotal sac retracts in response to cold hands and/or abrupt handling (yo-yo reflex).
   5. Bimanual digital rectal examination (DRE) may be used to evaluate the nonpalpable testis.

Diagnostic Tests
A. For a unilateral undescended testis without hypospadias, no laboratory studies are needed.
B. Hormone levels (testosterone) may be obtained if both testes are nonpalpable.
C. Karyotype to rule out chromosomal abnormalities is not routinely recommended in unilateral undescended testis, although it is recommended with bilateral nonpalpable testes, or at least one undescended testicle and proximal hypospadias.
D. Ultrasonography of the abdomen may have limited added value.
E. CT of the abdomen should be avoided.
F. Genetic testing should be considered for those with proximal hypospadias and at least one undescended testicle.

Differential Diagnoses
A. Anorchia (complete absence).
B. Retractile testis.
C. Ectopic testis.
D. Ambiguous genitalia: In male-appearing genitals, at least one testis must be palpated; if not, ambiguous genitalia cannot be eliminated. A deep cleft in the scrotum (bifid scrotum) is usually associated with other genitourinary (GU) anomalies or ambiguous genitalia.
E. Tumour: A hard, enlarged, painless testicle may indicate a tumour.

Plan
A. General interventions:
   1. Refer all children with cryptorchidism by 1 year of age to a surgeon for evaluation.
   2. Surgery (orchiopexy) is usually indicated between 6 and 18 months of age.
B. Pharmacological therapy: Hormonal therapy is carried out by a specialist.

Follow-Up
A. Follow up with surgeon as recommended per surgeon.
B. Monitor the client's testicles at each well-child visit.

Consultation/Referral
A. A mass that does not transilluminate or reduce with gentle pressure is likely to be an incarcerated hernia. This is a surgical emergency.
B. Refer the client for urologic recommendations regarding surgery.

Individual Considerations
A. Pediatrics:
   1. Testicular cancer screening should be done during and after puberty.
   2. Examine a child in the tailor's position or with the child sitting on a chair or examination table with legs in "frog position," kneeling, or standing. Note: If the child sits cross-legged, it abolishes the reflex of the cremaster muscle.
   3. Examine adolescents while standing and straining.
   4. Examination of an adolescent includes evaluation of maturation described by Tanner.
B. Adults:
   1. Males who have undescended testicles may have an increased risk of developing breast cancer and developing testicular germ cell cancers. Eleven percent of testicular cancers are seen in those with undescended testicles.
   2. Men with a history of undescended testes have an increased incidence of infertility (lower sperm counts, sperm of lower quality, and low fertility rates).
   3. Testicular torsion is 10 times higher in undescended testes. Torsion of an intra-abdominal testis can present as an acute abdomen.

Bibliography
American Urological Association. (2014a, April). *Evaluation and treatment of cryptorchidism: AUA guideline*. Retrieved from https://www.auanet.org/education/guidelines/cryptorchidism.cfm

Braga, L. H., Lorenzo, A. J., & Romao, R. L. P. (2017). Canadian Urological Association-Pediatric Urologists of Canada (CUA-PUC) guideline for the diagnosis, management, and followup of cryptorchidism. *Canadian Urological Association Journal, 11*(7), E251–E260. doi:10.5489/cuaj.4585

Ogunyemi, O. (2015, December 11). Testicular torsion. *Medscape*. Retrieved from http://emedicine.medscape.com/article/2036003-overview

Sachdeva, K. (2016, June 3). Testicular cancer. *Medscape*. Retrieved from http://emedicine.medscape.com/article/279007-overview

Urinary Incontinence (UI)

Cheryl A. Glass, Debbie Gunter, and Kristie A. D. Morydz

Definition
A. Urinary incontinence (UI) is the involuntary loss of urine severe enough to have unpleasant social or hygienic consequences. UI is diagnosed primarily on history; inquire about UI at every interview. UI is a symptom of an underlying disease process in most cases; some cases are reversible with appropriate treatment.
B. Incontinence is not considered a part of normal aging. Morbidity related to incontinence includes urinary tract infections (UTIs), indwelling catheters, falls/fractures, sleep interruption, social withdrawal, and depression.
C. Successful toileting depends on ready access to facilities, motivation to remain dry, mobility and manual dexterity, and the cognitive ability to recognize/react to the urge to void.
D. UI can be divided into the following categories: functional, urge, overflow, stress, and mixed. Each category has a unique etiology, pathophysiology, symptoms, and management.

Incidence/Prevalence
A. Ten percent of Canadians are estimated to have urinary incontinence.
B. UI is common in children. Daytime urinary continence normally occurs by age 4 years. Successful day-and-night continence is generally achieved by age 5 or 7 years:
    1. Up to 20% of children aged 4 to 6 years have an occasional daytime wetting. Three percent have urinary accidents more than two times per week.
    2. Daytime incontinence, a wetting accident at least once every two weeks, decreases with age in the pediatric population.
    3. Overactive bladder (OAB) in children has also been associated with other symptoms, including nocturnal enuresis, constipation, fecal incontinence, a history of UTIs, and poor toilet facilities.
C. The incidence of women identified with the definition of any leakage at least once in the last year ranges from 25% to 51%. The incidence is reported to be 10% when identified with weekly urinary leakage.
D. The prevalence of UI in men is approximately half that of women. The incidence of UI is affected by treatment of prostate disease. Men with incontinence have a higher risk of institutionalization compared with men without UI.
E. The elderly are more frequently affected with UI; 6% to 10% percent of admissions to long-term care facilities are related to incontinence.

Pathogenesis
UI can be caused by pathologic, anatomic, or physiological factors and differs by type of incontinence.
A. Functional incontinence: Loss of urine because of the inability to get to the bathroom, either caused by problems of mobility or cognition.
B. Urge incontinence/OAB: Inability to delay voiding after the sensation of fullness is perceived. Common causes are detrusor hyperactivity or hyperreflexia associated with disorders of the lower urinary tract, tumours, stones, uterine prolapse, cystitis, urethritis, or impaired bladder contractility. Central nervous system disorders, such as stroke, dementia, parkinsonism, or spinal cord injury, also can be causative factors.
C. Overflow incontinence: Loss of urine associated with an overdistension of the bladder. Common causes are anatomic obstruction by an enlarged prostate, a prolapsed cystocele, acontractile bladder caused by diabetes, spinal cord injury, multiple sclerosis, or suprasacral cord lesions.
D. Stress incontinence: Involuntary loss of urine during coughing, sneezing, laughing, bending over, or other physical activity that increases intra-abdominal pressure. Prostate surgery is the most common cause of stress incontinence in men.
E. Mixed incontinence: Combination of stress and urge incontinence in which the bladder outlet is weak and the detrusor is overactive.

Predisposing Factors
A. Age for both males and females.
B. Female: 85% of cases are in women.
C. Increased parity.
D. Previous genitourinary (GU) surgeries (e.g., prostate surgery, hysterectomy).
E. Restricted mobility.
F. Menopause.
G. Infections.
H. Chronic illnesses (e.g., diabetes).
I. Fecal impactions.
J. Excessive urinary output.
K. Delirium.
L. Dementia.
M. Neurologic disorders (e.g., stroke, spinal cord injury).
N. Variety of medications (e.g., antihypertensive medicines, diuretics, sedatives).
O. Pelvic trauma (e.g., episiotomy, forceps delivery).
P. Obesity.
Q. Sleep apnea.
R. Depression.
S. High-impact exercise.

Common Findings
A. Urgency: Sudden and compelling desire to pass urine.
B. Urge incontinence: Involuntary leakage accompanied by urgency with the following precipitating factors:
    1. Hearing running water.
    2. Placing hands in water.
    3. Trying to unlock the door when returning home.
    4. Exposure to a cold environment.
C. Stress incontinence: Involuntary leakage with the following precipitating factors:
    1. Exertion.
    2. Sneezing/coughing.
    3. May experience leakage with little or no activity.
D. OAB: Symptoms may occur with or without urge incontinence:
    1. Urgency.
    2. Frequency.
    3. Nocturia.

Other Signs and Symptoms
A. Mixed incontinence: Urge and stress leakage.

B. Experiencing leakage with little or no activity.
C. Continuous leakage (i.e., dribbling).
D. Daytime frequency.
E. Nocturia: Up one or more times a night to void.
F. Slow urine stream, intermittent stream, or hesitancy.
G. Need to strain to start, maintain, or improve voiding.
H. Incomplete emptying sensation.
I. Children exhibit holding maneuvers to postpone voiding or suppress urgency:
  1. Standing on tiptoes.
  2. Forcefully crossing legs (Vincent's curtsy).
  3. Squatting with hand or heel pressed to the perineum.

Subjective Data
A. Question the client regarding the onset, duration, and severity of the incontinence:
  1. Do you ever leak urine/water when you don't want to?
  2. Do you ever leak urine when you cough, laugh, or exercise?
  3. Do you ever leak urine on the way to the bathroom (urgency)?
  4. Do you ever use pads, tissue, or cloth in your underwear to catch urine?
B. Elicit situations when UI is worse, when it is improved, and what stimuli are associated with increasing UI (high fluid intake, high caffeine intake, agitation).
C. Review whether the female client is pre- or postmenopausal.
D. Review other lower urinary tract symptoms (LUTS) such as nocturia.
E. Review the client's history of bowel function (e.g., fecal incontinence). If constipation is a problem, abdominal pressure from a large retained stool can cause symptoms, including retention.
F. Review medications, including over-the-counter (OTC) drugs and herbals:
  1. Do not prescribe a muscarinic medication with clients when they are currently on other medications with anticholinergic properties.
G. Preview previous continence therapy including surgical treatments.
H. Review the impact of incontinence on quality of life, including work impairment, sexual dysfunction, activities of daily living, sleep, recreational activity, social interaction, and depression.
I. Assess whether the elderly client has incontinence despite toileting.
J. Review sexual function.
K. Review history and previous treatment for prostate disease.
L. Review other comorbid medical diagnoses such as neurologic disabilities, narrow-angle glaucoma, and diabetes:
  1. Do not prescribe a muscarinic medication in a client with narrow-angle glaucoma unless approved by the treating ophthalmologist.
  2. Use caution when prescribing antimuscarinic for OAB with a frail client.
M. What is the diabetic client's blood glucose average?

Physical Examination
Both sexes:
A. Check temperature (if infection is suspected), pulse, blood pressure (BP), and respiration.
B. Inspect:
  1. Look for evidence of cardiac overload: Pedal oedema.
C. Auscultate:
  1. Lungs for evidence of fluid overload: Rales.
D. Palpate:
  1. Abdomen for masses, fullness over bladder, and tenderness.
E. Neurologic examination:
  1. Assess cognitive and functional status, including mobility, transfers, manual dexterity, and ability to toilet in the elderly.
  2. Screen for depression.
  3. Assess for any change in sensation of the perineal area:
    a. Ask the client if they feel pressure in the bladder or rectal area when they need to urinate or defecate.
    b. Ask the client if they can feel when they are wiping.
    c. During the physical exam, assess for perineal sensation.

Females:
A. Inspect:
  1. Assess perineal skin for irritation, thinning, vaginal atrophy, and vaginal discharge.
B. Palpate:
  1. Perform a bimanual pelvic examination for prolapse, masses, or tenderness.
  2. Perform rectal examination for sphincter tone, masses, and fecal impaction.
C. Perform pelvic examination:
  1. Remove the top blade of the speculum and evaluate the vaginal wall support.
  2. Ask the woman to cough to reevaluate the vaginal wall support.

Males:
A. Inspect:
  1. Inspect the glans penis for abnormalities in urethral meatus. (Hypospadias may cause postvoid dribbling.)
  2. Uncircumcised men should be evaluated for phimosis and balanitis.
B. Palpate:
  1. Perform rectal examination for sphincter tone, masses, fecal impaction, prostate size, and contour.
  2. Palpate the scrotum to evaluate masses.
  3. Evaluate the presence of an inguinal hernia because straining with a partial urinary obstruction can worsen an inguinal hernia.

Diagnostic Tests
The history, physical examination, and urinalysis are sufficient to guide initial therapy. Other tests include the following:
A. Urine culture and sensitivity if infection is suspected.
B. Urine cytology if haematuria or pelvic pain is present.
C. Cystometry. See Section II: Procedure: "Cystometry: Bedside."
D. Postvoid residual (PVR) by catheterization or ultrasound. A PVR of <50 mL is considered adequate emptying and >200 mL is considered inadequate, suggesting either detrusor weakness or obstruction. Indications for PVR:
  1. Men with mild to moderate lower urinary symptoms.
  2. Men with OAB (urgency).
  3. Persons with spinal cord injury or Parkinson's disease.
  4. Persons with prior episodes of urinary retention.
  5. Persons with severe constipation.
E. A serum prostate-specific antigen (PSA) should be considered.
F. Routine urodynamic testing is not recommended.

G. Cystoscopy is not required for incontinence; however, it is indicated for haematuria.

Differential Diagnoses

Eight reversible causes of transient incontinence can be remembered by using the mnemonic: DIAPPERS.

Delirium
Infection (urinary)
Atrophic urethritis and vaginitis
Pharmacologicals
Psychological disorders, especially depression
Excessive urine output
Restricted mobility
Stool impaction

Plan

A. General interventions:
   1. Functional UI: Therapy is directed at the cause of the condition, such as overdiuresis, inability to go to the toilet, or poor access to toilet facilities.
   2. Behavioural interventions should be reviewed:
      a. A bladder diary (see Table 12.2) may provide information on usual timing and circumstances of UI.
      b. Timed scheduled voiding and/or prompted caregiver scheduled toileting.
      c. Bladder training by systematic ability to delay voiding through the use of urge of inhibition.
      d. Stress incontinence: Kegel perineal exercises may improve UI by 30% to 90%. Exercises using graduated vaginal cones or weights induce pelvic muscle tone and strength, reducing UI.
      e. Overflow UI: Crede's method is used for expressing the bladder, by applying pressure with the hands placed in the suprapubic area after voiding to assist in emptying.
      f. Intermittent catheterization is an option frequently used after other measures have failed or overflow UI.
      g. Weight loss is suggested for obese clients.
      h. Dietary changes including elimination of bladder irritants: caffeine, citrus/acidic foods, alcohol, and carbonated drinks.
      i. Avoid constipation. Discuss measures to prevent constipation.
      j. Reduce excessive fluid intake, with no fluid intake three to four hours before bedtime if nocturia is a problem.
▶ B. Client teaching: *Refer to Client Teaching Guide: Urinary Incontinence (Women).*
C. Other alternatives:
   1. Surgical treatment is based on the cause of incontinence.
   2. Continence pessaries may benefit women with stress UI.
   3. Electrical stimulation may be prescribed to inhibit bladder instability and improve striated and levator contractility and efficiency.
   4. Treatment of concomitant constipation is an important step in the treatment of incontinence.
   5. Treatment of vaginal atrophy is another important step in the treatment of incontinence.
   6. Injection of botulinum toxin (BTX) is an option for the treatment of urge incontinence in selected clients.
   7. Transurethral bulking agents injected into the submucosal tissues of the urethra or bladder neck are an option for women and men with UI caused by benign prostatic hypertrophy (BPH).
   8. Indwelling catheters are not recommended as a management strategy for OAB.
D. Pharmacological therapy:
   1. Use of anticholinergic and antispasmodic drugs to decrease reflex bladder contractions and increase bladder capacity (contraindicated in uncontrolled narrow-angle glaucoma, urinary retention, or gastric retention):
      a. Oxybutynin chloride.
      b. Tolterodine tartrate: Not recommended for children.
      c. Fesoterodine: Not recommended for children
      d. Trospium: Not recommended for children.
      e. Darifenacin: Not recommended for children.
      f. Solifenacin: Not recommended for children.
   2. Alpha-adrenergic antagonists stimulate urethral smooth muscle contraction:
      a. Imipramine: Used for childhood enuresis.
   3. Beta-3 adrenergic agonist: Mirabegron (Not recommended in children).
   4. No medications have been approved for stress incontinence.
   5. For postmenopausal women, vaginal oestrogen may restore urethral mucosa; use the same type, dosage, and client selection criteria as with oestrogen therapy (OT). Systemic oestrogen should not be prescribed for UI.

Follow-Up

A. Follow-up is based on the type and cause of UI.

Consultation/Referral

A. Refer to a specialist for incontinence with abdominal and/or pelvic pain or haematuria in the absence of a UTI, or when surgical treatment is desired.
B. Refer for urodynamic testing, which is considered the gold standard. Testing requires special equipment and training.
C. Refer to a gynecologist or urology clinic practitioner experienced in fitting a continence pessary.
D. Refer to a urologist for haematuria and/or risk factors of bladder cancer.

Individual Considerations

A. Pregnancy: Stress incontinence is frequently associated with pregnancy and is treated with pelvic exercises.
B. Pediatrics:
   1. UI is most often experienced as enuresis.
   2. UI in previously bladder-controlled children requires a thorough workup and referral to a pediatrician.
   3. Any child with a suspected neurologic abnormality should be evaluated for an occult neurologic lesion.
   4. Dysfunctional voiding is often associated with a psychological comorbidity or behavioural issues.
C. Geriatrics:
   1. Incontinence in the elderly is a risk factor for falls. Many falls occur en route to the bathroom, especially at night.
   2. Incontinence increases social isolation and depression.

▶ Client Teaching Guides are available at https://connect.springerpub.com/content/reference-book/978-0-8261-9498-5

TABLE 12.2 Bladder Control Diary

Your Daily Bladder Diary. This diary will help you and your health-care team figure out the causes of your bladder control trouble. The "sample" line shows you how to use the diary. Use this sheet as a master for making copies that you can use as a bladder diary for as many days as you need.

Your name: _____

Date: _____

Time	Drinks		Trips to the Bathroom		Accidental Leaks	Did You Feel a Strong Urge to Go?	What Were You Doing at the Time?
	What kind?	How much?	How many times?	How much urine? (circle one)	How much? (circle one)	Circle one	Sneezing, exercising, having sex, lifting, etc.
Sample	Coffee	2 cups	✓ ✓	(sm) med lg	sm (med) lg	Yes (No)	Running
6–7 a.m.				sm med lg	sm med lg	Yes No	
7–8 a.m.				sm med lg	sm med lg	Yes No	
8–9 a.m.				sm med lg	sm med lg	Yes No	
9–10 a.m.				sm med lg	sm med lg	Yes No	
10–11 a.m.				sm med lg	sm med lg	Yes No	
11–12 noon				sm med lg	sm med lg	Yes No	
12–1 p.m.				sm med lg	sm med lg	Yes No	
1–2 p.m.				sm med lg	sm med lg	Yes No	
2–3 p.m.				sm med lg	sm med lg	Yes No	
3–4 p.m.				sm med lg	sm med lg	Yes No	
4–5 p.m.				sm med lg	sm med lg	Yes No	
5–6 p.m.				sm med lg	sm med lg	Yes No	
6–7 p.m.				sm med lg	sm med lg	Yes No	
7–8 p.m.				sm med lg	sm med lg	Yes No	
8–9 p.m.				sm med lg	sm med lg	Yes No	
9–10 p.m.				sm med lg	sm med lg	Yes No	
10–11 p.m.				sm med lg	sm med lg	Yes No	
11–12 midnight				sm med lg	sm med lg	Yes No	
12–1 a.m.				sm med lg	sm med lg	Yes No	
1–2 a.m.				sm med lg	sm med lg	Yes No	
2–3 a.m.				sm med lg	sm med lg	Yes No	
3–4 a.m.				sm med lg	sm med lg	Yes No	

(continued)

TABLE 12-2 Bladder Control Diary (continued)

Time	Drinks		Trips to the Bathroom		Accidental Leaks	Did You Feel a Strong Urge to Go?	What Were You Doing at the Time?
	What kind?	How much?	How many times?	How much urine? (circle one)	How much? (circle one)	Circle one	Sneezing, exercising, having sex, lifting, etc.
4–5 a.m.				○ ○ ○	○ ○ ○	Yes No	
5–6 a.m.				○ ○ ○	○ ○ ○	Yes No	

I used _____ pads today. I used _____ diapers today (write number).
Questions to ask my health-care team:
_____
_____

Let's Talk About Bladder Control for Women is a public health awareness campaign conducted by the National Kidney and Urologic Diseases Information Clearinghouse (NKUDIC), an information dissemination service of the National Institute of Diabetes and Digestive and Kidney Diseases (NIDDK), National Institutes of Health.

Source: Adapted from National Kidney and Urologic Diseases Information Clearinghouse, National Institutes of Health. (n.d.). *Kidney disease.* Retrieved from www.niddk.nih.gov/health-information/health-topics/urologic-disease/urinary-incontinencewomen/pages/insertb.aspx

3. Functional incontinence is common in older adults with arthritis or Parkinson's or Alzheimer's diseases. Clients are unable to hold their urine until they reach the bathroom and undress. A toileting program usually assists in this situation.
4. Durable medical equipment, such as a bedside commode, should be considered.
5. Antimuscarinic medications may increase confusion.

Bibliography

Bettez, M., Tu le, M., Carlson, K., Corcos, J., Gajewski, J., Jolivet, M., & Bailly, G. (2012). 2012 update: guidelines for adult urinary incontinence collaborative consensus document for the Canadian urological association. *Canadian Urological Association Journal = Journal de l'Association des urologues du Canada*, 6(5), 354–363. doi:10.5489/cuaj.12248

Clemens, J. Q. (2013, February 6). Urinary incontinence in men. *UpToDate.* Retrieved from http://www.uptodate.com/contents/urinary-incontinence-in-men?topicKey=PC%2F14611

DuBeau, C. E. (2013, January 29). Epidemiology, risk factors, and pathogenesis of urinary incontinence. *UpToDate.* Retrieved from www.uptodate.com/contents/epidemiology-risk-factors-and-pathogenesis-of-urinary-incontinence?topicKey=PC%2F6875

Gormley, E. A., Lightner, D. J., Burgio, K. L., Chal, T. C., Clemens, J. Q., Culkin, D. J., & Vasavada, S. P. (2014, May). Diagnosis and treatment of overactive bladder (non-neurogenic) in adults: AUA/SUFU guideline. *American Urological Association.* Retrieved from www.auanet.org/content/media/OAB_guideline.pdf

Nepple, K. G., & Cooper, C. S. (2015, June 19). Etiology and clinical features of bladder dysfunction in children. *UpToDate.* Retrieved from www.uptodate.com/contents/etiology-and-clinical-features-of-bladder-dysfunction-in-children?topicKey=PEDS%2F6580

Vasavada, S. (2015, October 27). Urinary incontinence. *Medscape.* Retrieved from http://emedicine.medscape.com/article/452289-overview

Urinary Tract Infection (Acute Cystitis)

Cheryl A. Glass, Debbie Gunter, and Kristie A. D. Morydz

Definition

A. Urinary tract infection (UTI) is an infection of the urinary bladder. UTI is defined as the presence of at least 100,000 organisms per millilitre of urine in an asymptomatic client or more than 100 organisms per millilitre of urine with accompanying pyuria (greater than seven white blood cells [WBCs] per millilitre) in a symptomatic client. Asymptomatic bacteriuria (ASB) when left untreated is a risk factor for acute cystitis (40%) and pyelonephritis in 25% to 30% in pregnancy.
B. UTIs can be divided anatomically into upper and lower tract (cystitis) infections. For a discussion of upper tract infection, see the section "Pyelonephritis." in this chapter.
C. UTIs may be considered uncomplicated or complicated:
　1. An uncomplicated UTI is noted in a healthy person with a normal urinary tract system and may be treated with oral antibiotics.
　2. A UTI noted in a person with a structural or functional urinary tract system or in a person who is immunocompromised is considered complicated. It may require parental therapy until afebrile.

Incidence/Prevalence

A. Incidence depends on age and gender. The prevalence of UTI in males varies according to age:
　1. Young men aged 15 to 50 years rarely develop a UTI.
　2. The incidence of a UTI in geriatric males may be as high as in geriatric females (up to 15%).
B. In children, the incidence varies by age and gender. A UTI is the most common cause of fever of unknown origin in pediatrics.
C. More than 50% of women will have one UTI in their lifetime:
　1. Prevalence for females increases by 1% per decade and 2% to 4% throughout childbearing years.
　2. The incidence of UTIs in pregnancy ranges from 4% to 7%. In pregnancy, the increased incidence is related to both hormonal influence and anatomic changes that increase the risk of urinary stasis and vesicoureteral reflux.
　3. By age 30 years, approximately 50% of women have experienced symptoms of a UTI.

Pathogenesis

A. Bacteria ascend from the perineum through the urethra. The greater susceptibility of younger women and girls is related to a shorter urethra. In older women, it is related to oestrogen-mediated dilation of the urethra.

B. The normal male urinary tract has many natural defenses to infection. The greater susceptibility of elderly males is related to problems with the prostate and other urologic disease and can be linked to the instrumentation required for therapy.
C. Gram-negative bacilli are the most common pathogens; 80% to 90% of cases are related to coliform bacteria (*Escherichia coli*). It originates from fecal floras that colonize the periurethral area.
D. Other gram-negative bacteria include *Klebsiella pneumoniae* or *Proteus mirabilis*. *Staphylococcus saprophyticus* (gram-positive coccus) accounts for about 10% to 15% of UTIs.
E. Other pathogens include *Enterobacter, Pseudomonas, Enterococci*, and *Staphylococci*.
F. The incubation period depends on the pathogen.

Predisposing Factors
A. Female (until elderly, then equal frequency in males and females).
B. Pregnancy.
C. Poor hygiene.
D. Trauma.
E. Instrumentation.
F. Sexual intercourse.
G. Oral contraceptive or diaphragm use.
H. Female client diagnosed with diabetes (there is no increased risk for diabetic males).
I. Anomalies of the genitourinary (GU) tract.
J. Neurologic factors.
K. Vesicourethral reflux.
L. Obstruction: Stones.
M. Foreign bodies.
N. Bubble baths and hot tubs.
O. Douching.
P. Anal intercourse.
Q. HIV.
R. Uncircumcised penis.
S. Catheterization.
T. Nosocomial infection.
U. Phimosis.

Common Findings
A. Burning on urination.
B. Frequency.
C. Cloudy or bloody urine.
D. Urgency.
E. UTI in infants and children:
  1. Vague symptoms with or without fever.
  2. Gastrointestinal symptoms (vomiting and diarrhea).
  3. Frequent voiding.
  4. Incontinence.
  5. Dysuria.
  6. Suprapubic, abdominal, or lumbar pain.
F. Geriatrics:
  1. May not present with classic symptoms.
  2. Fever.
  3. Incontinence.
  4. Mental confusion.

Other Signs and Symptoms
A. Asymptomatic.
B. Frequency, dysuria, bladder spasms, suprapubic discomfort, urgency, and nocturia.
C. Suprapubic pain.
D. Fever.
E. Costovertebral angle (CVA) tenderness.
F. Haematuria.

Subjective Data
A. Review the onset, course, and duration of symptoms.
B. Does the client have fever and chills or back or flank pain (unilateral or bilateral)?
C. Are there any other genital problems such as herpes lesions or vaginal discharge?
D. Review the associated factors: Sexual intercourse (specifically review for anal intercourse), douching, or bubble bath.
E. Ask female clients if they use appropriate hygiene practices after urination and bowel movements (BMs):
  1. Wiping from front to back.
  2. Frequent changes of hygienic products.
  3. Handwashing.
F. Is the client pregnant? If not, what type of birth control does she use?
G. Is there any history of previous UTIs? How often, and how were they treated? Were any tests performed in a workup by a urologist?
H. How much liquid or water does the client drink every day? Note the amount of caffeine.
I. In older men, review the strength of the urinary flow, dribbling, hesitancy, and so forth.
J. In the postmenopausal woman, review whether she has a known prolapse and/or vaginal atrophy. Does she use any systemic or local oestrogen medications?
K. Is there any history of other medical diseases including diabetes or sickle cell disease?
L. Review for the presence of neurologic disorders including spinal cord injury or multiple sclerosis.
M. Does the client require self-catheterization?

Physical Examination
A. Check temperature, blood pressure (BP), pulse, and respiration. The absence of a fever does not exclude the presence of an infective process.
B. Inspect:
  1. General observation of general appearance for discomfort before and during examination.
C. Auscultate:
  1. Heart and all lung fields.
D. Palpate:
  1. Palpate the abdomen: Kidneys, masses; assess for suprapubic tenderness.
  2. Palpate the back; note CVA tenderness.
  3. Check for inguinal lymph node enlargement.
  4. Palpate the suprapubic area.
E. Percuss:
  1. The bladder and the CVA area for tenderness.
F. Females:
  1. Pelvic examination:
    a. Inspect external genitalia for lesions, Bartholin's gland cysts, irritation, and discharge.
    b. Milk urethra for discharge.
    c. Assess rectal area.
    d. Speculum examination: Evaluate vaginal vault for discharge, cervicitis, and inflammation; evaluate for atrophic vaginal changes and torn tissue.
    e. Bimanual examination: Check for cervical motion, tenderness, and masses.
G. Males:
  1. Inspect the penis/urinary meatus for phimosis, lesions, signs of inflammation, and discharge. Retract the foreskin (if present) and assess for hygiene and smegma.
  2. Palpate the testes and epididymides for inflammation, tenderness, and masses.

3. Rectal examination is mandatory in males: Check for swollen and tender prostate. In clients with suspected acute bacterial prostatitis, palpation should be very gentle because of the potential for bacteraemia.

Diagnostic Tests

The diagnosis of a UTI can often be made based on a focused history and the presenting symptoms.

A. Urinalysis: Clean-catch urinalysis may be performed. However, catheterization or suprapubic aspiration may be necessary depending on the client's age and condition. Examples include pediatrics, elderly, obese, microscopic haematuria or for functionally impaired clients. Catheterization should be reserved for clients with an obstruction or for those who cannot cooperate or collect a clean-catch urine specimen. The percutaneous bladder aspiration is used for young children and infants.

Urinalysis dipstick findings:

1. Appearance: Should be clear. Cloudy urine may indicate presence of pyuria, pus, blood, cells, phosphate, or lymph fluid.
2. Odour: Usually faint aromatic odour; ammonia odour indicates *Proteus*, related to food changes; offensive odour indicates bacterial infection.
3. pH: Normal is around 6 (acid); may normally vary from 4.6 to 7.5. Greater than 7.5 may indicate infection.
4. Specific gravity: Reflects the kidney's ability to concentrate urine and the body's hydration or dehydration status. Normal is 1.005 to 1.025.
5. Colour: Shows concentration; usually yellow or amber:
  a. Straw colour = dilute urine.
  b. Dark colour = concentrated (dehydrated).
  c. Red or red–brown, to bloody = transfusion reaction, drugs, and bleeding lesions.
  d. Yellow brown = bile duct disease, jaundice.
  e. Dark brown or black = melanoma or leukemia.
6. Positive leukocyte esterase and nitrates indicate infection.

A negative urine dipstick does not rule out an infection.

B. Microscopic examination of urine findings: White blood cells (WBCs) greater than two to five; WBC/high-power microscope field (HPF); bacteria; positive Gram stain for cocci or rods, yeast, and blood indicates infection.

C. Urine culture and sensitivity:
1. Positive culture standard is 10^5 colony forming units; symptomatic females, 10^2; symptomatic males, 10^3.
2. Screening for asymptomatic bacteria is recommended for clients in pregnancy, for elderly males with documented prostatic or urologic abnormalities, for clients with a recent catheterization, and for clients with known stones or documented structural abnormalities.

D. Culture for sexually transmitted infection (STI) if suspected.
E. Wet prep for female, if indicated.
F. Imaging:
1. Ultrasound (especially useful in children).
2. Conventional voiding cystourethrography.
3. Urodynamic evaluation.

Differential Diagnoses

A. UTI: Watch for systemic symptoms of pyelonephritis.
B. Vaginal or pelvic infection.
C. Prostatitis or epididymitis: Tender, enlarged prostate; tender testicle or scrotum.
D. Bladder tumour.
E. Interstitial cystitis (IC).
F. Urinary calculi.
G. Benign prostatic hypertrophy (BPH): Changes in urinary stream and nocturia.
H. Overactive bladder (OAB)/urge incontinence.
I. Pelvic organ prolapse.
J. Irritant urethritis.
K. Consider the possibility that chronic, asymptomatic infections are a potential source of disseminated infection, such as endocarditis. This is particularly likely in the male client with prostate disease and infection requiring instrumentation.

Plan

A. General interventions:
1. Treatment of acute cystitis is aimed at identifying the underlying cause and initiating treatment as soon as possible.
2. If antibiotic therapy is initiated, stress the importance of taking all medication as directed, even if symptoms improve before the end of treatment.

B. Client teaching: *Refer to Client Teaching Guide: Urinary Tract Infection (Acute Cystitis).*
1. Provide client teaching sheet.

C. Dietary management:
1. Instruct the client to increase fluids and drink at least one large glass of liquid every hour.
2. Instruct the client to avoid foods that irritate the bladder: caffeine, alcohol, tomatoes, citrus, and spicy foods.
3. Encourage the client to drink cranberry juice to help fight bladder infections. If the client dislikes the taste of plain cranberry juice, have him or her mix it 1:1 with another juice, such as orange juice.

D. Pharmacological therapy:
1. Antibiotics: 3-day course may be efficacious and is less expensive than the traditional 7- to 10-day course of therapy for uncomplicated infections.
2. The first-line antibiotic depends on the specific bacteria found on culture. Empiric antimicrobial therapy should cover all likely pathogens.
3. First-line therapy:
  a. Nitrofurantoin monohydrate/macrocrystals.
  b. Trimethoprim/sulfamethoxazole (use when bacterial resistance is <20% and client has no allergy).
  c. Fosfomycin—reserved for when other first-line options are not appropriate.
4. Second-line therapy:
  a. Ciprofloxacin.
  b. Ciprofloxacin extended-release.
  c. Levofloxacin.
  d. Cephalexin.
5. Alternative therapy:
  a. Amoxicillin-clavulanate.
6. Urinary analgesic if needed:
  a. Phenazopyridine HCl: Educate the client that this drug turns urine orange.
7. First-line treatments for UTI or pyelonephritis in pregnancy:
  a. Nitrofurantoin.
  b. Amoxicillin:

c. Amoxicillin-clavulanate.
   d. Cephalexin.
   e. Fosfomycin.
8. Children younger than 2 years are usually treated for 7 to 14 days; children older than 2 years who are afebrile and without abnormalities of the urinary tract or have previous episodes of UTIs are usually treated for five days:
   a. Amoxicillin-clavulanate—assess rates of resistance.
   b. Sulfonamide-trimethoprim-sulfamethoxazole.
   c. Cephalosporin-cefixime—risk of severe cutaneous adverse reactions (SCAR).
9. Antibiotics that should not be used in pediatrics or pregnancy include the following:
   a. Fluoroquinolones are not used in children because of potential concerns about sustained injury to developing joints.
   b. Fluoroquinolones (Category Class C) are contraindicated during pregnancy because of auditory and vestibular toxicity in the fetus.
   c. Tetracyclines should not be used in pregnancy (Category Class D) or in children because of tooth staining.
   d. Nitrofurantoin is contraindicated in pregnant clients at term, during labour, and during delivery.
10. Consider prophylactic therapy for clients with chronic conditions/recurrent infections:
    a. Low-dose antibiotics daily for three to six months.
    b. Self-start antibiotics.
    c. Postcoital antibiotics.
11. Quinolones, cephalosporins, and macrolides should be reserved for complicated or resistant infections.
12. Vaginal oestrogen should be considered in postmenopausal women with urogenital atrophic changes.

Follow-Up
A. Routine posttreatment urinalysis/culture is not indicated in asymptomatic clients.
B. Have the client return if symptoms do not resolve at the end of treatment.
C. Have the client return if the symptoms reoccur within two weeks of treatment for a urine culture. Retreatment with a seven-day course of antibiotics using a different agent should be considered.
D. Two UTIs in girls and one UTI in boys should trigger an evaluation to rule out an obstruction, vesicoureteric reflux, and dysfunctional voiding. UTI in children who are severely ill with vomiting and dehydration requires hospitalization and IV antibiotics.

Consultation/Referral
A. Refer all children with more than one UTI to a specialist.
B. Young men do not have UTIs very often; a urologic workup may be needed if etiology, such as an STI, cannot be determined.
C. Clients with bacteriuria are also more likely to have identifiable abnormalities on an intravenous pyelography (IVP), including small kidneys, delayed excretion, calyceal dilation and blunting, ureteral reflux, stones, and obstructive lesions.
D. Consultation with a urologist is essential in all forms of prostatitis or in all but the most clear-cut cases of acute scrotum.

Individual Considerations
A. Women:
   1. Recurrent infections are common in females.
   2. Repeat urine culture and sensitivity after an antibiotic course is complete (approximately two to four weeks after therapy is completed).
   3. If the client is perimenopausal and has two or fewer UTIs a year, consider client-initiated therapy to start when symptomatic. Consider topical estradiol cream for atrophic vaginitis. If the client has three UTIs a year, prescribe a prophylactic single-dose regimen after intercourse. If infections are not related to intercourse, consider urine cultures every two months, with extended antibiotic therapy.
B. Pregnancy:
   1. The incidence of pyelonephritis in pregnancy is 1% to 2%. Most cases develop as a consequence of undiagnosed or inadequately treated lower UTI.
      a. In the presumptive diagnosis of pyelonephritis in pregnancy, ultrasound of the kidneys and urinary tract should be considered.
   2. Approximately 75% to 80% of pyelonephritis cases occur on the right side, with a 10% to 15% incidence on the left side. A small percentage of cases are bilateral.
   3. Group B *Streptococcus* (GBS) colonization has important implications during pregnancy, contributing to maternal pyelonephritis and preterm birth. Intrapartum transmission may lead to neonatal GBS infection:
      a. Women with documented GBS bacteriuria in the current pregnancy should be treated at the time of labour or rupture of membranes with appropriate intravenous (IV) antibiotics for the prevention of early-onset neonatal GBS disease.
      b. Asymptomatic women with urinary GBS in pregnancy should not be treated with antibiotics for the prevention of adverse maternal and perinatal outcomes.
      c. Women with documented GBS bacteriuria should not be rescreened by genital tract culture or urinary culture in the third trimester, as they are presumed to be GBS colonized.
   4. Current guidelines recommend universal vaginal and rectal screening in all pregnant women at 35 to 37 weeks' gestation rather than treatment based on risk factors.
   5. A urine culture screening is recommended for all pregnant women at their first prenatal visit.
   6. Suppressive antibiotic therapy should be instituted in pregnant clients who develop acute cystitis, recurrent or persistent ASB, or pyelonephritis.
   7. Clients with sickle cell hemoglobinopathies are at increased risk of UTI and should be screened more aggressively, possibly benefiting from antibiotic prophylaxis.
   8. Antibiotics that should not be used during pregnancy include the following:
      a. Tetracyclines (adverse effects on fetal teeth/bones and congenital defects).
      b. Quinolones (congenital defects).
      c. Trimethoprim in the first trimester (facial defects and cardiac abnormalities).
      d. Sulfonamides in the last trimester (kernicterus).
      e. Aminoglycosides (permanent ototoxicity in the fetus).
C. Pediatrics:
   1. Tetracyclines should not be given to children because of tooth staining.

2. Fluorinated quinolones may produce cartilage toxicity.
3. Antibiotic therapy includes amoxicillin, cephalosporins, trimethoprim, and nitrofurantoin.
4. Children diagnosed with recurrent UTIs should be referred and assessed for sexual abuse.

D. Geriatrics:
1. Clients may not have classic symptoms. Consider UTI if the client presents with increased urinary incontinence (UI), fever, and mental confusion.

Bibliography

American Academy of Pediatrics. (2011, September, reaffirmed in 2014). Urinary tract infection: Clinical practice guideline for the diagnosis and management of the initial UTI in febrile infants and children 2 to 24 months. *Pediatrics, 128*, 595–610. doi:10.1542/peds.2011-1330

Beahm, N. P., Nicolle, L. E., Bursey, A., Smyth, D. J., & Tsuyuki, R. T. (2017). The assessment and management of urinary tract infections in adults: Guidelines for pharmacists. *Canadian Pharmacists Journal, 150*(5), 298–305. doi:10.1177/1715163517723036

Brusch, J. (2016, March 22). Prevention of urinary tract infections. *Medscape*. Retrieved from http://emedicine.medscape.com/article/2040239-overview#a1

Gormley, E. A., Lightner, D. J., Burgio, K. L., Chal, T. C., Clemens, J. Q., Culkin, D. J., & Vasavada, S. P. (2014, May). Diagnosis and treatment of overactive bladder (non-neurogenic) in adults: AUA/SUFU guideline. *American Urological Association*. Retrieved from www.auanet.org/content/media/OAB_guideline.pdf

Grabe, M., Bjerklund-Johansen, T. E., Botto, H., Cek, M., Naber, K. G., Pickard, R. S., & Wullt, B. (2013). Guidelines on urological infections. *European Association of Urology*. Retrieved from www.uroweb.org/guidelines/online-guidelines

Johnson, E. (2015, May 6). Urinary tract infections in pregnancy. *Medscape*. Retrieved from http://emedicine.medscape.com/article/452604-overview

Zaccardi, J. E. (2013, January 16). Managing UTIs in women. *Clinical Advisor*. Retrieved from http://www.clinicaladvisor.com/features/managing-utis-in-women/article/276373/2

Varicocele

Cheryl A. Glass, Debbie Gunter, and Kristie A. D. Morydz

Definition

A. Varicocele is engorgement of the internal spermatic veins above the testes. This vascular abnormality is a cause of decreased testicular function. Some varicoceles are easy to identify and may be surgically corrected. The presence of a varicocele does not mean that surgical correction is a necessity.

Incidence/Prevalence

A. Varicocele may occur in 15% to 20% of normal males; 80% to 90% of cases occur on the left side. Up to 35% to 40% of men with a palpable left-sided varicocele may actually have bilateral varicoceles that are identified on physical examination.

B. Right-sided varicocele is uncommon and can indicate retroperitoneal malignancy. Varicocele is the leading known cause of male infertility (40%). Decreased sperm counts, infertility, and testicular atrophy occur in 65% to 75% of varicocele cases. There is no correlation between the size of the varicocele and the degree of infertility.

Pathogenesis

A. The exact pathophysiologic mechanisms for varicoceles are not fully identified. Varicoceles may be because of valvular incompetence or elevated hydrostatic pressure in the spermatic veins. Testicular temperature elevation also appears to play a role in varicocele-induced dysfunction. **New varicoceles in older men may be secondary to renal tumours.**

Predisposing Factor

A. Varicoceles generally manifest at the time of puberty.

Common Findings

A. Asymptomatic.
B. Infertility.
C. Pain or discomfort in the scrotum.

Other Signs and Symptoms

A. Pain or aching and heaviness in the scrotum.
B. Feels like "worms"; scrotum may have bluish discolouration.

Subjective Data

A. Note the onset, course, and duration of symptoms. When was the varicocele first noted?
B. Has the scrotum enlarged? If there is enlargement, over what time span? Does it collapse with lying or sitting down?
C. Is there any pain or discomfort?
D. Has there been any history of infertility?

Physical Examination

A. Check vital signs and temperature as indicated.
B. Inspect:
1. The examination should be done when the client is lying or standing in a warm room. Warm temperature promotes relaxation of the scrotum.
2. Examine the general appearance of the penis; note scrotal size, shape, and rugae. Varicocele tends to collapse with the client sitting or supine.
3. Transilluminate the scrotum to visualize the varicocele.
4. A large varicocele can easily be identified by inspection.

C. Palpate:
1. Palpate each side of the scrotum for testicular size, presence of varicocele (Valsalva maneuver performed while the client stands helps to reveal a small varicocele), and absence of vas deferens:
   a. A moderate-size varicocele can be identified by palpation without having the client perform the Valsalva maneuver.
2. Palpate the spermatic cord between the thumb and forefingers while the client performs a Valsalva maneuver:
   a. A small varicocele is identified only when the client bears down, increasing the intra-abdominal pressure.
   b. Varicocele should significantly diminish in size when the client assumes the supine position.
3. Evaluate whether the varicocele can be reduced while the client is supine.
4. Palpate the abdomen for hernias, masses, and tenderness.
5. Rectal examination: Palpate the prostate and seminal vesicles for tenderness and other signs of infection.

D. Auscultate: Listen over the scrotum to assess bowel sounds to rule out hernia.

Diagnostic Tests

A. Scrotal ultrasound with a high-resolution colour-flow Doppler is the diagnostic method of choice when clinical

examinations are equivocal, but are not indicated for standard evaluation.
B. Semen analysis times two, if indicated.
C. CT to evaluate retroperitoneal pathology (e.g., renal cell carcinoma) for:
  1. Sudden onset of varicocele.
  2. Single right-sided varicocele.
  3. Any varicocele that is not reducible in the supine position.

Differential Diagnoses
A. Varicocele classifications:
  1. Grade I (small): Palpable only on Valsalva maneuver, which increases intra-abdominal pressure and therefore impedes drainage and increases the varicocele size.
  2. Grade II (medium): Palpable when standing and bearing down (Valsalva maneuver).
  3. Grade III (large): Visible on inspection alone.
  4. Subclinical: Not palpable, vein >3 mm on ultrasound; Doppler reflux on Valsalva maneuver.
B. Hernia.
C. Epididymitis.
D. Hydrocele.
E. Testicular tumour: Consider retroperitoneal tumour, especially if presenting symptoms have a sudden onset.

Plan
A. General interventions:
  1. Urologic consultation for diagnosis and possible surgery. Surgery should be considered when all of the following conditions are met:
    a. Palpable varicocele on physical examination:
    b. Couples with known infertility.
    c. Female has normal fertility or potential treatable cause of infertility.
    d. Male partner has abnormal semen parameters or abnormal results from sperm function tests.
B. Client teaching:
  1. If discomfort is present, an athletic supporter should be tried.
  2. If surgery is not indicated, no other interventions are needed.
C. Pharmacological therapy: None is recommended.

Follow-Up
A. After surgery, no follow-up is necessary if the client is taught scrotal self-examination.
B. If no surgery is performed, the client should be taught self-examination and instructed to return for pain or change in size and shape. *Refer to Client Teaching Guide: Testicular Self-Examination.*
C. Adolescents with varicoceles should be followed with annual objective measurements of testis size and/or semen analyses in order to detect the earliest sign of varicocele-related testicular injury.

Consultation/Referral
A. Refer the client to a urologist for surgical evaluation. Varicocelectomy is recommended in cases of pain and infertility, and it may be offered in the preadolescent to ensure proper testicular development.

Individual Considerations
A. Adults:
  1. New onset varicocele in older male may indicate a renal tumour.
B. Pediatrics:
  1. The young client with a varicocele should be followed every six months or yearly to see how the testis is growing.

Bibliography
Rovito, M. J., Cavayero, C., Leone, J. E., & Harlin, S. (2015). Interventions promoting testicular self-examination (TSE) performance: A systematic review. *American Journal of Men's Health*, *9*(6), 506–518. doi:10.1177/1557988314555360

The Testicular Cancer Resource Center. (2012, December 5). *How to do a testicular self examination*. Retrieved from http://tcrc.acor.org/tcexam.html

White, W. M. (2015, December 3). Varicocele. *Medscape*. Retrieved from http://emedicine.medscape.com/article/438591-overview

▶ Client Teaching Guides are available at https://connect.springerpub.com/content/reference-book/978-0-8261-9498-5

13 Obstetrics Guidelines

ANTEPARTUM

Preconception Counselling: Identifying Clients at Risk

Jill C. Cash, Susan Drummond, Kate Burkholder, Julie Johnson, and Susan Prendergast

A woman's health before conception influences her ability not only to conceive, but also to maintain pregnancy and to achieve a healthy outcome. Some women are unaware that their medical conditions, medications, occupational exposure, or social practices may have negative consequences in the earliest weeks of pregnancy, before the pregnancy test is positive. They do not know that organogenesis begins around 17 days after fertilization. Steps to provide the ideal environment for the developing foetus are most likely to be effective if they precede the traditional initiation of prenatal care.

The goal of preconceptional care is to reduce perinatal mortality and morbidity. Targeting only self-referred women who are planning their next conception or women referred with risk factors can result in a significant number of missed opportunities for primary prevention. Nurses working with women of childbearing age and their families have a responsibility to promote reproductive health during every health encounter. In Canada, the unintended pregnancy rate is nearly 64%; approximately 82% of teen pregnancies are unintended.

The preconception interview is the time to review primary care health issues. Topics of discussion should include status on immunizations; determination of hepatitis status; assessment of rubella immunity; Pap smears; cultures for sexually transmitted diseases (STDs); and reviewing history for chronic diseases, such as diabetes mellitus, hypertension, and lupus.

When discussing preconception plans, the client's history, as well as that of her partner, should be evaluated for poor health habits (alcohol, smoking, and drug use), exposure to toxic substances (radiation and chemicals), multiple sexual partners (risk of HIV, hepatitis, and sexually transmitted infections [STIs]), and racial or ethnic origin. Preconceptional evaluation should include the following:

A. Maternal age: Preeclampsia occurs at the extreme of ages, insulin-dependent diabetes increases with maternal age, and the risks of Down syndrome and other chromosomal abnormalities increase with age. Advanced maternal age is defined as 35 years of age at delivery. The Society of Obstetricians and Gynaecologists of Canada (SOGC) recommends counselling on genetic testing options for women of advanced maternal age.

B. Universal carrier screening is available for women who desire to know if they are carriers for an autosomal recessive disorder such as Tay–Sachs disease, sickle cell anaemia, or cystic fibrosis. Ideally, this blood test should be done preconceptionally, but it can be performed at any time during the pregnancy. If the screening test is positive, the woman's partner can then be tested.

C. Social issues: Screen all woman in all health-care settings for intimate partner violence (IPV). Research indicates that IPV often begins in pregnancy; this violence may increase in severity and frequency throughout pregnancy and also in the postpartum period. Screening for IPV should be done only if the partner is not present. Information (e.g., community, social, and legal resources) should be shared with the client. The immediate safety of the client and any children should be assessed. Based on this assessment, a safety plan should be discussed and developed with the client.

D. Financial issues: Discuss insurance, maternity benefits, work–leave policy, and contingency plans for lost wages because of pregnancy complications with the client.

E. Environmental and occupational considerations: Routine assessment of hobbies and home and employment environments may identify exposures that have been associated with adverse reproductive consequences that can be minimized in the preconceptual period.

F. Foetal effects are dependent on dose(s) and gestational age at exposure related to the following:

  1. Radiation: Foetal effects include microcephaly, intellectual disability, eye anomalies, intrauterine growth retardation (IUGR), and visceral malformations. Lead aprons should be used to protect the client from any radiation exposures.

  2. Heavy metals: Mercury exposure is related to brain damage and neuromuscular defects. Lead exposure is related to increased spontaneous abortion, low birth weight, brain damage, and increased premature rupture of membranes (PROM). Cadmium is retained by the foetal liver and kidney and is also associated with foetal craniofacial defects. Nickel is associated with neonatal deaths.

  3. Pesticides: Occupations at risk of pesticide exposure include, but are not limited to, the following: Ranch and farm workers (including migrant workers); gardeners (home and professional); groundskeepers; florists; structural pest control workers; hunting and fishing guides; health-care workers who deal with contamination; and people employed in pesticide production, mixing, and application. Dioxin is associated with an increased rate of spontaneous abortion, myelomeningocele, and limb defects. The pesticides dichlorodiphenyltrichloroethane (DDT) and dichlorodiphenyldichloroethylene (DDE) are associated with increased abortion, prematurity, low birth weight, and pregnancy-induced hypertension (PIH).

4. Other: Carbon monoxide is associated with increased stillbirths, neurologic deficits, seizures, spasticity, and retarded psychomotor development. Ozone is associated with increased spontaneous abortion and increased structural defects. Anaesthetic gases are associated with increased abortion, birth defects, low birth weight, and infertility.

G. Infectious diseases: See Chapter 15, Sexually Transmitted Infections Guidelines, and Chapter 16, Infectious Disease Guidelines.

H. Medications: Assess and minimize the risk of exposure to medications by reviewing the client's use of prescription and nonprescription drugs. Provide the client with information on the safest choices and the need to avoid drugs associated with foetal risks. Identify all prescription and nonprescription medications taken by the mother and partner to assess for risks to the foetus associated with current medications. Teratogenic defects linked to certain medications may include cleft lip and palate, congenital heart disease, microcephaly, caudal dysplasia, and caudal regression syndrome.

I. Medical problems: Health assessment of potential risk not only to the foetus but also to the woman, should she become pregnant, should be discussed. Care must be taken to identify and counsel all women whose life expectancy could be markedly reduced by pregnancy or whose foetus would have a high likelihood of complications. For example, women with known cardiac problems, epilepsy, transplanted organs, or uncontrolled diabetes and hypertension should be counselled about the risks associated with pregnancy.

1. Diabetes: Researchers have demonstrated a dose-related response between glycosylated haemoglobin (haemoglobin A1Cc) during the first trimester of pregnancy and the incidence of congenital defects: The better the glycaemic control, the lower the risk of birth defects. The preconceptional plan for diabetes includes the following:

   a. Change all clients on oral agents to insulin therapy before pregnancy is attempted:
      i. Achieve strict plasma glucose control. The SOGC and Diabetes Canada recommend self-glucose monitoring during pregnancy with the following glucose levels to be met:
         1) Fasting: ≤5.3 mmol/L.
         2) Preprandial glucose values <5.3 mmol/L.
         3) One-hour postprandial glucose levels <7.8 mmol/L.
         4) Two-hour postprandial glucose levels <6.7 mmol/L.
         5) Nighttime glucose levels should not drop below 60 mg/dL. Care should be taken to avoid hypoglycemia during pregnancy.
      ii. Aim for haemoglobin A1C 6.1% to 6.5 %.
      iii. Assess the client for vasculopathy, neuropathy, nephropathy, and retinopathy.
      iv. Refer the client for genetic and nutritional counselling.
      v. Enhance the woman's knowledge of diabetes during pregnancy.

J. Nutrition: Dietary evaluation and recommendations of alternatives that may benefit the foetus's development are important components of preconceptional counselling. Evaluation of nutritional status should include assessment of the appropriate weight for the client's height as well as a discussion of eating habits such as vegetarianism, fasting for religious or personal reasons, eating disorders, and the use of megavitamins. Discuss food hygiene and implications for foodborne infections. SOGC recommends folic acid for women with multiples, obesity of BMI >35, preexisting diabetes, previous infant with neural tube defects, and those taking anticonvulsants.

K. Obstetric considerations: Preconceptional reproductive history is an important tool for identifying factors that may be amenable to intervention. Review term, preterm, aborted (elective, spontaneous, and therapeutic) pregnancies, as well as a short history on living children. Review the gestational age at delivery of each neonate and any pregnancy and delivery complications. Preterm labour (PTL) has a 30% recurrence risk, and preeclampsia has a 5% to 65% recurrence rate in subsequent pregnancies. The higher rates are among those with severe features of the disease. In some instances, after preconceptual and genetic counselling, the couple may decide to forego pregnancy or to use assisted reproductive technologies such as donor eggs and/or sperm.

L. Recurrent loss: The workup and counselling for recurrent losses include evaluation for a uterine defect (septal or bicornuate uterus or uterus didelphys), endocrine problem (luteal phase defect or hypothyroidism), chromosomal defect, or presence of antiphospholipid syndrome. Antiphospholipid syndrome is defined as the presence of maternal anticardiolipin antibodies and/or lupus anticoagulant in association with recurrent pregnancy loss, thrombotic events, and/or thrombocytopaenia. Approximately 10% of women with unexplained recurrent pregnancy loss test positive for anticardiolipin antibodies and/or lupus anticoagulant. In the nonpregnant client, thrombosis of a single vessel is the most common complication associated with antiphospholipid syndrome.

M. Lifestyle: Queries regarding a woman's social lifestyle history should seek to identify behaviours and exposures that may compromise reproductive outcome. Although environmental exposures are a frequent concern of couples considering pregnancy, women should be informed that, in general, maternal use of alcohol, tobacco, and other mood-altering drugs is more hazardous for a foetus than most other lifestyle choices:

1. Alcohol: Alcohol is a known teratogen. There is no safe limit of alcohol use during pregnancy. Women should be informed that prenatal alcohol consumption is a preventable cause of birth defects and intellectual disability. Research indicates that as many as 73% of 12- to 34-year-old women expose their foetuses to alcohol at some time during pregnancy. Administer TWEAK screening tool for alcohol use (www.perinatalservicesbc.ca).

2. Smoking: Foetal effects of smoking are also related to the dose–response effect. Smoking is associated with an increase in bleeding in pregnancy (abruption and placenta previa), IUGR, preterm birth, low birth weight, stillbirth, respiratory distress in the neonate, and sudden infant death syndrome (SIDS). Counsel the client on smoking cessation. Suggestions of ways to quit include tapering the use of nicotine (tapering and brand switching to lower tar and nicotine), monitoring smoking behaviour, setting a contract to quit smoking, identifying

social support or a buddy, and restricting area(s) such as a no-smoking zone. Give the client positive reinforcement for behaviour change and cessation of the use of tobacco.

3. **Substance use:** If substance exposure is complicated by addiction, structured recovery programs are usually needed to effect behavioural change. Substance use/abuse is teratogenic to the foetus, and cessation of all substances is imperative before, during, and after pregnancy.

N. **Exercise:** Exercise and recreational activities should be reviewed and discussed relative to safety, including the use of bike helmets, avoiding strenuous exercise, and hyperthermia. The SOGC recommends that maternal heart rate (for pregnant women) not exceed 140 beats per minute (bpm). If the woman is not currently exercising, walking and swimming can be suggested. Heat exposure appears to be teratogenic. Use of saunas or hot tubs and high fevers in the first trimester have been associated with an increased risk of NTDs.

O. **Immunization:** The SOGC and Centers for Disease Control and Prevention (CDC) suggest a review of immunizations and strategies to update these prepregnancy. The following immune status should be reviewed:
1. Influenza.
2. Tdap (tetanus, diphtheria, and pertussis).
3. Varicella.
4. MMR (measles, mumps, and rubella).
5. Human papillomavirus (HPV).
6. Hepatitis A and B status.

P. **Mental health:** Maternal perinatal anxiety and worry are common; therefore, various screening tools such as Patient Health Questionnaire (PHQ9) and generalized anxiety disorder (GAD7) should be considered.

Preconception counselling helps to identify high-risk clients who need intensive care during pregnancy and delivery, and it identifies women who need referral for medical management, nutritional counselling, genetic counselling, or behaviour modification. Prescribe a prenatal vitamin daily for any woman considering pregnancy.

Bibliography

Compendium of Pharmaceuticals and Specialties. (2018). *Ergotamine maleate*. Retrieved from https://www.e-therapeutics.ca/
De-Regil, L. M., Peña-Rosas, J. P., Fernández-Gaxiola, A. C., & Rayco-Solon, P. (2015). Effects and safety of periconceptional oral folate supplementation for preventing birth defects. *Cochrane Database of Systematic Reviews*, 2015(2), CD007950. doi:10.1002/14651858.CD007950.pub3
Jovanovic, L., Savas, H., Mehta, M., Trujillo, A., & Pettitt, D. J. (2011). Frequent monitoring of A1C during pregnancy as a treatment tool to guide therapy. *Diabetes Care*, 34(1), 53–54. doi:10.2337/dc10-1455
Morbidity and Mortality Weekly Trend. (2013). *Preterm births—United States 2006–2010*. Retrieved from www.cdc.gov/mmwr/preview/mmwrhtml/su6203a22.htm
Nettina, S. (Ed.). (2013). *Lippincott manual of nursing practice* (10th ed.). Philadelphia, PA: Wolters Kluwer Health/Lippincott Williams & Wilkins.
O'Connor, D., Blake, J., Bell, R., Bowen, A., Callum, J., Fenton, S., . . . Rossiter, M. (2016). Canadian consensus on female nutrition: Adolescence, reproduction, menopause, and beyond. *The SOGC, Journal of Obstetrics and Gynecology Canada*, 38(6), 508–554. doi:10.1016/j.jogc.2016.01.001
Ontario Public Health Association. (2014). *Shift-Enhancing the health of Ontarians: A call to action for preconception health promotion and care*. Toronto, ON, Canada: Author.
Wilson, R. D. (2015). Pre-conception folic acid and multivitamin supplementation for the primary and secondary prevention of neural tube defects and other folic acid-sensitive congenital anomalies. *Journal of Obstetrics and Gynaecology Canada*, 37(6), 534–549. doi:10.1016/S1701-2163(15)30230-9
Wilson, R. D. (2018). Woman's pre-conception evaluation: Genetic and fetal risk considerations for counselling and informed choice. *Journal of Obstetrics and Gynaecology Canada*, 40(7), 935–949. doi:10.1016/j.jogc.2017.07.024

Routine Prenatal Care

Jill C. Cash, Susan Drummond, Kate Burkholder, Julie Johnson, and Susan Prendergast

Initial Prenatal Visit

The initial prenatal visit is a very important visit. A comprehensive health history is obtained; blood is drawn for baseline prenatal laboratory values to be established; and depending on the time, the physical examination may also be performed. Many practitioners have the client return in two weeks to perform the physical examination because of the amount of time needed for the history and collecting blood for laboratory tests. Another variation is to obtain the baseline lab tests (except ABO group and RH factor) after the first trimester (to avoid unnecessary testing in the event the client should have a miscarriage).

The initial visit is also a time for teaching the pregnant client. Literature and brochures on health promotion (i.e., breast self-examination, dietary recommendations, exercise, and smoking cessation) and information regarding the normal changes, discomforts, and concerns during pregnancy should be provided. Each province has a maternity/antepartum program that guides assessment, data collection and documentation, and client teaching. After-hours contact information should also be provided, along with contact information for labour and delivery. Reassure the client that as the pregnancy progresses, you will answer questions she may have; however, outside resources may also be beneficial for the client and her family. Encourage the client to enroll in childbirth education, sibling classes (if applicable), breastfeeding classes, and any other classes of interest to her and her partner.

Important information to cover is the client's medical and surgical history (including previous obstetric history), family genetic history, psychiatric disorders, contraception history, medications taken since the last menstrual period, menstrual history, social habits (smoking, substance abuse, and alcohol), environmental exposures (job, hobbies, etc.), exposure to abuse (mental, physical, and sexual), and sources of social support and health promotion (immunizations up to date, etc.).

Laboratory tests that are ordered at the initial examination include the following: Complete blood count (CBC), rubella and varicella titre, HIV (with the client's consent), syphilis (rapid plasma reagin [RPR] or Venereal Disease Research Laboratory [VDRL]), chlamydia and gonorrhea (urine or cervical), HBsAg, ABO group and RH factor, antibody screen, tuberculosis testing, urine culture and sensitivity, and bacterial vaginosis screen.

Optional tests include haemoglobin A1C, sickle cell screening, thyroid profile, and hepatitis C. Another test performed with the physical examination is a Pap smear; the SOGC states that cultures or urine and/or Pap smear (if not tested in the last 3 years) be obtained. Further optional tests include ferritin, to rule out anaemia; Tay–Sachs screen, if either partner is or may be of Ashkenazi Jewish (AJ) descent or an AJ carrier; HPLC (high-pressure liquid chromatography), for thalassemia; and haemoglobinopathy carrier screening for all women except those who are of Japanese, Korean, Indigenous, or Northern European Caucasian descent. Additional tests may be ordered throughout the pregnancy:

A. 15 to 20 weeks' gestation: Maternal serum multiple marker screening (quad screen; optional test per client wishes and father of baby and other family history).

B. 18 to 20 weeks' gestation: Obstetric ultrasonography.

C. 24 to 28 weeks' gestation: Screen all women for gestational diabetes through client history or clinical risk factors. Perform a 50 g glucose challenge; if abnormal, then 75 g oral glucose tolerance test (GTT). The alternate is a one-step approach of a 75 g oral GTT. According to Diabetes Canada, a diagnosis of GDM is made if one plasma glucose value is abnormal (fasting >5.1 mmol/L; 1 hour >10/0 mmol/L; 2 hours > 8.5 mmol/L.

D. 35 to 37 weeks' gestation: Vaginal culture for Group B *Streptococcus* infection. The Society of Obstetricians and Gynaecologists of Canada (SOGC) recommends universal screening for Group B *Streptococcus* infection at 36 weeks' gestation.

Neural Tube Defects

In about 90% of cases, neural tube defects (NTDs) are not expected on the basis of past history. NTDs are associated with multifactorial causes, including environmental factors, undernutrition (lack of folic acid), chromosomal defects, maternal hyperthermia, diabetes, clomiphene citrate induction, and maternal obesity.

Although white flour, ready-to-eat cereals, and fortified pasta and cornmeal in Canada contain folic acid, folic acid supplement at least one month before conception and during the first trimester of pregnancy is recommended. Women who have had a child with an NTD require higher doses of folic acid. The recurrence risk of NTD is 15% without the use of preconceptional doses of folic acid.

Genetic Screening

Genetic screening is recommended for all women. Genetic counselling for discussion of testing options is recommended if the mother is 35 years or older at the time of delivery, or if she has a family history of any abnormal genetic disorders such as Down's syndrome. The parents choose whether they would like to have genetic testing performed to evaluate the foetus for abnormal chromosomes. Although protocols vary across provinces, the following tests can be performed for genetic screening:

A. Chorionic villus sampling (CVS): Performed at 10 to 12 weeks' gestation.
B. Amniocentesis: Performed at 15 to 18 weeks' gestation.
C. Amniocentesis can also be performed to assess for spinal cord defects. The amniocentesis can detect elevated protein levels (alpha-foetoprotein and the presence of acetylcholinesterase) in the amniotic fluid that is present in the event of a spinal cord defect. Therefore, if performing an amniocentesis, information regarding genetic makeup and spinal cord defects can both be determined during the single procedure of the amniocentesis.
D. Noninvasive prenatal screening: Cell-free DNA from the foetus is found in maternal serum and can lead to prenatal identification of pregnancies at high risk of trisomy 13, 18, and 21, as well as detecting gender. This screen is a maternal blood test and can be done as early as 10 weeks. A positive screen should be confirmed with a diagnostic test such as CVS or amniocentesis.

Routine Prenatal Visits

The routine schedule of appointments includes a visit every 4 weeks until 28 weeks' gestation, every 2 weeks until 36 weeks' gestation, and then weekly until delivery.

A. Each visit should document the following:
  1. Weight.
  2. Blood pressure (BP).
  3. Fundal height, foetal heart tones, and foetal movement (should be detected by the client by 20 weeks).
  4. Urine: Protein and glucose.

B. Each visit should evaluate and discuss possible problems of pregnancy, such as preterm labour (PTL), vaginal bleeding, and so on. A few questions to ask at each visit include the following:
  1. Have you had any blurred vision, spots before your eyes, or epigastric pain?
  2. Have you had any headaches? If so, evaluate and note source of relief.
  3. Have you had any nausea or vomiting? If so, note source of relief.
  4. Have you had any abdominal pain, contractions, backache, pelvic pressure, or other pain?
  5. Have you had any vaginal bleeding, discharge, or leakage of fluid?
  6. Evaluate foetal movement, noting when movement was first felt (quickening) and daily foetal movement.
  7. Evaluate social support at home and in the work environment.
  8. Assess for substance use/abuse. If the client smokes, ask about current habits. Using a harm reduction approach, teach the client the effects of smoking on herself and the foetus (bleeding, intrauterine growth retardation [IUGR], and increased risk of miscarriage), and encourage smoking cessation. Screening tools such as TWEAK or CAGE can be used.
  9. Assess nutrition and dietary intake of recommended calories during pregnancy. Inquire if prenatal vitamins and folic acid are tolerated.
  10. Ask the client about her routine exercise program aiming for 150 minutes per week and tolerance of increased exercise during pregnancy.

Bibliography

American, A., Riley, L., Stark, A. R., Kilpatrick, S. J., & Riley, L. E. (2012). *Guidelines for perinatal care* (7th ed.). Elk Grove Village, IL: American College of Obstetricians and Gynecologists.

American College of Obstetricians and Gynecologists. (2005, September). The importance of preconception care in the continuum of women's health care. *ACOG Committee Opinion*, (313). reaffirmed 2015.

American College of Obstetricians and Gynecologists. (2010, August). Moderate caffeine consumption during pregnancy. *ACOG Committee Opinion*, (462). reaffirmed 2015.

American College of Obstetricians and Gynecologists. (2015a, September). Nausea and vomiting of pregnancy. *ACOG Practice Bulletin*, (153).

American College of Obstetricians and Gynecologists. (2015b, December). Obesity in pregnancy. *ACOG Practice Bulletin*, (156).

Black, A., Guilbert, E., Hassan, F., Chatziheofilou, I., Lowin, J., Jeddi, M., . . . Trusssell, J. (2015). The cost of unintended pregnancies in Canada: Estimating direct cost, role of imperfect adherence, and the potential impact of increased use of long-acting reversible contraceptives. *Journal of Obstetrics and Gynaecology Canada*, 37(12), 1086–1097.

Cash, J. C. (2014). Assessment of the childbearing woman. In J. Weber & J. Kelley (Eds.), *Health assessment in nursing* (5th ed., pp. 665–692). Philadelphia, PA: Lippincott-Raven.

Centers for Disease Control and Prevention. (2010). Prevention of perinatal Group B streptococcal disease. Revised guidelines from CDC. *Morbidity and Mortality Weekly Report*, 59(RR10), 1–32.

Compendium of Pharmaceuticals and Specialties. (2018). *Ergotamine maleate*. Retrieved from https://www.e-therapeutics.ca/

De-Regil, L. M., Peña-Rosas, J. P., Fernández-Gaxiola, A. C., & Rayco-Solon, P. (2015). Effects and safety of periconceptional oral folate supplementation for preventing birth defects. *Cochrane Database of Systemic Reviews*, 2015(2), CD007950. doi:10.1002/14651858.CD007950.pub3

Early Prenatal Care Summary and Checklist for Primary Care Providers. (2016, October). Retrieved from www.perinatalservicesbc.ca

Hale, T. W. (2014). *Medications and mother's milk* (16th ed.). Amarillo, TX: Hale

Jovanovic, L., Savas, H., Mehta, M., Trujillo, A., & Pettitt, D. J. (2011). Frequent monitoring of A1C during pregnancy as a treatment tool to guide therapy. *Diabetes Care*, 34(1), 53–54. doi:10.2337/dc10-1455

Nettina, S. (Ed.). (2013). *Lippincott manual of nursing practice* (10th ed.). Philadelphia, PA: Wolters Kluwer Health/Lippincott Williams & Wilkins.

O'Connor, D., Blake, J., Bell, R., Bowen, A., Callum, J., Fenton, S., . . . Rossiter, M. (2016). Canadian consensus on female nutrition: Adolescence, reproduction, menopause, and beyond. *The SOGC, Journal of Obstetrics and Gynecology Canada, 38*(6), 508–554. doi:10.1016/j.jogc.2016.01.001

Wilson, R. D. (2015). Pre-conception folic acid and multivitamin supplementation for the primary and secondary prevention of neural tube defects and other folic acid-sensitive congenital anomalies. *Journal of Obstetrics and Gynaecology Canada, 37*(6), 534–549. doi:10.1016/S1701-2163(15)30230-9

Wilson, R. D. (2018). Woman's pre-conception evaluation: Genetic and fetal risk considerations for counselling and informed choice. *Journal of Obstetrics and Gynaecology Canada, 40*(7), 935–949. doi:10.1016/j.jogc.2017.07.024

Anaemia, Iron Deficiency

Jill C. Cash, Susan Drummond, Kate Burkholder, Julie Johnson, and Susan Prendergast

Definition

A. Anaemia in pregnancy results from decreased serum iron. The iron-binding capacity is increased. Red blood cells (RBCs) are microcytic and hypochromic. The Guidelines and Protocols Advisory Committee, Iron Deficiency—Investigation and Management, Ministry of Health Services, British Columbia defines anaemia as the following:
- First trimester: Haemoglobin of <110 g/L.
- Second trimester: Haemoglobin <104 g/L.
- Third trimester: Haemoglobin <110 g/L.

Incidence/Prevalence

A. Anaemia is a common medical complication of pregnancy. Iron-deficiency anaemia constitutes 75% to 95% of pregnancy-related anaemias. The World Health Organization (WHO) estimates that 30% of reproductive-age women are anaemic and that over 40% of pregnant women globally have anaemia. This poses a global health problem.

Pathogenesis

A. Increased demand for iron during pregnancy occurs because of increased maternal blood volume. Haemoglobin (Hgb) and haematocrit (Hct) decrease during the first and second trimesters because of a greater expansion of plasma volume relative to the increase in RBC mass and usually increase during the third trimester when plasma expansion has ceased.

B. Another 0.5 to 1.0 mg/d of iron is needed for lactation. During most pregnancies, diet alone does not provide the necessary iron.

Predisposing Factors

A. Failure to take oral iron, often because of inability to tolerate oral iron supplements or financial constraints.
B. Socioeconomic status and nutritional status.
C. Multiple gestation increases iron requirement and may contribute to increased blood loss at delivery.
D. Diet high in phosphorus or foods such as tea, coffee, milk, soy, or carbonated beverages.
E. Alcoholism.
F. Low-iron and low-protein diet, eating nonfood items (pica), vegetarianism, veganism.
G. Not eating foods that help with absorption of iron (orange juice, broccoli, and strawberries).
H. History of gastrointestinal surgery (e.g., gastrectomy) or proton pump inhibitor (PPI) medications may cause iron malabsorption.
I. Chronic bleeding during pregnancy: Placenta previa, marginal sinus separation of placenta, haemorrhoidal bleeding, regular blood donors, frequent epistaxis, or chronic haematuria.
J. Short intervals between pregnancies.
K. Race: African Canadian females.
L. Age: Teenage girls.

Common Findings

A. Tiredness.
B. Inability to take prenatal vitamins because of nausea.
C. Bleeding problems (see section "Predisposing Factors").
D. Pica and pagophagia.

Other Signs and Symptoms

A. Fatigue.
B. Pale mucous membranes and skin.
C. Tachycardia.
D. Shortness of breath.
E. Lightheaded, syncopal.
F. Weakness.
G. Headache.
H. Alopecia.
I. Angular cheilitis.
J. Atrophic glossitis.
K. Koilonychias (spoon nails).
L. Restless legs syndrome.

Subjective Data

A. Elicit the onset, duration, and course of presenting symptoms.
B. Elicit information about the client's "typical" dietary intake for meals and snacks, and review pica (eating clay, starch, ice, and other nonnutritive substances).
C. Review the client's intake of prenatal vitamins and supplemental iron. How often does she take iron? Elicit the reason for skipping the supplemental iron (nausea, constipation), if applicable.
D. Review the client's history of gastrointestinal surgeries; irritable bowel syndrome (IBS); and inflammatory bowel diseases such as Crohn's disease, colitis, or celiac disease.
E. Review the client's history for any type of anaemia and previous treatment, including blood transfusions and frequency of blood donation (no more than twice per year).
F. Review pregnancy history for closely spaced pregnancies (two in a calendar year) and multiple gestation.
G. Review the client's intake of medications for the use of ASA and other nonsteroidal anti-inflammatory drugs (NSAIDs) and PPI medications.

Physical Examination

A. Check pulse and BP: Note postural hypotension and tachycardia.
B. Inspect General appearance:
   1. Inspect the skin, mucous membranes, and conjunctivae for pallor.
   2. Observe the mouth and tongue: Note atrophy of papillae and smooth, beefy red appearance of tongue with anaemia.
   3. Note dryness of skin. Inspect texture of nails (brittle, spoon-shaped, concave); inspect the hair for brittleness.
C. Palpate the abdomen for masses; assess fundal height.
D. Auscultate the heart for systolic flow murmurs; auscultate lungs.

Diagnostic Tests
A. Blood work: Hgb/Hct:
1. First trimester: Haemoglobin of <110g/L.
2. Second trimester: Haemoglobin <104 g/L.
3. Third trimester: Haemoglobin <110 g/L.

B. Peripheral blood smear: Note microcytic and hypochromic RBCs on peripheral smear.
C. Sickle cell screen, if applicable.
D. Serum iron: Low with anaemia.
E. Iron-binding capacity: High iron-binding capacity with anaemia.
F. Transferrin: Saturation <15%.
G. Stool for occult blood, if applicable.
H. Emesis for presence of blood, if applicable.

Differential Diagnoses
A. Normal physiological anaemia of pregnancy: During normal pregnancy, concentrations of erythrocytes and Hgb usually fall because of the greater increase in plasma volume (increased by 45%) relative to the increase in erythrocyte volume (increased by 25%).
B. Megaloblastic anaemia: This condition is commonly associated with iron-deficiency anaemia and is rarely seen alone. May be seen with other deficiencies such as folate, B12, hypothyroidism, and chronic kidney disease.
C. Haemolytic anaemia: Sickle cell anaemia, thalassaemia, hereditary spherocytosis, and erythrocyte enzyme deficiency.
D. Aplastic anaemia: Bone marrow failure.
E. Haematologic malignancies: Leukaemia and lymphoma.
F. Clotting factor or other haemostatic deficiencies: von Willebrand's disease, idiopathic thrombocytopaenia (ITP), and disseminated intravascular coagulation (DIC).

Plan
A. Do initial evaluation of Hgb and Hct at first prenatal visit; repeat at 24- to 28-week blood draw with diabetes testing. Treat if inadequate iron stores (ferritin) and reassess in 2 to 3 weeks.
B. Diet counselling and nutrition consultation:
1. Advise the client to take supplemental iron in addition to prenatal vitamins. If she is unable to tolerate prenatal vitamins, suggest a children's chewable vitamin.
2. Encourage the client to continue iron supplementation through the first month postpartum and throughout breastfeeding.

C. Client teaching.
D. Pharmacological therapy:
1. Prophylaxis: Oral iron supplements are recommended for all gestations with elemental iron, or ferrous sulphate. Time-release tablets may help, but are more expensive.
2. Most prenatal vitamins contain supplemental iron. Therefore, if the woman is taking vitamin supplements, she may need only a lower dosage of iron supplement. Nausea and vomiting occur in 20% to 25% of clients. These side effects are dose related. Have the client alter times of administration of the iron supplement to determine when the iron is best tolerated. To enhance tolerance, start with a lower dose and gradually increase after four to five days. Take on empty stomach or to minimize GI symptoms after meals, Take with vitamin C–rich foods or beverages or ascorbic acid tabs to aid in absorption.
3. Treatment: With iron-deficiency anaemia, three times the prophylactic dose of iron should be given,.
4. Intramuscular (IM) or intravenous (IV) iron may be ordered for the small proportion of clients who do not tolerate oral iron because of gastrointestinal complaints, malabsorption syndrome, or noncompliance with the oral iron regimen.

Follow-Up
A. Carry out routine prenatal and postpartum follow-up care. When the client begins taking the recommended dose of supplemental iron, the RBC response can be measured in two weeks by an elevation in her reticulocyte count.
B. Repeat Hct after four to six weeks of therapy.
C. If no improvement is seen in reticulocyte count or Hct after four weeks of therapy and the client has been compliant, another cause of anaemia should be investigated.

Consultation/Referral
A. Consider consult with a specialist if Hgb is <90 g/L or Hct is ≤27% and does not improve with the aforementioned treatments.

Bibliography
American College of Obstetricians and Gynecologists. (2008, July). Anemia in pregnancy. *ACOG Practice Bulletin*, (95). reaffirmed 2015.
Anemia Review Panel. (2014). *Anemia guidelines for family medicine* (2014th ed.). Toronto, ON, Canada: MUMS Guidelines.
Auerbach, M., & Landy, H. (2018). Anemia in Pregnancy. *UpToDate*. Retrieved from www.uptodate.com
Guidelines and Protocols Advisory Committee. (2010, June). Iron deficiency—Investigation and management. Retrieved from https://www2.gov.bc.ca/gov/content/health/practitioner-professional-resources/bc-guidelines
Iron Deficiency Anemia Clinical Practice Guideline. (2018, March). *Toward optimized practice*. Retrieved from http://www.topalbertadoctors.org/cpgs/
Nettina, S. (Ed.). (2013). *Lippincott manual of nursing practice* (10th ed.). Philadelphia, PA: Wolters Kluwer Health/Lippincott Williams & Wilkins.
O'Connor, D., Blake, J., Bell, R., Bowen, A., Callum, J., Fenton, S., . . . Rossiter, M. (2016). Canadian consensus on female nutrition: Adolescence, reproduction, menopause, and beyond. *The SOGC, Journal of Obstetrics and Gynecology Canada*, 38(6), 508–554. doi:10.1016/j.jogc.2016.01.001

Gestational Diabetes Mellitus

Jill C. Cash, Susan Drummond, Kate Burkholder, Julie Johnson, and Susan Prendergast

Definition
A. Gestational diabetes mellitus (GDM) is defined as "glucose intolerance first recognized in pregnancy" (CDG, 2018, p. S256).

Incidence/Prevalence
A. It is estimated that up to 6% of births in Canada are complicated by diabetes mellitus (DM) and approximately 90% of these cases represent women with GDM. GDM usually resolves after pregnancy.

Pathogenesis
A. Insulin antagonism caused by the placental hormones leads to gestational diabetes. As greater amounts of these hormones are produced with advancing gestation, the diabetogenic effect of pregnancy becomes more pronounced, reaching significant levels in the second trimester. Women with GDM are at risk of later development of type 1 and, more commonly, type 2 diabetes. GDM may actually be the expression of pregnancy-induced stresses on carbohydrate metabolism in the genetically predisposed client. It is estimated that up to 50% of women with GDM will develop

DM within approximately 25 years of the pregnancy. Some women have undiagnosed type 2 diabetes before pregnancy.

Predisposing Factors
A. Members of any of the following ethnic groups:
  1. African.
  2. Arab.
  3. Asian.
  4. Hispanic.
  5. Indigenous.
  6. South Asian.
B. Maternal age >35 years.
C. Obesity (body mass index [BMI]) >30).
D. Polycystic ovary syndrome.
E. Previous birth of an infant >4 kg.
F. Prediabetes.
G. Gestational diabetes in a previous pregnancy.
H. Parent or sibling with diabetes.

Common Findings
A. Common complaints of hyperglycaemia include polydipsia, polyuria, fatigue, and blurred vision. However, gestational diabetes is often asymptomatic.

Other Signs and Symptoms
A. Glycosuria.
B. Size of foetus greater than average for gestational age.
C. Frequent candidal infections.
D. Rapid weight gain.

Potential Complications
A. Ketoacidosis:
  1. May develop in GDM.
  2. More common in insulin-dependent diabetes.
  3. May develop with glucose levels as low as 11.09 mmol/L.
  4. May be present in an undiagnosed diabetic woman receiving beta-mimetic agents (such as terbutaline) for tocolysis or steroids to enhance foetal lung maturity. Foetal mortality rate is 10% in women who come to the hospital in diabetic ketoacidosis (DKA). Glucose and ketones cross the placenta.
  5. Management hinges on timely, aggressive volume resuscitation and correction of maternal metabolic derangements.
B. Polyhydramnios.
C. Increased risk of neonatal morbidity, such as hypoglycaemia, hyperbilirubinemia, polycythaemia, respiratory distress because of delayed lung maturity, and/or traumatic birth injury related to shoulder dystocia, which is associated with macrosomia.
D. Increased risk for stillbirth—risk is related primarily to poor glycaemic control.

Subjective Data
A. Review previous pregnancy history for two or more spontaneous abortions, previous stillbirths, or unexplained neonatal deaths.
B. Review birth weight (macrosomia) and gestational age of previous children.
C. Review previous pregnancy history for polyhydramnios and/or congenital anomalies.
D. Review the client's history for a predisposition to infections, especially urinary tract infections (UTIs) and candidal vaginitis and for family history of diabetes.
E. Review previous pregnancy history for gestational diabetes, diet restrictions, and need for insulin therapy.

Physical Examination
A. Check blood pressure (BP), pulse, and weight.
B. Inspect: Perform speculum examination for wet prep, if indicated.
C. Palpate: Check the client's fundal height each visit after 12 weeks' gestation.
D. Auscultate foetal heart tones after 10 to 12 weeks' gestation.

Screening/Diagnostic Tests
Women who have risk factors for diabetes or with a history of GDM should be screened during the first trimester using the glycosylated haemoglobin (haemoglobin A1C). Universal screening for all women is recommended between 24 and 28 weeks' gestation:
A. Perform "two-step" one-hour 50 g (nonfasting) OGTT followed by a three-hour 75 g (fasting) OGTT for positive results or "one-step" two-hour 75 g (fasting) OGTT.
B. Urine dipstick for glucose: Early glycosuria needs further evaluation (i.e., haemoglobin A1Cc, GDM screen as earlier).
C. Ultrasonography if foetal size is greater than average for gestational date to rule out twins, and polyhydramnios.

Differential Diagnoses
A. Gestational diabetes:
  1. DM (type 1).
  2. DM (type 2).

Plan
A. General interventions:
  1. Diabetes Canada (2018) recommends that all pregnant women be screened for diabetes.
    a. Diabetes mellitus screen (DMS): "Two-step" 1-hour 50 g (nonfasting) oral GTT followed by a two-hour 75 g oral glucose tolerance test (OGTT) for positive results.
      i. Administer 50 g oral glucose load (fasting not required).
      ii. Draw blood for glucose assessment 1 hour after glucose load is given.
      iii. Typically performed between 24 and 28 weeks' gestation; performed earlier if the client has glycosuria, risk factors, advanced maternal age, or if foetal size is greater than average for gestational date by fundal height measurement.
      iv. Abnormal result is a glucose level >7.8 mmol/L.
      v. Follow up all abnormal results with a two-hour GTT.
      vi. Abnormal result is as follows: (a) Fasting = >5.1 mmol/L; (b) one hour plasma glucose (PG) = >10.6 mmol/L; and (c) 2 hour PG = >9.0 mmol/L client.
      vii. If one abnormal value, diagnosis is gestational diabetes.
    b. "One step" two-hour 75 g OGTT:
      i. Draw fasting blood glucose first.
      ii. Administer 75 g glucose load.
      iii. Draw blood for glucose assessment at one and two hours after glucose load is given.
      iv. Plasma or serum glucose results.
        1) Fasting = >5.1 mmol/L.
        2) One hour = >10.0 mmol/L.
        3) Two hours = 8.5 mmol/L.

v. If one abnormal value, diagnosis is gestational diabetes.
Note: "One-step" two-hour 75 mg OGTT may be performed instead of the "two-step" approach.
2. Antepartum testing:
   a. For women with well-controlled GDM, it is suggested that more frequent foetal assessment should be considered with either the nonstress test (NST) or biophysical profile (BPP) beginning at 32 to 34 weeks.
   b. For women with insulin-dependent gestational diabetes or whose condition is not well controlled, weekly testing with either the NST or BPP beginning at 32 weeks is recommended. If a client's diabetes is poorly controlled, consider foetal assessment earlier and more frequently.
3. Serial ultrasonography:
   a. Evaluate foetal growth, estimate foetal weight, and detect polyhydramnios and malformations.
   b. Repeat at 4- to 6-week intervals to assess growth.
   c. Due to the increased risk of stillbirth, shoulder dystocia, and cesarean section for women with GDM, induction of labour should be offered at 38 to 40 weeks' gestation based on glycaemic control and presence of other comorbid factors.
4. Postpartum contraception:
   a. Low-dose oral contraceptives (OCs) may be used in women with GDM who do not have other risk factors.
   b. Rate of subsequent diabetes in OC users is not significantly different from those who do not use OCs.
   c. Consider serial measurement of total cholesterol, low-density lipoprotein, high-density lipoprotein, and triglycerides.
5. Notify nursery staff of perinatal diabetes history, especially if the client has a history of insulin-dependent diabetes, so that the neonate can be carefully monitored for hypoglycemia.

B. Client teaching: GDM requires intensive client and family education to help reduce perinatal complications:
1. Exercise:
   a. If the client had an active lifestyle before pregnancy, encourage her to continue a program of exercise approved for pregnancy, such as walking or swimming for 20 minutes per day.
   b. Upper extremity exercise in previously sedentary women with GDM may improve glycaemic control.
2. Instruct the client in self-monitoring blood glucose.
   a. Have her take measurement pre- or postprandially, or both. Preprandial values are typically taken if on insulin. Fasting and postprandial values may be taken if the client is diet controlled. Diabetes Canada blood glucose guidelines for women with GDM are the following:
      i. Fasting and before meals: <5.3 mmol/L.
      ii. One hour after meals: <7.8 mmol/L.
      iii. Two hours after meals: <6.7 mmol/L.
      The haemoglobin A1C goal is <7%.
   b. If the client is taking multiple doses of insulin, she may need to take measurements more frequently.

C. Dietary management: All women who are living with diabetes during pregnancy should be supported by a multidisciplinary team including registered dietician, diabetic nurse educator, birth care provider, and possibly endocrinologist. Women living with diabetes should be encouraged to eat a healthy, well-balanced diet and to monitor weight gain as per the Institute of Medicine Guidelines by prepregnancy BMI.

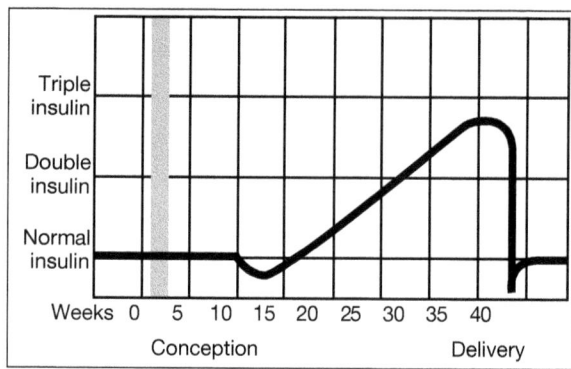

FIGURE 13.1 Insulin requirement during pregnancy.

D. Pharmacological therapy:
1. Insulin therapy is recommended if dietary management does not achieve glycaemic targets within one to two weeks. Two-hour postprandial values should be <6.7 mmol/L.
2. Oral antidiabetic medications, metformin and glyburide, are being used as second- and third-line agents, respectively. Metformin inhibits hepatic gluconeogenesis and glucose absorption and stimulates glucose uptake in peripheral tissues. Glyburide results in increased insulin secretion and insulin sensitivity at the tissue level.
3. Insulin therapy must respond to the changing insulin requirements during pregnancy. Women with relatively simple insulin programs when not pregnant may require more complex regimens as the pregnancy progresses.
4. Intensive insulin therapy (as opposed to conventional therapy) is often required in pregnancy.
5. Human insulin is preferred to animal or synthetic insulin.
6. The blood glucose values should be evaluated at least weekly to adjust to the client's changing needs.

Follow-Up
A. Weekly evaluation of blood glucose.
B. Foetal assessment:
C. For women who develop diabetes during pregnancy, give the client a 75 g glucose load to evaluate for the development of type 2 diabetes at the return postpartum visit at six weeks after delivery. These women should be screened at least every three years from then on. Encourage lifestyle changes to prevent the development of diabetes (Figure 13.1).

Consultation/Referral
A. Consult or comanage the client with a specialist as indicated and if GDM is not controlled by diet and exercise.
B. Refer to a registered dietitian for nutritional education and support for carbohydrate counting and to assist the client with dietary and lifestyle changes needed for tight glucose control.

Bibliography
American College of Obstetricians and Gynecologists. (2013, August). Gestational diabetes mellitus. *ACOG Practice Bulletin*, (137). reaffirmed 2015.
American College of Obstetricians and Gynecologists. (2015, December). Obesity in pregnancy. *ACOG Practice Bulletin*, (156).
American Diabetes Association. (2016). Standards of medical care in diabetes—2016. *Diabetes Care, 39*(Suppl. 1), S4–S5. doi:10.2337/dc16-S003

Bell, R., Glinianaia, S. V., Tennant, P. W., Rankin, J., & Bilous, R. W. (2012). Peri-conception hyperglycaemia and nephropathy are associated with risk of congenital anomaly in women with pre-existing diabetes: A population-based cohort study. *Diabetologia, 55*, 936–947. doi:10.1007/s00125-012-2455-y

Black, A., Guilbert, E., Hassan, F., Chatziheofilou, I., Lowin, J., Jeddi, M., . . . Trusssell, J. (2015). The cost of unintended pregnancies in Canada: Estimating direct cost, role of imperfect adherence, and the potential impact of increased use of long-acting reversible contraceptives. *Journal of Obstetrics and Gynaecology Canada, 37*(12), 1086–1097.

Feig, D., Berger, H., Donovan, L., Godbout, A., Kader, T., Keely, E., & Sanghera, R. (2018). Diabetes and pregnancy. *Canadian Journal of Diabetes, 42*, S255–S282. doi:10.1016/j.jcjd.2018.04.006

Jovanovic, L., Savas, H., Mehta, M., Trujillo, A., & Pettitt, D. J. (2011). Frequent monitoring of A1C during pregnancy as a treatment tool to guide therapy. *Diabetes Care, 34*(1), 53–54. doi:10.2337/dc10-1455

Nettina, S. (Ed.). (2013). *Lippincott manual of nursing practice* (10th ed.). Philadelphia, PA: Wolters Kluwer Health/Lippincott Williams & Wilkins.

Preeclampsia

Jill C. Cash, Susan Drummond, Kate Burkholder, Julie Johnson, and Susan Prendergast

Definition

Preeclampsia (antiquated term *toxaemia*) is hypertension with proteinuria that develops during pregnancy and lasts or develops up to 6 weeks' postpartum. In the absence of proteinuria, any of the following can establish the diagnosis: New-onset thrombocytopaenia, impaired liver function, renal insufficiency, pulmonary oedema, or visual or cerebral disturbances.

Hypertension is defined as the following:
A. Either a systolic blood pressure (BP) >140 mmHg or a diastolic BP >90 mmHg or both or, an increase from the client's normal BP of 30 mmHg systolic or diastolic or both. The values must be elevated on at least two separate occasions at least 4 hours apart. Severity of hypertension is not necessarily associated with the severity of preeclampsia.
B. Eclampsia, or the occurrence of grand mal seizures, in a client with preeclampsia.
C. Chronic hypertension in pregnancy is often complicated by superimposed preeclampsia.

Incidence/Prevalence

A. Hypertensive disorders are the most common medical complication of pregnancy, with a reported incidence of up to 10% worldwide. Incidence varies among different regions and countries. The risk of recurrent preeclampsia is between 5% and 70%. Women who develop severe features of preeclampsia before 30 weeks' gestation have the highest risk of preeclampsia in future pregnancies.

Pathogenesis

A. The aetiology of preeclampsia is unknown, although several theories exist. Generalized vascular endothelial damage is a hallmark of the pathophysiologic responses.

Predisposing Factors

A. Nulliparity.
B. Chronic hypertension.
C. Age extremes (< 18 years and > 35 years).
D. Race (black women are at higher risk).
E. Diabetes mellitus.
F. Renal disease.
G. Family history of preeclampsia in a sister or mother.
H. Previous pregnancy with preeclampsia.
I. Multiple gestation.
J. Hydatidiform mole.
K. Obesity.

Common Findings

A. Headache unrelieved by analgesics.
B. Right upper quadrant (RUQ) pain.
C. Severe heartburn unrelieved by antacids.
D. Nausea and vomiting.
E. Oedema: Peripheral and/or facial.
F. Visual disturbances.
G. Photophobia.

Other Signs and Symptoms

A. Hypertension (BP of 140 mmHg systolic or greater or 90 mmHg diastolic or greater that occurs after 20 weeks' gestation in a woman without a previous history of hypertension).

First-trimester signs of preeclampsia need ultrasonographic evaluation for the presence of a gestational trophoblastic disease (molar pregnancy) as well as the other differential diagnoses.

B. Proteinuria: Urinary excretion of 0.3 g protein or greater in 24-hour urine specimen.
C. Brisk deep tendon reflexes (DTRs) or clonus.

Potential Complications

A. Multiple organ involvement.
B. HELLP syndrome (haemolysis, elevated liver enzymes, and low platelets).
C. Eclampsia, which may lead to maternal demise.
D. Foetal complications: Intrauterine growth retardation (IUGR), oligohydramnios, abruptio placenta.

Subjective Data

A. Elicit information about headaches, their onset and duration, the progression of headache, and/or other symptoms.
B. What part of the head hurts? Differentiate headache from sinus headache. Note severity and any relief measure tried (acetaminophen, massage, sleep).
C. Is the headache "new"? Does the client have a previous history of migraines? Is this like a previous migraine?
D. What are other concurrent symptoms: Nausea, vomiting, RUQ pain, and visual changes?
E. Question the client about oedema. If oedema is present, has it significantly worsened over the past few days? Has she been able to wear rings up to this point? Has she had to wear different shoes because of pedal oedema?
F. What are the client's usual weight and today's weight (on the same scales)? Has she gained more than 1 kg in one week?
G. Ask specifics about RUQ pain, sometimes identified as "severe heartburn." Note the duration, severity, and relief measures tried. Have the client point to the area of discomfort (midsternum or under right breast).
H. Are there any visual disturbances, such as black dots she can't see through?
I. Review other gastrointestinal symptoms such as diarrhoea, abdominal pain, and gallbladder attack.
J. Review for signs of fever and thyroid storm.
K. Review the client's history for seizures.

Physical Examination

A. Check temperature, BP, pulse and respirations, weight, and foetal heart tones.
B. Inspect:
  1. Check pedal, hand, and facial oedema.
  2. Check fundal height.
C. Palpate:
  1. The abdomen, noting any hepatosplenomegaly and RUQ tenderness to the palpation.
  2. The lower extremities for pitting oedema.
D. Percuss:
  1. Gently check for liver enlargement.
  2. Perform neurologic examination for hyperreflexia: Check DTR and clonus.
E. Auscultate:
  1. The heart and lungs.
  2. The foetal heart tones.

Diagnostic Tests

A. Complete blood count (CBC) and platelets.
B. Liver profile (alanine aminotransferase [ALT] and aspartate aminotransferase [AST]).
C. Renal workup:
  1. Uric acid, serum creatinine, and urine protein.
  2. Urine culture if proteinuria is present to rule out urinary tract infection (UTI).
  3. Collect 24-hour urine for total protein and creatinine clearance.
D. Ultrasonography, if indicated, to rule out IUGR and/or oligohydramnios.

Differential Diagnoses

A. Gestational hypertension.
B. Hyperemesis gravidarum.
C. Infection: Appendicitis, gastroenteritis, pyelonephritis, glomerulonephritis, hepatitis, and pancreatitis.
D. Acute fatty liver of pregnancy.
E. Systemic lupus erythematosus.
F. Haemolytic uraemic syndrome.
G. Hepatic encephalopathy.
H. Gastrointestinal disorder: Peptic ulcer and heartburn.
I. Thrombotic or idiopathic thrombocytopaenia purpura (ITP).
J. Gallbladder disease.
K. Chronic hypertension.
L. Thyroid storm.

Plan

A. General interventions:
  1. Any client with an elevated BP should be reassessed in the lateral recumbent position, using proper cuff size, after the client is allowed to relax for several minutes before BP measurement.
  2. If the client's BP begins to rise above baseline values:
    a. Advise the client to maintain a modified bed rest schedule (stop working).
    b. Recommend frequent BP evaluation at home.
    c. See the client weekly or biweekly for further maternal and neonatal assessment; administer nonstress test (NST) and take biophysical profile (BPP) if appropriate.
  3. If hypertension and proteinuria are present, refer the client to an obstetrician or perinatologist for further assessment and management. She may need immediate admission to the hospital for inpatient management or delivery.
  4. If the client has a grand mal seizure, the primary consideration is to protect her. Monitor seizure type and duration. Call for immediate transport to the hospital labour and delivery unit. Place the client in the lateral recumbent position following the seizure.
  5. Immediately transfer the client to a hospital for eclampsia after stabilization.
B. Client teaching:
  1. Educate the client regarding her diagnosis and the importance of controlling her BP to prevent complications.
  2. Stress the importance of bed rest and foetal surveillance with NST or BPP to closely monitor the client and her foetus to reach the goal of a safe, healthy delivery.
  3. Discuss dietary recommendations for pregnancy. Salt restriction does not stop swelling and high BP problems in pregnancy.
C. Pharmacological therapy:
  1. Diuretics are *not* prescribed during pregnancy for oedema.
  2. Angiotensin-converting enzyme (ACE) inhibitors and angiotensin II receptor blockers (ARBs) are not recommended during pregnancy because of the teratogenic effects on the foetus that may occur, such as renal dysgenesis and/or foetal death.
  3. Methyldopa is commonly used during pregnancy to control chronic or superimposed hypertension during pregnancy.
  4. Inpatient therapy is determined by a specialist and may include the following:
    a. Magnesium sulphate for seizure prophylaxis.
    b. Hydralazine or labetalol are first-line antihypertensive agents if a client's diastolic BP is >110 mmHg.
    c. Corticosteroids may be given to enhance foetal lung maturity before delivery in clients between 24 and 34 weeks' gestation and may be considered in clients between 23 and 24 weeks' gestation.
    d. In preeclampsia with severe features, therapy may include cervical ripening agents, such as prostaglandins or misoprostol, and/or oxytocin induction of labour.
    e. Narcotics may be used for severe headaches.
    f. Diazepam and phenytoin are not recommended for seizures in pregnancy. There is increased risk of recurrent seizures.

Follow-Up

A. The only "cure" for preeclampsia is delivery. See the client one week after delivery for BP assessment, or sooner if symptoms persist.

Consultation/Referral

A. If the client is diagnosed with preeclampsia, refer her to a specialist for continued care and delivery.

Bibliography

American College of Obstetricians and Gynecologists. (2015, December). Obesity in pregnancy. *ACOG Practice Bulletin*, (156).

American College of Obstetricians and Gynecologists Task Force on Hypertension in Pregnancy. (2013). *Hypertension in pregnancy*. Washington, DC: American College of Obstetricians and Gynecologists.

Barton, J. R., & Sibai, B. M. (2008). Prediction and prevention of recurrent preeclampsia. *Obstetrics & Gynecology, 112*(2 Pt. 1), 359–372. doi:10.1097/AOG.0b013e3181801d56

Nettina, S. (Ed.). (2013). *Lippincott manual of nursing practice* (10th ed.). Philadelphia, PA: Wolters Kluwer Health/Lippincott Williams & Wilkins.

Preterm Labour

Jill C. Cash, Susan Drummond, Kate Burkholder, Julie Johnson, and Susan Prendergast

Definition
A. Preterm labour (PTL) is labour that produces documented cervical changes after 20 weeks and before 37 completed weeks of gestation.

Incidence/Prevalence
A. PTL occurs in approximately 8% of births in Canada and precedes approximately 70% of the preterm births.

Pathogenesis
A. Infection and ischaemia are common causes of PTL. Infection may originate from several sites, including the bladder, kidney(s), cervix, uterus, gastrointestinal tract, and upper respiratory tract. Ischaemia may be caused by decreased oxygen delivery to the uterus because of maternal hypoxia, hypovolemia, or vena caval compression. Overdistension of the uterus in the presence of polyhydramnios or multiple gestation may cause PTL symptoms. However, in most cases, the cause is unknown.

Predisposing Factors
A. Previous PTL or preterm delivery.
B. Premature rupture of membranes (PROM).
C. Uterine anomalies, surgery, and fibroids.
D. Multiple gestation.
E. History of second-trimester abortion(s).
F. Incompetent cervix.
G. History of cone biopsy.
H. Recurrent urinary tract and kidney infections.
I. Polyhydramnios.
J. Macrosomic foetus.
K. Maternal age extremes.
L. Placenta previa.
M. Abruptio placentae.
N. Poor nutritional status and low prepregnancy weight.
O. Maternal dehydration.
P. Maternal race (occurs more frequently in African American population).
Q. Low socioeconomic status.
R. Inadequate prenatal care.
S. Anaemia.
T. Substance use/abuse (smoking, drug, and alcohol).
U. Vaginal infection.
V. Presence of foetal fibronectin, a protein produced by the trophoblast and other foetal tissues, has been noted in cervical–vaginal secretions between 24 and 34 weeks' gestation in a subgroup of women who are at increased risk for preterm birth.
W. Short cervical length.
X. Short interpregnancy interval.

Common Findings
A. Abdominal pain or cramping.
B. Low backache.
C. Increase or change in vaginal discharge, "gush" of fluid, loss of mucus plug, and bloody show or vaginal spotting.
D. Diarrhoea.
E. "Something's not right."

Other Signs and Symptoms
A. Pelvic pressure.
B. Contractions or period-like cramps.

Subjective Data
A. Elicit information about the onset, frequency, duration, and course of cramps/contractions; presence or absence of backache; how long these symptoms have existed; and whether symptoms began subsequent to a certain event or activity. What, if anything, makes these symptoms better or worse?
B. Question the client about colour, odour, consistency, and amount of vaginal discharge or bleeding: Was there a spot the size of a quarter or a loonie? Has she been wearing a perineal pad? How often does she have to change the pad? Is the pad soaked with blood when she changes it?
C. For foetuses older than 18 weeks' gestation, question the client about frequency of foetal movements.
D. Question the client about urinary frequency and the presence of urgency or dysuria.
E. Question the client about recent sexual activity (i.e., has there been recent intercourse?).
F. If the client complains of diarrhoea, ask her if she has a fever and if anyone else in the family is ill.

Physical Examination
A. Check temperature, blood pressure (BP), and foetal heart tones.
B. Inspect: Note general appearance of discomfort.
C. Palpate:
   1. Abdomen: Note presence, frequency, intensity of uterine contractions, and resting tone. Measure fundal height.
   2. Back: Check for costovertebral angle (CVA) tenderness.
D. Auscultate the heart and lungs.
E. Sterile speculum examination: Evaluate rupture of membranes and vaginal discharge or bleeding. If meconium-stained amniotic fluid is noted, immediately consult a specialist and transfer the client to a hospital. Note whether meconium is thin or thick (thick meconium may be associated with breech presentation).
F. Bimanual examination: If membranes are not ruptured, perform gentle bimanual examination: Note cervical dilation, effacement, station, and cervical position.
G. Cervical examination during pregnancy: Do not perform a digital examination of the cervix if membranes are ruptured without active labour.

Diagnostic Tests
A. White blood cell (WBC), if indicated.
B. Urine dipstick for ketones, leukocyte, esterase, protein, and nitrite.
C. Evaluate vaginal discharge for pH with phenaphthazine (nitrazine) tape.
D. Check ferning if discharge is nitrazine positive or if PROM is suspected.
E. Wet prep, if indicated.
F. Cervical cultures for sexually transmitted diseases (STDs).
G. Cervical and rectal culture for Group B *Streptococcus*.
H. Foetal fibronectin, where available. Candidates for foetal fibronectin testing must meet the following criteria:
   1. Intact foetal membranes.
   2. Cervical dilation < 3 cm.

3. Gestational age 22 and 0/7th weeks to 34 6/7th weeks.
4. Nothing in the vagina in the preceding 24 hours.
I. Urine culture.
J. Ultrasonography: Foetal biometry and dating, cervical length, amniotic fluid volume, biophysical profile (BPP), placental location, foetal presentation, ruling out foetal anomalies.
K. Electronic foetal monitoring for contractions.

Differential Diagnoses
A. Braxton Hicks contractions with no cervical change.
B. Incompetent cervix.
C. PROM.
D. Low back muscle strain.
E. Pyelonephritis or urinary tract infection (UTI).
F. Placenta previa.
G. Abruptio placentae.
H. Gastroenteritis.
I. Vaginal infection.
J. Maternal dehydration.
K. Ketoacidosis.

Plan
A. General interventions:
   1. Regular uterine contractions with cervical dilation or effacement, with pressure on the lower uterine segment, strongly indicates PTL.
   2. If the cervix is dilated more than 3 cm with contractions upon presentation, the client is probably having PTL. Consult with a specialist for hospital admission and tocolysis candidacy.
   3. If the client is symptomatic with a positive foetal fibronectin test, consult with a specialist for maternal transfer to a hospital equipped to care for preterm infants.
B. Second trimester: If the client shows signs and symptoms of PTL, consider diagnosis of incompetent cervix. Refer the client to a specialist for ultrasonography for cervical length and possible cerclage placement.
C. Outpatient management:
   1. Education.
   2. Bed rest.
   3. Tocolysis therapy.
   4. Prophylactic treatment against infection.
   5. Administer corticosteroids to enhance foetal lung maturity if < 34 weeks' gestation. Observe the client for contractions in the office or have her use a uterine monitoring system at home.
   6. Foetal fibronectin testing, where available, using Society of Obstetricians and Gynecologists (SOGC) Guidelines.
D. Inpatient management of PTL:
   1. Observation, possibly with intravenous (IV) hydration.
   2. Cervical cerclage, if appropriate.
   3. Prophylactic treatment against infection (Group B *Streptococcus* until urine and cervical culture results are available).
   4. Parenteral tocolysis either to stop PTL or delay delivery long enough to allow transfer to a facility with the ability to care for preterm infants. According to numerous clinical studies, predelivery administration of magnesium sulphate reduces the occurrence of cerebral palsy, and therefore, may be the first-line treatment for parenteral tocolysis in the hospital setting.
   5. Administer corticosteroids to enhance foetal lung maturity if < 34 weeks.
   6. Transport the client to a perinatal centre for neonatal care.
E. Client teaching.
F. Pharmacological therapy:
   1. Tocolytics are generally prescribed from 24 to 34 weeks' gestation and may be considered between 23 and 24 weeks' gestation. Maintenance therapy with tocolytics is generally ineffective although short-term use is recommended mainly to allow for the administration of antenatal steroids and transfer of woman to appropriate care centre.
   Note: Recently, the Food and Drug Administration (FDA) posted warnings cautioning against the use of maintenance oral terbutaline during pregnancy because of lack of efficacy and potential maternal cardiac risks and death; it should not be prescribed on an outpatient basis. Injectable terbutaline may be used on a short-term basis (48–72 hours) in a hospital setting.
   2. Corticosteroids.
      a. Steroids are given to enhance lung maturity in the foetus if birth is expected to occur within seven days.
      b. A single rescue course may be considered if the antecedent treatment was given more than two weeks prior and the client is judged to be likely to deliver within the next week.

Follow-Up
A. Depending on the clinical scenario, the client may need to be seen weekly or biweekly. Foetal fibronectin test may be repeated every two weeks, but positive results alone should not be used to exclusively direct management. Repeat cultures as indicated, discontinuing antibiotics if cultures are negative. Encourage close phone contact with the client regarding questions or concerns.

Bibliography
American College of Obstetricians and Gynecologists. (2012, October). Prediction and prevention of preterm birth. *ACOG Practice Bulletin*, (130). reaffirmed 2016.
American College of Obstetricians and Gynecologists. (2016, October). Management of preterm labor. *ACOG Practice Bulletin*, (159).
Centers for Disease Control and Prevention. (2010). Prevention of perinatal Group B streptococcal disease. Revised guidelines from CDC. *Morbidity and Mortality Weekly Report*, 59(RR10), 1–32.
Kuhrt, K., Smout, E., Hezelgrave, N., Seed, P. T., Carter, J., & Shennan, A. H. (2016). Development and validation of a tool incorporating cervical length and quantitative fetal fibronectin to predict spontaneous preterm birth in asymptomatic high-risk women. *Ultrasound in Obstetrics & Gynecology: The Official Journal of the International Society of Ultrasound in Obstetrics and Gynecology*, 47(1), 104–109. doi:10.1002/uog.14865
Morbidity and Mortality Weekly Trend. (2013). *Preterm births—United States 2006–2010*. Retrieved from www.cdc.gov/mmwr/preview/mmwrhtml/su6203a22.htm
Nettina, S. (Ed.). (2013). *Lippincott manual of nursing practice* (10th ed.). Philadelphia, PA: Wolters Kluwer Health/Lippincott Williams & Wilkins.

Pyelonephritis in Pregnancy

Jill C. Cash, Susan Drummond, Kate Burkholder, Julie Johnson, and Susan Prendergast

Definition
A. Pyelonephritis is an infection in one or both kidneys, usually involving the entire urinary tract. Pyelonephritis may evolve into acute respiratory distress syndrome (ARDS) in pregnancy.

Incidence/Prevalence
A. The incidence of pyelonephritis in pregnancy is 1% to 2%. Most cases develop as a consequence of undiagnosed or inadequately treated lower urinary tract infection (UTI). Approximately 75% to 80% of pyelonephritis cases occur on the right side, with a 10% to 15% incidence on the left side. A small percentage of cases are bilateral.

Pathogenesis
A. *Escherichia coli* is the main pathogen in pyelonephritis, though *Klebsiella pneumoniae* and *Proteus* species are also important causes of infection. Occasionally, highly virulent gram-negative bacilli, such as *Pseudomonas, Enterobacter*, and *Serratia*, are responsible (more commonly noted in immunocompromised clients). Gram-positive Group B *Streptococcus* may also be responsible. Anaerobes are unlikely pathogens in pyelonephritis except in cases of chronic obstruction or instrumentation.

Predisposing Factors
A. Pregnancy: Because of pregnancy-related anatomic changes in the urinary tract, such as dilated ureters caused by smooth muscle relaxation and pressure on the bladder from the enlarging uterus, the immunosuppression of pregnancy may also contribute.
B. History of UTI, cystitis, and pyelonephritis.
C. Sickle cell disease.

Common Findings
A. Fever.
B. Chills.
C. Flank pain or tenderness.
D. Urinary frequency or urgency.
E. Haematuria and dysuria.

Other Signs and Symptoms
A. UTI is associated with urinary frequency, urgency, and dysuria; hematuria; and suprapubic pain:
    1. Chemical reactions to deodorant or douches can affect urination.
    2. Clients with frequent pyelonephritis may *not* complain of frequency and dysuria.
B. Pyelonephritis is associated with fever, palpitations, dizziness, backache, and urinary frequency:
    1. Haematuria may be present, especially if the client has a history of a previous kidney stone.
    2. Dysuria is not always present in upper tract infections.
C. Abdominal pain and uterine contractions, risk of preterm labour (PTL) and birth.
D. Shortness of breath (SOB).

Potential Complications
A. Sepsis and septic shock.
B. ARDS: Mortality rate—50% to 70%.
C. Pulmonary embolus, usually presents as sudden-onset costovertebral angle (CVA) tenderness.

Subjective Data
A. Elicit information on the onset, duration, and progression of symptoms.
B. Elicit problems with voiding. Ask the client about urinary frequency, urgency, and dysuria.
C. Ask the client whether she has experienced preterm contractions.
D. Ask whether the client is complaining of fever or chills.
E. Ask the client whether her urine has a bad odour.
F. Ask the client whether she has felt more tired than usual.
G. Ask the client whether she has felt more nauseated than usual or whether she has been vomiting.
H. Does the client have a backache? Note location (unilateral or bilateral) and what, if anything, makes the backache better or worse.
I. Review the client's history for sickle cell disease, if appropriate; has she been tested?
J. Review prenatal history for recurrent UTIs, previous pyelonephritis, and any abnormalities of the genitourinary (GU) tract.

Physical Examination
A. Check temperature, pulse, respirations, and blood pressure (BP): Fever >38°C, tachycardia, tachypnea, and hypotension are associated with sepsis, septic shock, and ARDS.
B. Inspect: Note general appearance for respiratory distress.
C. Palpate:
    1. Back: Check CVA tenderness (right CVA tenderness is more common in pregnancy).
    2. Abdomen:
        a. Palpate for uterine tenderness and contractions.
        b. Palpate for suprapubic tenderness.
D. Auscultate:
    1. The lungs and heart.
    2. The foetal heart rate (FHR).
E. Bimanual examination: Check for cervical dilation.

Diagnostic Tests
A. Complete blood count (CBC) with differential or white blood cell (WBC): Leukocytosis with left shift on differential seen.
B. Blood culture, if indicated.
C. Respiratory function:
    1. Pulse oximetry, if indicated.
    2. Arterial blood gases (ABGs), if indicated.
D. Renal function:
    1. Urinalysis:
        a. Check urinalysis for WBCs, red blood cells (RBCs), leukocyte esterase, and/or nitrites.
        b. Glucosuria may be normal in pregnancy because of decreased tubular capacity to reabsorb glucose. If it is consistently noted, further testing is needed.
        c. Proteinuria is *not* normal during pregnancy. All cases warrant further investigation.
    2. Urine culture and sensitivity: >100,000 colonies per millilitre indicates UTI.
    3. Intravenous pyelogram (IVP), if indicated.
    4. Renal ultrasonography, if indicated.

Differential Diagnoses
A. Cystitis.
B. Urethritis.
C. Urethral stricture.
D. Genital infection.
E. Chorioamnionitis.
F. Septic abortion.
G. Postpartum endometritis.
H. Muscular strain.
I. Pulmonary embolus.
J. Severe upper respiratory tract infection.
K. Postprocedural dysuria or urinary frequency (i.e., following bladder catheterization or cystoscopy).
L. Chemical irritants.
M. Postpartum septic pelvic thrombophlebitis.
N. Renal calculi.

Plan

A. General interventions:
  1. Rule out other sources of infection.
  2. Assess for PTL.
B. Client teaching.
C. Dietary management:
  1. Advise the client to eat a regular diet as tolerated.
  2. Encourage her to drink eight to ten glasses of water a day.
  3. Warn the client to avoid beverages with caffeine. Cranberry juice (100%) and cranberry and blueberry capsules can be useful for urinary tract problems but do not replace pharmacological management.
D. Pharmacological therapy:
  1. First-line treatment: Broad-spectrum antibiotic coverage until cultures and sensitivity results are back:
    a. Nitrofurantoin.
    b. Amoxicillin.
    c. Augmentin.
  2. If dysuria is present: Phenazopyridine. Warn the client that phenazopyridine turns urine orange.
  3. Alternative medications:
    a. Cephalexin.

Follow-Up

A. Once antibiotic therapy is initiated, most clients have a decrease in symptoms within 48 hours. By the end of 72 hours, almost 95% of clients are afebrile and asymptomatic. Stress to clients the importance of completing the course of antibiotics regardless of the absence of symptoms.
B. The most likely causes of treatment failure are a resistant microorganism or obstruction; common causes of obstruction in pregnancy are urolithiasis or compression of the ureter by the gravid uterus.
C. Repeat a urine culture at a two-week follow-up visit.
D. Recurrence rates are very high. After the initial antibiotic therapy course is completed, consider a daily prophylactic dose of an antibiotic, such as nitrofurantoin, for recurrent infections.
E. Clients receiving prophylactic antibiotics should have their urine screened for bacteria at each subsequent office visit and be questioned about the recurrence of symptoms.
F. If no prophylactic treatment is undertaken, obtain a urine culture if symptoms recur or if urine dipstick is positive for leukocyte esterase or nitrites.

Bibliography

Centers for Disease Control and Prevention. (2010). Prevention of perinatal Group B streptococcal disease. Revised guidelines from CDC. *Morbidity and Mortality Weekly Report, 59*(RR10), 1–32.

Nettina, S. (Ed.). (2013). *Lippincott manual of nursing practice* (10th ed.). Philadelphia, PA: Wolters Kluwer Health/Lippincott Williams & Wilkins.

Vaginal Bleeding: First Trimester

Jill C. Cash, Susan Drummond, Kate Burkholder, Julie Johnson, and Susan Prendergast

Definition

Vaginal bleeding during the first trimester of pregnancy may range from spotting to massive haemorrhage (spontaneous miscarriage). Types of spontaneous miscarriage are the following:

A. Threatened miscarriage: Vaginal bleeding with absent or minimal pain *and* a closed, long, thick cervix.
B. Inevitable miscarriage: Vaginal bleeding with pain and cervical dilation and/or effacement.
C. Spontaneous miscarriage: The nonviable products of conception are expelled from the uterus spontaneously.
D. Vaginal bleeding may also be related to ectopic pregnancy, implantation of the pregnancy, or cervical inflammation/infection.

Incidence/Prevalence

A. Vaginal bleeding is a common event in pregnancy. Spontaneous miscarriage, a primary concern in the first trimester, occurs in about 30% of all pregnancies; most occur before the 16th week. Ectopic pregnancy occurs in one of every 200 pregnancies; 75% of pregnancies occurring after failure of tubal sterilization are likely to be ectopic.

Pathogenesis

A. Spontaneous miscarriage: The pathogenesis varies according to cause. In most cases, it is caused by embryonic death, with resultant decrease in hormone levels and subsequent sloughing of the uterine decidua. Many embryonic deaths occur because of chromosomal abnormalities that are incompatible with life.
B. Ectopic pregnancy: Fertilized ovum is implanted outside of the uterus, most commonly in the fallopian tube.

Predisposing Factors

A. Spontaneous miscarriage: In most cases, the cause is unknown:
  1. Advanced maternal age (occurs more often in older women), suggesting that a genetic abnormality in the ovum may contribute.
  2. Abnormal uterine environment.
  3. Systemic disease.
  4. Weight extremes: Body mass index (BMI) <18.5 or > 25).
  5. Immunologic deficiencies.
  6. Substance use, including caffeine, alcohol, cigarettes, and cocaine.
  7. Trauma.
  8. Previous spontaneous miscarriage.
B. Ectopic pregnancy: There are many reasons for ectopic pregnancy, including previous damage or scar tissue in the fallopian tube, which blocks movement of the fertilized ovum (frequently caused by pelvic inflammatory disease, tubal surgery for infertility, or bilateral tubal ligation) and also in vitro fertilization.

Common Findings

A. Spontaneous miscarriage: Vaginal bleeding occurs that may or may not be associated with cramping or uterine contractions. When a pregnancy is greater than eight weeks' gestation, the presence of uterine bleeding, uterine contractions, and/or pain are the indications of a threatened miscarriage until proven otherwise.
B. Ectopic pregnancy: Vaginal bleeding and pelvic pain occur soon after the first missed period; the client may be unaware of pregnancy. Sudden, acute, localized abdominal pain is associated with fallopian tube rupture.

Other Signs and Symptoms

A. Threatened miscarriage: Slight bleeding may be present over several weeks; cramping; no passage of tissue; positive pregnancy symptoms present, including nausea, vomiting, fatigue, breast tenderness, and urinary frequency.

B. Inevitable miscarriage: Moderate to profuse vaginal bleeding occurs. Tissue may or may not be passed, uterine cramps or abdominal pain occur, and symptoms of pregnancy may be decreased or absent.
C. Incomplete miscarriage: Moderate to profuse vaginal bleeding, sometimes for several weeks, occurs; reports of passage of tissue; painful uterine cramping or "contractions" present; and symptoms of pregnancy often absent.
D. Complete miscarriage: Client experiences profuse bleeding, passage of tissue and large clots, abdominal cramping, or uterine contractions.
E. Ectopic pregnancy: Amenorrhoea or irregular vaginal bleeding; abdominal pain is usually present, may be unilateral or generalized, and in extreme cases may be associated with vertigo and syncope; shoulder pain, with irritation of phrenic nerve, may be present. Anxiety or palpitations are often noted.

Subjective Data
A. Elicit information about the onset, duration, and progression of symptoms.
B. Ask the client about vaginal bleeding. When did it start? Is it continuous bleeding, "like a period," or is it spotting? How much bleeding has occurred? How many pads have been saturated? What is the size of the blood spots? Determine the amount of bleeding: How much blood is on menstrual pad? (a) scant amount: <2.5 cm diameter; (b) light amount: <10 cm diameter; (c) moderate amount: <15 cm diameter; (d) heavy amount: Saturates the pad within one hour.
C. What is her current method of birth control? Was the birth control method used consistently? Has she had a tubal ligation, or has she recently used an intrauterine contraceptive device (IUD)?
D. Ask the client the first day of her last menstrual period to date the pregnancy. Did she have a positive pregnancy test? If so, when?
E. Does she have a history of ectopic pregnancy, pelvic inflammatory disease, or fertility assistance?
F. Question the client regarding the presence or absence of abdominal and/or back pain. If present, is it a continuous discomfort, or is it intermittent cramping? Was the onset sudden? How severe is the pain?
G. Is she experiencing shoulder pain? This may be referred pain from phrenic nerve irritation because of intraperitoneal bleeding.

Physical Examination
A. Check temperature, pulse, respirations, and BP: Note postural hypotension and tachycardia. Haemodynamic instability may be noted in cases of profuse bleeding; assess vital signs and be alert for hypotension, tachycardia, tachypnea, and/or laboured breathing.
B. Inspect:
  1. Note general overall appearance of discomfort or pain before, during, and after examination.
  2. Examine menstrual pad to determine amount of bleeding, if available.
C. Palpate:
  1. Perform abdominal examination for rebound tenderness, masses, softness, tenderness, or abdominal wall distension. Sudden, acute, localized abdominal pain with signs of internal haemorrhage suggest rupture of the fallopian tube.
  2. Palpate uterine size. Measure fundal height for consistency with pregnancy dates. If fundal height suggests pregnancy has advanced beyond first trimester, bleeding may be caused by abruption, placenta previa, or rupture of membranes with heavy bloody show.
  3. Check iliopsoas and obturator muscle tests.
D. Auscultate the heart, lungs, and bowel sounds to rule out other abdominal problems.
E. Pelvic examination:
  1. Perform sterile speculum examination: Assess colour and amount of bleeding. Tissue and the products of conception may be noted at cervical os or in vaginal vault. Assess for Chadwick's sign. The entire foetus may be noted in the vaginal vault; tissues that remain in the uterus may include portions of foetal membranes or placenta. Look for vaginitis/cervicitis and other signs and symptoms of infection that could be causing the bleeding.
  2. Bimanual examination: Check Hegar's sign; elicit this sign cautiously as a false-positive result may be related to a rough examination. Evaluate cervical dilation; cervical motion tenderness, often present with ectopic pregnancy; and a bulging cul-de-sac, which represents a haemoperitoneum. Adnexal mass is present in 50% of ectopic pregnancies.

Diagnostic Tests
A. Pregnancy test: Quantitative serum beta human chorionic gonadotropin (HCG); serial tests at least 48 hours apart, making sure to perform test at same lab for accurate results.
B. CBC with differential and platelet count.
C. ABO group and RH factor, antibody screen, and crossmatch if indicated.
D. Prothrombin time (PT) and partial thromboplastin time (PTT).
E. Doppler ultrasonography for foetal heart tones, for foetuses > 11 weeks.
F. Ultrasonography: Transvaginal and/or abdominal.

Differential Diagnoses
A. First-trimester vaginal bleeding secondary to the following:
  1. Threatened miscarriage.
  2. Inevitable miscarriage.
  3. Incomplete miscarriage.
  4. Complete miscarriage.
  5. Septic miscarriage.
  6. Ectopic pregnancy: There is a strong suspicion of ectopic pregnancy or fallopian tube rupture if symptoms present with a history of fallopian tube damage (i.e., tubal surgery for infertility, previous ectopic pregnancy), pelvic infection, or IUD use.
  7. Hydatidiform mole.
  8. Anovulatory bleeding with an antecedent period of amenorrhoea.
  9. Benign or malignant genital tract lesion.
  10. Menstrual bleeding.
  11. Genital trauma.
  12. Advanced pregnancy with placenta previa or abruptio placentae.
  13. Salpingitis.
  14. Appendicitis.
  15. IUD-related symptoms.
  16. Pelvic inflammatory disease.

Plan
A. General interventions: Stabilize maternal condition and then determine the cause of bleeding.

1. Threatened miscarriage: Expectant management. Bed rest is often prescribed. Symptoms either subside, leading to normal gestation, or worsen, leading to inevitable miscarriage. If bleeding persists without leading to spontaneous miscarriage, the client should be evaluated frequently, usually on a weekly basis, by means of ultrasonography to assess foetal viability. The client should avoid intercourse and should not use tampons to absorb bleeding.
2. Inevitable miscarriage: Care may include expectant management or preparation for dilation and curettage (D&C).
3. Incomplete miscarriage: Prepare for suction and possible D&C.
4. Complete miscarriage: If abortion is complete and the products of conception are delivered with complete membranes present and cessation of bleeding has occurred, no surgical intervention is indicated. In these cases, the tissue specimens must be carefully examined for completeness. Send all specimens to the laboratory for further examination. If there is any question regarding complete passing of the placenta, do serial quantitative HCGs until back to nonpregnant levels.
5. Ectopic pregnancy: Consult with a specialist regarding possible medical management with methotrexate or refer the client to a specialist for surgical intervention. The specialist may perform culdocentesis to assess for haemoperitoneum. If the client is in shock, resuscitation with IV fluids should be started immediately by means of two large-bore angiocatheters. Intravenous (IV) fluids, such as lactated Ringer's solution or normal saline, should be infused at a rapid rate. The client is taken to the operating room, where the indicated procedure is one that controls haemorrhage in the shortest period of time. Salpingectomy and/or hysterectomy may be included.
B. Pharmacological therapy:
1. RhO (D) immune globulin should be administered to any Rh-negative client.
2. Acetaminophen or ibuprofen as needed for discomfort.
3. Ectopic pregnancy: Methotrexate is a folic acid antagonist that has been used to inhibit the growth of trophoblastic cells. This chemotherapy is the first-line treatment for ectopic pregnancy when surgery is contraindicated, or in the management of postoperative persistent trophoblast. Refer the client to a specialist to evaluate her for methotrexate or operative intervention. In most cases, operative intervention is required.

Follow-Up

A. Threatened miscarriage: Follow the client weekly to assess for interval growth and presence of foetal cardiac motion. Instruct the client on menstrual pad count.
B. Spontaneous miscarriage: Once the uterine contents have been evacuated, follow up with a six-week post-miscarriage visit, unless the situation warrants an earlier follow-up visit. Contraception needs to be discussed with the client. Advise her that it is best to wait for two or three menstrual cycles before becoming pregnant again.
C. Ectopic pregnancy: Once the ectopic pregnancy has been removed, the client should be seen in two to six weeks for a postoperative examination, unless the situation warrants an earlier follow-up visit. If methotrexate is used, do serial quantitative HCGs until they return to nonpregnant levels.

Consultation/Referral

A. Consult with a specialist if the client has any frank bleeding, signs of foetal compromise, or maternal shock, or if the cause of bleeding cannot be determined.

Bibliography

American College of Obstetricians and Gynecologists. (2008, June). Medical management of ectopic pregnancy. *ACOG Practice Bulletin*, (94). reaffirmed 2014.
American College of Obstetricians and Gynecologists. (2016, October). Premature rupture of membranes. *ACOG Practice Bulletin*, (160).
Barash, J. H., Buchanan, E. M., & Hillson, C. (2014). Diagnosis and management of ectopic pregnancy. *American Family Physician*, 90(1), 34–40.
Nettina, S. (Ed.). (2013). *Lippincott manual of nursing practice* (10th ed.). Philadelphia, PA: Wolters Kluwer Health/Lippincott Williams & Wilkins.

Vaginal Bleeding: Second and Third Trimesters

Jill C. Cash, Susan Drummond, Kate Burkholder, Julie Johnson, and Susan Prendergast

Definition

Bright or dark red vaginal bleeding during the second or third trimester (more than 12 weeks' gestation) may be painless, or it may be associated with uterine contractions or severe abdominal pain. Antepartum bleeding (uterine bleeding after 20 weeks' gestation that is unrelated to labour and delivery) occurs in 4% to 5% of pregnancies. Common causes of bleeding include the following:
A. Low-lying placenta: The edge of the placenta grows into the area of the lower uterine segment near the cervical os.
B. Placenta previa: Implantation of the blastocyst occurs in the lower uterine segment, followed by placental growth. Eventually, the placenta may partially or completely cover the cervix.
C. Abruptio placentae: Partial or premature separation of the placenta takes place.
D. Uterine rupture: Complete uterine rupture extends through the entire uterine wall, and the uterine contents are extruded into the abdominal cavity. Incomplete rupture extends through the endometrium and myometrium, but the peritoneum remains intact. This occurs almost exclusively during labour and/or delivery.
E. Uterine dehiscence: Separation of an old surgical scar.
F. Bloody discharge is *not* normal before 37 weeks' gestation unless associated with recent sexual intercourse or pelvic examination. Light spotting or bleeding may be caused by recent sexual intercourse, preterm labour (PTL), rupture of membranes, or cervicitis. *Note*: The evaluation of vaginal bleeding before 20 weeks is similar to that in the first trimester.

Incidence/Prevalence

A. Placenta previa: Approximately 1:200 pregnancies, more common in parous women.
B. Abruptio placenta: Approximately 1:250 pregnancies.
C. Uterine rupture: If uterus is unscarred, incidence is approximately 1:6000 to 1:20,000 pregnancies. If uterus has a scar (usually from a previous caesarean section), incidence varies depending on the type and location of the prior uterine incision. If the prior incision was low transverse, the incidence is approximately 0.7% to 2.0% and if the prior incision was classical, the incidence is approximately 1% to 2%.

Pathogenesis

A. Placenta previa: The pathogenesis of placenta previa is unknown. One hypothesis is that the presence of suboptimal endometrium in the upper uterine cavity because of previous surgery or pregnancies promotes implantation of trophoblast in or toward the lower uterine segment. Another hypothesis is that a particularly large placental surface area, as in multiple gestation or in response to reduced uteroplacental perfusion, increases the likelihood that the placenta will cover or encroach upon the cervical os.
B. Abruptio placenta: Abruptio placenta is initiated by bleeding into the decidua basalis. The decidua then splits, and the placenta is sheared off. Blood may move into and through the myometrium, leading to a boardlike uterus.
C. Uterine rupture: Uterine rupture may occur from uterine injury because of previous surgery or trauma.

Predisposing Factors

A. Placenta previa: Late fertilization with delayed implantation, previous uterine scar, advanced maternal age, multiple gestation, large placenta, previous placenta previa, and smoking.
B. Abruptio placenta: Hypertension (chronic, gestational, or preeclampsia), cocaine use, trauma, high parity, sudden decompression of overdistended uterus (i.e., when membranes rupture), smoking, chorioamnionitis, abdominal trauma, and cephalic version.
C. Uterine rupture: Multiparity, previous uterine incision, tetanic contractions, or prolonged labour, especially with excessive use of oxytocin.

Common Findings

A. Placenta previa: Painless vaginal bleeding, usually in amounts of spotting to frank haemorrhage. Bleeding occasionally is accompanied by cramping or uterine contractions. A "gush" of fluid associated with sudden onset of massive vaginal bleeding may be reported. Painless vaginal bleeding should be treated as a placenta previa until proven otherwise.
B. Abruptio placentae: Firm, tender uterus; high-frequency, low-amplitude uterine contractions:
  1. Marginal abruption: Vaginal bleeding may be absent or minimal and bright red; there may be some old, dark blood. Abdominal pain is usually mild.

Frank vaginal bleeding with abdominal pain should be treated as an abruption until proven otherwise.

  2. Moderate abruption: Vaginal bleeding may be moderate or absent. Abdominal pain is usually significant and associated with contractions.
  3. Severe abruption: Vaginal bleeding may be moderate, severe, or absent. Abdominal pain is severe. The client may have a concealed placental abruption without vaginal bleeding.
C. Uterine rupture: Vaginal bleeding is moderate, severe, or absent. The client may experience a sudden onset of extreme abdominal pain (commonly at the previous uterine scar site).

Other Signs and Symptoms

A. External foetal monitor (EFM) tracings: May exhibit characteristics that are associated with anaemia or hypoxemia such as decreased or absent variability, bradycardia, tachycardia, recurrent late or prolonged decelerations, or a sinusoidal pattern.
B. Placenta previa: Uterine resting tone is usually relaxed. Foetal status at first examination is usually stable. Recurrence of bleeding is common. First bleeding episode in placenta previa is rarely significant. Second or third bleeding episode is often associated with significant vaginal bleeding.
C. Abruptio placentae: Rupture of membranes reveals blood-stained fluid:
  1. Marginal abruption: Uterine resting tone is usually relaxed. Foetal status on the foetal monitor at first examination is usually stable. Labour progresses rapidly with vaginal bleeding or large amounts of bloody show.
  2. Moderate abruption: Uterine resting tone is hypertonic. At first examination, the foetus is usually alive. Foetal heart rate (FHR) may exhibit characteristics that are associated with hypoxemia or anaemia such as decreased/absent variability, tachycardia, bradycardia, recurrent late or prolonged decelerations, or sinusoidal patterns. Labour progresses rapidly with vaginal bleeding or large amounts of bloody show.
  3. Severe abruption: Uterine resting tone is hypertonic or "boardlike." At first examination, the foetus may be dead. If the foetus is alive, EFM is consistent with hypoxemia or anaemia as listed earlier.
D. Uterine rupture: Uterine resting tone may be normal or hypertonic. At first examination, foetus is frequently dead or FHR pattern is consistent with hypoxemia or anaemia as listed earlier.

Subjective Data

A. Elicit information about the onset, duration, and progression of vaginal bleeding. When did it start? Is it continuous bleeding, "like a period," or is it spotting?
B. Ask: How much bleeding has occurred? How many pads have been saturated? What is the size of the blood spots, the size of a quarter or a loonie?
C. Elicit information regarding the presence or absence of abdominal pain. If present, review the onset, duration, and progression of pain. Is it a continuous discomfort or intermittent cramping? How severe is the pain? Did it have a sudden onset?
D. Is the client experiencing shoulder pain? This is likely to be referred pain from phrenic nerve irritation because of intraperitoneal bleeding.
E. Elicit the first day of client's last menstrual cycle, to date pregnancy.
F. Ask the client whether she feels the baby move, if >18 weeks' gestation, and if the movement has been normal this day.

Physical Examination

A. Check temperature, pulse, respirations, and blood pressure (BP); include FHR:
  1. A pregnant client does not demonstrate signs and symptoms of hypovolemic shock until she has lost 30% of her circulating volume.
  2. Prepare the client for emergency transport to a hospital even if she is haemodynamically stable.
B. Inspect: Inspect the client's general appearance related to discomfort and pain. Observe bleeding characteristics and pooling.
C. Palpate:
  1. Check for palpable foetal parts on abdominal wall; note foetal movement.
  2. Palpate the uterus for relaxed or hypertonic uterus. Check for contractions. If present, note frequency, duration, and intensity to palpation.

D. Auscultate:
  1. The abdomen: Check foetal heart tones or EFM for baseline and periodic FHR patterns.
  2. The maternal heart and lungs.
E. Perform sterile speculum examination to look for the source of bleeding. Do not perform vaginal bimanual examination until previa is ruled out.

Diagnostic Tests

A. Complete blood count (CBC) and platelets.
B. Prothrombin time (PT), partial thromboplastin time (PTT), and fibrinogen.
C. ABO group and RH status, and type and crossmatch if indicated.
D. Foetal cell stain, Kleihauer–Betke test; foetal cell stain can determine the amount of foetal blood in the maternal circulation.
E. Determine if RhO(D) immune globulin (RhoGAM) is indicated.
F. Ultrasonography.
G. Nonstress test (NST)/electronic foetal monitoring.

Differential Diagnoses

A. Placenta previa.
B. Abruptio placentae.
C. Uterine rupture.
D. Ruptured vasa previa.
E. Rupture of membranes.
F. Normal bloody show.
G. Rectal haemorrhoidal bleeding.

Plan

A. General interventions:
  1. Tocolysis may be considered if the client has no active haemorrhage and reassuring FHR pattern.
  2. If significant vaginal bleeding is present, the primary goal is to maintain oxygen delivery to the mother and foetus while preparing them for transport. Interventions include maternal positioning to avoid vena caval compression; administering supplemental oxygen; initiating large-bore intravenous (IV) line; delivery of fluid bolus of normal saline or lactated Ringer's solution; keeping a flow sheet of vital signs, assessments, actions, and responses; maintaining continuous recording of FHR and uterine activity on an electronic foetal monitor; and providing emotional support and anticipatory guidance.
  3. If vaginal bleeding is minimal and home management is being considered, discuss risks with the client and assess her ability to maintain bed rest. Also assess client's access to transportation in case of a major bleeding episode. Consider the distance from the client's home to the nearest hospital.
B. Pharmacological therapy for preterm placenta previa with preterm contractions:
  1. Tocolysis options:
    a. Terbutaline sulphate.
    b. Indomethacin: Should not be given after 32 weeks' gestation, and duration of indomethacin therapy should not exceed 72 hours.
    c. The client may be admitted to an antepartum unit for parenteral tocolysis such as magnesium sulphate.
  2. Antenatal steroids may be given if preterm delivery is a possibility within the next week and the estimated gestational age (EGA) is < 34 weeks:
    a. Betamethasone.
    b. Dexamethasone.
    c. Either regimen may be repeated once a week.
  3. If the client is Rh-negative, give RhO(D) immune globulin (RhoGAM) intramuscular (IM) by injection after each vaginal bleeding episode:
    a. Full-dose RhO(D) IM immune globulin, which is adequate.

Follow-Up

A. Follow-up depends on client diagnosis and whether client hospitalization is needed.

Consultation/Referral

A. Consult a specialist for all clients noted to have second- and third-trimester vaginal bleeding.
B. Consult with a specialist if the client has any frank, bright red bleeding; signs of foetal compromise or maternal shock; or if the cause of bleeding cannot be determined and/or treated by the practitioner.

Bibliography

American College of Obstetricians and Gynecologists. (2014, July). Antepartum fetal surveillance. *COG Practice Bulletin*, (145).
Nettina, S. (Ed.). (2013). *Lippincott manual of nursing practice* (10th ed.). Philadelphia, PA: Wolters Kluwer Health/Lippincott Williams & Wilkins.

POSTPARTUM

Breast Engorgement

Jill C. Cash, Susan Drummond, Kate Burkholder, Julie Johnson, and Susan Prendergast

Definition

A. Breast engorgement is swollen, tender breasts caused by overfilling of milk, increased blood flow, and fluids in the breasts.

Incidence/Prevalence

A. Breast engorgement may affect 40% of postpartum mothers.

Pathogenesis

A. *Primary engorgement* is the result of distension and stasis of the vascular and lymphatic circulations occurring two to four days following delivery. It is prompted by the decrease in progesterone levels after the placenta is delivered.
B. *Secondary engorgement* occurs because of distension of the lobules and alveoli with milk as lactation is established. It may occur from excessive stimulation of milk production via pumping, taking medications to increase milk supply, or decreased milk extraction from not feeding the baby as often. Without stimulation by suckling and removal of milk, secretion of prolactin decreases and milk production decreases and finally ceases.

Predisposing Factors
A. Engorgement often develops if early feedings are not frequent enough, suckling is inefficient, or breastfeeding is not conducted in a relaxing atmosphere. Engorgement is more likely to develop sooner and more intensely in mothers who have breastfed a prior child.

Common Findings
A. Swollen, tender breasts.
B. Discomfort when breastfeeding.
C. A low-grade fever lasting between 4 and 16 hours.

Other Signs and Symptoms
A. Pain, tenderness, and redness in one area of the breast are associated with mastitis.
B. Physical examination should not be focused just on breast symptoms but should include a general ruling out of other potential problems such as coexistent urinary tract infection (UTI).

Subjective Data
A. Elicit the onset, duration, and course of symptoms. Review the frequency of breastfeeding and/or use of a breast pump. Is the client still breastfeeding, or has she stopped because of the discomfort?
B. Exclude other causes of fever, such as UTI, wound infection, and red streaks on one or both breasts, to rule out mastitis.
C. Quantify pain symptoms and relief measures, including heat packs, ice packs, breast binder, and analgesics such as acetaminophen.

Physical Examination
A. Check temperature, blood pressure (BP), and pulse.
B. Inspect: Examine the breasts for erythemic streaks. Check the episiotomy or abdominal incision, if indicated.
C. Palpate:
  1. Examine the breasts for tenderness, hardness, warmth, and lumps.
  2. Palpate axilla for lymphadenopathy.
  3. Check back for costovertebral angle (CVA) tenderness.

Diagnostic Tests
A. Tests generally are not indicated for breast engorgement.
B. Urine culture or wound culture, if applicable.

Differential Diagnoses
A. Mastitis.

Plan
A. General interventions:
  1. Encourage the client to take analgesics before breastfeeding and continue breastfeeding.
  2. Encourage ice packs for discomfort and frequent breastfeeding. There should be *no stimulation* to the breasts other than that provided by the baby when nursing, and the client should take analgesics for discomfort. Reassure her that engorgement is temporary and usually resolves within 24 to 48 hours.
B. Client teaching:
  1. Educate the client regarding milk production and let-down reflex.
  2. Advise the client to breastfeed frequently to reduce chances of engorgement.
  3. Provide reassurance and support for the client to continue breastfeeding through this temporary period of discomfort. Engorgement may last two to three days before milk supply meets demand; continuation of breastfeeding will resolve discomfort and problems.
  4. Educate the client on proper latch and how to identify efficient milk transfer.
C. Pharmacological therapy: Acetaminophen or ibuprofen 30 to 45 minutes before breastfeeding and as needed.

Follow-Up
A. Follow-up may not be required for engorgement. If suspected or confirmed mastitis, advise follow-up.
B. Lactation consultation, if indicated.

Individual Considerations
A. Pregnancy loss: It is imperative to discuss breast care and engorgement with women who have a second-trimester termination of pregnancy, have a stillbirth, or experience a neonatal loss.

Bibliography
Hale, T. W. (2014). *Medications and mother's milk* (16th ed.). Amarillo, TX: Hale.

Nelson, D. B., Freeman, M. P., Johnson, N. L., McIntire, D. D., & Leveno, K. J. (2013). A prospective study of postpartum depression in 17 648 parturients. *Journal of Maternal–Fetal & Neonatal Medicine: The Official Journal of the European Association of Perinatal Medicine, the Federation of Asia and Oceania Perinatal Societies, the International Society of Perinatal Obstetricians, 26*(12), 1155–1161. doi:10.3109/14767058.2013.777698

Nettina, S (Ed.). (2013). *Lippincott manual of nursing practice* (10th ed.). Philadelphia, PA: Wolters Kluwer Health/Lippincott Williams & Wilkins.

Endometritis

Jill C. Cash, Susan Drummond, Kate Burkholder, Julie Johnson, and Susan Prendergast

Definition
A. Endometritis is an infection of the endometrium (the interior lining of the uterus) that occurs postpartum. Endometritis is the most common cause of puerperal fever in obstetrics.

Incidence/Prevalence
A. The incidence of endometritis has been noted to be as high as 38.5% after caesarean section; the incidence is 1.2% after vaginal delivery.

Pathogenesis
During labour and delivery, endogenous cervicovaginal flora enter the uterine cavity. Onset is usually three to five days after delivery, unless it is caused by beta-haemolytic *Streptococcus*, in which case the onset is earlier and more precipitous. Infection is usually polymicrobial in nature. Undiagnosed or unsuccessfully treated infection of the endomyometrium can progress to involve the entire uterus and may spread to accessory pelvic structures. The main pathway for spread of the infection is the broad ligament. Sources of bacteria may be any one or a combination of the following:
A. Endogenous vaginal bacteria, usually pathogenic only when tissue is damaged:
  1. Beta-haemolytic *Streptococcus*.
  2. *Streptococcus viridans*.
  3. *Neisseria gonorrhoeae*.
  4. *Gardnerella*.

B. Contamination by normal bowel bacteria:
1. *Clostridium perfringens.*
2. *Escherichia coli.*
3. *Proteus mirabilis.*
4. *Aerobacter aerogenes.*
5. *Enterococcus.*
6. *Pseudomonas aeruginosa.*
7. *Klebsiella pneumoniae.*

C. Contamination from environment; *Staphylococcus* is a common organism.

Predisposing Factors

A. Operative delivery: Caesarean section is the major predisposing factor for pelvic infection. The most important determinant of infection for clients undergoing caesarean delivery is the duration of labour.
B. Intrapartum: Prolonged rupture of membranes; numerous vaginal examinations in labour; use of internal monitoring devices during labour; use of instruments in delivery; prolonged labour; and intrauterine manipulation, such as internal rotation or manual removal of placenta, can all lead to endometritis.
C. Postpartum: Retained placental fragments or membranes, improper perineal care, and host resistance also predispose a client to infection.
D. Anaemia: This probably represents a marker for poor nutrition.
E. Obesity.

Common Findings

A. "Feeling ill" with fever or chills.
B. Muscle aches.
C. Headache.
D. Uterine pain and tenderness.
E. Foul-smelling lochia.

Other Signs and Symptoms

A. Fever (38ºC–40ºC).
B. Subinvolution.
C. Atonic uterus.
D. Abnormalities of lochia:
   1. May be scant and odourless if anaerobic infection.
   2. May be moderately heavy, malodourous, bloody, or seropurulent if aerobic infection.
E. Tachycardia.

Subjective Data

A. Elicit the onset, duration, and course of symptoms.
B. Review the colour, odour, and amount of lochia.
C. Review the client's pain or discomfort and the relief measures used.
D. Review other body symptoms to rule out other infections such as urinary tract infection (UTI), breast engorgement, or mastitis.
E. Review labour and delivery events for complications (see section "Predisposing Factors").

Physical Examination

A. Check temperature, pulse, and blood pressure (BP): The client may be tachycardic with heart rate of 100 to 140 beats per minute (bpm).
B. Inspect: Observe colour, amount, and odour of lochia. Check abdominal incision, if applicable. Check the perineum for lacerations, breakdown of incision, redness, and drainage.
C. Palpate:
   1. The abdomen; check uterine tenderness.
   2. The back; check CVA tenderness.
D. Auscultate the heart and lungs.
E. Speculum examination: Inspect the cervix for lacerations, drainage, or redness.
F. Bimanual examination: Check for cervical motion tenderness; palpate adnexa for masses and tenderness; note "heat" of the pelvis.

Diagnostic Tests

A. Complete blood count (CBC) with differential.
B. Blood and urine cultures.
C. Cervical cultures, to rule out a sexually transmitted infection (STI), if indicated.
D. Wet prep, if indicated.

Differential Diagnoses

A. Sexually transmitted diseases (STDs) such as chlamydia, gonorrhoea, or trichomoniasis.
B. UTI/pyelonephritis.
C. Pneumonitis.
D. Extreme breast engorgement: "Milk fever."
E. Wound infection.

Plan

A. General interventions for mild cases:
   1. Instruct on proper hygiene. Teach the client techniques to prevent infection (perineal area, incision site, and breast).
   2. Acetaminophen for fever as needed.
B. Client teaching.
C. Pharmacological therapy:
   1. Antibiotic therapy:
      a. Augmentin.
      b. Doxycycline if the client is allergic to penicillin and not breastfeeding.
      c. Cephalexin if the client is allergic to penicillin and is breastfeeding.
      d. Rocephin/ceftriaxone with flagyl 500 mg (if breastfeeding, pump and dispose of breast milk during treatment).
   2. If uterus is boggy and/or bleeding is excessive: Ergonovine maleate. (Do not give if the client is hypertensive.)
D. For more serious cases (moderate to severe), send the client to the nearest acute care facility for evaluation and treatment; all but mild cases of endometritis should be treated parenterally:
   1. Clindamycin plus gentamicin.
   2. Ampicillin is added if enterococcal infection is suspected or if no improvement occurs by 48 hours. Continuing treatment with oral antibiotics is not necessary when receiving intravenous therapy.

Follow-Up

A. Call the client in 24 to 48 hours to evaluate her status.
B. Instruct the client to call if symptoms do not resolve within 24 hours or if they worsen.

Consultation/Referral

A. Consult with specialist if symptoms do not resolve, if they worsen within 24 hours, or if the client's temperature does not go below 100.0ºF after 48 hours on antibiotics. If no significant improvement is seen within two to three days, the client may need to be admitted to the hospital.

Bibliography

American College of Obstetricians and Gynecologists. (2015, December). Obesity in pregnancy. *ACOG Practice Bulletin*, (156).

Mackeen, A. D., Packard, R. E., Ota, E., & Speer, L. (2015). Antibiotic regimens for postpartum endometritis. *Cochrane Database of Systematic Reviews*, (2), CD001067. doi:10.1002/14651858.CD001067.pub3

Nettina, S. (Ed.). (2013). *Lippincott manual of nursing practice* (10th ed.). Philadelphia, PA: Wolters Kluwer Health/Lippincott Williams & Wilkins.

Secondary Postpartum Haemorrhage

Jill C. Cash, Susan Drummond, Kate Burkholder, Julie Johnson, and Susan Prendergast

Definition

A. Secondary postpartum haemorrhage is blood loss of 500 mL or more after the first 24 hours of delivery and within six weeks of delivery.

Incidence/Prevalence

A. Incidence is approximately 0.5% to 2% of women in developed countries.

Pathogenesis

A. Haemorrhage may result from retained placental fragments, subinvolution of the uterus, intrauterine infection, or inherited coagulation defects.

Predisposing Factors

A. Abnormally adherent placenta.
B. Prolonged rupture of membranes leading to infection.
C. Overdistended uterus from multiple gestation, and polyhydramnios.
D. Haematoma.

Common Findings

A. Heavy red bleeding or slow reddish-brown oozing.
B. Abdominal pain.
C. Loss of appetite.
D. Fatigue; cannot get enough rest and is unable to complete self-care and infant-care activities.

Other Signs and Symptoms

A. Lochia rubra is bright red discharge immediately after delivery (one to three days) and may contain a few small clots. A continuous trickle of bright red blood suggests a laceration of the cervix or vagina. Saturation of one peri-pad in < 15 minutes (two pads in 30 minutes, or rapid pooling of blood under the buttocks) is considered excessive bleeding and requires immediate attention.
B. Foul odour: Lochia should not be malodourous. Lochia usually has a "fleshy" odour.
C. Boggy uterus: Check the consistency of the uterus, whether it is firm or boggy. If atony is present, support the lower uterine segment and massage the uterus or do bimanual compression.
D. Faintness.
E. Tachycardia.
F. Hypotension.

Subjective Data

A. Elicit the onset, duration, and course of symptoms.
B. Elicit the amount and colour of lochia, including the size of blood clot(s).
C. Review symptoms of infection, including fever and malodourous lochia.
D. Review labour and delivery events, including the date of delivery, use of forceps or vacuum, weight of baby, manual removal of placenta, complications, and postpartum course.
E. Review pregnancy for predisposing factors such as multiple gestation and polyhydramnios (as noted earlier).

Physical Examination

A. Check temperature, blood pressure (BP), pulse, and respirations.
B. Inspect:
　1. Note colour and amount of vaginal bleeding.

Lochia may appear heavier when the woman first stands up because the lochia pools in the vagina while she is recumbent. Once the pooled blood is discharged, lochia flow should return to normal.

　2. Inspect episiotomy or abdominal incision.
C. Palpate:
　1. Check for consistency of uterus, massaging uterus if boggy.
　2. Express clots, if applicable.
　3. By two weeks postpartum, the uterus should have involuted and once again be a "pelvic organ."
　4. Check abdominal tension.
D. Speculum examination: Assess cervical lacerations.
E. Bimanual examination: Rule out retroperitoneal haemorrhage.

Diagnostic Tests

A. Complete blood count (CBC) with differential.
B. If bleeding is not under control, type and crossmatch blood.
C. Coagulation test if disseminated intravascular coagulation (DIC) is suspected.
D. Blood cultures to rule out infection.

Differential Diagnoses

A. Late postpartum bleeding.
B. Normal postpartum bleeding.
C. Postpartum infection.

Plan

A. General interventions:
　1. Perform uterine massage: Support the lower uterine segment during massage to prevent uterine prolapse.
　2. Give intravenous (IV) hydration for hypovolemic shock: Hypotension, tachycardia, and faintness.
　3. Hospitalization is usually required for postpartum haemorrhage.
　4. Encourage breastfeeding (if applicable) to increase uterine contraction.
　5. Advise the client to rest and increase oral fluids.
B. Pharmacological therapy:
　1. First-line treatment: Ergonovine maleate. **Do not give if the client is hypertensive.**
　2. For severe haemorrhage:
　　a. Oxytocin.
　　b. Ergonovine maleate if the client has no history of hypertension. Advise the client to take full course of it even if bleeding stops.
　　c. Hemabate.
　　d. Misoprostol.

e. Continue bimanual compression and notify a specialist.

3. If infection is suspected or confirmed, antibiotics are prescribed.

Follow-Up
A. Reevaluate the client 1 week from the date of discharge from the hospital.
B. Repeat haematocrit (Hct)/CBC at postpartum visit.
C. The client may need iron-replacement therapy if not already prescribed. If stable at 1-week follow-up visit, have the client return in 4 to 6 weeks postpartum for routine postpartum examination.

Consultation/Referral
A. Immediately consult or refer the client to a specialist for possible hospitalization for dilation and curettage (D&C).

Bibliography
Abdul-Kadir, R., McLintock, C., Ducloy, A. S., El-Refaey, H., England, A., Federici, A. B., . . . Winikoff, R. (2014). Evaluation and management of postpartum hemorrhage: Consensus from an international expert panel. *Transfusion, 54*(7), 1756–1768. doi:10.1111/trf.12550
American College of Obstetricians and Gynecologists. (2006, October). Postpartum hemorrhage. *ACOG Practice Bulletin,* (76). reaffirmed 2015.
Nettina, S. (Ed.). (2013). *Lippincott manual of nursing practice* (10th ed.). Philadelphia, PA: Wolters Kluwer Health/Lippincott Williams & Wilkins.

Mastitis

Jill C. Cash, Susan Drummond, Kate Burkholder, Julie Johnson, and Susan Prendergast

Definition
A. Mastitis is an infection of breast tissue with the potential for abscess formation.

Incidence/Prevalence
A. Mastitis has been estimated to occur in 2% to 10% of breastfeeding mothers. Less than 1% of these require hospitalization. Symptoms seldom appear before the end of the first week postpartum and are most often seen during the first 2 months postpartum.

Pathogenesis
A. During the period of lactation, the breast changes from an essentially nonfunctioning organ to a complex functioning organ of the body. The developing multiductal system becomes a rich environment for the growth of bacteria. The most common offending organism is *Staphylococcus aureus* (95%). The immediate source of the organisms that cause mastitis is almost always the nursing infant's nose and mouth.

Predisposing Factors
Invasion of bacteria in the presence of breast injury, including the following:
A. Bruising from rough manipulation (pumping) or failing to break the neonate's attachment to the areola and nipple before removing from breast.
B. Prolonged breast engorgement.
C. Milk stasis in a duct.
D. Cracking or fissures of the nipple.
E. Poor handwashing.

Common Findings
A. Breast engorgement, usually bilateral.
B. Pain in the breast, usually unilateral.
C. Fever.
D. Red streak(s).
E. Flu-like symptoms: Body aches, headache, malaise, and chills.

Other Signs and Symptoms
A. Fever 37.8°C to 40.0°C, rapid rise.
B. Exquisitely tender breast tissue.
C. Hard mass in the breast.
D. Tachycardia and tachypnea.
E. Axillary lymphadenopathy.

Subjective Data
A. Elicit the onset, duration, and course of symptoms.
B. Note the frequency and length of time of the feeding or pumping.
C. Are there any red streaks on the breasts?
D. Are the nipples cracked and bleeding?
E. Quantify pain symptoms, relief measures tried, and results.
F. Review other symptoms to rule out other infections such as wound infection, episiotomy breakdown, and urinary tract infection (UTI).

Physical Examination
A. Check temperature, blood pressure (BP), pulse, and respirations.
B. Physical examination should not be focused only on breast symptoms, but should include a general ruling out of other potential problems such as coexistent UTI or endometritis.
C. Inspect:
   1. Visually inspect breasts.
   2. Observe breastfeeding for adequacy of latch, suck, swallow, jaw glide, and any clicking.
   3. Check episiotomy or abdominal incision to rule out infection.
D. Palpate:
   1. Perform breast examination.
   2. Palpate lymph modes of the neck and axilla.
   3. Palpate the abdomen.
   4. Check costovertebral angle (CVA) tenderness.
E. Auscultate: Heart and lungs.

Diagnostic Tests
A. Treatment is usually initiated based on symptoms and examination.
B. Complete blood count (CBC): Leukocytosis in peripheral smear.
C. White blood cell (WBC), culture and sensitivity of breast milk to identify bacteria for persistent signs of infection or if antibiotic treatment is unsuccessful.
D. Urine or wound cultures, if applicable.
E. Ultrasound considered if breast is not responding to treatment to evaluate for breast abscess.

Differential Diagnoses
A. Breast engorgement: Bilateral presentation of breast discomfort.
B. Breast abscess: Discharge of purulent exudate from nipple, masses, or reddened areas that develops a bluish hue of the skin over the area of abscess.

C. Viral syndrome.
D. Inflammatory breast cancer.

Plan
A. General interventions: Encourage self-care and support. Advise the family to assist the client with self-care and infant care during this acute period. The woman may feel extremely ill for the first 24 to 48 hours of therapy and may find it difficult to continue breastfeeding, self-care, and newborn care activities.
B. Client teaching:
   1. Advise the client to continue to breastfeed or pump to maintain milk supply.
   2. Stress the importance of continuation of breastfeeding or pumping despite infection.
   3. Inform the client that the breast milk is not infected and it is safe for the newborn to continue to breastfeed. The infection is localized to the breast tissue and will respond quickly with antibiotic therapy.
C. Dietary management:
   1. There are no dietary restrictions.
   2. Have the client increase fluid intake with increased temperature (at least 10–12 glasses a day).
   3. Encourage her to eliminate caffeine, if possible, or use in moderation.
D. Pharmacological therapy:
   1. First-line treatment: Antibiotics:
      a. Dicloxacillin.
   2. Alternative drug therapy:
      a. Cephalexin.
      b. Concerning methicillin-resistant *Staphylococcus aureus* (MRSA), trimethoprim/sulfamethoxazole, or clindamycin. Linezolid may also be used.
      c. For a severe infection, inpatient treatment with vancomycin should be used.
   3. Advise the client to complete the full course of antibiotics even if symptoms improve sooner.
   4. Candidal vaginitis may develop secondary to antibiotic therapy. The client should be aware of the signs, symptoms, and treatment plan if it should occur. Use the probiotics *Lactobacillus fermentum* or *Lactobacillus salivarius* with use of antibiotics.
   5. Acetaminophen or ibuprofen for pain management.
   6. The client may require pain medication if acetaminophen or ibuprofen is not effective. Use acetaminophen with codeine phosphate or other narcotic as needed for pain.

Follow-Up
A. Evaluate the client in 48 hours if a breast abscess is suspected; assess need for surgical consultation.

Consultation/Referral
A. Consult a specialist if a breast abscess is suspected, for persistent signs of infection, or if antibiotic treatment is unsuccessful. Treatment of a breast abscess may include surgical incision and drainage of the abscess.
B. Notify the baby's provider if mastitis is diagnosed.

Bibliography
Nettina, S. (Ed.). (2013). *Lippincott manual of nursing practice* (10th ed.). Philadelphia, PA: Wolters Kluwer Health/Lippincott Williams & Wilkins.

Postpartum Care: Six Weeks Postpartum Examination

Jill C. Cash, Susan Drummond, Kate Burkholder, Julie Johnson, and Susan Prendergast

History
A. Chart review:
   1. Antepartum course, including prenatal laboratory data: Pap smear, cervical cultures, maternal ABO group and RH factor, rubella and syphilis screen, and complete blood count (CBC).
   2. Intrapartum course: Length of labour, type of delivery, and any maternal complications.
   3. Neonatal course: Gestational age, weight, length, cord gases, admission to normal or intensive care nursery, length of stay in the intensive care nursery, and any neonatal complications.
   4. Immediate postpartum course: Postpartum recovery, any postpartum complications, laboratory data, and length of hospital stay.
B. Interval history:
   1. Number of weeks postpartum.
   2. General maternal health and well-being, including diet or appetite, bowel and bladder function, level of activity, sleep patterns, and pain or discomfort.
   3. Interval problems: Calls to health-care provider, visits to ED, fever, or illness.
   4. Adjustment and role adaptation to the baby: Motherhood, fatherhood, sibling rivalry, psychosocial assessment of depression, family support, housing or financial issues.
   5. Resumption of sexual activity: When, problems encountered, comfort measures used, and type of contraception used.
   6. Family planning: Previous method of contraception used, success of method, plans to resume contraception, and options for contraception.
   7. Status of infant: Breastfeeding or bottle feeding, consolability, sleep patterns, voiding, and stool patterns.
   8. Establishment of health-care follow-up: Well-baby appointments and immunizations with primary care provider and/or public health nurse; or follow-up with nurse practitioner or registered midwife.
C. Review of relevant systems:
   1. Breasts: Cracked or sore nipples, clogged ducts, engorgement, mastitis; breast care practiced.
   2. Bladder function: Stress incontinence, dysuria, urinary frequency, and flank pain.
   3. Bowel function: Constipation; discomfort, especially if the client has a history of third- or fourth-degree laceration; relief measures used and results.
   4. Perineum: Problems or discomfort at episiotomy site, problems with wound healing, and signs of infection.
   5. Lochia: Duration, type, odour, presence of clots; or resumption of menses: Date, duration, and amount.
   6. Abdomen: If caesarean delivery, healing of wound, signs of infection; exercises initiated.
   7. Legs: Varicosities, heat, swelling, and calf tenderness.

Physical Examination
A. Weight, blood pressure (BP), and pulse; temperature, if indicated.
B. Inspect:
   1. Examine breast: Examine nipple integrity; assess for drying, cracking, bleeding, blisters.

2. Examine legs for varicosities and signs of thrombophlebitis.
3. Examine perineum, healing of episiotomy or lacerations, and abnormalities of Bartholin's gland.
4. Inspect caesarean section incision for wound integrity and for signs of infection.

C. Auscultate the heart and lungs.
D. Palpate:
1. Abdomen for tenderness, masses, involution of uterus.
2. Breasts for masses, engorgement, inflammation.

E. Speculum examination: Note lesions or lacerations of cervix, discharge, signs of infection; obtain Pap smear.
F. Bimanual examination: Check for abnormalities of cervix, uterus, adnexa; status of involution; presence of cystocele or rectocele; and vaginal muscle tone.
G. Rectovaginal examination: Check for integrity of episiotomy or laceration if indicated.
H. Psychological examination:
1. See section "Postpartum Depression" for information on assessment of postpartum blues/postpartum depression.

Diagnostic Tests
A. Pap smear.
B. Other tests as indicated; CBC if anaemia or haemorrhage is documented or suspected.

Differential Diagnoses
A. Mastitis.
B. Postpartum blues.
C. Postpartum depression.

Plan
A. General interventions:
1. This visit may be the last contact the woman has with the health-care delivery system for some time. The practitioner should evaluate any problems and provide appropriate consultations, referrals, interventions, counselling, and teaching.

B. Client teaching:
1. Explain the necessity of routine gynaecologic examination.
2. Encourage regular aerobic, abdominal, and Kegel exercises.
3. Counsel the client on choice of contraception:
   a. Abstinence.
   b. Natural family planning, calendar method.
   c. Spermicides.
   d. Barrier methods: Condoms, cervical caps, diaphragm.
   e. Intrauterine devices.
   f. Oral contraceptives.
   g. Tubal ligation.
   h. Vasectomy.
   i. Depot medroxyprogesterone acetate (DMPA) injection.
   j. Contraceptive implants.
4. Explain the benefits of a healthy diet, especially if the client is breastfeeding.
5. Discuss breastfeeding, if applicable; answer any questions and address concerns.

C. Pharmacological therapy—only as indicated from earlier examination:
1. Contraception: See section "Contraception" in Chapter 14, Gynecologic Guidelines.

2. If infection is diagnosed, see section "Mastitis" or "Endometritis" in this chapter for treatment options.

Follow-Up
A. Administer rubella vaccination if the client has nonimmune status, administration of vaccine was missed in the hospital stay, and she has not had unprotected intercourse since delivery.
B. If a woman's physical examination and laboratory and Pap tests are normal, she does not require a physical for at least one year, depending on her individual risk factors.
C. Establish a plan for the woman to obtain Pap smear results (follow-up phone call or letter with results).
D. Each province has a postpartum program that guides assessment, data collection, and documentation and client teaching.

Bibliography
Black, A., Guilbert, E., Hassan, F., Chatziheofilou, I., Lowin, J., Jeddi, M., . . . Trussell, J. (2015). The cost of unintended pregnancies in Canada: Estimating direct cost, role of imperfect adherence, and the potential impact of increased use of long-acting reversible contraceptives. *Journal of Obstetrics and Gynaecology Canada, 37*(12), 1086–1097.

Hale, T. W. (2014). *Medications and mother's milk* (16th ed.). Amarillo, TX: Hale.

Nettina, S. (Ed.). (2013). *Lippincott manual of nursing practice* (10th ed.). Philadelphia, PA: Wolters Kluwer Health/Lippincott Williams & Wilkins.

O'Connor, D., Blake, J., Bell, R., Bowen, A., Callum, J., Fenton, S., . . . Rossiter, M. (2016). Canadian consensus on female nutrition: Adolescence, reproduction, menopause, and beyond. *The SOGC, Journal of Obstetrics and Gynecology Canada, 38*(6), 508–554. doi:10.1016/j.jogc.2016.01.001

Varney, H., Kriebs, J. M., & Gregor, C. L. (2013). *Varney's midwifery* (5th ed.). Sudbury, MA: Jones & Bartlett.

Postpartum Depression

Jill C. Cash, Susan Drummond, Kate Burkholder, Julie Johnson, and Susan Prendergast

Definition
A. Postpartum depression is a mood disorder characterized by unexplained tearfulness, sadness, irritability, and disturbances in appetite and sleep patterns; inability to care for self or baby; it usually presents within two weeks to three months postpartum.

Incidence/Prevalence
A. Reported incidence of postpartum depression in Canada is 7.5%.

Pathogenesis
A. It is believed that postpartum depression may be related to psychological, physiological, and cultural factors. The extreme hormonal changes that occur during the postpartum period may contribute. Postpartum thyroiditis is also a suspected factor. However, no confirmed biological cause has been found. Some authorities have suggested that the mother's feeling of "loss of control" over her own life is the underlying precipitating factor.

Predisposing Factors
The following may make a mother more likely to experience postpartum depression:
A. Preterm infant.
B. Multiple gestation.

C. History of postpartum depression or mental illness.
D. Social stressors: Dissatisfaction in the marriage, financial difficulties, and lack of support in the home.
E. Age younger than 20 years.
F. Single parent.
G. Poor relationship with the father of the baby.
H. Evidence of significant emotional problems in the past.
I. Having experienced separation from one or both parents during childhood or adolescence.
J. Having received poor parental support and attention in childhood or having limited social support in adulthood.
K. Low self-esteem.

Common Findings
A. Insomnia.
B. Poor appetite.
C. Tearfulness.
D. Fatigue.
E. Anxiety.
F. Headaches.
G. Difficulty concentrating or confusion.
H. Feelings of excessive guilt or worthlessness.
I. Possible suicidal ideations.

Other Signs and Symptoms
A. Mood swings.
B. Despondency, social withdrawal, and feeling of inadequacy.
C. Guilt.
D. Impaired memory.
E. Ambivalence about motherhood and baby.
F. Inability to care for self and baby.
G. Poor grooming of self and/or baby.

Subjective Data
A. Elicit the onset, duration, and course of symptoms.
B. Review the client's medical history for predisposing factors; see section "Predisposing Factors".
C. Question the client regarding her ability to care for her infant, herself, and other family members at home.
D. Review the amount of support in the home. Is she the primary caregiver? Are there any family members or friends who help in the household management, sibling childcare, and newborn care?
E. Does the client get out of bed and dress herself daily?
F. Does the client have thoughts of harming the infant, herself, or others?

Physical Examination
A. Check temperature, pulse, respirations, and BP.
B. Inspection: Note general overall appearance, including dress, make-up, neatness of hair, tearfulness, and apathy.
C. Observe her interaction with the baby: Tone of voice when talking to the baby, eye contact, and so on.

Diagnostic Tests
A. Administer the Edinburgh Postnatal Depression Scale: www.aap.org/en-us/advocacy-and-policy/aap-health-initiatives/practicing-safety/Documents/Postnatal%20Depression%20Scale.pdf.
B. Thyroid panel for diagnosis of depression.

Differential Diagnoses
A. Baby blues: Tearfulness, insomnia, fatigue, headaches, poor appetite, and so on; appearing between the birth and 14 postpartum days.
B. Postpartum psychosis: Extreme emotional lability, agitation, delusions, hallucinations, and sleep disturbances.
C. Postpartum panic disorder: Extreme anxiety, fear, tightness in the chest, and increased heart rate.
D. Postpartum obsessive-compulsive disorder: Obsessive thoughts of harming the child, exaggerated fear of being left alone with the infant, anxiety, depression, and/or unnecessarily vigilant protectiveness of the infant.
E. Bipolar disorder.

Plan
A. General interventions:
  1. Assess all clients for postpartum mood disorders at all postpartum contacts. See the Blues Questionnaire (Exhibit 13.1) for a sample assessment tool.
  2. Early assessment and treatment are very important. Symptoms that are not treated for several weeks may get progressively worse. Clients with severe depression, characterized by suicidal or homicidal ideation, aggressive behaviour, delusions, hallucinations, catatonia, poor judgment, or grossly impaired function, are typically hospitalized.
  3. Encourage involvement of the client's partner and immediate family members in the counselling sessions to assist them in learning ways to assist the client effectively.
B. Client teaching:
  1. Advise the client that she is not to blame for the condition. Its occurrence is not uncommon and successful treatment is likely.
  2. Discuss participation in a support group, interpersonal psychotherapy, or cognitive behavioural therapy.
  3. If antidepressants are prescribed, advise the client that the medication may take four to six weeks for peak effect. Review the benefits/risks/side effects of the medication prescribed. The risk of suicide may increase after beginning antidepressants; therefore, a follow-up appointment in one to two weeks is recommended.
C. Pharmacological therapy:
  1. Antidepressants may be ordered for women with moderate to severe symptoms of depression when physical and emotional functioning has been compromised. (Refer to the section "Depression" in Chapter 22, Psychiatric Guidelines.).
  2. Base selection of medication on whether or not the client is breastfeeding. Selective serotonin reuptake inhibitors (SSRIs) and tricyclic antidepressants are commonly used:
    a. Citalopram.
    b. Sertraline.
    c. Amitriptyline.

Follow-Up
A. If the client had risk factors for depression before delivery, a follow-up office visit three to four days after hospital discharge is suggested.
B. Frequent telephone contact, or several repeat visits, may be necessary during the course of the depression, until the symptoms have improved.

EXHIBIT 13.1 Blues Questionnaire

_____Days Postpartum _____Date: _____

Following is a list of words that newly delivered mothers have used to describe how they are feeling. Please indicate HOW YOU HAVE BEEN FEELING TODAY by ticking NO or YES. Then please mark the box that best describes how significant this difference is, if at all from your usual self.

	NO	YES		Much Less Than Usual	Less Than Usual	No Difference	More Than Usual	Much More Than Usual
Tearful			Is this					
Mentally tense			Is this					
Able to concentrate			Is this					
Low spirited			Is this					
Elated			Is this					
Helpless			Is this					
Finding it difficult to show your feelings			Is this					
Alert			Is this					
Forgetful, muddled			Is this					
Anxious			Is this					
Wishing you were alone			Is this					
Mentally relaxed			Is this					
Brooding on things			Is this					
Feeling sorry for yourself			Is this					
Emotionally numb, without feelings			Is this					
Depressed			Is this					
Overemotional			Is this					
Happy			Is this					
Confident			Is this					
Changeable in your spirits			Is this					
Tired			Is this					
Irritable			Is this					
Crying without being able to stop			Is this					
Lively			Is this					
Oversensitive			Is this					
Up and down in your mood			Is this					
Restlessness			Is this					
Calm, tranquil			Is this					

Source: Used with permission from The Royal College of Psychiatrists. Reprinted from Kennerley, H., & Gath, D. (1989). Maternity blues. I. Detection and measurement by questionnaire. *British Journal of Psychiatry, 155,* 356–362. Retrieved from http://bjp.rcpsych.org/content/155/3/356.long.

C. The risk of suicide may increase after beginning antidepressants; therefore, a follow-up appointment in one to two weeks is recommended.

D. Assess the client for suicidal ideation and child neglect at every contact.

Consultation/Referral

A. Assess the need to refer the client to a psychiatrist, psychologist, or family counsellor.

B. Refer to group therapy, interpersonal psychotherapy, and/or cognitive behavioural therapy.

C. Consult a psychiatrist about alternative treatments if no change in signs and symptoms is seen.

Resources

Postpartum Support International: www.postpartum.net (click on Canada in left column for resources)
Postpartum Support Line: 1-800-944-4773

Bibliography

Kennerley, H., & Gath, D. (1989). Maternity blues. I. Detection and measurement by questionnaire. *British Journal of Psychiatry, 155,* 356–362. Retrieved from http://bjp.rcpsych.org/content/155/3/356.long

Nelson, D. B., Freeman, M. P., Johnson, N. L., McIntire, D. D., & Leveno, K. J. (2013). A prospective study of postpartum depression in 17 648 parturients. *Journal of Maternal–Fetal & Neonatal Medicine: The Official Journal of the European Association of Perinatal Medicine, the Federation of Asia and Oceania Perinatal Societies, the International Society of Perinatal Obstetricians, 26*(12), 1155–1161. doi:10.3109/14767058.2013.777698

Nettina, S. (Ed.). (2013). *Lippincott manual of nursing practice* (10th ed.). Philadelphia, PA: Wolters Kluwer Health/Lippincott Williams & Wilkins.

Public Health Association of Canada. Retrived from https://www.canada.ca/en/public-health/services/publications/healthy-living/pregnancy-women-mental-health-canada.html

Wound Infection

Jill C. Cash, Susan Drummond, Kate Burkholder, Julie Johnson, and Susan Prendergast

Definition
A. Infection may occur at the site of caesarean section incision, episiotomy, or genital tract laceration. Most wound infections become clinically apparent five to six days after delivery.

Incidence/Prevalence
A. Rates of infection after caesarean delivery range from five to 30 times greater than vaginal delivery.

Pathogenesis
A. A variety of organisms may be responsible. Examples include *Staphylococcus* or *Streptococcus* species and gram-negative organisms, gram-positive cocci, and *Bacteroides* and *Clostridium* species.

Predisposing Factors
A. Obesity.
B. Anaemia.
C. Malnutrition.
D. Smoking.
E. Diabetes.
F. Substance abuse.
G. Susceptible to infection.
H. Poor hygiene.
I. Lower socioeconomic status.
J. Lack of preoperative prophylactic antibiotics.

Common Findings
A. Redness, heat, swelling, and tenderness at site.
B. Foul-smelling drainage.
C. Elevated temperature.

Other Signs and Symptoms
A. Fever and chills.
B. Oedema.
C. Foul-smelling discharge and pus.

Subjective Data
A. Elicit the onset, duration, and course of symptoms.
B. Review medical history (see section "Predisposing Factors"); antepartum history for complications such as diabetes; intrapartum complications for prolonged rupture of membranes, fever in labour, use of internal monitoring devices, length of labour, or frequent cervical examinations.
C. Question the client regarding hygiene at the wound site since delivery, including the frequency of changing peri-pads, use of sitz baths, and showering.
D. Question the client regarding drainage from the wound or episiotomy, noting colour, amount, and odour.
E. Review signs and symptoms of breast engorgement and urinary tract infection (UTI).
F. Review vaginal delivery for third- and fourth-degree episiotomy.

Physical Examination
A. Check temperature, pulse, respirations, and blood pressure (BP).
B. Examination should not be limited to the incision site. A complete physical examination is needed to evaluate breasts, lungs, haematomas, and concurrent UTIs.
C. Inspect:
   1. Examine the incision site (episiotomy or abdomen) for drainage, redness or oedema, and intactness.
   2. Inspect bilateral breasts, assessing for erythema, oedema, swelling.
   3. Inspect vagina, assessing episiotomy site, lacerations, and haematoma. Evaluate appearance of the lochia.
D. Palpate:
   1. Perform breast examination.
   2. Palpate suture line (episiotomy or abdomen). Probe incision with cotton-tipped swab to evaluate for haematoma, cellulitis, and/or pus.
   3. Palpate all abdominal quadrants.
   4. Palpate the vagina to rule out concealed haematoma.
E. Auscultate the heart and lungs.
F. Percuss the back to assess costovertebral angle (CVA) tenderness.

Diagnostic Tests
A. Complete blood count (CBC) with differential.
B. Blood culture (optional).
C. Culture of infected area.
D. Urinalysis, culture, and sensitivity, if indicated.

Differential Diagnoses
A. Wound infection.
B. Impending dehiscence. If serosanguinous drainage is noted after the first 24 hours, dehiscence is possible.
C. Episiotomy breakdown.

Plan
A. General interventions:
   1. The wound may need to be opened and cleaned.
   2. For an infection at a caesarean section site, wound irrigation and dressing changes several times a day may be necessary.
   3. Home health referral may be needed.
B. Client teaching:
   1. Instruct client on self-care for episiotomy or caesarean section incision site. Instructions on cleaning episiotomy/caesarean incision site should be reinforced.

C. Dietary management:
  1. No dietary restrictions are recommended; encourage the client to eat well-balanced meals. Increase protein in the diet for wound healing.
  2. Instruct the client to increase fluid intake; have her drink at least 10 to 12 glasses of liquid a day.
D. Pharmacological therapy:
  1. Clavulin.
  2. Clindamycin: Safe for breastfeeding.
  3. Cefoxitin: Safe for breastfeeding.
  4. Acetaminophen when required for elevated temperature.

Follow-Up
A. Reevaluate the client in 48 hours to assess wound healing.

Consultation/Referral
A. Consult a specialist for evaluation and possible surgical closure.

Bibliography
American College of Obstetricians and Gynecologists. (2015, December). Obesity in pregnancy. *ACOG Practice Bulletin*, (156).

Nettina, S. (Ed.). (2013). *Lippincott manual of nursing practice* (10th ed.). Philadelphia, PA: Wolters Kluwer Health/Lippincott Williams & Wilkins.

14 Gynecologic Guidelines

Amenorrhoea

Rhonda Arthur and Julia Blake

Definition
Amenorrhoea is the absence of menstruation when menstrual periods should occur:
A. Primary amenorrhoea:
  1. No menstrual period by age 14 years in the absence of growth or development of secondary sexual characteristics.
  2. No menstrual period by age 16 years regardless of the presence of normal growth and development with the appearance of secondary sexual characteristics.

B. Secondary amenorrhoea: No menstrual period for six months in a woman who usually has normal periods, or for a length of time equal to three-cycle intervals in a woman with less-frequent cycles.

Incidence/Prevalence
A. Amenorrhoea in a woman who has had menstrual periods is quite common at some time during her reproductive life. Amenorrhoea that is a result of agenesis of part of the reproductive system or a chromosomal anomaly is quite rare. See the following for the incidence of each cause.

Pathogenesis
A. Physiological: Pregnancy, breastfeeding, and menopause.
B. Disorders of the central nervous system (CNS) (hypothalamic): Hypothalamic amenorrhoea is the most common cause of amenorrhoea (28%). There is a deficiency in pulsatile secretion of gonadotropin-releasing hormone (GnRH). Examples include a stressful lifestyle (10%); weight loss, as in anorexia or bulimia (10%); extreme exercise; medications, such as hormones, as in postpill amenorrhoea; hypothyroidism (10%); and major medical disease, such as Crohn's disease or systemic lupus erythematosus (SLE).
C. Disorders of the outflow tract or uterine target organ: Abnormalities in the systems of this compartment are uncommon. Examples include Asherman's syndrome from inadvertent endometrial ablation during dilation and curettage (D&C; causes 7% of amenorrhoea); and agenesis or structural anomalies of the uterus, tubes, or vagina.
D. Disorders of the ovary: Examples include abnormal chromosomes, such as Turner's syndrome (0.5%); normal chromosomes (10%), such as in gonadal dysgenesis or agenesis (there may be no or very delayed Tanner stage); premature ovarian failure (POF); premature menopause, before the age of 40 years; effect of radiation or chemotherapy; and polycystic ovarian (PCO) disease.
E. Disorders of the anterior pituitary: Examples include prolactin tumours (7.5%).

Predisposing Factor
A. The disorder can affect any female between the ages of 14 and 55 years.

Common Findings
A. "I haven't had a period in months"; "I have periods only a few times each year."
B. "I have nipple discharge."
C. "I am 16 years old and have never had a menstrual period."

Other Signs and Symptoms
A. Irregular, infrequent menstrual periods.
B. Galactorrhoea.
C. Pregnancy.
D. Excessive hair growth.

Subjective Data
A. Review complete menstrual history, including age of onset, duration, frequency, regularity, and dysmenorrhoea.
B. Review the client's pregnancy history.
C. Review the client's contraception history.
D. Note other medications the client is taking, such as hormones or antidepressants.
E. Ask the client if she has had a major medical disease or treatment, such as chemotherapy for a childhood cancer.
F. Inquire about any breast discharge.
G. Review the client's weight pattern.
H. Ask the client to describe her physical self-image. Does she consider herself obese or fat?
I. Review sources of stress in her life.
J. Discuss exercise pattern and history.

Physical Examination
A. Check height, weight, blood pressure (BP), and pulse.
B. Inspect:
  1. Note overall appearance. Look at the neck (thyroid). Inspect the breast/genitalia for Tanner staging. See Appendix C, Tanner's Sexual Maturity Stages.
  2. Skin assessment: Check for central hair growth, which is androgen-responsive. Areas to inspect for coarse hair include the upper lip, chin, sideburns, neck, chest, lower abdomen, and perineum.
C. Palpate:
  1. The neck for thyroid enlargement.
  2. The abdomen for enlarged organs or uterine enlargement compatible with pregnancy.

D. Auscultate:
  1. Auscultate the heart and lungs.
  2. If pregnancy is suspected, consider auscultating for foetal heart tones.
E. Pelvic examination:
  1. Inspect external genitalia. Note pubic hair pattern for Tanner staging. Note any lesions, masses, or discharge.
  2. Speculum examination: Inspect vagina and cervix. Note bluish colour, which is Chadwick's sign with pregnancy.
  3. Bimanual examination: Palpate for softening of the cervical isthmus, which is Hegar's sign for pregnancy. Palpate for size of uterus and for adnexal masses.

Diagnostic Tests

A. Urine: Pregnancy test.
B. Serum:
  1. Serum human chorionic gonadotropin (HCG).
  2. Thyroid-stimulating hormone (TSH), to rule out thyroid disease.
  3. Prolactin: normal <25 mcg/L (often referenced as 25ng/mL).
  4. Follicle-stimulating hormone (FSH):>40 international units (IU)/L indicates ovarian failure.
  5. Luteinizing hormone (LH): FSH ratio to rule out polycystic ovaries.
C. Vaginal and/or pelvic ultrasonography.
D. Genetic testing/karyotype analysis in primary amenorrhoea.

Differential Diagnoses

A. Pregnancy.
B. Constitutional delay.
C. Hypothyroidism.
D. Polycystic ovary syndrome (PCOS).
E. POF, or early menopause.
F. Perimenopause.
G. Pituitary adenoma.
H. Androgen insensitivity syndrome.

Plan

A. General interventions:
  1. If laboratory values are normal, proceed to progesterone challenge test to rule out hypothalamic amenorrhoea.
  2. If the client is pregnant, counsel regarding pregnancy and begin antepartum care.
  3. If other laboratory information points to an underlying cause for amenorrhoea, treat as appropriate.
▶ B. Client teaching: *Refer to Client Teaching Guide: Amenorrhoea.*
C. Pharmacological therapy:
  1. Progesterone challenge:
    a. Micronized progesterone.
    b. Positive test is any vaginal bleeding. Withdrawal bleeding should occur within seven to 10 days after finishing the medicine. A late vaginal bleed may be associated with ovulation.
    c. In the absence of galactorrhoea, with a normal prolactin level, normal TSH, and positive progesterone challenge, further evaluation is unnecessary.

All anovulatory clients require therapeutic management. There is a risk of endometrial cancer with unopposed oestrogen. There is a short latent period in progression from a normal endometrium to atypia to cancer, even in a young woman.

    d. A negative withdrawal bleed may be associated with PCOS.
  2. Progesterone therapy for hypothalamic amenorrhoea:
    a. Medroxyprogesterone acetate.
    b. Low-dose oral contraceptive pills.
    c. Clomiphene citrate for women desiring pregnancy.
    d. Hormone replacement therapy (HRT) for perimenopausal women.

Follow-Up

A. Reproductive age: The client should return after six months of treatment with progesterone or oral contraceptive pills. Discontinue the hormones and assess for return of normal periods. If this does not occur, reinstitute progesterone or oral contraceptive therapy.
B. Perimenopausal: Maintain hormonal therapy. The client should return annually.

Consultation/Referral

A. Refer the client to a specialist if there is no withdrawal bleeding from the progesterone challenge. The problem is either with the outflow track, which is rare, or with the ovarian production of oestrogen or hypothalamic production of gonadotropins. This is usually beyond the scope of the nurse practitioner.
B. Refer the client to a specialist if her prolactin level is elevated (>25 mg/mL) for further workup to rule out pituitary adenoma.

Individual Considerations

A. Adolescence:
  1. Rule out pregnancy. Then determine whether primary or secondary amenorrhoea. Refer the client to a specialist for primary amenorrhoea.
  2. For secondary amenorrhoea, complete assessment and evaluation. Assess stress/emotional status, nutritional status, and exercise routine.
  3. Refer to a specialist if there is no withdrawal bleeding from progesterone challenge test.
  4. Refer for evaluation and treatment as indicated for eating, exercise, or psychiatric disorders.
B. Older adults:
  1. Irregular menses and amenorrhoea are common during perimenopause. Provide anticipatory guidance and instructions regarding the need for contraceptive use until menopause is confirmed.

Bibliography

Faucher, M. A., & Schuiling, K. D. (2013). Normal and abnormal uterine bleeding. In K. D. Schuiling & F. E. Likis (Eds.), *Women's gynecologic health* (2nd ed., pp. 609–646). Burlington, MA: Jones & Bartlett.

▶ Client Teaching Guides are available at https://connect.springerpub.com/content/reference-book/978-0-8261-9498-5

Atrophic Vaginitis

Rhonda Arthur and Julia Blake

Definition
A. Atrophic vaginitis is inflammation of the vaginal epithelium due to a lack of oestrogen support. Anything that lowers oestrogen levels after puberty can result in a loss of vaginal thickness and rugosity and a decrease in the elasticity of the vaginal tissues.

Incidence/Prevalence
A. Atrophic vaginitis is very common. It may occur in three stages of a woman's life: preadolescence, when breastfeeding a baby, and postmenopause.

Pathogenesis
A. Oestrogen maintains the vaginal pH in an acidic range. Lack of sufficient oestrogen promotes an increase in vaginal pH that supports the development of bacterial infections. Oestrogen loss also results in a decrease in vaginal glycogen and a thin-walled epithelium, promoting friability and inflammation.

Predisposing Factors
A. Preadolescence.
B. Breastfeeding.
C. Postmenopause.
D. Ovarian failure.

Common Findings
A. Vaginal dryness, irritation, and/or bleeding.
B. Dyspareunia.
C. Dysuria.

Other Signs and Symptoms
A. Postcoital bleeding.
B. Thin vaginal discharge.
C. Vaginal itching.

Subjective Data
A. Question the client regarding onset, duration, and course of symptoms.
B. Is this a new problem? If so, review the use of a new soap, laundry detergent, or hygiene products.
C. Describe the colour, amount, and odour of vaginal discharge or bleeding.
D. Determine existence of coexisting vasomotor symptoms, such as hot flashes.
E. Is the client experiencing dysuria, urinary frequency, vulvar dryness and itching, or dyspareunia? With dyspareunia, question the client whether the discomfort is due to irritation or pain with deep penetration, or both.
F. Determine whether the client is breastfeeding and for what length of time.
G. Ask the client the date of her last menses and if she is having irregular cycles. Determine whether the client had a hysterectomy with oophorectomy or ovarian failure.
H. Review the number of the client's sexual partners and any new sexual practices.
I. Review the client's current medications, including antidepressants.
J. Explore whether she has stopped hormone replacement therapy (HRT).
K. Has the client tried any self-help measures? Was there any relief?
L. When was the last Papanicolaou (Pap) smear, and what were the results?

Physical Examination
A. Check temperature, pulse, and respirations.
B. Inspect: Observe the client generally for discomfort before, during, and after examination.
C. Palpate:
　1. Back: Check for costovertebral angle (CVA) tenderness.
　2. Abdomen: Note suprapubic tenderness.

Pelvic Examination
A. Inspect:
　1. Examine external genitalia for friability, erythema, lesions, condyloma, and amount and colour of discharge.
　2. Sparse and brittle pubic hair, shrinking of the labia minora, and inflammation of the vulva may be noted in menopausal women.
　3. The vulva may appear erythematous, and there may be labial oedema.
　4. Excoriation may be present if the woman has complained of pruritus.
B. Palpate: "Milk" urethra for discharge to rule out infection.
C. Speculum examination:
　1. Check rugae, friability of vaginal epithelium, and colour and amount of discharge; evaluate cervix for lesions, friability, and erythema.
　2. Typical atrophic symptoms on inspection: Thin, friable vaginal epithelium; decreased or absent vaginal rugae; scant vaginal discharge.
D. Bimanual examination:
　1. Check for cervical motion tenderness (CMT), uterine size, and position (if no hysterectomy).
　2. Check adnexa for masses.

Diagnostic Tests
A. Routine hormone measurements to evaluate menopause status are not routinely indicated.
B. Urine culture, if applicable.
C. Vaginal pH; normal pH range in premenopausal women is 4 to 4.5. Reduced levels of oestrogen increase vaginal pH.
D. Pap smear with maturation index. (Vaginal wall maturation index evaluation is controversial.)
E. Wet prep, if applicable:
　1. Multiple white blood cells (WBCs) indicate inflammation, may show increased bacteria, and may have decreased lactobacillus, suggesting atrophic vaginitis.
　2. Test should be negative for *Trichomonas*. Bacterial vaginosis (BV): Whiff test should be negative.
F. Cultures for gonorrhoea and chlamydia, if applicable.
G. Ultrasound for uterine lining thickness if applicable (<4 or 5 mm suggests loss of oestrogenic stimulation).
H. Endometrial biopsy, if indicated.

Postmenopausal vaginal bleeding must be thoroughly investigated to rule out the possibility of endometrial hyperplasia or endometrial cancer.

Differential Diagnoses
A. Trauma.
B. Foreign body in the vagina.
C. Urinary tract infection (UTI).
D. Vaginitis from infective cause: fungus, bacteria, or virus.
E. Contact irritation: latex (condom), spermicide, lubricant.
F. Menopause.

Plan
A. General interventions:
   1. Treat any underlying infections (gonorrhoea, chlamydia, vaginitis), as diagnosed.
B. Client teaching:
   1. *Refer to Client Teaching Guides: Atrophic Vaginitis and Dyspareunia (Pain With Intercourse).*
   2. Preadolescent girls have amelioration of symptoms with increase of endogenous oestrogen as puberty approaches.
   3. Women should be reassured that this problem is physical, not emotional.
   4. Discuss the benefits of regular sexual activity to decrease problems of atrophic vaginitis. An important reason for decreased sexual activity is unavailability of a partner. Masturbation also facilitates the natural resumption of the production of lubricating secretions by the body. Decline in sexuality is influenced by culture and attitudes as well as physical problems.
   5. Symptomatic relief of dryness during sexual activity may be obtained with the use of water-soluble lubricants and adequate foreplay.
   6. Vaginal moisturizer may be applied for relief of symptoms.
   7. Discuss pregnancy prevention and inform that perimenopausal symptoms do not ensure lack of fertility.
C. Pharmacological therapy:
   1. Calamine lotion may be applied externally for local symptomatic relief.
   2. Oestrogen therapy (OT):
     a. Vaginal hormonal therapy:

Absolute contraindications for use of OT also apply to use of topical oestrogen (breast cancer, active liver disease, history of recent thromboembolic event). Vaginal oestrogen creams are systemically absorbed. As with the use of oral and transdermal oestrogen, a progestin must be administered to women who have an intact uterus, secondary to the risk of endometrial hyperplasia or cancer.

       i. Conjugated oestrogen (not for daily use if the client has an intact uterus).
       ii. Estradiol hemihydrate (not for daily use if the client has an intact uterus).

Vaginal oestrogen creams should not be used as a lubricant before intercourse as the hormone can be absorbed through a partner's skin.

       iii. Estradiol; the need for continued treatment should be assessed at each 90-day interval. Maximum duration of continual therapy is two years.
     b. Oral oestrogen replacement therapy:
       i. Conjugated oestrogen (plus medroxyprogesterone).
       ii. See the section "Menopause" in this chapter for other regimens of HRT.

For long-term OT, consider use of oral or patch methods of delivery if the client shows additional symptoms of hypo-oestrogenaemia (i.e., hot flashes, night sweats).

Follow-Up
A. Breastfeeding women should be reevaluated following weaning, especially if symptoms persist (i.e., alternate aetiology is suspected).
B. Postmenopausal women should be evaluated for additional aetiologies (i.e., endometrial hyperplasia) if vaginal bleeding persists beyond three to six months following a treatment.
C. The client should return to clinic one to two months after beginning oral or vaginal drug therapy; the client then needs to be seen in three to six months to check side effects, blood pressure (BP), and response to therapy.
D. Perform Pap smears and physical examination per client health history or risks and guidelines.

Consultation/Referral
A. If bleeding is a symptom in a postmenopausal woman, the practitioner must rule out bleeding of uterine origin. If there is any doubt, consultation for endometrial biopsy or dilation and curettage (D&C) must be obtained.

Individual Considerations
A. Breastfeeding women:
   1. Breastfeeding women have amelioration of symptoms as weaning progresses unless an alternate aetiology exists.
B. Postmenopausal women:
   1. Evaluate the client for other risks of hypo-oestrogenaemia, such as cardiovascular disease and osteoporosis. Continuous systemic oestrogen replacement therapy may be indicated.
   2. Vaginitis in the postmenopausal woman is rarely due to any of the organisms responsible for vaginitis in the premenopausal woman (unless she has new sexual partners). Candidiasis, trichomoniasis, and BV are uncommon after the menstruating years.

Bacterial Vaginosis (or Gardnerella)

Rhonda Arthur and Julia Blake

Definition
A. Bacterial vaginosis (BV) is an infection of the vagina caused by an alteration in the normal flora of the vagina, with an increase in anaerobes and Gram-negative bacilli as well as a decrease in the *Lactobacillus* flora.

Incidence/Prevalence
A. BV is one of the most common vaginal infections in women of childbearing age and is common in pregnant women. It is not considered exclusively a sexually transmitted infection (STI).

▸ Client Teaching Guides are available at https://connect.springerpub.com/content/reference-book/978-0-8261-9498-5

Pathogenesis

A. The main aetiologic agent in BV is an increase in anaerobes in the vagina. The reason why this occurs is unknown, but is associated with having multiple sexual partners, douching, lack of condom use, and lack of vaginal lactobacilli. When the normal lactobacilli of the vagina decrease, the vaginal pH is increased. The organisms present in BV cause the level of vaginal amines to be high. These amines are volatilized when the pH is increased, causing the characteristic "fishy" odour.
B. Bacterial vaginitis is primarily polymicrobial, and the pathogens seen include *Bacteroides* species, *Peptostreptococcus* species, *Eubacterium* species, *Mobiluncus* species, *Gardnerella*, and *Mycoplasma hominis*. The incubation period is unknown.

Predisposing Factors

A. History of STIs.
B. Multiple sexual partners.
C. Intrauterine device (IUD) use.
D. Factors that change the normal vaginal flora:
  1. Hormonal changes (menses, pregnancy).
  2. Medications: oral contraceptive use and antibiotic therapy.
  3. Foreign bodies in the vagina (tampons, IUDs), semen, and douching.

Common Findings

A. Vaginal discharge (thin, white, gray, or milky).
B. Fishy vaginal odour.
C. Postcoital odour.

Other Signs and Symptoms

A. Asymptomatic.
B. Increase in odour after menses.
C. Occasional itching and burning.

Subjective Data

A. Elicit onset, duration, and course of presenting symptoms.
B. Review any changes in the characteristics and colour of vaginal discharge. Does the client's partner(s) have any symptoms?
C. Review any symptoms of pruritus, perineal excoriation, burning; signs of urinary tract infection (UTI).
D. Review medication and medical history.
E. Determine whether the client is pregnant; note the date of last menstrual period (LMP).
F. Question the client for a history of STIs or other vaginal infections.
G. Review previous infection, treatment, compliance with treatment, and results.
H. Note the last intercourse date.
I. Elicit information about possible foreign body.
J. Review use of vaginal deodorants or sprays, scented toilet paper, tampons, pads, and douching habits.
K. Review change in laundry detergent, soaps, and fabric softeners.
L. Review use of tight restrictive clothing, tight jeans, and nylon panties.
M. Review history for seizures and anticoagulant therapy.

Physical Examination

A. Check temperature, pulse, and respirations.
B. Inspect: Examine external vulva and introitus for discharge, irritation, fissures, lesions, rashes, and condyloma.
C. Palpate:
  1. Palpate the abdomen for masses or tenderness. Note enlarged or tender inguinal lymph nodes.
  2. Palpate the external perineal area for vulvar masses.
  3. "Milk" the urethra for discharge.
  4. Check for costovertebral angle (CVA) tenderness.
D. Pelvic examination:
  1. Inspect:
    a. Note the colour, amount, and odour of discharge.
    b. Inspect the cervix:
      i. BV is a vaginosis rather than a vaginitis. There is usually little or no inflammation of the vaginal epithelium associated with BV.
      ii. BV is associated with a pink, healthy cervix; "strawberry cervix" is seen with cervicitis due to *Trichomonas vaginalis*.
      iii. A red, oedematous, friable cervix is seen with *Chlamydia trachomatis*.
  2. Speculum examination:
    a. Inspect sidewalls for adhering discharge.
    b. The clinical diagnosis of BV requires the presence of three of the following four signs:
      i. Homogeneous, white, adherent vaginal discharge may be present.
      ii. Vaginal fluid pH >4.5. For accurate pH, take smear for testing from the lateral walls of the vagina, not from the cervix.
      iii. A fishy, amine-like odour from vaginal fluid before or after mixing it with 10% KOH (positive whiff test). Semen releases the vaginal amines; therefore, there is an increase in odour after intercourse.
      iv. Presence of "clue cells" (squamous vaginal epithelial cells covered with bacteria, causing a stippled or granular appearance and ragged, "moth-eaten" borders) or coccobacilli forms both in the fluid and adheres to the epithelial cells.
  3. Bimanual examination: Check for cervical motion tenderness (CMT) and adnexal masses. BV may be a risk factor for pelvic inflammatory disease (PID).

Diagnostic Tests

A. Gram stain (considered the gold standard).
B. BV can be diagnosed by use of clinical criteria; three of the following four are needed to make clinical diagnosis (Amsel's diagnostic criteria [DC]):
  1. Vaginal pH: >4.5 with BV; normal vaginal pH range is 4 to 4.5.
  2. Clue cells on microscopic examination.
  3. Homogeneous, thick white discharge that coats the vaginal walls.
  4. A fishy odour of the vaginal discharge before or after the addition of 10% KOH (wet prep with 10% KOH and normal saline prep); microscopic examination of vaginal secretions should always be done.
C. Herpes culture, if indicated.
D. Urinalysis and culture, if indicated.

Differential Diagnoses

A. Vulvovaginal candidiasis.
B. Trichomoniasis.
C. Gonorrhoea.
D. Chlamydia.
E. Presence of foreign body.
F. Normal physiological discharge.

Plan

A. General interventions:
1. Inform the client regarding other modalities for treating BV. These methods include the following:
   a. Vinegar and water douches: One tablespoon of white vinegar in one pint of water. Douche one to two times a week.
   b. *Lactobacillus acidophilus* culture.
   c. Garlic suppositories: One peeled clove of garlic wrapped in a cloth dipped in olive oil, inserted vaginally overnight and changed daily.

B. Client teaching:
1. *Refer to Client Teaching Guide: Bacterial Vaginosis.*
2. BV is not considered an STI.

C. Pharmacological therapy:
1. First-line treatment:
   a. Metronidazole.
   b. Metronidazole gel:
      i. Metronidazole gel is less expensive, easier to use, and associated with greater compliance.
      ii. Side effects of metronidazole include sharp, unpleasant metallic taste in the mouth; furry tongue; central nervous system (CNS) reactions, including seizures; and urinary tract disturbances. Advise clients to avoid alcohol while taking metronidazole and 24 hours after completing the medication, or they will experience the severe side effects of abdominal distress, nausea, vomiting, and headache.
      iii. Metronidazole may prolong prothrombin time in clients taking oral anticoagulants.
   c. Clindamycin 2% cream.
2. Other medications if the client is unable to use oral metronidazole:
   a. Clindamycin.
   b. Metronidazole gel.

Clindamycin cream is oil based and may weaken latex condoms for at least 72 hours after terminating therapy.

3. Special considerations: Pregnancy.
BV has been associated with adverse pregnancy outcomes; therefore, all symptomatic pregnant women and asymptomatic women at high risk for preterm delivery require treatment:
   a. Metronidazole.
   b. Clindamycin.

Follow-Up

A. Nonpregnant women: No follow-up is recommended unless indicated. Recurrence is common.
B. Pregnancy: High risk for preterm delivery; pregnant women should be reevaluated one month after treatment.
C. Immunocompromised women: Recommendations for treatment of BV in females infected with HIV are the same as for noninfected clients.
D. Partners: Consider treatment of the client's partner(s) in women with recurrent disease.

Consultation/Referral

A. Refer the client to a specialist for recurrence that is unresponsive to therapies.

Individual Considerations

A. Pregnancy:
1. Clindamycin cream may be associated with increased adverse events in newborns and should not be used during the second half of pregnancy.

B. Partners:
1. Routine treatment of a client's partner(s) is not recommended at this time because it does not influence relapse or recurrence rates.

Bibliography

Centers for Disease Control and Prevention. (2015). *Sexually transmitted diseases treatment guidelines: Bacterial vaginosis*. Retrieved from http://www.cdc.gov/std/tg2015/bv.htm

van Schalkwyk, J., Yudin, H. M., & Infectious Disease Committee. (2015). Vulvovaginitis: Screening for and management of trichomoniasis, vulvovaginal candidiasis, and bacterial vaginosis. *Journal of Obstetrics and Gynaecolgy Canada*, 37(3), 266–274.

Bartholin's Cyst or Abscess

Rhonda Arthur and Julia Blake

Definition

A. The Bartholin's glands are small, round, nonpalpable, mucus-secreting organs. They are located bilaterally in the posterolateral vaginal orifice. Obstruction of the duct causes the gland to swell with mucus and form a Bartholin's cyst. The cause of obstruction is usually unknown but may be due to mechanical trauma, thickened mucus, neoplasm, stenosis of the duct, or infectious organisms not limited to sexually transmitted infections (STIs). The cyst may become infected, resulting in an abscess. Cysts develop more commonly in younger women, and occurrence decreases with aging; therefore, it is important to rule out neoplasm in women older than 40 years experiencing Bartholin's cyst.
B. The majority of women with Bartholin's cyst are asymptomatic, but large cysts can cause pressure and interfere with walking and sexual intercourse. Abscesses generally develop rapidly over a two- to three-day period and are painful. Some abscesses may spontaneously rupture and often reoccur.

Predisposing Factors

A. History of STIs.
B. Local trauma.

Common Findings

A. Cysts can be asymptomatic and found incidentally on physical examination.
B. Localized pain/irritation.
C. Dyspareunia.
D. Difficulty walking or sitting due to oedema.

Subjective Data

A. Elicit onset, duration, and course of presenting symptoms.
B. Review any changes in the characteristics and colour of vaginal discharge. Does the client's partner(s) have any symptoms?
C. Review any symptoms of pruritus, perineal excoriation, burning; signs of urinary tract infection (UTI).
D. Review the client's medication and medical history.

E. Determine whether the client is pregnant; note the date of last menstrual period (LMP).
F. Question the client for a history of STIs or other vaginal infections.
G. Review previous infection, treatment, compliance with treatment, and results.
H. Note last intercourse date.

Physical Examination
A. Inspect:
   1. Examine external vulva and introitus for discharge, irritation, fissures, lesions, and rashes. Bartholin's cyst will appear as a round mass usually near the vaginal orifice causing vulvar asymmetry.
B. Palpate:
   1. Bartholin's glands. Cysts are usually unilateral, tense, nontender, and without erythema. An abscess is usually unilateral, tense, erythematous, and painful on palpation.

Diagnostic Tests
A. Culture and sensitivity of purulent abscess fluid.
B. Cervical culture for STI (*Neisseria gonorrhoeae* and *Chlamydia trachomatis*).
C. Excisional biopsy in women older than 40 years.

Differential Diagnoses
A. Neoplasm.
B. STI.
C. Sebaceous cyst.

Plan
A. General interventions:
   1. Reassurance is indicated for women younger than 40 years with asymptomatic cysts. Incision and drainage (I&D) is often required for symptomatic cysts and abscesses. Because cysts and abscesses often reoccur, surgery to create a permanent opening from the duct to the exterior is often the definitive treatment. Two such surgical methods are placement of a Word catheter or marsupialization. Referral is indicated for I&D and other surgical interventions if the provider is not experienced with the procedures.

Women older than 40 years must be referred for surgical exploration and excision biopsy.

B. Client teaching:
   1. Reassure women younger than 40 years that asymptomatic cysts do not need intervention. Rapidly enlarging cysts that are painful or obstruct the vaginal orifice need to be reevaluated.
   2. Warm sitz baths three or four times a day may encourage spontaneous rupture of abscess and provide comfort.
C. Pharmacological therapy:
   1. Abscesses are treated with an antibiotic that covers methicillin-resistant *Staphylococcus aureus* (MRSA), such as trimethoprim/sulphamethazone or amoxicillin/clavulanate plus clindamycin.

Follow-Up
A. Follow up with provider if not improved in three to seven days.
B. Report to care provider if symptoms reoccur.

Consultation/Referral
A. Refer the client for recurrence that is unresponsive to therapies.

Individual Considerations
A. Older adults:
   1. Refer women older than 40 years with cyst for excisional biopsy.
B. Pregnancy: Treatment with antibiotics is recommended due to the risk of complicated infection. Avoid the use of trimethoprin/sulphamethazone during pregnancy. Refer to obstetrics and gynaecology (OB/GYN) for recurrence.

Bibliography
McNeeley, S. G. (2014, July). *Merck manual: Bartholin gland cysts*. Rahway, NJ: Merck Publishing. Retrieved from http://www.merckmanuals.com/professional/gynecology-and-obstetrics/benign-gynecologic-lesions/bartholin-gland-cysts

Breast Pain (Mastalgia)

Rhonda Arthur and Julia Blake

Definition
A. Benign breast disorders such as mastalgia, mastodynia, and fibrocystic breast changes are characterized by lumps or pain. The lumps may be a physiological nodularity, a ropy thickening, or distended, fluid-filled cysts that are mobile. The pain may be cyclic or noncyclic, and it may be unilateral or bilateral.

Incidence/Prevalence
A. This is a very common problem. Fifty percent or more of menstruating women experience breast pain. Two-thirds of breast pain is cyclic and occurs in women in their 30s; one-third is noncyclic and may occur in women at any age, but it tends to occur in women closer to menopause.

Pathogenesis
A. Dysplastic, benign histologic changes occur in the breast, such as hyperplasia of the breast epithelium, adenosis microcysts and macrocysts, duct ectasia, and apocrine metaplasia.

Predisposing Factors
A. Menstruation (related to hormonal changes).
B. Certain medications (combination oral contraceptives [COCs], hormone therapy, antidepressants, and others).
C. Ingesting substances containing methylxanthines (coffee, tea, chocolate, and cola drinks). Methylxanthines have been noted to contribute to breast pain by clinical observation only.
D. Pregnancy.

Common Findings
A. "My breasts are painful, particularly just before my period."
B. "I have lumps in my breasts, and they hurt."

Other Signs and Symptoms
A. Tender breasts with palpation.
B. Ropelike masses, usually bilateral, with mobile, well-circumscribed masses that are cystic or rubbery.

Subjective Data

A. Elicit history of pain. Note onset, duration, location, and relation to menstrual period. Ask: Is pain constant or intermittent?
B. What has the client tried to alleviate the pain? Note what has worked, such as nonsteroidal anti-inflammatory drugs (NSAIDs).
C. Note the client's family history of breast pain, lumps, or cancer.
D. Has there been trauma, such as being hit or having a rough experience during sex?
E. Do her breasts hurt during or after exercise, such as running, aerobics, soccer, or basketball?
F. Does she wear a good, supportive, properly fitted bra generally and for sports?
G. Has she had any breast surgery or biopsy?
H. Note medication history such as oral contraceptives.

Physical Examination

A. Inspect:
　1. Examine the breasts and note masses, dimples, changes in the skin, and changes in the way the nipples are pointed while the client is in the sitting position with arms in neutral position in lap, above the head, or pressing in on hips.
B. Palpate:
　1. The breasts; look for hard, fixed, or cystic masses in the breast, under the nipple, in the tail of the breast, and in the axilla. Use a standardized breast examination technique. Compress the nipple for discharge. Measure masses, and describe them in the client's record. Use a clock face to describe their location.

Diagnostic Tests

A. Mammogram: May be difficult to interpret in women younger than 35 years.
B. Ultrasonography to differentiate cystic from solid masses.
C. MRI is useful for detecting tissues with increased blood flow, but limited by false-positive results.
D. Fine-needle aspiration and biopsy.
E. Excisional biopsy for solid lumps.
F. Pregnancy test (as indicated).

Differential Diagnoses

A. Fibrocystic breast changes with mastalgia.
B. Benign breast masses: Fibroadenoma and duct ectasia.
C. Nipple discharge: Duct ectasia, prolactin-secreting pituitary tumours.
D. Pain: Costal chondritis, chest wall muscle pain, neuralgia, herpes zoster infection, and fibromyalgia.
E. Heart: Angina pectoris.
F. Gastrointestinal (GI): Gastro-oesophageal reflux disease.
G. Psychological: Anxiety and depression.

Plan

A. General interventions:
　1. Reassure the client. Use the term *fibrocystic changes* rather than *fibrocystic disease* to stress the functional nature of the problem. Stress that the pain is real, but not caused by a disease state.
B. Client teaching:
　▶ **1.** *Refer to Client Teaching Guide: Fibrocystic Breast Changes and Breast Pain.*
　2. Teach the client breast self-examination. Encourage monthly breast self-examination. Continue clinical breast examinations annually.
　3. "Lumpiness" that varies with the menstrual cycle is not abnormal. Breasts may normally be of different sizes. It is a change that is significant.
　4. Consider changing the dose or discontinuing hormone replacement therapy (HRT) for women on HRT with mastalgia.
　5. Symptomatic measures to relieve discomfort:
　　a. Good supportive bra, properly fitted. Adolescents whose breasts are maturing and perimenopausal women whose bodies are changing are two groups who often wear improperly fitted bras.
　　b. Local heat or ice application (whatever works best)
C. Pharmacological therapy:
　1. First-line therapy for mastalgia is topical NSAIDs.
　2. Diuretic: Spironolactone premenstrually.
　3. Oral contraceptive pills: Low-dose oestrogen pills are recommended.
　4. Anti-oestrogen treatment:
　　a. Danazol *Note*: Doses <400 mg daily may not inhibit ovulation. The client must use a barrier contraceptive or intrauterine device (IUD) contraceptive measure. Although the side effect profile is significant, long-term symptomatic relief and histologic changes may be achieved.

Follow-Up

A. Young women with fibrocystic changes need to be seen after one to two months of pharmacological therapy to assess for complications and efficacy.
B. Women with atypical hyperplasia on biopsy need close follow-up every three to six months by a specialist.

Consultation/Referral

A. Consult or refer the client to a specialist when breast masses are identified.
B. Consult with a specialist and refer the client to a surgeon if findings include a suspicious mammographic study, an abnormal needle biopsy, or a solid mass per ultrasonogram.

Individual Considerations

A. Pregnancy:
　1. Consider blocked duct or mastitis with treatment as indicated.
B. Adults:
　1. Mammography screening for women at average risk, according to the American Cancer Society: Mammography is offered annually for women from ages 40 to 64 years, and women should be informed of the risks, benefits, and limitations of regular screening. Women aged 45 to 54 years should have an annual mammogram. Women aged 55 years and older should switch to a mammogram every two years but be offered the choice to continue yearly screening.
　2. Care should be individualized considering potential risks, benefits, and limitations of screening. High-risk women may benefit from additional screening, including earlier initiation of screening and additional screening modalities such as ultrasound and MRI.

3. When clinical breast examination, mammography, and needle-aspiration biopsy are used, breast cancer detection rates are 93% to 100%.
C. Geriatrics:
1. Breast pain should be worked up as possible cancer.
D. Partners:
1. Pain may inhibit sexual activity involving the breast.

Bibliography

Aliotta, H. M., & Schaeffer, N. J. (2013). Breast conditions. In K. D. Schuiling & F. E. Likis (Eds.), *Women's gynecologic health* (2nd ed., pp. 377–401). Burlington, MA: Jones & Bartlett.

Rosolowich, V., Saettler, E., & Szuck, B. (2006). Mastalgia & Breast Disease Committee. *Journal of Obsterics and Gynaecology Canada, 28*(1), 49–60.

The Society of Obstetricians and Gynaecologist of Canada. (n.d.). *Breast pain.* Retrieved from https://sogc.org/publications-resources/public-information-pamphlets.html?id=31

Cervicitis

Rhonda Arthur and Julia Blake

Definition
A. Cervicitis is acute or chronic inflammation of the cervix that is visible to the examiner.

Incidence/Prevalence
A. Incidence is unknown due to multiple aetiologies.

Pathogenesis
A. Acute cervicitis is primarily due to infection from the following organisms:
  1. Bacteria:
     a. *Chlamydia trachomatis.*
     b. *Neisseria gonorrhoeae.*
     c. Mycoplasma.
     d. Ureaplasma.
  2. Viruses:
     a. Herpes simplex virus type 2 (HSV-2).
     b. Human papillomavirus (HPV).
  3. *Trichomonas vaginalis.*
B. Chronic cervicitis is primarily due to the following:
  1. Trauma occurring during childbirth or instrumentation.
  2. Infection (see earlier).
  3. Presence of foreign bodies (i.e., intrauterine devices [IUDs]).

Predisposing Factors
A. Vaginal delivery.
B. Cervical procedures: laser, loop, or other excision procedures.
C. IUD.
D. Sexually transmitted infections (STIs).

Common Findings
A. Copious mucopurulent vaginal discharge.
B. Postcoital bleeding.

Other Signs and Symptoms
A. Asymptomatic; may be found on routine gynaecologic examination.
B. Thick, yellow vaginal discharge.
C. Dysuria.
D. Dyspareunia.
E. Vulvovaginal irritation or pruritus.

Subjective Data
A. Determine onset, duration, and course of symptoms. Is there any dyspareunia, pelvic pain, fever, or urinary symptoms?
B. Determine characteristics of the vaginal discharge.
C. Review the client's history of STIs.
D. Review the client's sexual history to include number of partners and partner symptoms (if any), use of sex toys, and sexual lifestyle.
E. Note the last Papanicolaou (Pap) smear and results. Has the client ever had an abnormal Pap; if so, how was it treated?
F. Note date of last menstrual period (LMP), use of contraception, and type(s) of contraception.
G. If the client has recently been pregnant, review her records for cervical cerclage, vaginal delivery with cervical laceration, or other complications.

Physical Examination
A. Check temperature, pulse, and respirations.
B. Inspect:
  1. Observe generally for discomfort before, during, and after examination.
  2. Observe the external vulva for Bartholin's gland enlargement (Bartholin's gland abscess is due primarily to infection by chlamydia), lesions, irritation, fissures, and condyloma.
  3. Note colour, amount, and odour of vaginal discharge.
C. Palpate:
  1. Back: Note costovertebral angle (CVA) tenderness.
  2. Abdomen: Palpate for enlarged or tender inguinal lymph nodes.
D. Pelvic examination:
  1. Speculum examination:
     a. Inspect cervix for inflammation and ectropion. Cervical ectropion is found in 15% to 20% of healthy young women (especially in teens and with the use of oral contraceptives). It represents columnar epithelium that is found farther out on the ectocervix, causing the cervix to appear granular and red. Presence of cervical erosion, however, suggests advanced cervical pathology. A "strawberry cervix" (petechiae) is highly suggestive of *T. vaginalis.*
     b. Check cervix for friability and bleeding when the cervix is touched with a cotton-tipped swab.
     c. Assess the vagina and cervix for leukoplakia, lesions, polyps, and discharge.
     d. Assess vaginal walls for discharge and rugae.
     e. Vesicular or ulcerated cervical lesions warrant testing for syphilis and/or chancroid.
  2. Bimanual examination:
     a. Check cervical motion tenderness (CMT), adnexal masses, uterine size, consistency, and tenderness.
     b. Milk urethra for discharge.
     c. Palpate Bartholin's glands.

Diagnostic Tests
A. White blood cell (WBC), if indicated.
B. Consider testing for syphilis (rapid plasma reagin [RPR] or Venereal Disease Research Laboratory [VDRL] test).
C. Wet prep.
D. Cervical cultures for gonorrhoea and chlamydia.
E. Pap smear.
F. Urine culture and sensitivity, if indicated.
G. Herpes culture, if indicated.

Differential Diagnoses
A. Chlamydia.
B. Gonorrhoea.
C. Bartholin's gland abscess.
D. Cervical neoplasm.
E. Cervical polyps.
F. HSV-2.
G. Urinary tract infection (UTI).
H. Cervical ulceration, or erosion, from trauma: fingernail, cervical biopsy, postpartum, or sex toys.
I. Pelvic inflammatory disease (PID)

Plan
A. General interventions:
   1. Clients whose culture is negative generally respond to a round of doxycycline therapy, which is the first-line treatment for nonchlamydial, nongonorrhoeal cervicitis.
B. Client teaching:
   1. Women should be encouraged to obtain routine care and Pap smear evaluations per guidelines.
   2. Client should have no sexual intercourse for one week and avoid reinfection by abstaining from intercourse until sexual partners are adequately treated.
   3. Avoid tampons and douches until antibiotics are completed.
   4. Give the client a teaching sheet. *Refer to Client Teaching Guide: Cervicitis.*
C. Pharmacological therapy:
   1. First-line treatment for chlamydia: azithromycin or doxycycline. Treat all partners.
   2. First-line treatment for gonorrhoea: gentamicin plus either a single dose of azithromycin or doxycycline 100 mg orally twice a day for seven days.
   3. First-line treatment for HSV: acyclovir.
   4. First-line treatment for *trichomonas*: metronidazole. Clients should be cautioned to avoid alcohol consumption during and 24 hours after the completion of oral metronidazole due to a disulfiram-like reaction (nausea, vomiting, headache, cramps, and flushing).
   5. First-line treatment for UTI: See the section "Urinary Tract Infection (Acute Cystitis)" in Chapter 12, Genitourinary Guidelines.

Follow-Up
A. Recommend "test of cure": Return for repeat testing three months after treatment because of high rates of reinfection.
B. Follow up with Pap smear as mandated by guidelines.

Consultation/Referral
A. Refer the client for suspected neoplasm and for cervicitis unresponsive to treatment.
B. If the cervix has a suspicious lesion, the client should be referred for colposcopy and/or biopsy regardless of cytology results. On physical examination, the cervix may be oedematous and erythematous and may show exposed columnar epithelium. It may be friable. Reddened areas of the cervix may be seen around the cervical os. The irregularity and friability sometimes differentiate them from eversion; other times colposcopy is required to make the distinction.

Individual Considerations
A. Pregnancy:
   1. Cervical inflammation is common in early pregnancy.
   2. If an STI is diagnosed, nonteratogenic pharmacological therapies must be implemented.
B. Partners:
   1. A positive STI result warrants treatment of each sexual partner.

Bibliography
American Cancer Society. (2016). *What are the key statistics about cervical cancer?* Retrieved from http://www.cancer.org/cancer/cervicalcancer/detailedguide/cervical-cancer-key-statistics

American College of Obstetricians and Gynecologists. (2013). *New guidelines for cervical cancer screening.* Retrieved from http://www.acog.org/-/media/For-Patients/pfs004.pdf?dmc=1&ts=

Canadian Task Force on Preventive Health Care. (2013). Recommendations on screening for cervical cancer. *Canadian Medical Association Journal*, 185(1), 35–45.

Einstein, M. H., & Cox, J. T. (2013). Update on cervical disease. *ObG Management*, 25(5), 42–49.

Massad, L. S., Einstein, M. H., Huh, W. K., Katki, H. A., Kinney, W. K., Schiffman, M., & Lawson, H. W. (2013). 2012 updated consensus guidelines for the management of abnormal cervical cancer screening tests and cancer precursors. *Journal of Lower Genital Tract Disease*, 17(5 Suppl. 1), S1–S27.

Public Health Agency of Canada. (2017). *Canadian guidelines on sexually transmitted infections.* Retrieved from https://www.canada.ca/content/dam/phac-aspc/documents/services/publications/healthy-living/gonorrhea-alternate-treatment/alternate-treatmemt-gonorrhea-07-2017.pdf

Contraception

Rhonda Arthur and Julia Blake

Definition
A. Contraception is the intentional prevention of pregnancy by either or both sexual partners. Contraception can be mechanical, chemical, or surgical and is either reversible or nonreversible. Considerations in counseling regarding contraceptive choices include cost, efficacy, safety, and personal considerations such as personal belief systems and ability to use selected method.

Incidence/Prevalence
A. Women frequently visit primary care providers to request contraception and family planning education. In Canada, the most common methods of contraception are oral contraceptives (44%) and condoms (54%). The average age of oral contraceptive users was 26 years, especially among single, nulliparous, Canadian-born women. Consistent use of a reliable and effective contraceptive method can greatly reduce the unintended pregnancy rate. Easy access and education regarding contraceptive use is a keystone in the prevention of unintended pregnancy.

Subjective Data
A. Review complete menstrual history, including age of onset, duration, frequency, regularity, and dysmenorrhoea. Review date of last menstrual period (LMP).
B. Review the client's pregnancy history.
C. Review the client's contraception and sexual history.
D. Note other medications the client is taking, including over-the-counter (OTC) medications and supplements.
E. Ask the client whether she has had a major medical disease, including hypertension, cardiovascular incident, thromboembolic disease, diabetes, migraine headaches, gallbladder disease, or liver disease.
F. Review substance abuse/use history.

G. Review childhood illness and immunization record.
H. Note allergies.
I. Review pertinent family medical history.

Physical Examination
A. Check height, weight, blood pressure (BP), pulse, and body mass index (BMI).
B. Inspect:
 1. Note overall appearance. Look at neck (thyroid). Inspect breast/genitalia for Tanner staging. See Appendix C, Tanner's Sexual Maturity Stages.
 2. Skin assessment: Check for central hair growth, which is responsive to androgens. Areas to inspect for coarse hair include the upper lip, chin, sideburns, neck, chest, lower abdomen, and perineum.
C. Palpate:
 1. Palpate the neck for thyroid enlargement.
 2. Palpate the abdomen for enlarged organs or uterine enlargement compatible with pregnancy.
 3. Perform breast examination, palpating for masses. Assess for nipple discharge.
 4. Palpate axilla for masses, and lymphadaenopathy.
D. Auscultate:
 1. Auscultate the heart and lungs.
 2. If pregnancy is suspected, consider auscultating for foetal heart tones.
E. Pelvic examination:
 1. Inspect external genitalia. Note pubic hair pattern for Tanner staging. Note any lesions, masses, or discharge.
 2. Speculum examination: Inspect vagina and cervix. Note any vaginal discharge. Obtain Pap smear and cervical/vaginal cultures as appropriate.
 3. Bimanual examination: Palpate the cervix and check for cervical motion tenderness (CMT). Palpate the size of the uterus and assess for adnexal masses.
 4. Consider rectal examination as indicated.

Diagnostic Tests
A. Urine: Pregnancy test as indicated/urinalysis as indicated.
B. Serum: Complete blood count (CBC) if indicated by history.
C. Pap smear according to Canadian Task Force on Preventive Health Care recommendations on screening for cervical cancer.
D. Vaginal/cervical cultures for sexually transmitted infections (STIs) as indicated.

Plan
A. General interventions:
 1. Review all methods of contraception available with the client and, if available, partner.
 2. Consider all aspects of the client's history and make recommendations as appropriate.
B. Client teaching:
 1. Review anatomy and physiology of the menstrual cycle and reproduction with all clients.
 2. Review the risks, benefits, costs, use, and efficacy of contraceptive methods. Review perfect use versus typical use of method selected.
 3. Review STI prevention and limitations of STI prevention as related to each method.
 4. Assist the client in selecting the most appropriate method of contraception with regard to cost, efficacy, health status of the client, ability to use correctly and consistently, and the client's personal values.
 5. Warning signs and information as to when to call the care provider should be given to all clients.
 6. All women of childbearing age should be educated on the availability and proper use of emergency contraceptives. *Refer to Client Teaching Guide: Contraception: How to Take Birth Control Pills (for a 28-Day Cycle).*
 7. Provide all clients information on the prevention of STIs.

Methods of Contraception
A. Abstinence: Refraining from sexual intercourse:
 1. Advantages: Easy and no cost. Perfect use offers protection against STIs and pregnancy.
 2. Disadvantages: User-dependent.
B. Barrier methods:
 1. Male condom:
  a. Advantages: Male condoms are easily accessible (OTC with no prescription needed) and relatively inexpensive. Condoms do not require daily intervention and offer some protections against STIs.
  b. Disadvantages: Male condoms are technique dependent for efficacy. Breakage and spillage can occur. Some condoms are made from latex, and those with latex allergies need to be aware and carefully check the label for latex content. Nonlatex condoms are available. Male condoms are intended for one-time use only.
  c. Efficacy with perfect use of male condoms: Approximately two in 100 women will become pregnant each year. With typical use of male condoms, approximately 15 in 100 women will become pregnant each year.
 2. Female condom:
  a. Advantages: Female condoms are easily accessible (OTC with no prescription needed) and relatively inexpensive. Condoms do not require daily intervention and offer some protections against STIs.
  b. Disadvantages: Female condoms are technique dependent for efficacy. Slippage and spillage can occur. The female condom is intended for one-time use only and may be inserted up to eight hours before intercourse.
  c. Efficacy with perfect use of the female condom: Approximately five in 100 women will become pregnant each year. With typical use of the female condom, approximately 21 in 100 women will become pregnant each year.
 3. Diaphragm:
  a. Advantages: Diaphragms are nonhormonal and can be used for years with proper care. May be inserted up to six hours before intercourse.
  b. Disadvantages: Diaphragms must be properly fitted by an experienced health-care provider and are user controlled. Placement is crucial to contraceptive benefit and spermicide must be used. Must be removed within 24 hours due to risk of toxic shock syndrome (TSS). The client must have fit checked after childbirth and weight gain or loss. Urinary tract infections (UTIs) may be more frequent in diaphragm users, and some women may experience sensitivity or allergy to spermicide. Avoid use during menses.

▶ Client Teaching Guides are available at https://connect.springerpub.com/content/reference-book/978-0-8261-9498-5

  c. Efficacy with perfect use of the diaphragm: Six in 100 women will become pregnant each year. With typical use of the diaphragm, 16 in 100 women will become pregnant each year.
 4. Cervical cap:
  a. Advantages: Cervical caps are nonhormonal and can be used for years with proper care. The cervical cap may be inserted and left in place up to 48 hours.
  b. Disadvantages: Cervical caps must be properly fitted by an experienced health-care provider and are user controlled. Placement is crucial to contraceptive benefit and spermicide must be used. Must be removed within 48 hours due to risk of TSS. Some caps are made of latex and are not appropriate for latex-allergic clients. Some women may experience sensitivity or allergy to spermicide. Avoid use during menses.
  c. Efficacy with use of the cervical cap is similar to the diaphragm.
 5. Vaginal sponge:
  a. Advantages: The vaginal sponge is a nonhormonal OTC polyurethane sponge that releases the spermicide nonoxynol-9. It can be used for multiple acts of intercourse over 24 hours.
  b. Disadvantages: The vaginal sponge is user-controlled. Some women may experience sensitivity or allergy to the spermicide. Avoid use during menses.
  c. Efficacy with perfect use of the vaginal sponge: Among parous women, 20 in 100 will become pregnant each year, and nine nulliparous women will become pregnant each year. With typical use, 32 in 100 parous women and 16 nulliparous women will become pregnant each year.
C. Surgery:
 1. Male sterilization:
  a. Advantages: Sterilization is a very effective form of contraception. User does not have to remember to do anything before intercourse, and it is not user-dependent. Sterilization is permanent.
  b. Disadvantages: Sterilization involves a surgical procedure. Insurance may not cover the cost of the procedure.
  c. Efficacy with perfect use of male sterilization; 0.1 in 100 women will become pregnant each year. With typical use of male sterilization 0.15 in 100 women will become pregnant each year.
 2. Female sterilization is the second most often used contraceptive method in the United States:
  a. Advantages: Sterilization is a very effective form of contraception. User does not have to remember to do anything before intercourse, and it is not user-dependent. Sterilization is permanent.
  b. Disadvantages: Sterilization involves a surgical procedure. If pregnancy does occur, there is a higher incidence of ectopic pregnancy. Insurance may not cover the cost of the procedure.
  c. Efficacy with both perfect and typical use of female sterilization: 0.5 in 100 will become pregnant each year.
D. Intrauterine device (IUD):
 1. Hormonal:
  a. Advantages: Hormonal IUDs are a very effective form of contraception and may be left in place for five years. User does not have to remember to use before intercourse. These may reduce menstrual flow.
  b. Disadvantages: Risks of any IUD include uterine perforation, increased spontaneous abortion, ectopic pregnancy, and pelvic pain and infection. IUD must be inserted by a qualified health-care professional. IUD may be spontaneously expelled.
  c. Efficacy with both perfect and typical use: 0.2 in 100 will become pregnant each year.
 2. Nonhormonal:
  a. Advantages: Nonhormonal IUDs are a very effective form of contraception and may be left in place for 10 years. User does not have to remember to use before intercourse.
  b. Disadvantages: Risks of any IUD include uterine perforation; increased spontaneous abortion, ectopic pregnancy, and pelvic pain and infection. Nonhormonal IUD must be inserted by a qualified health-care professional. IUD may be spontaneously expelled.
  c. Efficacy with perfect use of the nonhormonal IUD: Six in 1,000 women will become pregnant each year. With typical use of the nonhormonal IUD, 8 in 1,000 women will become pregnant each year.

Women who are not appropriate candidates for an IUD include those with recent pelvic infections, anatomical uterine abnormalities, and pregnancy. Caution should be exercised when considering an IUD in women who have multiple sexual partners; pelvic inflammatory disease (PID); immunosuppression; undiagnosed, irregular, or heavy menstrual bleeding; abnormal Pap smear; and difficulty obtaining follow-up care. See World Health Organization's IUD Toolkit at www.k4health.org/toolkits/iud.

E. Pharmacological therapy:
 1. Progestin-only pills (POPs; also known as mini pills):
  a. Advantages: The POP is a safe hormonal alternative for women who cannot take oestrogen. It is preferred to combined oral contraceptives (COCs) for lactating women as it is not as likely to decrease milk supply. POPs are rapidly reversible and controlled by women.
  b. Disadvantages: The POP cannot be taken if the client has any contraindications to progestin use. POPs are less effective than COCs and must be taken daily at the same time, requiring strict adherence to regime.
  c. Efficacy with perfect use of POPs: Three in 1,000 women per year will become pregnant. With typical use, 80 in 1,000 women per year will become pregnant.
 2. Injection long-acting depot medroxyprogesterone acetate (DMPA):
  a. Advantages: Easy to use. The user only has to remember the injection every three months. May decrease vaginal bleeding. DMPA is a safe hormonal alternative for women who cannot take oestrogen.
  b. Disadvantages: Women cannot use DMPA if they have any contraindications to progesterone use. May cause amenorrhoea or irregular vaginal bleeding. May cause increased weight gain. Requires routine (three-month) visits to the provider's office for intramuscular (IM) injections. DMPA does not provide protection against STIs. DMPA is associated with reversible decreased bone mineral density.

c. Efficacy with perfect use of DMPA: Three in 1,000 women per year will become pregnant. With typical use, 30 in 1,000 women per year will become pregnant.
d. DMPA should be administered during the first five days of the menstrual cycle, or postpartum before resumption of intercourse (preferably after lactation has been established). If this is not possible or if a woman is late for injection, administer pregnancy test and have the client use condoms for at least one week after injection.

3. Combined oestrogen/progesterone contraceptives: Combined oestrogen/progesterone contraceptives come in three delivery methods: oral pills, a transdermal patch, and a vaginal ring. Advantages and disadvantages and efficacy are similar regarding hormones, but there are some differences in the delivery methods:
    a. Advantages: Combined contraceptives are easy to use, convenient, rapidly reversible, and controlled by women. The transdermal patch is only changed weekly, and the vaginal ring is left in place for three weeks. In addition to predictable menses, combined contraceptives decrease menstrual flow and length of menses.
    b. Disadvantages: Dependent on user, and oral pills must be taken daily. Exposure to hormones may not be suitable for certain women based on health status and risk. See absolute and relative contraindications that are not appropriate for some women in a prescriber's reference guide. Smoking in conjunction with use of combined contraceptive increases cardiovascular risk and should be considered. Does not protect against STIs. Other medications, such as anticonvulsants and antibiotics, may interfere with effectiveness of combined hormonal contraceptives and should be considered in prescribing.
    c. Efficacy with perfect use of combined hormonal contraceptive: Three in 1,000 women per year will become pregnant. With typical use, 80 in 1,000 women per year will become pregnant.
    d. Prescribing considerations: Oral contraceptives come in combination extended cycle, combination monophasic, combination biphasic, combination triphasic, and progestin-only formulations. Side effects can be managed in consideration of pill composition. See prescribing reference guides such as the *Monthly Prescribing Reference* at www.empr.com. General considerations for pill selection include age, health history/status, and the client's preference. Because POPs are highly sensitive to consistency in timing, reserve prescriptions of them for women who have contraindications to oestrogen. Alternatives for COCs should be considered in women older than 35 years who smoke due to increased risks of thrombolytic events. In asymptomatic adolescents, it is acceptable to prescribe COCs without an initial pelvic examination. For adolescents or anyone who may have difficulty remembering to take a daily pill, consideration should be given to prescription of the vaginal ring, patch, or other methods. See the office's prescriber's reference for complete information on safety side effects and contraindications.
    e. Absolute contraindications to oestrogen therapy (ET):
        i. Acute liver disease.
        ii. Cerebral vascular or coronary artery disease, myocardial infarction (MI), or stroke.
        iii. History of or active thrombophlebitis or thromboembolic disorders.
        iv. History of uterine or ovarian cancer.
        v. Known or suspected cancer of the breast.
        vi. Known or suspected oestrogen-dependent neoplasm.
        vii. Pregnancy.
        viii. Undiagnosed, abnormal vaginal bleeding.
    f. Relative contraindications to ET:
        i. Active gallbladder disease.
        ii. Familial hyperlipidaemia.

4. Spermicide (foam, film, gel, tablets, and suppositories):
    a. Advantages: Spermicide is a nonhormonal OTC preparation and contains nonoxynol-9. It is inexpensive and easily accessible.
    b. Disadvantages: Spermicide is user controlled and, if not used consistently, will lead to contraception failure. Some may experience sensitivity or allergy to spermicide. Spermicide has a high failure rate.
    c. Efficacy with perfect use of spermicide: 18 in 100 women will become pregnant each year. With typical use of spermicide, 29 of 100 women will become pregnant each year.

F. Natural family planning (NFP):
   1. Advantages: NFP is nonhormonal. It has no cost and is easy to use.
   2. Disadvantages: NFP is user controlled and depends on regularity of cycle and avoidance of intercourse. Can be complex for user and has a high failure rate. Does not protect against STIs.
   3. Efficacy with use: With typical use of the fertility awareness method, 25 in 100 women will become pregnant each year.

Additional information, training, and client teaching may be found at the following websites: Association of Reproductive Health Professionals (www.arhp.org/Publications-and-Resources/Quick-Reference-Guide-for-Clinicians/choosing/Fertility-awareness), Institute for Reproductive Health (www.irh.org), and Planned Parenthood (www.plannedparenthood.org).

G. Withdrawal:
   1. Advantages: Withdrawal is nonhormonal, inexpensive and easily accessible.
   2. Disadvantages: Withdrawal is user controlled. Withdrawal has a high failure rate and does not protect against STIs.
   3. Efficacy with use: With typical use of withdrawal method, 85 in 100 women will become pregnant each year.

Follow-Up

A. The client should return three months after initiation of oral contraceptives, ring, and patch to assess blood pressure, use, side effects, and satisfaction. Then yearly visits are recommended for health maintenance.
B. Clients on DMPA injections should return every three months for follow-up injection and weight evaluation and then yearly for health maintenance.
C. Clients with a diaphragm should return for refitting with change in weight or postpartum and for routine health maintenance.

Consultation/Referral
A. If the contraceptive method selected is one the practitioner is not experienced in providing (diaphragm, implant, IUD, or surgical sterilization), refer to an experienced appropriate provider.

Individual Considerations
A. Adults:
  1. Discontinue COCs for women aged 35 years and older who smoke.
  2. Increased age and obesity increase risk of venous thromboembolism with the use of COCs. COCs should be prescribed with caution and alternative contraceptives should be considered.
  3. The health-care provider should continue to assess for chronic conditions and medication use and weigh risks and benefits of selected methods.
  4. Provide anticipatory guidance regarding the need to use contraceptives until menopause is confirmed to prevent unintended pregnancy.

B. Adolescents:
  1. A pelvic examination is not required and should not become a barrier to access to contraception. Long-acting reversible contraceptives and methods that require less-frequent dosing (patch, ring) promote adherence and continuation and should be encouraged in teens.
  2. Education and counseling regarding pregnancy and STI prevention are essential.
  3. Many clients have mobile phones with reminder apps that assist in compliance with contraceptive use.

Bibliography
Black, A., & Guildert, E. (2015). Canadian contraception consensus (part 1 of 4). *Journal of Obstetrics and Gynaecology Canada, 37*(10), S1–S28.

Guttmacher Institute. (2015). *Contraceptive use in the United States.* Retrieved from http://www.guttmacher.org/fact-sheet/contraceptive-use-united-states

ParaGard. (2014). *Prescribing information.* Retrieved from http://www.paragard.com/Pdf/ParaGard-PI.pdf

Rotermann, M., Dunn, S., & Black, A. (2015). *Oral contraceptives use among women aged 15 to 49: reults from the Canadian Health Measure Survey.* Retrieved from https://www150.statcan.gc.ca/n1/pub/82-003-x/2015010/article/14222-eng.htm

Zieman, M., Hatcher, R. A., Trussell, J., Nelson, A. L., Cates, W., Hatcher, R. A., & Allen, A. Z. (2015). *Managing contraception for your pocket.* Tiger, GA: Bridging the Gap Foundation.

Dysmenorrhoea

Rhonda Arthur and Julia Blake

Definition
Dysmenorrhoea is painful uterine cramping felt primarily in the lower abdomen but also in the lower back and upper thighs.

A. Primary dysmenorrhoea: Not associated with pelvic pathology; usually associated with ovulatory cycles. Occurs on the first or second day of the menstrual period; usually worse the first day; affects teens and women in their 20s; is often associated with prostaglandin-induced symptoms of diarrhoea, nausea, vomiting, and/or headache.

B. Secondary dysmenorrhoea: Painful uterine contractions due to a pathologic aetiology such as endometriosis or pelvic inflammatory disease (PID). Primarily occurs in women in their 20s, 30s, and 40s.

Incidence/Prevalence
A. Primary dysmenorrhoea is very common, affecting up to 90% of young women to some extent at some time. Dysmenorrhoea frequently leads to absenteeism from work or school and impacts social and sports activities. The incidence of endometriosis is 8% to 30% of women of reproductive age.

Pathogenesis
A. Primary dysmenorrhoea is due to myometrial contractions that are caused by prostaglandins in the secretory endometrium. The prostaglandins cause uterine ischaemia through platelet aggregation, vasoconstriction, and dysrhythmic contractions.

B. Secondary dysmenorrhoea is associated with pathologic conditions such as endometriosis, cervical stenosis, tumours, adhesions, adenomyosis, myomas, polyps, infection (PID), intrauterine device (IUD)-retained products of conception, or nongynaecological causes. The pain of secondary dysmenorrhoea may also be unrelated to menses.

C. In endometriosis, there are islands of endometrium found on peritoneal surfaces of the bladder, broad ligaments, fallopian tubes, ovaries, bowel, and cul-de-sac, as well as distant sites on the abdominal wall, vagina, lung, or other sites.

Predisposing Factors
A. Female.
B. Reproductive age.
C. Normal menstrual function.
D. Cervical stenosis, possibly.

Common Findings
A. "I have painful periods."
B. "My menstrual cramps are terrible, particularly the first day of my cycle."
C. "My cramps are so bad I feel sick to my stomach and have diarrhoea."

Other Signs and Symptoms
A. History of menstrual cramps just before the onset of the menstrual period and for the first 24 to 48 hours.
B. Pain beginning earlier; associated with intercourse, defecation, and urination; and lasting throughout the menstrual period is associated with endometriosis or adenomyosis.
C. Acute pain may be associated with infection (PID) or ectopic pregnancy.

Subjective Data
A. Obtain a complete menstrual history: age at menarche; frequency, duration, and regularity of periods; amount of flow in number of perineal pads or tampons used.
B. Ask the client about the location of the pain; note radiation and associated symptoms such as nausea, vomiting, or diarrhoea.
C. Is pain rhythmic or spasmodic (primary) or steady (secondary)?
D. How old was the client when the pain began? Primary dysmenorrhoea usually begins two to three years after menarche.
E. Inquire about the type of contraception used.
F. Obtain obstetric history.
G. Is the pain related to the menstrual period, or does it occur before or independent of the menstrual period?

H. Does the client have dyspareunia?
I. Does she have urinary tract infection (UTI) symptoms?
J. What treatments have been tried, and which were effective?

Physical Examination

A. Check height and weight, temperature, blood pressure (BP), and pulse.
B. Inspect:
  1. Examine the general body habitus for female adipose distribution on the buttocks and thighs.
  2. Note breast development (see Appendix C, Tanner's Sexual Maturity Stages).
  3. Observe the abdomen for distension.
C. Palpate and percuss:
  1. Examine the abdomen for masses or tenderness.
D. Auscultate:
  1. The heart and lungs.
  2. Abdomen for bowel sounds.
E. Pelvic examination:
  1. Inspect the external genitalia for pubic hair pattern, lesions, discharge, and odour.
  2. Palpate the external genitalia for masses or areas of tenderness.
F. Speculum examination: Inspect the cervix and vagina for discharge, lesions, ectropion, cervical erosion, and IUD string.
G. Bimanual examination:
  1. Palpate the vagina and cul-de-sac areas for tenderness or masses.
  2. Check the cervical position, mobility, and pain with mobility.
  3. Check uterine size, mobility, shape, regularity, masses, position, and tenderness.
  4. Check the adnexa for masses (cystic or solid) and tenderness.
  5. A normal pelvic examination is a significant finding in primary dysmenorrhoea and often in endometriosis.

Diagnostic Tests

Primary dysmenorrhoea is often diagnosed by history, including symptoms and timing in menstrual cycle and pelvic examination. If secondary dysmenorrhoea is suspected and additional information is required, the care provider may consider the following diagnostic tests:
A. Consider pelvic ultrasonography to rule out pelvic pathology.
B. Laboratory studies: urinalysis, haemoglobin (Hgb), haematocrit (Hct), and white blood cell (WBC).
C. Consider vaginal and cervical cultures for chlamydia and gonorrhoea, if infection is suspected.
D. Pregnancy test as indicated.
E. Papanicolaou (Pap) smear per guidelines.

Differential Diagnoses

A. Complication of pregnancy: missed or incomplete abortion or ectopic pregnancy.
B. Endometriosis or adenomyosis.
C. Ruptured ovarian cyst.
D. Infection: endometritis, salpingitis, PID, or pelvic adhesions.
E. Fibroid tumours.
F. Adhesions.
G. UTI.
H. Bowel disease: Irritable bowel disease or inflammatory bowel disease.

Plan

A. General interventions:
  1. Support client concerns and identify reality of discomfort. Identify primary source of pain if other diagnoses exist.
B. Client teaching:
  1. *Refer to Client Teaching Guides: Dysmenorrhoea and Contraception: How to Take Birth Control Pills.*
  2. Educate the client about the physiology of menstruation.
  3. Teach the client that endometriosis is one of the leading causes of infertility.
  4. Encourage activity and exercise, such as walking or swimming.
  5. Advise warm baths or heating pads to help relieve some pain.
C. Pharmacological therapy:
  1. Nonsteroidal anti-inflammatory drugs (NSAIDs) are first-line treatment:
    a. They inhibit prostaglandin synthesis in the endometrium, thus decreasing uterine cramping. There is also an analgesic effect.
    b. The fenamates have been the most effective, followed by the propionic acid derivatives.
    c. The drugs should be started as the menstrual period begins. It is no longer considered the standard of care to begin the drugs a few days before the onset of the menstrual period.
    d. Prostaglandin inhibitors relieve dysmenorrhoea in 80% of women.
    e. Take NSAIDs with food to avoid gastrointestinal (GI) upset and irritation.
  2. First-line treatments for dysmenorrhoea:
    a. NSAIDs:
      i. Arylacetic acid derivatives: Naproxen sodium.
      ii. Propionic acid derivatives: Ibuprofen. These are over-the-counter (OTC) medications.
      iii. Anthranilic acid derivatives: Mefenamic acid. The treatment maximum is two to three days.
      iv. Benzeneacetic acid derivatives: Diclofenac potassium.
    b. Hormonal control:
      i. Oral contraceptive pills: Any combination pill is efficacious. Consider extended cycle dosing to prevent having monthly periods.
      ii. Vaginal ring.
      iii. Depot medroxyprogesterone acetate (DMPA) injections.
      iv. Hormonal IUDs.
  3. First-line treatments for endometriosis:
    a. NSAIDs.
    b. Oral contraceptive pills.
    c. With gynaecology specialist consultation or referral, danazol.
    d. With gynaecology specialist consultation or referral, gonadotropin-releasing hormone (GnRH) agonists such as leuprolide acetate and goserelin acetate.

▶ Client Teaching Guides are available at https://connect.springerpub.com/content/reference-book/978-0-8261-9498-5

Follow-Up
A. Have the client return in three months. Encourage the client to undergo the treatment for three months to determine the effectiveness.

Consultation/Referral
A. If dysmenorrhoea does not respond to NSAIDs or oral contraceptives, consult with a gynaecology specialist for further workup to determine the source of the pain.
B. Consider consultation with obstetrics and gynaecology (OB/GYN) for laparoscopy or hysteroscopy to diagnose endometriosis or adhesions. Laser may be used to destroy endometrial implants or to lyse adhesions.

Individual Considerations
A. Pregnancy: Uterine contractions in pregnancy could be preterm labour.
B. Adolescents:
  1. Remember that endometriosis can occur in this age group. It is not an extremely rare finding.
C. Adults:
  1. Endometriosis can be a disabling condition interfering with work and sexual relationships. It may continue into the perimenopausal period.

Bibliography
Burnett, M., & Lernyre, M. (2017). Primary dysmenorrhea consensus guideline. *Journal of Obstetrics and Gynaecology Canada, 39*(7), 585–595.
Osayande, A. S., & Mehulic, S. (2014). Diagnosis and initial management of dysmenorrhea. *American Family Physician, 89*(5), 341–346.

Dyspareunia

Rhonda Arthur and Julia Blake

Definition
A. Dyspareunia is genital or pelvic discomfort associated with sexual intercourse (entry or deep penetration) and interferes with sexual satisfaction. Dyspareunia may be superficial, relating to vulvar and vaginal pain, or it may be deep, relating to deep, pelvic pain. Vaginismus is the involuntary (often painful) contraction of the pelvic floor muscles in response to pressure or attempted penetration.

Incidence/Prevalence
A. Vaginismus occurs in 1% to 6% of women and dyspareunia occurs in 8% to 22% of postmenopausal women.

Pathogenesis
Physical and psychosocial aetiologies have been identified:
A. Physical causes:
  1. Vulvovaginal anomalies:
     a. Thick hymen.
     b. Short vagina.
     c. Vaginal agenesis.
     d. Vaginal septum.
  2. Organic dyspareunia:
     a. Episiotomy scars.
     b. Bartholin's gland cyst.
     c. Vulvar dystrophy.
     d. Inflammation or infection, sexually transmitted infection (STI).
     e. Vulvovaginal cancer.
  f. Pelvic disease:
     i. Pelvic inflammatory disease (PID).
     ii. Uterine or ovarian tumours.
     iii. Adenomyosis.
     iv. Pelvic scarring or adhesions versus endometriosis.
  3. Musculoskeletal anomalies:
     a. Disc disease.
     b. Myofascial pain.
     c. Coccygodynia.
  4. Extensive prolapse or organ displacement.
  5. Urethral syndrome or other urinary tract disorders.
  6. Vulvodynia.
  7. Gastrointestinal (GI) anomalies:
     a. Constipation.
     b. Irritable bowel syndrome (IBS).
     c. Inflammatory bowel disease (IBD).
     d. Anorexia.
  8. Hormonal factors:
     a. Hypo-oestrogenaemia causing atrophic vaginitis.
     b. Breastfeeding.
     c. Menopause.
B. Psychosocial causes:
  1. Childhood molestation.
  2. Fear of pain, infection, or pregnancy.
  3. Pelvic congestion syndrome.
  4. Poor partner communication.
  5. History of sexual assault, including date rape.
  6. Previous trauma during intercourse.
  7. Domestic violence.

Presentation
A. Irritation or burning with intercourse.
B. Lack of vaginal lubrication.
C. Pain with vulvar or vaginal contact.
D. Pain with deep penetration.
E. Postcoital bleeding.

Other Signs and Symptoms
A. Vulvar pain.
B. Vaginal pain or burning.
C. Vaginal dryness.

Subjective Data
A. Review the onset, duration, and course of presenting symptoms, including precise location and timing of pain during intercourse.
B. Review the client's medical or surgical history for physical causes (see the section "Pathogenesis").
C. Ask: How often does pain occur (with every intercourse, near periods, or in certain sexual positions)? What relief measures have been tried? Is there improvement with using extra lubrication? How much relief was obtained with each measure?
D. Obtain a complete sexual history, including the following:
  1. Sexual practices.
  2. Sexual satisfaction or orgasm.
  3. Perception of partner satisfaction.
  4. Age at first coitus.
  5. History of sexual abuse, molestation, rape.
  6. Perceptions regarding sexuality.
  7. Number of sexual partners and preferences.
  8. Time spent on foreplay.
  9. History of recent delivery and breastfeeding.

10. Age at onset of puberty, date of last menses, and cycle history.
11. Current method of birth control and satisfaction with method; previous methods and why they were discontinued.
12. Presence of vaginal discharge, odour, dysuria, or other physical symptoms before or after intercourse.
13. Medications, including prescription and over-the-counter (OTC) drugs.
14. Can the woman insert a tampon without pain?

Physical Examination
A. Check temperature, pulse, respirations, and blood pressure (BP).
B. Inspect: Observe generally for discomfort before, during, and after examination.

Look for signs of physical or sexual abuse, cuts, bruises, and lacerations. For pain greatest on deep penile penetration, suspect PID, ovarian cyst, endometriosis, pelvic adhesions, relaxation of pelvic support, or uterine fibroids.

C. Auscultate:
　1. The abdomen for bowel sounds in all quadrants. Auscultation of the abdomen should precede any palpation or percussion due to the changes in intensity and frequency of sounds after manipulation.
D. Palpate:
　1. Palpate the abdomen for masses; check for suprapubic tenderness.
　2. Examine the back, assess range of motion. Observe for evidence of disc disease, myofascial pain, and coccygodynia. Palpate for costovertebral angle (CVA) tenderness.
E. Pelvic examination:
　1. Inspect: Perform perineal examination for atrophic vaginitis. Atrophic vaginitis presents as red, shiny, smooth vagina (loss of rugae); vaginal thinning; decreased elasticity of vaginal tissues. Vulvar inflammation may be present. Assess discharge and rugae for hormonal support.
　2. Evaluate the client for vulvovaginitis. Perform vulvar examination for Bartholin's gland enlargement, fissures, condyloma, and herpes. Inspect for anatomic variants: narrowed introitus, congenital malformations (septum), and pelvic relaxation (cystocele and rectocele).
F. Speculum examination: Inspect for cervicitis, friability, and discharge. If the woman can insert a tampon without pain, a mechanical obstruction is unlikely.
G. Bimanual examination: Check cervical motion tenderness (CMT); adnexal masses; and uterine size, consistency, and position.
H. Rectovaginal examination: Palpate uterosacral ligaments for pain and nodularity and other signs of PID and endometriosis. In cases of rectal trauma, cultures may be needed to rule out STIs if anal intercourse is practiced.

Diagnostic Tests
A. **Wet prep to rule out candidiasis, trichomoniasis, and bacterial vaginosis (BV).**
B. Cervical cultures for chlamydia, gonorrhoea.
C. Viral cultures of lesions, if any.
D. Urine culture, if applicable.
E. Pelvic ultrasonography, if indicated.
F. **Stool culture, if applicable.**
G. Sedimentation rate, if indicated by physical.

Differential Diagnoses
A. See section "Pathogenesis."

Plan
A. General interventions:
　1. Detailed physical examination after a thorough history.
　2. Clients should be encouraged to involve their partner(s) in assessment, diagnosis, and treatment of dyspareunia.
　3. A secure, trusting relationship must be established with the care provider before many clients feel comfortable discussing sexuality issues. Continuity with one provider is essential.
　4. Clients with dyspareunia should be evaluated for multiple aetiologies. Treat underlying pathologies such as musculoskeletal anomalies, pelvic infection, urinary tract infection (UTI), sexually transmitted diseases (STDs), hormonal deficiencies, and GI aetiologies (see specific chapters for treatment plans and drug therapy).
B. Client teaching:
　1. *Refer to Client Teaching Guide: Dyspareunia (Pain With Intercourse).*
C. Pharmacological therapy:
　1. Refer to specific chapter for therapies related to aetiology.
　2. Vulvodynia: Consider the use of topical agents applied to the vulva or vestibule, antihistamine therapy, and/or tricyclic antidepressants.
　　a. Lidocaine 5% gel applied to vulva, vestibule, and fourchette.
　　b. Diphenhydramine or 0.1% triamcinolone acetonide cream pruritus.
　　c. Amitriptyline.

Follow-Up
A. Perform test of cure for all diagnosed infections, if indicated (see specific infection and therapy).
B. Refer to follow-up plans for specific aetiology.

Consultation/Referral
A. Refer the client to a gynaecologist for removal of cysts, endometriomas. Laparoscopy is indicated if endometriosis, adhesions, or an adnexal mass is suspected.
B. Refer the client to a gynaecologist for vulvovaginal anomalies, including thickened hymen, shortened vagina, and vaginal agenesis; vaginal dilator therapy may be tried.
C. Refer the client for sexual therapy consultation for continued complaints without an identifiable physical cause.

Individual Considerations
A. Pregnancy or postpartum:
　1. Sexual intercourse may continue throughout pregnancy unless there is pain, bleeding, preterm labour, or premature rupture of the membranes. Alternate positions should be suggested by the provider. Sexual intercourse may resume in the postpartum period when the bleeding has decreased or stopped, incision or episiotomy is healed, and the woman is comfortable upon finger insertion and test of vaginal discomfort.

▶ Client Teaching Guides are available at https://connect.springerpub.com/content/reference-book/978-0-8261-9498-5

2. Breastfeeding causes hormonal changes that may produce a menopause-like state, and extra lubrication is usually required.
B. Partners:
1. Encourage the client to have partner(s) participate in sexual health counseling.

Bibliography
Kumar, K., & Robertson, D. (2017). Superficial dyspareunia. *Canadian Medical Association Journal, 189*(24), E836

Emergency Contraception (EC)

Rhonda Arthur

Definition
A. Emergency contraception (EC) is a prospective method of pregnancy prevention when unprotected intercourse or birth control failure occurs.

Incidence/Prevalence
A. One in nine sexually active women report using EC, with the highest use rate among women aged 20 to 24 years. The intent is to increase the use of EC to reduce the number of unintended pregnancies and thus reduce the number of abortions and deliveries of truly unwanted children.

Pathogenesis
A. Hormones in oral contraceptive pills temporarily disrupt ovarian hormone production and cause an absent or dysfunctional luteal phase hormone pattern. This results in an out-of-phase endometrium that is unsuitable for implantation. Hormone disruption may likewise interfere with fertilization and cause disordered tubal transport. Hormones or minerals (copper) in an intrauterine device (IUD) cause an inflammatory response to occur, which make the endometrium unsuitable for implantation and interfere with fertilization and transport.

Predisposing Factors
A. Failure of other means of birth control, including broken condom, dislodged diaphragm or cervical cap, expelled IUD, or lost or forgotten pills.
B. Rape.
C. Unprotected intercourse.

Common Findings
A. "I'm worried that I might get pregnant because the condom broke."
B. "My diaphragm slipped."
C. "I went on vacation and forgot my pills."

Other Signs and Symptoms
A. Unprotected intercourse.

Subjective Data
A. Elicit a menstrual history. When was the client's last menstrual period (LMP)? Are her periods regular?
B. What form of contraception was used, if any?
C. Has the client experienced any early signs of pregnancy? If so, discuss.
D. Ask about early symptoms of pregnancy, such as frequency of urination, nausea, breast tenderness, and late or missed period.
E. Ask the client about her feelings or plans if she should get pregnant.

Physical Examination
A. Check blood pressure, pulse, and weight.
B. Inspect abdomen for enlargement compatible with pregnancy.
C. Palpate abdomen for uterine size; if fundus is palpable, measure for fundal height.
D. Auscultate:
1. Heart and lungs.
2. Abdomen. If the uterus is enlarged and is measured to be >11 weeks' gestation, attempt to hear foetal heart tones with foetal Doppler.
E. Pelvic examination:
1. Inspect the external genitalia for lesions; note female pubic hair pattern.
2. Speculum examination: Observe for bluish colour of cervix (Chadwick's sign). Observe vaginal discharge; note colour and odour.
3. Bimanual examination: Palpate the cervix for softening associated with early pregnancy. Palpate uterine size.

Diagnostic Tests
A. Pregnancy test: Urine or serum human chorionic gonadotropin (HCG).

Differential Diagnoses
A. Unprotected intercourse, potential for pregnancy.
B. Pregnancy.
C. Dysfunctional uterine bleeding (DUB).
D. Amenorrhoea from anovulation.
E. Polycystic ovary syndrome (PCOS).
F. Perimenopause.

Plan
A. General interventions:
1. Review the client's past medical history, contraceptive history, date of LMP, estimated date of ovulation, date of unprotected intercourse, and number of hours since the first and most recent unprotected intercourses.
2. Discuss the likely risk of pregnancy.
3. Explore the client's feeling about continuing pregnancy.
4. Decide whether a physical examination and pregnancy test are needed if there is a possibility of a pregnancy from the previous month.
B. Client teaching:
1. *Refer to Client Teaching Guides: Emergency Contraception—Levonorgestrel* or *Emergency Contraception—Ulipristal Acetate* based on selected method.
2. Discuss options, risks, failure rates, necessary follow-up, alteration of menstrual period, and warning signs of complications.
3. Discuss interim plan for contraception.
4. Advise the client to take oral contraceptive pills as prescribed or have an IUD inserted within 96 hours of unprotected intercourse.
5. Treatment is most effective if taken within 72 hours for progestin–oestrogen methods and within 120 hours for a progestin antagonist.
6. Treatment is not effective in an already established pregnancy.

▶ Client Teaching Guides are available at https://connect.springerpub.com/content/reference-book/978-0-8261-9498-5

7. Educate the client about the possibility of menstrual cycle disturbance with the next menstrual period.
8. If menstrual bleeding does not begin within three weeks, evaluate for possible pregnancy.
9. EC is not associated with an increased incidence of abnormal outcome of pregnancy, should pregnancy not be averted. EC does not always work.
10. This is not to be used as a primary contraceptive method.
11. Have prescription or pack of pills available for an emergency situation.
12. The IUD should be used only for women at low risk for pelvic inflammatory disease (PID) and when the woman intends to continue use of the IUD for contraception.

C. Pharmacological therapy:

Choosing the best method for EC should be based on the day and time of unprotected intercourse; body mass index (BMI); breastfeeding; and recent (within five days) use of pill, patch, or ring:

1. IUD—Most effective and can be used up to 120 hours after unprotected intercourse:
   a. Copper IUD must be inserted within five to seven days after ovulation in a cycle when unprotected intercourse has occurred. The advantage is that the IUD may be left in place for continuing contraception for 10 years.
   b. Mechanism of action: Two ideas have been proposed:
      i. IUD leads to endometrial changes that prohibit implantation.
      ii. The copper ions have a direct toxic effect on the embryo.
2. EC oral formulations:
   a. Levonorgestrel emergency contraceptive, commonly called "morning after pill." These progestin-only ECs are available unrestricted as over-the-counter (OTC) medicines. Less effective for women with a BMI >25 and may not be effective for women with a BMI >30:
      i. Levonorgestrel should be taken as soon as possible after unprotected sex (no later than 72 hours).
   b. Using a standard packet of oral contraceptives: Two doses of a combination of ethinyl estradiol and levonorgestrel, 12 hours apart. Table 14.1 provides the equivalent dosing that may be used as an emergency contraceptive:
      i. Method must be used within 72 hours of unprotected intercourse. Treatment is most effective if taken within 12 to 24 hours.
      ii. Side effects of nausea and vomiting with EC are common. Take each dose with food. Take antiemetic, dimenhydrinate, 30 minutes before dose of medication.
      iii. If vomiting occurs within one to three hours of taking a dose, take another dose.
      iv. Educate the client about common side effects, such as breast tenderness, abdominal pain, headache, and dizziness.

Follow-Up

A. Have the client return in three to four weeks if she does not have a menstrual period. If she has a menstrual period, recommend that she return in one month to assess contraceptive use and offer options.

Consultation/Referral

A. Consult a specialist if there is no withdrawal bleed within four weeks.
B. Consult or refer the client to a specialist if necessary to insert IUD.
C. Clients have access to EC at pharmacies across Canada, with a prescription required only in Quebec.

Special Considerations

A. Pregnancy: There is no increased incidence of anomalies if pregnancy does occur.

Bibliography

Afaxys, Inc. (2015). *Ella full prescribing information*. Retrieved from http://www.ellanow.com/pdf/ella-full-prescribing-information.pdf
Guttmacher Institute. (2015). *Contraceptive use in the United States*. Retrieved from http://www.guttmacher.org/fact-sheet/contraceptive-use-united-states
Planned Parenthood. (2014). *Morning-after pill (emergency contraception)*. Retrieved from http://www.plannedparenthood.org/learn/morning-after-pill-emergency-contraception
Women's Capital Corporation. (2015, August). *PlanB one-step*. Retrieved from http://planbonestep.com

TABLE 14.1 Emergency Contraception

Progestin-Only Emergency Contraceptive Pill			
Directions for progestin-only pills: Take one dose within 72 hours of intercourse			
Brand	Number of Pills per Dose	Ethinyl Estradiol (mcg)/Dose	Levonorgestrel (mg)/Dose
Plan B One-Step	One pill	0	1.5
Next Choice One Dose	One pill	0	1.5
COC Pills for Emergency Contraception			
Directions for COC pills: Take first dose within 72 hours and repeat dose in 12 hours			
Brand	Number of Pills per Dose	Ethinyl Estradiol (mcg)/Dose	Levonorgestrel (mg)/Dose
Yuzpe	Two white pills	100	0.50
Min-Ovral	Four white pills	120	0.60
Alesse	Five pink pills	100	0.50

COC, combined oral contraceptive.

Endometriosis

Rhonda Arthur and Julia Blake

Definition
A. Endometriosis is ectopic endometrial tissue that exhibits hormonal responsiveness but is located outside the uterine cavity. Bleeding from this ectopic endometrial tissue causes pelvic inflammation and scarring, resulting in chronic pelvic pain and infertility. Endometrial lesions have been found in the vagina, gastrointestinal (GI) tract (especially the sigmoid colon), thoracic cavity, limbs, and gallbladder.

Incidence/Prevalence
A. The true incidence of endometriosis is unknown. Ranges of 5% to 30% have been cited. Positive family history (mother or sister) increases the risk 10-fold. Endometriosis does not have a higher incidence for any particular race or socioeconomic group.

Pathogenesis
A. Retrograde menstruation is the most popular theory for the aetiology of endometriosis. Menses are suspected of "flowing backward" through the fallopian tubes, resulting in the "seeding" of endometrial tissue outside the uterus.

Predisposing Factors
A. Positive family history, mother and/or sister.
B. History of progressive dysmenorrhoea.
C. History of prolonged uninterrupted menstrual cycles; first pregnancy at a late age.
D. Limited or no prior use of hormonal contraceptives.

Common Findings
A. Pain before period.
B. Pain with intercourse.
C. Pain with bowel movements; may include constipation from the fear or pain of having a bowel movement (dyschezia).
D. Vaginal spotting and bleeding.

Other Signs and Symptoms
A. Dyspareunia and/or pain that radiates to the thigh.
B. Chronic, noncyclic pelvic pain.
C. Abnormal vaginal bleeding: Premenstrual spotting and dysfunctional uterine bleeding (DUB).
D. Other bowel symptoms: Diarrhoea and rectal bleeding.
E. Urinary symptoms: Dysuria, urgency, and haematuria.

Subjective Data
A. Review the onset, duration, and course of complaints.
B. Question the client regarding menstrual history: Interval and duration of menstrual cycles and history of dysmenorrhoea.
C. Question the client regarding former use of hormonal contraceptives, including levonorgestrel, birth control pills, medroxyprogesterone, and progesterone.
D. Question the client regarding change in bowel patterns or habits or pain with defecation.
E. Question the client regarding incidence of dyspareunia.
F. Note the client parity and/or history of infertility.

Physical Examination
A. Check temperature, pulse, respirations, and blood pressure.
B. Inspect:
  1. Note general appearance for discomfort before, during, and after examination.
  2. Perform detailed external genitalia examination.
C. Auscultate:
  1. Abdomen for bowel sounds in all quadrants. Auscultation of the abdomen should precede any palpation or percussion due to the changes in intensity and frequency of sounds after manipulation.
D. Palpate:
  1. Palpate abdomen for masses.
  2. Check for suprapubic tenderness.
  3. Back: Check for costovertebral angle (CVA) tenderness.
E. Pelvic examination:
  1. Speculum examination: Inspect the cervix for cervicitis; friability; and discharge colour, odour, and amount. Note any cutaneous lesions of the vagina, cervix, and perineum that resemble "powder burn or chocolate spots." Laparoscopic findings frequently reveal "powder burn" lesions of endometrial implants along the uterosacral ligament, pelvic peritoneum, ovaries, sigmoid colon, and other pelvic organs.
  2. Bimanual examination: Check for cervical motion tenderness (CMT), adnexal masses; check uterine size, consistency, position, and mobility.

The most common indicator of endometriosis is a fixed retroverted uterus with nodularity felt along the uterosacral ligaments. Palpation of endometrial implants may result in exquisite pain for the client.

  3. Rectovaginal examination: Palpate uterosacral ligaments for pain and nodularity. Evaluate for masses and polyps of rectum. A rectal examination is done because the uterus is often fixed in a retroverted position due to endometriosis. The endometrial nodules present on the posterior uterine wall, cul-de-sac, and uterosacral ligament may be distinguished better rectally.

Diagnostic Tests
There are no specific diagnostic tests for endometriosis. Definite diagnosis is done by laparoscopy:
A. Serum beta human chorionic gonadotropin (HCG) to rule out ectopic pregnancy.
B. White blood cell (WBC) to rule out infection.
C. Cervical culture for chlamydia or gonorrhoea, to rule out sexually transmitted infection (STI) and pelvic inflammatory disease (PID).
D. Urine culture, if indicated.
E. Transvaginal ultrasonography, to rule out cysts and masses.
F. GI series or barium enema, if indicated.

Differential Diagnoses
A. Dysmenorrhoea.
B. Ovarian cysts.
C. PID.
D. Premenstrual syndrome (PMS).
E. Mittelschmerz.
F. Trauma.

G. Appendicitis.
H. Pregnancy: normal, missed abortion, or ectopic.
I. GI or genitourinary (GU) complaints: Diverticular disease, spastic colon, or urinary tract infection (UTI).

Plan
A. General interventions:
   1. After surgical confirmation, the practitioner may comanage endometriosis with a specialist.
B. Client teaching:
   1. Treatment goals include prevention of disease progression, alleviation of pain, and establishment or restoration of fertility. Treatment options include the following:
      a. Observation alone.
      b. Medical therapy or pharmacological therapy.
      c. Referral or consultation for laparoscopic therapy, including laser vaporization and removal of adhesions.
   2. Continuation or recurrence of pelvic pain may necessitate assisting the woman to manage her chronic pelvic pain and dysmenorrhoea with nonsteroidal anti-inflammatory drugs (NSAIDs) therapy and/or other non-narcotic chronic pain therapies, such as visualization and biofeedback.
   3. Hysterectomy and bilateral salpingo-oophorectomy are the only definitive cures for women who do not wish to conserve their reproductive capacity. This should be considered only as a last resort for failed conservative treatment.
C. Pharmacological therapy: Diagnosis must first be confirmed by laparoscopy:
   1. Mild endometriosis:
      a. Combined oral contraceptive (COC) pills are considered the first-line therapy. If the client experiences pain during the week of withdrawal bleeding, she may take active pills continuously, omitting the placebo pills of the "off week."

Combination oral contraceptives are being used to produce a state of pseudopregnancy that should induce regression of the disease.

   b. Medroxyprogesterone acetate, norethindrone acetate, or megestrol acetate, or a long-acting progestin.
   2. Moderate to severe endometriosis:
      a. Gonadotropin-releasing hormone (GnRH) agonist:
         i. Leuprolide acetate, goserelin.

Use of a GnRH agonist, which acts to suppress ovulation, can result in side effects, including hot flashes, mood changes, and other menopausal symptoms. Use is restricted to six months to avoid decrease in bone density. Expense of this therapy may preclude its use.

   b. Danazol:
      i. Use of danazol, which acts to produce anovulation and hypogonadotropism, can result in androgenic side effects, including acne, hirsutism, weight gain, and voice changes that may not be reversible.
   c. With specialist consultation or referral, GnRH agonists such as leuprolide acetate and goserelin acetate:
      i. Other side effects, which are reversible, include decreased breast size, atrophic vaginitis, dyspareunia, hot flashes, and emotional liability.

Follow-Up
A. Clients must return monthly while receiving GnRH agonist or danazol therapies to assess for symptom relief and side effect profile.

Consultation/Referral
A. The workup, evaluation, and medications for endometriosis are expensive. Refer to a gynaecologist for initial management. A prudent approach is recommended with a conservative treatment option; evaluate the results before trying another.
B. Refer the client for a surgical consultation for definitive diagnosis. Endometriosis may be suspected based on symptoms and physical examination. It cannot, however, be confirmed unless actually visualized by laparoscopy.

Individual Considerations
A. Pregnancy:
   1. Infertility may be a presenting symptom. Treatment may, therefore, be focused on endometriosis abatement and fertility support.

Resource
The Endometriosis Network Canada: https://endometriosisnetwork.com/

Female Sexual Dysfunction

Nancy Pesta Walsh and Julia Blake

Definition
A. Any persistent problem with desire, sexual response, or function, which may affect the client and her relationship, and occurs for at least six months. It is classified into subtypes:
   1. Desire disorder: Lack of interest or desire (most common).
   2. Arousal disorder: Inability to become aroused during sexual activity; absent or reduced genital sensations.
   3. Orgasm disorder: Delay, absence, or decreased intensity of orgasm:
      a. Primary: The client has never had an orgasm.
      b. Secondary: The client has achieved orgasm in the past, but is unable to achieve orgasm at the time of presentation.
   4. Pain disorder: Genitopelvic pain/penetration disorder (formerly dyspareunia and vaginismus). This is described as pelvic or vulvovaginal pain during vaginal penetration, anxiety, and/or fear related to the thought of vaginal penetration, or marked tightening of pelvic floor muscles during vaginal penetration.

Incidence/Prevalence
A. Affects an estimated 22% to 43% of women worldwide, and 14% of women aged 45 to 64 years. Only 12% have diagnosable disorders. This includes women who report issues with sexual desire (64%), arousal difficulty (31%), and pain (26%).

Pathogenesis

A. Multiple models exist to describe the phases of normal sexual function:
   1. Masters and Johnson—consists of the stages of excitement, plateau, orgasm, and resolution.
   2. Kaplan and Leif—consists of desire, excitement, and orgasm.
   3. Basson—consists of emotional intimacy, sexual stimuli, psychological factors, and relationship satisfaction.

B. Sexual dysfunction includes various biological, psychological, and social components:
   1. Biological factors include aging; medical conditions such as diabetes and hypertension; and declining testosterone or oestrogen.
   2. Psychological factors include depression or anxiety, history of sexual abuse, childhood trauma, personality disorders, body image disorders, and perceived stress.
   3. Social factors include cultural or religious values, relationship issues, career issues, financial hardship, and household responsibilities.

C. Diagnosis is made based on the *Diagnostic and Statistical Manual of Mental Disorders* Fifth Edition (*DSM-5*; American Psychiatric Association, 2013) and requires the following: Symptoms must be present for a minimum of six months; a woman experiences personal distress; symptoms are not a result of substance or medication use, or medical conditions; and symptoms are not related to a nonsexual medical disorder.

D. Orgasm disorders can be caused by neurologic and/or vascular disease such as spinal cord injury, diabetes, or multiple sclerosis.

Predisposing Factors

A. Emotional:
   1. Depression.
   2. Mood disorders.
   3. Poor body image.
   4. Low self-esteem.
   5. Fatigue.
   6. Stress.

B. Poor health status:
   1. Spinal cord injury.
   2. Diabetes.
   3. Premature ovarian failure (POF).
   4. Trauma.

C. Partner relationship issues.

D. Medications that are associated with low sexual desire in women:
   1. Serotonin-specific reuptake inhibitors (SSRIs).
   2. Anxiolytics.
   3. Antihistamines.
   4. Anticholinergics.
   5. Calcium channel blockers.
   6. Angiotensin-converting enzyme (ACE) inhibitors.
   7. Oral contraceptives.
   8. Anticonvulsants.
   9. Opiates.
   10. Illicit drugs.

E. History of sexual abuse may contribute to low desire.

F. Advancing age:
   1. Menopausal women are affected more frequently. Low sexual desire may result from decreasing hormone levels, specifically testosterone and oestrogen levels. Low oestrogen levels are also linked to vulvovaginal atrophy and dyspareunia, both of which may decrease sexual desire in women.

Common Findings

A. Women:
   1. Absence of orgasm.
   2. Pain during vaginal penetration.
   3. Difficulty relaxing pelvic floor muscles to allow vaginal penetration.

B. Both sexes:
   1. Lack of interest or desire (most common).
   2. Inability to become aroused.
   3. Pain with intercourse.

C. Men: Presentation for men is specifically discussed in Chapter 11, Gastrointestinal guidelines.

Other Signs and Symptoms

A. Vaginal discharge.
B. Vulvar itching.
C. Vulvar pain, described as stinging, burning, irritation, raw sensation.

Subjective Data

A. Include full medical, gynaecologic, and sexual history, using open-ended questions:
   1. Assess the client for signs of depression, anxiety, and sexual concerns.
   2. Review the medication list with the client. Specifically ask about the types of medications that may contribute to low sexual desire:
      a. SSRIs.
      b. Anxiolytics.
      c. Antihistamines.
      d. Anticholinergics.
      e. Calcium channel blockers.
      f. ACE inhibitors.
      g. Oral contraceptives.
      h. Anticonvulsants.
      i. Opiates.
      j. Illicit drugs.
   3. Assess for medical conditions that contribute to sexual dysfunction, which may include the following:
      a. Chronic diseases (cardiovascular disease, diabetes, kidney or liver failure).
      b. Neurologic disorders.
      c. Hormone imbalances.
      d. Alcoholism.
      e. Elicit drug use.
      f. Evaluate for causes of pelvic pain: Vaginal dryness, vaginal discharge, or vaginal infectious causes (such as sexually transmitted infections [STIs], yeast infections, or pelvic inflammatory disease [PID]).
   4. Evaluate for history of previous pelvic disorders or surgery (fibroids, endometriosis, malignancy, uterine/bladder prolapse, or episiotomy).
   5. Evaluate for the degree of distress that this may cause the client.

B. The use of self-report screening tools is recommended to identify women with low sexual desire. These tools may include the following:
   1. Decreased Sexual Desire Screener: Found at www.obgynalliance.com/files/fsd/DSDS_Pocketcard.pdf
   2. Brief Sexual Symptom Checklist for Women May be downloaded from www.researchgate.net/figure/277610474_fig1_Figure-2-The-modified-Brief-Sexual-Symptom-Checklist-for-Women-BSSC-W
   3. Female Sexual Function Index: Found at www.fsfiquestionnaire.com

Physical Examination
A. Check blood pressure (BP), pulse, and respirations.
B. Inspect:
   1. Thyroid for presence of nodules.
   2. Breasts for presence of nipple discharge if history warrants.
   3. Skin for hirsutism, acne, alopecia, and truncal obesity may indicate hyperandrogenism.
C. Palpate.
   1. Thyroid for presence of nodules.
   2. May palpate breasts for presence of nipple discharge if history warrants.

Pelvic Examination
A. Inspect:
   1. Examine external genitalia for erythema, lesions, atrophy, or unusual discharge.
   2. Inspect for vulvar dermatoses, such as lichen sclerosus or lichen planus. Lichen sclerosus may look like white skin discolourations or wrinkled patches of skin. Severe cases may have bleeding or ulcerated lesions. Lichen planus may look like purple-coloured lesions or bumps with flat tops. Thin white lines or blisters may appear over the lesions.
   3. Inspect for pelvic floor prolapse and pelvic floor muscle contraction.
B. Palpate external genitalia for presence of pain.
C. Speculum examination:
   1. Assess for atrophy (common in postmenopausal women), pelvic floor muscle strength, masses, prolapse, and deep pelvic pain.
D. Bimanual examination:
   1. Check for cervical motion tenderness (CMT), uterine size, and position.
   2. Check adnexa for masses or tenderness.

Diagnostic Tests
A. Laboratory tests should be performed as indicated by the history and physical examination for any medical conditions that may contribute to low desire.
B. Pap smear, STI testing, wet prep.
C. Serum testing may include thyroid function tests and prolactin levels.
D. Androgen levels and testosterone levels alone are unreliable, unless you suspect a hyperandrogenic condition, as evidenced by hirsutism, acne, alopecia, and truncal obesity.
E. Transvaginal ultrasound may be warranted if pelvic pain upon examination.

Differential Diagnoses
A. Arousal disorder.
B. Desire disorder.
C. Orgasm disorder.
D. Pain disorder.
E. Vulvar dermatoses, such as lichen planus or lichen sclerosis.
F. Vaginal atrophy.
G. Infectious issues, such as STIs, candidiasis, or bacterial vaginosis (BV).
H. Depression or anxiety.
I. Cardiovascular disease.
J. Diabetes.
K. Thyroid disorder.
L. Neurologic disorder.
M. Hormonal imbalance.

Plan
A. General interventions:
   1. Set realistic goals for treatment.
   2. Empower women to take an active role in treatment plan. Encourage discussion about anatomy and sexual function, allowing the women to ask questions as they are comfortable.
   3. Office-based therapy may be useful for providers who wish to include this in their practice. The Permission, Limited Information, Specific Suggestion, Intensive Therapy (PLISSIT) model is one office-based counseling model detailed as follows:
      a. Permission: Women are given permission for full discussion of the topic.
      b. Limited Information: The provider gives educational information on sexual function and sexual dysfunction in the form of handouts or videos.
      c. Specific Suggestion: The provider gives very specific advice tailored to each client and her presenting issues.
      d. Intensive Therapy: The provider makes a referral for individual or couples' therapy.
B. Client teaching:
   1. Educate about normal anatomical and sexual functions.
   2. Encourage healthy lifestyle behaviours of diet, exercise, avoiding tobacco, and minimizing stress.
   3. Educate clients about the use of vaginal lubricants and moisturizers to assist with vaginal dryness or dyspareunia.
C. Pharmacological therapy is considered when nonpharmacological interventions are not successful:
   1. Vaginal oestrogen for the treatment of vaginal atrophy.

Follow-Up
A. As determined by the history and physical examination findings and diagnoses made. Women placed on medications should follow up one month after initiating and have routine follow-up at three- to six-month intervals to determine if continuation of the medication is necessary.
B. Postmenopausal women with vaginal bleeding should follow up immediately.

Consultation/Referral
A. Refer to any therapist who specializes in sexual problems:
   1. Counseling may include sex therapy or cognitive behavioural therapy (CBT).
B. May refer to pelvic floor therapist for treatment of genitopelvic pain disorders, once other medical conditions have been treated.

Individual Considerations
A. Use of opposing progestin is not necessary when using lowest dose oestrogens, though use of oestrogen should be the lowest possible effective dose for the shortest duration.
B. Clients with a history of breast cancer: Although risk is low, consult with the client's oncologist before initiating vaginal oestrogen.

Resources
The Sex Information & Education Council of Canada, 235 Danforth Avenue, Suite 400, Toronto, ON, M4K 1N2, www.sieccan.org
Canadian Menopause Society, Suite 103 - 1089 West Broadway, Vancouver, British Columbia, V6H 1E5, https://www.sigmamenopause.com

Bibliography

Chasson, S. (2013). Female sexual dysfunction. In K. D. Schuiling & F. E. Likis (Eds.), *Women's gynecologic health* (2nd ed., pp. 405–421). Burlington, MA: Jones & Bartlett.

Hilz, M. (2015). Assessment and treatment of male and female sexual dysfunction. *Journal of the Neurological Sciences, 357*(1), 498–499.

Ishak, W. W., & Tobia, G. (2013). *DSM-5 changes in diagnostic criteria of sexual dysfunctions*. Retrieved from http://www.omicsonline.org/dsm-5-changes-in-diagnostic-criteria-of-sexual-dysfunctions-2161-038X.1000122.php?aid=18508

Kingsberg, S. A., & Woodard, T. (2015). Female sexual dysfunction: Focus on low desire. *Obstetrics and Gynecology, 125*(2), 477–486.

Latif, E. Z., & Diamond, M. P. (2013). Arriving at the diagnosis of female sexual dysfunction. *Fertility and Sterility, 100*(4), 898–904.

The North American Menopause Society. (2016). *Vagina and vulvar comfort: Lubricants, moisturizers, and low-dose vaginal estrogen*. Retrieved from http://www.menopause.org/for-women/-em-sexual-health-menopause-em-online/effective-treatments-for-sexual-problems/vaginal-and-vulvar-comfort-lubricants-moisturizers-and-low-dose-vaginal-estrogen

The PLISSIT Model of Sex Therapy. (n.d.). Retrieved from https://coad7404.files.wordpress.com/2014/06/plissitanonsmodel.pdf

Thomas, H. N., & Thurston, R. C. (2016). A biopsychosocial approach to women's sexual function and dysfunction at midlife: A narrative review. *Maturitas, 87*, 49–60.

Wright, J. J., & O'Connor, K. M. (2015). Female sexual dysfunction. *Medical Clinics of North America, 99*(3), 607–628.

Infertility

Rhonda Arthur and Julia Blake

Definition

A. Infertility is defined as the inability to conceive within 12 months of unprotected intercourse. Many clinicians use a six-month time frame if the woman is 35 years of age and older.

B. A woman who has never been pregnant or a man who has never initiated a pregnancy is said to have "primary infertility."

C. If a previous pregnancy has been achieved and the couple is unable to conceive a subsequent pregnancy, the term "secondary infertility" is applied.

Incidence/Prevalence

A. It is estimated that approximately 16% of couples in Canada experience infertility. Infertility can be traced to either man, woman, or a combination of both, where the cause is three times out of 10 in men and four times out of 10 in women. Pelvic inflammatory disease (PID) is the leading cause of infertility in the world. About 10% of infertility is unexplained.

Pathogenesis

Infertility may occur in the male (approximately 35%) or female (approximately 55%). Evaluate both partners for:

A. Infrequent intercourse.
B. Interpersonal problems.
C. Medical causes (see Table 14.2).

Predisposing Factors

A. Predisposing factors depend on the aetiology.

Common Findings

A. The common complaint is an inability to achieve pregnancy despite frequent acts of intercourse.

Other Signs and Symptoms

A. Dependent on the pathogenesis and history.

Subjective Data

A. Obtain a complete health history, including the following:
    1. Age of both partners.
    2. General health of both partners.
    3. Complete pregnancy history of the female:
        a. Number of pregnancies: Term and preterm.
        b. Vaginal deliveries or caesarean sections.
        c. Recurrent miscarriages, gestational age(s).
        d. Stillbirths.
        e. Dilation and curettage (D&C) for abortions or miscarriages.
        f. Cerclage for incompetent cervix.
    4. Paternity history of the male:
    5. Length of infertility, including prior workup, if any.
    6. Coital history:
        a. Frequency.
        b. Timing and adequacy.
        c. Use of lubricants; some may be spermicidal.
        d. Postcoital habits: douching or voiding.
    7. Adequacy of intercourse:
        a. Penetration of the vagina.
        b. Ejaculation by the male.

B. Obtain a complete menstrual history, including the following:
    1. Age at puberty.
    2. Regularity of cycles.
    3. Discomfort during menses.
    4. Date of last menstrual period (LMP).

C. Obtain a complete gynaecologic history, including the following:
    1. Contraceptive use.
    2. Medical and surgical interventions:
        a. D&C.
        b. Laparoscopy or endometriosis.
    3. Anomalies.

D. Take a complete nutritional and exercise history; note eating disorders:
    1. Anorexia nervosa.
    2. Bulimia.

E. Review female and male reproductive tract infections and treatments for past and present partners.

F. Review each individual's habits:
    1. Smoking: How much, how often, and how long.
    2. Drugs: How much, how often, and how long for each drug.
    3. Alcohol: How much, how often, and how long.
    4. Use of saunas or hot tubs.
    5. Exercise, including cycling.

G. Take a complete medication history, specifically review for the following:
    1. Antihypertensives.
    2. Antidepressants.
    3. Antipsychotics.
    4. Antiulcer agents or antacids.
    5. Muscle relaxants.

H. Review for exposure to toxic chemicals, radiation, or known teratogens:
    1. Military war exposure.
    2. Employment exposure.
    3. Residential exposure:
        a. Microwaves.
        b. Pesticides.

I. Inquire about diethylstilbestrol (DES) exposure in utero (for either partner).

J. Review for symptoms of thyroid dysfunction:
    1. Weight gain or loss.

TABLE 14.2  Pathogenesis of Infertility

Male Pathogenesis	Female Pathogenesis

A. Faulty sperm production:
  1. Azoospermia from:
    a. Cancer therapy.
    b. Adult mumps.
    c. Sertoli-cell-only syndrome.
    d. Hypogonadism.
    e. Retrograde ejaculation.
  2. Oligospermia from:
    a. Varicocele.
    b. Small testicular size.
B. Reproductive tract anomaly:
  1. Blocked vas deferens.
  2. Varicocele.
  3. Congenital obstruction of epididymis.
C. Klinefelter's syndrome.
D. Physical and chemical agents' exposure:
  1. Coal tar.
  2. Radiation.
E. Endocrine disorders:
  1. Diabetes.
  2. Low serum testosterone.
  3. Pituitary tumours.
  4. Hyperprolactinaemia.
F. Testicular infection.
G. Injury to reproductive organs/tract.
H. Nerve damage/neurologic disease: Spinal cord injury.
I. Impotence/erectile difficulty: Performance anxiety.
J. Premature ejaculation.
K. Early withdrawal.
L. Lifestyle factors:
  1. Drugs.
  2. Smoking.
  3. Alcohol.
  4. Malnutrition.
M. Antispermatozoa antibodies.
N. Medications:
  1. Antihypertensives.
  2. Antidepressants.
  3. Antipsychotics
  4. Anti-ulcer agents/antacids.
  5. Muscle relaxants.
	A. Advanced maternal age.
	B. Disorder of ovulation/hypothalamic dysfunction:
	  1. Anovulation.
	  2. Amenorrhoea.
	  3. Polycystic ovary triad:
	    a. Acne.
	    b. Obesity.
	    c. Hirsutism.
	  4. Premature ovarian failure:
	    a. Autoimmune.
	    b. Idiopathic.
	    c. Cancer therapy.
	  5. Luteal phase insufficiency.
	  6. Prolactinoma.
	C. Ovarian factors:
	  1. Cysts or tumour.
	  2. Irradiation.
	D. Tubal disorders/damage/blocked:
	  1. PID.
	  2. *Chlamydia trachomatis*.
	  3. Postpartum infection.
	  4. Pelvic trauma (motor vehicle accident).
	  5. Inflammatory bowel disease.
	  6. Endometriosis.
	  7. Adhesions.
	E. Uterine pathology:
	  1. Congenital anomalies: Duplication.
	  2. Septate.
	  3. Fibroids.
	  4. IUD.
	  5. Asherman's syndrome.
	  6. Synechiae.
	F. Cervical factors:
	  1. Anatomic abnormalities (hood).
	  2. Previous cervical surgery (i.e., conization, which leads to mucus depletion).
	  3. Hostile cervical mucus.
	  4. Presence of sperm antibodies in the cervix.
	  5. Infections.
	G. Lifestyle factors:
	  1. Drugs.
	  2. Smoking.
	H. Vaginal factors:
	  1. Intact hymen.
	  2. Septum.
	  3. Absent vagina.
	  4. Infection:
	    a. *Trichomonas*.
	    b. *Candida*.
	    c. Chlamydia.
	    d. Mycoplasma.
	    e. BV.
	    f. Gonorrhoea.
	    g. *Streptococci*.
	I. Medications: Oral contraceptives.
	J. Medical problems:
	  1. Lupus.
	  2. Hypothyroidism.
	  3. Diabetes.
	  4. Antiphospholipid syndrome.

BV, bacterial vaginosis; IUD, intrauterine device; PID, pelvic inflammatory disease.

2. Change of bowel habits.
3. Intolerance to heat or cold.
4. Appetite changes.
K. Review for systemic diseases:
1. Cardiac.
2. Collagen vascular diseases.
3. Diabetes.
L. Assess the psychosocial context of the infertility, including personal, emotional, and economic factors; family pressures for children; expectations; timing of pregnancy; consideration of adoption; and stress from failure to conceive.

Signs and Symptoms
A. See the section "Pathogenesis" and information obtained in the section "Subjective Data" regarding past medical history.
B. History of not being able to get pregnant over the past six to 12 months is noted.

Physical Examination
Male
A. Check temperature, pulse, respirations, and blood pressure (BP). Obtain height, weight, and body mass index (BMI).
B. Inspect:
1. Note general signs and appearance of underandrogenization: decreased body hair, gynaecomastia, and eunuchoid proportions.
2. Test the client's visual field for possible mass lesion.
3. Examine the penis for hypospadias. Observe urethra for discharge.
C. Percuss: Check deep tendon reflexes (DTRs) for signs of hypothyroidism.
D. Palpate:
1. Neck: Examine thyroid.
2. Genitals: Examine the scrotum for testicular size, absence of vas deferens, and presence of varicocele.
E. Rectal examination: Check prostate and seminal vesicles for tenderness and other signs of infection.

Valsalva's maneuver performed while the client stands helps to reveal small varicocele. Varicocele feels like "a bag of worms" with bluish discolouration visible through the scrotum. Approximately 23% to 30% of infertile males have a varicocele (usually present on the left side). No treatment is necessary if the semen analysis is normal.

Female
A. Check temperature, pulse, respirations, and BP.
B. Inspect:
1. Examine breasts for the presence of nipple discharge.
2. Note general signs and appearance of polycystic ovary syndrome (PCOS).

PCOS triad includes acne, obesity, and hirsutism.

C. Auscultate: Abdomen for bowel sounds in all quadrants. Auscultation of the abdomen should precede any palpation or percussion due to the changes in intensity and frequency of sounds after manipulation.
D. Palpate:
1. Neck: Examine the thyroid.
2. Abdomen: Note tenderness and masses.
3. Back: Check for costovertebral angle (CVA) tenderness.
E. Percuss: Check DTRs.
F. Pelvic examination:
1. Inspect: Perform detailed external peritoneal examination for signs of infection; lesions; or anomalies of clitoris, labia, Skene's gland, Bartholin's gland, vulva, and perineum.
2. Speculum examination:
   a. Observe length of vagina, position and characteristic of cervix, and any anomalies.
   b. Sound the uterus and cervix for stenosis. Observe the characteristics of cervical mucus: Thin and watery or thick and cloudy, odour, or evidence of infection.
3. Bimanual examination: Check uterine size, consistency, contour, mobility, cervical motion tenderness (CMT), and adnexal masses.

A fixed, immobile uterus determined on bimanual examination indicates the presence of pelvic scarring resulting from conditions such as endometriosis and PID.

4. Rectovaginal examination: Palpate uterosacral ligaments for pain and nodularity; evaluate masses and polyps of the rectum.

Diagnostic Tests
A. Male factor: Semen analysis.
B. Female (ovarian) factor:
1. Basal body temperature (BBT).
2. Serum progesterone measured midway through luteal phase: Serum progesterone >40 nmol/L indicates ovulation.
3. Urinary luteinizing hormone (LH) for surge.
4. Follicle-stimulating hormone (FSH): A high FSH, >40 international units (IU)/L, indicates ovarian failure.
5. Thyroid-stimulating hormone (TSH).
6. Serum prolactin.

When nipple discharge is present, check serum prolactin and TSH to rule out hyperprolactinaemia and hypothyroidism.

C. Pelvic or uterine factor:
1. Hysterosalpingogram (HSG); also done for tubal factor.
2. Transvaginal ultrasonography.
3. Laparoscopy.
D. Other tests:
1. Papanicolaou (Pap) smear with maturation index.
2. Cultures for gonorrhoea and chlamydia.
3. Pregnancy test, if amenorrhoea is present.
4. Complete blood count (CBC), erythrocyte sedimentation rate (ESR).
5. Mycoplasma culture.
6. Wet mount.

Differential Diagnoses
A. Sexual dysfunction.
B. Hypothyroidism.
C. Hypothalamic dysfunction: Amenorrhoea.
D. Hyperprolactinaemia.
E. Menopause.
F. Ovarian failure.
G. PCOS.
H. Asherman's syndrome.

I. Tubal occlusion.
J. Antisperm antibodies.
K. Endometriosis.
L. Oligo-ovulation.
M. Uterine anomalies: Fibroids, synechiae, and septa.
N. Pelvic adhesions.

Plan
A. General interventions:
   1. Semen analysis is the first step in an infertility workup. Semen analysis should be performed in a reputable laboratory. If the first evaluation is abnormal, it should be repeated one time. Normal semen analysis includes the following:
      a. Sperm count: >20×10^6 per ejaculate.
      b. Volume: 1.5 to 5 mL.
      c. Motility: >50%.
      d. Morphology: >50% at one hour.
      e. Liquefaction: 20 to 30 minutes after collection.
   2. The male physical examination is generally done if semen analysis is abnormal.
   3. The male should always be evaluated first, before a long and expensive female evaluation is begun.
   4. Female evaluation:
      a. BBT: Followed for several months to evaluate ovulation. Some clients' temperatures dip just before the day of ovulation and then rise. Ovulation and the development of the corpus luteum manifest as an increase in BBT by 0.3°C to 0.6°C above the client's baseline temperature (LH surge). The BBT provides presumptive evidence of normal oocyte production and related hormonal change, as well as guidance for the frequency and timing of intercourse.
      b. Endometrial biopsy: Sampling of the uterine lining late in the luteal phase. The test is scheduled 10 days after the BBT increase, or two to three days before the onset of the next menses. A normal secretory endometrium and the absence of inflammation indicate that implantation is feasible.
      c. HSG (performed in radiology): Evaluates tubal patency and rules out uterine anomalies. The HSG should be scheduled for the interval between cessation of menstrual flow and ovulation to avoid retrograde flow of menstrual tissue into the tubes and the abdominal cavity.
      d. Laparoscopy: Diagnostic if used as the final screening examination for infertility. Performed by a gynaecologist, it is usually done in the first two weeks of the menstrual cycle to ensure that the client is not pregnant. Direct visualization of the pelvic organs provides data about degree of adhesion formation, presence of endometriosis or fibroids, and the possibility of surgical repair of damaged tubes.
B. Client teaching:
   1. Infertile couples often require extensive counselling, including grief counselling for failure to achieve pregnancy.
   2. Teach the client to take BBT measurements.
C. Pharmacological therapy:
   1. Treatment depends on causative factor(s).
   2. Prescription medications must be supervised by a specialist because of possible complications, such as ovarian hyperstimulation.

Follow-Up
A. Follow-up depends on causative factor(s).

Consultation/Referral
A. Consultation and referral are required for special testing, surgery, and assisted reproductive therapy.
B. Immediate referral to a specialist is necessary for ovarian hyperstimulation.

Individual Considerations
A. Older adults:
   1. Advancing age increases the risk of age-related infertility. Women aged 35 years and older should be referred to a fertility specialist if unsuccessful in conceiving after six months.
   2. Women aged 40 years and older should be referred as soon as possible for assisted reproductive therapy.

Bibliography
American College of Obstetricians and Gynecologists. (2015). *Gynecologic problems: Treating infertility.* Retrieved from http://www.acog.org/-/media/For-Patients/faq137.pdf?dmc=1&ts=

Centers for Disease Control and Prevention. (2015). *National center for health statistics: Infertility.* Retrieved from http://www.cdc.gov/nchs/fastats/infertility.htm

Government of Canada. (2013). *Fertility.* Retrieved from https://www.canada.ca/en/public-health/services/fertility/fertility.html

Olshanky, E. (2013). Infertility. In K. D. Schuiling & F. E. Likis (Eds.), *Women's gynecologic health* (2nd ed., pp. 443–465). Burlington, MA: Jones & Bartlett.

Menopause

Rhonda Arthur and Julia Blake

Definition
A. Physiologic or natural menopause is the cessation of menses for 12 consecutive months due to the loss of ovarian follicular activity. Natural or physiologic menopause is a retrospective diagnosis recognized 12 months after the final menses. Natural menopause is generally experienced in women between 45 and 55 years of age.
B. Natural menopause before the age of 40 years is considered premature.
C. Premature ovarian failure (POF) is the full or intermittent loss of ovarian function before the age of 40 years. POF is thought to be caused by genetics, autoimmune disorders, or surgical or chemical interventions.
D. Induced menopause is the abrupt cessation of menses related to chemical or surgical interventions.
E. Perimenopause is caused by fluctuations in ovarian function in the years preceding menopause. The average onset is usually in a woman's 40s, but may occur earlier. Due to fluctuations in ovarian function, pregnancy may still occur and unintended pregnancy should be avoided. Perimenopausal symptoms often last several years, with the average duration being five years.

Incidence/Prevalence
A. As of 2017, the number of women in Canada who are older than 50 years is 7,232,687, which makes up 39% of the female population and 20% of the overall population.

Pathogenesis
A. Physiologic menopause is due to failure of ovarian follicular development and ovarian hormone depletion. The major endocrine changes include the decreasing negative feedback on the hypothalamic–pituitary system with increasing follicle-stimulating hormone (FSH) and luteinizing

hormone (LH). When the ovaries cease to produce oestrogen, they become unable to respond to FSH, resulting in the cessation of ovulation and menstruation.

Common Findings
A. Insomnia.
B. Absence of menses.
C. Urogenital atrophy:
   1. Vaginal dryness.
   2. Dyspareunia.
   3. Dysuria/frequency.
D. Vasomotor symptoms such as hot flashes/night sweats.
E. Intermenstrual or postcoital spotting/bleeding should be evaluated for pathologic causes.

Subjective Data
A. Determine onset, duration, and course of presenting symptoms.
B. Obtain complete medical history, including medications, and assess for risk of osteoporosis, cardiovascular disease, and breast and endometrial cancer.
C. Obtain complete gynaecologic history, including menarche, interval, and duration of menstrual cycles; history of dysmenorrhoea; and pregnancy history. Question the client regarding sexual history and contraceptives used (condoms, pills, diaphragm, or intrauterine devices [IUDs]), and frequency of method used.
D. What is the client's current menstrual pattern? Does she think she is pregnant?
E. Review associated symptoms (hot flashes, insomnia, genitourinary symptoms); onset, timing, duration, and impact on daily life.
F. Assess for mood swings and dysphoria.

Physical Examination
A. Check temperature, pulse, respirations, and blood pressure (BP).
B. Inspect: Observe general overall appearance and obtain height, weight, and body mass index (BMI).
C. Auscultate:
   1. Heart.
   2. Lungs.
   3. Abdomen: Auscultation of the abdomen should precede any palpation or percussion due to the changes in intensity and frequency of sounds after manipulation.
D. Percuss the abdomen for organomegaly.
E. Palpate:
   1. Palpate thyroid gland.
   2. Perform clinical breast examination.
   3. Palpate groin for lymphadenopathy.
   4. Palpate the abdomen for masses.
F. Pelvic examination:
   1. Inspect: Examine vulva for Bartholin's gland enlargement, fissures, condyloma, herpes, pelvic relaxation, and atrophy.
   2. Palpate: "Milk" the urethra for discharge.
   3. Speculum examination: Inspect for cervicitis and friability. Evaluate vaginal discharge and bleeding for colour, amount, and odour. Perform cultures and Papanicolaou (Pap) test as indicated.
   4. Bimanual examination:
      a. Check cervical motion tenderness (CMT); evaluate the size, contour, mobility, and tenderness of the uterus. An enlarged or irregular uterus requires additional evaluation.

Over time, it is normal for the postmenopausal uterus to decrease in size.

      b. Palpate the adnexa for tenderness and masses.

Ovaries should not be palpable in postmenopausal women and require further evaluation if masses or ovaries are appreciated.

   5. Rectovaginal examination: Examine stool for occult blood in women older than 50 years.

Diagnostic Tests
A. Consider thyroid-stimulating hormone (TSH).
B. Consider qualitative beta human chorionic gonadotropin (HCG).
C. Complete blood count (CBC) if excessive vaginal bleeding.
D. Obtain Pap smear as indicated.
E. Endometrial biopsy as indicated for intermenstrual spotting or vaginal bleeding after menopause.
F. Transvaginal ultrasonography for enlarged or irregular uterus.
G. Additional screening as indicated, such as mammogram, haemoccult, cholesterol, and bone mineral density.
H. FSH >40 international units (IU)/L is consistent with menopause; however, fluctuations in FSH and 17–2 estradiol (E2) may make use of these markers unreliable and are no longer recommended for determining menopausal status.

Differential Diagnoses
A. Anaemia.
B. Cardiac abnormalities.
C. Leukaemia or other cancer.
D. Menstrual irregularity for any cause of secondary amenorrhoea.
E. Pregnancy.
F. Psychosomatic illness.
G. Thyroid disorders.

Plan
A. General interventions:
   1. Provide reassurance as to the cause of the absence of menses.
B. Client teaching:
   1. Discuss common symptoms of menopause.
   2. Provide education regarding healthy lifestyle changes: regular exercise, weight control, smoking cessation, limiting use of drugs and alcohol, and stress reduction.
   3. Encourage a healthy diet rich in vitamin D and calcium. Supplement diet with calcium supplements:
      a. Vitamin D supplements: Consider vitamin D serum screening and, if deficient, treat accordingly. See section "Vitamin D Deficiency" in Chapter 21, Rheumatological Guidelines.
   4. Encourage water-soluble vaginal lubricants as needed for vaginal dryness. See section "Atrophic Vaginitis."
   5. Avoid warm environments, caffeine, alcohol, spicy food, and emotional upset; these may trigger hot flashes.
   6. Encourage sleep hygiene and adequate rest.
   7. Discuss the risks and benefits of hormone replacement therapy (HRT).

TABLE 14. Hormone Replacement Therapy

Name	Active Ingredient
Oestrogen Sequential or Continuous Combined	
Premarin	Conjugated oestrogen
CES	Conjugated oestrogen
Congest	Conjugated oestrogen
PMS-conjugated oestrogens	Conjugated oestrogen
Estragyn	Esterified oestrogen
Estrace	Micronized estradiol
Ortho-est	Estropipate
Progestin Only for Sequential Regimen	
Apo-medroxy	Medroxyprogesterone
Medroxy 5	Medroxyprogesterone
Provera	Medroxyprogesterone
Prometrium	Micronized progesterone
Progestin Only for Continuous Combined Regimen	
Medroxy 2.5	Medroxyprogesterone
Provera	Medroxyprogesterone
Combination Packet for Continuous Combined Regimen	
Premplus	0.625 mg conjugated equine oestrogen and 2.5 mg medroxyprogesterone
Activelle	1 mg 17-beta estradiol and 0.5 mg norethindrone

PMS, premenstrual syndrome.

8. Assess and manage women at increased risk for osteoporosis according to current osteoporosis guidelines.
9. Assess and treat cardiac risk factors, including hypertension and lipids, as indicated.
▶ 10. Give the client the relevant teaching guide. *Refer to Client Teaching Guide: Menopause.*

C. Pharmacological therapy:
1. HRT:
   a. All women should be counseled regarding the risk, benefits, limitations, and potential increased risks of HRT. Benefits of HRT include the reduction of hot flashes, insomnia, night sweats, vaginal dryness, mood swings, and depression. Although HRT does reduce the risk of bone loss and fracture, due to potential risks and effective alternative treatments for osteoporosis, it is not recommended for the treatment of osteoporosis (see section "Osteoporosis/Kyphosis/Fracture" in Chapter 21, Rheumatological Guidelines). Risks of HRT include venous thromboembolism and breast cancer. Long-term unopposed oestrogen therapy (ET) increases the risk of endometrial cancer. Potential areas of concern with the use of HRT include gallbladder disease and cardiovascular events. The provider should carefully screen and educate the client before initiating HRT.
   b. Oestrogen and progesterone are recommended for the treatment of moderate to severe vasomotor symptoms and moderate to severe vulvar and vaginal atrophy symptoms. For women with an intact uterus, progesterone is used with ET to reduce the risk of endometrial hyperplasia and cancer. Postmenopausal women without an intact uterus generally are not prescribed progesterone and are treated with oestrogen alone.
   c. Oral HRT may be given either sequentially or continuously. The sequential regimen is given daily, with progesterone given on days 1 to 12 of the month. It is common to have withdrawal bleed with this regimen. An alternative to this is the continuous regimen, in which both oestrogen and progesterone are taken daily.
2. Transdermal oestrogen.
3. Transvaginal oestrogen (see Tables 14.3–14.5).
4. Absolute contraindications to use of ET also apply to use of oral and topical oestrogen (breast cancer, active liver disease, and/or history of recent thromboembolic event). Vaginal oestrogen creams are systemically absorbed. As with the use of oral and transdermal oestrogen, a progestin must be administered to women who have an intact uterus, secondary to the risk of endometrial hyperplasia or cancer.
5. Absolute contraindications to ET:
   a. Acute liver disease.
   b. Cerebral vascular or coronary artery disease, myocardial infarction (MI), or stroke,
   c. History of or active thrombophlebitis or thromboembolic disorders.
   d. History of uterine or ovarian cancer.
   e. Known or suspected cancer of the breast.

▶ Client Teaching Guides are available at https://connect.springerpub.com/content/reference-book/978-0-8261-9498-5

TABLE 14.4 Transdermal Replacement Therapy

Delivery	Name
Transdermal patch	Climara
	Estalis 140/50
	Estalis 250/50
Gel-Pump	Divigel 0.1%
Gel-Pump	Estrogel

TABLE 14.5 Transvaginal Replacement Therapy

Delivery	Name
Cream	Estragyn cream
	Premarin
Ring	Estring
Vaginal tablet	Vagifem
IUD	Mirena

IUD, intrauterine device.

   f. Known or suspected oestrogen-dependent neoplasm.
   g. Pregnancy.
   h. Undiagnosed, abnormal vaginal bleeding.
6. Relative contraindications to ET:
   a. Active gallbladder disease.
   b. Familial hyperlipidaemia.
7. Absolute contraindications to progesterone therapy:
   a. Active thrombophlebitis or thromboembolic disorders.
   b. Acute liver disease.
   c. Known or suspected cancer of the breast.
   d. Pregnancy.
   e. Undiagnosed, abnormal vaginal bleeding.

Educate the client to notify the care provider if unusual vaginal bleeding, calf pain, chest pain, shortness of breath, haemoptysis, severe headaches, visual disturbances, breast pain, abdominal pain, or jaundice occur while being prescribed HRT.

D. Nonhormonal pharmacological therapy for vasomotor symptoms: (see complete prescribing reference or package insert for dosing, titration, contraindications, and side effects.).
   1. Antidepressants:
      a. Fluoxetine.
      b. Venlafaxine.
      c. Paroxetine.
      d. Desvenlafaxine.
      e. Citalopram.
      f. Escitalopram.
   2. Anticonvulsant:
      a. Gabapentin.
   3. Antihypertensive:
      a. Clonidine: For nonhormonal pharmacological therapies, review prescribing literature for side effects, titrations, and discontinuation regimens.
   4. Belladonna, ergotamine tartrate, and phenobarbital:
      a. For nonhormonal pharmacological treatment of vasomotor symptoms, review prescribing literature for side effects, titrations, and discontinuation regimens.
E. Nonprescription remedies/herbals:
   1. Many nonprescription remedies are currently available for the treatment of menopausal symptoms. These remedies include isoflavones (soy and red clover), black cohosh, dong quai, evening primrose oil (EPO), ginseng, licorice, and vitamins E and C.
   2. The provider should review with the client the lack of standardization and evidence regarding the safety and efficacy of these products. Currently, results from the research have been insufficient to support or refute the use of these remedies for the treatment of menopausal symptoms.

Follow-Up

A. Follow up for three to six months to assess a response to treatment, and then yearly for physical examination, Papanicolaou (Pap) smear, and lipid panel as indicated.
B. Consider discontinuation of HRT in five years based on client response and risks and benefits.

Consultation/Referral

A. Consult a gynaecologist if the client experiences symptoms resistant to treatment or vaginal bleeding from an unknown source.

Bibliography

Alexander, I. M., & Andrist, L. C. (2013). Menopause. In K. D. Schuiling & F. E. Likis (Eds.), *Women's gynecologic health* (2nd ed.). Burlington, MS: Jones & Bartlett.

The Society of Obestricians and Gynaecologist of Canada. (2014). *Managing menopause*. Retrieved from https://sogc.org/wp-content/uploads/2014/09/gui311CPG1505Erev.pdf

Statistics Canada. (2018). *Population estimates on July 1st by age and sex*. Retrieved from https://www150.statcan.gc.ca/t1/tbl1/en/tv.action?pid=1710000501&pickMembers%5B0%5D=1.1&pickMembers%5B1%5D=2.3

Pap Smear Screening Guidelines and Interpretation

Rhonda Arthur and Juila Blake

The Papanicolau (Pap) smear is a sample of cells taken from the cervix for cytologic evaluation. The Pap smear is a screening test designed to increase detection and treatment of precancerous and early cancerous lesions, and to decrease morbidity and mortality from cases of invasive cervical cancer.

In Canada, approximate 1,550 new cases of cervical cancer will be diagnosed annually. It is estimated that one in 426 will die of cervical cancer. Cervical cancer is the seventh most common cancer in women. There has been a 50% reduction in cervical cancer deaths over the last 30 years due to the use of Pap smear screening.

The following are risk factors for development of cervical cancer:
A. Early age at first intercourse: Younger than 18 years.
B. Multiple sexual partners: More than three in a lifetime.
C. High parity.
D. Lower socioeconomic status.
E. Advanced age.
F. Compromised immune system: Infection with HIV.
G. Smoking.
H. Male partner with a history of multiple partners or sexually transmitted infections (STIs).
I. History of STI, especially human papillomavirus (HPV).

Sexually transmitted agents, particularly the HPV strains 16, 18, 31, 33, 39, and 42, are strongly associated with the development of cervical cancer. HPV DNA is present in 93% of cervical cancer and precursor lesions.

J. Diethylstilbestrol (DES) exposure in utero.
K. Cervical dysplasia: The risk of carcinoma is 100 times greater in women with dysplasia than in those with a normal cervix.

The Pap smear should include sampling from both the ectocervix and the endocervix to be considered "adequate for interpretation." The ectocervix is the cervical portion extending outward from the external cervical os. The endocervix extends upward from the external os to the internal os, where the cervical epithelium meets the uterine endometrium.

Cervical epithelium is composed of squamous and columnar cells. Squamous epithelium, appearing smooth and pink, lines the vagina and continues upward to cover variable amounts of the ectocervix. Columnar epithelium, darker red and more granular in appearance, lines the endometrium and continues downward to the cervix, lining the endocervical canal. The boundary between squamous and columnar epithelium is called the squamocolumnar junction (or transformation zone) and may occur anywhere on the ectocervix or endocervix.

The squamocolumnar junction may regress at various times as a result of hormonal variation, particularly with sexual activity and during pregnancy, through processes known as epidermidalization and squamous metaplasia. Epidermidalization is an upward growth of squamous cells that replace columnar cells. Squamous metaplasia is the differentiation of columnar cells into squamous cells. The area between the original and new squamocolumnar junction is called the transformation zone. When columnar epithelium is visible on the ectocervix, appearing as a granular, red area, it is referred to as eversion, ectropion, or ectopy. This is often seen in pregnancy or with oral contraceptive use.

Cervical cancer is a progressive disease with a number of histologically definable stages. Invasive cancer of the cervix and its precursors are detectable by cytology before becoming symptomatic and before gross clinical signs appear. When symptoms are present, they usually include (in order of frequency) postcoital spotting; intermenstrual bleeding, especially after exertion; and increased menstrual bleeding. Clients with invasive cancer may experience serosanguineous or yellowish vaginal discharge, which may be foul smelling and intermixed with blood.

Advanced disease may cause urinary or rectal symptoms, including bleeding. On speculum examination, advanced lesions appear as necrotic ulcers; in invasive disease they may extend upward or protrude into the vagina.

Bethesda System

The 2001 Bethesda System (classification system used to interpret cytologic findings) was updated in 2014. It includes the following information:
A. Specimen type:
　1. Conventional versus liquid-based preparation versus other.
B. Adequacy of the specimen:
　1. Satisfactory for evaluation.
　2. Presence or absence of endocervical or transformational zone components.
　3. Quality indicators, such as obscuring blood or inflammation.
　4. Unsatisfactory for evaluation and specific reason.
C. General categorization:
　1. Negative for intraepithelial lesion or malignancy.
　2. Other, such as endometrial cells in women older than 45 years.
　3. Epithelial cell abnormality: See section "Interpretation/result" that follows.

If an infection is indicated as a Pap smear finding, evaluate the client and treat her accordingly. Pap smears are not diagnostic of vaginal or cervical infection. Institute therapy for infections confirmed through the use of wet prep and/or cultures as guided by cytologic reading. For example, if Candida is identified on Pap smear results, evaluate the client in the office, confirm finding, and treat the client with appropriate antifungal therapy.

D. Interpretation/result:
Negative for intraepithelial lesion or malignancy (optional to report):
　1. Nonneoplastic cellular variations.
　2. Reactive cellular changes associated with the following:
　　a. Inflammation.
　　b. Radiation.
　　c. Intrauterine device (IUD).
　3. Organisms:
　　a. *Trichomonas vaginalis*.
　　b. Fungal organisms.
　　c. Shift in flora suggestive bacterial vaginosis (BV).
　　d. Cellular changes consistent with herpes simplex virus (HSV).
　　e. Cellular changes consistent with cytomegalovirus.
　4. Other:
　　a. Endometrial cells (in a woman 45 years or older).
E. Epithelial cell abnormalities:
　1. Squamous cell abnormalities:
　　a. Atypical squamous cells of undetermined significance (ASCUS): Indicates some abnormality but the cause is unclear (infection common).
　　b. Atypical squamous cells—high grade (ASC-H): Cannot exclude high-grade squamous intraepithelial lesion.
　　c. Low-grade squamous intraepithelial lesion (LSIL): Indicates HPV, mild dysplasia, or cervical intraepithelial neoplasia (CIN) I.
　　d. High-grade squamous intraepithelial lesions (HSILs): Moderate and severe dysplasia, carcinoma in situ or CIN II, and CIN III
　　e. Squamous cell carcinoma.

2. Glandular cell:
      a. Atypical:
         i. Endocervical cells (not otherwise specify [NOS] or specify in comments).
         ii. Endometrial (NOS or specify in comments).
         iii. Glandular (NOS or specify in comments).
      b. Atypical:
         i. Endocervical cells favor neoplastic.
         ii. Glandular cells favor neoplastic.
      c. Endocervical adenocarcinoma in situ.
      d. Adenocarcinoma:
         i. Endocervical.
         ii. Endometrial.
         iii. Extrauterine.
         iv. NOS.
F. Other malignant neoplasms: Specify.
G. Adjunctive testing.
H. Computer-assisted interpretation of cervical pathology.
I. Educational notes and comments appended to cytology report (optional).

Recommendations

According to the Canadian Task Force on Preventive Health Care, the Society of Obstetricians and Gynaecologists of Canada, The Society of Gynaecologic Oncology of Canada, and the Society of Canadian Colposcopists guidelines, all women should begin cervical cancer screening at the age of 25 years. Women younger than 25 years should not be screened regardless of the age of sexual initiation. Screening should be performed every three years. No woman should be screened annually. Highlights of the recommendations include the following:

A. Begin screening at the age of 25 years.
B. Women from ages 25 to 29 years should have conventional or liquid-based cytology every three years.
C. Women from ages 30 to 69 years should have conventional or liquid-based cytology every three years or, to extend testing time, use conventional or liquid-based cytology.
D. Stop screening at age older than 70 years only if the last three Pap tests in the last 10 years were negative. Negative history includes having three consecutive negative cytology results or two consecutive tests with cotesting results in the past five years for the client.
E. Continued regular screening is recommended for women who have had a history of CIN II, CIN III, or adenocarcinoma.
F. Posthysterectomy: Stop screening for total hysterectomy. However, if the client had a history of high-grade lesions before surgery, then cytology screening every three years for the next 20 years is recommended.
G. HPV vaccination screen according to age-specific recommendation.
H. Women who have a high-risk medical history (immunocompromised, HIV positive, DES-exposed in utero, or a history of cervical cancer) are not included in the updated routine guidelines.

The National Advisory Committee on Immunization recommends routine vaccination of females aged 9 to 45 years with three doses of HPV2, HPV4, or HPV9 vaccine and states the series can be started as young as 9 years of age. Catch-up vaccination is recommended for adolescents and young adults aged 13 to 26 years. Males aged 9 to 26 years are indicated for HPV4 or HPV9 as three separate doses.

Client education regarding the prevention of cervical cancer by avoiding exposure to HPV should include reduction or elimination of high-risk activities. These high-risk activities include having sexual intercourse at an early age, having multiple sexual partners, having partners with multiple partners, and having sex with uncircumcised males. Use of condoms can reduce the risk of HPV as well as other STIs. Smoking cessation can also reduce the risk of cervical cancer. Identification and treatment of precancerous lesions can reduce the risk of invasive cervical cancer, so screening according to Canadian Task Force on Preventive Health Care guidelines should be encouraged.

Treatment Modalities

Treatment is instituted based on the severity of the lesion and the presence of pathology within the columnar epithelium of the endocervix. Treatment options include the following:
A. Observation and repeat cytology.
B. Cryotherapy.
C. Loop excision of the transformation zone.
D. Laser of the transformation zone.
E. Cold-knife conization.
F. Observation and repeat cytology.

Bibliography

Centers for Disease Control and Prevention. (2015). *Human papillomavirus*. Retrieved from http://www.cdc.gov/hpv/parents/vaccine.html

Government of Canada. (2016). *Updated recommendatins on human papillomavirus vaccines: 9-valent HPV vaccine and clarification of minimum intervals between doses in the HPV immunization schedule*. Retrieved from https://www.canada.ca/en/public-health/services/publications/healthy-living/9-valent-hpv-vaccine-clarification-minimum-intervals-between-doses-in-hpv-immunization-schedule.html

Government of Canada. (2017). *Cervical cancer*. Retrieved from https://www.canada.ca/en/public-health/services/chronic-diseases/cancer/cervical-cancer.html

Nayar, R., & Wilbur, D. C. (2015). The Pap test and Bethesda 2014. "The reports of my demise have been greatly exaggerated" (after a quotation from Mark Twain). *Acta Cytologica*, *59*(2), 121–132.

Pelvic Inflammatory Disease (PID)

Rhonda Arthur and Julia Blake

Definition

A. Pelvic inflammatory disease (PID) is an inflammation caused by an infection of the upper genital tract. This inflammation can involve the uterine endometrium (endometritis), fallopian tubes (salpingitis), ovaries (oophoritis), broad ligament or uterine serosa (parametritis), and the pelvic vascular system or pelvic connective tissue.

Incidence/Prevalence

A. Annual incidence is difficult to obtain due to difficulty in definitive diagnosis and reporting.
B. PID is the leading cause of infertility in the world.

Pathogenesis

A. PID is caused by organisms that ascend from the vagina and cervix into the uterus. Menses facilitates gonococcal invasion of the upper genital tract as the luteal phase stimulates gonococcal growth and the cervical mucus barrier is removed. Infection and inflammation spread throughout the endometrium to the fallopian tubes. From there, they extend to the ovaries and peritoneal cavity.
B. The most common organisms cultured from clients with PID are *Chlamydia trachomatis, Neisseria gonorrhoeae, Mycoplasma hominis, Ureaplasma urealyticum*, Bacteroides,

Peptostreptococcus, Escherichia coli, and some endogenous aerobes and anaerobes.
C. The incubation period varies with the infective organism.

Predisposing Factors
A. Age: Rates of PID are higher for women at younger ages. It is highest in the younger than 30-year-old age group (70% incidence under the age of 25 years). Teens are particularly susceptible because they have an immature immune system and larger zones of cervical ectopy with thinner cervical mucus.
B. Sexual activity: Women with multiple sexual partners are three times more likely to develop PID, when compared to women with only one partner.
C. Intrauterine devices (IUDs): IUDs can lead to an iatrogenic development of PID and can promote the spread of vaginal or cervical organisms into the uterus by means of the IUD string.
D. History of PID.
E. Menstruation: Supports the development and spread of PID. Women who are not currently menstruating have a decreased risk.
F. History of invasive procedures: These procedures may result in iatrogenic PID. PID is usually seen within four weeks of the procedure (dilatation and curettage [D&C], IUD insertion, hysterosalpingogram [HSG], and vacuum curettage abortion).
G. There is an increased incidence of PID in African Americans and ethnic minority women and women in lower socioeconomic groups.
H. Cigarette smoking.
I. Frequent vaginal douching.

Common Findings
A. Lower abdominal pain.
B. Fever or chills.
C. Increased vaginal discharge.
D. Nausea and vomiting.
E. Low back pain.

Other Signs and Symptoms
A. Asymptomatic; vague and nonspecific symptoms.
B. Minimal to severe pelvic pain.
C. Right upper quadrant pain (25%).
D. Abnormal vaginal bleeding.

Subjective Data
A. Determine onset, duration, and course of presenting symptoms.
B. Review the character of vaginal discharge (if any); history of recent dysmenorrhoea and/or dyspareunia; any intestinal or bladder symptoms.
C. Question the client regarding sexual history: current number of sexual partners; current or most recent sexual activity; and contraceptive used (condoms, pills, diaphragm, or IUD) and frequency of method used.
D. Question the client as to whether her current sexual partner has experienced any symptoms.
E. What is the client's current menstrual pattern? Does she think she is pregnant? When did the pain begin in relation to her cycle?
F. Review prior pelvic or abdominal surgeries and procedures (HSG, abortion) and when they were done.
G. Review the history and quality of pain: how long, bilateral or unilateral, what makes it better, and what makes it worse (intercourse, Valsalva's maneuver with bowel movement, activity).

Physical Examination
A. Check temperature, pulse, respirations, and blood pressure (BP).
B. Inspect: Observe general overall appearance for discomfort before, during, and after examination.
C. Auscultate abdomen for bowel sounds in all quadrants. Auscultation of the abdomen should precede any palpation or percussion due to the changes in intensity and frequency of sounds after manipulation.
D. Percuss the abdomen for organomegaly.
E. Palpate:
  1. Palpate the groin for lymphadenopathy.
  2. Palpate the abdomen for masses.
  3. Palpate the levator ani muscle left and right, the urethra, and the trigone of the bladder.
  4. Perform rebound, involuntary guarding, and jar tests. The jar test is performed by intentionally hitting or jarring the examination table and watching for a pain response. Pelvic discomfort is exacerbated by the Valsalva maneuver, intercourse, or movement. Abdominal or pelvic pain with PID is usually bilateral. About 25% of clients complain of right upper quadrant (RUQ) pain; the pain usually occurs within seven to 10 days of menses, remains continuously, and is most severe in the lower quadrants.
F. Pelvic examination:
  1. Inspect: Examine the vulva for Bartholin's gland enlargement, fissures, condyloma, herpes, and pelvic relaxation.
  2. Palpate: "Milk" the urethra for discharge.
  3. Speculum examination: Inspect for cervicitis and friability. Evaluate vaginal discharge and bleeding for colour, amount, and odour. Lower abdominal or pelvic pain is the most common symptom of PID and typically is moderate to severe; however, many women may have subtle or mild symptoms that are not readily recognizable as PID, including abnormal bleeding, dyspareunia, or vaginal discharge.
G. Bimanual examination:
  1. Check cervical motion tenderness (CMT); evaluate the size, contour, mobility, and tenderness of the uterus.
  2. Palpate the adnexa for tenderness and masses. Classic PID presentation is lower abdominal and adnexal tenderness and CMT (chandelier sign). The pelvic area may feel hot.
H. Rectovaginal examination: Assess for adnexal thickening and masses.

Diagnostic Tests
A. Complete blood count (CBC) with differential; white blood cell (WBC) >10,500 cell/mm^3.
B. Sedimentation rate or C-reactive protein (CRP).
C. Quantitative beta human chorionic gonadotropin (HCG).
D. Rapid plasma reagin (RPR), hepatitis B surface antigen, and HIV if indicated.
E. Cultures for gonorrhoea and chlamydia.
F. Endometrial biopsy.
G. Transvaginal ultrasonography.
H. Laparoscopy, by referral.

Because of the extreme risk of ectopic pregnancy, always test the client for quantitative beta HCG even if she claims her menses are regular and she is using reliable contraception. Cultures must always be done; lab work (such as HIV) may be done as indicated depending on the client's history and presentation. Eliciting data in the health history about hysterectomy, previous appendectomy, abortions, and procedures such as HSG may provide exclusionary diagnoses.

I. Diagnostic criteria (DC) for clinical diagnosis of PID:
  1. Minimal criteria: Empiric treatment for PID should be initiated in sexually active women at risk for sexually transmitted diseases (STDs) if they are experiencing one of the following with no other cause identified:
      a. Lower abdominal tenderness.
      b. Adnexal tenderness.
      c. CMT.
  2. Additional routine criteria (one or more of the following support diagnosis of PID):
      a. Oral temperature >38.3°C.
      b. Abnormal cervical or vaginal discharge.
      c. Elevated erythrocyte sedimentation rate (>20 mm/hr).
      d. Elevated CRP.
      e. Laboratory documentation of cervical infection with *N. gonorrhoeae* or *C. trachomatis*.
  3. Elaborate criteria for diagnosing PID:
      a. Histopathologic evidence of endometritis on endometrial biopsy.
      b. Tubo-ovarian abscess on ultrasound or radiologic tests.
      c. Laparoscopic abnormalities consistent with PID.

Differential Diagnoses

A. Gynaecologic factors:
  1. Ectopic pregnancy.
  2. Pelvic endometriosis.
  3. Dysmenorrhoea.
  4. Adenomyosis.
  5. Functional ovarian cysts.
  6. Endometrial polyps or fibroid.
  7. Pelvic relaxation.
  8. Anatomic abnormalities.
B. Gastrointestinal (GI) factors:
  1. Acute appendicitis.
  2. Irritable bowel syndrome (IBS).
  3. Ulcerative colitis, Crohn's disease.
  4. Diverticulitis.
  5. Hernia.
C. Genitourinary factors:
  1. Cystitis, urethritis interstitial cystitis.
  2. Ureteral obstruction.
  3. Carcinoma of bladder.
D. Musculoskeletal factors:
  1. Myofascial pain.
  2. Pelvic floor myalgia.
  3. Spinal injuries or degenerative disease.
E. Neurologic factor: Nerve entrapment syndrome.

Plan

A. General interventions:
  1. A low threshold is needed for diagnosis of PID because of the risk of damage to reproductive health. Early treatment with the use of antibiotics of an upper genital tract infection is imperative. Other causes of lower abdominal pain, such as IBS and endometriosis, are not likely to be impaired by empiric antibiotic therapy. The risk of ectopic pregnancy is six to 10 times greater with women with PID compared with uninfected women.
  2. Antibiotic therapy should be instituted promptly, based on clinical diagnosis without awaiting culture results, to minimize the risk of progression of the infection and risk of transmission of the organisms to other sexual partners.
  3. If a woman with an IUD in place is diagnosed with PID, the IUD does not need to be removed. The woman should receive recommended treatment. If there is no improvement in 48 to 72 hours, the health-care provider should consider removing the IUD.
  4. Ambulatory clients should be monitored closely and reevaluated within three days of initiating antibiotic therapy. A decrease in pelvic tenderness should be observed within three to five days of initiation of therapy; if not, additional evaluation is warranted.
B. Client teaching: *Refer to Client Teaching Guide: Pelvic Inflammatory Disease.*
  1. Male sexual partners (and all partners) of clients with PID must be examined, cultured when possible, and treated empirically for presumptive gonorrhoeal and chlamydial infection.
  2. Women who do not use any contraception are at the greatest risk. Transmission of sexually transmitted infections (STIs) can be minimized with effective use of barrier contraceptives. Spermicides prevent infection with chlamydia and gonorrhoea. The use of nonoxynol-9 is protective against *N. gonorrhoeae, Treponema palladium, Trichomonas,* herpes simplex virus (HSV), and *Candida.*
  3. Oral contraceptive pills are associated with an increase in chlamydia detection in the cervix, and they protect against symptomatic PID.
C. Pharmacological therapy (see Table 14.6):
  1. Dilute ceftriaxone with 1% lidocaine without epinephrine to reduce discomfort.

Follow-Up

A. Because of the high risk of reinfection, many clinicians recommend reevaluation in four to six weeks after completion of therapy. Clients with positive cultures for gonorrhoea and chlamydia should be recultured in seven to 10 days after completing therapy. "Test of cure" is necessary.
B. Hepatitis B immunization should be initiated in previously unvaccinated persons.

Consultation/Referral

Consult a gynaecologist if the client diagnosis is atypical, evidence for a presumptive diagnosis is present, or hospitalization is required. General criteria for hospitalization are the following:
A. Diagnosis is uncertain.
B. Pelvic or tubo-ovarian abscess is suspected.
C. IUD in situ.
D. The client is pregnant.
E. The client is an adolescent or is believed to be incapable of adhering to outpatient regimen.
F. Outpatient therapy fails; the client is not better in 48 to 72 hours.
G. The client cannot be reevaluated in 48 to 72 hours.

▶ Client Teaching Guides are available at https://connect.springerpub.com/content/reference-book/978-0-8261-9498-5

TABLE 14.6 Canadian Guidelines on Sexually Transmitted Infections: Recommendations for Treating Pelvic Inflammatory Disease

Inpatient Therapy	Ambulatory Therapy
Regimen Aa Cefoxitin *plus* doxycycline. This regimen is continued for at least 24 hours after clinical improvement and followed by doxycycline to complete 14-day total course. **Regimen Ba** Clindamycin **Plus** Gentamicin. This regimen is continued for at least 24 hours after significant clinical improvement is demonstrated, and it is followed by doxycycline to complete a 14-day total course. Alternatively, clindamycin may be given to complete a 14-day total course.	**Regimen A** Ceftriaxone for 14 days or cefoxitin concurrently once *plus* doxycycline for 14 days or other parenteral third-generation cephalosporin (e.g., ceftizoxime or cefotaxime) *plus* doxycycline **With or Without** Metronidazole **Regimen B** Ofloxacin for 14 days plus/minus metronidazole for 14 days or levofloxacin plus/minus metronidazole for 14 days metronidazole for 14 days

Note: For women or their partners who cannot tolerate doxycycline, erythromycin may be used for 10 to 14 days. When tubo-C is present, many clinicians use clindamycin because it provides more effective anaerobic coverage than doxycycline.

H. The client is HIV positive.
I. There is generalized peritonitis or severe illness.
J. The client cannot tolerate oral medication therapies.
K. Surgical emergencies cannot be ruled out.

Individual Considerations
A. Pregnancy:
   1. Fluoroquinolones are generally contraindicated for pregnant and nursing mothers.
   2. Pregnant women with suspected PID should be hospitalized and treated with parenteral antibiotics.
B. Paediatrics:
   1. Fluoroquinolones are generally contraindicated for children and adolescents younger than 18 years.
C. Partners:
   1. Sexual partners should be evaluated and treated for STIs.

Bibliography
Centers for Disease Control and Prevention. (2015). *Sexually transmitted diseases treatment guidelines: Pelvic inflammatory disease*. Retrieved from http://www.cdc.gov/std/tg2015/pid.htm
Government of Canada. (2016). *Canadian guidelines on sexually transmitted infections – management and treatment of specific syndromes – Pelvic Inflammatory Disease (PID)*. Retrieved from https://www.canada.ca/en/public-health/services/infectious-diseases/sexual-health-sexually-transmitted-infections/canadian-guidelines/sexually-transmitted-infections/canadian-guidelines-sexually-transmitted-infections-22.html

Premenstrual Syndrome (PMS) and Premenstrual Dysphoric Disorder (PMDD)

Rhonda Arthur and Julia Blake

Definition
A. Premenstrual syndrome (PMS) is a psychoneuroendocrine disorder with a constellation of symptoms that occur in the luteal phase, days 18 to 21, and interfere with a woman's life. This is followed by a symptom-free period. Moderate to severe forms of premenstrual distress are now classified in the American Psychiatric Association's (APA) 2013 *Diagnostic and Statistical Manual of Mental Disorders* (*DSM-5*; 2013) as premenstrual dysphoric disorder (PMDD).

Incidence/Prevalence
A. Virtually every menstruating woman experiences some symptoms sometimes. Twenty percent of menstruating women have symptoms serious enough to interfere with their lives, but only 2% to 5% of premenopausal women experience PMDD. Symptoms occur more commonly in women in their 30s and 40s.

Pathogenesis
A. The basis of PMS and PMDD is presumably hormonal. During the luteal phase, progesterone levels increase and oestrogen levels decrease, causing a shift in the ratio of these hormones, which contributes to the symptoms experienced during PMS. These hormones are also known to interact with neurotransmitters in the brain, such as serotonin, and these interactions are thought to cause some of the symptoms experienced, such as mood changes and pain thresholds, during PMS and PMDD.

Predisposing Factor
A. Females of reproductive age.

Common Findings
A. Symptoms are temporally related to the menstrual cycle, beginning during the last week of the luteal phase and remitting after the onset of menses.
B. The diagnosis of PMDD requires symptoms to be present in most menstrual cycles over the last year. At least five of the following symptoms including one of the first four listed must be present:
   1. Affective lability, for example, sudden onset of being sad, tearful, irritable, or angry (mood swings).
   2. Persistent and marked anger or irritability.
   3. Marked anxiety or tension.
   4. Markedly depressed mood and feelings of hopelessness.
   5. Decreased interest in usual activities.

6. Easily fatigued or a marked lack of energy.
7. Subjective sense of difficulty in concentrating.
8. Hypersomnia or insomnia.
9. A subjective sense of being overwhelmed or out of control.
10. Marked change in appetite, overeating, or specific food cravings.
11. Physical symptoms such as breast tenderness, headaches, oedema, abdominal bloating, joint or muscle pain, and weight gain.

Other Signs and Symptoms
A. The symptoms interfere with work, usual activities, or relationships.
B. The symptoms are not an exacerbation of another psychiatric disorder.
C. "I've got PMS; I'm so miserable."
D. Feelings of irritability and emotional lability.

Subjective Data
A. Obtain a complete menstrual history:
  1. Age at menarche; frequency, duration, and regularity of periods.
  2. Ask about premenstrual symptoms that are physical: Weight gain, oedema, acne, nausea, vomiting, constipation, backache, headache, migraine, syncope, breast tenderness, breast enlargement, hot flashes, paresthesia of hands or feet, aggravation of convulsive disorder, increased appetite, food cravings (sweets, salt, or food in general), and fatigue.
  3. Ask about premenstrual symptoms that are emotional: Irritability, emotional lability, anxiety, depression, crying, palpitations, fatigue, aggression, lethargy, and sleep disturbances.
  4. Ask particularly about the timing of the symptoms. When do the symptoms begin and end in relationship to the menstrual period? Has the client kept a calendar of symptoms?
B. Ask about symptoms of dysmenorrhoea. Some women confuse menstrual cramps and PMS.
C. Note type of contraception the client uses.
D. Review her obstetric history, if applicable.
E. Elicit the types of treatment the client has tried and efficacy of treatment.
F. Ask the client about the amount and type of exercise she gets. Women with PMS often get little exercise.

Physical Examination
A. Check height, weight, and blood pressure (BP).
B. Inspect:
  1. Note overall appearance.
  2. Inspect thyroid.
C. Palpate:
  1. The neck, noting thyroid enlargement or nodules.
  2. The abdomen, noting enlargement, masses, or tenderness.
D. Auscultate the heart, lungs, and abdomen.
E. Pelvic examination (if indicated):
  1. Inspect the external genitalia for pubic hair pattern, lesions, or discharge.
  2. Speculum examination: Check for discharge and lesions.
  3. Bimanual examination: Check for size, mobility, shape, and tenderness of the uterus and adnexal area.
  4. No physical abnormality or changes are consistent with PMS.

Diagnostic Tests
PMS is diagnosed primarily based on the pattern of symptoms; however, the following diagnostic test should be considered if indicated:
A. Pap smear according to guidelines.
B. Screen for sexually transmitted infections (STIs), if indicated.
C. Thyroid-stimulating hormone (TSH).
D. Screen for psychiatric disorders as indicated.

Differential Diagnoses
A. Major depression.
B. Dysmenorrhoea.
C. Substance abuse.
D. Perimenopausal symptoms.
E. Sexual dysfunction.
F. Fibromyalgia.
G. There are rarely major medical problems, but hypothyroidism, hyperthyroidism, anaemia, and autoimmune disorders (such as systemic lupus erythematosus [SLE]) must be kept in mind.

Plan
A. General interventions:
  1. Have the client keep a menstrual calendar or diary for at least three months to document occurrence of symptoms in the luteal phase.
  2. Symptomatic treatments: Treatment must be individualized.
B. Client teaching: *Refer to Client Teaching Guide: Premenstrual Syndrome:*
  1. Diet: Have the client eat six small meals a day to even out glucose load. Have her avoid caffeine to decrease irritability and facilitate sleep. Encourage her to avoid simple sugars and eat complex carbohydrates to provide a slow, steady source of energy. She should decrease intake of salt, sugar, and fat. Avoid caffeine and alcohol.
  2. Activity: Instruct the client to increase exercise, preferably aerobic exercise. Suggest exercising every day (walking, swimming, and stretching). Encourage at least 30 minutes of aerobic exercise most days of the week. Encourage stress reduction activities such as imagery or yoga, cognitive behavioural therapy (CBT), support or counselling groups. Encourage smoking cessation as well as adequate sleep and rest.
C. Pharmacological therapy:
  1. Nonsteroidal anti-inflammatory drugs (NSAIDs) for relief of muscular aches, headaches, and menstrual cramps. Follow directions for the particular NSAIDs, whether over-the-counter (OTC) or prescription.
  2. Minerals:
    a. Magnesium.
    b. Calcium 1.
    c. Chromium.
    d. Zinc.
  3. Vitamins are used to decrease anxiety and irritability, food cravings, painful breasts, depression, fatigue, and lethargy:
    a. Vitamin B6 (limited benefit).
    b. Vitamin E (limited benefit).

TABLE 14.7 Medications Used With PMS

Drug	Purpose
Diuretics Spironolactone	Decreases oedema peripherally and, perhaps, centrally
Antidepressants Fluoxetine Paroxetine Sertraline hydrochloride	Decreases depression and anxiety and improves mood
Antianxiety Drugs	Decreases anxiety
Miscellaneous Drugs Bromocriptine mesylate Oral contraceptive pills Danazol	Used to decrease tenderness; works slowly Evens the hormonal milieu, blocks ovulation Has anti-oestrogenic effects. *Consult with a specialist.*

PMS, premenstrual syndrome.

4. Herbals and biotanics:
   a. Vitex Agnus-Castus (Chaste Tree Berry).
   b. Evening primrose oil (mixed results on effectiveness). This oil contains vitamin E; therefore, do not have the client take additional vitamin E.
5. See Table 14.7 for other therapies used for PMS.

Follow-Up
A. Follow up every three to four months to assess or alter treatment and/or therapy.

Consultation/Referral
A. Consult a specialist if symptoms are severe or not relieved by first-line measures.

Individual Considerations
A. Partners:
   1. Encourage the client to have her partner come to a visit. Partner education and support are helpful.

Bibliography
American College of Obstetricians and Gynecologist. (2015). *Gynecologic problems: Premenstrual syndrome (PMS)*. Retrieved from http://www.acog.org/-/media/For-Patients/faq057.pdf

Association of Reproductive Health Professionals. (2008). *Managing premenstrual symptoms*. Retrieved from http://www.arhp.org/uploadDocs/QRGPMS.pdf#search=%22premenstrual%22

Taylor, D., Schuiling, K. D., & Collins Sharp, B. A. (2013). Menstrual cycle pain and disorders. In K. D. Schuiling & F. E. Likis (Eds.), *Women's gynecologic health* (2nd ed., pp. 573–607). Burlington, MA: Jones & Bartlett.

Vulvovaginal Candidiasis

Rhonda Arthur and Julia Blake

Definition
A. Candidiasis (also known as moniliasis) is a common, yeast-like fungal infection of the vulva and vagina. In 90% of the cases, the cause is *Candida albicans* infection.

Incidence/Prevalence
A. Approximately 75% of all women have at least one episode of candidiasis. It is estimated that 50% of these women have recurrences. Yeast has been identified with circumcised males, but symptomatic complaints are more common with uncircumcised males.

Pathogenesis
A. Multiple fungal species cause candidiasis, including *C. albicans* (90%), *Candida tropicalis*, *Torulopsis glabrata* (10%), *Candida parapsilosis*, and *Candida krusei*.
B. *C. albicans*, *C. tropicalis*, or *T. glabrata* are part of the normal flora of the mouth, gastrointestinal (GI) tract, and vagina. They may become pathogenic with changes in the vaginal pH that encourage the overgrowth of the fungus.
C. The incubation period is 96 hours.

Predisposing Factors
A. Diabetes.
B. Systemic antibiotic use.
C. Pregnancy.
D. Oral contraceptive pill use.
E. Obesity.
F. Warm climate.
G. Immunocompromised.
H. HIV.
I. Wearing tight, restrictive clothing.
J. Corticosteroid use.
K. Tub bathing.
L. Frequent use of hot tubs or whirlpools.

Common Findings
A. Thick white "cheesy" vaginal discharge.
B. Itching, mild to intense vulvar pruritus.
C. Vaginal or vulvar irritation, red, and swollen.
D. Discomfort during and after sexual intercourse.

Other Signs and Symptoms
A. Vulvar excoriation.
B. Vaginal swelling or inflammation.
C. Burning with urination.
D. Burning with or during intercourse.
E. Increased symptoms near menses.

Subjective Data
A. Determine onset, course, and duration of symptoms; note whether the infection is first occurrence, recurrent, persistent, or chronic.
B. Obtain medication history; include antibiotics, steroids, and birth control pills.
C. Review the client's past medical history, and review systems for evidence of diabetes, HIV, or any immunocompromise.

D. Review hobbies that include the use of hot tubs, whirlpools, or tight exercise clothing.
E. Review the client's history of wearing polyester underwear, wearing underwear to bed, or wearing tight jeans.
F. Review previous treatment, self-treatment measures, and compliance with previous treatments.
G. Determine whether the client is pregnant; note first day of last menstrual period (LMP).
H. Review sexual activity and partners. Do the partner(s) have any of the same symptoms, "jock itch," or oral candidiasis?
I. Review the use of vaginal deodorants or spray, scented toilet paper, tampons, pads, and douching.
J. Has there been any change in soaps, laundry detergent, or fabric softeners?
K. Review diet for high sugar content.

Physical Examination
A. Check temperature, pulse, and blood pressure (BP).
B. Inspect:
   1. Inspect the vulva for inflammation, fissures, lesions, excoriation, rashes, and condyloma.
   2. Examine the hairline and skin folds for inflammation, irritation, or skin breakdown.
   3. Note skin changes that suggest secondary bacterial infection (erythema, drainage).

Inflammation that spares the skin folds is consistent with contact irritation. Inflammation that is within the skin folds suggests candida.

C. Palpate:
   1. Perform external examination for enlarged or tender inguinal lymph nodes, vulvar masses, and lesions.
   2. Back: Assess for costovertebral angle (CVA) tenderness.
D. Pelvic examination:
   1. Inspect: Observe side walls of vagina. Note amount, smell, and colour of the discharge.

Typical discharge with Candida *is adherent to vaginal side walls and characteristically thick, white, and curdlike (resembles cottage cheese). Side walls may exhibit erythema. The discharge has a musty odour.*

   2. Speculum examination: Inspect the cervix for discharge and friability.
   3. Bimanual examination: Check for cervical motion tenderness (CMT). Palpate for the size of the uterus and for adnexal masses or tenderness.

Diagnostic Tests
A. Wet prep with 10% KOH and normal saline prep.

Yeast hyphae and/or spores are determined by microscopic examination of vaginal discharge prepared with 10% KOH or normal saline. A positive whiff test indicates bacterial vaginosis (BV).

B. Test discharge with nitrazine paper.

The pH with candidiasis remains in the normal range of <4.5.

C. Consider two-hour glucose testing.
D. Consider testing for gonorrhoea and chlamydia.
E. Herpes culture, if lesions present.
F. Urinalysis and culture, if indicated.

Differential Diagnoses
A. Vulvar dystrophy.
B. BV.
C. Chlamydia.
D. Gonorrhoea.
E. Trichomonas.
F. Herpes simplex virus type 2 (HSV-2).
G. Chemical vaginitis.
H. Normal physiological discharge.

Plan
A. General interventions:
   1. Although vaginal candidiasis is treated using over-the-counter (OTC) products, encourage clients with initial presenting symptoms to have an evaluation to rule out other vaginal infections before self-treatment.
   2. Consider treating partners.

Although candidiasis is not considered a sexually transmitted infection (STI), it can be sexually transmitted. The partner should be treated in cases of recurrent infections, even if the partner is asymptomatic.

   3. For recurrent infections, consider fasting and two-hour postprandial glucose tests for chronic yeast infections.
   4. Consider testing for HIV for chronic yeast infections.
   5. Preventive care therapies:
      a. *Acidophilus* capsules, especially two to three days before menses.
      b. Vitamin C to increase vaginal acidity.
      c. Daily yogurt douches or intravaginal applicator full of yogurt twice a day for a week. Have the client use *plain yogurt* with active cultures.
B. Client teaching:
   1. Clients should be encouraged to present for evaluation whether, after appropriate therapy has been instituted, they continue to have symptoms.
   2. Treatment should continue even during menstruation.
C. Pharmacological therapy:
   1. Vaginal antifungal creams: Mild cases may respond to three days of therapy; severe cases may require 10 to 14 days. Some of these preparations are available in vaginal suppository form for a one- or three-night regimen with proven efficacy.
      a. Clotrimazole.
      b. Miconazole.
      c. Terconazole.
      d. Terconazole vaginal antifungal cream is not available OTC. Imidazole drugs (miconazole, clotrimazole, econazole, and butoconazole) are not as effective for non–C. albicans infections as are triazole compounds.
   2. Oral antifungal agents:
      a. Fluconazole: If treatment is not successful, prescription may be refilled one time; if it is still unsuccessful, consider treating the client's partner and/or glucose testing for diabetes.

    b. Nystatin.
    c. Ketoconazole.

Follow-Up
A. The client who presents with recurrent candidiasis should be evaluated for HIV and/or other immunocompromised aetiologies and diabetes.
B. If fasting and two-hour blood glucose testing is normal, other options for recurrent candidiasis include treatment with clotrimazole one applicator every other week for two months. If the client remains symptom-free, reduce treatment to once each month, in the week before her menstrual period.
C. If recurrent candidiasis persists, request laboratory typing of *Candida* for *T. glabrata* or *C. tropicalis*. If confirmed, treat with prescription of gentian violet-treated tampons.

Consultation/Referral
A. Consult or refer the client to a specialist if there is no response to the previous treatments and/or in presence of concurrent systemic disease.

Individual Considerations
A. Pregnancy:
    1. Pregnancy may lead to an increase in vulvovaginal candidiasis because of the increased glycogen content of the vagina and to the stimulatory effects of oestrogen and progesterone on candidal growth. OTC antifungal creams are appropriate for use in this population if there is no rupture of membranes.
    2. Candidiasis may be transmitted from infected mother to newborn at delivery.
B. Partners:
    1. Partners should be evaluated if the client presents with recurrences. OTC antifungal creams are appropriate for use in this population.

Bibliography
van Schalkwyk, J., Yudin, H. M., & Infection Disease Committee. (2015). Vulvovaginitis: Screening for and management of trichomoniasis, vulvovaginal candidiasis, and bacterial vaginosis. *Journal of Obstetrics and Gynaecolgy Canada, 37*(3), 266–274.

15 Sexually Transmitted Infections Guidelines

General Approach to Sexually Transmitted Infections

Kristen Heise and Luisa Barton

The approach to working with clients with sexually transmitted infections (STIs) should be nonjudgmental. Simple terms and sex-positive language should be used.

Subjective Data
A. Ask questions regarding any symptoms related to STIs, both genital and systemic, such as vaginal, urethral, or anal discharge; pruritus; dysuria; dyspareunia; abnormal vaginal bleeding; abdominal pain; testicular pain; rashes; lesions; fever; weight loss; and lymphadenopathy.
B. Inquire regarding personal risk factors and prevention, such as condom use, vaccination against human papillomavirus (HPV), hepatitis B, and, in the case of individuals at risk, hepatitis A.
C. Inquire regarding knowledge of increased risk of exposure to STIs. Have you had contact with an individual with a known STI?

STI Risk Assessment
Inquire about the following:
A. Are you experiencing any symptoms that you are concerned may be related to an STI?
B. Are you presently sexually active or have you been sexually active in the past?
C. Are your partners now or in the past male, female, both, trans or identify as other?
D. What types of sexual activity do you engage in (e.g., oral, vaginal, and/or anal activity, and for each, receptive or penetrative)?
E. If you have a regular partner, how long have you been sexually active together? Are there any concerns about this relationship(s) (e.g., abuse, coercion, and violence)?
F. How many partners have you had sexual contact with in the last two months? One year?
G. When was the last sexual contact? Was a condom used? What type of sexual activity?
H. What are you doing to avoid pregnancy? Do you or your partner use any type of birth control?
I. How often do you and your partner use condoms? What percentage of the time do you use condoms? What influences your choice to use condoms or not?
J. Have you ever been tested for STIs? If yes, when was the last time?
K. Have you ever had an STI in the past? If yes, what and when?
L. Do you have a specific sexual contact of concern?
M. Do you or your partners use injection drugs or other drugs?
N. Do you have any tattoos or piercings that were done without sterile equipment?
O. Have you had sexual encounters with individuals from a country other than Canada? If yes, where and when?
P. Have you ever had anonymous sexual partnering (e.g., Internet, party, and bathhouse)?
Q. Sex trade worker or client: Have you ever traded sex for money, drugs, shelter, or food? Have you ever paid for sex?
R. Sexual abuse: Have you ever been forced to have sex? Have you ever been sexually abused? If yes, when and by whom?
S. Homelessness or street involvement: Do you have a home? Where do you sleep?

Specific to Females
A. Are you using any form of contraception?
B. When was your last Pap test? What were the results? Do you have a history of abnormal Pap tests? If yes, explain.
C. When was your last menstrual period?
D. Have you ever been pregnant? If yes, what was/were the outcome(s) (e.g., live births, abortions, miscarriages)?

Note: Any individual with potential risk factors for STIs should have a more detailed history completed. Other risk factors should be explored, such as drug use; if yes, What drugs do you use? How often do you use these drugs? Have you ever/do you share drug paraphernalia?

Objective Data
A. Examine for systemic signs of STIs: weight loss, fever, and lymphadenopathy.
B. Examine joints for effusion and swelling.
C. Inspect all mucocutaneous regions: pharynx, vulva/vagina, and perianal for lesions, discharge, and inflammation.

Male-Specific Exam
A. Palpate testicles to assess epididymis.
B. If foreskin present, retract to inspect glans for lesions, discharge, and inflammation.
C. If discharge noted by individual, have examiner or individual "milk" urethra to evaluate more closely the discharge.
D. Examine for lymphadenopathy (palpate inguinal nodes).

Note: Consider anoscopy (or digital rectal exam) if the individual practiced receptive anal intercourse *and* has rectal symptoms.

Female-Specific Exam
A. Inspect external genitalia (labia majora, minora, clitoris, urethral opening, vaginal opening, and perineum) for genital discharge, lesions, inflammation, and lymphadenopathy (palpate inguinal nodes).

B. Perform a perianal inspection: discharge, lesions, inflammation.
C. Perform a speculum examination to visualize the vaginal walls and the cervix: Search for inflammation, sores, or lesions on the walls and note the cervix for smoothness, lesions, and colour and examine for discharge endocervically or vaginally.
D. Perform a bimanual pelvic exam to assess uterus for size, shape, and position and any cervical motion tenderness, and adnexa for tenderness or masses (if present, note size, shape, and consistency). A bimanual may not be required if asymptomatic.
E. Abdomen: Palpate for masses or tenderness and rebound tenderness.

Bibliography

Anti-infective Review Panel. (2013). *Anti-Infective guidelines for community-acquired infections*. MUMS Clearing House.
Borhart, J., & Birnbaumer, D. M. (2011). Emergency department management of sexually transmitted infections. *Emergency Medicine Clinics of North America, 29*(3), 587–603. doi:10.1016/j.emc.2011.04.008
Centers for Disease Control and Prevention. (2015a). *Incidence, prevalence, and cost of sexually transmitted infections in the United States*. Retrieved from https://www.cdc.gov/std/stats/sti-estimates-fact-sheet-feb-2013.pdf
Centers for Disease Control and Prevention. (2015b). *Sexually transmitted diseases treatment guidelines, 2015*. Retrieved from https://www.cdc.gov/std/tg2015
Government of Canada. (2018). *Public health agency of Canada—Canadian guidelines on sexually transmitted infections*. Retrieved from https://www.canada.ca/en/public-health/services/infectious-diseases/sexual-health-sexually-transmitted-infections/canadian-guidelines/sexually-transmitted-infections.html
Kao, T., & Manczak, M. (2013). Family influences on adolescents' birth control and condom use, likelihood of sexually transmitted infections. *Journal of School Nursing, 29*(1), 61–70. doi:10.1177/1059840512444134
Mark, H., Jordan, E. T., Cruz, J., & Warren, N. (2012). What's new in sexually transmitted infection management: Changes in the 2010 guidelines from the Centers for Disease Control and Prevention. *Journal of Midwifery & Womens Health, 57*(3), 276–284. doi:10.1111/j.1542-2011.2012.00179.x
O'Connor, C., & Shubkin, C. (2012). Adolescent STIs for primary care providers. *Current Opinion in Pediatrics, 24*(5), 647–655. doi:10.1097/MOP.0b013e328357bf86
Public Health Agency of Canada. (2017). *Canadian guidelines on sexually transmitted infections: Treatment of N. gonorrhoeae in response to the discontinuation of spectinomycin: Alternative treatment guidance statement*.
Richardson, K. K., & Shannon, M. T. (2012). STI screening and treatment in pregnancy. *Nurse Practitioner, 37*(12), 30–37. doi:10.1097/01.NPR.0000422203.95229.ee

Chlamydia

Jill C. Cash, Robertson Nash, Kristen Heise, and Luisa Barton

Definition
Chlamydia is a sexually transmitted infection (STI).

Incidence/Prevalence
The World Health Organization (WHO) estimates 50 million cases worldwide, with more than 4 million cases annually. In Canada, between 2010 and 2015, chlamydia rates increased by 16.7% and were highest among females and young adults. The prevalence of chlamydia can be much higher in certain populations. For example, Indigenous communities have a higher prevalence compared to urban Canadian street youth.

Pathogenesis
Chlamydia trachomatis is an intracellular bacterium with parasitic properties. It is transmitted by sexual contact or perinatally when a vaginal delivery occurs through an infected birth canal.

Predisposing Factors
A. History of STIs.
B. Multiple sexual partners.
C. Early age at first coitus.
D. Unprotected intercourse.

Common Findings
A. Up to 80% of those infected are asymptomatic.
B. Mucopurulent cervical, vaginal, or urethral discharge.
C. Dysuria.
D. Urinary frequency and urgency.
E. Pelvic pain (dull or severe).
F. Abnormal vaginal bleeding.
G. Dyspareunia.
H. Testicular pain.

Other Signs and Symptoms
A. Cervical friability.
B. Cervical motion tenderness (CMT).
C. Uterine and/or adnexal tenderness.

Subjective Data
Refer to General Approach to STIs.

Physical Examination
Refer to General Approach to STIs.

Diagnostic Tests
A. Nucleic acid amplification tests (NAATs) are preferred to culture for diagnosis of *Chlamydia trachomatis*. NAAT tests for both male and female urogenital specimens are collected via clean-catch urine for males and females or vaginal swab for females. NAAT swabs for pharyngeal and rectal sites are available in some laboratories. NAAT is the more sensitive method, whereas culture is more specific. A culture is preferred for medico-legal purposes but NAAT is suitable in most cases. It is important to obtain a thorough sexual history from the client and to screen all orifices used during sexual contact (including oropharynx and rectum). Always consult with your local laboratory concerning specimen storage and transport requirements.
B. Other techniques for obtaining specimens include culture, antigen detections, and genetic probes, which are less sensitive but may be appropriate for certain situations.

Differential Diagnoses
A. Gonorrhoea.
B. Urethritis.

Plan
A. General interventions for symptomatic clients:
   1. Collect samples immediately for timely treatment. Consider testing for other STIs such as gonorrhoea, trichomoniasis, and HIV.
   2. Empirical treatment: People presenting with signs and symptoms of chlamydia and/or gonorrhoea should be tested and treated for both infections at the time of presentation to clinic for care. NAAT swabs should be collected from all orifices exposed to sexual contact, and urine should also be collected and tested. Absent antibiotic allergies, these clients should be treated with ceftriaxone and azithromycin.
B. Client teaching:
   1. Discuss with the client the need for partner notification and treatment. As per the Public Health Agency of

Canada (PHAC), notification is recommended for any partner with whom the client has had sexual contact within the last 60 days, and if no sexual partner in the last 60 days, trace back to the last sexual partner.

2. Stress the importance of completing the treatment regimen.

3. Advise the client to avoid sexual intercourse during treatment and for seven days following the last day of antibiotic treatment for the individual and his or her partner(s).

C. Pharmacological therapy for confirmed infections:
  1. In cases in which the presence of *C. trachomatis* is demonstrated by NAAT and *Neisseria gonorrhoeae* is not present, the PHAC recommends the following:
     a. Azithromycin.
     b. Doxycycline.
  2. Alternative regimen:
     a. Ofloxacin OR
     b. Erythromycin.

Follow-Up
A. The PHAC recommends that a test of cure is not routinely indicated if a recommended treatment is taken, and symptoms and signs have resolved and there is no reexposure to an untreated partner, except where compliance is suboptimal, alternative treatment was used, for all prepubertal children, and for all pregnant individuals.

B. Repeat testing is recommended for all positive chlamydia individuals at six months posttreatment, as reinfection is high.

Consultation/Referral
A. Consult or refer the client to a specialist when treatment with the recommended dosage fails if client noncompliance and reexposure have been ruled out.

Individual Considerations
A. Pregnancy:
  1. Doxycycline and quinalones are contraindicated during pregnancy and for lactating women.
  2. All pregnant women diagnosed with chlamydial infection should be retested in three to four weeks following the treatment.

The PHAC recommends the following medications for pregnant women and nursing mothers (urethral, endocervical, and rectal infections):
  a. Amoxicillin OR
  b. Erythromycin OR
  c. Azithromycin, single dose, if poor compliance is expected.

B. Paediatrics.

The need to treat infants <6 weeks of age for *C. trachomatis* can be avoided by screening pregnant women and treating before delivery. Doxycycline is contraindicated in children under 9 years of age. Quinolone's safety for children has not been established.
  1. Infants first week of life to 1 month: erythromycin.
  2. Greater than 1 month to <9 years: azithromycin. Alternatives: erythromycin OR sulfamethoxazole.
  3. 9 to 18 years: Doxycycline OR azithromycin, in a single dose if poor compliance is expected. Alternatives: erythromycin OR sulfamethoxazole.

C. Adults: Untreated or long-standing chlamydial infection in women may lead to infertility, pelvic inflammatory disease (PID), ectopic pregnancy, chronic pelvic pain, epididymo-orchitis, and Reiter syndrome in both men and women.

Bibliography
Centers for Disease Control and Prevention. (2015a). *Chlamydia*. Retrieved from www.cdc.gov/std/chlamydia/default.htm

Centers for Disease Control and Prevention. (2015b). *Reported STDs in the United States: 2014 national data for chlamydia, gonorrhea, and syphilis*. Retrieved from www.cdc.gov/std/stats14/std-trends-508.pdf

Government of Canada. (2018). *Canada communicable disease report: Chlamydia*. Retrieved from https://www.canada.ca/en/public-health/services/reports-publications/canada-communicable-disease-report-ccdr/monthly-issue/2018-44/issue-2-february-1-2018/article-3-chlamydia-2010-2015.html

Gonorrhoea

Jill C. Cash, Robertson Nash, Kristen Heise, and Luisa Barton

Definition
Gonorrhoea is a bacterial sexually transmitted infection (STI). Although most commonly seen in both male and female urogenital organs, *Neisseria gonorrhoeae* can thrive in both the oropharynx and rectum. It is important to complete a thorough sexual history of all clients presenting with concern for exposure to an STI.

Incidence/Prevalence
The World Health Organization (WHO) estimates 2.5 million cases worldwide. In Canada, gonorrhoea is a reportable infection. In 2015, there were 19,845 cases of gonorrhoea reported in Canada, corresponding to a rate of 55.4 cases per 100,000 population and a 65.4% increase from 2010 (33.5 cases per 100,000 population). Males had consistently higher rates than females (70.2 per 100,000 vs. 40.6 per 100,000 in 2015) and the rates of gonorrhoea in males also increased at a faster rate (85.2% vs. 39.5% in 2010–2015). Rates among adults 60 years and older increased faster than rates among younger people, although the highest rates were among those 15 to 29 years of age. The Northwest Territories, Nunavut, and Yukon had the highest gonorrhoea rates in 2015.

Pathogenesis
N. gonorrhoeae, a gram-negative diplococcus, is the causative organism. The infection begins with adherence of *N. gonorrhoeae* to the mucosal cells in the genitourinary tract or endocervix. The incubation period is typically 2 to 5 days for urethritis and 5 to 10 days for cervical infection. Rectal and pharyngeal infections are usually asymptomatic. Transmission during vaginal birth is possible and may result in conjunctivitis and blindness in neonates.

Predisposing Factors
A. History of STIs, including HIV.
B. Multiple sexual partners.
C. Early age at first coitus.
D. Sexual contact with a person with a confirmed or suspected gonococcal infection.
E. Unprotected sex with a resident of an area with high gonorrhoea burden and/or high risk of antimicrobial resistance.
F. Sex workers and their sexual partners.
G. Sexually active youth <25 years of age.
H. Street-involved youth and other homeless populations.
I. Men who have unprotected sex with men.

Common Findings
A. Dysuria.
B. Yellow, white, or mucoid urethral discharge in males.
C. Greenish, irritating vaginal discharge in females.
D. Menstrual irregularities.
E. Pelvic pain.
F. Fever.

Other Signs and Symptoms
A. Asymptomatic.
B. Uterine or adnexal tenderness.
C. Mucopurulent discharge from endocervix.
D. Polyarthralgia.
E. Necrotic skin lesions.

Subjective Data
Refer to General Approach to STIs.

Physical Examination
Refer to General Approach to STIs.

Diagnostic Tests
A. Nucleic acid amplification tests (NAATs) are preferred to culture for diagnosis of *N. gonorrhoeae* as it is more sensitive and specific. However, culture is strongly recommended, because it allows for testing of antimicrobial susceptibility and is preferred in symptomatic individuals and as a test of cure for suspected treatment failure, for symptomatic men who have sex with men (MSM), in the case of sexual abuse/sexual assault (rectal, pharyngeal, and vaginal), to evaluate pelvic inflammatory disease (PID), and if the infection was acquired in countries or areas with high rates of antimicrobial resistance. It is important to obtain a thorough sexual history from the client and to screen all orifices used during sexual contact (including oropharynx and rectum).
B. Consult with the laboratory for specific instructions on enhancing pathogen survival.
C. During the septic joint stage, gonococci can be recovered from the joint by aspiration for culture.
D. For persons diagnosed with gonorrhoea, testing should also be performed for chlamydia, syphilis, and HIV.

Differential Diagnoses
A. Chlamydia.
B. Arthritis (rheumatoid or osteoarthritis).

Plan
A. General interventions:
1. Offer screening to asymptomatic sexually active individuals with risk factors for gonorrhoea.
2. Report positive test results to the local public health department.
3. Empirical treatment: People presenting with signs and symptoms of gonorrhoea should be tested and treated for both gonorrhoea and chlamydia at time of presentation to clinic for care. NAAT swabs should be collected from all orifices exposed to sexual contact, and urine should also be collected and tested.
B. Client teaching:
1. Stress the importance of completing the medication regimen.
2. Discuss with the client the need for partner notification, testing, and empirical treatment. Notification is recommended for any partner with whom the client has had sexual contact within 60 days of the onset of symptoms or date of specimen collection. Local public health may assist in partner notification.
3. Repeat screening is recommended at six months post-treatment.
4. Follow-up cultures for test of cure from all positive sites should be done three to seven days after the completion of therapy in particular situations (e.g., pharyngeal infections).
C. Pharmacological therapy:
Public Health Agency of Canada (PHAC) recommendation:
1. Ceftriaxone OR Ceftriaxone plus Azithromycin
2. If ceftriaxone is not available, cefixime plus azithromycin, OR
3. For clients with severe allergy to cephalosporins, azithromycin plus gentamicin.
4. Azithromycin is preferred over the alternative of doxycycline.
5. The PHAC and WHO advises that quinolones should no longer be used for treatment of gonorrhoea due to the increased bacterial resistance. Thirty-nine percent of Canadian isolates tested in 2015 were resistant.

Follow-Up
A. A test of cure is recommended only when first-line therapy is not used and in other specific clinical situations, including infection in pregnancy and pharyngeal gonorrhoea.
B. All individuals should be closely monitored for treatment failure.
C. Reinforce treatment of all sexual partners within the past 60 days of diagnosis.
D. Providers are advised to report all treatment failures to the local public health department.
E. All clients treated with an alternative regimen should have a test of cure (from all positive sites), using cultures taken three to seven days after the completion of therapy. If NAAT is the only choice for test of cure, it should be done two to three weeks after treatment to avoid false-positive results due to the presence of nonviable organisms. Repeat screening for individuals with a gonococcal infection is recommended six months posttreatment.

Consultation/Referral
A. Consult with or refer to a specialist if treatment with the recommended dosage fails and client noncompliance and re-exposure have been ruled out.

Individual Considerations
A. Pregnancy:
1. Pregnant women with *N. gonorrhoeae* infections should be treated with ceftriaxone plus azithromycin.
2. If the client is unable to tolerate penicillin, consult with infectious disease specialist.
3. Presumed or diagnosed coinfections with chlamydia should be treated with azithromycin.
B. Adults:
1. Untreated or long-standing gonorrhoeal infection in women can lead to infertility.
2. For clients with allergies to cephalosporins, azithromycin is recommended.
C. Paediatrics:
1. Ophthalmia neonatorum prophylaxis—perinatal exposure to the mother's infected cervix during birth can cause a gonococcal conjunctivitis, which can lead to

blindness if left untreated. Accordingly, the PHAC recommends a single application of erythromycin (0.5%) in each eye of an infant at birth.

2. Sexual abuse should be considered. Suspect chlamydia for conjunctivitis if the infant is 30 days old or younger.

    a. Treatment: If is the presence of *N. gonorrhoeae* is confirmed, treatment with ceftriaxone plus azithromycin OR cefixime plus azithromycin.

Bibliography

Centers for Disease Control and Prevention. (2015a). *Gonorrhea*. Retrieved from www.cdc.gov/std/gonorrhea/default.htm

Centers for Disease Control and Prevention. (2015b). *Reported STDs in the United States: 2014 national data for chlamydia, gonorrhea, and syphilis*. Retrieved from www.cdc.gov /std/stats14/std-trends-508.pdf

Government of Canada. (2018b). *Canada communicable disease report: Gonorrhea*. Retrieved from https://www.canada.ca/en/public-health/services/reports-publications/canada-communicable-disease-reportccdr/monthly-issue/2018-44/issue-2-february-1-2018/article-1-gonorrhea-2010-2015.html

Ontario Agency for Health Protection and Promotion, Public Health Ontario. Ontario Agency for Health Protection and Promotion, Public Health Ontario. (2013). *Guidelines for testing and treatment of gonorrhea in Ontario*. Toronto, ON, Canada: Queen's Printer for Ontario.

World Health Organization, Department of Reproductive Health and Research. (2012). *Global action plan to control the spread and impact of antimicrobial resistance in* Neisseria gonorrhoeae. Retrieved from http://www.who.int/reproductivehealth/publications/rtis/9789241503501/en/index.html

Herpes Simplex Virus Type 2

Jill C. Cash, Robertson Nash, Luisa Barton, and Kristen Heise

Definition

A. Herpes simplex is a lifelong, recurring viral disease, which is transmitted by direct contact with the secretions or mucosa of an infected individual who is shedding the virus. The virus is usually characterized by painful vesicular lesions that form an ulcer, crust over, and then dry without scarring.

Incidence/Prevalence

A. According to the World Health Organization (WHO), more than 500 million people worldwide have herpes simplex type 2. A 2013 study released by Statistics Canada found that one in seven Canadians aged 14 to 49 years may be infected with HSV-2 with more than 90% of them possibly unaware of their status.

Pathogenesis

A. Herpes simplex virus (HSV) is the causative organism. HSV-1 produces oral lesions, and HSV-2 produces genital lesions, although genital lesions can be caused by HSV-1 and vice versa. Kissing, sexual contact, vaginal delivery, and autoinoculation are all possible routes of transmission. The virus remains dormant, and outbreaks can be stimulated by several factors, including stress, illness, sunlight exposure, sexual intercourse, and menstruation. Transmission of the virus can also occur during periods of asymptomatic viral shedding. Recurrences may be preceded by prodromal symptoms such as tingling, burning, or itching in the area a few minutes to several days before lesions appear.

Predisposing Factors

A. Early age at first coitus.
B. Multiple sexual partners.
C. History of STIs.

Common Findings

A. Dysuria.
B. Pruritus.
C. Burning.
D. Swelling sensation.

Other Signs and Symptoms

A. Primary episode:
    1. Painful, itchy, vesicular, ulcerated, or crusted oral or genital lesion, singly or in clusters.
    2. Flu-like syndrome: Fever, chills, headache, malaise, and myalgia with tender lymphadenopathy.
B. Recurrent episode: Less painful lesions and little or no systemic symptoms. Recurrent lesions in the same location as the previous outbreak is a significant clinical clue that the lesions are herpetic.

Subjective Data

Refer to the General Approach to STIs.

Physical Examination

Refer to the General Approach to STIs.

Diagnostic Test

A. Viral culture:

Clinical diagnosis is often reliable, but confirmation with viral culture should be attempted. Vesicles should be unroofed or crust removed for most reliable sample.

    1. The most common method used to confirm HSV diagnosis is culture, as it is sensitive (70% from ulcers and 94% from vesicles) and permits typing of HSV. Nucleic acid amplification test (NAAT) is more sensitive than culture and 100% specific but has not yet replaced culture for routine diagnosis in Canada.
    2. Viral isolation: Obtain vesicular fluid by swabbing the lesion with a cotton- or Dacron-tipped applicator.
    3. Place the applicator in appropriate viral transport medium before drying.
    4. Refrigerate until ready for transport.
B. Serology: HSV-specific glycoprotein G2 (HSV-2) and glycoprotein G1 (HSV-1). Pap smear is not a sensitive test for HSV-2.

Differential Diagnoses

A. Primary syphilis.
B. Chancroid.
C. Lymphogranuloma venereum.
D. Folliculitis.
E. Candidal fissure.
F. Vestibular vulvitis.
G. Mucocutaneous manifestations of Crohn's disease.

Plan

A. General interventions:
    1. Culture samples immediately to begin treatment.
B. Client teaching:
    1. Advise clients to abstain from sexual activity during prodrome or while lesions are present.
    2. Condom use should be encouraged when sexually active but may not protect 100% against transmission because of location of lesions or asymptomatic shedding.

3. Individuals need to inform their sexual partners that they have HSV and supportive counselling, possibly including the partner, is useful.
4. Advise individuals that episodic antiviral therapy may shorten the duration of recurrent outbreaks and suppressive antiviral therapy can reduce the frequency and severity of recurrences, reduce asymptomatic viral shedding, and have psychological benefit to the individual.

C. Pharmacological therapy: The Public Health Agency of Canada (PHAC) recommends the following treatment regimens:
1. Primary episode: Acyclovir, valacyclovir, OR famciclovir.
2. Recurrent episode: Begin during prodrome, as early as possible or at least within 72 hours of symptoms with valacyclovir and within five days for acyclovir and famciclovir.
3. Daily suppressive therapy: Acyclovir, famciclovir, OR valacyclovir.

Clients receiving daily suppressive therapy of acyclovir should use the lowest dose that provides relief from symptoms. Suppressive therapy has been shown to reduce frequency of recurrences by 75% in clients with more than six recurrences per year. It does not eliminate symptomatic or asymptomatic viral shedding or the potential for transmission.

4. Topical antivirals offer minimal clinical benefit and their use is not recommended.
5. Individuals can be provided with a supply of medication or a prescription so that self-initiation of treatment can occur immediately upon symptom presentation.

Follow-Up
A. Follow-up is not recommended unless it is warranted by clinical presentation. Supportive counselling is an important component of managing individuals with HSV.

Consultation/Referral
A. Consult or refer to a specialist when there is prolonged ulceration unresponsive to therapy.

Individual Considerations
A. Adults:
1. Diagnosis is most often made via clinical presentation. Although viral testing is available, empiric treatment is recommended, versus testing and treating (see the section "Other Signs and Symptoms").
2. Clients with HIV may have outbreaks of HSV lesions anywhere on their body. Do not limit diagnosis based on the physical location of lesions.
3. Clients presenting with HSV-1/HSV-2 lesions should be tested for HIV and other STIs.
4. Failure to isolate HSV does not mean that the client does not have HSV.

B. Pregnancy:
1. Transmission of genital herpes from an infected pregnant client to the neonate is high, approximately 30% to 50%, when herpes is acquired during the last trimester or near delivery. The risk of transmission is much lower for pregnant clients who have a history of HSV or first acquire the virus during the first half of the pregnancy.
2. All pregnant clients should be questioned and screened for HSV when they are admitted to the hospital for delivery. All women with recurrent genital herpes lesions present at the onset of labour should undergo caesarean section delivery to decrease the risk of transmission of the herpes virus to the neonate.
3. Acyclovir and valacyclovir is category B for pregnancy and considered safe to use during pregnancy. These medications can be used for treatment as well as for suppression during pregnancy. According to the Society of Obstetricians and Gynaecologists of Canada (SOGC), women with known recurrent genital HSV infection should be offered acyclovir or valacyclovir suppression at 36 weeks' gestation to decrease the risk of clinical lesions and viral shedding at the time of delivery and therefore decrease the need for caesarean section.
4. Culture lesions if outbreak occurs. Lesion must be crusted for seven days for vaginal delivery to be an option; otherwise, a caesarean delivery is recommended to avoid transmission of virus to newborn.
5. Pregnant women without genital herpes should be advised to avoid intercourse during the third trimester with partners known or suspected of having genital herpes.
6. Acyclovir allergy: No effective alternatives to acyclovir have been identified.

C. Partners: Symptomatic partners should be evaluated and treated in the same manner as any client with genital lesions.

D. Paediatrics:
1. Transmission of HSV from mother to infant during birth is possible. In all cases of suspected neonatal or congenital HSV infection, the SOGC recommends an early consultation with a paediatrician.
2. A paediatric infectious diseases expert is highly recommended.

E. Geriatric:
1. Genital herpes is rarely seen in the elderly. Recurrent infection of the buttocks region is not uncommon, especially in females.

Bibliography
American College of Obstetricians and Gynecologists Committee on Practice Bulletins. American College of Obstetricians and Gynecologists Committee on Practice Bulletins. (2007). ACOG Practice Bulletin. Clinical management guidelines for obstetrician-gynecologists. No. 82 June 2007 reaffirmed in 2016. Management of herpes in pregnancy. *Obstetrics and Gynecology, 109*(6), 1489–1498.

Centers for Disease Control and Prevention. (2015). *Genital herpes—CDC fact sheet*. Retrieved from https://www.cdc.gov/std/herpes/stdfact-herpes.htm

Human Papillomavirus

Jill C. Cash, Robertson Nash, Luisa Barton, and Kristen Heise

Definition
The human papillomavirus (HPV) is a sexually transmitted infection (STI). Condyloma acuminata, genital warts, and venereal warts are other names for HPV.

Incidence/Prevalence
As HPV is one of the most common STIs, it is estimated that more than 70% of sexually active Canadian men and women will have a sexually transmitted HPV infection at some point in their lives.

Pathogenesis
The HPV, a slow-growing DNA virus of the papovavirus family, is the causative organism. More than 70 strains of the

virus have been identified, and types 6 and 11 are most associated with genital warts. Types 16, 18, 31, 33, and 35 are of high risk and are associated with cervical neoplasia. Warts may appear as early as one to two months after exposure, but most infections remain subclinical.

Predisposing Factors
A. Early first coitus.
B. Multiple sexual partners.
C. History of transmitted infections.

Common Findings
A. Painless genital "bumps" or warts.
B. Pruritus.
C. Bleeding during or after coitus.
D. Malodourous vaginal discharge.
E. Dysuria.

Other Signs and Symptoms
A. Wart-like growths on genital area that are elevated and rough or flat and smooth.
B. Lesions occurring singly or in clusters, from <1 mm to cauliflower-like aggregates.
C. Papillomas that are pale pink in colour.

Subjective Data
Refer to the General Approach to STIs.

Physical Examination
A. Inspect:
  1. Inspect external genitalia, perineum, and anus for lesions.
  2. Females, speculum examination: Inspect vaginal walls and cervix for lesions.
  3. Application of 3% acetic acid whitens lesions (not diagnostic).

Diagnostic Tests
A. Visual identification is adequate in most cases.
B. Cytology: Pap smears are useful for screening. The following Pap results are all suggestive of HPV:
  1. Atypical squamous cells of undetermined significance (ASCUS): Results are borderline.
  2. Atypical squamous cells–cannot exclude HSIL (ASC-H): Results are borderline, but may indicate something more serious.
  3. Low-grade squamous intraepithelial lesion (LSIL): Results suggest mildly abnormal cellular changes on the cervix.
  4. High-grade squamous intraepithelial (HSIL): Results suggest more serious cell changes in the cervix.
C. Histology: Colposcopy with directed biopsy is diagnostic for subclinical lesions, dysplasia, and malignancy.
D. DNA typing: Determination of specific strains is useful in diagnosing subclinical infections (the test is costly and false negatives occur) and it is not recommended for women under the age of 30.

Differential Diagnoses
A. Condylomata.
B. Molluscum contagiosum.
C. Carcinoma.

Plan
A. General interventions: Make diagnosis promptly to begin treatment.
B. Client teaching:
  1. Explain to the client that therapy eliminates visible warts but does not eradicate the virus. No therapy has been shown to be effective in eradication of HPV. Ablation of warts may decrease viral load and transmissibility.
  2. Advise the client to abstain from genital contact while lesions are present.
C. Pharmacological therapy:
  1. Therapy is not recommended for subclinical infections (absence of exophytic warts).
  2. Trichloroacetic acid (TCA) 80% to 90% solution applied weekly to visible warts by clinician until warts resolve. If unresolved after six applications, consider other therapy.
  3. Podophyllum resin 10% to 25% in tincture of benzoin compound applied weekly to visible warts by clinician until warts resolve.
    a. Application of petroleum jelly on surrounding skin may be used for protection of unaffected areas.
    b. Advise the client to wash off resin after four hours. If unresolved after six applications, consider other therapy.
  4. Apply TCA 80% to 90% to the warts and allow to dry weekly by clinician until warts resolve.
  5. Podofilox, 0.5% solution for home treatment, applied to visible warts by the client twice daily for three consecutive days, followed by four days without treatment. The cycle is repeated up to four times.
  6. Imiquimod 5% cream applied to wart at bedtime, left on for 6 to 10 hours, then washed with mild soap. Use daily, three times a week (Monday, Wednesday, and Friday), until wart resolves or up to 16 weeks.
D. Medical/surgical management: Cryotherapy, electrodesiccation, electrocautery, carbon dioxide laser, and surgical excision are options to be considered for clients with large or extensive lesions or refractory disease. When available, the treatment of choice is cryotherapy: the application of liquid nitrogen directly to the warts.

Follow-Up
A. Short-term follow-up is not recommended if the client is asymptomatic after treatment.
B. Cervical screening guidelines do not recommend more frequent Pap smears for women with external warts.
C. Long-term follow-up should include annual Pap smears and pelvic examinations. Encourage the client to self-examine genitalia.

Consultation/Referral
A. Consult or refer the client to a specialist when lesions persist after six consecutive treatments or when cervical or rectal warts are diagnosed.

HPV Vaccines
A. There are several HPV vaccines available or in use in Canada, including bivalent, quadrivalent, and nine-valent. Nine-valent provides protection against an additional five HPV types that cause an additional 14% of anogenital cancers. These vaccines are approved for use in females 9 to 45 years of age, and males aged 9 to 26.

B. For both girls and boys, vaccine administration may start at as young as 9 years of age. The vaccine is recommended for girls and young women aged between 9 and 26 years. For males, the vaccine is recommended for those between 9 and 26 years of age.
C. Administration for children 9 to 11 years of age should be two doses of intramuscular (IM) vaccine, with the second dose given between 6 and 12 months following the first dose. Administration for children of 15 years of age or greater is via a three-dose series of IM injections, with the second dose given 1 to 2 months after the first and the third given 6 months after the first.

Individual Considerations
A. Pregnancy: Podophyllum and podofilox are contraindicated during pregnancy.
B. Partners:
  1. Treatment is recommended if visible lesions are present.
  2. Testing sex partners for HPV is not recommended.
  3. Sex partners are likely to share HPV. In most cases, the virus is likely to clear without associated health concerns. The risk of HPV warts and cancers increases greatly when the infection does not clear and becomes chronic.
  4. Consistent condom usage can lower the chances of acquisition and transmission of HPV virus. However, the virus can infect areas not protected by condoms (i.e., female anus during vaginal intercourse and buccal mucosa during oral sex).
C. Adolescents: Education regarding gardasil vaccine is recommended for youth 9 to 25 years of age for prevention of acquiring the HPV. The vaccination may help to prevent contracting four of the viruses (types 6, 11, 16, and 17) that increase the risk of cervical cancer for women.
D. Geriatric:
  1. Verrucous carcinoma and vulvar intraepithelial neoplasia (VIN) can be indistinguishable from condyloma. Older women are more likely to have VIN or carcinoma.
  2. Diagnosis is made by biopsy; colposcopy is strongly advised.
  3. Immunocompetence should be investigated in new or recurrent condyloma.

Bibliography
Centers for Disease Control and Prevention. (2015). *Genital HPV infection—Fact sheet*. Retrieved from https://www.cdc.gov/std/hpv/stdfact-hpv.htm
Government of Canada. (2017). *HPV*. Retrieved from https://www.canada.ca/en/public-health/services/infectious-diseases/sexual-health-sexually-transmitted-infections/human-papillomavirus-hpv.html

Syphilis

Jill C. Cash, Robertson Nash, Luisa Barton, and Kristen Heise

Definition
Syphilis is a sexually transmitted infection (STI) characterized by distinct primary, secondary, and tertiary stages that occur over several years or decades. Latent or inactive periods occur between the stages. Early latent is less than one year after infection; late latent is more than one year after infection. Syphilis is considered a reportable infection in Canada.

Incidence/Prevalence
From 2010 to 2015, the rate of infectious syphilis in Canada increased by 85.6%, from 5.0 to 9.3 cases per 100,000 population. In 2015, a total of 3321 cases of infectious syphilis were reported, mainly in males (93.7%), among whom the rate was 17.5 cases per 100,000 males versus 1.2 per 100,000 females. The rate also increased faster among males in 2010 to 2015, a 90.2% increase versus 27.8% among females. Individuals aged 20 to 39 years had the highest rates. Individuals of Indigenous ethnicity are disproportionately affected by syphilis in some geographic areas of Canada, particularly in some areas experiencing outbreaks of infectious syphilis.

Pathogenesis
A. *Treponema pallidum*, a spirochaete bacterium, is the causative organism that infects the mucous membrane.

Predisposing Factors
A. History of STIs, specifically past HIV and syphilis.
B. Multiple sexual partners.
C. Injection drug users.
D. Sex trade work.
E. Men who have sex with men (MSM).

Common Findings
A. Genital lesion, generalized rash involving palms and soles, mucous patches, and condyloma latum are common.

Other Signs and Symptoms
A. Primary syphilis:
  1. Chancre that is painless or minimally painful.
  2. Round, indurated lesion with little or no purulent exudate.
  3. Regional bilateral lymphadenopathy.
B. Secondary syphilis:
  1. Generalized maculopapular rash that is nonpruritic and copper coloured, on palms or soles; may be erythematous or scaly.
  2. Mucous patches; painless, white, mucous membrane lesions.
  3. Generalized lymphadenopathy; flu-like syndrome, including fever, headache, sore throat, and malaise.
  4. Patchy alopecia.
C. Tertiary syphilis:
  1. Gumma: Locally destructive granulomatous tumours involving various organs or systems; commonly seen on liver but can occur on other organs (heart, brain, skin, bone, and testes).
  2. Cardiovascular: Aortic involvement, aneurysms, and valve insufficiency.
  3. Neurologic: Tabes dorsalis and general paresis.
D. Latent syphilis: Asymptomatic.

Latent phase syphilis manifests itself after treatment failure or no history of treatment. Spirochaete can lie dormant for years.

E. Congenital syphilis: Symptoms range from asymptomatic to fatal.

Subjective Data
Refer to the General Approach to STIs.

Physical Examination
A. Check temperature, pulse, respirations, and blood pressure.

B. Inspect:
   1. Inspect the skin; note lesions and rashes.
   2. Observe the head; note patchy alopecia.
   3. Examine the mouth and throat; note lesions.
   4. Inspect the genital and rectal area; note lesions and rashes.
C. Palpate the lymph nodes (neck, supraclavicular, axillary, epitrochlear, and inguinal regions).
D. Auscultate heart and lungs.
E. Neurologic examination:
   1. Assess sensory functioning.
   2. Test cranial nerves, first through 12th.

Diagnostic Tests

There are two types of tests available for use in the diagnosis and management of syphilis—nontreponemal and treponemal—and knowledge of both is essential. Nontreponemal tests, such as the rapid plasma reagin (RPR), assess for biomarkers typically created by spirochaetes. These tests are inexpensive, rapid, and easy to perform. In addition, the results are reported as titres, which facilitate monitoring the status of the infection. These are not antibody tests, however. Therefore, it is possible to have a false positive due to several conditions, including autoimmune disease, HIV, pregnancy, older age, and intravenous drug use.

Treponemal tests, such as the treponemal pallidum particle agglutination (TP-PA), are antibody tests. Although more accurate than nontreponemal tests, treponemal tests are more expensive. A further complication of using treponemal tests as screening tools is that a treponemal test is positive for life once a person has had syphilis. Used in isolation, treponemal tests do not reveal whether an infection is active.

Interpretation of treponemal test findings is done in conjunction with findings from nontreponemal tests. Specifically, a fourfold drop in an initial nontreponemal titre indicates successful treatment of syphilis, that is, 1:64 to 1:4. In some cases, titres remain persistent over extended periods (more than two to three years); these individuals are referred to as sero-fast.

The introduction of treponemal enzyme immunoassays (EIAs) may provide a more sensitive screening test for syphilis and are now commercially available for use in some laboratories in Canada. Although EIA is highly sensitive, the test can lack specificity and in some jurisdictions may be followed by a confirmatory test (usually another treponemal-specific test). Syphilis testing algorithms vary across Canada and it is therefore recommended that you check with your laboratory regarding local testing protocols.

Evaluate for other STIs for clients presenting with syphilis.
STI, sexually transmitted infection.

A. Serology: Nontreponemal tests:
   1. Venereal Disease Research Laboratory (VDRL) test.
   2. RPR tests.
   3. HIV: Due to the increased likelihood of false-positive nontreponemal tests in people with HIV, all HIV-infected clients with a positive nontrepomenal test should be followed with a treponemal test, as per section "Diagnostic Tests."

Results are reactive (positive) or nonreactive (negative). Titres correlate with active disease and should be quantitative. These tests are equally valid but cannot be compared because of titre differences (RPR is slightly higher than VDRL). All reactive results require confirmation with treponemal tests.
RPR, rapid plasma regain; VDRL, Venereal Disease Research Laboratory.

B. Serology: Treponemal tests:
   1. Fluorescent treponemal antibody absorption (FTA-ABS) test.
   2. Microhemagglutination assay for antibody to *T. pallidum* (TP-PA; MHA-TP).

Once FTA-ABS for antibody to Treponema pallidum, VDRL, and RPR are reactive, these tests usually remain reactive for life.
FTA-ABS, fluorescent treponemal antibody absorption; RPR, rapid plasma reagin; VDRL, Venereal Disease Research Laboratory.

C. Cerebrospinal fluid (CSF) culture to detect neurosyphilis.
D. Microscopy: *T. pallidum* cannot be seen with light microscopy; dark-field microscopic examination of the serous exudate from lesions is the definitive test for syphilis. Properly equipped labs with specially trained personnel must be available for this test.

Differential Diagnoses
A. Herpes simplex virus (HSV).

Plan
A. General interventions: Staging of the disease may be difficult but guides management decisions.
B. Client teaching:
   1. Advise the client to abstain from sexual activity until treatment is completed.
   2. Inform the client of Jarisch–Herxheimer reaction (fever, headache, and myalgia) that may occur within the first 24 hours of treatment. Antipyretics may be prescribed.
   3. Discuss the importance of partner notification.
   4. Stress the importance of complying with the follow-up regimen.
C. Pharmacological therapy:
   1. Primary syphilis, secondary syphilis, early latent syphilis:
      a. Adults: Benzathine penicillin G.
      b. Paediatrics: Benzathine penicillin G.
   2. Late latent syphilis, latent syphilis of unknown duration, late syphilis (manage with expert consultation):
      a. Adults: Benzathine penicillin G.
      b. Paediatrics: Benzathine penicillin G.
   3. Neurosyphilis (manage with expert/specialist consultation):
      a. Adults: Aqueous crystalline penicillin G.
      b. Adults: Procaine penicillin.
      c. Paediatrics: Penicillin desensitization, then treatment with recommended regimen.
   4. Primary syphilis, secondary syphilis, latent syphilis, late latent syphilis in (nonpregnant) client with penicillin allergy: Doxycycline or tetracycline.
   5. Latent syphilis of unknown duration, late syphilis: Treat with aforementioned medications for infections of less than one-year duration. If greater than one year, treat with aforementioned medications for four weeks.

6. For pregnant clients with penicillin allergy, penicillin treatment after desensitization is recommended for the following reasons:
   a. Penicillin is effective for preventing transmission and treating the infected fetus.
   b. Doxycycline and tetracycline are contraindicated in pregnancy.
   c. Erythromycin may not cure the infected fetus.

Follow-Up
A. Primary and secondary syphilis: Clinical and serologic examinations should be conducted at 6, 12, and 24 months. Absence of fourfold decrease in RPR titre at three months is indicative of treatment failure.
B. Latent syphilis: Clinical and serologic examinations should be conducted at 6, 12, and 24 months. Absence of fourfold decrease within 12 to 24 months is indicative of treatment failure.
C. Tertiary syphilis: Minimal evidence regarding follow-up exists. Follow-up largely depends on nature of lesions.
D. Neurosyphilis: CSF examination should take place every six months until cell count is normal.

Consultation/Referral
A. Consult or refer the client to a specialist when the recommended treatment fails and client noncompliance and reexposure have been ruled out, or when neurosyphilis is diagnosed.

Individual Considerations
A. Pregnancy:
   1. Draw blood samples for RPR/VDRL from all prenatal clients.
   2. Women in communities with high prevalence of syphilis and/or with high-risk behaviour should be tested twice during the third trimester: Once at 28 to 32 weeks, and again at delivery.
   3. Any woman having a fetal death at >20 weeks should be tested for syphilis.
   4. Administer appropriate regimen of penicillin for the client's stage of syphilis. Consider a second dose of penicillin one week after the initial treatment.
   5. Clients who are allergic to penicillin should be desensitized and treated with penicillin during pregnancy.
   6. Follow-up: Perform serologic tests monthly until adequacy of treatment has been ensured.
   7. The Jarisch–Herxheimer reaction may predispose women to premature labour or fetal distress if treatment occurs in the second half of the pregnancy. Advise these clients to immediately seek medical attention if they experience uterine contractions or changes in fetal movement.
   8. All pregnant women diagnosed with syphilis should be offered HIV screening.
B. Paediatrics:
   1. Congenital syphilis is caused by untreated infection or treatment failure in the mother.
   2. Refer the client to an infectious disease specialist for consultation.
   3. Medication therapy: See the section "Pharmacological Therapy."
C. Partners: Identify at-risk partners who have had sexual contact with the client within these time frames:
   1. Primary syphilis: Three months plus duration of symptoms.
   2. Secondary syphilis: Six months plus duration of symptoms.
   3. Early latent syphilis: One year.
D. Geriatric:
   1. Dementia, tremors, and pupillary changes are the result of long-term untreated syphilis.
   2. The CSF should be tested using the FTA-ABS test. The VDRL is usually not adequate.
   3. Syphilis is uncommon in the elderly in developed countries; however, it is very common worldwide.

Bibliography
Centers for Disease Control and Prevention. (2015). *Reported STDs in the United States: 2014 national data for chlamydia, gonorrhea, and syphilis*. Retrieved from www.cdc.gov/std/stats14/std-trends-508.pdf
Government of Canada. (2015). *Syphilis*. Retrieved from https://www.canada.ca/en/public-health/services/reports-publications/canada-communicable-disease-report-ccdr/monthly-issue/2018-44/issue-2-february-1-2018/article-2-syphilis-2010-2015.html

Trichomoniasis

Jill C. Cash, Robertson Nash, Luisa Barton, and Kristen Heise

Definition
Trichomoniasis is a sexually transmitted infection (STI). Nonsexual transmission by means of fomites is possible but rare.

Incidence/Prevalence
Globally, it is considered the most common nonviral STI, with an estimated 170 million cases reported annually. Trichomoniasis is not a reportable infection in Canada; therefore, the incidence of this STI is unavailable. Trichomoniasis is associated with an increased risk of HIV acquisition and transmission in women.

Pathogenesis
A. *Trichomonas vaginalis*, a flagellated protozoan, is the causative organism.

Predisposing Factors
A. History of STIs.
B. Multiple sexual partners.

Common Findings
A. Copious, yellow–green, or watery gray vaginal discharge.
B. Vaginal odour.
C. Dysuria.
D. Dyspareunia.
E. Postcoital spotting or bleeding.
F. Abdominal discomfort.
G. Pruritus.

Other Signs and Symptoms
A. Asymptomatic in 10% to 50% of clients.
B. Perineal irritation.
C. Erythema of vulva and punctate haemorrhages and friability of cervix ("strawberry cervix").

Subjective Data
Refer to General Approach to STIs.

Physical Examination
Refer to General Approach to STIs.

Diagnostic Tests
A. Wet prep: Perhaps the most common diagnostic tool, intended to visualize presence of motile, flagellated trichomonads. Increased number of white blood cells (WBC) (>0.10 per high-power field) may be present. According to the Public Health Agency of Canada (PHAC), wet mount microscopy, antigen detection, and nucleic acid hybridization assays are available, but are less sensitive.
B. It is best detected by antigen testing using vaginal swabs collected and evaluated by immunoassay or nucleic acid amplification test.
C. Culture is more sensitive that wet prep for trichomoniasis.
D. Pap smear: Report may include trichomonads, but sensitivity is low.
   1. If trichomonads are noted on Pap smear, the client should be reexamined and diagnosis confirmed with a wet prep.
E. Vaginal pH is usually >4.5.
F. The potassium hydroxide/wet prep "whiff test" may be positive.

Differential Diagnoses
A. Bacterial vaginosis.
B. Vulvovaginal candidiasis.
C. Chlamydia.
D. Gonorrhoea.
E. Pelvic inflammatory disease.
F. Foreign-body vaginitis.

Plan
A. General interventions: Prompt diagnosis helps to initiate treatment.
B. Client teaching:
   1. Advise the client to abstain from sexual activity until treatment is complete.
   2. Advise the client to avoid alcohol consumption during and 24 hours after metronidazole treatment due to the possible disulfiram effect from the medication.
   3. Inform the client that urine may darken in colour during treatment.
   4. Inform the client of a possible metallic taste in the mouth during treatment.
C. Pharmacological therapy:
   1. First-line treatment: Metronidazole. Advise clients that alcohol and alcohol-containing products should be avoided at least 24 to 48 hours after the last dose of metronidazole is taken.
   2. Expected cure rate from either regimen is 95% if partner is also treated.
   3. Treatment failure: Repeat metronidazole.
   4. Metronidazole gel is unlikely to achieve therapeutic levels in the urethra or perivaginal glands. It is a considerably less efficacious treatment than oral preparations and is not recommended for use.

Follow-Up
A. Test of cure following treatment with metronidazole is not recommended.

Consultation/Referral
A. Should treatment with metronidazole fail in a client felt to be adherent with medication and not subject to reinfection, consult with or refer client to a specialist for assessment of metronidazole susceptibility.

Individual Considerations
A. Pregnancy: Trichomoniasis may be associated with premature rupture of the membranes, preterm birth, and low birth weight. Metronidazole is not contraindicated during pregnancy or breastfeeding but it does enter the breast milk and may affect its taste.
   1. Symptomatic: Metronidazole. It is unclear whether treatment will improve pregnancy outcomes.
   2. Lactation: Metronidazole. Discontinue breastfeeding during and 24 hours after treatment. Pumping and discarding milk is recommended.
   3. Asymptomatic: Some guidelines suggest that treatment can be deferred or is not recommended.
B. Partners: Recommended treatment is metronidazole.
C. Geriatric:
   1. Uncommon pathogen in postmenopausal women.
   2. Symptoms are vulvar irritation with discharge.
   3. Diagnose with wet prep.
   4. Treat with metronidazole.
D. Clients with HIV:
   1. Screen all women at first visit and annually for trichomoniasis. Treatment for trichomoniasis—same as for HIV-negative individuals.

Bibliography
Society of Obstetricians and Gynecologists of Canada. (2015). *Vulvovaginitis: Screening for and management of trichomoniasis, vulvovaginal candidiasis, and bacterial baginosis.* Retrieved from https://sogc.org/wp-content/uploads/2015/03/gui320CPG1504E.pdf

16 Infectious Disease Guidelines

Cat Scratch Disease (CSD)

Cheryl A. Glass, Jill C. Cash, and Jocelyn T. Whittier

Definition
A. Cat scratch disease (CSD) is a lymphatic infection occurring three to 14 days after a dermal abrasion from a cat scratch. Infection causes unilateral regional adenitis; however, CSD manifestations may also include visceral organ, neurologic, and ocular involvement. There are two phases of symptoms:
   1. Oroya fever: Symptoms include fever, headache, muscle aches, abdominal pain, and severe anaemia.
   2. Verruga peruana: Symptoms include skin lesions/nodular growths that then emerge as red to purple vascular lesions. The lesions are prone to bleeding and ulceration.

Incidence/Prevalence
A. CSD occurs worldwide. The prevalence of CSD in Canada is unknown as it is not a reportable disease. More than 90% of cases have had a history of recent contact with cats, often kittens, which are usually healthy. Multiple cases have been observed in families, presumably resulting from contact with the same animal. There is no documentation of human-to-human transmission. Persons who are immunocompromised are more susceptible to the systemic manifestations. Dissemination to the liver, spleen, eyes, or central nervous system (CNS) occurs in 5% to 14% of individuals.
B. Most cases, 70% to 90%, of CSD occur in the fall and winter months in Canada.
C. CSD is more common in clients younger than 21 years.
D. Approximately 1% of diagnosed cases have no history of an animal scratch.

Pathogenesis
A. *Bartonella henselae* is considered to be responsible for most cases of CSD. *B. henselae* is a fastidious, slow-growing, Gram-negative bacterium. Most transmission occurs from feline bites or scratches as well as cat licking to nonintact skin. About 40% of cats carry *B. henselae* at some time in their lives. Other vectors that may be involved in the transmission of *B. henselae* to humans include dogs, monkeys, Ixodes ticks, and fleas from cats or kittens.
B. The incubation period for lesions to appear is seven to 12 days after abrasion; lymphadenopathy appears to 50 days (median = 12 days) after appearance of the primary lesion.

Predisposing Factors
A. Exposure to domestic and outside cats.
B. Immunocompromised.

Common Findings
A. Swollen lymph glands (regional lymph node, groin, axillary, and cervical areas). The predominant sign is regional lymphadenopathy in an otherwise healthy person.
B. Low-grade fever.
C. Body aches.
D. Fatigue.
E. Anorexia.

Other Signs and Symptoms
A. A skin papule appears three to 10 days after inoculation, often found at the presumed site of inoculation. The papule progresses through the erythematous, vesicular, and popular crusted stages. The papules are generally nonpruritic.
B. Headache.
C. Extreme fatigue (anaemia).
D. Abdominal pain in the presence of hepatosplenomegaly.
E. Arthropathies of the knee, wrist, ankle, and elbow.
F. Visual:
   1. Unilateral eye redness/conjunctivitis is the most common ocular manifestation.
   2. Loss of vision.
   3. Visual disturbances.
   4. Ocular pain (e.g., foreign-body sensation).
   5. Serous discharge.
G. Central nervous:
   1. Changes in level of consciousness (LOC).
   2. Persistent high fever.
   3. Seizures within six weeks of lymphadenopathy.
H. Cardiac:
   1. Murmur.
   2. Dyspnoea.

Subjective Data
A. Review onset and duration of symptoms.
B. Elicit the history of abrasion caused by a kitten/cat or other vectors.
C. Ask the client about other symptoms, such as low-grade fever and body aches.
D. Rule out other illness with review of symptoms (such as pharyngitis and mononucleosis).
E. Ask about visual loss (painless, unilateral visual loss is present with neuroretinitis).
F. Has the client had a febrile seizure?

Physical Examination
A. Check temperature, pulse, respirations, and blood pressure (BP).
B. Inspect:

1. Examine the skin for scratches, bite marks, erythema, or rash.
2. Conduct an ear, nose, and throat examination.
3. Conduct an eye examination if indicated:
   a. Visual examination: Snellen chart.
   b. Funduscopic examination:
      i. The optic disc appears oedematous.
      ii. Exudates frequently surround the macula.
      iii. The funduscopic examination may need to be deferred if photophobia is present.
C. Auscultate heart and lungs.
D. Palpate:
   1. Palpate lymph nodes: Preauricular, cervical, axillary, epitrochlear, and inguinal nodes. Unilateral tender lymph nodes (usually singular) are palpable near the scratch site. The area around the affected lymph nodes is typically tender, warm, erythematous, and indurated.
   2. Abdomen to rule out organomegaly.
   3. Breasts: Examine, if indicated. Mastitis is rare.

Diagnostic Tests

A. Usually none; CSD is often diagnosed by history and physical examination alone. Presenting symptoms may indicate further testing, including the following:
1. Complete blood count (CBC) with differential.
2. Sedimentation rate.
3. Bartonella antibody testing.
4. Disseminated polymerase chain reaction (PCR) assay.

B. Warthin–Starry silver impregnation stain of lymph node, skin, or conjunctival tissue.
C. Biopsy of lymph node (when malignancy is suspected).
D. Culture and sensitivity of any aspirated fluid or blood cultures. Cultures should be held for 21 days since *B. henselae* is a slow-growing bacterium. Trench fever, Carrion's disease, and endocarditis can also be diagnosed with serology.
E. Abdominal ultrasound or CT in the presence of hepatomegaly, splenomegaly, or hepatosplenomegaly on physical examination.
F. The cat-scratch skin test is no longer recommended.

Differential Diagnoses

A. Infectious mononucleosis.
B. Kawasaki disease (KD).
C. Lyme disease.
D. Malignancies that involve lymph nodes such as lymphoma/Hodgkin's disease.
E. Fever of unknown origin (FUO).
F. Trench fever.
G. Carrion's disease.
H. Endocarditis.

Plan

A. General interventions:
   1. Management is usually the treatment of symptoms. CSD is self-limiting with slow resolution in two to four months.
   2. Prescribe analgesics for pain.
   3. Rest is advised.
   4. Ice may be applied to the affected nodes.
   5. About 10% of nodes will suppurate and require aspiration. However, lymph node aspiration is not recommended unless to relieve severe pain. During aspiration, the needle should be moved around in several locations because microabscesses often exist in multiple septated pockets. Incision and drainage are not recommended because of the potential of chronic sinus tract formation.
B. Client teaching:
   1. The lymphadenopathy usually regresses within two to four months but may persist for up to one year.
   2. Client education on cats includes the following:
      a. People should avoid playing roughly with cats.
      b. Stray cats should not be handled by children or immunocompromised people.
      c. Testing cats is not recommended. Cats do not need to be removed or destroyed.
      d. Always cleanse animal bites or scratches immediately with soap and water to prevent or reduce the transmission of CSD.
      e. Control fleas (fleas have been found to have *B. henselae*).
   3. If there are any signs of an infection after a cat bite/scratch, the client should be seen by his or her healthcare provider.
   4. Disease is not contagious: There is no person-to-person transmission.
   5. No vaccination is currently available.
C. Pharmacological therapy:
   1. Antibiotic therapy is not essential for clients with normal immune systems. Symptoms are usually self-limiting.
   2. Acetaminophen as needed.
   3. Nonsteroidal anti-inflammatory drugs (NSAIDs) as needed.
   4. Oral corticosteroids for individuals with atypical symptoms.
   5. Antibiotics may be prescribed if the client is acutely ill with systemic symptoms, particularly immunocompromised individuals; with haepatosplenomegaly, visual, cardiac, or neurologic symptoms; or with large, painful adenopathy:
      a. Azithromycin for treatment of lymphadenitis.
      b. Clarithromycin may be used as an alternative to azithromycin for lymphadenitis.
      c. Rifampin may be used as an alternative for lymphadenitis.
      d. Trimethoprim-sulphaamethoxazole may be used as an alternative for lymphadenitis.
      e. For haepatosplenic disease and prolonged fever, use rifampin for 10 to 14 days and add a second agent such as:
         i. Azithromycin.
         ii. Gentamicin.
      f. Neurologic disease/neuroretinitis: Clients diagnosed with neuroretinitis or neurologic disease should be prescribed doxycycline plus rifampin. Consult with an infectious disease specialist. Consult with the ophthalmologist since the client will require close monitoring and adjunctive corticosteroid therapy for six weeks may be required.
      g. Endocarditis: The optimal antibiotic therapy and optimal duration of therapy for *Bartonella* endocarditis are unknown. Consult with an infectious disease specialist.

Follow-Up

A. Reevaluate the client in approximately six to eight weeks if mild symptoms.
B. Reevaluate in 10 days if placed on antibiotics.
C. CSD is not a reportable disease in Canada.

Consultation/Referral

A. Complications are rare; refer the client to specialists as required (e.g., infectious disease, neurologist, cardiologist, and ophthalmologist) if infection is systemic or unresponsive to antibiotics:
  1. Hearing loss.
  2. Neurologic disability.
  3. Digit or limb amputations.
  4. Skin scarring.
B. Clients diagnosed with neuroretinitis should be referred to an ophthalmologist for comanagement.
C. Infectious disease consult should be ordered for clients diagnosed with serious infections such as trench fever, Carrion's disease, and endocarditis.

Individual Considerations

A. Paediatrics:
  1. If neuroretinitis is diagnosed in children <8 years of age, treatment should include azithromycin or trimethoprim-sulphamethoxazole in place of doxycycline.

Bibliography

Centers for Disease Control and Prevention. (2014). *Cat-scratch disease.* Retrieved from www.cdc.gov/healthypets/diseases/cat-scratch.html

Centers for Disease Control and Prevention. (2015). *Bartonella infection (cat scratch disease, trench fever, and Carrion's disease). For Health-Care Providers.* Retrieved from www.cdc.gov/bartonella/clinicians/index.html

Government of Canada. (2011, August 19). *Pathogen safety data sheets. Infectious substances: Bartonella henselae.* Retrieved from https://www.canada.ca/en/public-health/services/laboratory-biosafety-biosecurity/pathogen-safety-data-sheets-risk-assessment/bartonella-henselae.html

Spach, D., & Kaplan, S. (2018). Treatment of cat scratch disease. *UpToDate.* Retrieved from www.uptodate.com

Cytomegalovirus (CMV)

Cheryl A. Glass, Jill C. Cash, and Jocelyn T. Whittier

Definition

A. Cytomegalovirus (CMV) is in the herpesvirus family, which includes varicella-zoster virus (chickenpox) and infectious mononucleosis (Epstein–Barr virus [EBV]). Differences in CMV genotypes may be associated with differences in virulence. CMV is responsible for a viral infection with a high rate of asymptomatic excretion. Shedding of the virus takes place intermittently. CMV can be isolated in cell culture from urine, pharynx, respiratory secretions, human milk, tears, saliva, semen, cervical secretions, and body fluids such as blood and amniotic fluid. Cytomegalic cells can be found in tissue, including the lung, liver, kidney, intestine, adrenal gland, and the central nervous system (CNS).
B. CMV persists in latent form after a primary infection, and reactivation can occur years later, particularly under conditions of immunosuppression, transplantation, and pregnancy. CMV is one of the TORCH infections (toxoplasmosis, other [e.g., hepatitis and syphilis], rubella, CMV, and herpes infections).
C. The most common illness caused by CMV is retinitis.

Incidence/Prevalence

A. CMV is found worldwide in all ages, races, and ethnic groups. Seropositivity increases with age, ranging from 40% to 100% depending on geography, cultures, child-rearing practices, and socioeconomic status. Approximately 50% of blood donors have been exposed to CMV, and 10% carry CMV in white blood cells (WBCs). The incidence of horizontal transmission of CMV occurring in settings such as day care ranges from 10% to more than 80% from the exposure to saliva and urine. Another increase in CMV is noted in adolescence secondary to sexual activity.
B. CMV is the most common congenital infection in Canada. The incidence of congenital vertical transmission of CMV ranges from 0.2% to 2.5%. Most newborns appear normal and are asymptomatic; however, 5% to 15% of congenitally infected newborns will have symptoms at delivery. Prenatal CMV infections occur from contact with maternal cervicovaginal secretions during delivery or from breast milk ingestion. Preterm infants are at greatest risk of acquiring CMV from breast milk.
C. Combination antiretroviral therapy (ART) has reduced the risk of CMV in people with HIV by 75%.
D. The risk of CMV is the highest in HIV clients when their CD4 cell counts are below 50 cells/μL. CMV is rare if the CD4 count is >100 cells/μL.
E. The most common illness caused by CMV is retinitis.

Pathogenesis

A. Human CMV, a DNA virus, is a member of the herpesvirus group. This virus is transmitted both horizontally (by direct person-to-person contact with virus-containing secretions) and vertically (from mother to infant before, during, or after birth). Infections have no seasonal correlation.
B. The incubation period for horizontally transmitted CMV infections in households is unknown. Primary CMV infection usually manifests itself within four to seven weeks and may persist as long as 16 to 20 weeks after initial infection. CMV disease is most likely 30 to 60 days after transplant.
C. CMV remains in a person for life; there is no treatment that will permanently eliminate CMV infection.

Predisposing Factors

A. Exposure to young children (especially those in day-care centers).
B. Sexual contact (cervicovaginal secretions and semen).
C. Blood transfusions: Clients with impaired immune function (e.g., bone marrow and organ transplant recipients, premature babies) are at risk for CMV infection from contaminated transfused blood.
D. Hospital or occupational exposure: Universal precautions are considered adequate to prevent transmission of CMV within hospitals. Nosocomial transmission from person-to-person has not been documented. Isolation is not recommended.
E. Pregnancy: Pregnant health-care workers are not restricted from caring for CMV-infected clients and should follow universal precautions.
F. Transplacental transmission.
G. Ascending infection from the cervix.
H. Tissue or organ transplantation.
I. Household spread among family members; a young child is most frequently the index case.
J. Breast milk.

Common Findings

A. Mononucleosis-like syndrome.
B. Fever.
C. Overwhelming fatigue.
D. Pharyngitis.
E. Ulcerative lesions in the mouth.

F. Loss of vision (retinal detachment may occur in up to 50%–60% in the first year after diagnosis).

Other Signs and Symptoms

A. Mothers: Asymptomatic or mononucleosis-like syndrome.
B. Fetuses:
  1. Intrauterine growth retardation (IUGR)/small for gestational age.
  2. Nonimmune hydrops fetalis.
  3. Microcephaly noted on ultrasound.
  4. Intracerebral calcification.
C. Infants after congenital exposure:
  1. Asymptomatic.
  2. Skin:
    a. Jaundice at birth.
    b. Petechiae and purpura of the skin.
  3. Haepatosplenomegaly.
  4. Anaemia.
  5. Thrombocytopaenia.
  6. Eyes: Chorioretinitis, retinal haemorrhage, optic atrophy.
  7. Seizure disorders.
  8. Feeding difficulties.
D. Children with congenital exposure:
  1. Asymptomatic.
  2. Development: Developmental delays, learning disability, and intellectual disability.
  3. Ears: Progressive hearing loss (usually unilateral). Universal hearing screening programs may identify some of the otherwise asymptomatic infants.
  4. Loss of vision.
E. Adults:
  1. Visual changes: Floaters or loss of visual fields on one side.
  2. Retinitis.
  3. Arthralgias.
  4. Nausea, abdominal cramping, and vomiting (includes haematemesis).
  5. Prolonged fever.
  6. Mild haepatitis.
  7. Headache.
  8. Gastritis presents with abdominal pain and colitis presents as a diarrhoeal illness. CMV may infect the gastrointestinal (GI) tract from the oral cavity through the colon. The typical manifestation of disease is ulcerative lesions. In the mouth, these may be indistinguishable from ulcers caused by herpes simplex virus (HSV) or aphthous ulceration.
F. Immunocompromised persons:
  1. Bacterial: Pneumonia, retinitis, myocarditis, and aseptic meningitis.
  2. Anaemia.
  3. Thrombocytopaenia.

Subjective Data

A. Review onset of presenting signs and symptoms, and their duration.
B. Review the client's history for recent upper respiratory infection (URI) and mononucleosis-like symptoms.
C. Elicit information concerning contact with any person known to be CMV infected.
D. Review history for other family members with similar symptoms.
E. Ask the client about any occupational exposure.
F. Review the client's exposure to children in day-care centers.
G. Review recent blood transfusions and/or organ transplantation.
H. Determine the client's history for risk factors or presence of HIV:
  1. If known HIV, does the client know his or her last viral load CD4 count?
  2. Is the client taking ART? When were the antivirals started?
I. Ask family members if the client has been confused, lethargic, or withdrawn or has exhibited personality changes (CMV encephalitis, dementia).

Physical Examination

A. Check temperature, pulse, respirations, blood pressure (BP), and weight (document serial weight loss).
B. Inspect:
  1. Inspect skin for jaundice and petechiae.
  2. Evaluate age-appropriate developmental tasks.
  3. Conduct a detailed eye examination:
    a. CMV infection may appear as yellow–white areas with perivascular exudates and haemorrhage, having a "cottage cheese and ketchup" appearance at either the periphery or the center of the fundus:
      i. Differentiating suspected CMV retinitis and cotton wool spots is essential. Cotton wool spots appear as small, fluffy white lesions with indistinct margins and are not associated with exudates or haemorrhages.
    b. Evaluate field of vision.
  4. Perform ear, nose, and throat examination.
C. Auscultate heart and lungs.
D. Palpate:
  1. The abdomen, noting organomegaly.
  2. Pregnancy: Palpate fundal height and evaluate for suspected IUGR.
E. Neurologic examination:
  1. Assess all cranial nerves.
  2. Sensation (deficits may occur without loss of vibratory sense and proprioception).
  3. Deep tendon reflexes (DTRs).
  4. Motor skills and coordination.
  5. Gait.
  6. Conduct hearing test.

Diagnostic Tests

A. Viral culture of specimen from urine, cervix, vagina, nasopharynx, and saliva:
  1. Viral culture is the best means of diagnosing acute CMV infections although it does not distinguish between primary and recurrent disease. Urine contains high titres of the virus because CMV is relatively stable in urine.
B. Complete blood count (CBC) with differential: Differential WBC count reveals increased lymphocytes, many of which are atypical.
C. Total direct and indirect serum bilirubin.
D. Liver function: Alanine aminotransferase (ALT) and aspartate aminotransferase (AST).
E. Serology for CMV immunoglobulin G (IgG) and immunoglobulin M (IgM): Only the recovery of the virus from a target organ provides unequivocal evidence that the disease is caused by CMV infection. However, a fourfold or greater rise in IgG-specific antibody titre is usually considered evidence of acute infection.

F. Immunocompromised clients, especially transplant recipients, may be monitored for viral surveillance weekly using surrogate markers for viraemia (polymerase chain reaction [PCR]).
G. Chest x-ray if indicated.
H. CT scan if indicated to evaluate abnormalities of the brain in the presence of an abnormal neurologic examination, seizures, and microcephaly.
I. Sensorineural hearing evaluation.

Differential Diagnoses
A. Other TORCH infections.
B. HIV.
C. Viral: autoimmune haepatitis or haepatitis A to E.
D. Enteroviruses.
E. Fever of unknown origin (FUO).

Plan
A. General interventions:
  1. Provide support for the client and family.
  2. Contact social services if long-term support will be required for these infants/families.
  3. Rest is vital.
B. Client teaching:
  1. Clients with splenomegaly should avoid activity that may increase the risk of injury to the spleen (e.g., contact sports, heavy lifting).
  2. Mothers infected with CMV should be discouraged from breastfeeding because CMV is secreted in breast milk. CMV-specific IgM antibodies are present in only 80% of clients with primary CMV infections and in 20% of clients with recurrent infections; therefore, a negative result does not exclude the diagnosis of CMV.
  3. Isolation is not required.
  4. Use universal precautions, especially good handwashing.
  5. Do not share eating or drinking utensils, drinks, or food with toddlers or young children.
  6. Educate about the importance of ART in treating CMV:
     a. Clients with CMV retinitis may require lifelong suppressive therapy to prevent blindness. Vision loss will not return to pre-CMV status.
     b. Report visual deterioration immediately.
C. Pharmacological therapy:
  1. First-line treatment: Ganciclovir is the treatment for CMV retinitis in adults and children older than three months; treatment is divided into an induction and a maintenance phase:
     a. The safety of ganciclovir in pregnancy has not been established.
     b. Clients receiving ganciclovir should have blood counts monitored closely due to dose-dependent bone marrow suppression. Monitor for leukopaenia, neutropaenia, anaemia, or thrombocytopaenia. Growth factors may be necessary.
     c. The dose should be decreased in clients with impaired renal function. Monitor creatinine.
     d. Although ganciclovir has appeared to be beneficial in the treatment of some congenitally infected infants, its use is controversial and is considered mainly for high-risk clients with severe congenital CMV.
  2. Alternative drug therapy foscarnet:
     a. Used in ganciclovir-resistant CMV retinitis and herpes simplex disease.
     b. Use in children is limited; safe dose has not been established.
     c. The safety of foscarnet in pregnancy has not been established.
     d. Foscarnet is nephrotoxic. Meticulous attention must be paid to renal function. Small changes in creatinine require new calculation of dose for renal clearance. Obtain a 24-hour serum creatinine at baseline and discontinue if serum creatinine is <0.4 ml/min/kg.
     e. Clients must be well hydrated.
  3. Cidofovir:
     a. Treatment is divided into an induction and a maintenance phase.
     b. Probenecid is given on the day of the intravenous (IV) infusion in order to reduce the renal uptake of cidofovir.
  4. CMV immunoglobulin intravenous: For more information, refer to the Canadian Immunization Guide: www.canada.ca/en/public-health/services/publications/healthy-living/canadian-immunization-guide-part-5-passive-immunization.html#p5a4b.
  5. Immune globulin (Ig) or CMV hyperimmune globulin may be utilized for passive immunoprophylaxis, especially in bone marrow and organ transplant recipients, to help develop antibodies and protect against CMV infection.
  6. CMV vaccines are currently in clinical trials.

Follow-Up
A. Retinitis is the most common manifestation of CMV disease; clients with CNS, GI, or pulmonary disease should be assessed with a dilated retinal examination to detect subclinical retinal disease.
B. The client should be seen for reports of excessive bruising or bleeding, jaundice, or abnormal CNS functioning.
C. Monitor CBC, serum creatinine, and electrolytes (especially calcium and magnesium) every week.
D. Congenital CMV is reportable to provincial/territorial Medical Officers of Health in most provinces/territories in Canada.

Consultation/Referral
A. Consultation with an infectious diseases specialist is indicated for acute infection, especially for immunocompromised clients.
B. Antivirals have many adverse effects and are best managed by an infectious disease specialist who has experience using these drugs.
C. Consultation with a haematologist is needed in severe cases, especially with haemolytic anaemia and thrombocytopaenia.
D. Consultation with a neurologist is indicated for meningitis, encephalitis, polyneuritis, and Guillain–Barré syndrome.
E. Consultation with an ophthalmologist is needed on an emergent basis for a dilated retinal examination due to the risks of blindness. Serial dilated retinal examinations should be done after ART induction therapy and monthly thereafter.
F. Consultation with a perinatologist is indicated for pregnant clients. Evaluation may include ultrasonography, amniocentesis, and percutaneous umbilical blood sampling (PUBS).
G. Refer to a gastroenterologist for an endoscopic evaluation with tissue biopsies.

Individual Considerations

A. Pregnancy:
   1. Routine maternal screening for CMV infection is not recommended during pregnancy. Laboratory tests that are currently available generally cannot conclusively determine whether a primary CMV infection has occurred during the pregnancy.
   2. Between 40% and 50% of pregnant women are immune to CMV, with a higher prevalence of immunity in lower socioeconomic populations.
   3. Susceptible pregnant women have a 2% to 2.5% risk of acquiring primary CMV during pregnancy. Those with prior immunity have a 1% chance of reactivation of latent infection.
   4. Amniocentesis for PCR to detect CMV DNA is the preferred diagnostic approach for detecting the infected fetus.
   5. Recovery of CMV from the cervix or urine of women at or before the time of delivery does not warrant a cesarean section.

B. Perinatal transmission of CMV occurs by four routes:
   1. In utero transplacental infections.
   2. Ascending infections from the cervix.
   3. Exposure to infected secretions from the lower genital tract during delivery.
   4. Ingestion of infected breast milk.

Because CMV is spread by intimate contact with infectious secretions, handwashing after exposure to secretions is particularly important for pregnant health-care workers.

C. Paediatrics:
   1. Routine screening for CMV is not recommended for internationally adopted children.
   2. Up to half of all neonates exposed to CMV in the lower genital tract during delivery become infected. Intrapartum or postpartum CMV acquisition does not result in adverse outcomes or sequelae except in very-low-birth-weight infants. Viral excretion from intrapartum or postpartum exposure begins at three to nine weeks of life; thus, the initial viral cultures are negative.
   3. The child with congenital CMV infection should not be treated differently from other children and should not be excluded from school or childcare institutions as the virus is frequently found in many healthy children.
   4. Sensorineural hearing loss is the most common sequelae following congenital CMV infection. Evaluate for hearing loss at each paediatric visit.

D. Adults:
   1. Occupational exposure: Risk often appears to be greatest for child-care personnel who care for children younger than two years.
   2. Routine serologic screening for child-care staff is not currently recommended.
   3. Pregnant personnel who may be in contact with CMV-infected clients should be counseled regarding the risk of acquiring CMV infection and about the need to practice good hygiene, particularly handwashing. There is no need for routinely transferring personnel to other work situations.

E. Geriatrics:
   1. CMV colitis can be life threatening for the immunocompromised older client with chronic renal disease.
   2. Monitor for symptoms such as bloody diarrhoea. Consider colonoscopy with biopsy for diagnosis.

Bibliography

Akhter, K. (2015). Cytomegalovirus. *Medscape*. Retrieved from www.emedicine.medscape.com/article/215702-overview

American College of Obstetricians and Gynecologists. (2015). Practice Bulletin no. 151: Cytomegalovirus, parvovirus B19, varicella zoster, and toxoplasmosis in pregnancy. *Obstetrics & Gynecology (Serial Online), 125*(6), 1510–1525.

Friel, T. J. (2017). Epidemiology, clinical manifestations, and treatment of cytomegalovirus infection in immunocompetent adults. *UpToDate*. Retrieved from www.uptodate.com

Government of Canada. (2011, April 19). *Pathogen safety data sheets. Infectious substances: Cytomegalovirus*. Retrieved from www.canada.ca/en/public-health/services/laboratory-biosafety-biosecurity/pathogen-safety-data-sheets-risk-assessment/cytomegalovirus.html

Government of Canada. (2019, February 25). *Canadian immunization guide: Part 5–Passive immunization. Cytomegalovirus immune globulin*. Retrieved from https://www.canada.ca/en/public-health/services/publications/healthy-living/canadian-immunization-guide-part-5-passive-immunization.html#p5a4b

Ontario Hospital Association & Ontario Medical Association. (2017). *Cytomegalovirus surveillance protocol for Ontario hospitals*. Retrieved from https://www.oha.com/Documents/Cytomegalovirus%20Protocol%20Revised%20May%202017.pdf

Savva, G. M., Pachnio, A., Kaul, B., Morgan, K., Huppert, F. A., Brayne, C., & Moss, P. A. (2013). Cytomegalovirus infection is associated with increased mortality in the older population. *Aging Cell, 12*, 381–387. doi:10.1111/acel.12059

Encephalitis

Cheryl A. Glass, Jill C. Cash, and Jocelyn T. Whittier

Definition

Encephalitis is the inflammation of cerebral tissue caused by viral agents or other toxins. The syndrome of acute encephalitis shares many clinical features with acute meningitis. Clients with either syndrome present with fever, headache, and altered states of consciousness. In most cases of encephalitis, there is some concomitant meningeal inflammation, in addition to the cephalitic component, a condition commonly referred to as meningoencephalitis.

Incidence/Prevalence

A. Incidence is unknown. Japanese encephalitis (JE) occurs in annual epidemics in Asia during the rainy season. The prevalence of JE (arbovirus) is related to ecologic and climatic conditions that affect the natural transmission cycles during summer months (June–September). A vaccine is available.

B. Arboviruses (Eastern or Western equine, St. Louis, and West Nile virus [WNV]) cause disease when mosquitoes are active, whereas walking in the woods or marshy areas with high tick populations might suggest other viral encephalitides such as Colorado tick fever (may be found in western Rockies in Canada) or nonviral aetiologies such as Lyme disease or Rocky Mountain spotted fever (RMSF).

C. Herpes encephalitis has the highest morbidity and mortality of the common viral encephalitides and may occur at any time. The mortality rate for untreated clients is 70%; <5% of survivors have normal neurologic function. Herpes simplex virus (HSV) type 1 is the most common cause of sporadic encephalitis. The most important viral aetiology to rule out is HSV, because this clinical entity is usually fatal if left untreated. Survival and recovery from neurologic sequelae are related to the mental status at the time of acyclovir initiation.

D. Encephalopathy is the most common central nervous system (CNS) manifestation of HIV infection, occurring in 65% of clients with HIV/AIDS.

E. Mortality depends on the aetiological agent. Morbidity related to the severity of sequelae also varies according to the causative agent.

Pathogenesis
A. Encephalitis may occur as a secondary infection from mumps, varicella (chickenpox), rubella, rubeola, rabies, herpes simplex types 1 and 2, Epstein–Barr virus (EBV), HIV, and influenza. Postinfectious encephalitis, in contrast to viral encephalitis, typically occurs either as the initial infection is resolving or may appear following subclinical illness that was not appreciated by the client.
B. The incubation period depends on the pathogen.
C. Tick-borne diseases include Russian spring–summer encephalitis and Powassan encephalitis.

Predisposing Factors
A. Military personnel and travelers.
B. Age extremes are highest risk.
C. Exposure to vectors:
   1. Mosquitoes.
   2. Ticks.
   3. Bats.
   4. Raccoons.
   5. Feral dogs/cats.
   6. Sandflies.
D. HIV positive.
E. Herpes.
F. Rodent-borne arenavirus: Exposure to the secretions of mice, rats, and hamsters.
G. Occupational exposure:
   1. Laboratory workers.
   2. Health-care workers.
   3. Veterinarians.
H. Recreational activities (e.g., camping, hunting).
I. Recent vaccination.

Common Findings
A. Severe headache: A person with encephalitis has a severe headache throughout the entire head. Over the course of about 48 hours, the person may show a lack of energy and then lapse into a coma.
B. Stiff neck.
C. Mental changes: Altered mental status, altered behaviour, and personality changes.
D. Decreased level of consciousness (LOC).
E. Fever.

Other Signs and Symptoms
A. CNS symptoms:
   1. Nuchal rigidity.
   2. Irritability.
   3. Hemiparesis: Weakness or paralysis on one side of body.
   4. Flaccid paralysis: Consider WNV infection.
   5. Seizures.
   6. Exaggerated deep tendon reflexes (DTRs).
   7. Ataxia.
   8. Nystagmus.
B. Photosensitivity.
C. Swollen or protruding eyes.
D. Malaise.
E. Nausea and/or vomiting.
F. Dysphagia with rabies.
G. Parotitis: Consider mumps encephalitis.
H. Maculopapular rash.
I. Tremors.

Subjective Data
A. Review the onset, duration, and course of all symptoms.
B. Rule out recent history of chickenpox, rubeola, herpes, or other infections.
C. Ask the client about recent travel and vaccines.
D. Question the client regarding recent mosquito or animal bites (rule out rabies).
E. Elicit a detailed sexual history.
F. Does the client have HIV?
G. Ask about recent recreational activities, including camping, spelunking, or hunting.

Physical Examination
A. Check temperature, pulse, respirations, and blood pressure (BP).
B. Inspect:
   1. Observe general overall appearance.
   2. Conduct an eye examination.
   3. Examine the skin for rash, vesicles, or bites:
      a. Maculopapular rash is seen in approximately half of clients with WNV.
      b. Grouped vesicles in a dermatomal pattern suggest varicella zoster.
      c. Classic herpetic skin lesions suggest herpes encephalitis.
   4. Assess dehydration status.
   5. Observe for seizure activity.
   6. Observe for tremors of the eyelids, tongue, lips, and extremities, which may suggest the possibility of St. Louis encephalitis (found in the United States year-round) or West Nile encephalitis.
C. Auscultate:
   1. Lungs and monitor breathing pattern.
   2. Heart.
D. Palpate:
   1. The lymph nodes: Preauricular, posterior auricular, submental and sublingual, anterior cervical chains, and supraclavicular nodes.
   2. The mastoid bone.
E. Neurologic examination:
   1. Assess LOC.
   2. Assess the client for personality changes.
   3. Assess for meningeal signs:
      a. Signs of meningeal irritation include nuchal rigidity.
      b. Positive Brudzinski's and Kernig's signs:
         i. Brudzinski's sign: Place the client supine and flex the head upward. Resulting flexion of hips, knees, and ankles with neck flexion indicates meningeal irritation (see Figure 16.1).
         ii. Kernig's sign: Place the client supine. Keeping one leg straight, flex the other hip and knee to a bent knee to form a 90-degree angle. Slowly extend the lower leg. This places a stretch on the meninges, resulting in pain and spasm for the hamstring muscle. Resistance to further extension can be felt (see Figure 16.2).
   4. Check DTRs (exaggerated and/or pathologic reflexes).

Diagnostic Tests
A. Complete blood count (CBC) with differential, electrolytes, glucose, urea, and creatinine.

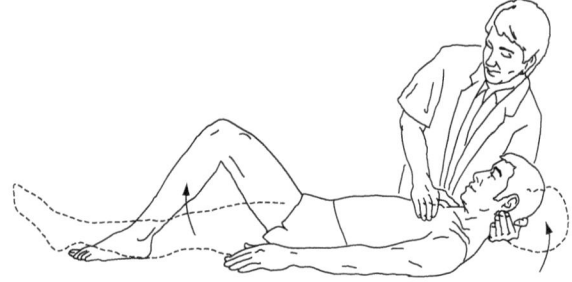

FIGURE 16.1 Brudzinski's sign.

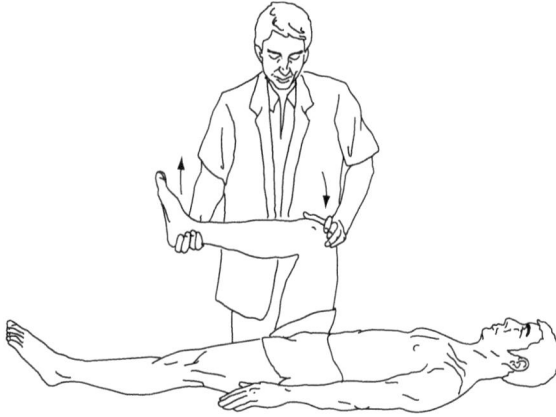

FIGURE 16.2 Kernig's sign.

B. Polymerase chain reaction (PCR) tests for viruses.
C. Serology for arboviruses.
D. Lumbar puncture for the following:
  1. Protein (elevated).
  2. Glucose (usually normal).
  3. White cell count (increased).
  4. Red cell count (usually negative in a nontraumatic tap).
  5. Culture (viral and bacterial): Detection of virus-specific IgM antibody in cerebrospinal fluid (CSF) is diagnostic.
E. EEG.
F. CT scan: Useful to rule out space-occupying lesions or brain abscess.
G. MRI: Sensitive for detecting demyelination.
H. Brain scan: Imaging studies (CT scan, MRI, and brain scan) may be normal early; later, nonspecific abnormalities are seen.
I. Stool or throat cultures may be helpful if enteroviruses are suspected.
J. Skin lesions and urine may be cultured for herpes simplex and cytomegalovirus (CMV).
K. Brain biopsy is the diagnostic standard.

Differential Diagnoses
A. WNV.
B. St. Louis virus.
C. Chickenpox.
D. Measles: rubeola or rubella.
E. Herpes.
F. Rabies.
G. Influenza.
H. Mumps.
I. Meningitis.
J. Brain abscess.
K. Tuberculosis.
L. Syphilis.
M. Intracranial haemorrhage.
N. Trauma.
O. Toxic ingestion.
P. Fungal meningitis.
Q. RMSF/tick-borne diseases.
R. Cerebral bacterial infections.
S. Toxoplasmosis.
T. Lyme disease.
U. Cat scratch disease.
V. CMV.
W. Nonparalytic poliomyelitis.

Plan
A. General interventions: If encephalitis is suspected, hospitalization is recommended for further diagnostic studies and evaluation.
B. Client teaching:
  1. Prevention of vector-borne encephalitis involves mosquito and tick avoidance, use of insect repellents, and vaccination.
  2. The JE vaccine is an inactivated vaccine derived from infected mouse brain and is recommended for expatriates living in Asia and for certain travelers. It is also recommended for the following:
    a. Persons who will be residing in areas where JE virus is endemic or epidemic.
    b. Travelers planning prolonged stays (>30 days) in endemic areas during the transmission season, especially with activities such as bicycling, camping, or other unprotected outdoor activities in rural areas.
  3. If rabies is suspected, the domestic animal should be observed for 10 days to detect rabid behaviour. If there is no indication of rabies, the animal should be immunized. Animals that show rabid behaviour or wild animals should be sacrificed and their brains submitted to the local health department for pathology testing. Prophylactic rabies vaccine is available to travelers going to at-risk countries staying in rural areas or working with animals.
C. Pharmacological therapy:
  1. Empiric treatment for HSV-1 should always be initiated as soon as possible if the client has encephalitis without explanation, due to the high mortality and morbidity. Acyclovir is used for treatment.
  2. Antibiotics for bacterial aetiology.
  3. Anticonvulsants for seizures.
  4. Other pharmacological therapies depend on specific causal agent.
  5. Initiate short courses of corticosteroids to control brain oedema.
  6. If rabies is suspected: Human rabies immune globulin should be given.

Follow-Up
A. Follow-up varies and is specific to causal agent.
B. Long-term management of clients with neurologic sequelae includes rehabilitation services, home care, or nursing home placement for convalescent care.

Consultation/Referral
A. Refer the client to hospital. Consultations include a neurologist, infectious diseases specialist, and neurosurgeon for managing elevated intracranial pressure.

Individual Considerations

A. Adult travelers: Advise client to take insecticide-treated mosquito bed nets and aerosol insecticide sprays to reduce the risk of mosquito bites at day and night, respectively.
B. For current information regarding the JE vaccine, refer to the Canadian Immunization Guide:
www.canada.ca/en/public-health/services/publications/healthy-living/canadian-immunization-guide-part-4-active-vaccines/page-11-japanese-encephalitis-vaccine.html.
C. Geriatrics:
  1. Elderly clients may be at risk for severe disease.
  2. WNV encephalitis occurs primarily in clients older than 65 years.
  3. Encephalitis should be considered in all elderly clients who have progressive mental confusion.
  4. Herpes simplex encephalitis in the elderly may present in an atypical fashion:
    a. Progressive amnestic cognitive disorder.
    b. Behavioural changes.
    c. Progressive mental confusion.
    d. Focal neurologic deficits, which mimic stroke.

Bibliography

Gluckman, S. (2017). Viral encephalitis in adults. *UpToDate*. Retrieved from www.uptodate.com/contents/viral-encephalitis-in-adults
Government of Canada. (2016, September 1). *Canadian immunization guide: Part 4-Active vaccines. Japanese Encephalitis Vaccine*. Retrieved from https://www.canada.ca/en/public-health/services/publications/healthy-living/canadian-immunization-guide-part-4-active-vaccines/page-11-japanese-encephalitis-vaccine.html

H1N1 Influenza A

Cheryl A. Glass, Jill C. Cash, and Jocelyn T. Whittier

Definition

A. H1N1 influenza A (swine flu) is an influenza A virus that causes a highly contagious respiratory disease. H1N1 has been reported worldwide and was designated a phase 6 global pandemic status by the World Health Organization (WHO) in 2009. Influenza causes approximately 12,200 hospitalizations and 3,500 deaths annually in Canada.
B. Persons with flu-like symptoms should promptly contact their health-care providers. If an antiviral is warranted (confirmed influenza on polymerase chain reaction [PCR] and requiring hospitalization), it should ideally be started within 48 hours from the onset of symptoms. Viral pneumonia is the primary sign of clinical deterioration.

Incidence/Prevalence

A. The WHO declared the 2009 H1N1 pandemic over as of August 2010. However, this strain of flu still continues to circulate with other seasonal flu strains.

Pathogenesis

A. H1N1 is a new subtype of influenza A virus that is spread by human-to-human transmission. The swine flu is also transmitted pig-to-person; however, persons cannot be infected with the H1N1 virus from consuming pork.
B. The primary mode of transmission is through exposure to viral strain respiratory secretions from respiratory droplets (coughing or sneezing) and direct contact of contaminated surfaces. H1N1 is also noted to be spread through contaminated diarrhoeal stools.
C. The infectious period is considered to be one day before the onset of fever until 24 hours after fever ends.

Predisposing Factors

A. Age:
  1. Children younger than five years, especially those younger than two years.
  2. Adults 25 to 64 years who have medical conditions that place them at high risk for influenza-related complications.
  3. Adults aged 65 years or older.
B. Pregnant women.
C. Women up to two weeks postpartum.
D. Crowded conditions.
E. Institutions such as nursing homes.
F. Occupational exposure: teachers and health-care workers.

Common Findings

A. Clinical manifestations of H1N1 influenza depend on the age and previous experience with the influenza virus. Rapid-onset respiratory illness is the most common complaint:
  1. Cough.
  2. Sore throat.
  3. Dyspnoea/wheezing.
  4. Rhinorrhoea.
B. Abrupt onset of fever and/or chills (temperature of 37.8°C or greater).
C. Headache.
D. Body aches.
E. Altered mental status.
F. Children:
  1. Apnoea.
  2. Tachypnoea.
  3. Cyanosis.
  4. Dehydration.
  5. Extreme irritability.
  6. Febrile seizure.

Other Signs and Symptoms

A. Joint pain.
B. Diarrhoea (common with H1N1).
C. Vomiting (common with H1N1).

Subjective Data

A. Review the onset, course, and duration of symptoms, especially fever and respiratory symptoms.
B. Review symptoms of other family members or coworkers who are also ill. Is the onset of acute febrile respiratory illness within seven days of close contact with a person with a confirmed case of H1N1?
C. If pregnant, establish gestational age.
D. Review for recent travel location and use of cruise ships/planes.
E. Evaluate living conditions for exposure risks.
F. Is the client a smoker?
G. Review all medications, including over-the-counter (OTC) and herbal products. Has the client taken any medications for the symptoms?
H. Does the client have a history of asthma or chronic obstructive pulmonary disease (COPD)?
I. Is the client immunocompromised (e.g., HIV, transplant recipient, chemotherapy)?
J. What other medical comorbidities, such as diabetes, does the client have?

Physical Examination

A. Check temperature, pulse, respirations, and blood pressure (BP).

B. Inspect.
   1. Observe general overall appearance for pallor and for any respiratory distress.
   2. Assess hydration status inspecting skin turgor and mucous membranes.
   3. Conduct an eye, ear, nose, and throat examination.
   4. Children:
      a. Observe for seizure activity.
      b. Note level of activity (playful vs. lethargic).
C. Auscultate:
   1. Lung fields: Observe for wheezing and crackles.
   2. Heart.
D. Palpate:
   1. Neck.
   2. Lymph nodes: preauricular, posterior auricular, submental and sublingual, anterior cervical chain, and supraclavicular nodes.
E. Neurologic examination:
   1. Assess level of consciousness (LOC).
   2. Assess for nuchal rigidity.
   3. Assess for meningeal signs:
      a. Signs of meningeal irritation include nuchal rigidity.
      b. Positive Brudzinski's and Kernig's signs (see Figures 16.1 and 16.2):
         i. Brudzinski's sign: Place the client supine and flex the head upward. Resulting flexion of both hips, knees, and ankles with neck flexion indicates meningeal irritation.
         ii. Kernig's sign: Place the client supine. Keeping one leg straight, flex the other hip and knee to a bent knee to form a 90 degree angle. Slowly extend the lower leg. This places a stretch on the meninges, resulting in pain and spasm for the hamstring muscle. Resistance to further extension can be felt.

Diagnostic Tests

Testing is not necessary for all clients who present with influenza-type symptoms:
A. Rapid influenza antigen testing.
B. Respiratory swab for H1N1 testing for detection by real-time reverse transcriptase PCR.
C. Viral culture.
D. Complete blood count (CBC) with differential (not a required test).
E. Imaging (rule out complications):
   1. Chest x-ray.
   2. CT chest imaging for complications, if indicated clinically.

Differential Diagnoses
A. Influenza:
   1. Influenza A (H1, H2, or H3 haemagglutinins with N1 or N2 neuraminidase subtypes).
   2. Influenza B (less antigenic changes than influenza A).
   3. Influenza C (acute respiratory illnesses in children and more rarely in adults).
   4. Avian flu (H5N1 and H7H9).
B. Pneumonia.
C. Bronchitis.
D. Mononucleosis.
E. Respiratory syncytial virus (RSV).
F. Early HIV.
G. Severe acute respiratory syndrome (SARS).
H. Meningitis.

Plan
A. General interventions:
   1. Management usually focuses on treatment of symptoms and is supportive:
      a. Bed rest.
      b. Increased fluids.
      c. Antipyretics and analgesics for fever and myalgias.
      d. Encourage clients to stay home (self-isolate) if they become ill and avoid touching the eyes, nose, and mouth.
   2. Community precautions:
      a. Avoid close contact with those who are sick.
      b. Wash hands often or use alcohol-based hand gels.
      c. Use of face masks may be advisable or required.
      d. Droplet precautions should be used and maintained for seven days after onset of illness or until symptoms have resolved.
B. Pharmacological therapy:
   1. Coverage for the H1N1 swine flu is now included in the seasonal influenza vaccination currently available in Canada: an inactivated quadrivalent influenza vaccine (QIV), a live attenuated influenza vaccine (QLAIV), and five trivalent inactivated influenza vaccines (TIV). The influenza vaccine should be administered as prophylaxis before flu season (generally October to March). All clients older than 6 months should be encouraged to receive an annual flu vaccine, including pregnant women. The vaccine protection is generally achieved two weeks after vaccination and immunity lasts less than one year. Egg allergy is not a contraindication for influenza vaccination:
      a. The live attenuated influenza vaccine is available as a nasal mist is available for target age populations for use in children older than 2 years of age to the age of 59 years. Children aged 2 to 8 years who have never received an influenza vaccine require a second dose four weeks later.
      b. Children 6 to 23 months require an initial dose and a second dose four weeks later if they have never received an influenza vaccine before.
      c. Ages 2 years and older one dose, annually.
      d. Ages 65 years and over one dose, annually.
      e. For current information regarding the influenza vaccine, refer to the Canadian Immunization Guide.
   2. Antiviral therapy:

Antivirals started within the first 48 hours confer the greatest benefit.

   a. For current information, refer to *The use of antiviral drugs for influenza: Guidance for practitioners*.
   b. Neuraminidase inhibitors oseltamivir and zanamivir are used for both treatment and chemoprophylaxis of the H1N1 influenza A virus.
   c. The WHO recommends that clients with underlying medical conditions and pregnant women should receive treatment with oseltamivir or zanamivir as soon as possible after symptom onset without waiting for laboratory test results.
   d. Antiviral therapy recommendations vary by type of influenza, age group, renal function, and risk factor. In order to prescribe the most current antiviral therapy, refer to Government of Canada, Influenza (flu) for Health Professionals:
      www.canada.ca/en/public-health/services/diseases/flu-influenza/health-professionals.html#s6.

e. Oseltamivir should not be administered with an QLAIV within two weeks before or 48 hours after treatment.

3. Acetaminophen or ibuprofen as needed for fever and myalgia.

4. Health-care providers should refrain from recommending cough suppressants and OTC cough medicines for young children because of associated morbidity and mortality. The Centers for Disease Control and Prevention (CDC) noted in 2009 that, in response to safety concerns, manufacturers of cough and cold medications for children voluntarily changed labels stating that the medications should not be used for children younger than 4 years of age.

Follow-Up
A. Schedule a follow-up visit within seven to 10 days if symptoms do not improve.
B. Monitor client for pulmonary and neurologic complications.
C. The local and state health departments are the point of contact for information about current influenza activity.

Consultation/Referral
A. Refer the client to a neurologist for any complications.

Individual Considerations
A. Pregnancy:
  1. Pregnancy predisposes the client to an increased risk for influenzal pneumonia.
  2. Flu vaccine may be given to clients in high-risk populations. Because of the risk of influenzal pneumonia, it is recommended that pregnant women be vaccinated.
  3. Immunization of pregnant women is considered safe at any stage of pregnancy.
  4. Zanamivir is the first-line antiviral for pregnancy because of limited systemic absorption.
  5. Oseltamivir is used in pregnancy for women with asthma secondary to a higher risk for complications.
  6. Both oseltamivir and zanamivir are pregnancy category C drugs.
  7. Breastfeeding is not contraindicated during influenza.
B. Paediatrics:
  1. Influenza A/H1N1 vaccine should be offered/administered before flu season (as early as September) to children with asthma and chronic lung problems or those who are immunosuppressed.
  2. Infants who are ill with H1N1 influenza A should continue to breastfeed.
  3. ASA should not be given to children and young adults with viral illnesses before 21 years of age due to the increased risk of Reye's syndrome.
  4. Reye's syndrome has been associated primarily with influenza B, but it is also associated with influenza A infections.
  5. Amantadine hydrochloride and rimantadine hydrochloride are not effective against H1N1 infections and are not U.S. Food and Drug Administration (FDA) approved for use in children younger than 1 year.
C. Adults: Persons with high-exposure occupations, such as teachers, health-care workers, police, and firefighters, should consider yearly immunization. Vaccine should be offered/administered to persons with chronic metabolic diseases, renal dysfunction, HIV infection, and immunosuppression.

Resource
CDC: www.cdc.gov/flu/professionals
Government of Canada website: https://www.canada.ca/en/public-health/services/diseases/flu-influenza/health-professionals.html

Bibliography
Thorner, A. (2016). Treatment and prevention of pandemic H1N1 influenza ("swine influenza"). *UpToDate*. Retrieved from www.uptodate.com

Influenza (Flu)

Cheryl A. Glass, Jill C. Cash, and Jocelyn T. Whittier

Definition
Influenza is a common, acute, viral infection that is a self-limiting, febrile illness of the respiratory tract. Illness is spread person-to-person primarily by respiratory secretions that can be spread from infected persons through sneezing, coughing, talking, and self-inoculation of secretions through direct contact routes. Influenza is one of the top 10 causes of death in the Canada and the United States when it occurs with pneumonia.

Incidence/Prevalence
Epidemics occur yearly, primarily in the winter months, in both the northern and southern hemispheres. Travelers should be reminded that the flu season is different by hemisphere and can occur on cruise ships. Attack rates may be as high as 10% to 20% of the population. Mortality is highest in the geriatric population older than 65 years, except during pandemics, when 50% of influenza deaths occur in individuals younger than 65 years. Extraordinarily high attacks have occurred in the institutionalized and semiclosed populations.

Pathogenesis
A. Influenza A and B are viruses that have the ability to undergo periodic antigenic changes of their envelope glycoproteins, the haemagglutinin and neuraminidase. Among influenza A viruses that infect humans, there are three major subtypes of haemagglutinins (H1, H2, and H3) and two subtypes of neuraminidases (N1 and N2). Influenza A outbreaks typically start abruptly, peak over two to three weeks, and last approximately two to three months. H1N1 (swine flu) is an influenza A virus.
B. The avian flu was the N5N1 and H7N7 viral infection associated with recent exposure to dead or ill poultry. Following exposure, the incubation period for human H5N1 infection is seven days or less. Clusters of human-to-human transmission of avian flu had a typical incubation period of three to five days.
C. Influenza B outbreaks are generally less extensive and less severe. Outbreaks associated with the B virus have been reported in schools, military camps, nursing homes, and cruise ships.
D. *Haemophilus influenzae* is a gram-negative coccobacillus. *H. influenzae* is an invasive bacterial disease that can cause meningitis, otitis media, sinusitis, epiglottitis, septic arthritis, occult febrile bacteraemia, cellulitis, pneumonia, and empyema; occasionally, this virulent organism causes neonatal meningitis.
E. The incubation period for *H. influenzae* is between 18 and 72 hours to five days after exposure. The exact period of communicability for *H. influenzae* is unknown, but it may be for as long as the organism is present in the upper respiratory tract.

Predisposing Factors

The primary mode of spread is via exposure to viral strain respiratory secretions from respiratory droplets (coughing or sneezing) and direct contact of contaminated surfaces.
A. Adults:
 1. Aged older than 65 years (dependent on the viral strain).
 2. Pregnancy.
 3. High-exposure jobs: Teachers, health-care workers, police, and firefighters.
 4. Recent illnesses or state that has lowered resistance (stress, excessive fatigue, poor nutrition).
 5. Immunosuppression from drugs, illness, or chronic illness (transplant recipients, lung disease, heart disease, rheumatoid arthritis).
 6. Crowded living conditions, including military camps and institutions such as nursing homes.
 7. Travel in endemic areas.
 8. Avian flu: Exposure to dead or ill poultry.
B. Paediatrics:
 1. Chronic pulmonary disease, including bronchopulmonary dysplasia/chronic lung disease, asthma, cystic fibrosis, or any condition that compromises the respiratory function.
 2. Congenital heart disease or abnormalities.
 3. Children younger than five years.

Common Findings

A. Clinical manifestations of influenza depend on age and previous experience with the influenza virus. Children cannot verbalize symptoms such as myalgias and headache. Respiratory symptoms may be less prominent at the onset of illness in children and adults.
B. Rapid-onset respiratory illness is the most common complaint.
C. Abrupt onset of fever and/or chills (children tend to run higher fevers).
D. Joint pain.
E. Headache.
F. Conjunctivitis (avian flu).

Other Signs and Symptoms

A. Upper respiratory congestion (watery eyes, clear nasal drainage, headache, sore throat, and hoarseness).
B. Malaise or fatigue.
C. Anorexia.
D. Swollen lymph nodes.
E. Nonproductive cough (persisting for weeks).
F. Muscle aches.
G. Gastrointestinal (GI) symptoms (children tend to have more nausea, vomiting, and poor appetite).
H. Febrile seizures.
I. Otitis media.

Subjective Data

A. Review the onset, course, and duration of symptoms, especially myalgia and malaise.
B. Query the client when his or her last flu vaccination was received.
C. Review symptoms of other family members or coworkers who are also ill.
D. Check immunization status. For children, note whether *H. influenzae* b (Hib) vaccination is up-to-date.
E. Review for recent travel location and use of cruise ships/planes.
F. Evaluate living conditions for exposure risks.
G. Is the client a smoker?
H. Review all medications, including over-the-counter (OTC) and herbal products. Has the client taken any medications for the symptoms?
I. Does the client have a history of asthma or chronic obstructive pulmonary disease (COPD)?
J. Is the client immunocompromised (e.g., HIV, transplant recipient, chemotherapy)?
K. What other medical comorbidities, such as diabetes, does the client have?

Physical Examination

A. Check temperature, pulse, respirations, and blood pressure (BP):
B. Inspect:
 1. Observe overall appearance for pallor and for any respiratory distress.
 2. Assess hydration status.
 3. Conduct an eye, ear, nose, and throat examination.
 4. Children:
  a. Observe for seizure activity.
  b. Note level of activity (playful vs. lethargic).
C. Auscultate:
 1. Lung fields: Observe for wheezing and crackles.
 2. Heart.
D. Palpate:
 1. Neck.
 2. Lymph nodes: preauricular, posterior auricular, submental and sublingual, anterior cervical chain, and supraclavicular nodes.
E. Neurologic examination:
 1. Assess level of consciousness (LOC).
 2. Assess for nuchal rigidity.
 3. Assess for meningeal signs:
  a. Signs of meningeal irritation include nuchal rigidity.
  b. Positive Brudzinski's and Kernig's signs (refer to Figures 16.1 and 16.2):
   i. Brudzinski's sign: Place the client supine and flex the head upward. Resulting flexion of both hips, knees, and ankles with neck flexion indicates meningeal irritation.
   ii. Kernig's sign: Place the client supine. Keeping one leg straight, flex the other hip and knee to a bent knee to form a 90-degree angle. Slowly extend the lower leg. This places a stretch on the meninges, resulting in pain and spasm for the hamstring muscle. Resistance to further extension can be felt.

Diagnostic Tests

Usually none is required. However, if the client appears ill, consider the following:
A. Complete blood count (CBC; white blood cells [WBC]).
B. Viral RNA cultures: Obtain during the first 72 hours of illness because the quality of virus shed subsequently decreases rapidly. There is some evidence that a throat sampling yields an improved specimen. Nasopharyngeal secretions obtained by swab or aspirate should be placed in an appropriate transport medium for culture.
C. Rapid antigen test (usually less sensitive in the detection of influenza A than the polymerase chain reaction [PCR]; a negative rapid diagnostic test should be confirmed with a viral culture or other means).
D. Monospot test (monospot test is negative with the flu and positive with mononucleosis).

E. Chest x-ray (only if pneumonia is suspected).
F. Sputum culture (complications only).
G. Lumbar puncture (complications only).
H. Rapid plasma reagin (RPR) test (for high-risk HIV factors): Negative RPR to rule out syphilis.
I. PCR assay (can differentiate between influenza subtypes; it offers high sensitivity and specificity but is not readily available for clinical use).

Differential Diagnoses
A. Influenza:
  1. Influenza A (H1, H2, or H3 haemagglutinins with N1 or N2 neuraminidase subtypes).
  2. Influenza B (less antigenic changes than influenza A).
  3. Influenza C (acute respiratory illnesses in children and more rarely in adults).
  4. Avian flu (H5N1 and H7H9).
  5. H1N1 (swine flu).
B. Pneumonia.
C. Bronchitis.
D. Mononucleosis.
E. Respiratory syncytial virus (RSV).
F. Early HIV.
G. Severe acute respiratory syndrome (SARS).
H. Meningitis.

Plan
A. General interventions:
  1. Management is usually treatment of symptoms.
  2. Encourage flu vaccine for clients in susceptible populations before flu season.
  3. *H. influenzae*, including both type B and non–type B infection and cases in fully or partially immunized children, are reportable in Canada. See Chapter 1, Health Maintenance Guidelines, for Hib immunization information.
  4. Influenza-associated deaths are reportable provincially/territorially in Canada.
  5. Clients should expect to have a persistent cough and malaise after initial acute phase. Health-care providers should refrain from recommending cough suppressants and OTC cough medicines for young children because of associated morbidity and mortality. The Centers for Disease Control and Prevention (CDC) noted in 2009 that, in response to safety concerns, manufacturers of cough and cold medications for children voluntarily changed labels stating the medications should not be used for children younger than 4 years.
▶ B. lient teaching: *Refer to Client Teaching Guide: Influenza (Flu).*
C. Pharmacological therapy:

Influenza can alter the metabolism of certain medications, especially theophylline, possibly resulting in the development of toxicity from high serum concentrations.

  1. Acetaminophen as needed for fever.
  2. Nonsteroidal anti-inflammatory drugs (NSAIDs) are given as needed for body aches.
  3. Antivirals started within the first 48 hours confer the greatest benefit. Antiviral therapy recommendations vary by type of influenza, age group, renal function, and risk factor. In order to prescribe the most current antiviral therapy and for the most up-to-date recommendations, refer to the following:
  Government of Canada, Influenza (flu) for Health Professionals:
  www.canada.ca/en/public-health/services/diseases/flu-influenza/health-professionals-flu-influenza.html.
  Canadian Paediatric Society, *The use of antiviral drugs for influenza: Guidance for practitioners*: www.cps.ca/en/documents/position/antiviral-drugs-for-influenza.
  4. Zanamivir is not recommended for persons with underlying airway disease, including asthma or COPD.
  5. Vaccination:
    a. The Canadian Paediatric Society recommends annual influenza vaccination for all children aged 6 months to 18 years.
    b. For information regarding contraindications to vaccination, please access BC Centre for Disease Control, Communicable Disease Control Manual, Chapter 2, Immunization, Appendix C—Contraindications and Precautions for Immunization:
      www.bccdc.ca/resource-gallery/Documents/Guidelines%20and%20Forms/Guidelines%20and%20Manuals/Epid/CD%20Manual/Chapter%202%20-%20Imms/Appendix_C_ContraindicationsPrecautions.pdf.
    c. The vaccine should be administered in the autumn before the flu season, at least six weeks before the onset of the season.
    d. Immunization is the major means of influenza prevention. Each year the vaccine is produced with influenza strains. The vaccine may be trivalent or quadrivalent formulations.
    e. Two types of administration of the vaccine are available:
      i. Inactivated influenza vaccine (QIV), previously called trivalent inactivated vaccine (TIV), is administered intramuscularly (IM).
      ii. Quadrivalent live attenuated influenza vaccine (QLAIV) is administered intranasally.
      iii. A high-dose influenza vaccine is also available for adults older than 65 years.
    f. The recommended site of vaccination in adults and older children is the deltoid muscle. The anterolateral aspect of the thigh is the preferred site for flu vaccine for small children.
    g. Oseltamivir should not be administered with an QLAIV within two weeks before or 48 hours after treatment.

Follow-Up
A. Schedule a follow-up visit within seven to 10 days if symptoms do not improve.
B. Monitor the client for pulmonary and neurologic complications.
C. Local and provincial/territorial health departments are the points of contact for information about current influenza.

Consultation/Referral
A. Refer the client to a specialist or neurologist for any complications.

Individual Considerations
A. Pregnancy:

▶ Client Teaching Guides are available at https://connect.springerpub.com/content/reference-book/978-0-8261-9498-5

1. Pregnancy predisposes the client to an increased risk for influenzal pneumonia.
2. The flu vaccine may be given to clients in a high-risk population. Because of the risk of influenzal pneumonia, considerations should be given to vaccinating pregnant women when an epidemic threatens.
3. Immunization of pregnant women is considered safe at any stage of pregnancy. Inactivated vaccine is safe for breastfeeding mothers and their children.
4. Zanamivir is the first-line antiviral for pregnancy because of limited systemic absorption.
5. Oseltamivir is used in pregnancy for women with asthma secondary to a higher risk for complications.

B. Paediatrics:
1. Influenza vaccine should be offered/administered before flu season (as early as September) to children with asthma or chronic lung problems, or those who are immunosuppressed.
2. The most common paediatric complication of influenza is otitis media. However, in young infants, influenza can produce a sepsis-like picture and occasionally can cause croup or pneumonia.
3. ASA should not be given to children and young adults with viral illnesses before 21 years of age due to the increased risk of Reye's syndrome.
4. Reye's syndrome has been associated primarily with influenza B, but it is also associated with influenza A infections.

C. Adults: Persons with high-exposure occupations, such as teachers, health-care workers, police, and firefighters, should consider yearly immunization. Vaccine should be offered/administered to persons with chronic metabolic diseases, renal dysfunction, HIV infection, and immunosuppression.

D. Geriatrics:
1. Influenza vaccine is recommended yearly for clients over the age of 60 years. The vaccine should be offered to nursing home residents, especially those with a history of cardiopulmonary disease. Factors that contribute to more severe infections include decreased lung compliance and decreased respiratory muscle strength.
2. Pneumococcal pneumonia and influenza are significant causes of mortality and morbidity in the elderly.

Resource:
Government of Canada. (2018, October 25). *Flu (influenza): For health professionals.* Retrieved from https://www.canada.ca/en/public-health/services/diseases/flu-influenza/health-professionals-flu-influenza.html#s6

Bibliography
Canadian Paediatric Society. (2018a). *Caring for kids: Influenza vaccine.* Retrieved from www.caringforkids.cps.ca/handouts/influenza_vaccine

Canadian Paediatric Society. (2018b). *2017 results: Canadian paediatric surveillance program.* Retrieved from www.cpsp.cps.ca/uploads/publications/CPSP-2017-Results_1.pdf

Centers for Disease Control and Prevention. (2016a). *ACIP votes down use of LAIV for 2016–2017 flu season.* Retrieved from www.cdc.gov/media/releases/2016/s0622-laiv-flu.html

Centers for Disease Control and Prevention. (2016b). *Frequently asked flu questions 2016–2017 influenza season.* Retrieved from www.cdc.gov/flu/about/season/flu-season-2016-2017.htm

Centers for Disease Control and Prevention. (2016c). *Immunizations and pregnancy vaccines chart.* Retrieved from www.cdc.gov/vaccines/pregnancy/pregnant-women/index.html

Centers for Disease Control and Prevention. (2016d). *Influenza (flu).* Retrieved from www.cdc.gov/flu

Centers for Disease Control and Prevention. (2018, August 23). *Influenza (Flu). Information for health professionals.* Retrieved from www.cdc.gov/flu/professionals/index.htm

Dolin, R. (2018). Epidemiology of influenza. *UptoDate.* Retrieved from https://www.uptodate.com/contents/epidemiology-of-influenza

Government of Canada. (2018a, May 1). Public Health Agency of Canada. An Advisory Committee Statement (ACS), National Advisory Committee on Immunization (NACI). *Canadian Immunization Guide Chapter on Influenza and Statement on Seasonal Influenza Vaccine 2018-2019.* Retrieved from: https://www.canada.ca/en/public-health/services/publications/vaccines-immunization/canadian-immunization-guide-statement-seasonal-influenza-vaccine-2019-2020.html

Government of Canada. (2018b, October 25). *Flu (influenza): For health professionals.* Retrieved from: https://www.canada.ca/en/public-health/services/diseases/flu-influenza/health-professionals.html

Journal Watch Specialties. (n.d.). *FluMist: Intranasal flu vaccine.* Retrieved from infectious-diseases.jwatch.org/cgi/content/full/2003/808/3

Russell, K., Blanton, L., Kniss, K., Mustaquim, D., Smith, S., Cohen, J., & Burns, E. (2016). Update: Influenza activity—United States, October 4, 2015—February 6, 2016. *Morbidity & Mortality Weekly Report, 65*(6), 146–153. doi:10.15585/mmwr.mm6506a3

Sanfort, C., Pottinger, P., & Jong, E. (2017). *The travel and tropical medicine manual* (5th ed.). London: Elsevier.

Zachary, K. (2018). Treatment of seasonal influenza in adults. *UptoDate.* Retrieved from www.uptodate.com

Kawasaki Disease (KD)

Cheryl A. Glass, Jill C. Cash, and Jocelyn T. Whittier

Definition
A. Kawasaki disease (KD) is an acute febrile illness associated with generalized vasculitis. It was formerly known as mucocutaneous lymph node syndrome. KD has an incidence of 30 per 100,000 children under 5 years in Canada. It is the leading cause of acquired heart disease in children in North America. Death results from myocardial infarction with coronary occlusion due to thrombosis or progressive stenosis. Approximately 75% of fatalities occur within six weeks of the onset of symptoms, but myocardial infarction and sudden death can occur months to years after the acute episode.

B. Although a febrile seizure may occur, there is no evidence that links KD with autism or a long-term seizure disorder.

C. Long-term prognosis is unknown. Second episodes rarely occur in previously affected children. Cardiac problems are the primary cause of morbidity and mortality from pericardial effusion, myocarditis, aneurysms, ectasia (coronary artery larger than normal for the child's age), and myocardial infarction. Canadian guidelines align with the American Heart Association (AHA) guidelines, which stratify KD by its risk of myocardial infarction:
1. Risk Level I—normal coronary arteries on all imaging studies.
2. Risk Level II—transient coronary artery ectasia or dilation that resolves by eight weeks after disease onset.
3. Risk Level III—small to medium coronary artery aneurysms.
4. Risk Level IV—large (>6 mm) aneurysms and coronary arteries with multiple complex aneurysms without obstruction.
5. Risk Level V—coronary artery aneurysms with obstruction documented on angiography.

D. For children presenting with a rash and a persistent fever (greater than five days), the diagnosis of KD should be held at the forefront for workup for confirmation of KD secondary to the long-term cardiovascular sequelae. Diagnostic criteria: Diagnosis of typical syndrome requires fever of at least five days duration, plus four of the following:
1. Mucous membrane changes (red cracked lips and strawberry tongue).
2. Extremity changes.

3. Cervical lymphadenopathy of at least 1 cm in size is the least consistent feature of KD. When present, it tends to involve the anterior cervical nodes overlying the sternocleidomastoid muscle.
4. Rash.
5. Bilateral nonexudative conjunctivitis: Present in more than 90% of clients.

Incidence/Prevalence
A. Peak age of occurrence in the North America is between 18 and 24 months. Approximately 80% of clients are younger than 5 years. Children older than 8 years rarely have the disease. KD has been noted worldwide and affects all races. Approximately 2% of clients experience KD a second time months to years later.
B. Approximately one in five children will develop coronary artery aneurysms.
C. The risk of myocardial infarction is greatest the first two years after onset of KD.

Pathogenesis
A. Aetiology is unknown; it may be caused by viruses or bacteria such as Group A *Streptococci*. A microbial agent is favoured because of the disease's acute, self-limited course and community-wide outbreaks.
B. The incubation period is unknown.

Predisposing Factors
A. Age: children younger than age 5 years.
B. Gender: incidence higher in boys than in girls (2:1).
C. Asian and Pacific Island ancestry.
D. Siblings of children with KD (possibly genetic).
E. Epidemics generally occur during the winter and spring seasons.

Common Findings
A. Long-term fever (one to two weeks) that does not respond to antibiotics. The fever ranges from 38°C to above 40°C. Fever may rise and fall for up to three weeks.
B. Bilateral bulbar conjunctival injection without exudate.
C. Red, tender hands and soles of feet on days three to five-following fever.

Classic finding is swollen, indurated, erythematous, and tender palms. Desquamation of the fingers and toes occurs approximately one to two weeks after onset of the fever, and a deep groove may cross the nails (Beau's lines).

D. Cracked, red, dry lips; tongue may appear coated, slightly swollen, and look like a strawberry; mouth ulcers.
E. Irritability.
F. Decreased food/fluid intake.
G. One or more gastrointestinal symptoms (e.g., vomiting, diarrhoea, abdominal pain).
H. One or more respiratory symptoms (e.g., rhinorrhoea, cough).

Other Signs and Symptoms
A. Tachycardia (disproportionate to fever), gallop rhythms, and ECG changes, including sinus tachycardia, QRS/QT prolongation, diffuse T-wave inversions, ventricular arrhythmias, and atrioventricular (AV) conduction defects, are suggestive of myocarditis.
B. Pericarditis (often subclinical): Coronary aneurysms have been detected as early as three days after onset of symptoms, but in most cases they appear one to two weeks later. Carditis can occur at any time during the first three weeks of illness and generally resolves by six to eight weeks.
C. Polymorphous rash that may be maculopapular, scarlatiniform, morbilliform, erythema marginatum, or rarely vesiculopustular; frequently confluent in the perineum, where it undergoes desquamation. Rash involves the entire body, especially in the perineal region.
D. Swollen cervical lymph node(s). Client may have a singular enlarged lymph node, usually a cervical node, up to 1.5 cm.
E. Joint pain.
F. Weakness.
G. Urethritis with sterile pyuria (70% of cases).
H. Mild anterior uveitis (25%–50% of cases).
I. Arthritis or arthralgia.
J. Photophobia.

Subjective Data
A. Review onset, course, and duration of symptoms, especially fever.
B. Elicit the initial site of the rash and the progression to other body areas.
C. Determine whether the client has had any new medication and contact exposures.
D. Rule out other family members with similar symptoms.
E. Review the client's history for recent strep infection.
F. Take a thorough history of symptoms and medication or treatment type and duration.

Physical Examination
A. Check temperature, pulse, respirations, and blood pressure (BP).
B. Inspect:
  1. Inspect skin, especially hands, feet, and nails:
    a. Rash: polymorphous that may be maculopapular, scarlatiniform, morbilliform, erythema marginatum, or rarely vesiculopustular; frequently confluent in the perineum. (Bullae and pustules are not diagnostic of KD.).
    b. The rash involves the entire body; only the face is spared.
    c. Fine desquamation in the groin area can occur in the acute phase.
    d. Check the nail beds for detachment (periungal lifting) and transverse grooves across the finger and toenail beds (Beau's lines).
    e. Observe for facial swelling.
  2. Conduct a thorough eye examination:
    a. Bilateral bulbar conjunctival injection without exudate.
  3. Conduct a thorough ear and nose examination.
  4. Perform an oral examination:
    a. Red fissured lips with oedema.
    b. Tongue may appear coated and slightly swollen (generally in the first four to five days): strawberry tongue after the membrane is shed.
    c. Posterior pharynx and palate: erythematous.
  5. Check hydration status.
C. Auscultate:
  1. Heart: A persistent resting tachycardia and the presence of an S3 gallop are often noted.
  2. Lungs.
D. Palpate:
  1. Palpate the lymph nodes, especially the cervical area:

a. Primarily noted in the anterior cervical nodes overlying the sternocleidomastoid muscles.
b. Size: at least 1.5 cm.
c. Lymphadenopathy is the least common clinical symptom, but may be present and most prominent in an older child.
2. Check the joints for swelling and tenderness.
3. Males: Check for testicular swelling.
4. Evaluate for splenomegaly.

Diagnostic Tests

No laboratory study proves diagnosis; diagnosis rests on clinical features and exclusion of the other illnesses in the differential diagnosis:
A. Complete blood count (CBC) with differential: neutropaenia.
B. Erythrocyte sedimentation rate (ESR): elevated.
C. C-reactive protein (CRP): elevated.
D. Uric acid.
E. Platelet count: elevated platelet count (one week after onset).
F. Serum transaminase: elevated.
G. Serum albumin.
H. Specialty tests: quantitative serum immunoglobulins, antinuclear antibody (ANA), rheumatoid factor (RF), Venereal Disease Research Laboratory (VDRL) test, immune complexes, and complement levels.
I. Urinalysis: proteinuria and sterile pyuria.
J. Echocardiogram.
K. ECG.
L. Angiography may be needed.
M. Chest radiograph.

Differential Diagnoses

A. Streptococcal scarlet fever.
B. Rubeola.
C. Cat scratch fever.
D. Drug reaction.
E. Rocky Mountain spotted fever (RMSF).
F. Infectious mononucleosis.
G. Toxic shock syndrome.
H. Other febrile viral exanthemas.
I. Syphilis.
J. Lyme disease.
K. Juvenile rheumatoid arthritis.
L. Stevens–Johnson syndrome.
M. Staphylococcal scalded skin syndrome.
N. Adenovirus.

Plan

A. General interventions:
1. The most severe sequela is the development of a coronary artery aneurysm; therefore, prevention and early detection are important.
2. Initial therapy should be started within 10 days of illness, which reduces the risk of coronary artery aneurysm fivefold. Management is initially aimed at reducing inflammation.
3. Use of intravenous immunoglobulin (IVIG) therapy has drastically reduced the incidence and morbidity and mortality of cardiovascular aneurysm.
B. Client teaching:
1. Teach parents which signs and symptoms indicate when to contact the office: arthralgias, chest pain, and palpitations.
2. Disease is not communicable by means of person-to-person contact; therefore, clients do not need to be isolated from other family members.
C. Pharmacological therapy:
1. Canadian Paediatric Society (CPS) recommends the following: IVIG within the first seven to 10 days of the illness to shorten the duration of fever and decrease the frequency of coronary artery aneurysms and other abnormalities. **IVIG is considered the gold standard for treatment of KD**.
2. Up to 20% of clients who receive the IVIG single infusion and ASA may have a recurrent fever and require retreatment with IVIG within 24 to 48 hours of persistent fever.
3. The CPS recommends initial use of ASA until afebrile. The maximum ASA dose should not be exceeded. Then ASA should be given daily for six to eight weeks for its antiplatelet action.
4. ASA is continued until laboratory markers for acute inflammation (e.g., platelet count and ESR) return to normal, unless cardiac abnormalities are detected by echo.
5. ASA should be rapidly discontinued upon exposure to or sign of varicella or influenza due to the increased risk of Reye's syndrome.
6. Analgesic and antipyretic medications, such as acetaminophen or ibuprofen, as needed for pain and inflammation.
7. The role of glucocorticoids remains unclear for treatment of KD.
8. Scheduled routine immunizations of inactivated childhood vaccines may be given at recommended intervals except for live virus vaccines such as varicella-containing vaccines and measles for children who have received IVIG. Varicella and measles vaccination may be given for an outbreak if the child's exposure is high and as long as the vaccination is repeated in at least 11 months after administration of IVIG.
9. Ibuprofen should be avoided in children taking ASA because it may antagonize the antiplatelet effect of the ASA.

Follow-Up

A. The prognosis of clients following KD depends on the severity of cardiac involvement. Refer the client to a paediatric cardiologist for follow-up.

Consultation/Referral

A. Consult with a specialist if fever persists longer than five days and KD is suspected.
B. Refer all affected children to a paediatric cardiologist for coronary artery evaluation.
C. Long-term management of KD is based on the extent of coronary artery abnormalities—risk level.

Individual Considerations

A. Paediatrics:
1. Most children are hospitalized for diagnostic evaluation and supportive care. Older children with mild disease may be managed on an outpatient basis.
2. Yearly influenza vaccination is indicated in clients six months to 18 years of age who require long-term ASA therapy, because there is an increased risk for children taking ASA of development of Reye's syndrome.

3. Children should have limited physical activity during convalescence. Restrictions should be prescribed by the cardiologist.

Resources
AHA Scientific Statement: Diagnosis, treatment, and long-term management of KD. Available at: circ.ahajournals.org/content/110/17/2747.full.pdf+html

The Canadian Paediatric Surveillance Program: https://www.cpsp.cps.ca/uploads/publications/Highlights-kawasaki-disease.pdf

KD Foundation: www.kdfoundation.org

Bibliography
Gewitz, M. H., Baltimore, R. S., Tani, L. Y., Sable, C. A., Shulman, S. T., Carapetis, J., . . . American Heart Association Committee on Rheumatic Fever, Endocarditis, and Kawasaki Disease of the Council on Cardiovascular Disease in the Young. (2015). Revision of the Jones criteria for the diagnosis of acute rheumatic fever in the era of Doppler echocardiography: A scientific statement from the American Heart Association. *Circulation, 131*, 1806–1818. doi:10.1161/CIR.0000000000000205

Kawasaki Disease Foundation. (n.d.). Retrieved from https://kdfoundation.org/

Newburger, J. W., Masato, T., Burns, J. C., & Takahashi, M. (2016). Kawasaki disease. *Journal of the American College of Cardiology, 67*(14), 1738–1749. doi:10.1016/j.jacc.2015.12.073

O'Connell, J., & Sloand, E. (2013). Kawasaki syndrome and streptococcal scarlet fever: A clinical review. *Journal of Nurse Practitioners, 9*, 259–264.

Rowley, A. H., & Ryan. S. F. (2013). Kawasaki disease. *Clinician Reviews, 23*, 34–38. Retrieved from https://www.mdedge.com/clinicianreviews/article/82991/cardiology/kawasaki-disease

Succimarri, R., & Yeung, R. (2014). Kawasaki Disease: Hight index of suspicion needed in a febrile child. *Paediatrics and Child Health, 19*, 239–240. Retrieved from https://www.ncbi.nlm.nih.gov/pmc/articles/PMC4029235/

Sundel, R. (2016). Kawasaki disease: Clinical features and diagnosis. *UpToDate*. Retrieved from www.uptodate.com

Lyme Disease

Cheryl A. Glass, Jill C. Cash, and Jocelyn T. Whittier

Definition
A. Lyme disease is a multisystem infection that may be acute or chronic. Lyme disease is the leading vector-borne disease in the United States.

B. Morbidity from Lyme disease usually involves neurologic/cognitive dysfunction and rheumatic conditions, causing arthralgias. Approximately 15% to 55% of untreated or inadequately treated clients develop some post-Lyme disease symptoms. Posttreatment Lyme disease syndrome (PTLDS) includes cognitive disturbances, fatigue, joint/muscle pain, headaches, hearing loss, vertigo, mood disturbances, paresthesias, and difficulty sleeping.

C. Proposed criteria for PTLDS include the presence of fatigue, musculoskeletal pain, and/or cognitive difficulties within six months of the diagnosis and persistence of symptoms for at least six months after completion of accepted antibiotic therapy.

Incidence/Prevalence
A. Lyme disease is currently endemic in six provinces in Canada (British Columbia, Manitoba, Ontario, Quebec, New Brunswick, and Nova Scotia). There is a seasonal increase between the months of April and October; more than 50% of cases occur in June and July. In North America, the incidence is highest among children aged 5 to 9 years and in adults aged 45 to 54 years.

Pathogenesis
A. *Borrelia burgdorferi*, a spirochete bacterium, is the infectious agent and is carried by the *Ixodes* black-legged ticks and western black-legged ticks. Vector transmission is usually from the deer tick to humans. Rodents and pets can also harbour deer ticks.

B. The spirochete enters the bloodstream at the time of tick feeding. The incubation period is three to 32 days, or about one to three weeks after bite. Late manifestations occur several months to more than one year later.

Predisposing Factors
A. People of all ages are affected.
B. Recreational exposure:
  1. Hiking.
  2. Golfing.
  3. Hunting.
  4. Soccer.
C. Gardening.
D. Exposure to rodents such as field mice and domestic pets, which may also carry the ticks.

Common Findings
A. Flu-like symptoms.
B. Fatigue.
C. Headache.
D. Joint pain.

Other Signs and Symptoms
A. Stage 1: Acute (early localized):
  1. Rash: Erythema migrans.

About 80% of infected persons develop a characteristic expanding erythematous rash, erythema migrans. It usually begins as a red macule at the site of the tick bite and spreads out to form a large annular lesion with red secondary outer rings, an intense red outer border (measuring at least 5 cm), and some clearing at the site of the bite. Appearance is a "bull's-eye" shape. The lesion is generally painless and not pruritic.

  2. Body aches.
  3. Fever or chills.
  4. Swollen lymph nodes.
B. Stage 2: Disseminated infection (early disseminated):
  1. Malaise, debilitating fatigue.
  2. Headache.
  3. Photophobia.
  4. Mild neck stiffness.
  5. Joint or muscle pain.
  6. Migratory arthralgia.
  7. Rash: diffuse erythema.
  8. Itching.
  9. Transient heart block:
     a. In 5% to 10% of cases, clients have cardiac involvement: a transient heart block ranging from asymptomatic, first-degree atrioventricular (AV) block to complete heart block with fainting. Cardiac phase lasts three to six weeks.
  10. Bell's palsy:
     a. A unilateral or bilateral Bell's palsy is the most common cranial nerve deficit.
  11. Mild encephalopathy.

C. Stage 3: Chronic (late disease):
1. Prolonged arthritis:
   a. Approximately 60% of complaints evolve into frank arthritis. Onset of arthritis is variable but averages six months from the time of initial infection. The knee is the most common site and the pattern continues to be oligoarticular.
2. Chronic neurologic deficits.
3. Distal paresthaesia.
4. Radicular pain.
5. Memory loss.

Subjective Data

A. Review the onset, course, and duration of symptoms.
B. Ask the client about any recent outdoor activities, such as camping, hiking, gardening, or other activities. Less than half of the people infected remember a tick bite. A history of a tick bite is not necessary for diagnosis.
C. Have other family members had similar symptoms?
D. Review thorough history of medications.
E. Review any history of rash and course of spread.
F. Rule out late symptoms associated with Lyme disease, such as arthritis, memory loss, and distal paresthaesia.
G. Has the client been previously treated for Lyme disease or Rocky Mountain spotted fever (RMSF)?

Physical Examination

A. Check temperature, pulse, respirations, and blood pressure (BP).
B. Inspect:
1. Observe general overall appearance.
2. Observe rash pattern and type.
3. Inspect the skin; observe for target-like pattern (bull's-eye appearance).
C. Palpate:
1. Palpate the lymph nodes and mastoid bones.
2. Examine the joints for tenderness, swelling, and range of motion.
D. Auscultate heart and lungs.
E. Neurologic examination: Evaluate for signs of meningeal irritation by means of Brudzinski's sign and Kernig's signs (refer to Figures 16.1 and 16.2):
1. Brudzinski's sign: Place the client supine and flex the head upward. Resulting flexion of both hips, knees, and ankles with neck flexion indicates meningeal irritation.
2. Kernig's sign: Place the client supine. Keeping one leg straight, flex the other hip and knee to a bent knee to form a 90-degree angle. Slowly extend the lower leg. This places a stretch on the meninges, resulting in pain and spasm for the hamstring muscle. Resistance to further extension can be felt.

Diagnostic Tests

A. Complete blood count (CBC) with differential.
B. Sedimentation rate.
C. Serum antibody (enzyme-linked immunosorbent assay [ELISA]) testing for *B. burgdorferi* (not present for several weeks).
D. Western blot if ELISA is positive.
E. Lyme titre or culture for spirochete (after 20 days of signs and symptoms).
F. Arthrocentesis for joint effusion.
G. Polymerase chain reaction (PCR) testing.
H. Alanine aminotransferase (ALT) and aspartate aminotransferase (AST; may be mildly elevated).
I. Creatine phosphokinase.
J. Lumbar puncture indicated for the presence of manifestations of meningitis.

Differential Diagnoses

A. Insect or spider bite.
B. RMSF.
C. Cellulitis.
D. Arthritis.
E. Bacterial meningitis.
F. Chronic fatigue syndrome (CFS).
G. Viral syndrome.
H. Nummular eczema.
I. Tinea corporis (ringworm).

Plan

A. General interventions:
1. Prophylactic therapy after a tick bite is generally not advised. It takes 24 hours from the time of tick contact with the skin to transmit the spirochete.
2. Start prophylactic treatment with doxycycline for tick bites that are "swollen."
3. Wait for the development of symptoms (e.g., erythema migrans) and treat promptly if the client becomes symptomatic.
4. There is no evidence of the existence of "chronic Lyme disease." Some symptoms (fatigue, arthralgia, headaches) may last for several months; however, long-term antibiotic treatment has not proven to be effective and can contribute to a host of other adverse problems.
B. Client teaching:
1. *Refer to Client Teaching Guide: Lyme Disease and Removal of a Tick.*
2. Not all neurologic signs and symptoms may completely resolve (such as headache, photophobia, Bell's palsy, and third-stage symptoms).
3. Clients with active Lyme disease should not donate blood because spirochetaemia occurs in early Lyme disease. Clients who have been treated for Lyme disease in the past can be considered for blood donation.
4. Nonspecific symptoms may persist for months after treatment of Lyme disease; there is no evidence that the complaints represent ongoing active infection or need repeated antibiotics:
   a. Headache.
   b. Fatigue.
   c. Arthralgias.
C. Pharmacological therapy:
1. Early localized Lyme disease:
   a. Doxycycline: Caution client regarding photosensitivity.
   b. Amoxicillin.
   c. Cefuroxime.
2. Lyme carditis:
   a. Ceftriaxone.
   b. Penicillin.
3. Neurologic manifestations:
   a. Facial nerve paralysis: Use oral regimen for early disease for 21 to 28 days.
   b. Lyme meningitis:
      i. Ceftriaxone.
      ii. Penicillin.

▶ Client Teaching Guides are available at https://connect.springerpub.com/content/reference-book/978-0-8261-9498-5

c. Possible alternative for Lyme meningitis: doxycycline.
4. Lyme arthritis:
   a. Same oral regimen as early localized Lyme disease for a total of 28 days.
   b. Ceftriaxone.
   c. Penicillin.
5. Pregnant women:
   a. For localized early Lyme disease, amoxicillin.
   b. For disseminated early Lyme disease or any manifestation of late disease, penicillin G.
   c. For asymptomatic seropositivity, no treatment is necessary.
6. The Jarisch–Herxheimer reaction, with increased fever, chills, and malaise, can occur transiently when antibiotic therapy is initiated. Nonsteroidal anti-inflammatory drugs (NSAIDs) may be beneficial, and the antimicrobial agent should be continued.

Follow-Up
A. Follow-up depends on the stage of disease.
B. Repeat Lyme titre in one to two months to determine the need for continuation of antibiotic therapy.

Consultation/Referral
A. Referral to an infectious diseases specialist is indicated when the client with strong clinical evidence of Lyme disease fails to respond to prescribed antibiotics.
B. Consultation with an infectious diseases specialist is particularly important for those clients with refractory neurologic deficits or debilitating arthritis.
C. Consultation with a rheumatologist is needed for clients with persistent arthritis or fibromyalgia occurring after Lyme disease.

Individual Considerations
A. Pregnancy:
1. Maternal–fetal transmission of infection with subsequent injury to the fetus has been reported. Antibiotic treatment should be instituted promptly in symptomatic clients.
2. Tetracyclines are contraindicated in pregnancy. Otherwise, therapy is the same as for nonpregnant persons.
3. There is no causal relationship between maternal Lyme disease and congenital malformations.
4. There is no evidence that Lyme disease can be transmitted in breast milk.

B. Paediatrics:
1. Erythema migrans is the most common manifestation of Lyme disease in children.
2. Carditis occurs rarely in children.
3. The Canadian Paediatric Society (CPS) recommends that children not be exposed to products containing more than 10% N, N-diethyl-m-toluamide (DEET). The CPS recommends that insect repellents should not be applied to children younger than six months due to potential neurotoxicity; age six months to two years, no more than 10% DEET only once a day; age two to 12 years, no more than 10% DEET up to three times a day; and over 12 years, up to 30% DEET.
4. The CPS also recommends that insect repellents not be used around children younger than 6 months.
5. DEET repellent should not be applied to children's hands.
6. Lyme disease is a reportable disease in Canada.

Resources
American Lyme Disease Foundation: www.aldf.comlymedisease.org
American Lyme Disease Foundation. Lyme Disease Tick Map [Mobile application software]. Retrieved from www.aldf.com/lyme-disease
Canadian Paediatric Society: Lyme disease https://www.cps.ca/en/documents/position/lyme-disease-children
Government of Canada (2018, December 12). For health professionals: Lyme disease. https://www.canada.ca/en/public-health/services/diseases/lyme-disease/health-professionals-lyme-disease.html

Bibliography
Canadian Paediatric Society. (2018). *Insect repellents: How to protect your child from insect bites.* Retrieved from www.caringforkids.cps.ca/handouts/insect_repellents
Canadian Paediatric Society. (2019). *Lyme disease in Canada: Focus on children.* Retrieved from www.cps.ca/en/documents/position/lyme-disease-children
Centers for Disease Control and Prevention. (2015a). *Lyme disease.* Retrieved from www.cdc.gove/lyme/treatment/index.html
Centers for Disease Control and Prevention. (2015b). *Tick removal.* Retrieved from www.cdc.gov/ticks/removing_a_tick.html
Hu, L. (2018). Clinical manifestations of Lyme disease in adults. *UpToDate.* Retrieved from www.uptodate.com
Meyerhoff, J. O. (2014). Lyme disease. *Medscape.* Retrieved from emedicine.medscape.com/article/330178-overview
Sanchez, E., Vannier, E., Wormser, G. P., & Hu, L. T. (2016). Diagnosis, treatment and prevention of Lyme disease, human granulocytic anaplasmosis, and babesiosis: A review. *Journal of the American Medical Association, 315*(16), 1767–1777. doi:10.1001/jama.2016.2884
Sanfort, C., Pottinger, P., & Jong, E. (2017). *The travel and tropical medicine manual* (5th ed.). London, England: Elsevier.
Shapiro, E. D. (2016). Lyme disease: Clinical manifestations in children. *UpToDate.* Retrieved from www.uptodate.com
Wormser, R. J., Dattwyler, E. D., Shapiro, J. J., Halperin, A. C., Steere, A. C., Klempner, M. S., . . . Nadelman, R. B. (2006). The clinical assessment, treatment, and prevention of Lyme disease, human granulocytic anaplasmosis, and babesiosis: Clinical Practice Guidelines by the Infectious Diseases Society of America. *Clinical Infectious Disease, 43*(9), 1089–1134.

Meningitis

Cheryl A. Glass, Jill C. Cash, and Jocelyn T. Whittier

Definition
A. Meningitis is an acute inflammation of the meninges, or membranes lining the brain and spinal cord. A virus or noninfectious insult, such as blood in the subarachnoid space, causes aseptic meningitis. Three baseline clinical features have been independently associated with an adverse outcome: hypotension, altered mental status, and seizures.
B. Vaccines are available for three types of bacteria that cause meningitis:
1. *Neisseria meningitidis*: Polysaccharide or conjugate vaccines are available.
2. *Streptococcus pneumoniae*: pneumococcus vaccine.
3. *Haemophilus influenzae type b*: Hib vaccine.

C. Bacterial meningitis is a severe infection with associated complications including brain damage, hearing loss, neurologic/learning disabilities, and digit or limb amputations. Mortality rate varies in part with the organism and if it is a nosocomial or a community-acquired infection.

Incidence/Prevalence
In Canada, invasive bacterial meningitis had an average incidence of 0.58 cases per 100,000 population between 2006 and 2011. The incidence rates were highest among infants less than one year of age (average 7.35 cases per 100,000), followed by one- to four-year-olds (1.89 cases per 100,000), and 15- to 19-year olds (1.17 cases per 100,000). It is also

considered to be one of the top 10 infectious causes of death. It is estimated that meningococcal meningitis, which is the bacterial form, can cause severe brain damage and is fatal in 50% of cases that are not treated. The most common organisms causing bacterial meningitis are presented here.
A. Neonates:
1. Group B *Streptococcus* (GBS).
2. *Escherichia coli*.
3. *Listeria monocytogenes*.
B. Ages two to 18 years:
1. *N. meningitidis* with portal entry in the nasopharynx.
2. *S. pneumoniae*.
3. *H. influenzae* type b.
4. Remaining cases are caused by GBS and *L. monocytogenes*.
C. Adults up to age 60 years:
1. *S. pneumoniae*.
2. *N. meningitidis*.
3. *H. influenzae*.
4. *L. monocytogenes*.
5. GBS.
D. Adults 60 years and older:
1. *S. pneumoniae*.
2. *L. monocytogenes*.
3. *N. meningitidis*.

Acute meningitis due to infectious causes usually does not recur. However, a small number of clients with acute meningitis may develop recurrent attacks between intervals of good health. Chronic meningitis is arbitrarily defined as meningitis lasting four weeks or more.

Pathogenesis
A. An acute inflammation of the meninges can be caused by *S. pneumoniae*, GBS *H. influenzae, L. monocytogenes, N. meningitidis*, gonococci (rare), *Mycobacterium tuberculosis, E. coli*, pol herpes, Gram-positive anaerobes, and *Bacteroides*, and as a sequela of Lyme disease and varicella (chickenpox).
B. The incubation period is variable, depending on the pathogen, usually one to 10 days. Transmission occurs from person-to-person through droplets from the respiratory tract and requires close contact.

Predisposing Factors
A. Peak demographics:
1. Children four years of age or younger (the peak attack rate is younger than one year).
2. Adolescents.
3. Freshman college/university students living in dormitories.
B. Attendance at day care, school, camps, and the military.
C. Sequela of Lyme disease.
D. Odontogenic infection.
E. Sequela of otitis media, bacterial sinusitis, *H. influenzae* type B infection, and varicella.
F. Sickle cell disease, asplenia, Hodgkin's disease, and antibody deficiencies.
G. Review history for sexually transmitted and HIV infection.
H. Penetrating wound, head trauma, spinal tap, surgery, or anatomic abnormality.
I. Occupational exposure, such as laboratory personnel.
J. Travel exposure.
K. Maternal infection and fever at the time of delivery.
L. Lumbar epidural steroid injections.
M. Immunosuppression.

Common Findings
A. Classic triad:
1. Nuchal rigidity.
2. Fever.
3. Altered mental status.

Other Signs and Symptoms
A. Neonates or infants:
1. Decreased level of consciousness (LOC).
2. High-pitched cry.
3. Irritability, inconsolability.
4. Fever and/or temperature instability.
5. Poor feeding and/or vomiting.
6. Bulging fontanelles.
7. Seizures.
8. Respiratory distress syndrome.
9. Hypotonia.
B. Children or adults:
1. Sudden onset of a severe, constant headache affecting the entire head that worsens with movement; central nervous system (CNS) symptoms (nuchal rigidity, nausea and/or vomiting, confusion, lethargy, decreased LOC).
2. Fever or chills.
3. Backache.
4. Photophobia.
5. Difficulty swallowing.
6. Facial and eye weakness and sagging eyelids.
7. Seizures.
8. Rash: The type of rash (macular, maculopapular, petechial, or purpuric) is dependent on the virus/organism.
9. Anorexia.
C. Chronic meningitis: Usually have subacute onset of symptoms including fever, headache, and vomiting.

Subjective Data
A. Review the onset, course, and duration of symptoms, including a progressive petechial or ecchymotic rash.
B. Determine current or recent history of ear infections, upper respiratory infection (URI), sinus infection, and chickenpox exposure.
C. Ask the client about any recent dental procedures, extractions, and gum procedures.
D. Review the client's recent history of tick bite and any treatments.
E. Review the client's recent history of Hib immunization.
F. Evaluate a history of serious drug allergies.
G. Evaluate a history of recent head trauma/fracture.
H. Evaluate full history for ventriculoperitoneal shunt and other cranial surgery/procedures.
I. Review history for use of lumbar epidural steroid injections for pain.
J. Review all medications, including over-the-counter (OTC) and herbal products. Determine recent use of antibiotics.
K. Review for a history of illicit drug use, especially the intravenous (IV) route.
L. Review any recent travel locations.
M. Neonates: Review pregnancy, labour, and delivery history for treatment for GBS.

Physical Examination
A. Check temperature, pulse, respirations, and blood pressure (BP).

B. Inspect:
  1. Observe general overall appearance.
  2. Examine the skin for the presence of a petechial or ecchymotic rash.
  3. Complete an ear, nose, and throat examination.
  4. Examine mouth and teeth for dental diseases and disorders.
  5. Assess the client for dehydration.
  6. Observe the client for seizure activity.
  7. Assess level of pain.
  8. Inspect for cranial nerve palsies.
C. Auscultate:
  1. Lungs, monitor breathing pattern.
  2. Heart.
D. Palpate:
  1. Neck: Palpate the lymph nodes.
  2. Head: Palpate the fontanelle in children.
  3. Palpate the mastoid bones.
  4. Abdominal examination: haepatosplenomegaly.
E. Neurologic examination:
  1. Perform a complete neurologic examination.
  2. Evaluate for signs of meningeal irritation by means of positive Brudzinski's and Kernig's signs:
    a. Brudzinski's sign: Place the client supine and flex the head upward. Resulting flexion of both hips, knees, and ankles with neck flexion indicates meningeal irritation (refer to Figures 16.1 and 16.2).
    b. Kernig's sign: Place the client supine. Keeping one leg straight, flex the other hip and knee to a bent knee to form a 90degree angle. Slowly extend the lower leg. This places a stretch on the meninges, resulting in pain and spasm for the hamstring muscle. Resistance to further extension can be felt.

Diagnostic Tests

The definitive diagnosis is from bacteria isolated from cerebrospinal fluid (CSF) and the presence of elevated protein and low glucose in the CSF.

A. Lumbar puncture to obtain CSF for analysis:
  1. Gram stain.
  2. Absolute neutrophil count.
  3. CSF protein.
  4. CSF glucose.
  5. Culture and sensitivity.
  6. White blood cells (WBCs [pleocytosis]).
B. Laboratory tests:
  1. Complete blood count (CBC) with differential.
  2. Metabolic panel, including electrolytes, glucose, urea, and liver profile.
  3. Coagulation profile.
  4. Platelet count.
  5. Blood cultures × 2.
C. Cultures of petechial or purpuric lesion scraping and synovial fluid.
D. MRI or CT scan, with and without contrast (a screening CT is not necessary in the majority of the clients).

Differential Diagnoses

A. Meningitis:
  1. Bacterial aetiology.
  2. Viral aetiology.
  3. Fungal aetiology.
  4. Aseptic meningitis.
  5. Chronic meningitis.
B. Neonatal sepsis or pneumonia.
C. Lyme disease.
D. Herpes.
E. Dementia.
F. Gonorrhoea.
G. Otitis media.
H. Dental abscess.
I. Chickenpox.
J. Sinusitis.
K. Mastoiditis.
L. Intracranial abscess.
M. Encephalitis.
N. Subarachnoid haemorrhage.

Plan

A. General interventions:
  1. Treat aggressively because the progression of disease is often rapid. Antibiotic therapy should be initiated immediately after blood cultures are drawn and the results of the lumbar puncture if the clinical suspicion is high.
  2. Dexamethasone should be given shortly before or at the same time as the antibiotics if clinical/laboratory evidence suggests bacterial meningitis.
  3. Maintain hydration.
  4. In addition to standard precautions, droplet precautions are recommended until 24 hours after initiation of effective antimicrobial therapy.
  5. Chemoprophylaxis is warranted for people who have been exposed directly to a client's oral secretions through close social contact, such as sharing of toothbrushes or eating utensils as well as childcare and preschool contact within seven days before the onset of the disease in the index case. Throat and nasopharyngeal cultures are of no value in deciding who should receive chemoprophylaxis and are not recommended.
  6. Airline travelers with eight hours of contact seated directly next to an infected person should receive prophylaxis.
B. Client teaching:
  1. If a child suddenly develops a severely stiff neck along with fever and irritability, he or she needs medical help immediately.
  2. Advise close contacts of the client with meningococcal and *H. influenzae* meningitis that prophylactic treatment with rifampin may be indicated; they should check with their health-care providers or the local public health department.
C. Pharmacological therapy:
  1. Dexamethasone therapy should be considered when bacterial meningitis in infants and children (older than one month) is diagnosed or strongly suspected on the basis of the CSF tests, *H. influenzae type B* meningitis, and pneumococcal or meningococcal meningitis:
    a. Dexamethasone should be administered 15 to 20 minutes before the first dose of antibiotics.
  2. Antibiotic therapy: Broad-spectrum coverage should be initiated until culture results are available. The doses vary by the organism. All antibiotics should be administered IV for at least seven days. Empiric therapy may require adjustment after the culture results:
    a. Cefotaxime and ceftriaxone are commonly used as empiric therapy with *S. pneumoniae, N. meningitidis*, and *H. influenzae*. Vancomycin may be added to cefotaxime or ceftriaxone if renal function is normal until culture and susceptibility results are available.
    b. Listeria has traditionally been treated with ampicillin or penicillin G, and gentamicin may be added for its synergistic effect.

c. *Pseudomonas aeruginosa* is often resistant to most commonly used antibiotics. Ceftazidime has been the most consistently effective cephalosporin therapy.

3. Chemoprophylaxis in adults includes rifampin, ceftriaxone, ciprofloxacin, and azithromycin.

4. Vaccinations: For current information regarding meningococcal vaccinations, refer to the Canadian Immunization Guide:

www.canada.ca/en/public-health/services/publications/healthy-living/canadian-immunization-guide-part-4-active-vaccines/page-13-meningococcal-vaccine.html#p4c12t1.

Polysaccharide (alone or conjugate) meningococcal vaccines are licensed in Canada. Two types of vaccines protect against meningococcal serogroups A, C, W, and Y: meningococcal polysaccharide vaccine and meningococcal conjugate vaccine.

Follow-Up

A. Have the client return to the clinic in two to three days if conditions (e.g., otitis media) are not significantly improved with antibiotic therapy.

B. Follow-up is dependent on symptoms. Schedule a return visit after completion of antibiotics or two to three weeks after initial examination.

C. Sequelae associated with meningococcal disease occur in 11% to 19% of clients:
   1. Hearing loss.
   2. Neurologic disability.
   3. Digit or limb amputations.
   4. Skin scarring.

D. Invasive meningococcal disease is a reportable disease in Canada. All presumptive, probable, and confirmed cases should be reported.

Consultation/Referral

A. Neonate: Consult with a neonatologist if the client is younger than three months. Neonates need hospitalization.

B. Child: Consult with a paediatrician:
   1. Exceptions: localized, nonserious infections. Child should be active, playful, drinking, and voiding.
   2. The child needs immediate consultation with a paediatrician if lethargic and inconsolable.

Individual Considerations

A. Pregnancy:
   1. Advances in Labour and Risk Management (ALARM) lists the following indications for selective intrapartum chemoprophylaxis in GBS-positive women:
      a. Preterm labour and delivery.
      b. Preterm rupture of membranes.
      c. Rupture of membranes greater than 18 hours before delivery.
      d. Intrapartum fever.
      e. Multiple gestation.
      f. Previous offspring with invasive GBS disease.
   2. Maternal: Culture introital or vaginal and anorectal samples for GBS, using a selective medium such as Todd–Hewitt broth. Vaginal colonization of GBS occurs in 5% to 40% of pregnant women, of whom 40% to 70% transmit GBS to their offspring.
   3. The most significant problem associated with pregnancy is exposure of the fetus to GBS in the maternal genital tract. The Society of Obstetricians and Gynaecologists of Canada (SOGC) recommends universal perinatal screening for vaginal and rectal GBS colonization at 35 to 37 weeks' gestation.
   4. Treat clients with positive urine culture only because recolonization occurs frequently. Antibiotics should be administered to women in labour for preterm labour, premature rupture of membranes, positive GBS cultures (past or present), and preterm premature rupture of membranes in labour.

B. Paediatrics:
   1. Neonatal sepsis occurs in approximately 1% to 2% of cases. The incidence of invasive Hib disease in Canada after vaccine introduction is 0.08 cases per 100,000 population (2006–2012).
   2. Neonatal GBS infections *usually* present as early onset in the first two days of life and as late onset in newborns up to three months of age.
   3. The premature neonate is at the highest risk for development of symptomatic neonatal disease.
   4. Neonates often appear normal at delivery, only to develop a fulminant infection with rapid deterioration. Because of the severity and fulminant course of neonatal GBS infections, the primary focus is on preventing the vertical transmission of the organism.
   5. Infants up to two years old may have meningitis without a stiff neck.
   6. All infants with meningitis should undergo careful follow-up examinations, including tests for hearing loss and neurologic abnormalities.

C. Adults: Immunization with the pneumococcal vaccine has been shown to decrease the incidence of bacterial meningitis.

D. Geriatrics: increased mortality rate for these clients secondary to the comorbid conditions.

Bibliography

Advances in Labour and Risk Management. (2016). *Group B Streptococcus*. Retrieved from https://www.jogc.com/article/S1701-2163(18)30495-X/abstract

Canadian Paediatric Society. (2018). *2017 results: Canadian paediatric surveillance program*. Retrieved from www.cpsp.cps.ca/uploads/publications/CPSP-2017-Results_1.pdf

Centers for Disease Control and Prevention. (2015). *Meningococcal disease*. Retrieved from www.cdc.gov/meningococcal/about/prevention.html

Centers for Disease Control and Prevention. (2016). *Vaccine information statement: Meningococcal ACWY vaccines (MenACWY and MPSV4) VIS*. Retrieved from www.cdc.gov/vaccines/hcp/vis/vis-statements/mening.html

Domingo, P., Pomar, V., de Benito, N., & Coll, P. (2013). The spectrum of acute bacterial meningitis in elderly patients. *BMC Infectious Diseases, 13*, 108. doi:10.1186/1471-2334-13-108

Government of Canada. (2015, February 19). *Invasive Meningococcal disease: For health professionals*. Retrieved from https://www.canada.ca/en/public-health/services/immunization/vaccine-preventable-diseases/invasive-meningococcal-disease/health-professionals.html

Government of Canada. (2018a, November 18). *Canadian immunization guide: Part 4–Active Vaccines. Meningococcal vaccines*. Retrieved from: https://www.canada.ca/en/public-health/services/publications/healthy-living/canadian-immunization-guide-part-4-active-vaccines/page-13-meningococcal-vaccine.html

Government of Canada. (2018b, November 19). *Canada's Provincial and Territorial Routine (and Catch-up) Vaccination Routine Schedule Programs for Infants and Children*. Retrieved from: https://www.canada.ca/en/public-health/services/provincial-territorial-immunization-information/provincial-territorial-routine-vaccination-programs-infants-children.html

Hasbun, R. (2014). Meningitis. *Medscape*. Retrieved from emedicine.medscape.com/article/232915-overview

Hemmert, A. C., & Gilbreath, J. J. (2016). The current state of diagnostics for meningitis and encephalitis. *Medical Laboratory Observer, 48*(7), 12–14.

Sanfort, C., Pottinger, P., & Jong, E. (2017). *The travel and tropical medicine manual* (5th ed.). London: Elsevier.

Tunkel, A. R. (2018). Clinical features and diagnosis of acute bacterial meningitis in adults. *UpToDate*. Retrieved from www.uptodate.com

World Health Organization. (2015). *Meningococcal meningitis fact sheet*. Retrieved from www.who.int/mediacentre/factsheets/fs141/en/

Mononucleosis (Epstein–Barr)

Cheryl A. Glass, Jill C. Cash, and Jocelyn T. Whittier

Definition
A. Infectious mononucleosis is an acute, infectious viral disease caused by Epstein–Barr virus (EBV). EBV is also known as human herpesvirus 4. There are three classic symptoms: fever, pharyngitis, and lymphadenopathy. The spread is via intimate contact between susceptible persons and asymptomatic EBV shedders through the passage of saliva.
B. Oral shedding may occur for six months after the onset of symptoms before its latency phase.
C. The fatigue related to EBV may last several months.

Incidence/Prevalence
A. Antibodies to EBV have been demonstrated in all population groups with a worldwide distribution. Approximately 90% to 95% of adults are EBV seropositive. Incidence is unknown; it occurs primarily in adolescents and young adults. The peak incidence of infection is noted in the 15- to 24-year age range. The majority of clients with primary EBV recover uneventfully.

Pathogenesis
A. EBV, human herpesvirus 4, is the primary agent of infectious mononucleosis. EBV persists asymptomatically for life in nearly all adults and is associated with the development of B-cell lymphomas, T-cell lymphomas, and Hodgkin's lymphoma in certain clients.
B. The incubation period is 30 to 50 days, with an average of 11 days; it is communicable during the acute phase, which may be prolonged. Acute symptoms resolve in one to two weeks. Pharyngeal excretion may persist for up to 18 months following clinical recovery. It is estimated that once infected with EBV, the virus may be intermittently shed in the oropharynx for decades.
C. EBV has also been isolated both in the cervix and in male seminal fluid, suggesting the possibility of sexual transmission.
D. EBV has also been noted in breast milk.

Predisposing Factors
A. Age 12 to 40 years, with peak incidence between 15 and 24 years of age.
B. Exposure through oropharyngeal secretions (kiss, cough, shared food).
C. Roommates.
D. Intrafamilial transmission to siblings.

Common Findings
A. Infectious mononucleosis is characterized by the following triad of symptoms:
  1. Fever.
  2. Tonsillar pharyngitis (with exudate possibly having a white, gray–green, or necrotic appearance).
  3. Lymphadenopathy (usually posterior cervical chains, typically symmetric).

Other Signs and Symptoms
A. Fatigue: May be persistent and severe.
B. Generalized aches.
C. Appetite loss.
D. Headache.
E. Hepatosplenomegaly: Mild hepatitis is encountered in approximately 90% of individuals; splenomegaly is noted in approximately 50%. Jaundice is uncommon.
F. Otitis media (infants and children).
G. Abdominal complaints and diarrhoea (infants and children).
H. Upper respiratory symptoms (more prominent in young infants).

Subjective Data
A. Review signs, symptoms, and course and duration of symptoms, specifically the triad of pharyngitis, fever, and lymphadenopathy.
B. Assess the client for recent upper respiratory infection (URI) and sore throat.
C. Inquire about any contact with persons known to have mononucleosis and other infections such as strep infections.
D. Review the client's history for other family members with similar symptoms.
E. Carefully review medications. A mononucleosis syndrome with atypical lymphocytosis can be induced by drugs, including the following:
  1. Phenytoin.
  2. Carbamazepine.
  3. Antibiotics (e.g., isoniazid, minocycline).

Physical Examination
A. Check temperature, pulse, respirations, and blood pressure.
B. Inspect:
  1. Conduct ear, nose, and throat examination, especially tonsils and palate:
    a. Pharynx shows lymphoid hyperplasia, erythema, and oedema.
    b. Tonsillar exudates are present in about 50% of the cases.
    c. Tonsillar pillars may touch ("kissing tonsils") and may lead to airway compromise.
    d. Evaluate for petechiae at the junction of the hard and soft palate.
    e. Evaluate for oral hairy leukoplakia (OHL) on the lateral portions of the tongue. OHL appears as white corrugated painless plaques that cannot be scraped from the surface (EBV-related malignancies as well as HIV may present with OHL).
C. Auscultate heart and lungs.
D. Palpate:
  1. Lymph nodes, especially anterior and posterior cervical chains, axilla, and groin. Firm, tender, and mobile lymph nodes are indicative of mononucleosis; lymphadenopathy is usually symmetric and presents in the posterior cervical chain more than the anterior chain.
  2. Abdomen, especially the spleen. Splenomegaly is noted in 50% of cases. Haepatomegaly and tenderness are noted in 10% of cases.
E. Percuss abdomen, especially the spleen area.
F. Neurologic examination: Evaluate for facial nerve palsy or symptoms of meningitis. See section "Meningitis" in this chapter.

Diagnostic Tests

A. White blood cell (WBC) count with differential and a heterophile test.

A positive heterophile antibody test is diagnostic of EBV.

B. Throat swab for rapid strep; if negative, send for culture.
C. Monospot test is not recommended for general use. Results may reflect a false positive/negative result. Results do not confirm the absence of EBV infection since the heterophile antibodies detected by this test are often not present in children.
D. Viral capsid antigen (VCA):
   1. Anti-VCA immunoglobulin M (IgM): Appears early and disappears in four to six weeks.
   2. Anti-VCA immunoglobulin G (IgG): Appears in the acute phase of infection, peaks at two to four weeks, declines, and remains positive for a person's lifetime.
   3. EBV nuclear antigen: Performed by immunofluorescent test, not sensitive early in acute phase but appears two to four months after onset and remains positive for life.
   4. Elevated antibody levels are not diagnostic of recent infection and can be present for years.
E. Cold agglutinin titre is markedly elevated in the setting of haemolysis (>1:1,000).
F. Liver function tests: Abnormal liver function tests in a client with pharyngitis strongly suggest the diagnosis of infectious mononucleosis (80%–90% of cases have elevated liver enzymes).
G. Abdominal ultrasound is performed if indicated for splenomegaly.

Differential Diagnoses

A. Streptococcal pharyngitis (Group A beta-haemolytic *Streptococcus*).
B. Viral syndrome.
C. Hodgkin's disease.
D. Hepatitis.
E. Cytomegalovirus (CMV).
F. Secondary syphilis.
G. Chronic fatigue syndrome (CFS).
H. Acute HIV.
I. Toxoplasmosis.
J. Adenovirus.
K. Rubella.
L. Acute HIV.
M. Human herpesvirus type 6 (HHV-6; roseola).
N. HHV-7.

Plan

A. General interventions:
   1. Make certain that the client does not have an upper airway obstruction from enlarged tonsils and lymphoid tissue.
   2. Treat concurrent infections.
   3. Isolation is not required with good handwashing and prevention of the spread of pharyngeal secretions.
   4. Bed rest is unnecessary.
   5. There is no commercially available vaccine to prevent EBV infection.
   6. Splenic rupture is rare but potentially life threatening, occurring in one to two cases per 1,000. It occurs between the fourth and 21st day of symptomatic illness, but can be the presenting symptom. The typical manifestations are abdominal pain and/or a falling haematocrit.
B. Client teaching:
   1. *Refer to Client Teaching Guide: Mononucleosis.*
   2. Prolonged communicability may persist for up to one year.
C. Pharmacological therapy:
   1. Acyclovir is not recommended for infectious mononucleosis.
   2. Antibiotic therapy is reserved for concurrent infections such as streptococcal pharyngitis.
   3. Administer analgesics, such as acetaminophen or nonsteroidal anti-inflammatory drugs (NSAIDs), for fever, body aches, and malaise.
   4. Corticosteroids may be considered in the presence of overwhelming infections, including mononucleosis-related airway obstruction, or other complications, such as severe haemolytic or aplastic anaemia.

Follow-Up

A. Examine the client every one to two weeks.
B. Initial monospot test may be negative.
C. If splenomegaly is present, schedule an appointment to reevaluate the client before the release for contact sports. Splenomegaly puts clients at risk for rupture secondary to blunt trauma (e.g., sports and motor vehicle accidents).
D. Clients with the classic triad symptoms of mononucleosis should also have a diagnostic test for strep, since the presenting symptoms are so similar.

Consultation/Referral

A. Consult a specialist for marked tonsil enlargement and difficulty swallowing or symptoms lasting longer than two weeks. An emergent consultation with an otolaryngologist may be required.

Individual Considerations

A. Pregnancy: Intrauterine infection with EBV is rare.
B. Paediatrics: Primary EBV in young infants and children is common and frequently asymptomatic. Ampicillin and penicillin may cause morbilliform rashes.
C. Geriatrics: Older adults may not present with the classic triad of symptoms:
   1. Lymphadenopathy is not as common with older clients.
   2. Pharyngitis and myalgia are the most frequent complaints.
   3. Fever may be prolonged, lasting several weeks.

Bibliography

Aronson, M. D., & Auwaeter, P. G. (2016). Infectious mononucleosis in adults and adolescents. *UpToDate*. Retrieved from https://www.uptodate.com/contents/infectious-mononucleosis

Centers for Disease Control and Prevention. (2014). *About Epstein–Barr virus (EBV)*. Retrieved from www.cdc.gov/epstein-barr/about-ebv.html

Cunha, B. A. (2015). Infectious mononucleosis. *Medscape*. Retrieved from emedicine.medscape.com/article/222040-overview

Saccomano, S. J., & Ferrara, L. R. (2013). Infectious mononucleosis. *Clinician Reviews*, 23, 42–49. Retrieved from https://www.mdedge.com/clinicianreviews/article/81448/infectious-diseases/infectious-mononucleosis

Salvaggio, M. R. (2013). Human herpesvirus 6 infection differential diagnoses. *Medscape*. Retrieved from emedicine.medscape.com/article/219019-differential

Mumps

Cheryl A. Glass, Jill C. Cash, and Jocelyn T. Whittier

Definition
A. Mumps is an acute systemic viral illness. The viral illness is self-limited. Humans are the only natural host to the mumps virus. Mumps is highly contagious for clients who are not immune by vaccination or through maternal antibodies.
B. The hallmark sign of mumps is the unilateral swelling of one or more salivary glands. The parotid glands are typically involved unilaterally, then bilaterally. The swelling is visible under the ears and chin.
C. Mumps is spread by respiratory droplets, saliva, direct contact, or fomites. Current literature indicates that clients should be isolated for approximately five days from the onset of symptoms.
D. Central nervous system (CNS) involvement is the most common extrasalivary complication of mumps. Meningitis and encephalitis from mumps have a good prognosis and usually resolve with complete recovery.
E. There is no specific treatment for mumps except supportive therapy; mumps is most often treated on an outpatient basis.
F. Immunization: The vaccine is a live attenuated measles–mumps–rubella (MMR) vaccine or the measles–mumps–rubella–varicella (MMRV). For current information regarding mumps vaccination, refer to the Canadian Immunization Guide: Part 4—Active Vaccines—Mumps.
www.canada.ca/en/public-health/services/publications/healthy-living/canadian-immunization-guide-part-4-active-vaccines/page-14-mumps-vaccine.html.
For current information regarding routine schedules for vaccination in the provinces and territories, refer to:
www.canada.ca/en/public-health/services/provincial-territorial-immunization-information/provincial-territorial-routine-vaccination-programs-infants-children.html.
  1. Common side effects of the MMR vaccination include low-grade fever, skin rash, itching, hives, redness and swelling at the immunization site, and weakness.
  2. Severe adverse side effects of the MMR vaccination include seizures; encephalopathy; thrombocytopaenia; joint, muscle, and nerve pain; gastrointestinal (GI) disorders; and conjunctivitis.
  3. MMR vaccine may be given with other vaccines at different injection sites and given in separate syringes.

Incidence/Prevalence
A. Mumps occurs worldwide.
B. Males and females are affected equally with parotitis.
C. Symptomatic meningitis is more common in males (3:1 ratio over females).

Pathogenesis
A. Mumps is caused by the *Rubulavirus*, a specific RNA virus. *Rubulavirus* is in the genus *Paramyxovirus* and is a member of the Paramyxoviridae family. The *Rubulavirus* shares morphologic features with the human parainfluenza; however, there is no cross-immunity between the two.
B. Mumps shares characteristics with other paediatric illnesses, including measles and rubella.
C. Mumps has an incubation of 16 to 18 days. Incubation can be as early as seven days and as late as 23 days. Infectious period is approximately three days before to nine days after the onset of symptoms. The illness lasts an average of seven to 10 days.

Predisposing Factors
A. Lack of immunization.
B. International travel.
C. Immune deficiencies.
D. Age groups:
  1. Primary school ages.
  2. High school ages.
  3. College ages.
  4. Occupational exposure.
E. Crowded settings, such as day care and military bases.

Common Findings
A. Asymptomatic (20%–30%).
B. Prodromal symptoms may last three to five days and include the following:
  1. Low-grade fever.
  2. Headache.
  3. Anorexia.
  4. Malaise.
  5. Myalgias.
C. About 48 hours after the prodromal period, the most common symptom is parotitis (30%–40%) caused by the direct viral infection of the ductal epithelium:
  1. Unilateral initially, then bilateral parotitis:
     a. Tenderness/pain with pressure.
     b. Oedema (may last for 10 days).
  2. Males:
     a. Unilateral orchitis (uncommon in males under 10 years of age, but occurs in 33% of postpubertal males).
     b. Bilateral orchitis occurs only in about 10% of cases.
     c. Orchitis develops within one to two weeks of parotitis.
     d. High fever.
     e. Severe testicular pain accompanied by swelling and scrotal erythema.
     f. Nausea, vomiting, and abdominal pain with orchitis.
  3. Females: oophoritis (7%).
  4. Aseptic meningitis (usually presents within the first week after parotid swelling):
     a. Headache.
     b. Fever.
     c. Nuchal rigidity.
     d. Nausea and vomiting.

Other Signs and Symptoms
A. Earache on the same side as the parotitis.
B. Acute pancreatitis (5% incidence):
  1. Abdominal distention.
  2. Pain.
  3. Fever (usually low grade).
  4. Nausea and vomiting.
C. Thyroiditis.
D. Mastitis.
E. Encephalitis (five cases per 1,000 mumps cases).

Potential Complications
A. Meningitis.
B. Encephalitis.
C. Gonadal atrophy (20%–50% in postpubertal males).
D. Sterility (rare).
E. Guillain–Barré syndrome.
F. Sensorineural deafness (0.5–5 cases per 100,000 cases):
  1. Up to 20% is bilateral deafness.
  2. Often deafness is permanent.

G. Impaired renal function/glomerulonephritis.
H. Miscarriage if pregnant.

Subjective Data
A. Review the onset and duration of symptoms.
B. Rule out similar symptoms in other family members.
C. Review the client's immunization history.
D. Determine any new contact exposures.
E. Determine whether the client is pregnant.
F. Ask client to list all medications, including over-the-counter (OTC) and herbal products.

Physical Examination
A. Check temperature, pulse, respirations, and blood pressure (BP).
B. Inspect:
  1. Visually inspect the face, under/behind the ears, and chin for oedema.
  2. Conduct an ear, nose, throat, and mouth examination.
  3. Make a visual inspection of the scrotum.
C. Palpate:
  1. Palpate the parotid glands.
  2. Palpate the neck and lymph glands, especially the cervical chains.
  3. Palpate the abdomen.
  4. Gently palpate the scrotum.
D. Auscultate:
  1. Lungs (at risk for pneumonia).
  2. Heart (at risk for myocarditis).
E. Neurologic examination:
  1. Assess hearing (may be unilateral loss).
  2. Evaluate for signs of meningeal irritation by means of Brudzinski's and Kernig's signs. How to perform and note positive Brudzinski's and Kernig's signs (refer to Figures 16.1 and 16.2):
    a. Brudzinski's sign: Place the client supine and flex the head upward. Resulting flexion of both hips, knees, and ankles with neck flexion indicates meningeal irritation.
    b. Kernig's sign: Place the client supine. Keeping one leg straight, flex the other hip and knee to a bent knee to form a 90-degree angle. Slowly extend the lower leg. This places a stretch on the meninges, resulting in pain and spasm for the hamstring muscle. Resistance to further extension can be felt.

Diagnostic Tests
A. Serum amylase level increase supports the diagnosis.
B. Serum lipase.
C. Mumps immunoglobulin M (IgM) and immunoglobulin G (IgG; not required if the client has a classic presentation of parotitis).
D. Other tests as indicated for presenting symptoms of complications.

Differential Diagnosis
A. Cytomegalovirus (CMV).
B. Parainfluenza virus 1 and 3.
C. Influenza A.
D. HIV.
E. Bacterial infection.
F. Drug reaction.
G. Coxsackievirus.
H. Epstein-Barr virus (EBV).
I. Adenovirus.
J. Bacterial infections, particularly *Staphylococcus aureus*.

Plan
A. General interventions:
  1. There is no medication prescribed for the mumps.
  2. Symptomatic treatment recommended for comfort.
  3. Clients with complications, such as severe nausea/vomiting, may be hospitalized for intravenous (IV) hydration.
  4. Monitor for severe complications such as meningitis or pancreatitis. Hospitalization may be required.
  5. Notify the local public health department of active cases of the mumps.
B. Client teaching.
  1. The Canadian Paediatric Society recommends that infected children not attend school/childcare until five days after parotid swelling begins to subside.
  2. Stress universal precautions. The mumps virus can be found in the saliva, throat, and urine of the person infected:
    a. Practice good handwashing techniques.
    b. Use droplet precautions: Cover the mouth and nose with a tissue when coughing and sneezing and dispose of the tissue immediately.
    c. Do not share food or drink with the person with mumps.
  3. Encourage rest.
  4. Apply warm or cold packs to parotid gland for comfort.
  5. Add scrotal elevation/support and ice pack compresses.
C. Dietary management:
  1. There is no special diet for the mumps. However, one should avoid acidic fluids and liquids, such as orange juice. Acid-containing foods may cause pain and difficulty swallowing with parotitis.
  2. Encourage drinking of fluids.
D. Pharmacological therapy:
  1. Antiviral agents are not indicated for the mumps.
  2. Immunoglobulin has not been shown to be effective as a postexposure therapy.
  3. Analgesics, such as acetaminophen or ibuprofen, are prescribed for headache and parotitis.

Follow-Up
A. Follow-up is determined by client's needs, severity of symptoms, and the presence of complications.
B. Mumps is a reportable disease in Canada. Notify the local health department if mumps occurs in a childcare setting. Persons exempted from vaccination for medical, religious, or other reasons should be excluded for school/day care until at least 26 days after the onset of parotitis in the last person with mumps in the affected family.

Consultation/Referral
A. Consult with a specialist for evaluation and need for hospital admission for complications.

Individual Considerations
A. Pregnancy:
  1. There is no evidence that the mumps causes congenital abnormalities.
  2. Vaccinated women should avoid pregnancy for three months after immunization.

3. Termination of pregnancy is not indicated if the MMR vaccination is given during pregnancy.
B. Paediatric: Infants born to mothers who have mumps a week before delivery may have clinically apparent mumps at birth or mumps may develop in the neonatal period.

Bibliography

Albrecht, M. A. (2016). Epidemiology, clinical manifestations, diagnosis and management of mumps. *UpToDate*. Retrieved from http://www.uptodate.com/contents/epidemiology-clinical-manifestations-diagnosis-and-management-of-mumps

Canadian Paediatric Society. (2018). *2017 results: Canadian paediatric surveillance program*. Retrieved from www.cpsp.cps.ca/uploads/publications/CPSP-2017-Results_1.pdf

Centers for Disease Control and Prevention. (2016). *Immunizations and pregnancy vaccines chart*. Retrieved from www.cdc.gov/vaccines/pregnancy/pregnant-women/index.html

Defendi, G. L. (2014). Mumps. *Medscape*. Retrieved from reference.medscape.com/article/966678-overview

Government of Canada. (2018a, July 26). *Canadian immunization guide: Part 4-Active vaccines. Mumps vaccine*. Retrieved from https://www.canada.ca/en/public-health/services/publications/healthy-living/canadian-immunization-guide-part-4-active-vaccines/page-14-mumps-vaccine.html

Government of Canada. (2018b, November 19). *Canada's Provincial and Territorial Routine (and Catch-up) Vaccination Routine Schedule Programs for Infants and Children*. Retrieved from: https://www.canada.ca/en/public-health/services/provincial-territorial-immunization-information/provincial-territorial-routine-vaccination-programs-infants-children.html

National Vaccine Information Center. (n.d.). *Quick facts mumps*. Retrieved from www.nvic.org/vaccines-and-diseases/Mumps.aspx

Sanfort, C., Pottinger, P., & Jong, E. (2017). *The travel and tropical medicine manual* (5th ed.). London: Elsevier.

Parvovirus B19 (Fifth Disease, Erythema Infectiosum)

Cheryl A. Glass, Jill C. Cash, and Jocelyn T. Whittier

Definition

A. Parvovirus B19, also known as "fifth disease," is considered one of the TORCH (toxoplasmosis, other [e.g., hepatitis and syphilis], rubella, cytomegalovirus, and herpes) infections.
B. In children, parvovirus B19 can cause erythema infectiosum (EI), a mild febrile illness with rash. EI is also referred to as "fifth disease" since it represents one of six common childhood exanthems, each named in the order of dates they were first described. In contrast, clients with underlying haemolytic disorders can develop a transient aplastic crisis (TAC). Parvovirus B19 is an acute, communicable, viral infection that is spread by means of respiratory droplet and transplacental transmission. It can be associated with chronic haemolytic anaemia and, in pregnancy, has been associated with nonimmune fetal hydrops and fetal death in 2% to 6% of cases.
C. Parvovirus B19 is the only infectious cause of TAC in over 80% of clients with sickle cell disease.
D. The polyarthropathy associated with parvovirus B19 typically lasts one to three weeks; however, the arthritis may be prolonged and parvovirus should be considered in the differential diagnosis of newly diagnosed rheumatoid arthritis.
E. Parvovirus B19 rash may be confused with rubella.
F. There is no vaccine that can prevent parvovirus B19 infection.

Incidence/Prevalence

A. Parvovirus B19 is extremely common, but the true incidence is unknown. Parvovirus occurs worldwide. It is more common in children, and outbreaks are more usual in late winter and early spring. Up to 60% of the infections occur during school. Because <1% of teachers who are pregnant during EI outbreaks are expected to experience an adverse fetal outcome, exclusion of pregnant women from employment in childcare or teaching is not recommended.

Pathogenesis

A. Human parvovirus B19 belongs to the *Erythrovirus* genus within the Parvoviridae family. Human parvovirus B19 is a DNA virus with preference to erythroid precursor cells. The virus replicates in the erythroid progenitor cell of the bone marrow and blood, leading to inhibition of erythropoiesis, which can result in symptoms of anaemia. The parvovirus-associated rash is presumed to be at least partially immune mediated.
B. The incubation period for initial symptoms to develop is four to 14 days after exposure; the rash usually lasts five days, but it can last as long as 21 days. Parvovirus B19-specific immunoglobulin M (IgM) antibodies are detected at days 10 to 12 and can persist for up to five months. Rash and joint symptoms occur two to three weeks after acquisition of infection.
C. The annual seroconversion rate among pregnant women without parvovirus B19 is 1.5%.

Predisposing Factors

A. The only known host for parvovirus B19 is humans.
B. Exposure to school-aged (through junior high) and daycare populations.
C. Occupational exposure for teachers (20%), day-care workers and homemakers (9% each), and health-care workers.
D. Exposure to close contact or crowded conditions.

Common Findings

A. Clinical presentation is influenced by the infected individual's age and haematologic and immunologic status.
B. Approximately 25% of infected individuals are asymptomatic, and 50% have nonspecific flu-like symptoms of malaise, muscle pain, and fever.
C. Classic symptoms:
  1. Red rash on the face that spreads to the rest of the body. Erythematous, macular rash on cheeks produces "slap-cheek" pattern.
  2. Arthritis: Joint pain most frequently affects the hands, followed by the knees and wrists. Joint symptoms are more common in adults and may be the sole manifestation of infection. Joint pain is more common in women. The arthritis associated with acute parvovirus B19 infection does not cause joint destruction.
  3. Oedema.

Other Signs and Symptoms

A. Adults: Chronic arthropathy.
B. Children:
  1. Bright red rash on cheeks; may be confused with rubella.
  2. Maculopapular rash on trunk and extremities; may be pruritic.
  3. Circumoral pallor.
  4. Malaise.
  5. Headache.
  6. Sore throat and pharyngitis.

7. Conjunctivitis.
  8. Diarrhoea.
 C. Foetus:
  1. Nonimmune hydrops fetalis.
  2. Stillbirth.
  3. Anaemia.

Subjective Data
A. Review the onset, duration, and course of symptoms.
B. Elicit the initial site of rash and progression to other body areas; determine whether the rash is pruritic, especially on the soles of the feet.
C. Elicit job exposure for school teachers and day-care workers.
D. Determine whether the client is pregnant.
E. Determine whether the client has had any new medication or contact exposures.
F. Rule out other family members with similar symptoms.
G. Ask about pain in the joints (usually in the hands, feet, or knees).
H. Review all medications, including over-the-counter (OTC) and herbal products.

Physical Examination
A. Check temperature, pulse, respirations, and blood pressure.
B. Inspect:
  1. Observe rash pattern:
    a. Erythematous malar "slapped-cheek sign" rash on the face is the typical facial erythema. The facial rash is the most recognized feature.
    b. "Lacy"-patterned rash over the chest, back, buttocks, arms, and legs.
  2. Conduct an ear, nose, and throat examination.
C. Palpate:
  1. Blanch rash area: Rash over extremities blanches with pressure, heat or cold, and sunlight.
  2. Palpate spleen: Splenomegaly is a hallmark sign.
  3. Palpate lymph nodes: Enlarged lymph nodes, especially the posterior cervical nodes, are indicative of infection.
  4. Assess joints for tenderness, swelling, and range of motion.

Diagnostic Tests
A. Complete blood count (CBC) with differential: Hallmark laboratory finding is the dramatic decrease or absence of measurable reticulocytes.
B. Parvovirus IgG and IgM antibodies—approximately 30% to 60% of adults have positive antibodies.
C. Polymerase chain reaction (PCR) test.
D. Pregnancy test if necessary.
E. Fetal assessment:
  1. Ultrasonography to evaluate for fetal hydrops. Fetal ascites and pleural and pericardial effusions are evident on ultrasonogram (nonimmune hydrops fetalis).
  2. Percutaneous umbilical blood sampling (PUBS) to evaluate for fetal infection and anaemia may be performed.

Differential Diagnoses
A. Rubella.
B. Aplastic crisis.
C. Other viral infection.
D. Contact dermatitis.
E. Medication allergies.
F. Chronic anaemia.

Plan
A. General interventions:
  1. Management is usually supportive treatment of symptoms.
  2. Analgesics for joint pain.
  3. Antipyretics for temperature.
  4. Starch bath for pruritus.
  5. Self-limiting without treatment.
  6. Immunosuppressed clients respond well to intravenous immunoglobulin (IVIG).
  7. Aplastic crises may require transfusion.
B. Client teaching:
  1. Educate pregnant and immunocompromised clients to avoid exposure.
  2. Routine infection control practices minimize the risk of transmission, including handwashing and droplet precautions. Avoiding sharing food or drinks may partially prevent the spread of parvovirus B19.
  3. Disease is most communicable before rash; it is not communicable after rash outbreak.
C. Pharmacological therapy:
  1. Acetaminophen for fever.
  2. Nonsteroidal anti-inflammatory drugs (NSAIDs) for symptomatic relief.
  3. There is no vaccine to prevent parvovirus B19.

Follow-Up
A. None is recommended, as the disease is self-limiting for low-risk population.

Consultation/Referral
A. The incidence of acute parvovirus B19 in pregnancy is 3.3% to 3.8%. Refer pregnant clients to a perinatologist for fetal evaluation for acute exposure in pregnancy.
B. Consult or refer the client to an infectious disease specialist immediately for exposure of immunocompromised clients, who might require a blood transfusion.

Individual Considerations
A. Pregnancy:
  1. A positive (IgG) antibody and a negative (IgM) indicate maternal immunity, and the fetus is therefore protected from infection. A positive IgM antibody is consistent with acute parvovirus infection:
    a. If testing is negative for IgG and IgM after recent parvovirus exposure, PCR testing for maternal parvovirus B19 DNA should be performed.
  2. Parvovirus B19 is not teratogenic. Fetal risks are related to the trimester of exposure. Nonimmune hydrops fetalis occurs secondary to haemolysis and inadequate production of erythrocytes. Other risks include spontaneous abortion, intrauterine growth restriction, stillbirth, and neonatal death.
  3. Women who are diagnosed with acute infection beyond 20 weeks' gestation should receive periodic ultrasounds (although serial ultrasounds are commonly performed).
  4. Intrauterine blood transfusion may be performed if severe anaemia is confirmed.
  5. Delivery and postnatal management of the hydropic infant should occur in a tertiary care centre. The majority

of hydropic infants require respiratory assistance and mechanical ventilation.
B. Paediatrics:
1. Neonates who had hydrops attributed to parvovirus B19 in utero do not require isolation if the hydrops is resolved by delivery.
2. Most children born to mothers who develop parvovirus B19 infection in pregnancy do not appear to suffer long-term sequelae; the infection does not appear to cause long-term neurologic morbidity.
3. Children with abnormal red blood cells (RBCs) (sickle cell disease, hereditary spherocytosis, thalassaemia) can develop transient aplastic anaemia and may require multiple transfusions.
4. Children may attend childcare or school once the rash appears, since they are no longer contagious.
C. Adults:
1. Clients may have arthritis and arthralgias lasting months to years after exposure.
2. Adults may initially be asymptomatic.
3. Immunocompromised clients may develop severe, chronic anaemia.
4. Working women with young children may benefit from prenatal testing and limiting exposure in pregnancy.

Bibliography

American College of Obstetricians and Gynecologists. (2015). Practice Bulletin no. 151: Cytomegalovirus, parvovirus B19, varicella zoster, and toxoplasmosis in pregnancy. *Obstetrics & Gynecology (Serial Online), 125*(6), 1510–1525.
Canadian Paediatric Society. (2018). *2017 results: Canadian paediatric surveillance program.* Retrieved from www.cpsp.cps.ca/uploads/publications/CPSP-2017-Results_1.pdf
Centers for Disease Control and Prevention. (2015). *Fifth disease.* Retrieved from www.cdc.gov/parvovirusb19/fifth-disease.html
Jordan, J. A. (2013). Clinical manifestations and pathogenesis of human parvovirus B19 infection. *UpToDate.* Retrieved from www.uptodate.com/contents/clinical-manifestations-and-pathogenesis-of-human-parvovirus-b19-infection?topicKey=ID%2F8272
Riley, L. E., & Fernandes, C. J. (2016). Parvovirus B19 infection during pregnancy. *UpToDate.* Retrieved from www.uptodate.com

Rheumatic Fever

Cheryl A. Glass, Jill C. Cash, and Jocelyn T. Whittier

Definition

A. Acute rheumatic fever (ARF) is an autoimmune inflammatory process that occurs as sequelae of a Group A beta-haemolytic streptococcal (GABHS) tonsillopharyngitis. Rheumatic fever is a preventable disease through the detection and adequate treatment of streptococcal pharyngitis.
B. The individual who has had an attack of rheumatic fever is at very high risk of developing recurrences after subsequent GABHS pharyngitis and needs continuous antimicrobial prophylaxis to prevent such recurrences (secondary prevention). The most significant complication of ARF is rheumatic heart disease, which occurs after repeated bouts of acute illness.

Incidence/Prevalence

A. The incidence of rheumatic fever is 19 per 100,000 worldwide. In Canada, the incidence in the general population is lower (2–14 cases per 100,000) following ineffectively treated cases of GABHS upper respiratory infections (URIs). But in some of Canada's Indigenous communities, the incidence is 21.3 per 100,000, which is 75 times greater than the incidence in Canada's general population; this is attributed to late diagnosis, overcrowded housing, and inadequate health care in remote communities. ARF is most common among children five to 15 years of age. It is relatively rare in infants and uncommon in preschool-aged children. The incidence of first episodes falls steadily after adolescence and is rare after 30 years of age. The disease does not seem to have a major racial predisposition. About 20% of children diagnosed with rheumatic fever have a positive history of pharyngitis and only 35% to 60% recall having any upper respiratory symptoms within the preceding three months.
B. Cardiac involvement is the most serious complication. Morbidity due to congestive heart failure (CHF), stroke, and endocarditis is common among individuals with rheumatic heart disease, and annually, about 1.5% of persons with rheumatic carditis die of the disease. Mitral stenosis and Sydenham chorea are more common in females who have gone through puberty.

Pathogenesis

Rheumatic fever is caused by a preceding infection with GABHS and *Streptococcus pyogenes.* Nonsuppurative inflammatory lesions of the joints, heart, subcutaneous tissue, and central nervous system (CNS) characterize ARF. The incubation period is between one and five weeks as well as six months after GABHS pharyngitis.

Predisposing Factors

A. Group A pharyngitis, untreated or inadequately treated.
B. Age five to 15 years.
C. Crowded living conditions.
D. Occupational exposure: teachers, health-care providers, military personnel.
E. Most common in tropical countries.
F. Gender: More common in females.

Common Findings

A. Sore throat (generally of sudden onset), pain on swallowing.
B. Joint pain/arthralgias to frank polyarthritis is usually symmetrical and involves large joints such as the knees, ankles, elbows, and wrists. Joints feel warm, swollen, and inflamed. Polyarthritis is the most common manifestation. Both synovitis and periarticular inflammation occur, especially in the knees and ankles. There may be erythema of the overlying skin.
C. Fever varies from 38°C to 40°C.

Other Signs and Symptoms

A. Fatigue.
B. Appetite loss.
C. Sydenham chorea (more common in girls): Chorea, a CNS disorder lasting one to three months, is purposeless, involuntary, rapid movements often associated with muscle weakness, involuntary facial grimaces, speech disturbance, and emotional liability. Sydenham chorea usually resolves without permanent damage but occasionally lasts two to three years.
D. Subcutaneous nodules are firm, painless nodules that are seen or felt over the extensor surface of certain joints, particularly elbows, knees, and wrists; in the occipital region; or over the spinous processes of the thoracic and lumbar vertebrae. The skin overlying them moves freely and is not inflamed.
E. Erythema marginatum is an evanescent, nonpruritic, pink rash with pale centers and round or wavy margins; lesions vary greatly in size and occur mainly on the trunk and

extremities and are usually not seen on the face. Erythema is transient, migrates from place to place, and may be brought out by the application of heat.
F. Enlarged lymph nodes.
G. Headache.
H. Carditis: development of new heart murmurs, cardiomegaly, and CHF.
I. Pericarditis, pericardial friction rub, and/or pericardia effusion.
J. Aortic regurgitation, manifested by the following:
  1. Palpitations.
  2. Dyspnoea on exertion.
  3. Angina at rest.

Subjective Data
A. Review a recent history (one to three months) of sore throat and the onset, duration, severity, and treatment of symptoms.
B. Complete a drug history. Did the client finish the prescribed antibiotics? Does the client take ASA? Use of ASA can mask signs of inflammation and tends to prolong the course of the disease.
C. Assess the client for signs and symptoms of rheumatic and scarlet fever.
D. Discuss the client's history of heart problems, chest pain, or shortness of breath.
E. Evaluate the onset and complaints of chorea: fidgeting, clumsiness, uncoordinated erratic facial movements, including grimaces, grins, and frowns.
F. Tongue movements. Ask whether the movements and other symptoms disappear with sleep.
G. Review symptoms of joint pain.

Physical Examination
A. Check temperature, pulse, respirations, and blood pressure (BP).
B. Inspect:
  1. Inspect joints for swelling and warmth.
  2. Observe for signs of chorea (symptoms noted previously).
  3. Conduct a dermal examination, especially the trunk and proximal aspects of the extremities. Individual lesions of erythema marginatum are evanescent, moving over the skin in wavy patterns or with indented margins. The lesions may be macular and can develop and disappear in minutes, appearing to change shape while being examined.
  4. Complete an ear, nose, mouth, and throat examination. Evaluate tonsillopharyngeal erythema with or without exudates. Observe for beefy, red, swollen uvula.
C. Auscultate:
  1. Auscultate the heart. Note any heart murmur, pericardial friction rub, or effusion. Characteristic murmurs of acute carditis include the high-pitched, blowing, holosystolic, apical murmur of mitral regurgitation and a high-pitched, decrescendo, diastolic murmur of aortic regurgitation heard in the aortic area. The features of CHF include tachycardia, a third heart sound, rales, and oedema.
  2. All lung fields. Note shortness of breath.
D. Palpate:
  1. Neck lymph nodes.
  2. Extremities: Apical and radial pulses.
  3. Abdomen.
E. Neuromuscular examination for chorea:
  1. Have the client stick out his or her tongue for observation of a "bag of worms" when protruded.
  2. Have the client grip your hand; with chorea, the client will be unable to maintain a grip, rhythmic squeezing results.
  3. Observe for the spooning sign, a flexion at the wrist with finger extension when the hand is extended.
  4. Observe for the pronator sign, the palms turn outward when held above the head.

Diagnostic Tests
A. No single specific laboratory test can confirm the diagnosis of ARF. The throat culture remains the criterion for confirmation of GABHS infection:
  1. If a rapid antigen detection test is negative, obtain a throat culture.
  2. Because of the high specificity, a positive rapid antigen test confirms a streptococcal infection.
B. Erythrocyte sedimentation rate (ESR) is usually elevated at the onset of ARF.
C. C-reactive protein (CRP) is usually elevated at the onset of ARF.
D. ECG or echocardiography. *Note*: Prolonged PR interval.
E. Chest radiograph can reveal cardiomegaly and CHF.
F. Echocardiography may demonstrate valvular regurgitant lesions.
G. Tests that may rule out differential diagnoses include rheumatoid factor (RF), antinuclear antibody (ANA), Lyme serology, blood cultures, and evaluation for gonorrhoea.

Differential Diagnoses
A. Rheumatic fever: Jones criteria (updated in 2015):
  1. Requires two major criteria or one major plus two minor criteria to support the diagnosis of ARF in a client with evidence of a preceding GABHS infection.
  2. Clients with a history of ARF are at risk of repeat episodes of ARF with GABHS and more likely to have cardiac involvement. These clients require two major, one major plus two minor, or three minor criteria for the diagnosis of recurrent ARF. Criteria are as follows:
    a. Major criteria:
      i. Carditis (based on clinical criteria; 50%–70% seen).
      ii. Polyarthritis (35%–66% seen).
      iii. CNS involvement (Sydenham chorea—neurologic disorder exhibiting abrupt, nonrhythmic, involuntary movements, muscle weakness, emotional disturbance; rare in adults, seen in 10%–30%).
      iv. Erythema marginatum (uncommon, rare in adults, <6% seen).
      v. Subcutaneous nodules (uncommon, rare in adults, 0%–10% seen).
    b. Minor criteria:
      i. Arthralgia.
      ii. Fever.
      iii. Elevated ESR or CRP level.
      iv. Prolonged PR interval.
  3. There are three exceptions to the aforementioned criteria in which criteria do not need to be met for the diagnosis of ARF. Those three exceptions are the following:
    a. Chorea as only symptom.
    b. Indolent carditis for clients who present months after acute GABHS infection.
    c. Recurrent ARF for clients with a history of ARF-associated carditis or rheumatic heart disease.
  4. Criteria may also be modified for moderate- to high-risk populations.

B. Juvenile rheumatoid arthritis.
C. Rheumatoid arthritis.
D. Gonococcal arthritis.
E. Septic arthritis.
F. Sickle cell anaemia.
G. Infective endocarditis.
H. Leukaemia.
I. Gout.
J. Huntington's chorea.
K. Kawasaki disease (KD).
L. Systemic lupus erythematosus.
M. Lyme disease.
N. Reiter's syndrome.
O. Scarlet fever.

Plan

A. General interventions: Bed rest is a traditional part of ARF therapy and is especially important with carditis. Bed rest is needed throughout the acute illness and should continue until the ESR has returned to normal for two weeks.
B. Client teaching:
   1. Reinforce the need to take the complete prescribed course of antibiotics for strep infections.
   2. Adequate treatment for a streptococcal pharyngitis or skin infection is the best prevention against rheumatic fever. Strep infections are contagious, but rheumatic fever is not.
   3. Chorea is usually managed conservatively in a quiet, nonstimulatory environment. Valproic acid is the preferred agent if sedation is needed. Although there is no conclusive evidence of their efficacy, intravenous immunoglobulin (IVIG), steroids, and plasmapheresis have all been used successfully in refractory chorea.
   4. Diuretics are the mainstay of carditis/heart failure.
C. Pharmacological therapy:
   1. Antibiotic treatment in clients who present with ARF is necessary regardless of the throat culture results to minimize the possible transmission of the rheumatogenic streptococcal strain. First-line treatment is penicillin, but erythromycin or sulphadiazine may be used in clients who are allergic to penicillin. Use of long-acting intramuscular penicillin G avoids compliance problems of oral regimens:
      a. Benzathine penicillin G.
      b. Penicillin VK—first-line treatment for GABHS pharyngitis.
      c. Amoxicillin.
      d. Cephalexin.
      e. Clients with severe hypersensitivity to beta-lactam antibiotics.
         i. Azithromycin.
         ii. Clarithromycin.
         iii. Clindamycin.
   2. Codeine is the first-line analgesic for arthritis symptoms in adults. Morphine is the first-line analgesic in paediatric clients.
   3. ASA is the first-line anti-inflammatory therapy. It is used in clients with moderate to severe arthritis and carditis without heart failure. Treatment is administered for one to two weeks but may be administered for six to eight weeks.
   4. Cardiac involvement with confirmed rheumatic fever:
      a. Heart failure—antibiotics + diuretic + angiotensin-converting enzyme inhibitors + steroid therapy.
      b. Atrial fibrillation—antibiotics + digoxin.
      c. Valve leaflet or chordae tendineae rupture—antibiotics and full assessment for an emergent valve replacement.
   5. Severe chorea—antibiotics + anticonvulsants.
   6. Secondary antibiotic prophylaxis for procedures for chronic established changes of the heart valves.

Follow-Up

A. The test of cure is a negative throat culture.
B. Pharyngitis clients with a history of rheumatic fever and those who are symptomatic and have a household member with documented GABHS infection should receive immediate treatment without need for prior testing.
C. Prophylaxis for systemic bacterial endocarditis is no longer recommended except in high-risk clients. For more information, refer to www.inesss.qc.ca/fileadmin/doc/INESSS/Outils/Guides_antibio_II/endocardite_2012_web_EN.pdf.
D. The major complication is cardiac valve disease. Rheumatic fever accounts for the largest number of aortic regurgitation cases. Continuous streptococcus prophylaxis in clients with prior rheumatic fever is the major means of preventing cardiac sequelae.
E. The client with carditis should be followed every six months and by a cardiologist with an echocardiography every one to two years.

Consultation/Referral

A. Consult and comanage the client with an ear, nose, and throat (ENT) specialist if indicated for clients with intact tonsils and recurrent symptomatic strep infections for consideration of tonsillectomy.
B. Consultation with a cardiologist may be required to manage heart blocks and CHF.
C. Consultation with a neurologist or psychiatrist may be required to confirm the diagnosis of chorea and to assist in its management.

Individual Considerations

A. Paediatrics: highest risk group; rare in children younger than 5 years.
B. Adults:
   1. Cases are rare for clients older than age 40 years.
   2. Cases of arthritis following a streptococcal infection that are not supported by the Jones criteria are called post-streptococcal reactive arthritis. Many of these clients will have one major and two minor symptoms and are considered to have ARF.
C. Pregnancy:
   1. Penicillin G is pregnancy category B. Fetal risk is not confirmed in humans but has been shown in some studies in animals.
   2. Erythromycin is pregnancy category B.
   3. ASA products are pregnancy category D. As fetal risk has been shown in humans, use only if the benefits outweigh the risk to the fetus.

Bibliography

Armstrong, C. (2010). Practice guidelines: AHA guidelines on prevention of rheumatic fever and diagnosis and treatment of acute streptococcal pharyngitis. *American Family Physician, 81*(3), 346–359. Retrieved from www.aafp.org/afp/2010/0201/p346.html

Canadian Paediatric Society. (2018). *2017 results: Canadian paediatric surveillance program*. Retrieved from www.cpsp.cps.ca/uploads/publications/CPSP-2017-Results_1.pdf

Galloway, J., & Cope, A. P. (2015). The ying and yang of fever in rheumatic disease. *Clinical Medicine, 15*(3), 288–291. doi:10.7861/clinmedicine.15-3-288

Gewitz, M. H., Baltimore, R. S., Tani, L. Y., Sable, C. A., Shulman, S. T., Carapetis, J., . . . American Heart Association Committee on Rheumatic Fever, Endocarditis, and Kawasaki Disease of the Council on Cardiovascular Disease in the Young. (2015). Revision of the Jones criteria for the diagnosis of acute rheumatic fever in the era of Doppler echocardiography: A scientific statement from the American Heart Association. *Circulation, 131*, 1806–1818. doi:10.1161/CIR.0000000000000205

Gibofsk, A. (2016). Acute rheumatic fever: Clinical manifestations and diagnosis. *UpToDate*. Retrieved from www.uptodate.com

Gordon, J., Kirlew, M., Schreiber, Y., Saginur, R., Bocking, N., Blakelock, B., . . . Kelly, L. (2015). Acute rheumatic fever in First Nations communities in northwestern Ontario, Social determinants of health "bite the heart". *Canadian Family Physician, 61*(10), 881–886.

Government of Canada. (2018, November 19). *Canada's Provincial and Territorial Routine (and Catch-up) Vaccination Routine Schedule Programs for Infants and Children*. Retrieved from https://www.canada.ca/en/public-health/services/provincial-territorial-immunization-information/provincial-territorial-routine-vaccination-programs-infants-children.html

Pichichero, M. E. (2016). Complications of streptococcal tonsillopharyngitis. *UpToDate*. Retrieved from www.uptodate.com

Wallace, M. R. (2014). Rheumatic fever. *Medscape*. Retrieved from emedicine.medscape.com

World Heart Federation. (2014). *Rheumatic heart disease*. Retrieved from www.world-heart-federation.org

Rocky Mountain Spotted Fever (RMSF)

Cheryl A. Glass, Jill C. Cash, and Jocelyn T. Whittier

Definition

A. Rocky Mountain spotted fever (RMSF) is a systemic febrile illness with characteristic rash from the bite of an infected tick. It can involve the skin; central nervous, cardiac, and pulmonary systems; gastrointestinal (GI) tract; and muscles. Ticks need six to 10 hours of feeding to transmit RMSF; therefore, early discovery and removal of ticks is a preventative measure.
B. RMSF is a common tick-born disease; currently it is seen only in Western Canada. It is the most severe rickettsial illness.
C. Long-term sequelae are common with severe RMSF, including the following:
   1. Paraparesis.
   2. Hearing loss.
   3. Peripheral neuropathy.
   4. Seizures.
   5. Bowel incontinence.
   6. Cerebellar and vestibular dysfunction.
   7. Blindness.

Incidence/Prevalence

A. RMSF is the most common rickettsial infection in the United States, with the occurrence of 250 to 1,200 cases annually, and occurs throughout all the Americas; current Canadian data on incidence/prevalence are not available. In the United States, RMSF is seen in the southeastern and southern central states. Although RMSF is more common in rural and suburban locations, it does occur in urban areas. The incidence varies by geographic area. RMSF is more common in the spring and early summer in Canada and the United States, but it has been seen in the cold weather months in the southern United States.
B. People of all ages can be infected.
C. African Americans have a higher case-fatality rate.

Pathogenesis

A. *Rickettsia rickettsii* is the infectious agent and is transmitted by a tick vector. *Rickettsia* also infects rodents, squirrels, and chipmunks. Up to one-third of clients with proven RMSF do not recall a recent tick bite or tick contact. RMSF is not transmitted by person-to-person contact.
B. The incubation period is usually about one week, but it ranges from two to 14 days after the tick bite. It appears to be related to the size of the rickettsial inoculum.
C. Principal recognized vectors:
   1. *Dermacentor variabilis* (American dog tick).
   2. *Dermacentor andersoni* (Rocky Mountain wood tick).
   3. *Amblyomma americanum* (Lone Star tick).
   4. *Rhipicephalus sanguineus* (brown dog tick).

Predisposing Factors

A. Outdoor activities (e.g., hunting, hiking, and camping).
B. Tick bite: The tick must attach and feed for four to six hours before transmitting the infection.
C. Age is not a predisposing factor, but the disease is more common in children and young adults.
D. Exposure to heavy brush areas.
E. Contact with dogs and other animals with ticks.
F. Transmission has occurred on rare occasion by blood transfusion.
G. Blood transmission is rare.

Common Findings

In early phase, most clients have nonspecific signs and symptoms that may include the following:
A. Fever.
B. Sudden onset of severe headache.
C. Children may present with prominent abdominal pain that may be mistaken for acute appendicitis, cholecystitis, or bowel obstruction.
D. Rash (90%) usually occurs between days three to five of illness. The typical RMSF rash begins as a pink macu-lopapular eruption on the ankles and wrists. The rash then spreads both centrally and to the palms of hands and soles of the feet. By the fourth day, the rash spreads centripetally and becomes petechial and papular. Haemorrhagic, ulcerated lesions may follow. In a small percentage, onset of the rash is delayed (past five days) and/or is atypical (e.g., confined to one body region). Urticaria and pruritus are not characteristic of RMSF, and their presence makes the diagnosis unlikely.
E. Malaise.
F. Myalgias.
G. Nausea with or without vomiting.

Other Signs and Symptoms

A. Deep cough.
B. Oedema, especially in children.
C. Bleeding.
D. Conjunctivitis.
E. Retinal abnormalities.
F. ECG abnormalities.
G. Seizures.
H. Dehydration.

Subjective Data

A. Review the onset, course, and duration of symptoms.

B. Elicit information about a recent tick bite or removal.
C. Ask the client about any recent outdoor activities such as camping, hiking, and so on.
D. Rule out similar symptoms in other family members.
E. Review any history of rash and course of spread.
F. Elicit a history of mental or neurologic changes, including seizures.
G. Rule out other symptoms associated with Lyme disease, such as arthritis, memory loss, and distal paresthaesia.
H. Review the client's recent history of blood transfusion.

Physical Examination
A. Check temperature, pulse, respirations, and blood pressure (BP).
B. Inspect:
   1. Conduct an ear, nose, and throat examination.
   2. Inspect the skin, especially on the wrists, palms, ankles, and soles of the feet.
   3. Note the presence of petechiae.
   4. Conduct an eye examination and evaluate periorbital oedema and petechial conjunctivitis.
   5. Auscultate:
      a. Perform a complete heart evaluation.
      b. Auscultate all lung fields.
C. Palpate:
   1. All lymph nodes.
   2. The mastoid bones.
D. Neurologic examination:
   1. Assess level of consciousness (LOC).
   2. Evaluate the client for signs of meningeal irritation, such as nuchal rigidity and positive Brudzinski's and Kernig's signs (see Figures 16.1 and 16.2).

Diagnostic Tests
A. Antibody titres: A fourfold rise in antibody titre is the diagnostic gold standard for RMSF. Antibodies typically appear seven to 10 days after the onset of the illness.
B. Complete blood count (CBC) with differential.
C. Platelet count: As the illness progresses, thrombocytopaenia becomes more prevalent and may be severe.
D. Electrolytes.
E. Liver function studies.
F. Bilirubin.
G. Skin biopsy: 3-mm punch biopsy.
H. Lumbar puncture may be indicated.
I. Rickettsial blood cultures are highly sensitive and specific; however, they require specialized laboratories.

Differential Diagnoses
A. RMSF is commonly mistaken for an undifferentiated viral illness during the first few days of illness.
B. Viral meningitis.
C. Lyme disease.
D. Mononucleosis.
E. Atypical measles.
F. Viral hepatitis.
G. Parvovirus B19 (fifth disease).

Plan
A. General interventions:
   1. Early treatment is necessary; never delay initiation of antimicrobial treatment to confirm clinical suspicion of the disease. This is a life-threatening disease.
   2. Antibiotic therapy (see section "Pharmacological therapy"): If penicillin or a cephalosporin is administered empirically in the first few days of the illness, the subsequent rash may be incorrectly diagnosed as a drug reaction.
   3. Hospitalization should be considered for most clients, especially children.
B. Client teaching:
   1. Refer to Client Teaching Guide: Lyme Disease and Removal of a Tick.
   2. RMSF is not transmissible by person-to-person contact; therefore, isolation is not necessary.
   3. Relapse of the illness may occur; the client should report recurrence of symptoms immediately.
   4. Clients who report tick bites should be advised to inform their health-care provider if any systemic symptoms, especially fever and headache, occur in the following 14 days.
   5. All pets should be treated for ticks.
C. Pharmacological therapy:

The diagnosis of RMSF can rarely be confirmed or disproved in its early phase; the cornerstone of management is empiric therapy based on clinical judgment and the epidemiologic setting.

   1. First-line treatment: Doxycycline:
      a. Doxycycline may be given for critically ill clients.
      b. Doxycycline is the first-line treatment in adults except for pregnant women.
      c. Tetracyclines can cause dental staining when administered to children younger than eight years. Most experts consider the risk of morbidity from rickettsial diseases greater than the minimal risk of dental staining from one short course of doxycycline.
   2. Alternative drug therapy: Chloramphenicol:
      a. Chloramphenicol requires frequent serum platelet counts and complete blood counts (CBCs).
      b. Use of chloramphenicol should be considered only in rare cases, such as severe allergy to doxycycline or in pregnancy if the mother's life is in danger.
      c. Use of chloramphenicol is associated with a higher risk of fatal outcome.
   3. Prophylactic therapy with doxycycline or another tetracycline is not recommended following tick exposure.
   4. Severe doxycycline or tetracycline allergy in clients should be discussed with the client. Consider consulting with allergy/immunology specialist. If not life-threatening, administer doxycycline in a controlled setting or consult for rapid doxycycline desensitization with an allergy/immunology specialist. Anaphylactic reactions have been reported, but rare.
   5. Asymptomatic clients with seropositive results for tick-borne rickettsial disease should not be treated with antibiotics because antibodies may remain positive for several years after infection.

Follow-Up
A. See the client 24 to 48 hours after initial visit and again at the end of antibiotic therapy (unless following lab for chloramphenicol therapy). **RMSF progresses rapidly.** Approximately 10% of outpatients are subsequently admitted to the hospital.

▶ Client Teaching Guides are available at https://connect.springerpub.com/content/reference-book/978-0-8261-9498-5

B. The client must be seen for any alteration in mental status, stiff neck, severe headaches, nausea and vomiting, severe weakness, dizziness, or high fever.
C. Hospitalization is indicated in clients who are severely ill or have complications, such as seizures, hypotension, or marked gastrointestinal (GI) symptoms.
D. Several rickettsial diseases, including RMSF, are nationally notifiable diseases and should be reported to state and local health departments.

Consultation/Referral
A. Consult an infectious disease specialist for any suspected signs of RMSF, because the client is in danger of vascular collapse and disseminated intravascular collapse.
B. Consultation with an infectious disease specialist is advised.

Individual Considerations
A. Pregnancy: Tetracyclines should not be used in pregnancy. Limited data exist for the use of doxycycline during pregnancy. Data on the risks of treatment during pregnancy are unlikely to have a substantial teratogenic risk. Prophylactic use of tetracycline is not recommended. Chloramphenicol is an alternative for RMSF; however, precautions should be used for possible gray baby syndrome. Short-term (less than three weeks) use of doxycycline is considered safe during lactation.

Bibliography
Alberta Health Services. (2017). *Bugs & drugs. Pregnancy & lactation. Doxycycline*. Retrieved from http://www.bugsanddrugs.org/Home/Index/bdpage62B55D83D9294CF6AA576C8B045C139F
Biggs, H. M., Barton Behravesh, C., Bradley, K. K., Dahlgren, F. S., Drexler, N. A., Dumler, J. S., . . . Traeger, M. S. (2016). Diagnosis and management of tickborne Rickettsial diseases: Rocky Mountain spotted fever and other spotted fever group Rickettsioses, Ehrlichioses, and Anaplasmosis—United States. *Morbidity & Mortality Weekly Report, 65*(2), 1–44. doi:10.15585/mmwr.rr6502a1
Canadian Paediatric Society. (2018). *Insect repellents: How to protect your child from insect bites*. Retrieved from www.caringforkids.cps.ca/handouts/insect_repellents
Centers for Disease Control and Prevention. (2015). *Tick removal*. Retrieved from www.cdc.gov/ticks/removing_a_tick.html
Cunha, B. A. (2016). Rocky Mountain spotted fever. *Medscape*. Retrieved from emedicine.medscape.com/article/228042-overviewencephalitisandemedicine.medscape.com/article/234009-overview
Government of Canada. (2011, February 18). *iPathogen safety data sheets: Infectious substances–Rickettsia rickettsii*. Retrieved from www.canada.ca/en/public-health/services/laboratory-biosafety-biosecurity/pathogen-safety-data-sheets-risk-assessment/rickettsia-rickettsii.html
Salvaggio, M. R. (2013). Human herpesvirus 6 infection differential diagnoses. *Medscape*. Retrieved from emedicine.medscape.com/article/219019-differential
Sanfort, C., Pottinger, P., & Jong, E. (2017). *The travel and tropical medicine manual* (5th ed.). London: Elsevier.

Roseola (Exanthem Subitum)

Cheryl A. Glass, Jill C. Cash, and Jocelyn T. Whittier

Definition
Roseola is a benign viral illness. It is the most common exanthem in infants and young children aged one to three years. Roseola can often be diagnosed by its classic presentation of a sudden onset of a high fever, up to 40°C, lasting three to four days. The pink-red macules and papules on the trunk and extremities occur after the client's fever defervesces. The high fever associated with roseola often triggers a febrile seizure. Up to 15% of children will experience their first febrile seizure with roseola.

Incidence/Prevalence
A. Incidence is unknown; 90% of cases involve children younger than two years. Human herpesvirus type 6 (HHV-6) has been isolated in Kaposi sarcoma (caused by HHV-8), in which roseola may contribute to tumour progression. HHV-6 may facilitate oncogenic potential in lymphoma and has been associated with chronic fatigue syndrome (CFS).

Pathogenesis
A. HHV-6 is the causative organism. The two variants of HHV-6 are A and B. The genomes of HHV-6A/B have been sequenced. Nearly all primary infections in children appear to be caused by HHV-6B. In the primary infection, replication of the virus occurs in the leukocytes and the salivary glands. It is present in the saliva. HHV-6 and HHV-7 are spread by respiratory droplets. The communicable period is most likely during the febrile phase.
B. The incubation period is fivefive to 15 days.
C. Like other herpesviruses, HHV-6 remains latent in most clients who are immunocompetent. Following the acute primary infection, HHV-6 remains latent in lymphocytes and monocytes and has been found in low levels in many tissues. The HHV-6 virus is a major cause of morbidity and mortality in clients who are immunosuppressed, particularly in clients with AIDS and in those who are transplant recipients.

Predisposing Factors
A. Classic age: nine to 12 months (age range: two weeks to three years).
B. Attendance at daycare centers.
C. Transplacental infection in about 1% of cases.
D. Immunosuppression.

Common Findings
A. Primary infection with HHV-6 may be asymptomatic or it may cause the exanthem subitum/roseola syndrome.
B. Child with high fever (up to 40.6°C) for one to three days: Abrupt onset of fever followed by rose–pink maculopapular rash with rapid resolution of both is characteristic of roseola. Rash appears after fever is resolved.
C. Rose-pink rash on chest and body: Rash typically begins on the trunk or chest and spreads to the arms and neck, with mild involvement of face and legs; rash can last several hours to two days and fades quickly.
D. Characteristic enanthem (Nagayama spots) consists of erythematous papules on the mucosa of the soft palate and the base of the uvula (usually present on the fourth day).

Other Signs and Symptoms
A. Drowsiness.
B. Seizures (secondary to high fever).
C. Bulging anterior fontanelle (rare).
D. Encephalopathy (rare).
E. Irritability.
F. Mild diarrhoea.
G. Otitis media.
H. Respiratory distress.
I. Clients who are immunocompromised may have malaise and central nervous system (CNS) and other organ system involvement.

Subjective Data
A. Ask the parent or caregiver to describe the progression and colour of the rash, onset, and duration of all symptoms.
B. Ask about the client's temperature history and the treatments administered.
C. Review other symptoms, such as coryza, cough, sore throat, and watery eyes (rules out roseola).
D. Review family history of others with similar symptoms.
E. Review the client's history of febrile seizures.
F. Complete a drug history for possible allergic reaction.
G. Inquire regarding recent measles–mumps–rubella (MMR) immunization.

Physical Examination
A. Check temperature, pulse, respirations, and blood pressure (BP).
B. Inspect.
  1. Inspect the skin. Observe for the presence of erythematous pink–red 3- to 5-mm maculopapular rash on chest and body: Rash typically begins on the trunk or chest and spreads to the arms and neck, with mild involvement of face and legs.
  2. Observe the client for seizure activity.
  3. Conduct an ear examination for inflamed tympanic membranes to rule out otitis media.
  4. Observe for the presence of periorbital oedema, which is common in the febrile phase of infection.
  5. Conduct a nasal examination; coryza is generally not a presenting symptom of roseola.
  6. Conduct an oral/throat examination to evaluate for the presence of characteristic enanthem Nagayama spots appear as erythematous papules on the mucosa of the soft palate and the base of the uvula.
C. Auscultate:
  1. Heart.
  2. Lungs; cough may be present.
D. Palpate:
  1. The head and the anterior fontanelle (if applicable).
  2. The neck and the cervical, suboccipital, and postauricular lymph nodes.
E. Neurologic examination: Check for nuchal rigidity.

Diagnostic Tests
A. None is required unless the diagnosis is unclear.
B. Rule out testing:
  1. Complete blood count (CBC) with differential.
  2. Urinalysis and culture for urinary tract infection (UTI).
  3. Chest radiograph for pneumonia.
  4. Blood cultures.
  5. Cerebrospinal fluid (CSF) examination if indicated.
C. Skin biopsy (rarely performed unless the diagnosis is unclear and there are other complicating medical factors).

Differential Diagnoses
A. Allergic reaction.
B. Cytomegalovirus (CMV).
C. Rocky Mountain spotted fever (RMSF).
D. Fifth disease (parvovirus B19).
E. Scarlet fever.
F. Meningococcaemia.
G. Fever of unknown origin (FUO).
H. Pneumococcaemia.
I. Herpes simplex.
J. Otitis media.
K. Rubella.
L. Enterovirus.
M. Epstein–Barr virus (EBV).
N. Measles.

Plan
A. General interventions:
  1. Encourage fluids to prevent dehydration (e.g., oral rehydration solution, popsicles, and clear fluids).
  2. Monitor for lethargy, decreased fluid intake, cough, and irritability.
B. Client teaching:
  1. Treatment is supportive.
  2. Advise parents/care provider that controlling temperature and providing supportive care is essential.
  3. Discomfort and body aches are often related to fever.
C. Pharmacological therapy:
  1. At present, there is no antiviral therapy available for HHV-6 infection.
  2. Acetaminophen as needed for fever.
  3. Acute or chronic antiseizure medications are not recommended for infants who have had a febrile seizure secondary to roseola.

Follow-Up
A. None is required unless other problems occur; resolution is usually rapid.
B. See the client immediately for the following:
  1. Twitching or other signs of seizure.
  2. Refusal to drink liquids or signs of dehydration.
  3. Loud and persistent crying; does not stop when consoled.
  4. Listlessness and stiff neck.

Consultation/Referral
A. Consult and/or refer the client to a specialist if febrile seizures/neurologic signs are present.

Individual Considerations
A. Paediatrics: Children with roseola are often playful without change in appetite, even with high fever.

Bibliography
Canadian Paediatric Society. (2018). *2017 results: Canadian paediatric surveillance program*. Retrieved from www.cpsp.cps.ca/uploads/publications/CPSP-2017-Results_1.pdf
Tremblay, C., & Brady, M. T. (2016). Roseola infantum (exanthema subitum). *UpToDate*. Retrieved from www.uptodate.com
White, S. W. (2013). Roseola infantum. *Medscape*. Retrieved from emedicine.medscape.com/article/1133023-overview

Rubella (German Measles)

Cheryl A. Glass, Jill C. Cash, and Jocelyn T. Whittier

Definition
A. Rubella, also known as German measles and three-day measles, is primarily known as a childhood disease. Rubella is considered one of the TORCH (toxoplasmosis, other [e.g., hepatitis and syphilis], rubella, cytomegalovirus, and herpes) infections and is highly contagious. The disease is preventable by immunization. Passive immunity is acquired from birth to six months of age from maternal antibodies.
B. The goal of immunization is to prevent congenitally acquired rubella. Routine immunization is achieved by using

the measles–mumps–rubella (MMR) or the MMR combined with varicella (MMRV) vaccine. The rubella vaccine is a live attenuated virus.
C. Immunization schedule recommended by the Government of Canada:
   1. For current information regarding rubella vaccination, refer to the Canadian Immunization Guide: Part 4—Active Vaccines—Rubella:
      www.canada.ca/en/public-health/services/publications/healthy-living/canadian-immunization-guide-part-4-active-vaccines/page-20-rubella-vaccine.html.
   2. For current information regarding routine schedules for vaccination in the provinces and territories, refer to
      www.canada.ca/en/public-health/services/provincial-territorial-immunization-information/provincial-territorial-routine-vaccination-programs-infants-children.html.

Incidence/Prevalence
A. Rubella is no longer endemic in the Canada, as a result of an intensive vaccination campaign. In Canada, 26 cases were reported in 2018 and one of congenital rubella syndrome. Peak season for rubella is late winter and spring.
B. The rubella vaccination is given only in about half of the world's population. Congenital rubella syndrome causes 15% of all birth defects in Russia.
C. Congenital defects occur in up to 85% of infants if maternal rubella infection occurs during the first 12 weeks of gestation.

Pathogenesis
A. Rubella virus is an enveloped, positive-stranded RNA virus classified as Rubivirus in the Togaviridae family. Humans are the only source of infection. The virus is spread by nasopharyngeal, airborne respiratory droplets and transplacental routes.
B. The incubation period for postnatally acquired rubella ranges from 14 to 23 days (usually 16–18 days). It is communicable one week before and four days after rash and illness. The neonate born with congenital rubella is often highly infectious and should be isolated. Neonates may continue to shed the virus for one year or longer.

Predisposing Factors
A. Age five to nine years.
B. Transplacental transmission.
C. Never received rubella vaccine.
D. Attendance at schools and day-care centres.
E. Compromised immune system.

Common Findings
A. Low-grade fever.
B. Swollen glands: Posterior auricular, suboccipital, and posterior cervical lymphadenopathy is frequently present 24 hours before rash develops.
C. Rash: Light pink to red macular rash that starts on the face and moves down the body to the trunk. The facial rash clears as the extremity rash erupts. The macular lesions rapidly become papular lesions and fade in three to four days. Exanthematous lesions remain discrete and pink, in contrast with the rash of rubeola, which is deep red and becomes confluent (Koplik's spots). Exanthem of rubella is usually preceded by one to five days of prodrome symptoms and generally last three days, but may persist for as long as five days.

Other Signs and Symptoms
A. Headache.
B. Sore throat.
C. Mild coryza.
D. Cough.
E. Malaise.
F. Conjunctivitis.
G. Forchheimer spots in the soft palate.
H. Transient polyarthralgia and polyarthritis (older children, adolescents, and women).
I. Itching.
J. Asymptomatic.

Subjective Data
A. Review the onset, duration, and course of symptoms.
B. Rule out similar symptoms in other family members.
C. Review the client's immunization history (especially recent immunization of MMR or MMRV vaccines).
D. Determine any new medications or contact exposures.
E. Review any history of rash and the course of spread.
F. Determine whether the client is pregnant.
G. If a fever is present, has the client experienced a febrile seizure?

Physical Examination
A. Check temperature, pulse, respirations, and blood pressure (BP).
B. Inspect:
   1. Conduct an ear, nose, and throat examination.
   2. Inspect the mouth for Koplik's spots. Forchheimer spots are reddish spots on the soft palate seen during the prodrome or first day of the rash.
   3. Inspect the skin.
C. Auscultate heart and lungs.
D. Palpate: Check the lymph nodes, especially the anterior/posterior cervical chains in neck.

Diagnostic Tests
A. Blood or urine:
   1. Latex agglutination.
   2. Enzyme immunoassay (enzyme-linked immunosorbent assay [ELISA]).
   3. Passive haemagglutination.
   4. Fluorescent immunoassay tests.
B. Rubella titre (test initially and repeat two to four weeks after exposure).

Serologic rubella titre less than eight indicates nonimmunity. Rubella titre >1:32 indicates immunity from a past infection. A fourfold rise in the titre (about two weeks after exposure) indicates infection.

C. Pregnancy test if indicated.
D. Tissue culture of throat.

Differential Diagnoses
A. Rubeola.
B. Parvovirus.
C. Scarlet fever.
D. Allergic reaction, contact dermatitis.
E. Roseola.
F. Infectious mononucleosis.
G. Toxoplasmosis.

Plan

A. General interventions:
1. Primary prevention is through immunization.
2. Vaccinating adolescents and adults in college reduces the chance of outbreaks and helps to prevent congenital rubella syndrome.
3. Generally, the course is mild; however, rest is encouraged.
4. Treatment is supportive. Have the client increase oral fluid intake.
5. Reinforce respiratory and nasal discharge precautions (droplet precautions); encourage good handwashing.
6. Immunize clients preconceptually; advise them to use a method of birth control for at least four weeks or longer after immunization.
7. Rubella cases should be reported to the local health department.
8. Health-care professionals should be immunized.

B. Client teaching:
1. Client/children should not return to work or school for seven days after the onset of the rash.
2. Pregnant clients with documented rubella infection should be counseled about the risk of fetal infection and/or compromise.
3. Children with congenital rubella should be considered contagious until they are at least one year of age, unless nasopharyngeal and urine culture are negative consecutively for rubella virus; infection control precautions should be considered in children up to three years who are hospitalized for congenital cataract extraction.
4. Febrile seizures may occur in children 12 to 24 months of age.

C. Pharmacological therapy:
1. Acetaminophen for fever and headache.
2. Antihistamines: diphenhydramine for pruritus.
3. Limited data indicate that intramuscular immunoglobulin (Ig) may decrease clinically apparent shedding and the rate of viraemia significantly in exposed susceptible people. The absence of clinical signs in a woman who has received intramuscular Ig does not guarantee that infant infection is prevented.
4. Live-virus rubella vaccine administered within three days of exposure has not been demonstrated to prevent illness.
5. Glucocorticoids, platelet transfusion, and other supportive measures are reserved for clients with complications such as thrombocytopaenia or encephalopathy.

Follow-Up

A. The disease is self-limiting and has no sequelae (except congenital exposure).
B. Repeat titre three to four weeks after exposure.
C. Rubella is a reportable disease in Canada.

Consultation/Referral

A. Refer the client to an obstetrician if the client is pregnant.

Individual Considerations

A. Pregnancy:
1. Rubella infection has few consequences for an adult, but it presents significant problems for a fetus. Rubella's viral teratogenic effects include cardiovascular malformation, deafness, intellectual disability, cataracts, glaucoma, microcephaly, and microphthalmos.
2. If maternal infection occurs during the first trimester, 50% of the fetuses infected may abort or have complications. Approximately 30% to 50% of fetuses that acquire rubella in the first month of gestation suffer cardiac anomalies. Neural deafness is a common sequela when infection occurs in the second gestational month.
3. The rubella vaccine is a live, attenuated virus; therefore, it is *not* safe to give in pregnancy. Immunization may be given postpartum; instruct the client to avoid pregnancy for the next four weeks or longer. The rubella vaccine may be given to a woman if she is breastfeeding.
4. Routine prenatal screening for rubella immunity should be undertaken. If a woman is found to be susceptible, the rubella vaccine should be administered during the immediate postpartum period before discharge.

B. Paediatrics:
1. The infected neonate must be kept in isolation in the nursery. The neonate may continue to spread the virus for one year or longer.
2. Cardiac and eye defects are most frequent when maternal infection occurs before eight weeks' gestation; hearing loss and growth retardation are observed in maternal infections up to 16 weeks' gestation.
3. Other reported abnormalities include jaundice, hepatosplenomegaly, thrombocytopaenia, and dermal erythropoiesis (blueberry muffin lesions).

Bibliography

Canadian Paediatric Society. (2018). *2017 results: Canadian paediatric surveillance program.* Retrieved from www.cpsp.cps.ca/uploads/publications/CPSP-2017-Results_1.pdf

Centers for Disease Control and Prevention. (2016). *Immunizations and pregnancy vaccines chart.* Retrieved from www.cdc.gov/vaccines/pregnancy/pregnant-women/index.html

Edwards, M. S. (2016). Rubella. *UpToDate.* Retrieved from https://www.uptodate.com/contents/rubella

Government of Canada. (2016a, February 2). *For health professionals: Measles.* Retrieved from https://www.canada.ca/en/public-health/services/diseases/measles/health-professionals-measles.html

Government of Canada. (2016b, March 3). *Surveillance of rubella.* Retrieved from https://www.canada.ca/en/public-health/services/diseases/rubella/surveillance-rubella.html

Government of Canada. (2018a, July 26). *Canadian immunization guide: Part 4–Active vaccines. Rubella vaccine.* Retrieved from https://www.canada.ca/en/public-health/services/publications/healthy-living/canadian-immunization-guide-part-4-active-vaccines/page-12-measles-vaccine.html

Government of Canada. (2018b, November 19). *Canada's Provincial and Territorial Routine (and Catch-up) Vaccination Routine Schedule Programs for Infants and Children.* Retrieved from https://www.canada.ca/en/public-health/services/provincial-territorial-immunization-information/provincial-territorial-routine-vaccination-programs-infants-children.html

Government of Canada. (2019, February 27). *Canadian immunization guide: Part 4–Active Vaccines. Measles vaccine.* Retrieved from https://www.canada.ca/en/public-health/services/publications/healthy-living/canadian-immunization-guide-part-4-active-vaccines/page-12-measles-vaccine.html

Sanfort, C., Pottinger, P., & Jong, E. (2017). *The travel and tropical medicine manual* (5th ed.). London: Elsevier.

Rubeola (Red Measles)

Cheryl A. Glass, Jill C. Cash, and Jocelyn T. Whittier

Definition

A. Rubeola (red measles), also known as hard measles, is a highly communicable viral disease. The disease is preventable by immunization. Passive immunity is acquired from birth to between four and six months of age if the mother is immune before pregnancy. Immunity after measles infection is thought to be lifelong.

B. Modified measles occurs in clients who received the serum immunoglobulin (Ig) postexposure to the measles virus. The incubation period may be up to 21 days. Their symptoms are generally milder.

C. Atypical measles occurs in clients who had the original killed-virus measles immunization that has incomplete immunity. Their symptoms are similar to the clinical presentation for clients who have not been vaccinated and have initial exposure:

1. In Canada, before 1970, killed-virus vaccine was administered in two provinces; this practice was discontinued when it was found to cause atypical measles. Revaccination with live vaccines was recommended.
2. Live measles vaccine was licensed in Canada in 1963. By the early 1970s, publicly funded one-dose immunization programs, routinely given at 1one year of age, were introduced across the country.

D. In Canada, the measles vaccine is currently available in two formulations: the trivalent measles–mumps–rubella (MMR) vaccine and the measles–mumps–rubella–varicella (MMRV) vaccine:

For current information regarding measles vaccination, refer to the Canadian Immunization Guide: Part 4, Active Vaccines—Measles:

www.canada.ca/en/public-health/services/publications/healthy-living/canadian-immunization-guide-part-4-active-vaccines/page-12-measles-vaccine.html.

For current information regarding routine schedules for vaccination in the provinces and territories, refer to

www.canada.ca/en/public-health/services/provincial-territorial-immunization-information/provincial-territorial-routine-vaccination-programs-infants-children.html.

Incidence/Prevalence

A. According to the World Health Organization (WHO), red measles is the leading cause of vaccine-preventable deaths in children worldwide, with 110,000 deaths occurring globally in 2017. Most of those deaths occurred in children younger than 5 years. Measles vaccination resulted in an 80% drop in measles deaths between 2000 and 2017 worldwide. In 2017, the WHO reported that about 85% of the world's children received one dose of measles vaccine by their first birthday and between 2000 and 2017, measles vaccination prevented an estimated 21.1 million deaths worldwide. According to the WHO, red measles has made a resurgence, with 29 cases reported in Canada, 372 cases reported in the United States, and 41,000 cases in Europe (January to June 2018).

B. In temperate areas, the peak incidence of infection occurs during late winter and spring.

C. About 5% of all measles cases are due to vaccine failure.

D. There is an increased incidence in two populations: Children younger than five years and college students who have not been immunized.

E. Rubeola is rarely encountered in pregnancy; however, the reported mortality of congenital measles is 32%.

F. One in every 1,000 clients with measles will develop acute encephalitis. Most fatalities from measles are from respiratory tract complications or encephalitis.

G. Clients with defects in cell-mediated immunity (AIDS, lymphoma, or other malignancies) are at risk for severe, progressive measles infection.

H. A generalized immunosuppression that follows measles frequently predisposes clients to complications such as otitis media and bronchopneumonia. Laryngotracheobronchitis (croup) and diarrhoea occur more commonly in young children. Two rare neurologic syndromes are associated with measles:

1. Acute disseminated encephalomyelitis may occur soon after the initial clinical manifestations of measles have resolved.
2. Subacute sclerosing panencephalitis presents seven to 10 years after the initial infection.

Pathogenesis

A. Paramyxovirus (an RNA virus) is the causative agent and is spread by respiratory droplet, direct skin contact, or transplacental passage. The incubation period lasts seven to 14 days from exposure to onset. It is communicable a few days before fever to four days after rash appears. The measles virus replicates locally, spreads to regional lymphatic tissues, and is then thought to disseminate to other reticuloendothelial sites via the bloodstream.

B. The virus remains active and contagious in the air or on infected surfaces for up to two hours.

Predisposing Factors

A. Age less than five years and not immunized.
B. Schools: Those not immunized with two doses of MMR.
C. Late winter and early spring.
D. Transplacental passage; presents clinically in the first 10 days of life.
E. Crowded living conditions.
F. Measles has been attributed to poor nutritional status and vitamin A deficiency.

Common Findings

A. Suspected case: Febrile illness accompanied by a rash.
B. Clinical case: The client is usually very ill with a fever and the three Cs: cough, coryza, and conjunctivitis. The client generally recovers rapidly after the first three to four days:

1. Fever >38°C and often exceeding 40°C.
2. Respiratory symptoms: Coryza and cough. The cough may persist for one to two weeks after the measles infection.
3. Conjunctivitis.

C. Rash: Macular rash develops on the face and neck; then lesions become maculopapular and spread to the trunk and extremities in 24 to 48 hours. The rash may appear red brown or purple red at the hairline. The rash lasts four to seven days.

D. Koplik's spots on buccal mucosa: Koplik's spots are pathognomonic for measles—bluish-gray specks or "grains of sand" on a red base.

E. Probable case meets clinical case definition but is not linked epidemiologically to a confirmed case and lacks serologic or virologic proof of disease.

F. Confirmed case meets the laboratory criteria for measles or meets the clinical case definition and is epidemiologically linked to a confirmed case.

Other Signs and Symptoms

A. Loss of appetite.
B. Bronchitis.
C. Photophobia.
D. General lymphoid involvement.
E. Myalgia.
F. Pruritus.
G. Diarrhoea.

Subjective Data
A. Review the onset and duration of symptoms such as cough, conjunctivitis, coryza, and Koplik's spots.
B. Rule out similar symptoms in other family members.
C. Review the client's immunization history.
D. Determine any new medications or contact exposures.
E. Review any history of rash and the course of spread.
F. Elicit the presence of chest pain, ear pain, and confusion (signs of complications).
G. Determine whether the client is pregnant.
H. Review the client's history of tick bite (recent camping, hiking, and so forth).

Physical Examination
A. Check temperature, pulse, respirations, and blood pressure (BP).
B. Inspect:
  1. Conduct an eye examination: Nonpurulent conjunctivitis with lacrimation is not uncommon. Photophobia may be present.
  2. Conduct an ear examination: Otitis is a complication noted with the measles.
  3. Conduct a nasal examination: Coryza is one of the classic triad of symptoms.
  4. Conduct a throat examination: Pharyngitis encompasses all complications of the measles.
  5. Examine the mouth for Koplik's spots; they appear on buccal mucosa within 12 hours. Koplik's spots are tiny (1–3 mm) bluish-white spots on an erythematous base that cluster adjacent to the molars on the buccal mucosa. Koplik's spots often begin to slough when the exanthem appears.
  6. Conduct a dermal examination. The characteristic rash is maculopapular and blanches; it begins on the face and spreads centrifugally to involve the neck, upper trunk, lower trunk, and extremities. The lesions may become confluent, especially in the face, where the rash develops first. The palms and soles of the feet are rarely involved. Some petechiae may be present with the rash.
C. Auscultate lungs and heart.
D. Palpate:
  1. Palpate the neck and lymph nodes.
  2. Generalized lymphadenopathy and splenomegaly are uncommon.
E. Neurologic examination:
  1. Check for nuchal rigidity.
  2. Complete a Mental State Examination.

Diagnostic Tests
A. Serologic procedures are not routinely done; however, leukopaenia and T-cell cytopaenia often occur and thrombocytopaenia may also be seen.
B. Antibody titre at the onset of the rash; repeat antibody titre every three to four weeks:
  1. Rubeola immunoglobulin G (IgG) and immunoglobulin M (IgM) antibody levels. The WHO has recommended that the diagnosis of measles be confirmed with laboratory testing.
  2. Serum IgM alone is the standard test to confirm the diagnosis of measles. At least a fourfold increase in antimeasles antibody titre is indicative of infection.
C. Chest x-ray if indicated: may show interstitial pneumonitis.

Differential Diagnoses
A. During the prodromal period, measles may resemble a common cold, except a fever is present.
B. Rubella (German measles).
C. Roseola (exanthem subitum).
D. Rocky Mountain spotted fever (RMSF).
E. Scarlet fever.
F. Mononucleosis.
G. Drug reaction.
H. Kawasaki disease (KD).
I. Parvovirus B19.
J. Toxic shock syndrome.
K. Mycoplasma pneumoniae.
L. Respiratory viruses:
  1. Rhinoviruses.
  2. Parainfluenza.
  3. Influenza.
  4. Adenovirus.
  5. Respiratory syncytial virus (RSV).
M. Dengue fever should be ruled out for international travelers.

Plan
A. General interventions:
  1. Primary prevention is through immunization:
     a. In order for vaccination to be considered adequate for school outbreaks, two doses of measles vaccine must have been administered after the age of 12 months and separated by at least 28 days.
     b. Those who are properly vaccinated may reenter school immediately after vaccination.
     c. International travelers should receive one or two doses of the measles vaccine before travel.
  2. Encourage the client to rest.
  3. The client must be isolated four days from the onset of the rash, up to 21 days.
  4. Encourage respiratory and nasal discharge precautions. The cough may persist for up to two weeks after the measles.
  5. There is no specific treatment for rubeola:
     a. Otitis media and pneumonia, both due to bacterial superinfection, should be treated with appropriate antibiotics.
     b. Intravenous (IV) hydration may be required secondary to dehydration from diarrhoea or vomiting.
  6. Monitor the client for signs of complications.
B. Client teaching:
  1. Discuss with the client to avoid bright lights with photophobia; may need sunglasses.
  2. Reinforce the need to comply with immunization schedule.
C. Pharmacological therapy:
  1. Vitamin A is recommended by the WHO and the United Nations Children's Fund (UNICEF) to all children with measles in areas where vitamin A deficiency is prevalent or where the mortality from measles exceeds 1%. Vitamin A treatment can help prevent eye damage and blindness. It has been shown to reduce the number of deaths by 50%.
  2. Treatment for exposed persons:
     a. Give live measles vaccine if exposure was within 72 hours.
     b. Give Ig by intramuscular (IM) injection, to induce passive immunity and to prevent or modify symptoms, within six days of exposure for the following high-risk groups:
        i. Immunocompromised.
        ii. Infants six months to one year of age.
        iii. Infants younger than six months who are born to mothers without measles immunity.

iv. Pregnant women.
  c. If Ig dose exceeds 10 mL, divide dose into several muscle sites to reduce local pain.
  d. Do not give Ig with the live measles vaccine.
3. Live measles virus vaccine should be given (except in pregnant women) approximately three months after Ig administration as long as client is at least 15 months of age at that time and there is no contraindication to vaccination.
4. Children and adolescents with symptomatic HIV infection who are exposed to measles should receive Ig regardless of vaccination status.
5. Exposure to measles is not a contraindication to vaccination. Available data suggest that live measles virus vaccine, if given within 72 hours of measles exposure, provides protection in some cases. If the exposure does not result in infection, the vaccine should induce protection against subsequent measles infection.

Follow-Up
A. See the client daily for Mental State Examination and examination of chest to rule out complications such as encephalitis and pneumonia.
B. Follow-up is needed three to four days after the onset of exanthem.
C. Investigate immune status of the family and other immediate contacts; prescribe vaccine if necessary.
D. Rubeola is a reportable disease in Canada; one case is considered an outbreak.

Consultation/Referral
A. Refer the client to an infectious disease specialist if fever lasts over four days; this is indicative of complications. Hospitalization may be indicated for treatment of measles complications (e.g., bacterial superinfection, pneumonia, dehydration, or croup).

Individual Considerations
A. General:
  1. A history of anaphylaxis after ingestion of gelatin is associated with an increased risk of anaphylaxis from the MMR or measles vaccine. This history should warrant a skin test for gelatin allergy.
  2. Individuals with anaphylaxis, excluding contact dermatitis, from neomycin should not receive these vaccines because they contain a small amount of this antibiotic.
  3. A history of anaphylaxis after egg ingestion is *not* a contraindication to measles immunization.
B. Pregnancy:
  1. Susceptible pregnant women who are exposed to rubeola should receive the Ig (see section "Pharmacological Therapy") in an attempt to modify or prevent the infection.
  2. Although no increase in risk of birth defects has been observed in mothers who were given live measles or MMR vaccine during pregnancy, there is a theoretical risk of such events. Measles vaccine is a live attenuated vaccine and is contraindicated in pregnancy.
  3. Measles in the mother during delivery does not necessarily lead to measles in the neonate. Congenital measles (defined by the appearance of the measles rash within 10 days of birth) and postnatally acquired measles (rash appears within 14–30 days of birth) have been associated with a spectrum of illnesses ranging from mild to severe disease.
  4. Measles vaccine may be administered postpartum to nonimmune mothers.
C. Paediatrics:
  1. Ig should be given to infants delivered from mothers with measles in the last week of pregnancy or the first postpartum week.
  2. Children without evidence of measles immunity are recommended not to be admitted to school until the first dose of MMR has been administered.
  3. A childhood maintenance visit between 11 and 12 years of age is recommended to update vaccinations.
  4. Concern has been raised periodically about the possible link between receipt of MMR/MMRV and autism. A number of studies have now been performed that fail to demonstrate any such association.
  5. Paediatric immunization: Trivalent MMR vaccine should be used unless contraindicated in adults and children older than 12 months.

Bibliography
Canadian Paediatric Society. (2018). *2017 results: Canadian paediatric surveillance program*. Retrieved from www.cpsp.cps.ca/uploads/publications/CPSP-2017-Results_1.pdf
Centers for Disease Control and Prevention. (2015). *Measles (rubeola)*. Retrieved from www.cdc.gov/measles/hcp/
Centers for Disease Control and Prevention. (2016). *Immunizations and pregnancy vaccines chart*. Retrieved from www.cdc.gov/vaccines/pregnancy/pregnant- women/index.html
Chen, S. S. P. (2013a). Measles clinical presentation. *Medscape*. Retrieved from emedicine.medscape.com/article/966220-clinical
Chen, S. S. P. (2013b). Measles treatment & management. *Medscape*. Retrieved from emedicine.medscape.com/article/966220-treatment
Fiebelkorn, A. P., & Goodson, J. L. (2015). Measles (Rubeola). In G. W. Brunette (Ed.), *The yellow book: CDC health information for international travel 2016* (pp. 258–261). New York, NY: Oxford University Press. Retrieved from www.nc.cdc.gov/travel/yellowbook/2016/infectious-diseases-related-to-travel/measles-rubeola
Government of Canada. (2016, February 2). *For health professionals: Measles*. Retrieved from https://www.canada.ca/en/public-health/services/diseases/measles/health-professionals-measles.html
Government of Canada. (2018, November 19). *Canada's Provincial and Territorial Routine (and Catch-up) Vaccination Routine Schedule Programs for Infants and Children*. Retrieved from: https://www.canada.ca/en/public-health/services/provincial-territorial-immunization-information/provincial-territorial-routine-vaccination-programs-infants-children.html
Government of Canada. (2019, February 27). *Canadian immunization guide: Part 4–Active Vaccines. Measles vaccine*. Retrieved from https://www.canada.ca/en/public-health/services/publications/healthy-living/canadian-immunization-guide-part-4-active-vaccines/page-12-measles-vaccine.html
Katz, S. L., King, A., Varughese, P., De Serres, G., Tipples, G., Waters, J., & Members of the Working Group on Measles Elimination. (2004). Measles elimination in Canada. *Journal of Infectious Diseases, 189* (Suppl. 1), S236–S242.
Sanfort, C., Pottinger, P., & Jong, E. (2017). *The travel and tropical medicine manual* (5th ed.). London: Elsevier.
World Health Organization. (2016). *Measles fact sheet*. Retrieved from https://www.who.int/immunization/diseases/measles/en/

Scarlet Fever (Scarlatina)

Cheryl A. Glass, Jill C. Cash, and Jocelyn T. Whittier

Definition
A. Scarlet fever is an acute infectious disease with vascular response to bacterial exotoxin usually associated with Group A streptococcal (GABHS) pharyngitis. Scarlatina may be present with pharyngitis. Scarlet fever is known as scarlatina in older literature references.

B. Scarlet fever is a nonsuppurative (inflammation without pus) complication of Group A beta-hemolytic streptococcal (GABHS). Development of the scarlet fever rash requires prior exposure to *Streptococcus pyogenes*.
C. There is no vaccine available for the prevention of scarlet fever.

Incidence/Prevalence
Scarlet fever is uncommon in children younger than 2 years. Highest incidence is in children four to eight years of age. By the time children are 10 years old, 80% have developed lifelong protective antibodies against streptococcal pyrogenic exotoxins.

Pathogenesis
A. GABHS and some strains of *Staphylococcus* are spread by respiratory droplet means and occasionally by direct physical contact from infected wounds, skin, or burns.
B. The incubation period is 12 hours to four days. It is communicable during the incubation period and clinical illness (around 10 days) and is no longer infectious after 24 hours of antibiotic therapy.
C. Exotoxin-mediated streptococcal infections range from localized skin disorders (e.g., bullous impetigo) to the systemic rash of scarlet fever to the uncommon but highly lethal streptococcal toxic shock syndrome.

Predisposing Factors
A. Strep throat pharyngitis; family history of recurrent strep infections.
B. Direct physical contact with sputum or infected skin.
C. Crowded situations (e.g., schools, institutional settings) or unsanitary living conditions.
D. Occurs year-round but peaks in the winter and spring.
E. Age: Children five to 15 years of age.

Common Findings
A. Abrupt onset of fever.
B. Headache.
C. Sore throat.
D. Bright red rash.
E. Nausea and vomiting.
F. Pruritus follows with the desquamating rash.

Other Signs and Symptoms
A. Day 1: High fever (as high as 39°C–40°C), red sore throat, swollen tonsils (may have exudate), enlarged lymph nodes in neck, cough, and vomiting. Fever peaks by the second day and gradually returns to normal in five to seven days. Fever abates within 12 to 24 hours after initiation of antibiotic therapy.
B. Day 2: The characteristic rash appears 12 to 48 hours after onset of fever. Bright red rash on the face, except around the mouth. Bright red rash blanches on pressure, has a rough sandpaper texture, and appears first on flexor surfaces, then rapidly becomes more generalized. The rash lasts four to 10 days followed by desquamation of the hands and feet that disappears by the end of three weeks. Rash is typically present on the face, which usually has a flushed appearance with circumoral pallor. The rash is most marked in the skin folds. The rash often exhibits a linear petechial character in the antebital fossae and axillary folds, known as Pastia's lines.
C. Day 3: Strawberry tongue; rash on the body increases and then spreads to neck, chest, back, then the entire body. Strawberry tongue appears as a thick, white coat with hypertrophied red papillae 24 to 48 hours after infection.
D. Days 4 to 5: The white coating disappears from the tongue.
E. Day 6: Rash fades and skin begins to peel; continues for 10 to 14 days; the palms of the hands and the soles of the feet are usually spared.

Subjective Data
A. Ask the client/parent about the onset and progression of the rash, its colour and duration, and all other symptoms.
B. Review other symptoms related to complications, such as ear pain, chest pain, and oedema.
C. Review family history and possible contact with infected wounds or others with similar symptoms of pharyngitis.
D. Determine any new medications or contact exposures.
E. Determine whether the client is allergic to penicillin.
F. Review client's recent history of impetigo.

Physical Examination
A. Check temperature, pulse, respirations, and blood pressure (BP).
B. Inspect:
  1. Conduct an ear and nose examination.
  2. Inspect the mouth and throat:
    a. Exudative tonsillitis preceding scarlet fever is often accompanied by erythematous oral mucous membranes, along with petechiae, and punctuate red macules on the hard and soft palate and uvula (e.g., Forchheimer spots).
    b. Day 1 or 2, a white coating covers the dorsum of the tongue with reddened papillae projecting through white before becoming a strawberry red tongue.
    c. Distinctive facial finding: circumoral pallor.
  3. Inspect the skin:
    a. Note the texture of the rash: "sandpaper" quality secondary to small 1- to 2-mm papular elevations.
    b. The red rash starts on the head, with the soles of the feet and the palms spared.
    c. The rash is most marked in the skin folds of the inguinal, axillary, antecubital, and abdominal areas and about pressure points.
    d. The rash associated with scarlet fever may have a linear petechial characteristic known as Pastia's lines in the antecubital and axillary folds.
    e. The erythematous rash blanches with pressure.
    f. The rash desquamates with the fingers and toes most pronounced.
C. Auscultate heart and lungs.
D. Palpate:
  1. Abdomen for organomegaly.
  2. Lymph nodes in the neck: tender and bilateral cervical nodes noted.

Diagnostic Tests
A. Throat culture remains the criterion standard for confirmation of GABHS upper respiratory infection (URI). Vigorously swab the posterior pharynx, tonsils, and any exudates with a cotton or Dacron swab under strong illumination; avoid the lips, tongue, and buccal mucosa.
B. Rapid antigen detection testing via strep throat swab.
C. White blood cells (WBCs) in scarlet fever may increase to 12,000 to 16,000 per mm^3, with a differential up to 955 polymorphonuclear lymphocytes.

Differential Diagnoses

A. Scarlet fever: Staphylococcal scarlet fever can be differentiated from streptococcal scarlet fever in the following ways:
  1. There is no circumoral pallor or strawberry tongue with staphylococcal scarlet fever.
  2. The erythematous skin is often painful or tender with staphylococcal infection.
  3. Desquamation of the superficial epidermis occurs as with the streptococcal illness; if the superficial skin separates and sloughs after only a few days, the client should be classified as having scalded skin syndrome. Desquamation, one of the most distinctive features of scarlet fever, begins seven to 10 days after the resolution of the rash and may continue up to six weeks.

B. Kawasaki disease (KD): KD needs to be carefully differentiated from scarlet fever; KD has additional signs of conjunctivitis, cracking lips, and diarrhoea.
C. Rubeola.
D. Rubella.
E. Toxic shock syndrome.
F. Drug reaction.

Plan

A. General interventions:
  1. Have the client rest with no work or school. Clients should not return to work or school until they have completed a full 24 hours of antibiotics.
  2. Prepare the client for skin desquamation. The desquamating rash is self-limited but may take over two weeks for resolution. Skin emollients may be used.
  3. Throat cultures on other household members may be necessary.
  4. Acetaminophen for temperature and pain relief.

B. Client teaching: Reinforce the need to comply with full antibiotic treatment even if the symptoms resolve.
C. Pharmacological therapy:

The goal of antibiotic therapy is the prevention of acute rheumatic fever, acute glomerulonephritis, and other complications.

  1. Tetracyclines and sulfonamides should not be used.
  2. First-line treatment for streptococcal infections is penicillin by mouth or intramuscular(IM) injection. Azithromycin and erythromycin may be substituted for clients with penicillin allergies:
     a. Adults:
       i. Penicillin V.
       ii. Penicillin G benzathine.
       iii. Erythromycin.
     b. Children:
       i. Children younger than 12 years: penicillin V.
       ii. Children older than 12 years: penicillin V.
       iii. Children <27 kg: penicillin G benzathine.
       iv. Children >7 kg: penicillin G benzathine.
       v. Amoxicillin is often used in place of oral penicillin in children, since the taste of the oral suspension is more palatable.
       vi. Erythromycin for children with a penicillin allergy.
       vii. Azithromycin for children with a penicillin allergy.
  3. Antihistamines may be used to control pruritus that follows the desquamating rash.

Follow-Up

A. No follow-up is needed for clients with uncomplicated illnesses. Clients should return if they continue to have fever and increased throat or sinus pain.
B. Consider KD if fever persists more than four days.

Consultation/Referral

A. Refer the client to an ear, nose, and throat [ENT] or infectious disease specialist for complications, such as unresolved otitis media, sinusitis, bacteraemia, rheumatic fever, and glomerulonephritis.
B. Consult a dermatologist if the diagnosis is unclear.

Bibliography

Canadian Paediatric Society. (2018). *2017 results: Canadian paediatric surveillance program.* Retrieved from www.cpsp.cps.ca/uploads/publications/CPSP-2017-Results_1.pdf

O'Connell, J., & Sloand, E. (2013). Kawasaki syndrome and streptococcal scarlet fever: A clinical review. *Journal of Nurse Practitioners, 9,* 259–264.

Sotoodian, B. (2016). Scarlet fever. *Medscape.* Retrieved from www.medscape.com

Toxoplasmosis

Cheryl A. Glass, Jill C. Cash, and Jocelyn T. Whittier

Definition

A. Toxoplasmosis is caused by an intracellular protozoan parasite, *Toxoplasma gondii.* Cats are the primary host in which *T. gondii* can complete its reproductive cycle. Humans are the intermediate host. Toxoplasmosis is acquired through contact with infected cat faeces, by eating raw or undercooked meat, and by eating soil-contaminated fruit or vegetables. In less developed countries, contaminated unfiltered water is an important source of infection, as is a transfusion or organ transplantation from an infected donor (rare).

B. Emphasis should not be placed on prior exposure to cats, since clients can acquire toxoplasma without direct contact with felines. Toxoplasmosis is one of the TORCH (toxoplasmosis, other [e.g., hepatitis and syphilis], rubella, cytomegalovirus, and herpes) infections. Toxoplasmosis causes central nervous system (CNS) disease in clients with AIDS and has perinatal consequences. Latent infection can persist for the life of the host.

C. There are three genotypes of *T. gondii,* types I, II, and III. Genotype II is generally responsible for congenital toxoplasmosis in the United States.

D. There is no vaccination available for the prevention of toxoplasmosis.

Incidence/Prevalence

A. Toxoplasmosis has a worldwide distribution of 15% to 85% of adults with chronic infection. There is no association with cat ownership. Adults most commonly acquire toxoplasmosis by environmental exposure, that is, ingestion of infectious oocysts usually from soil contamination with feline faeces and with high prevalence in environments that are moist and hot.

B. Once a person is infected, the parasite lies dormant in neural and muscle tissue and will never be eliminated. Approximately 25% of all in Canadians are IgG positive from the past exposure.

C. The global annual incidence of congenital toxoplasmosis is approximately 190,100 cases, which poses a global health burden. The severity of congenital infection is dependent on

the gestational age at the vertical transmission. The greatest risk to the fetus is vertical transmission in the first trimester. Thirty percent of exposed fetuses acquire the infection; however, 85% of live infants appear normal at birth.
D. *T. gondii* is the third most common lethal foodborne disease.

Pathogenesis

A. *T. gondii* is the causative agent and an intracellular protozoan parasite. *T. gondii* is worldwide in distribution; cats, birds, and domesticated animals serve as reservoirs. *T. gondii* is recognized as a major cause of opportunistic infection in AIDS.
B. The incubation period is estimated to be on average seven days (four– to 21–day range).
C. Routine screening for toxoplasmosis in pregnancy is not currently recommended:
   1. Maternal toxoplasmosis infection is acquired orally.
   2. Fetal infection results from transmission of parasites via the placenta (vertical transmission).
   3. Neonatal infection may also occur during vaginal delivery.

Predisposing Factors

A. Food sources:
   1. Eating raw or undercooked meats, especially mutton, lamb, and pork.
   2. Drinking unpasteurized goat milk.
   3. Eating raw shellfish.
B. Exposure to contaminated soil or garden, kitty litter, and cats.
C. Immunocompromised state:
   1. HIV infection/AIDS.
   2. Cancer therapy.
   3. Transplant recipients.
   4. Prescribed immunosuppressive drugs.
D. *T. gondii* has been documented as being acquired from blood or blood product transfusion and organ (e.g., heart) or bone marrow transplant from a seropositive donor with latent infection.
E. Poor sanitary conditions.
F. Consumption of contaminated unfiltered water.
G. Occupational exposure:
   1. Working with meat.
   2. Landscaping.
H. Travel to underdeveloped country.

Common Findings

A. 80% to 90% of acute *T. gondii* infectious hosts are asymptomatic.
B. Bilateral, symmetrical, nontender cervical adenopathy.
C. 30% of symptomatic clients have generalized lymphadenopathy.

Other Signs and Symptoms

A. Usually subclinical infection:
   1. Fever.
   2. Arthralgia, malaise, and myalgia.
   3. Headache.
   4. Sore throat/pharyngitis.
   5. Skin rash: diffuse nonpruritic maculopapular rash.
   6. Hepatosplenomegaly.
   7. Chorioretinitis: ocular pain and loss of visual acuity (most frequent, permanent manifestation of toxoplasmic infection).

B. Pregnancy:
   1. Intrauterine growth retardation (IUGR) or low birth weight.
   2. Hydrocephaly.
   3. Microcephaly.
   4. Anaemia.
C. CNS toxoplasmosis:
   1. Headache, dull and constant, is an almost universal symptom of cerebral lesions in AIDS clients.
   2. Fever.
   3. Lethargy.
   4. Altered mental state.
   5. Seizures.
   6. Weakness.
   7. Hemiparesis.
   8. Cranial nerve disturbances.
   9. Sensory abnormalities.
   10. Movement disorders.
   11. Neuropsychiatric manifestations: Toxoplasmosis is a significant factor in the causation of intellectual disabilities and blindness.

Subjective Data

A. Review onset, course, and duration of symptoms.
B. Determine whether the client is pregnant.
C. Review presence of an indoor cat and contact with kitty litter.
D. Rule out other illnesses with review of symptoms such as pharyngitis (mononucleosis).
E. Elicit initial site of rash and progression to other body areas.
F. Determine any new medications and contact exposures.
G. Rule out other family members with similar symptoms.
H. Review HIV status.
I. Review ingestion of raw/rare or undercooked meats, raw shellfish, and unpasteurized goat milk.
J. Review recent travel to an underdeveloped country (untreated water).
K. Review occupational exposure.

Physical Examination

A. Check temperature, pulse, respirations, and blood pressure (BP).
B. Inspect:
   1. Conduct ear, nose, and throat examination and careful funduscopic examination.

A funduscopic examination may reveal yellow–white areas of retinitis with fluffy borders. Diagnosis of ocular toxoplasmosis is based on observation of characteristic retinal lesions in conjunction with toxoplasma-specific serum IgG or immunoglobulin M (IgM) antibodies.

   2. Complete a dermal examination.
C. Auscultate heart and lungs.
D. Palpate:
   1. Palpate all lymph nodes, especially cervical nodes. Lymph nodes are usually smaller than 3 cm in size and nonfluctuant.
   2. Abdomen.
   3. Joints, noting swelling, erythema, or pain with examination.
E. Neurologic examination: Conduct a Mental State Evaluation.

Diagnostic Tests

A. Enzyme-linked immunosorbent assay (ELISA) is the most commonly employed test due to overall performance and cost for toxoplasmosis IgG and IgM antibody titre. Maternal infections usually are confirmed by a fourfold rise in the serum IgG.
B. Serial titres: No single level of IgG antibody can be used to determine the duration of the infection. IgG-specific antibodies achieve peak concentration one to two months after exposure and remain positive indefinitely.
C. Complete blood count (CBC) with differential.
D. HIV (rule out).
E. Pregnancy test if indicated.
F. Culture: Tissue smears, tissue section, and body fluids for presence of *T. gondii* may be considered in neonates. It takes three to six weeks to confirm the diagnosis.
G. CT scan or MRI (usually superior to CT scan).

Differential Diagnoses

A. Epstein–Barr virus (EBV).
B. Cytomegalovirus (CMV [CMV retinitis]).
C. Cat scratch disease (CSD).
D. Tuberculosis (TB).
E. Syphilis.
F. Sarcoidosis.
G. Hodgkin's disease.
H. Lymphoma.
I. Viral syndrome.
J. HIV.
K. Mononucleosis.
L. *Pneumocystis carinii* pneumonia.
M. Varicella zoster.
N. Fungal infection of eye.

Plan

A. Client teaching: **Handwashing is the single most important measure to reduce transmission of *T. gondii*.**
▶ *Refer to Client Teaching Guide: Toxoplasmosis.*
B. Pharmacological therapy:
   1. Treatment is rarely necessary because most clinical illnesses resolve spontaneously; the exception is during pregnancy.
   2. Treatment is usually given for two to four weeks:
     a. Nonpregnant adults: One of two regimens is typically prescribed:
       i. Pyrimethamine *plus* sulphadiazine *plus* leucovorin calcium.
       ii. Pyrimethamine *plus* clindamycin *plus* leucovorin calcium.
     b. Pregnancy: Despite the lack of evidence of treatment efficacy, prenatal treatment is usually offered to pregnant women who are diagnosed with toxoplasmosis:
       i. Less than 18 weeks' gestation: Spiramycin alone continued until amniotic fluid polymerase chain reaction (PRC) results are obtained after 18 weeks of gestation, due to concerns of teratogenicity associated with pyrimethamine-sulphadiazine in early pregnancy.
       ii. After 18 weeks gestation: Pyrimethamine *plus* sulphadiazine until delivery if positive amniotic PRC or fetal ultrasound suggestive of congenital toxoplasmosis.
       iii. Leucovorin calcium is added during pyrimethamine and sulphadiazine administration to prevent bone marrow suppression.
     c. Children:
       i. Trimethoprim-sulphamethoxazole.
       ii. For children one month of age or older: Dapsone *plus* pyrimethamine *plus* leucovorin.
     d. Persons with compromised immune system:
       i. Trimethoprim *plus* sulphamethoxazole. May be considered as a nonpyrimethamine alternative for AIDS clients if unable to tolerate usual adult therapy noted previously.
       ii. Administering dapsone with pyrimethamine appears to provide effective chemoprophylaxis in HIV clients seropositive for *T. gondii* who have CD4 cell counts lower than 200. However, rash, fever, and haemolytic anaemia are common adverse effects, often necessitating cessation of therapy.
       iii. For AIDS clients, after primary therapy, lifelong prophylaxis for recurrence of toxoplasmosis is required for as long as they are immunosuppressed.

Follow-Up

A. Follow up in one week to evaluate for secondary complications.
B. Pyrimethamine is a folic acid antagonist that can cause dose-related bone marrow suppression with resultant anaemia, leukopaenia, and thrombocytopaenia. Sulphadiazine is another folic acid antagonist, works synergistically with pyrimethamine, and can cause bone marrow suppression and reversible acute renal failure. Clients should return for laboratory monitoring (CBC and platelet counts) weekly.

Consultation/Referral

A. Consultation is needed for all clients; comanage with a specialist.
B. Refer the client to an obstetrician if she is pregnant.
C. Ophthalmologist medication recommendation depends on the size of the eye lesion, the location, and the characteristics of the lesion (active acute vs. chronic not progressing).

Individual Considerations

A. Pregnancy:
   1. Routine prenatal screening is not the standard of care secondary to costs. Many women have antibodies before pregnancy that protect the fetus.
   2. Transplacental infection increases the incidence of first-trimester spontaneous abortion, IUGR, preterm birth, neonatal anomalies, and stillbirth.
   3. Pyrimethamine is a folic acid antagonist and should not be given in the first trimester.
   4. Sulphadiazine should not be given in the third trimester secondary to the increased incidence of jaundice in the neonate.
   5. Transmission of toxoplasmosis in breast milk has not been demonstrated. Pyrimethamine is excreted in breast milk; however, the World Health Organization (WHO) classifies it as compatible with breastfeeding and it has a category C risk in breastfeeding in Canada.
B. Paediatrics:
   1. Seventy percent to 90% of affected infants with congenital infection may be asymptomatic at birth or may

present with low birth weight, enlarged liver and spleen, jaundice, and anaemia.
   a. Signs of congenital toxoplasmosis at birth can include maculopapular rash, generalized lymphadenopathy, haepatomegaly, splenomegaly, jaundice, and thrombocytopaenia.
   b. Cerebral calcifications may be demonstrated by radiography, ultrasound, or CT of the head.
   c. Characteristic retinal lesions (chorioretinitis) develop in up to 85% of young adults after untreated congenital infection. Acute ocular involvement manifests as blurred vision.
   d. Ocular disease can become reactivated years after the initial infection in health and immunocompromised people.
   2. Complications including visual impairment from chorioretinitis or learning disabilities or intellectual disabilities that may develop several years later.
   3. Treatment consists of drug therapy for the first year of life (see section "Pharmacological therapy"), which appears to limit further CNS injury but does not reverse the prenatal damage already sustained by the neonate.
   4. Corticosteroids also may be administered to infants with chorioretinitis.
C. AIDS clients:
   1. Clients with AIDS who have antibodies to *T. gondii* and a CD4 count of 100 cells/mm³ should be considered at high risk for the development of clinical disease. Reactivation of latent infection in the CNS is a common HIV- and AIDS-related complication.
   2. Clients with a CD4 count less than 100 cells/mm³ should receive prophylaxis against toxoplasmosis.
   3. Serology in HIV-infected clients is used mainly to identify those at risk for developing toxoplasmosis. Therefore, all HIV-positive clients should be tested for the presence of IgG antibodies.

Bibliography

American College of Obstetricians and Gynecologists. (2015). Practice Bulletin no. 151: Cytomegalovirus, parvovirus B19, varicella zoster, and toxoplasmosis in pregnancy. *Obstetrics & Gynecology (Serial Online)*, *125*(6), 1510–1525.
Centers for Disease Control and Prevention. (2013). *Parasites—Toxoplasmosis (Toxoplasma infection)*. Retrieved from www.cdc.gov/parasites/toxoplasmosis
Many, A., & Koren, G. (2006). *The College4 of Family Physicians of Canada. Toxoplasmosis during pregnancy*. Retrieved from https://www.ncbi.nlm.nih.gov/pmc/articles/PMC1479740/
Paediatrics and Child Health. (1999). Common questions about the diagnosis and management of congenital toxoplasmosis. *Paediatric Child Health*, *4*(2), 137–141.
Sanfort, C., Pottinger, P., & Jong, E. (2017). *The travel and tropical medicine manual* (5th ed.). London: Elsevier.
Torgerson, P. R., & Mastroiacovo, P. (2013). The global burden of congenital toxoplasmosis: A systematic review. *Bulletin of the World Health Organization*, *91*(7), 501–508. doi:10.2471/BLT.12.111732

Varicella (Chickenpox and Shingles)

Cheryl A. Glass, Jill C. Cash, and Jocelyn T. Whittier

Definition

A. Varicella, commonly called chickenpox, is a viral disease with a vesicular rash that occurs in crops. It manifests as a generalized, pruritic, vesicular rash. Varicella-zoster virus (VZV) infection causes two clinically distinct forms of disease: varicella (chickenpox) and herpes zoster (shingles):
   1. Primary VZV results in the diffuse vesicular rash of chickenpox.
   2. VZV remains dormant in the sensory nerve roots for life. Reactivation of the virus is known as shingles:
      a. With shingles, the virus migrates along sensory nerve via dermatomes. The symptoms include pain, sensory loss, and neurologic complications.
      b. A diagnostic clue of shingles is sensory symptoms that do not cross the midline.
      c. Postherpetic neuralgia is a prolonged complication from shingles.
B. Varicella is considered one of the TORCH (toxoplasmosis, other [e.g., haepatitis and syphilis], rubella, cytomegalovirus, and herpes) infections. Varicella infection can be fatal for an infant if the mother develops varicella from five days before to two days after delivery. A newborn is protected for several months from chickenpox if the mother had the disease before or during pregnancy. Infant immunity diminishes in four to 12 months.
C. There are two available vaccines for the prevention of varicella. The measles–mumps–rubella–varicella (MMRV) and a monovalent varicella vaccine are currently available. The Canadian Paediatric Society recommends that the quadrivalent MMRV is preferred to giving two separate injections secondary to the additional pain and the risk of the child falling behind in his or her immunization schedule.
   1. For current information regarding varicella vaccination, refer to the Canadian Immunization Guide: Part 4, Active Vaccines—Varicella (chickenpox) vaccine:
      www.canada.ca/en/public-health/services/publications/healthy-living/canadian-immunization-guide-part-4-active-vaccines/page-24-varicella-chickenpox-vaccine.html#p4c23t1.
   2. For current information regarding routine schedules for vaccination in the provinces and territories, refer to
      www.canada.ca/en/public-health/services/provincial-territorial-immunization-information/provincial-territorial-routine-vaccination-programs-infants-children.html.
   3. Both the monovalent and the quadrivalent immunizations carry a risk of febrile seizures. A personal or family history of seizures is considered a precaution for the administration of the MMRV.

Incidence/Prevalence

A. Varicella occurs worldwide. Infants are generally protected in the first few months through passive immunity. The peak incidence shifting from children younger than 10 years to children between 10 and 14 years of age demonstrates the highest incidence following the implementation of universal immunization in 1995. Varicella tends to be more severe in adolescents, adults, and pregnant women. Haemorrhagic varicella is much more common among immunocompromised clients. Immunity is generally considered lifelong.
B. Varicella incidence has greatly declined since the chickenpox vaccine has become available in Canada. It is predicted that varicella deaths, outbreaks, and hospitalizations have been greatly reduced. In the prevaccine era, approximately 350,000 varicella cases and 1,500 to 2,000 varicella-related hospitalizations occurred each year in Canada. These cases were primarily healthy children up to 12 years of age.
C. After the primary infection, the risk of shingles increases with age. The lifetime risk of herpes zoster infection in Canada is one in three Canadians in their lifetime, with two-thirds of cases occurring in people over the age of 50 years and 10% in persons 65 years requiring hospitalization.
D. The incidence of congenital varicella is 1% to 2% if the maternal infection occurs before 20 weeks' gestation.

Pathogenesis

A. VZV, herpesvirus 3, is a member of the herpesvirus family. Humans are the only source of infection for this highly contagious virus, infecting over 90% of susceptible household contacts. Person-to-person transmission occurs primarily by direct contact with a client with varicella or zoster, and it occasionally occurs by airborne droplet spread, from respiratory secretions spread onto the conjunctival or nasal/oral mucosal, and from direct contact with vesicular zoster lesions. In utero infections also occur from transplacental passage of the virus during maternal varicella infection.
B. The incubation period is 14 to 16 days. It is communicable one to two days to one week before macular eruption and until lesions crust over (about one week).

Predisposing Factors

A. Exposure to someone with the varicella virus:
  1. Direct contact with skin lesions or by respiratory tract secretions.
  2. Direct contact with clients with shingles can induce chickenpox in susceptible health-care workers.
B. Compromised immune system.
C. Nosocomial transmission is well documented in paediatric units, but transmission is extremely rare in newborn nurseries.
D. Late winter and early spring.

Common Findings

A. Low-grade fever.
B. Mild malaise.
C. Skin lesions or rash: Characteristic rash is pruritic, vesicular exanthem occurring in crops that begin on the head and neck and progress to involve the trunk and extremities. Blisters collapse within 24 hours to one week and crust over to form scabs. Skin eruptions appear almost anywhere on the body, including the scalp; penis; and inside the mouth, nose, throat, and vagina.
D. Itching.
E. Myalgia one to four days before onset of rash.

Other Signs and Symptoms

A. Children may have a mild prodrome to bacterial infections.
B. Adults may develop varicella pneumonitis. (The risk of pneumonitis is higher in smokers than in nonsmokers.)
C. Cough.
D. Headache.
E. Respiratory symptoms: cough and chest discomfort. Respiratory symptoms usually develop shortly after cutaneous eruption. Respiratory failure in pregnancy can be rapid.
F. Abdominal pain lasting one to two days.

Subjective Data

A. Review the onset, duration, and course of symptoms.
B. Elicit exposure information when noting characteristic rash, the time it started, spread of the rash or lesions, and characteristic changes.
C. Review any pulmonary or nervous system problems, such as seizures, that occur as complications.
D. Determine whether the person has HIV, is immunocompromised, or is pregnant.
E. Determine the caregiver's immunity status to varicella.
F. Review the client's immunization history.
G. Review all medication, including over-the-counter (OTC) and herbal products.

Physical Examination

A. Check temperature, pulse, respirations, and blood pressure (BP).
B. Inspect:
  1. Conduct a dermal examination, especially the hairline.
  2. Inspect the buccal mucosa.
  3. Conduct an ear, nose, and throat examination and a detailed eye examination.
  4. Shingles: Note location of lesions; they usually involve only one to three dermatomes.
C. Auscultate heart and lungs.
D. Palpate neck and lymph nodes.

Diagnostic Tests

A. Diagnosis is usually determined by the appearance of the skin eruptions, and laboratory tests are not necessary.
B. Enzyme-linked immunosorbent assay (ELISA).
C. Tissue culture of vesicular fluid or tissue biopsy (requires up to a week for result).
D. Varicella immunoglobulin G (IgG) and immunoglobulin M (IgM): VZV-specific IgM is present within five days of onset of the rash and lasts four to five weeks. A significant increase in varicella IgG antibody by standard serologic assay can confirm a diagnosis retrospectively. These antibody tests are not as reliable in immunocompromised people.
E. Pregnancy test if indicated; if positive, order the following:
  1. Anti-VZV IgG to establish immunity.
  2. Tzanck smear of suspicious lesions.
  3. Culture lesion for herpes simplex.
F. Polymerase chain reaction (PCR) of vesicular swabs or scrapings, scabs for crusted lesions, or tissue biopsy.
G. Chest x-ray, if indicated, to rule out pneumonia.
H. Genotyping of the virus is available free of charge through a specialized Government of Canada reference lab, **Viral Exanthemata and STDs—Viral STI, Polyoma and Herpesviruses Unit**. The contact number is (204) 789-6024 or (204) 789-7042 and email phac. nml. vestd-lnm. evmts. aspc@canada.ca.

Differential Diagnoses

A. Herpes simplex.
B. Scabies.
C. Impetigo.
D. Coxsackievirus.
E. Insect or spider bite.
F. Drug reaction.
G. Secondary syphilis.
H. Measles.
I. Rubella.
J. Rocky Mountain spotted fever (RMSF).
K. Scabies.

Plan

A. General interventions:
  1. Avoid contact with persons infected with chickenpox. Clients with varicella should avoid contact with others. Health-care workers should be immune to varicella. Determine immunity status with varicella IgG antibody titre if status unknown.
  2. Strict isolation should be enforced. Varicella is contagious one week before outbreak and until the lesions crust over (about one week). Isolation is a precaution until the vesicles dry.

3. Order oatmeal baths for comfort. Spray starch may also be sprayed on lesions to assist with severe itching.
B. Client teaching:
1. *Refer to Client Teaching Guide: Chickenpox (Varicella).*
2. Lesions that can be covered pose little risk to a susceptible person because transmission usually occurs from direct contact with the fluid from the lesion. Clothing or a dressing should cover lesions until they have crusted.
3. Scarring can occur from secondary infection of lesions; encourage good handwashing and no scratching.
C. Pharmacological therapy:
1. **Children with varicella should not receive salicylates, such as ASA, or salicylate-containing products due to the increased risk of Reye's syndrome.** Acetaminophen may be used as needed for fever.
2. Acyclovir therapy is *not* recommended routinely for treatment of uncomplicated varicella in otherwise healthy children.
3. Acyclovir is recommended if it can be initiated within the first 24 hours after the onset of rash in the following groups:
   a. Otherwise healthy, nonpregnant individuals 13 years of age or older.
   b. Children older than 12 months with a chronic cutaneous or pulmonary disorder, and those receiving long-term salicylate therapy.
   c. Children receiving a short, intermittent, or aerosolized course of corticosteroids (if possible, discontinue corticosteroids).
4. If therapy can be initiated within the first 24 hours of rash onset, prescribe oral acyclovir. Clients on oral acyclovir should be well hydrated during therapy.
5. Acyclovir by intravenous (IV) infusion is recommended for treatment of immunocompromised clients and clients with serious complications such as varicella pneumonia or encephalitis.
6. Varicella-zoster immune globulin (VZIG) is no longer available. The only manufacturer of this product has ceased production.
7. Systemic antipruritic: diphenhydramine hydrochloride.
8. Varicella vaccine may be given in Canada as a live attenuated univalent varicella virus vaccine or in combination with the measles-mumps-rubella (MMR) vaccine. Children should receive two doses prior to school entry, but ideally at 12 and 18 months with at least three months between doses if univalent.
For current information regarding the vaccine, refer to the Canadian Immunization Guide:
   www.canada.ca/en/public-health/services/publications/healthy-living/canadian-immunization-guide-part-4-active-vaccines/page-24-varicella-chickenpox-vaccine.html#p4c23a1.
Refer to provincial or territorial vaccine guidelines at
   www.canada.ca/en/public-health/services/provincial-territorial-immunization-information/provincial-territorial-routine-vaccination-programs-infants-children.html.
9. Antihistamines are helpful in the symptomatic treatment of pruritus.
10. The use of corticosteroids for clients with shingles to prevent postherpetic neuralgia is controversial.
11. Treatment for postherpetic neuralgia includes gabapentin, pregabalin, tricyclic antidepressants, phenytoin, carbamazepine, cimetidine, and topical capsaicin.

Follow-Up
A. No follow-up is necessary in uncomplicated cases.
B. Have the client return to the office for any secondary skin infections, conjunctival involvement, central nervous system (CNS) problems such as encephalitis and meningitis, or pneumonia.

Consultation/Referral
A. Refer the client to a specialist if pregnant; varicella pneumonia in pregnancy is a medical emergency.

Individual Considerations
A. Pregnancy:
1. Varicella vaccine should not be administered to pregnant women:
   a. Women are advised not to get pregnant for at least one month following the varicella immunization.
   b. A pregnant mother or household member is not a contraindication for immunization for a child in the household.
2. When postpubertal females are immunized, pregnancy should be avoided for at least one month after immunization.
3. VZIG (VarIg): If a pregnant woman without evidence of immunity is exposed to varicella, VarIg should administered within 96 hours of significant exposure. Maternal therapy's aim is to reduce maternal morbidity; whether it protects the fetus is unknown. VZIG should also be given to newborns whose mothers developed varicella within five days before delivery or within 48 hours after delivery.
4. Maternal complications of active varicella infection may include preterm labour, encephalitis, and varicella pneumonia. Mortality rate in gravid females is 10%. The profound maternal hypoxia that occurs in varicella pneumonia is associated with increased risk of spontaneous abortion and stillbirth.
5. Fetal complications of active varicella infection may include intrauterine growth retardation (IUGR), limb reduction defects, and eye defects.
B. Paediatrics:
1. Varicella can develop between one and 16 days of life in infants born to mothers with active live varicella at delivery.
2. Neonates usually have no prodrome or mild signs and symptoms with slight malaise and low-grade fever. Neonatal varicella is a serious illness associated with up to a 25% mortality rate. Complications include conjunctival involvement, secondary bacterial infection, viral pneumonia, encephalitis, aseptic meningitis, myelitis, Guillain–Barré syndrome, and Reye's syndrome.
3. Children entering day-care facilities and schools should have received varicella vaccine or have evidence of immunity.
4. Children with varicella should not receive salicylates or salicylate-containing products, due to the risk for Reye's syndrome.
5. Children with varicella who have been excluded from childcare may return when all lesions have dried and crusted.
C. Adults:
1. Adult clients usually have a prodrome and more severe illness than children. Adults have a 25% increased risk of mortality.

▶ Client Teaching Guides are available at https://connect.springerpub.com/content/reference-book/978-0-8261-9498-5

2. Shingles (reactivated chickenpox) appears as grouped vesicular lesions distributed in one to three sensory dermatomes, sometimes accompanied by pain localized to the area. Systemic symptoms are few.
  3. A recommendation for varicella vaccination includes persons at high risk for exposure, which include adolescents and adults who live in households with children.

D. Immunocompromised: IV antiviral therapy is recommended for immunocompromised clients, including clients being treated with chronic corticosteroids. Therapy initiated early in the course of illness, especially within 24 hours of rash onset, maximizes efficacy. Oral acyclovir should not be used to treat immunocompromised children with varicella, because of poor bioavailability.

Bibliography

Albrecht, M. A. (2016). Vaccination for the prevention of shingles (herpes zoster). *UpToDate*. Retrieved from http://www.uptodate.com/contents/vaccination-for-the-prevention-of-shingles-herpes-zoster

American College of Obstetricians and Gynecologists. (2015). Practice Bulletin no. 151: Cytomegalovirus, parvovirus B19, varicella zoster, and toxoplasmosis in pregnancy. *Obstetrics & Gynecology (Serial Online), 125*(6), 1510–1525.

Anderson, W. E. (2014). Varicella-zoster virus. *Medscape*. Retrieved from https://emedicine.medscape.com/article/231927-overview

Canadian Paediatric Society. (2018). *2017 results: Canadian paediatric surveillance program*. Retrieved from www.cpsp.cps.ca/uploads/publications/CPSP-2017-Results_1.pdf

Centers for Disease Control and Prevention. (2012). *Summary of rationale for Varicella vaccination*. Retrieved from www.cdc.gov/vaccines/vpd-vac/varicella/rationale-vacc.htm

Centers for Disease Control and Prevention. (2016). *Immunizations and pregnancy vaccines chart*. Retrieved from www.cdc.gov/vaccines/pregnancy/pregnant-women/index.html

Government of Canada. (2018a, July 26). *Canadian immunization guide: Part 4–Active vaccines. Varicella (chickenpox) vaccine*. Retrieved from https://www.canada.ca/en/public-health/services/publications/healthy-living/canadian-immunization-guide-part-4-active-vaccines/page-24-varicella-chickenpox-vaccine.html

Government of Canada. (2018b, November 19). *Canada's Provincial and Territorial Routine (and Catch-up) Vaccination Routine Schedule Programs for Infants and Children*. Retrieved from: https://www.canada.ca/en/public-health/services/provincial-territorial-immunization-information/provincial-territorial-routine-vaccination-programs-infants-children.html

Government of Canada. (n.d.). *Guide to services. VZV genotyping*. Retrieved from http://cnphi.canada.ca/gts/proficiency-panel/11881?labId=1017

Sanfort, C., Pottinger, P., & Jong, E. (2017). *The travel and tropical medicine manual* (5th ed.). London: Elsevier.

West Nile Virus (WNV)

Cheryl A. Glass, Jill C. Cash, and Jocelyn T. Whittier

Definition

West Nile Virus (WNV) disease is a mosquito-borne viral illness caused by one of the most widely distributed arthropod-borne (arbovirus) viruses. WNV is a member of the genus *Flavivirus* group, meaning it is a single-strand RNA virus. WNV is transmitted from infected animal hosts, typically wild birds, to humans via the most common types of mosquitoes. Once a client recovers from WNV disease, he or she is thought to have a lifelong immunity to the disease. There is no immunization for WNV.

The two categories of WNV disease are nonneuroinvasive and neuroinvasive:

A. Nonneuroinvasive disease is less severe and often presents as a febrile illness.
B. Neuroinvasive disease leads to encephalitis, meningitis, and flaccid paralysis, and requires much more intensive treatment.

Incidence/Prevalence

A. WNV is a reportable disease in Canada. In Canada in 2018, 367 cases were reported occurring mainly in southern Alberta, Manitoba, Ontario, and Quebec.
B. Approximately 20,000 new cases occur in North America each year, with one in 150 clients developing severe neurologic disease; 3% to 15% of those developing severe neurologic disease will die.
C. WNV was first noted in North America in 1999. WNV is endemic in the Middle East, Africa, and Asia.
D. Human WNV infections usually begin in mid-summer and decline in September, correlating with peak mosquito activity. Mosquito bites are most likely to occur during peak feeding times, during dawn and dusk. Prolonged contact or multiple mosquito bites increase the risk of developing WNV.

Pathogenesis

A. Mosquitoes are infected with WNV when feeding on an infected animal host. Wild birds are the most common source of infection, although other animals, such as horses and chickens, can be animal hosts. The virus is delivered to the human via mosquito bite when the mosquito's saliva is deposited in the human skin cells. The virus replicates in the skin cells and migrates to the lymph nodes and various organs. Infected immune cells are able to transverse the blood–brain barrier and infect the brain parenchyma leading to encephalitis and meningitis. The typical incubation period for WNV is three to 14 days.

Predisposing Factors

A. Time of year: Late summer and early fall.
B. Region: living in or traveling to a region with a higher number of reported cases.
C. Work or recreational outdoor exposure.
D. Homelessness.
E. Age: Most likely to occur in children and young adults, with most serious disease occurring in the elderly and infants.

Common Findings

A. Nonneuroinvasive WNV:
  1. Up to 80% of persons are asymptomatic.
  2. Fever.
  3. Headache.
  4. Myalgia.
  5. Arthralgias.
  6. Fatigue.
  7. Gastrointestinal (GI) symptoms: Nausea, vomiting, and diarrhoea.
  8. Maculopapular rash: Usually noted on chest, back, and arms and occurs in 20% to 50% of clients. The presence of the rash represents a decreased risk of neuroinvasive disease.

Other Signs and Symptoms

A. Abdominal pain.
B. Eye pain.
C. Irregular heart rhythm.

Potential Complications

A. Meningitis: Stiff neck, photophobia, focal neurologic deficits, and higher fever (up to 104°F).

B. Encephalitis: Mental status changes, stupor, confusion, coma, movement disorders, focal neurologic deficits, personality changes, higher fever (up to 40°C), and seizures.
C. Flaccid paralysis: Cranial nerve palsy, vertigo, dysarthria, dysphagia, respiratory failure.
D. Other rare complications:
  1. Cardiac dysrhythmia.
  2. Myocarditis.
  3. Rhabdomyolysis.
  4. Optic neuritis.
  5. Uveitis.
  6. Chorioretinitis.
  7. Orchitis.
  8. Pancreatitis.
  9. Hepatitis.

Subjective Data
A. Review the onset, course, and duration of symptoms, especially fever, rash, headache, and myalgia.
B. Ask client to describe any neurologic symptoms, changes in mental status, stiff neck, photophobia, and seizures.
C. Review symptoms of other family members or coworkers who are also ill.
D. Ask the client to recall what activity brought about or preceded his or her symptoms.
E. Ask client what steps he or she has taken to treat symptoms at home.
F. Review the client's medical history for any chronic illnesses.
G. Review all medications, including over-the-counter (OTC) and herbal products.
H. Review history of mosquito bites and any preventive steps taken such as use of insect repellent:
  1. Outdoor work activities.
  2. Outdoor recreational activities.
  3. Review recent travel.
I. Evaluate living conditions for exposure risks.

Physical Examination
Clients presenting with neurological symptoms should be quickly assessed and referred to a neurologist for immediate evaluation of symptoms.
A. Check temperature, pulse, blood pressure (BP), and respirations.
B. Inspect:
  1. Observe general overall appearance noting weakness, difficulty breathing, or changes in affect, speech, or level of consciousness (LOC).
  2. Assess hydration status.
  3. Ophthalmic examination: Assess the presence of papilloedema.
  4. Inspect the face for muscle weakness or drooping.
  5. Dermal inspection for the presence of a maculopapular rash, especially on the abdomen, back, and arms.
  6. Children:
    a. Observe for seizure activity.
    b. Note LOC (playful vs. lethargic).
C. Auscultate:
  1. Heart for dysrhythmias.
  2. All lung fields for adventitious breath sounds.
D. Palpate:
  1. Skin for signs of dehydration—poor skin turgor.
  2. The neck and lymph nodes: preauricular, posterior auricular, submental and sublingual, anterior cervical chain, and supraclavicular nodes.
  3. Abdomen for tenderness and/or organomegaly.
E. Mental State and Neurologic Examination.
  1. Administer Mental State examination to look for confusion, stupor, and changes in LOC.
  2. Complete cranial nerve testing: Focus on visual fields, extraocular movement (EOM) of a transient downbeat nystagmus, facial muscle movement and strength, and gag reflex.
  3. Muscle strength testing and testing for sensation in all extremities.
  4. Test reflexes:
    a. Deep tendon reflexes (DTRs).
    b. Babinski reflex is performed by running the reflex hammer up the midline of the sole of the foot from heel to the base of the toes (both feet are tested):
      i. A normal reaction is for the toes to either remain still or curl downward.
      ii. A positive Babinski is noted when the big toe points upward and the other toes fan out, *except for infants*.
  5. Assess for meningeal signs:
    a. Signs of meningeal irritation include nuchal rigidity.
    b. Assess for positive Brudzinski's and Kernig's signs (refer to Figures 16.1 and 16.2).
    c. Brudzinski's sign: Place the client supine and flex the head upward. Resulting flexion of both hips, knees, and ankles with neck flexion indicates meningeal irritation.
    d. Kernig's sign: Place the client supine; keeping one leg straight, flex the other hip and knee to a bent knee to form a 90-degree angle. Slowly extend the lower leg. This places a stretch on the meninges, resulting in pain and spasm for the hamstring muscle. Resistance to further extension can be felt.

Diagnostic Tests
A. WNV immunoglobulin M (IgM) antibody capture enzyme-linked immunosorbent assay (MAC-ELISA) is the gold standard diagnostic test. A positive result would indicate WNV.
B. If there is concern that the illness could have been caused by another type of flavivirus, an additional test, the plaque reduction neutralization test, is used to identify false-positive MAC-ELISA test results.
C. Complete blood count (CBC) with differential, will show increased leukocytes.
D. For clients with neuroinvasive disease:
  1. Lumbar puncture—positive for WNV—will show pleocytosis, increased lymphocytes, increased protein, and normal glucose. The MAC-ELISA test should be performed on cerebrospinal fluid (CSF) when lumbar puncture is completed.
  2. Imaging: MRI of the brain and spinal cord is the preferred imaging test. MRI may show meningeal inflammation and bilateral lesions.
  3. EEG: May show generalized slowness.

Differential Diagnoses
A. Nonneuroinvasive WNV:
  1. Other viral causes of febrile illness.
B. Neuroinvasive WNV:
  1. Other viral causes of encephalitis: St. Louis equine encephalitis, California encephalitis, Western and Eastern encephalitis.

2. Acute poliomyelitis.
3. Postpolio syndrome.
4. Guillain–Barré syndrome.
5. Multiple sclerosis.
6. Vertebrobasilar stroke.

Plan

A. General interventions:
  1. WNV is a reportable disease in Canada. Special populations may be subject to follow-up.
  2. Care is primarily supportive, treating symptoms such as fever, nausea/vomiting, and diarrhoea.
  3. Neuroinvasive disease: Clients presenting with neurological symptoms should be quickly assessed and referred to a neurologist for immediate evaluation and treatment of acute symptoms.
B. Client teaching:
  1. Discuss expected signs and symptoms of WNV acute febrile illness with the client and family.
  2. Explain signs and symptoms requiring immediate medical evaluation (e.g., mental status changes, stiff neck, and neurological symptoms).
  3. Encourage the client to rest as needed. The client may expect fatigue to continue for up to three weeks.
C. Dietary management:
  1. There are no specific dietary recommendations for WNV.
  2. Encourage the client to drink plenty of fluids to prevent dehydration.
  3. If the client is experiencing nausea and vomiting, meals should be light and taken in smaller amounts more frequently.
D. Pharmacological therapy:
  1. Utilize supportive therapy such as acetaminophen for fever, antiemetics for nausea and vomiting, and antidiarrhoeal medications for diarrhoea.

Follow-Up

A. Follow-up is determined by the client's needs, severity of acute symptoms, and risk of complications.

Consultation/Referral

A. Neuroinvasive disease: Refer to neurologist immediately:
  1. For longer term relief from neuroinvasive disease, the client may benefit from a referral to a neuropsychologist, rehabilitation specialist, physical therapist, occupational therapist, and/or speech therapist.
B. Consider an infectious disease specialist if there is difficulty with identifying the infectious agent.

Individual Considerations

A. Pregnancy:
  1. There has been no causal relationship found between WNV during pregnancy and fetal abnormalities. A small number of infants born to women who developed WNV within three weeks before delivery were found to have symptomatic WNV disease shortly after birth.
  2. If WNV is diagnosed during the last few weeks of pregnancy, a detailed examination of the newborn should be completed and steps taken to monitor for signs and symptoms of the disease in the days and weeks after the birth.
  3. All cases of WNV in pregnant women should be reported to the health department so that the cases can be followed to determine the outcome of the pregnancies.
  4. The virus has been found in breast milk and, in rare cases, breastfeeding has been linked to development of WNV in infants. The benefits of breastfeeding outweigh the risks of WNV disease; therefore, mothers should be encouraged to breastfeed.
  5. Pregnant women can use insect repellent products containing up to 30% N-diethylmetatoluamide (DEET) without adverse effects.
B. Paediatrics:
  1. Infants are more likely to suffer a more serious illness with WNV. A thorough assessment and educating the parent to recognize important signs and symptoms are crucial.
  2. The Canadian Paediatric Society recommends that regarding insect repellent:
     - **Do not** apply to children younger than six months.
     - Age six months to two years—no more than 10% DEET once a day.
     - Age two to 12 years—no more than 10% DEET up to three times a day.
     - 12 years—up to 30% DEET as per recommendations on the product.
C. Geriatrics:
  1. Older adults are more likely to suffer more serious illness and are more likely to develop neuroinvasive disease. Close attention should be given to the Mental State Examination and neurologic examination of the elderly.

Bibliography

Canadian Paediatric Society. (2018a). *Insect repellents: How to protect your child from insect bites*. Retrieved from www.caringforkids.cps.ca/handouts/insect_repellents

Canadian Paediatric Society. (2018b). *2017 results: Canadian paediatric surveillance program*. Retrieved from www.cpsp.cps.ca/uploads/publications/CPSP-2017-Results_1.pdf

Centers for Disease Control and Prevention. (2015). *West Nile virus*. Retrieved from www.cdc.gov/westnile/index.html

Centers for Disease Control and Prevention. (2016). *West Nile virus neuroinvasive disease incidence by state—United States, 2015* (as of January 12, 2016). Retrieved from www.cdc.gov/westnile/statsmaps/preliminarymapsdata/incidencestatedate.html

Cunha, B. A. (2015). West Nile encephalitis. *Medscape*. Retrieved from www.emedicine.medscape.com

Farrar, F. (2013). West Nile virus: An infectious viral agent to the central nervous system. *Critical Care Nursing Clinics of North America, 25*(2), 191–203. doi:10.1016/j.ccell.2013.02.005

Government of Canada. (2018, December 24). *Surveillance of West Nile virus*. Retrieved from https://www.canada.ca/en/public-health/services/diseases/west-nile-virus/surveillance-west-nile-virus.html

Petersen, L. R. (2016). Epidemiology and pathogenesis of West Nile virus infection. *UpToDate*. Retrieved from www.uptodate.com

Salinas, J. D. (2016). West Nile virus. *Medscape*. Retrieved from emedicine.medscape.com

Sanfort, C., Pottinger, P., & Jong, E. (2017). *The travel and tropical medicine manual* (5th ed.). London: Elsevier.

Zika Virus Infection

Jill C. Cash and Jocelyn T. Whittier

Definition

A. Zika virus is an arthropod-borne virus that is transmitted by the *Aedes* species mosquito. The virus is in the same family as the dengue virus, yellow fever virus, Japanese encephalitis,

and West Nile virus. It was initially found in the rhesus monkey in 1947 and then detected in humans in 1952 in Uganda and Tanzania. The Zika virus infection has been documented in Africa, Southeast Asia, and the Pacific Islands, and has now spread to the Americas. Mosquito-borne transmission has not been reported in the United States; however, cases of infection have been reported in male and pregnant and nonpregnant female travelers who were exposed in other countries from the mosquito-borne illness. There are two Zika virus lineages, Asian and African. Currently, mosquitoes that transmit Zika are not established in Canada due to the climate.
B. Congenital microcephaly is a known pregnancy complication of Zika viral infection. Vertical transmission to the fetus occurs from the primary infected mother or can occur from the infected male to noninfected female.

Incidence/Prevalence
A. The first case of congenital microcephaly in the United States was reported in January 2016 in Hawaii, in which the pregnant woman had lived in Brazil during her pregnancy.
B. In Canada as of September 1, 2018, there have been 569 travel-related cases and four sexually transmitted cases. Since October 2015, when surveillance began in Canada, there have been 45 cases in pregnant women. Only five cases of Zika-associated severe microcephaly/congenital Zika syndrome have been detected to date in Canada.

Pathogenesis
A. Incubation period is unknown; however, it is thought to be within a few days to seven to 12 days.
B. The Zika virus is transmitted to humans by an infected mosquito that bites the person.
C. The virus is detected in urine, blood, semen, saliva, female genital secretions, breast milk, amniotic fluid, and cerebral spinal fluid.
D. The virus can be transmitted by maternal–fetal transmission, sex (vaginal, anal, and oral), blood transfusion, organ transplantation, and exposure in the laboratory from body fluids.

Predisposing Factors
A. Recent travel to Brazil or other countries at high risk for Zika virus. See the Government of Canada website for a list of high-risk areas: www.canada.ca/en/public-health/services/diseases/zika-virus/affected-countries-areas.html.
B. Exposure to body fluids from documented infected person.
C. Sexual contact with person confirmed with Zika virus.
D. Vertical transmission from infected mother.

Common Findings
Two or more of the following symptoms appear; symptoms may be mild and/or may not be recognized by the client:
A. Acute onset low-grade fever.
B. Maculopapular pruritic rash.
C. Arthralgia of small joints (hand and feet).
D. Conjunctivitis (nonpurulent).

Other Signs and Symptoms
A. Headache.
B. Malaise.
C. Retro-orbital (eye) pain.
D. Asthenia.
E. Less common symptoms may include gastrointestinal symptoms (nausea, vomiting, diarrhoea, abdominal pain, and mucous membrane ulcers).

Subjective Data
A. Inquire whether the client has traveled outside of the Canada in areas that are high risk for Zika virus, such as Brazil, Sint Eustatius, and Argentina. Refer to the Government of Canada website listed earlier.
B. Has the client had sexual contact with another person who could possibly be infected with the Zika virus? If so, were condoms used?
C. What are the client's current symptoms? When did symptoms begin and how have they progressed?
D. Has the client had low-grade fever, joint pain, headache, eye pain, muscle weakness?
E. Does the client have any gastrointestinal (GI) symptoms (nausea, vomiting, abdominal pain)?
F. Has the client noted any skin rash or irritation?
G. What has the client used for symptoms that have presented? Did the treatment(s) improve symptoms? Has the client taken any medications before the appointment to help with fever or pain?

Physical Examination
A. Check vital signs: Temperature, blood pressure (BP), pulse, respirations.
B. Inspect:
  1. Skin for rash. Note if maculopapular, pruritic rash is present.
  2. Eyes for erythema, drainage. Perform ophthalmic examination. Note eye pain.
C. Auscultate heart and lungs.
D. Palpate:
  1. Abdomen for tenderness, rebound tenderness, masses.
  2. Back for costovertebral angle (CVA) tenderness.
  3. Joint examination should be performed in hands, feet, and other joints in which the client is complaining of joint pain.
E. Neurological examination:
  1. Perform neurological examination if Guillain–Barré syndrome is suspected. See section "Guillain-Barré Syndrome" in Chapter 19, Neurological Guidelines, for assessment.

Diagnostic Tests
A. Complete blood count (CBC)—is usually normal.
B. The Government of Canada has issued two diagnostic tests for Zika virus: Zika immunoglobulin M (IgM) antibody capture enzyme-linked immunosorbent assay (MAC-ELISA) and Trioplex real-time reverse transcriptase polymerase chain reaction (PCR) assay. Only certain laboratory centers are qualified to run these complex tests. For a decision flow sheet as to when to test, refer to www.canada.ca/en/public-health/services/diseases/zika-virus/health-professionals.html#_Testing.
C. Zika virus is currently not a reportable disease in Canada.

Differential Diagnoses
A. Other viruses (e.g., dengue fever, parvovirus, rubella, enterovirus, adenovirus).
B. Group A *Streptococcus*.
C. Measles.

D. Malaria.
E. Leptospirosis.
F. Guillain–Barré syndrome.

Plan

A. General interventions:
   1. There is no vaccine or treatment available for Zika virus.
   2. Treatment is recommended for presenting symptoms such as low-grade fever, joint pain, and so on.
   3. Mosquito bite prevention is highly recommended to avoid this virus.
   4. Confirmation of the diagnosis is essential for proper care and management.
   5. Pregnant women should avoid traveling to areas at high risk for Zika virus.
   6. Sexual contact should be avoided with clients diagnosed with Zika virus.

B. Client teaching:
   1. *Refer to Client Teaching Guide: Zika Virus Infection.*
   2. Advise travelers to avoid going to areas that are high risk for Zika virus, such as Brazil. Refer to the Centers for Disease Control (CDC) website for a list of countries at risk for the Zika virus: www.CDC.gov.
   3. The *Aedes* mosquito is most active during daytime hours, but precautions must also be used at dusk and nighttime.
   4. Educate the client regarding preventive measures for the Zika virus:
      a. Advise clients to wear loose, long-sleeved, light-coloured clothing (shirts and pants) to avoid mosquito bites. Treat clothing with insecticide, such as permethrin.
      b. Apply insect repellent that contains N-diethylmetatoluamide (DEET) when outside.
      c. Apply insect repellent after sunscreen.
      d. If traveling in exposed areas, use mosquito bed nets while sleeping if areas are not screened in or screens are not used in windows. Treat bed nets with insecticide.
      e. Avoid mosquito insect breeding areas, such as standing water (pools, water-filled buckets, etc.). Empty out containers with standing water.
      f. Advise women to avoid becoming pregnant while traveling to high-risk areas as well as avoiding pregnancy up to eight weeks after travel.
   5. Practice safe sex, using condoms; or abstain from sexual activity with clients diagnosed with Zika virus.
   6. Pregnant women confirmed with the Zika virus should use condoms or abstain from sex for the duration of the pregnancy.
   7. Men with confirmed Zika virus should use condoms or abstain from sex for at least six months after the onset of the virus.
   8. Couples in which the man has traveled to a high-risk area but did not develop symptoms should use condoms or abstain from sex for at least eight weeks to prevent spreading potential virus.

C. Pharmacological therapy:
   1. There is no medication currently available for the prevention or the treatment of Zika virus.
   2. Use analgesics such as acetaminophen for the treatment of arthralgia and fever.
   3. Nonsteroidal anti-inflammatory drugs (NSAIDs) and ASA should be avoided due to the risk of dengue infection and risk of haemorrhage.

Follow-Up

A. Depending on symptoms, the client should be reevaluated in 24 to 48 hours either by office visit or phone.
B. If the client has myalgia, joint pain, and fever, or if symptoms worsen or new symptoms present, advise the client to return for a follow-up evaluation.
C. If the client begins having muscle weakness and/or symptoms of Guillain–Barré syndrome, the client should make a follow-up appointment immediately with the provider or go to the ED for evaluation. See section "Guillain–Barré Syndrome" in Chapter 19, Neurologic Guidelines, for assessment and client education.
D. Blood work that is sent to the laboratory for screening for the Zika virus may take up to three weeks for final interpretation of results. Advise the client that precautions should be taken while waiting on results.

Consultation/Referral

A. Consult with collaborating infectious disease specialist if a client presents with complaints relating to Zika virus.
B. Consider referral to infectious disease specialist for evaluation and management.

Individual Considerations

A. Paediatrics:
   1. Presenting symptoms in children may be the same as in adults. Other symptoms may include poor feeding, irritability, difficulty walking or bearing weight, and joint pain with active/passive movement of joint.
   2. Neurologic complications (brain ischaemia, myelitis, meningoencephalitis) have been documented in children who were exposed to the virus in utero.
B. Pregnancy:
   1. Congenital microcephaly and fetal loss have been reported in newborns exposed to the Zika virus in utero.
C. Adults:
   1. Guillain–Barré syndrome has been documented as a complication of Zika virus. Further evaluation is necessary if Guillain–Barré is suspected.

Bibliography

Basarab, M., Bowman, C., Aarons, E. J., & Cropley, I. (2016). Zika virus. *British Medical Journal, 352*, i1049. doi:10.1136/bmj.i1049

Canadian Paediatric Society. (2018a). *Insect repellents: How to protect your child from insect bites.* Retrieved from www.caringforkids.cps.ca/handouts/insect_repellents

Canadian Paediatric Society. (2018b). *2017 results: Canadian paediatric surveillance program.* Retrieved from www.cpsp.cps.ca/uploads/publications/CPSP-2017-Results_1.pdf

Centers for Disease Control and Prevention. (2016). *Zika virus.* Retrieved from www.cdc.gov/zika

Government of Canada. (2018a, February 26). *Zika Virus: Information for health professionals.* Retrieved from https://www.canada.ca/en/public-health/services/diseases/zika-virus/health-professionals.html

Government of Canada. (2018b, April 23). *For health professionals: Zika virus infection.* Retrieved from https://www.canada.ca/en/public-health/services/reports-publications/canada-communicable-disease-report-ccdr/monthly-issue/2018-44/ccdr-volume-44-1-january-4-2018/zika-virus-2015-2017.html

Government of Canada. (2019, February 7). *Zika Virus prevention and treatment recommendations.* Retrieved from https://www.canada.ca/en/public-health/services/publications/diseases-conditions/zika-virus-prevention-treatment-recommendations.html

Hilton, L. (2016). Zika virus: Top mosquito repellent recommendations. *Contemporary Pediatrics, 33*(6), 14–16.

Lockwood, C. J. (2016). Zika virus and microcephaly. *Contemporary OB/GYN, 61*(2), 6–9. Retrieved from https://www.contemporaryobgyn.net/modern-medicine-feature-articles/zika-virus-and-microcephaly

Lupton, K. (2016). Zika virus disease: A public health emergency of international concern. *British Journal of Nursing, 25*(4), 198–202. doi:10.12968/bjon.2016.25.4.198

O'Malley, P. A. (2016). Zika virus. *Clinical Nurse Specialist: The Journal for Advanced Nursing Practice, 30*(4), 194–197.

Oster, A. M., Russell, K., Stryker, J. E., Friedman, A., Kachur, R. E., Petersen, E. E., . . . Brooks, J. T. (2016). Update: Interim guidance for prevention of sexual transmission of Zika virus—United States, 2016. *Morbidity & Mortality Weekly Report, 65*(12), 323–325.

Palomo, A. M. (2016). Zika virus: An international emergency? *Journal of Public Health Policy, 37*(2), 133–135.

Petersen, E. E., Polen, K. D., Meaney-Delman, D., Ellington, S. R., Oduvebo, T., Cohn, A., . . . Rivera, M. (2016). Update: Interim guidance for health care providers caring for women of reproductive age with possible Zika virus exposure—United States, 2016. *Morbidity & Mortality Weekly Report, 65*(12), 315–322.

Plourde, A. R., & Bloch, E. M. (2016). A literature review of Zika virus. *Emerging Infectious Diseases, 22*(7), 1185–1192.

Sanfort, C., Pottinger, P., & Jong, E. (2017). *The travel and tropical medicine manual* (5th ed.). London: Elsevier.

World Health Organization. (2016, June 2). Fact sheet on Zika virus disease. *Weekly Epidemiological Record, 91*(24), 314–316.

17 Systemic Disorders Guidelines

Chronic Fatigue Syndrome (Systemic Exertion Intolerance Syndrome)

Julie Adkins and Daris Klemmer

Definition
A. Fatigue is one of the most common symptoms confronting the practitioner in an office practice. A client with chronic fatigue is characterized as having fatigue with multiple associated symptoms for longer than six months, during which time these symptoms, which are moderate to severe, have a profound impact on daily activities and occur over half the time. The fatigue is not relieved by rest.

Incidence/Prevalence
A. Fatigue accounts for 1% to 3% of visits to generalists as an isolated symptom or diagnosis. Psychiatric disorders are involved in <50% of cases. Chronic fatigue has a reported frequency in excess of 20%. Fatigue is seen four times more often in women than in men, and the highest prevalence in people aged 30 to 50 years is the typical age of onset, but it can affect people of all ages, including teens and children.

Pathogenesis
A. Fatigue is a sensitive but nonspecific indicator of underlying medical and/or psychological pathology. It is reportedly more often due to unknown cause or to psychiatric illness than to physical illness, injury, medications, drugs, or alcohol.

Predisposing Factors
A. Hyperthyroidism.
B. Hypothyroidism.
C. Cardiac disease: Congestive heart failure (CHF).
D. Neurally mediated hypotension.
E. Infections: Endocarditis, hepatitis.
F. Respiratory disorders: Chronic obstructive pulmonary disease (COPD) and sleep apnea.
G. Anemia.
H. Arthritis and related disorders.
I. Cancer.
J. Alcoholism.
K. Side effects from drugs such as sedatives and beta-blockers.
L. Psychological conditions such as insomnia, depression, anxiety, and somatization disorder.
M. Female gender.
N. Virus: Epstein–Barr virus and herpes virus—EBV increased in certain subsets of myalgic encephalomyelitis (ME)/chronic fatigue syndrome (CFS) clients.
O. Can be familial or inherited.

Common Findings
A. Extreme exhaustion lasting more than 24 hours after physical or mental exercises: key consideration in diagnosis of CFS.
B. Sudden onset of fatigue.
C. Unrefreshing sleep.
D. Loss of memory and concentration.
E. Joint pain that moves around without swelling, redness, or generalized pain.
F. Muscle fatigue.
G. Swollen lymph nodes in neck/armpits.

Other Signs and Symptoms
A. Headache with new pattern and intensity.
B. Overexertion.
C. Poor physical conditioning.
D. Stress.
E. Undernutrition and poor appetite.
F. Emotional/psychological problems: depression, anxiety, and somatization disorder.

Subjective Data
A. Review history for onset, duration, and course description of the fatigue.
B. Ask the client about significant losses, low self-esteem, and occurrence of crying spells and suicidal thoughts. High prevalence of depression and suicide is present in this client population.
C. Ask the client about a history of any abuse of hypnotic drugs, alcohol, or tranquilizers.
D. Review medications, both over-the-counter (OTC) and prescription drugs.
E. Review the client's medical history for cardiac, thyroid, and other medical conditions.
F. Review sleep and insomnia history.
G. Review history for family illness or factors such as a new baby.
H. Establish last menses to rule out pregnancy.
I. Review exercise patterns.
J. Review diet with 24-hour recall.
K. Elicit history of fever, night sweats, weight loss, and enlarged lymph node(s).

L. Inquire about recent major life changes, such as moving or a change in job.
M. Establish usual weight, and review recent weight gain or loss, over what period.
N. Review any recent infections, flu, or mononucleosis. Clients often present after acute viral illness; common infections include herpes/enterovirus.
O. Review history for high-risk sexual practices, intravenous drug use, or transfusion of blood products to rule out HIV exposure.
P. Obtain history of the client's daily living and working habits.

Physical Examination
A. Check temperature, pulse, respirations, blood pressure, and weight; check for postural hypotension.
B. Inspect:
  1. Observe general overall appearance.
  2. Skin: Conduct dermal examination for changes in pigmentation, purpura, dryness, rashes, jaundice, pallor, splinter haemorrhages, or petechiae.
  3. Eyes: Conduct a funduscopic examination to rule out abnormalities or systemic illness.
  4. Check sclerae for icterus.
  5. Throat: Inspect pharynx for petechiae at the junction of the hard and soft palates to rule out mononucleosis.
  6. Extremities: Inspect the joints for inflammation and peripheral oedema.
C. Auscultate:
  1. Heart.
  2. Lungs.
D. Percuss the abdomen for organomegaly, masses, ascites, and hepatic tenderness.
E. Palpate:
  1. Palpate the neck and examine the thyroid.
  2. Palpate all lymph nodes (neck, axilla, and groin) for size, degree of tenderness, and distribution.
  3. Complete clinical breast examination for masses.
  4. Examine the abdomen for organomegaly, masses, and ascites.
  5. Examine joints for tenderness, effusions, and erythema.
  6. Assess the genitalia/rectal area for masses and tenderness.
F. Neurologic examination.
G. Mental State Examination.

Diagnostic Tests
A. Complete blood count (CBC) with differential and peripheral smear.
B. Erythrocyte sedimentation rate (ESR).
C. Calcium, albumin, urea, and creatinine.
D. Glucose.
E. Transaminase (aminotransferase): Viral hepatitis is associated with elevation in transaminase.
F. HIV serum test.
G. Thyrotropin-stimulating hormone (progressive thyroid-stimulating hormone [TSH]) to rule out hyperthyroidism or hypothyroidism.
H. Heterophile test to rule out acute mononucleosis.
I. Monospot.
J. Epstein–Barr virus.
K. Sleep study if suspecting underlying sleep disorder.
L. Human chorionic gonadotropin (HCG).
M. Depression screening tool (i.e., Patient Health Questionnaire [PHQ 9]).

Differential Diagnoses
A. CFS. According to the 2015 Institute of Medicine Criteria, CFS must have the following three symptoms[a]:
  1. Decreased ability to engage in pre-illness activities such as work, social, educational, or personal activities. Must last six months, along with severe fatigue that is not improved with rest.
  2. Post exertional malaise.
  3. Unrefreshing sleep:
  Must have one of the two of the following symptoms:
    a. Cognitive impairment.
    b. Orthostatic intolerance.
B. Hypercalcemia.
C. Mild renal failure.
D. Early diabetes mellitus.
E. Hypothyroid or hyperthyroidism.
F. Cardiac disease.
G. Anaemia.
H. Anicteric hepatitis.
I. Connective tissue disease.
J. Immune hyperactivity.
K. Disturbed sleep.
L. Occult neoplasm.
M. Infection: History of fever, sweats, weight loss, and diffuse adenopathy. These symptoms also suggest HIV, especially with high-risk behaviours (see the section "Human Immunodeficiency Virus").
N. Fibromyalgia: Comorbid in 50% of individuals with CFS.

Plan
A. General interventions:
  1. Find out the client's view of his or her illness before proceeding with client education.
  2. Manage underlying disease.
  3. Managing CFS can be as complex as the illness itself. There is no cure and symptoms vary over time. Treating the most disruptive symptoms first is paramount and then monitoring medications and supplements, managing activities and exercise, and improving health and quality-of-life issues are the primary goals.
  4. Cognitive behavioural therapy and exercise therapy have been shown to be beneficial to the client.
  5. Evaluate the client for the possibility that he or she is confusing focal neuromuscular disease with generalized lassitude.
B. Client teaching:
  1. Discuss and review the evidence for the diagnosis, and offer a careful explanation of symptoms. Many clients think they have a medical problem producing fatigue symptoms.
  2. Review the diagnostic criteria for depression (see Chapter 22, Psychiatric Guidelines), and describe the neurochemical mechanisms by which depression leads to fatigue. Refer the client for individual counselling or group therapy.
  3. Review the idiopathic nature of CFS and its nonprogressive nature. Inform the client that it has a gradually improving clinical course and has the chance of full recovery. Symptoms are self-limited, usually clearing within 12 to 18 months. Research shows that people with chronic

---

[a] Retrieved from Institute of Medicine of the National Academies. *Beyond Myalgic Encephalomyelitis/CFS: Redefining an Illness*. Report brief, January 2015. Reprinted with permission from the National Academies Press, Copyright 2015 National Academy of Sciences.

fatigue symptoms for two years or less are more likely to improve than the person for whom it has taken more time to diagnose.
4. Encourage the client to begin a gentle exercise program and to engage in life's activities.
5. Provide nutritional education.
C. Pharmacological therapy: Need to consider comorbidities present.
  1. For postural hypotension:
    a. Increase dietary sodium.
    b. Antihypotensive agent: Fludrocortisone.
  2. Low-dose antidepressant therapy for disordered sleep—ensure sleep hygiene has been discussed.
    a. Amitriptyline HCl.
    b. Imipramine HCl.
    c. Doxepin HCl.
  3. Nonsteroidal anti-inflammatory drugs (NSAIDs) for symptomatic relief of myalgia, arthralgia, or headache—analgesics often are ineffective; tricyclics may be of benefit and can be used for insomnia.
  4. Correct anaemia with iron supplements, if applicable.

Follow-Up
A. Follow up in two weeks to re-evaluate status and then monthly, depending on signs and symptoms.
B. Follow up closely if the client is depressed.

Consultation/Referral
A. Consult a specialist if no improvement is seen with therapies. Emphasize the legitimacy of the client's symptoms and summarize the workup, its rationale, and its findings.
B. Refer the client to a mental health professional as indicated by depression and/or suicidality.

Individual Considerations
A. Adults:
  1. Fatigue is most often explained by common factors such as overexertion, poor physical conditioning, inadequate quantity or quality of sleep, obesity, undernutrition, stress, and emotional problems.
B. Paediatrics:
  1. Between 0.2% and 2.3% of children and adolescents suffer from CFS. It is more prevalent in adolescents than in younger children and is more likely to develop after an acute flu-like illness or mononucleosis. Gradual onset may also occur.

Resource
Fact sheets may be obtained with information about CFS at the National ME/FM Action Network www.mefmaction.com

Bibliography
Centers for Disease Control and Prevention. (2014). *Chronic fatigue syndrome (CFS)*. Retrieved from www.cdc.gov/cfs
Christley, Y. J., & Martin, C. R. (2012). Perinatal perspective on chronic fatigue syndrome. *British Journal of Midwifery, 20*(6), 389–393. doi:10.12968/bjom.2012.20.6.389
Eriksen, W. (2018). ME/CFS, case definition, and serological response to Epstein-Barr virus. A systematic literature review. *Fatigue: Biomedicine, Health & Behavior, 6*(4), 220–234. doi:10.1080/21641846.2018.1503125
Fosnocht, K., & Ende, J. (2018). Approach to the adult with fatigue. *UpToDate*. Retrieved from https://www.uptodate.com/contents/approach-to-the-adult-patient-with-fatigue
Institute of Medicine. (2015). *Beyond myalgic encephalomyelitis/chronic fatigue syndrome: Redefining an illness*. Washington, DC: National Academies Press.
Mayo Clinic. (2014). *Chronic fatigue syndrome*. Retrieved from www.mayoclinic.org
Towards Optimized Practice (TOP) ME/CFS Working Group. (2016). *Identification and symptom management of myalgic encephalomyelitis/chronic fatigue syndrome clinical practice guideline*. Edmonton, AB: Towards Optimized Practice. Retrieved from www.topalbertadoctors.org
Yancey, J., & Thomas, S. (2012). Chronic fatigue syndrome: Diagnosis and treatment. *American Family Physician, 86*(8), 741–746.

Fevers of Unknown Origin

Julie Adkins and Daris Klemmer

Definition
The criteria for fevers of unknown origin (FUO) are an illness of at least a three-week duration, fever >38.3°C on several occasions, and remaining undiagnosed after one week of study in the hospital. Because of cost factors and increased ability of outpatient evaluation, the criterion requiring one week of hospitalization is often bypassed.

Incidence/Prevalence
In adults, infections account for 30% to 40% of cases. Cancer accounts for 20% to 30% of cases of FUO. In children, infections are the most common cause of FUO, accounting for 30% to 50% of cases; cancer is a rare cause of FUO in children. Autoimmune disorders occur with equal frequency in adults and children. Infection, cancer, and autoimmune disorders combined account for 20% to 25% of FUO in clients who have been febrile for six months or longer. Various miscellaneous diseases account for another 25%. Approximately 50% of FUO remain undiagnosed but have a benign course, with symptoms eventually resolving. Between 5% and 51% of FUO cases defy diagnosis even after exhaustive studies. FUO are more often caused by an atypical presentation of a common condition than by a rare disorder; true FUO are rare.

Pathogenesis
There are five categories of causes of FUO:
A. Infection: Most common systemic infections are tuberculosis (TB) and endocarditis (now less common due to improved techniques for the isolation of organisms that cause this).
B. Neoplasms: Most common are lymphoma and leukaemia.
C. Autoimmune disorders: Most common are Still's disease, systemic lupus erythematosus (SLE), and polyarteritis nodosa.
D. Miscellaneous causes: These include hyperthyroidism, thyroiditis, sarcoidosis, Whipple's disease, familial Mediterranean fever, recurrent pulmonary emboli, alcoholic hepatitis, drug-related fever, factitious fever, and others.
E. Undiagnosed FUO.

Predisposing Factors
A. Upper respiratory infection.
B. Urinary tract infection.
C. Viral illnesses.
D. Drug allergy, especially to antibiotics.
E. Connective tissue disease.
F. TB.
G. HIV.
H. Parasite infection.

Common Findings
A. The client feels "sick all over," with malaise and fatigue.

B. The client has chills all over the body with high fever.

Other Signs and Symptoms
A. Tachycardia.
B. Sensation of warmth or flushing.
C. Piloerection.
D. Myalgias.
E. Mild inability to concentrate, confusion, delirium, or even stupor.
F. Labial/genital herpes simplex outbreak, or fever blisters.
G. Children: Seizures.

Subjective Data
A. Review the onset, course, and duration of symptoms. For children, Does the fever respond to antipyretics?
B. Review family, occupational, and social history: new hobbies; changes at work or at home; new events.
C. Review sexual practices, including monogamy and oral, rectal, and vaginal sexual habits; recreational habits; and any new changes.
D. Elicit information regarding use of drugs—both illicit (intravenous drug [IVD]) and recent antimicrobial/nonsteroidal anti-inflammatory drug (NSAIDS)/antipyretics.
E. Review whether the client has had this illness before. How was it treated?
F. Review travel during the last month.
G. Assess for changes in cognition.
H. Review the client's history for contact with any friends or family members who have been sick and do not seem to be getting any better.
I. Review the client's history for eating any undercooked meat and dietary changes during the past month.
J. Review the child's history specifically for febrile seizures.
K. Review for risk factors for thrombophlebitis (see Chapter 10, Cardiovascular Guidelines).
L. Dental issues (abscess).
M. Urinary tract concerns: Nocturia associated with prostatitis, flank pain (pyelonephritis).

Physical Examination
A. Check temperature, pulse, respirations, blood pressure, weight, and height.
B. Inspect:
  1. Conduct funduscopic examination to rule out retinopathy, Roth's spots, and choroidal tubercles.
  2. Examine the ears, nose, and throat. Inspect the mouth for gingivitis, obvious swelling, or palpable induration.
  3. Observe the skin and mucous membranes.
  4. Perform transillumination of sinus cavities for evidence of sinusitis.
  5. Inspect body for skin rashes (lesions/urticarial/erythema) or wounds.
C. Auscultate:
  1. Heart for murmurs and rubs: bradycardia can be associated with multiple infectious diseases.
  2. Lungs for rales, consolidation, and effusion.
D. Percuss:
  1. Sinuses for tenderness.
  2. Chest for consolidation.
  3. Abdomen.
E. Palpate:
  1. Neck, axilla, and groin for lymphadenopathy.
  2. Thyroid gland.
  3. Abdomen for organomegaly, masses, tenderness, guarding, rebound, suprapubic tenderness, and costovertebral angle (CVA) tenderness, Murphy's sign, McBurney's point, or Psoas sign, any evidence of peritoneal signs.
  4. Musculoskeletal system for bone or joint swelling, tenderness, increased warmth; check lower extremities for evidence of phlebitis, asymmetrical swelling, calf tenderness, and palpable cord.
  5. Elderly: Palpate scalp for tender arteries.
  6. Infants: Palpate fontanelles.
F. Neurologic examination:
  1. Assess for signs of meningeal irritation (Brudzinski's and Kernig's signs) and presence of focal deficits.
  2. Conduct Mental State Examination.
G. Genitorectal examination, if applicable:
  1. Female: Conduct pelvic examination for cervical discharge, adnexal masses, lesions, and pelvic inflammatory disease (PID) symptoms.
  2. Male: Conduct prostate and testicular examination for tenderness and masses; check penis for discharge, rash, and lesions.
  3. Both: Conduct rectal examination for discharge, tenderness, and masses; check stool for occult blood specimen.

Diagnostic Tests
A. Complete blood count (CBC) with differential and peripheral smear.
B. C-reactive protein (CRP) and progress to erythrocyte sedimentation rate (ESR) if suspecting inflammatory cause and CRP normal.
C. Urinalysis and urine culture: Send only if symptoms of lower urinary tract symptoms (LUTS) or >50 white blood cells (WBC) in urine.
D. Kidney function tests and glucose level.
E. Liver function test.
F. Three blood cultures from different sites drawn over period of several hours.
G. Targeted testing: Consider serology for suspected infections or pathology (refer to Chapter 16, Infectious Disease Guidelines). Suspected infections include Epstein–Barr virus, Q fever, Lyme disease or other tick-borne diseases, hepatitis, syphilis, and cytomegalovirus (CMV).
H. Suspected collagen disease: Antinuclear antibodies (ANAs) and rheumatoid factor.
I. Suspected TB: Tuberculin skin test, sputum, and urine cultures.
J. Immunologic studies: Enzyme-linked immunosorbent assay (ELISA), Western blot test, and antistreptolysin O (ASLO) titre.
K. Suspected mononucleosis: Heterophile antibody test.
L. Suspected Salmonella: Widal's test.
M. Suspected thyroiditis: Thyroid profile.
N. Suspected malaria or relapsing fever: direct examination of blood smears.
O. Imaging: Depends on suspected infection.
  1. Chest, sinus radiographic films.
  2. Gastrointestinal (GI) studies: Proctosigmoidoscopy, evaluate gallbladder function.
  3. Abdominal ultrasonography: Progress to CT abdomen and pelvis based on U/S results and client symptoms.
  4. MRI is better than CT scan for detecting lesions of the nervous system.
P. Suspected embolism: Ventilation–perfusion (V/Q) scan.
Q. Suspected endocarditis or atrial myxoma: Echocardiography.

R. Radionuclide studies: Gallium scan and radium-labeled immunoglobulin are useful in detecting infection and neoplasm.
S. Laparotomy in the deteriorating client if the diagnosis is elusive despite an extensive evaluation. Any abnormal finding should be aggressively evaluated: headache necessitates a lumbar puncture to rule out meningitis; biopsy any skin from an area of rash to look for cutaneous manifestations of collagen vascular disease or infection; enlarged lymph nodes should be aspirated or biopsied and examined for cytologic features to rule out neoplasm and sent for culture; liver/bone marrow/temporal artery should be biopsied if symptoms or previous diagnostic testing indicate need.

Differential Diagnoses
A. Systemic and localized infections.
B. Neoplasms.
C. Autoimmune disorders.
D. Thrombophlebitis.
E. Miscellaneous causes (see the section "Definition").

Plan
A. General interventions: Observe the client taking his or her own temperature to document the presence of a fever to make sure the temperature is not self-induced.
  1. Treatment should be directed toward the underlying cause once a diagnosis is made.
B. Client teaching:
  1. Instruct the client to keep a record of temperatures, preferably rectal, taken each evening, when elevations are most likely to occur.
  2. Reassure the client that there is nothing abnormal about temperatures in the range of 36.1°C to 37.5°F.
  3. Instruct the client on use of physical cooling aids, such as exposure of skin to cool ambient temperature, bedside fan, and sponging with cool water or alcohol.
  4. Explain to the client that immersion in an ice water bath may be indicated for hyperthermic emergencies.
C. Pharmacological therapy:
  1. Start therapeutic trials if a diagnosis is strongly suspected:
    a. Antituberculous drugs for TB.
    b. Tetracycline for brucellosis.
    c. If the client shows no clinical response in two weeks, stop therapy and reevaluate.
  2. Symptomatic antipyretic therapy: Salicylates or acetaminophen.

Follow-Up
A. Follow up in 24 to 48 hours or three to seven days, dependent on overall wellness and symptoms.
B. Indications for admission to the hospital: Fever remains elevated beyond 38.3° C (101°F) for weeks, and ambulatory diagnostic efforts have been unsuccessful.

Consultation/Referral
A. Consult with an infectious disease physician for diagnosis and comanagement if indicated.
B. Refer the client to a specialist (infectious disease) if unable to differentiate definitive diagnosis.

Individual Considerations
A. Pregnancy:
  1. Refer the client for prenatal consultation.
  2. High fevers early in the first trimester have been associated with an increase in neural tube defects.
  3. Maternal fevers may cause fetal tachycardia.
B. Paediatrics:
  1. Toxic-appearing infants and children should be hospitalized and given parenteral antibiotic therapy following prompt diagnostic testing that includes white blood cell (WBC); urinalysis; and cultures of blood, urine, and cerebrospinal fluid.
  2. Infants under 28 days regardless of appearance are generally hospitalized and given parenteral antibiotic therapy following prompt diagnostic testing with WBC, urinalysis, and cultures.
  3. ASA products should not be given to children due to the risk of Reye's syndrome.
  4. Consider inflammatory bowel disease in older children and adolescents.
C. Geriatrics:
  1. Common causes of FUO include TB, Hodgkin's lymphoma, and temporal arteritis.
  2. Elderly clients commonly present with nonspecific symptoms.

Bibliography
Bor, D. (2018). Approach to the adult with fever of unknown origin. *UpToDate*. Retrieved from http://www.uptodate.com/contents/approach-to-the-adult-with-fever-of-unknown-origin

Chan-Trak, K. (2015). Fever of unknown origin. *Medscape*. Retrieved from http://emedicine.medscape.com/article/217675

Eriksen, W. (2018). ME/CFS, case definition, and serological response to Epstein-Barr virus. A systematic literature review. *Fatigue: Biomedicine, Health & Behavior, 6*(4), 220–234. doi:10.1080/21641846.2018.1503125

Horowitz, H. (2013). Fever of unknown origin or fever of too many origins? *New England Journal of Medicine, 368*(3), 197–199. doi:10.1056/NEJMp1212725

Palazzi, D. (2017). Fever of unknown origin in children: Evaluation. *UpToDate*. Retrieved from https://www.uptodate.com/contents/fever-of-unknonw-origin-in-children-evaluation

Human Immunodeficiency Virus (HIV)

Beverly R. Byram and Daris Klemmer

Definition
A. Acquired immune deficiency syndrome (AIDS) is a chronic, life-threatening condition caused by HIV. HIV is a retrovirus that targets helper T (CD4) cells and contains a viral enzyme called reverse transcriptase that allows the virus to convert its ribonucleic acid (RNA) to DNA then integrate and take over the cell's own genetic material. Once taken over, the new cell begins to produce new HIV retrovirus. This process kills the CD4 cells that are the body's main defense against illness. This interferes with the body's ability to fight off infection. AIDS is the term used to define a severely compromised immune system.

Incidence/Prevalence
A. According to the Centers for Disease Control and Prevention (CDC), by the end of 2012, there were approximately 1.2 million persons living with HIV in the United States. Approximately 12.8% of those were unaware of their HIV status. In 2014, an estimated 45% of those living with HIV were African American, 29% Caucasian, and 23% Hispanic. Asians/Pacific Islanders and Indigenous peoples each represent 3%. The Public Health Agency of Canada estimates that approximately 71,300 (58,600–84,000) people are believed to be living with HIV/AIDS in Canada to the end of 2011,

about 25% of whom (14,500–21,500) were unaware of their HIV infection.
B. The largest population living with HIV comprises men having sex with men (MSM), followed by persons infected by high-risk heterosexual contact, those infected by intravenous drug users (IVDUs), and those exposed through both MSM and IVDU.
C. The widespread use of antiretroviral therapy (ART) has altered the course of HIV disease. In 2012, HIV was reclassified as a chronic illness. More than 50% of deaths in HIV-positive persons on highly active antiretroviral therapy (HAART) are related to conditions other than AIDS.
The Public Health Agency of Canada HIV Screening and Testing Guide has identified the following indications for HIV screening: individuals who request testing; those with symptoms and signs of HIV infection; clients with illnesses associated with a weakened immune system or a diagnosis of tuberculosis (TB); individuals engaging in unprotected anal or vaginal intercourse or use of shared drug equipment with a partner whose HIV status is known to be positive; victims of sexual assault and women who are pregnant or planning a pregnancy; and their partners as appropriate.
D. Due to the rapidity of changing technology and knowledge, refer to the CATIE website for the most recent statistics, testing, and treatment guidelines: www.catie.ca/en/pif/spring-2017/canadian-hiv-testing-and-prevention-guidelines.

Pathogenesis
A. HIV belongs to a subgroup of retroviruses called lentiviruses or "slow" viruses. The course of infection of the virus is characterized by a long interval between infection and the onset of serious symptoms. CD4 cells are the primary target of HIV.
B. Primary HIV infection is followed by a burst of viraemia during which the virus is easily detected in peripheral blood per HIV polymerase chain reaction (PCR) viral load (VL). During the "window period," the first two to six weeks following the infection, persons may test negative for the HIV antibody with the enzyme-linked immunosorbentassay (ELISA) and Western blot tests. During this time, the person can be highly infectious to sexual partners. In this time of early infection with high VL, CD4 count can decrease by 20% to 40%. Within two to four weeks after exposure to the virus, up to 70% of infected clients experience a flu-like illness related to acute infection. The immune system fights back to reduce the HIV levels with killer T cells (CD8) that attack and kill the infected cells. The client's CD4 cell count may rebound by 80% to 90%. A client can remain symptom-free for a long time, often years. During this time, there is low-level replication of HIV but an ongoing deterioration of the immune system. Enough of the immune system remains intact to prevent most infections. The client is infectious during this time.
C. The final phase of HIV occurs when a sufficient number of CD4 cells are destroyed and when production of new CD4 cells cannot match destruction. Clients exhibit fatigue, fever, and weight loss. This failure of the immune system leads to AIDS.
D. An HIV-infected person can live an average of 8 to 10 years before developing clinical symptoms. HIV disease is not uniformly expressed in all people. A small portion of clients develop AIDS and die within months of infection. Approximately 5% of infected clients, known as "long-term nonprogressors," have no signs of disease after 12 or more years.

E. Most AIDS-defining conditions are marked by a CD4 count of <200 cells or the appearance of one or more opportunistic infections (OIs). Bacteria, viruses, or fungi that would not cause illness in a healthy immune system cause OIs. These infections are often severe and sometimes fatal.

Predisposing Factors
A. Gay or bisexual men or prostitutes.
B. Needle sharing by IVDU.
C. Perinatal infection: Mother-to-child transmission.
D. Exposure of open wounds or mucous membranes to body fluids of infected person.
E. Recipients of transfusion of contaminated blood or blood products (rare since 1985).

Common Findings
A. Fatigue: Often severe.
B. Fever: Longer than one month, usually 38° to 40°C.
C. Night sweats: Drenching.
D. Anorexia.
E. Weight loss.
F. Rash.
G. Myalgias.
H. Headache in acute phase.
I. Painful mucotaneous ulcerations: Distinctive of HIV as usually NOT present in other viral presentations.
J. Pharyngitis.

Other Signs and Symptoms
A. Lymphadenopathy: Enlarged lymph nodes often involving at least two noncontiguous sites—usually develops within second week of illness.
B. Anaemia.
C. Neutropenia.
D. Thrombocytopaenia.
E. Cough.
F. Dyspnoea.
G. Asymptomatic whitish patches on sides of tongue: Hairy leukoplakia.
H. Thrush: Oral candidiasis.
I. Odynophagia: Oesophageal candidiasis, cytomegalovirus (CMV) esophagitis.
J. Chronic vaginal candidiasis.
K. Skin changes: Rashes, dry skin, and seborrhoeic dermatitis.
L. Purplish, nonblanching nodules found on the skin, mucous membranes, and viscera: Kaposi's sarcoma.
M. Muscle wasting.
N. Chronic diarrhoea: Longer than one month.
O. Hepatosplenomegaly.
P. Cardiomyopathy.
Q. Chronic bacterial infections, including community-acquired pneumonias (not common in acute phase).
R. TB (not common in acute phase).
S. Sexually transmitted infections (STIs).
T. Peripheral neuropathy.
U. Neurological: Headache and self-limiting encephalopathy.
V. Children: Failure to thrive.

Subjective Data
A. Review symptoms: Onset, course, and duration.
B. Ask about previous HIV testing, including dates and reasons for testing.

C. Past medical history: Hospitalizations, comorbidities, immunizations, normal weight, pain, chronic lymph node disorders, and any changes of skin overlying lymph nodes.
D. Past surgical history.
E. Sexual history: Number of partners in the past year, number of lifetime partners, any previous partner known to be HIV positive or have STIs, and any previous partner known to have been incarcerated:
   1. Women: History of abnormal Paps, contraception, and condom use with partner.
   2. Men: MSM, heterosexual, bisexual, receptive anal intercourse, and condom use.
F. Past mental health history: Past and current mental health diagnosis and treatment.
G. Substance use: Tobacco, alcohol, and drugs.
H. History of IVDU: Needle sharing and timing of last drug use.
I. Transfusion or blood product history before 1985.
J. Lived or traveled outside of Canada: When and for how long.
K. Assess the presence of persistent fever with no localizing symptoms.
L. Assess the client's support system: Who knows the diagnosis?

Physical Examination

A. Height, weight, blood pressure, pulse, respiratory rate, and temperature.
B. General observation: General appearance, including fat distribution signs of wasting.
C. Inspect:
   1. Skin: Evaluate for rashes, seborrhoea, folliculitis, moles, Kaposi's sarcoma, warts, herpes, dry skin, skin cancer, fungal infections, molluscum contagiosum, jaundice, and needle marks.
   2. Head and neck: Head, eyes, ears, nose, and throat (HEENT):
      a. Assess visual acuity.
      b. Retina examination for abnormal findings—cotton wool spots, and the like.
      c. Evaluate sclera for icterus.
      d. Oral examination for thrush, hairy leukoplakia, mucosal Kaposi's sarcoma, gingivitis, aphthous ulcers, and dental health.
D. Auscultate:
   1. Pulmonary auscultation for air movement and abnormal breath sounds.
   2. Cardiac evaluation for normal and abnormal heart sounds.
E. Palpate:
   1. Palpate the thyroid.
   2. Lymphatic evaluation of regional versus generalized swelling: Specific location, size, and texture of nodes.
   3. Palpate the abdomen to evaluate the presence of hepatosplenomegaly, masses, tenderness, pain, or rebound tenderness.
F. Rectal/vaginal examination:
   1. Both genders: Inspect for the presence of ulcers and warts in the vagina, perineum, and rectum.
   2. Females: Perform bimanual examination, Pap smear, obtain specimens for STI testing, and perform a digital rectal examination. Consider anal cytology if abnormal Pap smear.
   3. Males: Testicular examination, digital rectal examination, anal cytology if MSM.

G. Neurologic examination:
   1. Assess mental status.
   2. Assess cranial nerves, including gait, strength, deep tendon reflexes, evaluation of proprioception, vibration, pinprick, temperature, and sensation in distal extremities.
H. Psychiatric examination: Screen for depression.

Diagnostic Tests

A. Repeat HIV testing if the client does not have a confirmed lab copy of diagnosis.
B. Complete blood count (CBC), with differential, including platelets.
C. Complete chemistry profile.
D. Fasting lipid profile.
E. Venereal disease research laboratory (VDRL) test and rapid plasma reagin (RPR) test.
F. Serologies for toxoplasmosis.
G. CD4/CD8 cells and CD4/CD8 ratio.
H. HIV RNA VL.
I. HIV-resistance genotype and integrase strand transfer inhibitors (INSTI) genotype if under previous exposure.
J. HLA-B 5701 (risk of abacavir hypersensitivity reaction syndrome).
K. Hepatitis serologies: Hepatitis A virus (HAV) serology (antibody), hepatitis B virus (HBV) complete serology profile, and hepatitis C virus (HCV) serology (antibody).
L. Cultures for gonorrhoea/chlamydia (GC)/chlamydia/syphilis/trichomoniasis—anal, vaginal, and oral.
M. Urinalysis.
N. Pap smear.
O. Anal cytology with MSM: recommended for women with abnormal Pap smear.
P. TB screening: T-spot, QuantiFERON, or purified protein derivative (PPD). Chest X-ray yearly in case of a history of TB treatment. Refer to a TB clinic if screening is positive. Clinical Pearl: All HIV suspected cases should undergo STI testing, including syphilis, gonorrhoea, chlamydia, herpes, and hepatitis, plus anyone with recent positive STI should have HIV screening, and all STI testing should include HIV testing due to clients not being forthcoming about potential high-risk sexual behaviours.

Differential Diagnoses

A. Other diseases that lead to immune suppression or are related to symptoms.
B. Cancer.
C. Chronic infections.
D. Toxoplasmosis, other (syphilis, varicella-zoster, parvovirus B19), rubella, CMV, and herpes (TORCH) infections.
E. TB.
F. Endocarditis.
G. Infectious enterocolitis.
H. Bowel disorders: Antibiotic-associated colitis, inflammatory bowel disease, or malabsorptive symptoms.
I. Endocrine diseases.
J. Neuropathy.
K. Alcoholism.
L. Liver disease.
M. Renal disease.
N. Thyroid disease.
O. Vitamin deficiency.
P. Chronic meningitis.

Plan

Clinical Guidelines per British Columbia Centre for Excellence in HIV/AIDS cfenet.ubc.ca/therapeutic-guidelines/guidelines-management-acute-hiv-infections and the National Institutes of Health: AIDSinfo.NIH.gov.

A. General interventions:
  1. Refer and comanage the client with HIV/AIDS clinician.
  2. Identify and treat substance abuse.
  3. Explain to the client that at each visit you will review history, conduct a physical examination, and run laboratory studies to assess health status.
  4. Discuss health habits: Smoking, nutrition, exercise, and sexual health practices.
  5. Discuss treatment plan:
     a. HAART.
     b. Therapy for opportunistic infections (OIs) and malignancies.
     c. Prophylaxis for OIs: *Pneumocystis carinii* pneumonia (PCP) and mycobacterium avium complex (MAC) according to CD4 count.
     d. Managing side effects of medications and comorbidities.
     e. Immunizations.
B. Client teaching:
  1. Discuss living with HIV disease.
  2. Discuss transmission prevention strategies: Safer sex practices and condom use.
  3. Provide contact information for AIDS service organizations (ASOs).
  4. Discuss the client's concerns, including notification of sexual partner(s) and needle-sharing partner(s).
C. Discuss birth control and family-planning issues. Offer preconception counselling.
D. Pharmacological therapy:
  1. Treatment with HAART: Always consult with an HIV/AIDS specialist for treatment options.
     a. HAART: There are 25 individual medications from seven classes of drugs as well as 14 pills that are combinations of two to four of these medications. Medication selection should be based on known resistance patterns. The seven drug classes are:
        i. Nucleoside/nucleotide reverse transcriptase inhibitors (NRTIs).
        ii. Nonnucleoside reverse transcriptase inhibitors (NNRTIs).
        iii. Protease inhibitors (PIs).
        iv. INSTIs.
        v. Fusion inhibitors (FIs).
        vi. Entry inhibitors (EIs).
        vii. Pharmacokinetic enhancer.
        viii. Combination antiretrovirals.
     Recommendations for triple therapy induce a pharmacologically boosted PI, an INSTI, and two NRTIs: emtricitabine and tenofovir isoproxil fumarate (British Columbia Centre for Excellence in HIV/AIDS: Management of acute HIV Infections).
  2. Prophylaxis and treatment for OIs. May discontinue prophylaxis if sustained an immune reconstitution on HAART:
     a. PCP. Prophylaxis if CD4 count <200 or client has oral candidiasis:
        i. First line: Trimethoprim/sulfamethoxazole.
        ii. Alternatives: Dapsone, atovaquone, and aerosolized pentamidine.
     b. MAC prophylaxis if CD4 count is <75:
        i. First line: Zithromax.
        ii. Alternative: Clarithromycin.
  3. Managing side effects of HAART and complications of HIV therapy: Multiple complications of long-term HIV infection and treatment with HAART:
     a. Lipodystrophy syndrome, bone marrow suppression, cardiovascular disease, CNS side effects, gastrointestinal (GI) intolerance, hepatic failure, hepatoxicity, hyperlipidaemia, insulin resistance, diabetes, lactic acidosis/hepatic steatosis, nephrotoxicity, osteonecrosis, osteopaenia, peripheral neuropathy, nephrolithiasis, urolithiasis, crystalluria, hypogonadism, and psychiatric complications.
  4. Immunizations:
     a. Hepatitis A and B series: If not immune, recommended dosing as per renal failure.
     b. Tetanus.
     c. Pneumococcal vaccine.
     d. Yearly influenza vaccines.
     e. HPV vaccine series for women and men up to age 27 years.
     f. Enquire on drug coverage: Need for social work consult/compassionate coverage.

Follow-Up

A. Schedule return visit within four weeks after initial visit to discuss staging HIV/AIDS, living with HIV/AIDS, and to start HAART regimen.
B. PPD yearly unless there is a history of positive PPD, then yearly chest X-ray.
C. Pap smear:
  1. Initially, if normal, repeat in six months, then yearly if remains normal.
  2. If abnormal, follow the guidelines at www.colposcopycanada.org/guidelines.html.
D. Some clinicians advocate for anal Pap smears for men but there are no set guidelines at present.

Consultation/Referral

A. Refer the client to a specialist in HIV for management of continued care and pharmacological therapy.
B. Refer the client to a nutritionist for baseline evaluation and diet counselling.
C. Refer pregnant women to an obstetrician.
D. Ophthalmology examination yearly for CMV screening and vision changes.
E. Dental referral.
F. Hepatology referral if chronic, active hepatitis B and/or C.
G. Referral for support of social work/psychology due to increased depression/anxiety diagnosis with HIV/community resources/insurance and disability information.

Individual Considerations

A. Adults:
  1. Preconception counselling: Clinical Guidelines per National Institutes of Health—AIDSinfo.NIH.gov.
  2. Preconception counselling: The goal is to avoid transmission of HIV to partner and fetus. Use ovulation kits (basal body charts) to determine the most fertile time for pregnancy.
     a. Discordant couples:
        i. HIV-positive female and HIV-negative male:
           1) Self-insemination (methods: syringe, turkey baster, and cervical cap).

            2) Use of preexposure prophylaxis (PrEP) for HIV-negative partner.
        ii. HIV-positive male and HIV-negative female:
            1) Sperm washing/In vitro fertilization (IVF): Very expensive; often cost-prohibitive.
            2) HIV-positive male partner on HAART and HIV VL as close to undetectable as possible.
            3) Unprotected sex during ovulation times only and no other.
            4) Use of PrEP for uninfected partner.
        iii. HIV-positive male and HIV-positive female: Avoid superinfection:
            1) Both partners on HAART and VL as close to undetectable as possible.
            2) Unprotected sex during ovulation times only and no other.
B. Pregnancy: Clinical Guidelines per National Institutes of Health—AIDSinfo.NIH.gov.
    1. Antepartum:
        a. HAART starting at 10 to 12 weeks of gestation or maintaining treatment if already on pregnancy-approved HAART.
        b. Goal of therapy is undetectable HIV-VL.
        c. Efavirens should not be used in pregnancy during first trimester.
        d. Vaginal delivery can be offered if HIV-VL is <1000.
    2. Intrapartum:
        a. Continue oral HAART.
        b. Zidovudine.
        c. C-section if HIV-VL >1000.
    3. Postpartum:
        a. HAART for mother is continued depending on immunologic status.
        b. Infant receives zidovudine for the first four weeks of life if mother has undetectable HIV-VL. If mother's VL is unknown or the aforementioned is undetectable, the baby should receive combination therapy.
        c. Breastfeeding is contraindicated.
C. Paediatrics: Clinical Guidelines per National Institutes of Health—AIDSinfo.NIH.gov.
    1. Perinatal transmission in the United States has been reduced to <2% due to HAART.
    2. Infants born to HIV-infected mothers test positive for HIV antibody ELISA test. Transplacentally acquired antibody may persist in the child for up to 18 months.
    3. Clinical and laboratory evaluation of the child must be done postpartum. Initial HIV-RNA-VL testing should be done at birth, 14 to 21 days, 1 to 2 months, and 4 to 6 months postpartum.
    4. Children who are HIV positive from vertical transmission should be followed by paediatric infectious disease clinicians.
    5. All routine immunizations are recommended for HIV-infected children except for severely immunocompromised HIV-infected children who should not receive live-virus vaccines.
D. Prophylaxis:
    1. PrEP is a prevention method for HIV-negative partners.
        a. Emtricitabine/tenofovir is recommended for use as PrEP for heterosexual and MSM-HIV-negative partners:
        b. Those taking PrEP should be monitored for potential side effects.

    2. Postexposure prophylaxis (PEP): Clinical Guidelines per British Columbia Centre for Excellence in HIV/AIDS—www.cfenet.ubc.ca and the National Institutes of Health—AIDSinfo.NIH.gov.
        a. Depending upon exposure type and severity, postexposure ART should be started as quickly as possible and be taken for four weeks postexposure.
        b. Expert consultation should be obtained as quickly as possible.
        c. Follow with occupational health for regular clinical assessment and labs.
        d. Perform HIV testing: Baseline, six weeks, three months, six months, and one year.
        e. HIV testing with HIV-RNA-VL if an illness compatible with seroconversion illness occurs (fever, lymphadenopathy, pharyngitis, rash).
        f. Advise transmission precautions during first three to six months postexposure (use condoms, refrain from donating blood, discontinue breastfeeding).

Resources

British Columbia Centre for Excellence in HIV/AIDS http://www.cfenet.ubc.ca

CATIE Canada's Source for HIV and hepatitis C https://www.catie.ca/

Bibliography

The AIDS Infonet. (2013). *Factsheets*. Retrieved from www.aidsinfonet.org

AIDSmeds. (2012a, August 28). *Treatment for HIV & AIDS*. Retrieved from http://www.aidsmeds.com/list.shtml

AIDSmeds. (2012b, November 13). *Currently approved drugs for HIV: A comparative chart*. Retrieved from http://www.aidsmeds.com/articles/DrugChart_10632.shtml

American Academy of HIV Medicine. (2010). *Fundamentals of HIV medicine for the HIV specialist*. Washington, DC: Author. Retrieved from http://www.AAHIVM.org

The Body. (2016). *The complete HIV/AIDS resource*. Retrieved from http://www.thebody.com

The Body. (n.d.-a). *Approved HIV medications by class*. Retrieved from http://www.thebody.com/index/treat/classes.html

The Body. (n.d.-b). *First steps to HIV/AIDS treatment*. Retrieved from http://www.thebody.com/index/treat/first.html

The Body. (n.d.-c). *HIV/AIDS medication basics*. Retrieved from http://www.thebody.com/content/art40488.html

The Body. (n.d.-d). *HIV drug-drug interactions*. Retrieved from http://www.thebody.com/index/treat/interactions.html

The Body. (n.d.-e). *Side effects of HIV/AIDS and HIV medications*. Retrieved from http://www.thebody.com/index/treat/side_effects.html#general

Centers for Disease Control and Prevention. (2012, June). Monitoring selected National HIV prevention and care objectives by using HIV surveillance data-United States and 6 U.S. dependent areas-2010. *HIV Surveillance Supplemental Report*. Retrieved from https://www.cdc.gov/hiv/topics/surveillance/reports

Centers for Disease Control and Prevention. (2013a, January). *HIV testing trends in the United States, 2000–2011*. Retrieved from https://www.cdc.gov/hiv/pdf/testing_trends.pdf

Centers for Disease Control and Prevention. (2013b, April 15). *HIV surveillance report: Diagnoses of HIV infection in the United States and dependent areas, 2011*. Retrieved from https://www.cdc.gov/hiv/pdf/statistics_2011_HIV_Surveillance_Report_vol_23.pdf

Centers for Disease Control and Prevention. (2013c, November). *HIV in the United States: At a glance*. Retrieved from https://www.cdc.gov/hiv/basics/statistics.html

Centers for Disease Control and Prevention. (2013d, May 13). *HIV among African American gay and bisexual men*. Retrieved from https://www.cdc.gov/hiv/risk/racialethnic/bmsm/facts/index.html

Centers for Disease Control and Prevention. (2014b, December 11). *Recommendations for HIV Prevention with adults and adolescents with HIV*. Retrieved from https://www.cdc.gov/hiv/guidelines/personswithhiv.html

Centers for Disease Control and Prevention. (2016a). *HIV/AIDS statistics overview*. Retrieved from www.cdc.gov/hiv/statistics/overview

Centers for Disease Control and Prevention. (2016b). *Opportunistic infections*. Retrieved from www.cdc.gov/hiv/basics/livingwithhiv/opportunisticinfections.html

Centers for Disease Control and Prevention. (2016c). *Updated guidelines for antiretroviral postexposure prophylaxis after sexual, injection drug use, or other nonoccupational exposure to HIV—United States, 2016.* Retrieved from stacks.cdc.gov/view/cdc/38856

Günthard, H. F., Saag, M. S., Benson, C. A., del Rio, C., Eron, J. J., Gallant, J. E., . . . Volberding, P. A. (2016). Antiretroviral drugs for treatment and prevention of HIV infection in adults: 2016 recommendations of the International Antiviral Society-USA Panel. *Journal of the American Medical Association, 316*(2), 191–210. doi:10.1001/jama.2016.8900. Retrieved from https://www.iasusa.org/content/antiretroviral-drugs-treatment-and-prevention-hiv-infection-adults-2016-recommendations

International AIDS Society–USA. (n.d.). *Antiretroviral treatment of adult HIV infection.* Retrieved from https://www.iasusa.org/content/antiretroviral-drugs-treatment-and-prevention-hiv-infection-adults-2016-recommendations

Panel on Antiretroviral Guidelines for Adults and Adolescents. (2016, July 14). *Guidelines for the use of antiretroviral agents in HIV-1-infected adults and adolescents.* Washington, DC: Department of Health. Retrieved from https://aidsinfo.nih.gov/contentfiles/lvguidelines/AdultandAdolescentGL.pdf

Panel on Antiretroviral Therapy and Medical Management of HIV-Infected Children. (2016, March 1). *Guidelines for the use of antiretroviral agents in pediatric HIV infection.* Washington, DC: Department. Retrieved from https://aidsinfo.nih.gov/contentfiles/lvguidelines/pediatricguidelines.pdf

Panel on Opportunistic Infections in HIV-Infected Adults and Adolescents. (2013, May 7). *Guidelines for the prevention and treatment of opportunistic infections in HIV-infected adults and adolescents: Recommendations from the Centers for Disease Control and Prevention, the National Institutes of Health, and the HIV Medicine Association of the Infectious Diseases.* Society of America. Washington, DC: Department of Health and Human Services. Retrieved from https://aidsinfo.nih.gov/contentfiles/lvguidelines/adult_oi.pdf

Panel on Treatment of HIV-Infected Pregnant Women and Prevention of Perinatal Transmission. (2016, October 26). *Recommendations for use of antiretroviral drugs in pregnant HIV-1-infected women for maternal health and interventions to reduce perinatal HIV transmission in the United States.* Washington, DC: Department. Retrieved from http://aidsinfo.nih.gov/contentfiles/lvguidelines/perinatalgl.pdf

POZ.com. (n.d.). *HIV drug chart.* Retrieved from https://www.poz.com/drug_charts/hiv-drug-chart

Public Health Agency of Canada. (2012). *HIV screening and testing guide.* Ottawa: Author. Retrieved from http://www.phac-aspc.gc.ca

Sax, P. (2017). Acute and early HIV infection: Clinical manifestations and diagnosis. *UpToDate.* Retrieved from https://www.uptodate.com/contents/acute-and-early-HIV-infection-clinical-manifestations-and-diagnosis

Sax, P. (2018). Acute and early HIV infection: Treatment. *UpToDate.* Retrieved from https://www.uptodate.com/contents/acute-and-early-HIV-infection-treatment

U.S. Food and Drug Administration. (n.d.). *Antiretroviral drugs used in the treatment of HIV infection.* Retrieved from http://www.fda.gov/ForPatients/Illness/HIVAIDS/Treatment/ucm118915.htm

U.S. Preventive Services Task Force Recommendation Statement. (2013, April). *Screening for HIV.* Retrieved from http://www.uspreventiveservicestaskforce.org/uspstf13/hiv/hivfinalrs.htm

World Health Organization. (2012, July). *Guidance on oral pre-exposure prophylaxis (PrEP) for serodiscordant couples, men and transgender women who have sex with men at high risk for HIV: Recommendations for use in the context of demonstration projects.* Geneva, Switzerland: Author. Retrieved from http://www.who.int/hiv/pub/gidanceprep/en

Idiopathic (Autoimmune) Thrombocytopaenic Purpura

Julie Adkins and Daris Klemmer

Definition

A. Idiopathic thrombocytopaenic purpura (ITP) is an acquired thrombocytopaenia autoimmune disorder in which an immunoglobulin G (IgG) autoantibody is formed that binds to platelets, caused by autobodies against platelet antigens. The platelet count is <100,000 mm^3.
B. Three common types of ITP: (a) primary ITP is acquired due to autoimmune thrombocytopaenia leading to platelet destruction and platelet underproduction not triggered by an associated condition; (b) secondary ITP is associated with another condition (e.g., HIV, hepatitis C, systemic lupus, chronic lymphocytic leukemia [CLL]); (c) drug-induced immune ITP is due to drug-dependent platelet antibodies that cause platelet destruction, which must be distinguished from drug-induced bone marrow suppression.
C. Time elapsed since diagnosis: (a) newly diagnosed—up to three months since diagnosis; (b) persistent—3 to 12 months since diagnosis; (c) chronic—more than 12 months diagnosis.

Incidence/Prevalence

A. Acute ITP occurs commonly in childhood is frequently precipitated by a viral infection and usually resolves spontaneously. It is seen in children of 1 to 6 years of age and middle-aged adults of 30 to 40 years of age. There is a two-to-one female-to-male predominance. The adult form is usually a chronic disease (more than six months) and seldom follows a viral infection.

Pathogenesis

A. ITP results from production of antiplatelet antibodies, which leads to peripheral destruction and sequestration of platelets. It is not clear which antigen on the platelet surface is involved. Platelets are not destroyed by direct lysis. Destruction takes place in the spleen, where splenic macrophages with Fc receptors bind to antibody-coated platelets. The primary cause of long-term morbidity and mortality is haemorrhage, whether spontaneous or accident-induced trauma. Two common events are infections (usually viral) and systemic conditions that disrupt immune homeostasis (autoimmune disorder, lymphoid, or malignancy).

Predisposing Factors

A. Infections (cytomegalovirus [CMV], varicella, hepatitis C, HIV).
B. Chronic alcoholism.
C. Sepsis.
D. AIDS.
E. Immune disorders, such as systemic lupus erythematous (SLE).
F. Drug use.
G. CLL.
H. Pregnancy.

Common Findings

ITP can be asymptomatic:
A. Purple spots and bruises on skin.
B. Epistaxis.
C. Mouth and gum bleeding.
D. Fatigue and decreased quality of life.

Other Signs and Symptoms

A. Purpura, petechiae, and hemorrhagic bullae in the mouth—concerning for more severe bleeding.
B. Tendency to bleed easily—easy bruising.
C. Menorrhagia—abnormal heavy menstruation.
D. No systemic illness: The client feels well and is not febrile.

Subjective Data

A. Determine when the client or caregiver first noticed symptoms; note whether the symptoms have changed or progressed.
B. Rule out pregnancy as a cause of nosebleeds.

C. Ask whether the client is feeling well except for the bleeding or bruising.
D. Determine whether the client has a fever.
E. Obtain medication history for over-the-counter (OTC) and prescribed medications.
F. Determine the client's history of immune disorders, recent infections, alcoholism, and pregnancy.
G. Establish usual weight and any recent weight loss.
H. Discuss diet and use of herbal remedies, quinine, and walnuts.

Physical Examination
A. Check temperature, pulse, respirations, blood pressure, and weight.
B. Inspect:
 1. Observe general appearance.
 2. Conduct dermal examination for purpura and petechiae.
 3. Conduct eye examination; check sclera for haemorrhages.
 4. Examine the mouth for dental caries and poor hygiene, mouth petechiae, and haemorrhagic bullae.
C. Palpate:
 1. The abdomen, liver, and spleen.

Normally, the spleen should not be palpable.

 2. Palpate the cervical, axillary, and groin lymph nodes for adenopathy.
D. Percuss—assess for hepatosplenomegaly:
 1. Abdomen.
 2. Liver.
 3. Spleen.
E. Auscultate:
 1. Heart.
 2. Lungs.
 3. Abdomen for bowel sounds and bruits.

Diagnostic Tests
A. Platelet count.

The major concern during the initial phase is risk of cerebral haemorrhage when platelet count is <5000 platelets per microlitre.

B. IgG.

Increased levels of IgG appear on the platelet count in the presence of thrombocytopaenia.
IgG, immunoglobulin G.

C. Complete blood count (CBC) with differential and peripheral smear.

Peripheral smear shows normal WBCs and RBCs, platelets low in count with large size.

D. Bleeding time is prolonged.
E. Coagulation tests: Prothrombin time/international normalized ratio (PT/INR), partial thromboplastin time (PTT), and fibrinogen—usually normal. Platelet-associated antibodies may be detected—may not be needed if mild thrombocytopaenia but should be done for moderate to severe bleeding or planned invasive procedure.

Coagulation studies are normal.

F. Bone marrow aspiration, per specialist.

Bone marrow may appear normal or have increased megakaryocytes (early form of platelets) with thrombocytopaenia.

G. May consider thyroid-stimulating hormone (TSH) and *Helicobacter pylori*, dependent on symptoms.

Differential Diagnoses
Thrombocytopaenia may be produced in two ways: by abnormal bone marrow function or by peripheral destruction of platelets. It is also a diagnosis of exclusion.
A. Abnormal bone marrow function:
 1. Aplastic anaemia.
 2. Haematologic malignancies.
 3. Myelodysplasia: This can be ruled out only by examining the bone marrow.
 4. Megaloblastic anaemia.
 5. Chronic alcoholism.
B. Non–bone marrow disorders:
 1. Immune disorders:
  a. ITP.
  b. Drug induced from medications being taken.
  c. Secondary to CLL and SLE.
  d. Posttransfusion purpura.
 2. Hypersplenism resulting from liver disease.
 3. Disseminated intravascular coagulation (DIC).
 4. Thrombotic thrombocytopaenic purpura.
 5. Sepsis.
 6. Haemangiomas.
 7. Viral infection.
 8. AIDS.
 9. Pregnancy.
 10. Hypothyroidism.

Plan
A. General interventions: Signs of active bleeding indicate need for more urgent evaluation and therapy. If severe bleeding arrange for immediate referral to haematology for management advice, client may need urgent intravenous immunoglobulin (IVIG) or platelet transfusion (rare). Consider transfer to acute care facility for severe bleeding or critical platelet counts.
B. Client teaching:
 1. Instruct the client to avoid trauma. Advise that the client cannot participate in contact sports.
 2. Instruct the client to avoid salicylates and gingko biloba; they impair platelet function.
 3. Instruct client to update all immunizations.
 4. Prednisone therapy benefits:
  a. Prednisone increases platelet count by increasing platelet production.
  b. Long-term therapy may decrease antibody production.
  c. Bleeding often diminishes one day after beginning prednisone.
  d. Platelet count usually begins to rise within a week for most clients, and two-thirds will see response in two to five weeks; responses are almost always seen within three weeks.
  e. About 80% of clients respond to treatment and the platelet count usually returns to normal.

C. Medical or surgical management:
  1. Splenectomy is the most definitive treatment. Most adults ultimately undergo splenectomy.
  2. Splenectomy is indicated if clients do not respond to prednisone initially or require unacceptably high doses to maintain an adequate platelet count.
D. Pharmacological therapy:
  1. Initial treatment:
    a. Prednisone:
      i. High-dose therapy should be continued until the platelet count is normal (usually around one to two weeks) and the dose should then be gradually tapered.
      ii. In most clients, thrombocytopaenia recurs if prednisone is completely withdrawn.
      iii. High-dose therapy should not be continued indefinitely in an attempt to avoid surgery.
  2. Alternative drug therapy:
    a. High-dose IVIG is highly effective in rapidly raising the platelet count.
      i. This treatment is expensive, costing approximately $5000 or more.
      ii. The beneficial effect lasts two to six weeks.
      iii. This therapy should be reserved for emergency situations such as preparing a severely thrombocytopaenic client for surgery/procedure/severe bleeding.
    b. Thrombopoietin receptor agonists: Drugs that boost platelet production such as romiplostim and eltrombopag. The medications stimulate the bone marrow to produce more platelets. Side effects include headache, dizziness, nausea, and vomiting. There is also an increased risk of blood clots.
  3. Platelet transfusions are an option rarely used. Transfusions may be necessary in emergency situations along with intravenous methylprednisolone and intravenous immune globulin.
  4. Avoid ASA, nonsteroidal anti-inflammatory drugs (NSAIDs), warfarin, or gingko biloba, which interfere with platelet function and blood clotting.

Exogenous platelets survive no better than the client's own platelets. In many cases, platelets survive less than a few hours. This therapy is reserved for cases of life-threatening bleeding in which enhanced haemostasis for even an hour may be of benefit.

Follow-Up
A. The client must be monitored very closely. Perform daily to weekly platelet counts; frequency depends on the severity and course.
B. Prognosis for acute ITP: 80% respond and fully recover within two months; 15% to 20% progress to chronic ITP.
C. Prognosis for chronic ITP: 10% to 20% recover fully; remainder continue to have low platelet counts and may see a remission or relapse over time.
D. The principal cause of death from ITP is intracranial haemorrhage.

Consultation/Referral
A. After diagnosis, refer the client to a haematologist.

Individual Considerations
A. Pregnancy:
  1. Rule out hemolysis, elevated liver enzymes, low platelets (HELLP) syndrome, infection, and DIC as causes of thrombocytopaenia.
  2. There is an increased incidence of spontaneous abortions and haemorrhage at the time of delivery from genital tract injury.
  3. Antepartum management: Conduct fetal blood sampling and testing when the mother has a known history of ITP.
  4. Intrapartum management:
    a. Avoid fetal hypoxia, which can decrease the fetal platelet count.
    b. Avoid prolonged labour.
    c. Conduct continuous fetal monitoring.
    d. Epidural anaesthesia may be used if the platelet count is at least 100,000 cells per cubic millimetre.
  5. Postpartum management: Breastfeeding is not recommended because of the possible transmission of antiplatelet antibodies through breast milk.
B. Paediatrics:
  1. ITP is frequently precipitated by a viral infection.
  2. It usually has an acute course that is self-limited.
C. Geriatrics:
  1. ITP is uncommon in this population; there is usually another cause for low platelets in geriatrics.
  2. Persons older than 60 years must be evaluated for other causes such as myelodysplastic syndromes, acute leukemia, or bone marrow infiltration.
  3. Persons with ITP aged 70 years or older are at risk of spontaneous bleeding and adverse events of treatment.

Bibliography
George, J., & Arnold, D. (2018). Immune thrombocytopenia (ITP) in adults: Clinical manifestations and diagnosis. *UpToDate*. Retrieved from https://www.uptodate.com/contents/immune-throbocytopenia-(ITP)-in-adults-clincal-manifestations-and-diagnosis

Kahanov, L., Eberman, L. E., & Grammer, S. (2012). Diagnosis and treatment of idiopathic thrombocytopenic purpura. *International Journal of Athletic Therapy & Training, 17*(2), 25–28. doi:10.1123/ijatt.17.2.25

Kessler, C. (2015). Immune thrombocytopenic purpura (ITP). *Medscape*. Retrieved from emedicine.medscape.com

Mayo Clinic. (2016). *Idiopathic thrombocytopenia purpura (ITP)*. Retrieved from www.mayoclinic.org

Weiss, S. (2012). Oral involvement of systemic diseases. *Clinical Advisor for Nurse Practitioners, 15*(6), 25–30.

Iron-Deficiency Anaemia (Microcytic, Hypochromic)

Julie Adkins and Daris Klemmer

Definition
A. Microcytic anaemia is characterized by small, pale red blood cells (RBCs) and depletion of iron (Fe) stores. The haematocrit (Hct) is <41% in males, with a haemoglobin (Hgb) <13.5 g/dL. In females, the Hct is <37% with an Hgb <12 g/dL.

Incidence/Prevalence
A. Iron deficiency is the most common cause of anaemia worldwide; it is particularly prevalent in women of childbearing age. It is estimated to occur in 20% of adult women, 50% of pregnant women, and 3% of adult males in the United States.

Pathogenesis
A. Anaemia is acquired; it develops slowly and in stages. Iron loss exceeds intake so that stored iron is progressively

depleted. As stored iron is depleted, a compensatory increase in absorption of dietary iron and in the concentration of transferrin occurs. Iron storage can no longer meet the needs of the erythroid marrow; the plasma-transferring level increases and the serum iron concentration declines, resulting in a decrease in iron available for RBC formation.

Predisposing Factors

A. Increased requirement: Rapid growth (infants and adolescents); menstruation; pregnancy in the second and third trimesters; lactation.
B. Increased loss: Gastrointestinal (GI)—oesophagitis, erosive gastritis, peptic ulcer, inflammatory bowel disease (IBD), benign tumours, intestinal/stomach cancer, angiodysplasia, haemorrhoids, hookworm infestation, occult blood loss secondary to cow's milk protein–induced colitis, chronic or high-dose use of nonsteroidal anti-inflammatory drugs (NSAIDs)/salicylates; genitourinary (GU)—menorrhagia, chronic haematuria; haemolysis—intravascular haemolysis; other—regular blood donors, frequent epistaxis, haemorrhagic telangiectasia (rare). Overt bleeding most common cause of IDA.
C. Decreased absorption: Dietary factors—coffee, carbonated beverages, pica, pagophagia, nonhaem iron ingestion, GI—gastrectomy, duodenal bypass, bariatric surgery, *Helicobacter pylori*, celiac disease, atrophic gastritis, paediatric short bowel syndrome, IBD (Crohn's/colitis), chronic kidney disease.
D. Decreased intake: Elderly, alcoholism, diet (vegetarian/vegan/iron poor), low Socio-economic status (SES), malnutrition.

Common Findings

A. Fatigued all of the time.
B. Heart feels like it is racing, beating hard.
C. Out of breath on exertion.
D. Loss of appetite.
E. Nausea and vomiting.
F. Headaches throughout day.
G. Weak and dizzy.
H. Low work productivity/difficulty concentrating.

Other Signs and Symptoms

Clinical presentation depends on severity, client's age, and the ability of the cardiovascular and pulmonary systems to compensate for the decreasing oxygen-carrying capacity of the blood.

A. Initial: Exercise-induced dyspnoea and mild fatigue symptoms may be minimal until the client has significant anaemia.
B. As Hct falls, dyspnoea and fatigue increase:
 1. Malaise.
 2. Drowsiness.
 3. Sore tongue and mouth: Papillae, atrophic glottis.
 4. Skin pallor.
 5. Pale mucous membranes and conjunctiva, blue sclerae.
 6. Nails: Pale and brittle.
 7. Tachycardia.
 8. Palpitations.
 9. Tinnitus.
 10. Pica and pagophagia symptoms.
 11. Hair loss.
 12. Irritability and depression.
C. Severe anaemia
 1. Atrophic glossitis, cheilitis (lesions at the corner of the mouth).
 2. Koilonychia (thin concave fingernails with raised edges).
D. Children.
 1. Attention deficit hyperactivity disorder (ADHD)/hyperactivity.
 2. Breath holding.
 3. Growth restriction.
 4. Tiredness.
 5. Restlessness.
 6. Irritability.
 7. Cognitive and intellectual impairment.

Subjective Data

A. Inquire about onset, course, and duration of symptoms.
B. Ask the client about past history of GI bleeding.
C. Take careful history of GI complaints that might suggest gastritis, peptic ulcer disease, or other conditions that might produce GI bleeding.
D. Ask whether there has been a change in stool colour or bleeding from haemorrhoids.
E. In menstruating women, ask about blood loss during menses.
F. Ask about dietary intake of iron-rich foods and ask about dietary restrictions.
G. Inquire about pica habits, intake of nonfood items such as clay, dirt, detergent, and the like.
H. Obtain medication history, especially use of ASA and other NSAIDs.
I. Rule out history of anaemia, blood-clotting problems, sickle cell disease, glucose-6-phosphate dehydrogenase (G6PD) deficiency, or other hereditary haemolytic disease, screen for celiac disease.
J. Review occupation and activities with exposure to lead or lead paint.
K. Has the client experienced palpitations, chest pain, dizziness, or shortness of breath?

Physical Examination

A. Check temperature, pulse, respirations, blood pressure, and weight. Check for postural hypotension. Children: Plot weight, height, and head growth parameters on growth chart (see Table 17.1).
B. Inspect:
 1. Inspect general appearance; the client may be pale, lethargic, or without overt signs if anaemia is mild.

TABLE 17. **Normal Haemoglobin and Haematocrit Values for Children**

Age (Years)	Hgb (%)	Hct (%)
1–2	>11.0	>33.0
2–5	>11.2	>34.0
5–8	>11.4	>34.5
8–12	>11.6	>35.5
12–18	>12.0	>36.0

Hct, haematocrit; Hgb, haemoglobin.

2. Conduct eye examination; check conjunctivae for paleness and sclerae for blueness.
3. Examine oral mucosa, corners of the mouth (for cheilitis); note appearance of the tongue (atrophy of the papillae; smooth, shiny, beefy red appearance), angular stomatitis, pale gums, or atrophic glottis.
4. Examine the skin for dryness and perfusion.
5. Examine nails for brittleness, flattening, ridges, and concave or spoon shape.
6. Check for hair loss.

C. Auscultate:
1. Heart for systolic flow murmurs.

D. Palpate:
1. Abdomen for tenderness and enlargement of the liver and spleen.

E. Percuss:
1. Abdomen.

F. Rectal examination: Assess for masses, haemorrhoids, and/or obvious bleeding.

Diagnostic Tests

A. Initial;
1. Complete blood count (CBC) with differential and peripheral smear.
2. Serum ferritin level, serum iron, total iron-binding capacity (TIBC), reticulocyte count, RBC indices.
3. Serum iron concentration: Absent iron storage equals ferritin value <30 ng/mL.
4. Urinalysis:

Clinical Pearls: Investigating the underlying cause of Iron deficiency anemia (IDA) is as important as treating the IDA; stool for occult blood is of no benefit in investigating IDA; adults without an obvious source of blood loss and new diagnosis of IDA must be evaluated for occult gastric malignancy in the form of endoscopy.

B. Follow-up diagnostics, if indicated:
1. TIBC: Serum TIBC and serum ferritin rise.
2. Hct three to four weeks after treatment. Treatment should continue for at least four to six months after the Hct returns to normal.
3. GI series, if indicated.
4. Endoscope, if indicated.
5. Ultrasonography, if indicated.

Differential Diagnoses

A. Haemolytic diseases such as sickle cell and G6PD deficiency.
B. Inadequate intake of iron.
C. Any condition that causes acute or chronic blood loss.
D. Neoplasm.
E. Anaemia of chronic disease (thalassaemia, sideroblastic anaemias).
F. Lead poisoning.

Plan

A. General interventions:
1. Identify source of anaemia.
2. Discuss dietary sources of iron-rich foods.
3. Infants should be ingesting formula enriched with iron and iron-enriched cereals.

B. Client teaching:
1. Stress the importance of dietary intake of foods high in iron, which is absorbed better than most vitamins. Vitamin C increases absorption of iron. Suggest taking with a glass of orange juice or vitamin C supplement.
2. Provide iron supplements as indicated.
3. Encourage the client to stop smoking if applicable.

C. Pharmacological therapy:
1. Oral iron replacement.
    a. Adult.
        i. Begin six-month trial of ferrous sulphate. Food decreases iron delivery by 50%.
        ii. Iron supplement.
        iii. If the client has been prescribed an antacid, oral iron supplements should be taken two hours before or four hours after taking the antacid to avoid absorption interaction.
    b. Children:
        i. Liquid iron.
        ii. Chewable vitamin with an iron supplement for mild cases.
    c. **Clinical Pearls of Oral Iron Supplement:** Encourage clients to take iron in the morning (iron absorption decreased when hepcidin levels are highest, hepcidin peaks in the evening hours); take vitamin C supplement to maximize absorption; should NOT be taken with calcium products such as supplements, certain antacids, and dairy products such as milk, cheese, and yogurt, and NOT be taken with high oxalate food such as caffeine, tea, spinach, kale, and broccoli; can cause GI upset (nausea, vomiting, diarrhoea, constipation, metallic taste, dark stools)—if your client is experiencing this, consider starting lower dose and titrating upward, switch to liquid form in smaller doses, change preparation to smaller dosage, take iron with small snack or at bedtime (decreases absorption), could consider polysaccharide iron complex but is expensive and no better other iron salt formation.

2. Alternative drug therapy: Parenteral iron is indicated if the client cannot tolerate or absorb oral iron or if iron loss exceeds oral replacement:
    a. Iron dextran injection—Client needs test dose and observation prior to proceeding with first dose.
    b. Iron sucrose:
        i. Parenteral iron therapy is expensive.
        ii. It is associated with significant side effects: anaphylaxis, phlebitis, regional adenopathy, serum sickness-type reaction.
        iii. Dose is based on the client's weight.
        iv. Do not administer parenteral iron along with oral iron.
        v. Intramuscular (IM) iron should be avoided due to pain and staining at injection site, and variable absorption, plus known cases of development of sarcoma.

Follow-Up

A. Follow-up of adults is variable, depending on the source of blood loss. Manage signs of anaemia.
B. It is advisable to see the client after three to four weeks, both to monitor the haematologic response and to answer questions about the medication, which may result in improved compliance.
C. If the client's Hgb level has increased by 1.0 g/dL in three to four weeks, continue iron supplementation for an additional three to six months. The Hct should return to normal after two months of iron therapy. However, keep taking iron supplements for another 6 to 12 months to replace the body's iron storage in the bone marrow.

D. Determine the effectiveness of iron replacement therapy during the first two weeks of therapy by checking the reticulocyte count.

Consultation/Referral
A. Refer the client to hematology for the following:
   1. Hgb is not increased by 1.0 g/dL after one month of treatment, or client continues to decline.
   2. The therapeutic trial should not be continued beyond one month because the Hgb concentration has not increased and client compliance with recommended regimen is not a factor.
   3. There is a steady downward trend in Hct despite treatment.
   4. There is a significant drop in Hct over previous readings (rule out lab error first).
   5. Laboratory findings show Hgb <9.0 g/dL or Hct <27%. Suspect underlying inflammatory, infectious, or malignant disease.
B. Refer the client for nutrition consultation, if indicated.

Individual Considerations
A. Pregnancy:
   1. Check Hct at initial prenatal visit, 28 weeks, and 4 weeks after initiating therapy.
   2. Laboratory findings of Hgb >13 g/dL and Hct >40% may indicate hypovolaemia. Be alert for signs of dehydration and preeclampsia.
   3. Counsel the client on proper diet and refer her to a dietitian.
   4. Recommend 60–200 mg of elemental iron a day,
   5. If unable to tolerate vitamins, recommend children's chewable vitamins with iron.
B. Paediatrics:
   1. Place medication in back of mouth, and rinse mouth/brush teeth following administration to reduce staining of teeth.
   2. All infants must be on iron-fortified formula or breast milk.
   3. Inform caregiver not to give cow's milk to infants younger than 12 months old. Assess daily milk intake in children older than 1 and teach that too much milk intake decreases iron absorption.
   4. Educate parents about iron-rich foods that are age-appropriate: Cereals, bran, dried fruit, red meat, and beans.
   5. Obtain height and weight of infants and children, plot on growth chart, and compare with previous parameters.
   6. If required supplement with elemental iron with vitamin C,minimal amount of GI side effects.
C. Adults:
   1. Bleeding is the usual cause of anaemia in adults. In adult men and postmenopausal women, bleeding is usually from the GI tract.
   2. In premenopausal women, menstrual loss may be the underlying cause of anaemia.
   3. Smokers may have higher Hgb levels; therefore, anaemia may be masked if standard Hgb levels are used.

Bibliography
American Society of Hematology. (2016). *Iron deficiency anemia*. Retrieved from www.hematology.org

Friedman, J. J., Chen, Z., Ford, P., Johnson, C., Lopez, A., Shander, A., . . . van Wyck, D. (2012). Iron deficiency anemia in women across the life span. *Journal of Women's Health*, 21(12), 1282–1289. doi:10.1089/jwh.2012.3713

Grasso, P. (1973). Sarcoma after intramuscular iron injection. *British Medical Journal*, 2(5867), 667. doi:10.1136/bmj.2.5867.667

Greenberg, G. (1976). Sarcoma after intramuscular iron injection. *British Medical Journal*, 1(6024), 1508–1509. doi:10.1136/bmj.1.6024.1508-a

Short, M., & Domagalski, J. (2013). Iron deficiency anemia: Evaluation and management. *American Family Physician*, 87(2), 98–104.

Solomons, N., & Schumann, K. (2004). Intramuscular administration of iron dexetranis inappropriate for treatment of moderate pregnancy anemia, both in intervention research on underpriviledged women and in routine prenatal care provided by public health services. *American Journal of Clinical Nutrition*, 79, 1–3. doi:10.1093/ajcn/79.1.1

Towards Optimized Practice Iron Deficiency Anemia Committee. (2018 March). *Iron Deficiency Anemia clinical practice guideline*. Edmonton, AB: Toward Optimized Practice. Retrieved from http://www.topalbertadoctors.org

U.S. National Library of Medicine. (2013, March 12). *Iron deficiency anemia*. Retrieved from https://www.ncbi.nlm.nih.gov/pubmedhealth/PMHT0022011

Weiss, S. (2012). Oral involvement of systemic diseases. *Clinical Advisor for Nurse Practitioners*, 15(6), 25–30.

Lymphadenopathy

Julie Adkins and Daris Klemmer

Definition
Lymphadenopathy is the enlargement of a lymph node, manifested in benign, self-limiting diseases and in those that are incurable and fatal. Only small lymph nodes in the neck, axilla, and groin are palpable in normal individuals. Palpable nodes in other regions, or any node exceeding 0.5 cm in size, are potentially abnormal. The body has approximately 600 lymph nodes.

There are different categories of lymphadenopathy:
A. Localized adenopathy (one region).
B. Hilar adenopathy.
C. Generalized lymphadenopathy (more than one region).
D. Other lymphatic abnormalities that present in other ways, such as lymphangitis, lymphadenitis, and lymphoedema.

Incidence/Prevalence
A. Lymphadenopathy is a very common presenting symptom. Age is an important diagnostic factor: In clients younger than 30 years, the cause proves to be benign in 80% of cases; in clients older than age 50, the rate of benign disease falls to 40%. In primary care, clients with unexplained lymphadenopathy, approximately three-fourths of clients will present with localized lymphadenopathy and one-fourth with generalized lymphadenopathy. Lymphadenopathy in children is commonly caused by benign self-limiting diseases, such as viral disease.

Pathogenesis
A. Inflammation and infiltration are responsible for pathologic enlargement. Localized lymphadenopathy may represent the spread of disease from an area of drainage. The left supraclavicular node is referred to as the "sentinel" node, which is in contact with the thoracic duct and drains much of the abdominal cavity. The right supraclavicular node drains the mediastinum, lungs, and oesophagus. Generalized lymphadenopathy often results from infection, malignancy, hypersensitivity, and metabolic disease. Supraclavicular lymphadenopathy is commonly associated with high-risk malignancy, 34% to 50% of clients with this presentation found malignancy with increased numbers in those over 40 years.

Predisposing Factors
A. Factors posing high risk for HIV infection:
1. Homosexuality and bisexuality.
2. Intravenous drug abuse.
3. Haemophilia or other conditions requiring multiple transfusions.
4. Prostitution.
5. Haitian ancestry.

B. Occupational exposure.
C. History of pharyngitis, upper body infections (head and neck), or intraoral infection.
D. Exposure to animals: Cats, sheep, cattle, rodents, deer ticks.
E. Travel to the southwest United States, South America, Africa, Asia, India, and the Mediterranean.
F. Exposure to bird droppings.
G. Lacerations sustained from gardening.
H. Exposure to tuberculosis (TB).
I. History of sexual exposure resulting in sexually transmitted infections (STIs).
J. History of tobacco abuse.
K. Cancer.
L. Medications:
1. Anticonvulsant drugs that cause skin rash, fever, hepatosplenomegaly, and eosinophilia (e.g., phenytoin).
2. Certain antihypertensives: Hydralazine, captopril, atenolol.
3. Para-aminosalicylic acid, sulindac.
4. Certain antibiotics: Cephalosporins, penicillins, and sulphonamides.
5. Misc.: Gold, allopurinol, quinine, pyrimethamine.

Common Findings
A. Sore throat.
B. Fever.
C. Fatigue and malaise.
D. Loss of appetite.
E. Loss of weight.
F. Swollen, painless lumps in neck, axilla, supraclavicular, iliac, and inguinal areas.

Other Signs and Symptoms
A. May feel "good" except for finding enlarged lymph node.
B. Node location(s): For inguinal enlargement, rule out conditions that may resemble inguinal or femoral lymphadenopathy—Hernias; ectopic testicular, endometrial, or splenic tissue; lipomas; varices; and aneurysms. If inguinal area is painful and tender, it is most frequently caused by STIs.
C. Skin rash.
D. Bruising or petechiae.
E. Pruritus.
F. Erythema of skin or scalp.
G. Skin eruption.
H. Night sweats.
I. Abdominal pain, enlarged and tender abdomen.
J. Joint pain.

Subjective Data
A. A comprehensive and detailed history is necessary for diagnosis (see the section "Predisposing Factors").
B. Review the onset, course, and duration of symptoms.
C. What does the client note with respect to location, tenderness or painfulness, softness or hardness, and mobility of lymph nodes? Has the client noticed more than one enlarged lymph node?
D. Review the client's history of risky behaviours: IVD, alcohol use, sexual activity, HIV risks.
E. Review history for hobbies, specifically gardening and camping, and occupation (see the sections "Lyme Disease" and "Toxoplasmosis" in Chapter 16, Infectious Disease Guidelines).
F. Review medications: Prescription, over-the-counter (OTC), and herbal remedies.
G. Determine whether the client has a fever or a known valvular heart disease.
H. Review any other associated symptoms or signs.
I. Review any recent exposure to family and friends with infections. Has the client had recent immunizations?
J. Review recent dental problems or abscessed teeth.
K. Note whether the client is/was a smoker. If so, how much, for how long, and (if relevant) when did the client quit smoking?
L. Review the client's history for recent cat scratches (see the section "Cat Scratch Disease" in Chapter 16, Infectious Disease Guidelines).
M. Review the client's history for recent travel.
N. Review the client's history for new sexual partners, to rule out STIs.
O. Review usual weight and any recent weight loss, noting how much and over what period of time.
P. Elicit information about similar symptoms in the past, when they occurred, how they were treated (antibiotics, biopsy), and the success of the treatment.
Q. Elicit information about alcohol intake, noting how much, how long, and whether the client has quit and how long ago.
R. Document immunization history.

Physical Examination
Essential to take time to complete a THOROUGH physical examination
A. Check temperature, pulse, respirations, blood pressure, and weight.
B. Inspect:
1. Conduct a funduscopic examination.
2. Examine the eyes, ears, nose, and throat.
3. Conduct a dermal examination, and check mucous membranes for a primary inoculation site; this may be a clue to a diagnosis of cat scratch disease (CSD).

C. Auscultate:
1. Heart and lungs.

D. Palpate:
1. Palpate the abdomen.
2. Conduct a clinical breast examination. Palpate mass to determine if it is a lymph node, if applicable.
3. Palpate all nodal areas for localized and generalized lymphadenopathy:
   a. Hard, fixed nodes suggest metastasis, and a biopsy should be taken promptly. Size alone is not itself diagnostic, but any node larger than 3 cm suggests neoplastic disease.
4. Palpate the scalp in the elderly for the tender arteries of cranial arteritis.
5. Palpate the neck for thyroid gland tenderness or masses.
6. Musculoskeletal system examination:
   a. Assess and palpate for bone or joint swelling, tenderness, and increased warmth.
   b. Examine lower extremities for evidence of phlebitis: asymmetric swelling, calf tenderness, and palpable cord.

E. Percuss:
   1. Sinuses for tenderness, and transilluminate for evidence of sinusitis.
F. Genital–rectal examination:
   1. Conduct careful external evaluation for herpetic lesions, masses, discharge, erythema, chancroid, scabies, and pediculosis.
   2. Examine urethra for discharge.
   3. Note any folliculitis if the client regularly shaves/waxes the genital area.
   4. Female pelvic examination: Look for cervical discharge, cervical motion tenderness, adnexal tenderness, and mass or "heat" in the pelvis.
   5. Males: Examine the prostate and testicles for tenderness and masses, and the penis for discharge and rash.
   6. Examine the rectum for discharge, tenderness, masses, and fistulas.

Diagnostic Tests
Should be completed in stepwise approach based on concerns and high suspicion differential diagnoses.
A. **Generalized lymphadenopathy:**
Complete blood cell count and differential (CBCD), CXR, HIV serology, hepatitis serology (A, B, C), peripheral blood smear, basic chemistries (liver function tests, C-reactive protein [CRP], and kidney function tests), antinuclear antibody (ANA), Epstein–Barr virus (EBV) serology, blood cultures, syphilis serology, urethral/cervical smears, throat swab. If negative then progress to TB testing—CXR if not already done, TB skin testing.
B. **Concern for malignancy:** Should have imaging (ultrasound [US]/CT) and biopsy.
C. **Localized lympadenopathy:** CBCD and targeted testing based on risk factors, exposure, and high-suspicion differential diagnoses.
Clinical Pearl: In some clients with viral upper respiratory tract infection (URTI) and cervical lymphadenopathy, close clinical follow-up to ensure resolution may be appropriate as the lymphadenopathy should resolve with the viral illness; if persists then progress to further diagnostics. The prevalence of malignancy for clients referred from primary care providers was 17%.

Differential Diagnoses
A. There are four general categories for lymphadenopathy:
   1. Infections:
      a. Mononucleosis.
      b. AIDS or AIDS-related complex (ARC): Generalized adenopathy in an asymptomatic HIV-infected client indicates a high risk of progression to AIDS. The lymphadenopathy represents follicular hyperplasia in response to HIV infection.
      c. Toxoplasmosis.
      d. Secondary syphilis.
   2. Hypersensitivity reactions:
      a. Serum sickness.
      b. Phenytoin and other drugs.
   3. Metabolic diseases:
      a. Hyperthyroidism.
      b. Lipidoses.
   4. Neoplasia:
      a. Leukaemia.
      b. Hodgkin's disease, advanced stages.
      c. Non-Hodgkin's lymphoma.
B. Causes can be isolated by site of the enlarged nodes (see Table 17.2).

Plan
A. General interventions:
   1. Pay careful attention to nodal history and characteristics on physical examination.
   2. Make a careful assessment to establish the palpable mass is a lymph node. Chronicity alone is not always serious.

TABLE 17.2 Causes of Lymphadenopathy by Site of Enlarged Nodes

Anterior auricular	**Axillary**
Viral conjunctivitis	Breast malignancy
Trachoma	Breast infection
Posterior auricular	Upper extremity infection
Rubella	**Epitrochlear**
Scalp infection	Syphilis (bilateral)
Submandibular or cervical (unilateral)	Hand infection (unilateral)
Buccal cavity infection	**Inguinal**
Pharyngitis (can be bilateral)	Syphilis
Nasopharyngeal tumour	Genital herpes
Thyroid malignancy	Lymphogranuloma venereum chancroid
Cervical (bilateral)	Lower extremity or local infection
Mononucleosis sarcoidosis	**Any region**
Toxoplasmosis pharyngitis	Cat scratch fever
Supraclavicular (right)	Hodgkin's disease
Pulmonary malignancy	Leukaemia
Mediastinal malignancy	Metastatic cancer
Oesophageal/GI malignancy	Sarcoidosis
Supraclavicular (left)	Granulomatous infections
Intra-abdominal malignancy	**Hilar adenopathy**
Renal malignancy	Sarcoidosis (unilateral or bilateral)
Testicular or ovarian malignancy	Fungal infection (histoplasmosis, coccidioidomycosis)
	Lymphoma (unilateral or bilateral)
	Bronchogenic carcinoma (unilateral or bilateral)
	Tuberculosis (unilateral or bilateral)

GI, gastrointestinal.

B. Client teaching: As indicated by the particular disease process causing the lymphadenopathy.
C. Pharmacological therapy: Dependent on the diagnosis.

Follow-Up
A. Follow the client closely to evaluate resolution of lymphadenopathy and disease process.
B. Follow-up depends on the diagnosis.

Consultation/Referral
A. Admission may be useful if a period of observation is needed.
B. Refer the client to a specialist after initial workup, if indicated.
C. Refer the client to an oncologist or an oncologic surgeon if the client is suspected of having a malignancy, to consider the need for biopsy or best approach to obtaining a tissue diagnosis.

Individual Considerations
A. Paediatrics:
  1. Palpable nodes in the anterior cervical triangle of the neck are common in children and usually suggest infection as a cause.
  2. Kawasaki disease is seen among children and young adults; it is also known as mucocutaneous lymph node syndrome (see Chapter 16, Infectious Disease Guidelines).
B. Adults:
  1. Hodgkin's lymphoma is one of the most common cancers of young adults.
C. Geriatrics:
  1. Regional lymphadenopathy occurs often when carcinomas metastasize to lymph nodes in the elderly.

Bibliography
Eriksen, W. (2018). ME/CFS, case definition, and serological response to Epstein-Barr virus. A systematic literature review. *Fatigue: Biomedicine, Health & Behavior, 6*(4), 220–234. doi:10.1080/21641846.2018.1503125

Ferrer, R. (2018). Evaluation of peripheral lymphadenopathy in adults. *UpToDate*. Retrieved from https://www.uptodate.com/contents/evaluation-of-peripheral-lymphadenopathy-in-adults

Kanwar, V. (2016). Lymphadenopthy. *Medscape*. Retrieved from www.emedicine.medscape.com

Motyckova, G., & Steensma, D. (2012). Why does my patient have lymphadenopathy or splenomegaly? *Hematology/Oncology Clinics of North America, 26*(2), 395–408. doi:10.1016/j.hoc.2012.02.005

Park, S., Kang, J., Roh, J., Huh, H., Yeo, J., & Kim, D. (2013). Secondary syphilis presenting as a generalized lymphadenopathy: Clinical mimicry of malignant lymphoma. *Sexually Transmitted Diseases, 40*(6), 490–492. doi:10.1097/OLQ.0b013e3182897eb0

Pernicious Anaemia (Megaloblastic Anaemia)

Julie Adkins and Daris Klemmer

Definition
A. Pernicious anaemia is a megaloblastic, macrocytic, normochromic anaemia caused by a deficiency of intrinsic factor in the gastric juices produced by the stomach, which results in malabsorption of vitamin B12 necessary for DNA synthesis and maturation of red blood cells (RBCs). There is production of abnormally large and oval red cells with a mean corpuscular volume in excess of 100 fL (femtolitres). The anaemia can be severe, with haematocrit (Hct) as low as 10% to 15%.

Incidence/Prevalence
A. Pernicious anaemia is common in people of Northern European descent. Both sexes are equally affected. It usually occurs in the fifth and sixth decades of life; it is rarely seen in persons younger than 35 years, but it can occur in individuals in their 20s. There is an increased incidence in those with other immunologic disease (diabetes mellitus [DM] type 1, vitiligo, thyroid, and adrenal insufficiency).

Pathogenesis
A. Pernicious anaemia is possibly due to an autoimmune reaction involving the gastric parietal cell that results in non-production of intrinsic factor and atrophy of gastric mucosa. Vitamin B12 deficiency can result from inadequate intake, impaired absorption, increased requirements as in pregnancy, or faulty utilization. Poor intake is rare, occurring most often in strict vegetarians or vegans: the vitamin is found primarily in meat, poultry, shellfish, eggs, and dairy products.

Predisposing Factors
A. People of Northern European descent.
B. Ages 50 to 60 years.
C. Immunologic disease.
D. Loss of parietal cells following gastrectomy.
E. Overgrowth of intestinal organisms.
F. Crohn's disease.
G. Ileal resection or abnormalities.
H. Fish tapeworm.
I. Congenital enzyme deficiencies.
J. Diet: Strict vegetarian or vegan.
K. Medications such as aminosalicylate sodium.
L. Alcoholism.
M. Hashimoto's thyroiditis.
N. Addison's disease, Graves' disease, myasthenia gravis, or type 1 diabetes.

Common Findings

Classic presentation involves sore tongue and numbness and tingling in the extremities, hands, or feet.

A. Weakness/fatigue and dizziness.
B. Tongue is sore, red, and shiny due to loss of papillae, may have mouth ulcers.
C. Numbness, burning, tingling sensation of arms or legs.
D. Feel heart "jumping out of skin."
E. Oedema of lower extremities.
F. Anorexia.
G. Diarrhoea if associated with gastrointestinal (GI) as underlying conditions.
H. Irritability.

Other Signs and Symptoms
A. Dyspnoea on exertion.
B. Pallor if severe.
C. Fatigue.
D. Tachycardia/palpitations.
E. Exercise intolerance.
F. Angina.
G. Glossitis.
H. Mucositis.
I. Peripheral paraesthesia.
J. Palpitations.
K. Abdominal tenderness, organomegaly.
L. Mood impairment/depression.

M. Irritability.
N. Cognitive changes/slowing.
O. Advanced stages: Dementia and spinal cord degeneration; chest pain and shortness of breath (SOB).

Subjective Data
A. Inquire about onset, duration, and course of presenting symptoms.
B. Ask the client to describe usual bowel habits. Has there been any blood in stools?
C. If GI complaints are present, inquire about presence of red, burning tongue; abdominal complaints; and/or presence of diarrhoea or constipation.
D. If neurologic complaints are present, inquire about the presence of pins and needles paraesthesia and weakness, unsteadiness due to proprioceptive difficulties, lethargy, and fatigue.
E. Inquire about dietary intake, using a 24-hour recall.
F. Ask about alcohol consumption: How much? How long?
G. Obtain medication history: Over the counter (OTC) and prescription drugs.
H. Obtain past medical history, specifically if the client has a history of gastrectomy, resection of ileum, or other GI disorders.
I. Review usual weight and recent loss.

Physical Examination
Focus on four areas: GI/derm/lymphadenopathy/hepatosplenomegaly.
A. Check temperature, pulse, respirations, blood pressure, weight, and height for children; plot on graph.
B. Inspect:
  1. Observe general, overall appearance; observe walking.
  2. Conduct oral examination for characteristic red, shiny tongue.
  3. Conduct dermal and eye examinations for colour: Affected clients are slightly icteric.
  4. Evaluate the look of the person related to age: Affected clients show premature aging or graying.
C. Auscultate:
  1. Heart sounds and lungs.
  2. The abdomen for bowel sounds.
D. Palpate:
  1. Palpate the abdomen for masses.
  2. Evaluate pedal oedema.
E. Percuss:
  1. The abdomen for tenderness and organomegaly.
F. Neurologic examination:
  1. Assess deep tendon reflexes (DTRs) and mental status.
  2. Assess for paraesthesia involving hands and feet.
  3. Observe for gait disturbances.
  4. Ask the client to perform finger-to-nose test. Poor finger–nose coordination may be seen.
  5. Observe Romberg's test. Elicit Babinski's sign. Positive Romberg's and Babinski's signs may be present.
  6. Assess for memory loss. Differentiate among mild forgetfulness, dementia, or altered thought processes.

Diagnostic Tests
Focus on stepwise approach dependent on differential diagnoses of high suspicion:
A. Complete blood count (CBC) with differential and peripheral smear: Macroovalocytes and hypersegmented neutrophils may be present on peripheral blood smear. (They are absent in the setting of concurrent iron deficiency.)
B. Serum vitamin B12 level:<100 pg/mL.
C. Serum folic acid levels, serum iron, serum ferritin, and total iron-binding capacity (TIBC).
D. Serum intrinsic factor antibody.
E. Lactate dehydrogenase (LDH).
F. Urinalysis.
G. Stool for occult blood: Consider for GI malignancy concerns.
H. GI radiographic studies.
I. Gastric analysis: Achlorhydria is found on stimulation testing.
J. Bone marrow aspiration.
K. A woman with low B12 levels may have a false-positive Pap smear due to vitamin B12 effects on the epithelial cells.

Differential Diagnoses
Differential diagnosis of anaemia by red cell morphology can be undertaken (mean corpuscular volume [MCV], mean corpuscular haemoglobin concentration [MCHC]). Common causes of each type of anemia are as follows:
A. Normochromic, normocytic: Normal MCV = 80 to 100, MCHC = 32% to 36%:
  1. Aplastic anemia.
  2. Chronic disease.
  3. Early iron deficiency.
  4. Haemolysis.
  5. Haemorrhage.
B. Microcytic: MCV = 50 to 82, MCHC = 24 to 32:
  1. Chronic disease.
  2. Iron deficiency.
  3. Thalassaemia.
C. Macrocytic: MCV >100, MCHC >36:
  1. Antimetabolites.
  2. Folic acid deficiencies.
  3. Vitamin B12 deficiencies.
  4. Chronic alcoholism.

Plan
A. General interventions:
  1. Most common method of determining vitamin B12 deficiency is by serum vitamin B12 assay.
  2. Most common method of demonstrating folate deficiency is by measurement of serum folic acid levels.
  3. Red cell indices and peripheral smear should be done to determine classification of anemia to facilitate workup.
  4. Red cell distribution width (RDW) determination can assist in detecting red cell heterogeneity previously available only by examination of the peripheral smear. The RDW determination overcomes the problems of detecting coexisting microcytic and macrocytic anaemias.
B. Client teaching:
  1. Neurologic symptoms usually improve with treatment; however, some neurologic deficits may not be reversible.
C. Pharmacological therapy:
  1. Vitamin B12:
    a. Decrease the frequency and administer a total of 2000 mg during the first six weeks of therapy (weekly for one month).
    b. Maintenance treatment requires lifelong administration depending on B12 levels.
    c. Intranasal cyanocobalamin—not an option until in remission.
  2. Concomitant iron supplementation during first month of therapy. Rapid blood cell regeneration increases iron requirements and can lead to iron deficiency.

Follow-Up

A. The client must be seen in two weeks to determine response to treatment: Increased reticulocyte count and increased Hct; diminution in neurologic signs and symptoms.
B. Evaluate the client monthly when giving vitamin B12 injections.
C. Endoscopy every five years is used to rule out gastric carcinoma. People with pernicious anaemia may have gastric polyps and are more likely to develop gastric cancer and gastric carcinoid tumours.
D. Check the client every six months for Hct, and check his or her stool for occult blood.
E. Hct value rises 4% to 5% per week in uncomplicated cases.

Consultation/Referral

A. Refer the client to a dietitian.
B. Rapid reticulocytosis should be seen following treatment; it peaks in 7 to 10 days.

Individual Considerations

A. Pregnancy:
   1. Lactovegetarians and ovolactovegetarians do well in pregnancy.
   2. Vegan women should take vitamin B12 supplements during pregnancy and lactation.
B. Paediatrics:
   1. Congenital disorder usually seen before 3 years of age.
C. Adults:
   1. Disorder rarely seen in clients younger than age 35 years.
D. Geriatrics:
   1. Disorder most commonly is seen in the geriatric population.
   2. Follow up elderly clients with assessment of cardiovascular symptoms 48 hours after initiating therapy.
   3. Rapid blood cell regeneration increases iron requirements and can lead to iron deficiency.

Bibliography

Brown, H. (2013). Managing pernicious anemia. *Independent Nurse, 18*(02), 22–24.

Schrier, S. (2017). Macrocytosis/Macrocytic Anemia. *UpToDate*. Retrieved from https://www.uptodate.com/contents/macrocytosis-macrocytic-anemia Please put in Pernicious Anemia

Stabler, S. (2013). Clinical practice: Vitamin B12 deficiency. *New England Journal of Medicine, 368*(2), 149–160. doi:10.1056/NEJMcp1113996

U.S. National Library of Medicine. (2013, March 12). *Pernicious anemia*. Retrieved from https://www.ncbi.nlm.nih.gov/pubmedhealth/PMHT0022012

Weiss, S. (2012). Oral involvement of systemic diseases. *Clinical Advisor for Nurse Practitioners, 15*(6), 25–30.

18 Musculoskeletal Guidelines

Neck and Upper Back Disorders

Julie Adkins, Wanda Emberley-Burke, and Valda Duke

Definition
A. Nonspecific disorders: Self-limited, usually benign disorders with unclear etiology, such as regional upper back and neck pain and shoulder pain adjacent to the neck. Pain can occur as a result of injury or through strain or poor posture over time.
B. Degenerative disorders: Sonsequences of aging or repetitive use, or a combination thereof, such as degenerative disc disease and osteoarthritis (OA).
C. Potentially serious neck or upper back disorders: Fractures, dislocation, infection, tumour, progressive neurologic deficit, or cord compression. Examples include muscle strains, overuse injuries, sports injuries, auto accidents; all can result in muscular irritation of the shoulder girdle, causing upper back pain.
D. There are three general types of neck pain:
　1. Acute—lasts less than four weeks.
　2. Subacute—lasts 4 to 12 weeks.
　3. Chronic—lasts three months or longer.
E. There are seven vertebrae of the cervical spine that surround the spinal cord and canal. The neck includes skin, neck muscles, arteries, lymph nodes, thyroid gland, parathyroid gland, esophagus, larynx, and trachea. Any condition affecting these tissues of the neck can cause neck pain.

Incidence/Prevalence
A. The prevalence of neck and upper back disorders is unknown. Neck pain is common among adults but can occur at any age. In the course of a year, 25% of Canadians reported that neck and shoulder pain were most prevalent among repetitive stress injuries. Adults reporting neck pain also may experience limitations of activities of daily living. Among Canadians who suffer from chronic pain, 5.4% reported the neck as the primary anatomical site of the pain. Neck pain can range from being a mild nuisance to excruciating pain. The pain can go away in a few days or weeks or more, or constantly radiate to other body parts. Neck pain and upper back disorders can cause headaches or occipital neuralgia.

Pathogenesis
Cervical strain is the irritation and spasm of the upper back and cervical muscles. The upper portion of the trapezius and the levator scapulae muscles, rhomboid major and minor muscles, and the long cervical muscles are most often affected. Neck pain can be identified by location:

A. C1 and C2: At the top of the cervical spine, these control the head; irritation may cause headaches.
B. C3 and C4: These regulate the diaphragm, which is instrumental in breathing. C4 can radiate pain to the lower neck and shoulder.
C. C5: If this is impinged or irritated, shoulder pain and weakness can affect the top of the upper arms.
D. C6: If this impinged or irritated, weakness can affect the biceps and the wrists. Pain, tingling, and numbness can radiate through the arm to the thumb.
E. C7: Compression here causes weakness of the back of the upper arm or pain that can radiate down the back of the arm and into the middle finger.
F. C8: Compression here causes weakness with the handgrip as well as numbness and tingling down the arm to the little finger.

Predisposing Factors
A. Whiplash-like injuries.
B. Cervical strain.
C. Cervical arthritis.
D. Holding your head in a forward posture or odd position.
E. Sleeping on a pillow too high or too flat.
F. Stress/tension.
G. Lack of ergonomically correct workspace design.

Common Findings
A. Aching neck.
B. Tightness and tenderness in neck area.
C. Stiffness and tightness in shoulders.
D. Stiff neck and a headache on awakening.

Other Signs and Symptoms
A. Limited range of motion (ROM).
B. Back pain—guarding with cervical motion.
C. Numbness in upper extremities.
D. Muscle weakness.

Subjective Data
A. What are presenting symptoms? Note pain, numbness, weakness, or stiffness.
B. Was there any type of injury, either recently or in the past?
C. Is the pain located primarily in the neck, upper back, or shoulder? Is there any radiation noted?
D. How do these symptoms limit the client's activity?
E. How long can the client sit, stand, walk, or do overhead work?
F. Is the client able to lift? If so, how much weight is bearable? Compare with normal weight.

G. How long has the client had these symptoms?
H. How have the symptoms evolved, from the beginning of discomfort until now?
I. If the client has a previous history of a similar or the same pain, what therapy was used in the past and what were the results?
J. Does the client have any medical or psychological problems?
K. Does the client have marked upper extremity weakness?
L. Does the client have pain that wakes them from sleep?
M. Does the client have any fatigue, swollen joints, or fever?

Physical Examination

Infection may include severe cervical spasms (nuchal rigidity), elevated temperature, chills, hypotension, and tachycardia.
A. Check temperature, blood pressure, and pulse.
B. Inspect: Observe stance, gait, and spine alignment. Note the client's coordination and use of extremities.
C. Auscultate heart and lungs.
D. Palpate:
   1. Palpate trigger points in upper back, paracervical and rhomboid muscles.
   2. Palpate for any bony tenderness in neck, shoulders, and upper back.
   3. Perform ROM tests.
   4. Assess the client for reduced ipsilateral and contralateral bending of the neck.
   5. Check for fracture, or inability to move the neck due to pain, and severe cervical midline vertebral pain. Note tenderness, the client holding head for stability; look for possible neurologic deficits.
E. Assess deep tendon reflexes (DTRs) bilaterally.
   1. Biceps reflex tests fifth and sixth cervical nerve root.
   2. Brachioradialis reflex tests fifth and sixth cervical nerve root.
   3. Triceps reflex tests seventh and eighth cervical nerve root.
F. Shoulders: Test muscle strength in shoulders. Ask client to shrug shoulders against resistance. Test abduction of upper extremities.
G. Elbows: Abduction, elbow flexion, or supination tests fourth and fifth cervical discs.
H. Wrists: Check for weakness of radial wrist extension, indicating fifth and sixth cervical disc problems. Check for weakness of elbow extension and ulnar wrist flexion, indicating seventh cervical nerve impairment. Check weak finger abduction and adduction, indicating seventh and eighth cervical nerve impairment.
I. Measure circumference at forearm and upper arm for muscle atrophy. Dominant arm is 0.6 cm greater than non-dominant arm.
J. Sensory: Test light touch, pinprick, pressure sensations in forearm and hand. Possible cervical spinal cord compromise is indicated by paraesthesia of upper extremities, weakness of upper or lower extremities, and difficulty walking.
K. Percuss back, spine, and neck areas. Tumour is indicated by tenderness to vertebral percussion and cachexia.

Diagnostic Tests

A. Nontraumatic neck pain should have radiographic studies performed on clients with the following criteria:
   1. Age more than 50 years with new symptoms.
   2. Concern of infection.
   3. Unexplained symptoms, such as weight loss, fever, or chills.
   4. Neurologic symptoms that continue to progress.
   5. Concern or history of malignancy.
B. Radiology of cervical spine. Testing may include the following:
   1. X-ray: Recommended for nontraumatic pain in all clients older than 65 years with new symptoms or symptoms that suggest systemic aetiology. Review client with uncomplicated subacute neck pain (four to twelve weeks duration) with or without arm pain as well as clients with persistent neck pain (>12 weeks) with or without arm pain.
   2. MRI: Recommended if symptoms are worsening or signs of neurologic disease, symptoms longer than six weeks, or concern over malignancy or infection.
   3. CT scan of spine is primary investigation for high-risk clients on an emergency basis.
   4. Myelogram.
   5. Electromyography (EMG): More useful for pain experienced in extremities than in the neck.
   6. Nerve conduction studies: Evaluates nerve damage.
   7. Bone scan.

Differential Diagnoses

A. Regional neck pain.
B. Cervical strain.
C. Cervical arthritis.
D. Cervical nerve root compression with radiculopathy.
E. Rotator cuff tendinitis.
F. Rotator cuff tendon tear.
G. Postlaminectomy syndrome.
H. Spinal stenosis.
I. Torticollis, which that may be present at birth or caused by injury or disease.
J. Cervical neoplastic causes or bone tumour.

Plan

A. General interventions:
   1. Correct posture and lifestyle modifications (e.g., exercise and strengthening) are imperative for the client to remain free of pain. Client education and therapy depend on individual diagnosis.
B. Client teaching:
   1. Teach the client to use local applications of cold packs during the first three days of acute pain and hot pack applications thereafter.
   2. Encourage the following changes in lifestyle:
      a. Sitting straight with shoulders held high.
      b. Sleeping with the head and neck aligned with the body and a small pillow under the neck.
      c. Driving with shoulders slightly shrugged, using arm rests.
      d. Avoiding carrying objects with a strap over shoulders.
      e. Ergonomic positioning of computer screens.
   3. Encourage daily stretching exercises, including shoulder roll, scapular pinch, and neck stretches.
   4. Encourage physiotherapy treatment, dependent on diagnosis.
   5. Have the client perform ROM exercises daily.
   6. Advise the client to avoid extremes of ROM, prolonged periods in one position, and any other aggravating activity.
   7. Explain relaxation techniques and stress reduction.
   8. Advise that massage may be useful to help relax muscles in back and neck, *if applicable*.

C. Pharmacological therapy:
  1. Nonprescription medications: Acetaminophen, topical pain relief patches, muscle rubs. Avoid narcotics as they may be harmful and ineffective.
  2. Prescription medications—muscle relaxants for nighttime use:
    a. Cyclobenzaprine: Use for periods longer than two to three weeks is not recommended. Dosing should be considered for clients with liver impairment and/or elderly clients. Advise clients that driving and the use of machinery is not recommended while taking this medication. A short nighttime course is recommended for severe pain with caution for daytime use. Clients may even benefit from a single-dose use at nighttime. Client must be made aware of overuse risks.
    b. Carisoprodol: Daily, as needed. Precautions should be given for no driving or use of machinery while taking this medication. Use caution in clients with compromised liver and/or kidney function. Carisoprodol should not be used for longer than two to three weeks.
  3. Trigger injections of cortisone and anaesthetics may be used as necessary. These injections may be used for short-term relief; there is insufficient evidence to support injections as monotherapy.

Follow-Up
A. Evaluate the client after two weeks of conservative treatment. If pain continues after two to three weeks despite adequate therapy, order radiology and physiotherapy. Treatment options include ultrasonography, massage, and gentle cervical traction beginning at 5 pounds for 5 to 10 minutes once a day. A cervical collar is contraindicated and may hamper recovery.

Consultation/Referral
A. Consult or refer the client to a specialist if there is still no improvement after adequate time for healing and no relief is noted with physiotherapy and medications.

Individual Considerations
A. Adults: Neck and upper back problems are more commonly seen in adults.
B. Paediatrics: Sports are the primary cause for head and neck/spinal injuries in children. Football, soccer, cheerleading, hockey, and gymnastics are the sports most commonly seen in athlete head/spinal injuries.
C. Geriatrics: Use prescribing literature for guidance. Consider using lower-dose medications for older clients. Long-term medications should also be taken into consideration for interactions between medications.

Bibliography
Bickley, L. S., & Szilaygi, P. G. (2017). *Bates' guide to physical examination and history taking* (12th ed.). Philadelphia, PA: Lippincott Williams & Wilkins.

Bussieres, A., Stewart, G., Al-Zoubi, F., Decina, P., Descarreaux, M., Hayden, J., ... Ornelas, J. (2016). The treatment of neck pain-associated disorders and whiplash associated disorders: A clinical practice guideline. *Journal of Manipulative & Physiological Therapeutics, 39*(8), 523–564. doi:10.1016/j.jmpt.2016.08.007

Bussieres, A., Taylor, J., & Peterson, C. (2008). Diagnostic imaging practice guidelines for musculoskeletal findings in adults: An evidence-based approach. Part 3: Spinal Disorders. *Journal of Manipulative and Physiological Therapeutics, 31*(1), 33–88. doi:10.1016/j.jmpt.2007.11.003

Dains, J. E., Baumann, L. C., & Scheibel, P. (2015). *Advanced health assessment and clinical diagnosis in primary care* (5th ed.). Toronto, ON, Canada: Mosby.

Gross, A. R., Paquin, J. P., Dupont, G., Blanchette, S., Lalonde, P., Cristie, T., ... Cervical Overview Group. (2016). Exercises for mechanical neck disorders: A Cochrane review update. *Manual Therapy, 24*, 25–45. doi:10.1016/j.math.2016.04.005

Gray, J. (Ed.). (2011). *Therapeutic choices* (6th ed.). Ottawa, ON, Canada: Canadian Pharmacists Association.

Hall, H., McIntosh, G., Alleyne, J., & Cote, P. (2015). Pain in the neck. *Journal of Current Clinical Care, 5*(1), 24–33. doi:10.1016/j.math.2016.04.005

Hirsch, B. P., Webb, M. L., Bohl, D. D., Fu, M., Buerba, R. A., Gruskay, J. A., & Gracer, J. N. (2014). Improving visual estimates of cervical spine range of motion. *American Journal of Orthopedics, 43*(11), 261–265. Retrieved from https://www.amjorthopedics.com/

Javanshir, K., Amiri, M., Mohseni Bandpei, M. A., De las Penas, C. F., & Rezasoltani, A. (2015). The effect of different exercise programs on cervical flexor muscles dimensions in patients with chronic neck pain. *Journal of Back & Musculoskeletal Rehabilitation, 28*(4), 833–840. doi:10.3233/BMR-150593

Joyey, R. (2011). The prevalence of chronic pain in Canada. *Pain Research Management, 16*(6), 445–450. Retrieved from https://www.hindawi.com/journals/prm/

Jun Ho, K., Han Suk, L., & Sun Wook, P. (2015). Effects of the active release technique on pain and range of motion of patients with chronic neck pain. *Journal of Physical Therapy, 27*(8), 2461–2464. doi:10.1589/jpts.27.2461

Kovacs, F. M., Seco, J., Royuela, A., Melis, S., Sánchez, C., Díaz-Arribas, M. J., ... Abraira, V. (2015). Patients with neck pain are less likely to improve if they experience poor sleep quality: A prospective study in routine practice. *Clinical Journal of Pain, 31*(8), 713–721. doi:10.1097/AJP.0000000000000147

Murphy, K. A., Spence, S. T., McIntosh, C. N., & Connor Gorber, S. K. (2006). *For the Population Health Impact of Disease in Canada (PHI). Health State Descriptions for Canadians: Musculoskeletal Diseases.* (Catalogue no. 82-619- MIE2006003). Ottawa: Statistics Canada.

Schopflocher, D., Taenzer, P., & Joyey, R. (2011). The prevalence of chronic pain in Canada. *Pain Research Management, 16* (6), 445–450. Retrieved from https://www.hindawi.com/journals/prm/

Steill, I. G., Clement, C. M., McKnight, R. D., Brison, R., Schull, M. J., Rowe, B. H., ... Wells, G. A. (2003). Canadian C-Spine Rule versus the NEXUS low-risk criteria in clients with trauma. *New England Journal of Medicine, 349*, 2510–2518. doi:10.1056/NEJMoa031375

Xie, P., Qin, B., Yang, F., Yu, T., Yu, J., Wang, J., & Zheng, H. (2015). Lidocaine injection in the intramuscular innervation zone can effectively treat chronic neck pain caused by MTrPs in the trapezius muscle. *Pain Physician, 18*(5), E815–E826. Retrieved from https://www.painphysicianjournal.com/index

Plantar Fasciitis

Julie Adkins, Wanda Emberley-Burke, and Valda Duke

Definition
Plantar fasciitis is an inflammatory condition in the plantar fascia (foot) that causes pain in the arch of the foot and radiates to the heel. The plantar fascia connective tissue runs across the bottom of the foot and connects the bottom of the tuberosity of the calcaneous to the heads of the metatarsal bones.

Incidence/Prevalence
Plantar fasciitis is the most common cause of heel pain in Canada. Plantar fasciitis is seen in both men and women; it is common in middle-aged people.

Pathogenesis
Repetitive small tears in the plantar fascia causing collagen breakdown at the medial tubercle of the calcaneus.

Predisposing Factors
A. Athletes: Overuse injury from running.
B. Tight or weak muscles/tendons (Achilles tendon, heel cord, gastrocnemius, and soleus muscle).

C. Poor arch support/improper footwear (poor support in shoes).
D. Anatomic abnormalities (low arch support, flat foot, high arch, tibial torsion, overpronated foot, leg-length discrepancy, forefoot varus, and thinning of fat pad).
E. Overweight/obesity.

Common Findings
A. Severe, stabbing foot pain in the bottom of the foot, especially first thing in the morning.
B. Burning pain when walking.
C. Stiffness in foot/heel.
D. May be worse in the morning, improve during the day, and then get painful at the end of the day.
E. Increased foot pain with walking after long periods of standing or sitting.

Other Signs and Symptoms
A. Both heels may be affected.
B. Pain is located at the medial tubercle of the calcaneus, medial of the longitudinal arch.
C. Heel spurs may or may not be present.
D. Pain worsens with standing for long periods of time.

Subjective Data
A. Ask the client when pain began, when it occurs, and how long it lasts.
B. Does pain occur with walking, running, and standing?
C. Is the pain constant or stabbing? Rate pain on a pain scale of 1 to 10.
D. Locate pain site; does pain radiate into toes or leg?
E. Ask the client what makes the pain better or worse.

Physical Examination
A. Check pulse and blood pressure.
B. Inspect:
  1. Examine feet bilaterally.
  2. Note swelling, discoloration, or rash.
  3. Observe gait.
C. Auscultate heart and lungs.
D. Palpate:
  1. Palpate both feet, noting point tenderness. Point tenderness will be noted over insertion on medial heel (calcaneus medial tubercle).
  2. Perform passive dorsiflexion of toes and ankle. Have the client stand on tips of toes to see if this elicits pain.

Diagnostic Tests
A. X-ray may be performed but is often normal and not needed. Perform if tumour, spur, or stress fracture is suspected.
B. MRI should be ordered if thickening of proximal plantar fascia is noted or rupture of proximal fascia suspected.

Differential Diagnoses
A. Heel pain.
B. Heel spur.
C. Arthritis.
D. Stress fracture.

Plan
A. General interventions:
  1. Conservative treatment includes avoiding long periods of standing for the next six to eight weeks.
  2. Proper foot care and support recommended.

B. Client teaching:
  1. Shoe arch supports are imperative for relief. Consider obtaining custom-made foot orthotics. New shoes may provide this support, or additional arch supports may be needed to insert into the shoe to provide adequate support.
  2. Suggest getting proper shoe fitting for running if the client is an athlete.
  3. The client should avoid walking on hard surfaces and never go barefoot, even indoors. Avoid wearing sandals and flip-flops.
  4. Ice therapy may help with pain control and swelling.
  5. For severe cases, a corticosteroid lidocaine injection directly into the most tender area on the sole of the foot may be helpful.
  6. Exercises;
    a. Roll foot arch under the ball of the foot, using a tennis ball or a frozen bottle of water or a towel, for 20 to 30 minutes each evening to help stretch the plantar fascia.
    b. Perform calf stretches against a wall; leaning forward against the wall and extending one leg behind you and one leg in front of you, stretch the leg, and reverse.
  7. Encourage client to seek treatment from a physiotherapist.
C. Pharmacological therapy: Nonsteroidal anti-inflammatory drugs (NSAIDs) such as ibuprofen and/or naproxen for pain relief.

Follow-Up
A. Recommend follow-up in four weeks following the treatment. Pain should slowly improve with aggressive treatment management. The client must be compliant with instructions given for improvement. May take 6 to 12 months for complete resolution.
B. Complications of foot, knee, hip, or back problems may occur if change of gait occurs to minimize pain with walking.
C. If pain worsens, consider diagnostic workup (e.g., MRI). X-rays are not typically indicated related to nonbone-related causality. In rare cases, an ultrasound or a bone scan may be indicated.

Consultation/Referral
A. Refer to a podiatrist if conservative therapy fails after six weeks. If nerve entrapment is suspected, referral to a specialist is warranted.

Individual Considerations
A. None.

Bibliography
American Orthopedic Foot and Ankle Society. (2016). *Plantar fasciitis*. Retrieved from www.aofas.org/footcaremd/conditions/ailments-of-the-heel/pages/plantar-fasciitis.aspx

Bickley, L. S., & Szilaygi, P. G. (2017). *Bates' guide to physical examination and history taking* (12th ed.). Philadelphia, PA: Lippincott Williams & Wilkins.

Blahd, W., Poinier, A. C., Thompson, E. G., Husney, A., Romito, K., & Chalmers, G. W. G. (2017). Plantar fasciitis. *HealthLink BC*. Retrieved from https://www.healthlinkbc.ca/health-topics/hw114458

Bussieres, A., Taylor, J., & Peterson, C. (2008). Diagnostic imaging practice guidelines for musculoskeletal findings in adults: An evidence-based approach. Part 3: Spinal Disorders. *Journal of Manipulative and Physiological Therapeutics, 31*(1), 33–88. doi:10.1016/j.jmpt.2007.11.003

Dains, J. E., Baumann, L. C., & Scheibel, P. (2015). *Advanced health assessment and clinical diagnosis in primary care* (5th ed.). Toronto, ON, Canada: Mosby.

Gray, J. (Ed.). (2011). *Therapeutic choices* (6th ed.). Ottawa, ON, Canada: Canadian Pharmacists Association.

Kalaci, A., Cakici, H., Hapa, O., Yanat, A. N., Dogramaci, Y., & Sevinç, T. T. (2009). Treatment of Plantar fasciitis using four different local injection modalities: A randomized prospective clinical trial. *Journal of the American Podiatric Medical Association, 99*(2), 108–113. doi:10.7547/0980108

Karls, S. L., Snyder, K. R., & Neibert, P. J. (2016). Effectiveness of corticosteroid injections in the treatment of plantar fasciitis. *Journal of Sport Rehabilitation, 25*(2), 202–207. doi:10-1123/jsr.2014-0234

Mayo Clinic. (2014). *Plantar fascitis*. Retrieved from www.mayoclinic.org

Podolsky, R., & Kalichman, L. (2015). Taping for plantar fasciitis. *Journal of Back & Musculoskeletal Rehabilitation, 28*(1), 1–6. doi:10.3233/BMR-140485

Shashua, A., Flechter, S., Avidan, L., Ofir, D., Melayev, A., & Kalichman, L. (2015). The effect of additional ankle and midfoot mobilizations on Plantar fasciitis: A randomized controlled trial. *Journal of Orthopaedic & Sports Physical Therapy, 45*(4), 265–272. doi:10.2519/jospt.2015.5155

Zhou, B., Zhou, Y., Tao, X., Yuan, C., & Tang, K. (2015). Classification of calcaneal spurs and their relationship with plantar fasciitis. *Journal of Foot and Ankle Surgery: Official Publication of the American College of Foot and Ankle Surgeons, 54*(4), 594–600. doi:10.1053/j.jfas.2014.11.009

Sciatica

Julie Adkins, Wanda Emberley-Burke, and Valda Duke

Definition
Sciatica is a sharp or burning pain, usually associated with numbness that radiates down the posterior or lateral leg, that can result in neurosensory and/or motor deficits. Sciatica indicates abnormal function of the lumbosacral nerve roots or one of the nerves in the lumbosacral plexus.

Incidence/Prevalence
Ninety percent of the Canadian population see their primary healthcare practitioner for back pain; 65% are diagnosed with nonspecific lower back pain, while sciatica accounts for 11%. The most common cause of sciatica is herniated discs, 95% of which occur at the L4 to L5 or L5 to S1 level.

Pathogenesis
A. Pressure on the nerve from a herniated disc, from bony osteophytes, a compression fracture, trauma, or any other extrinsic pressure (e.g., pelvic mass or epidural process, "wallet sciatica"), causes progressive sensory, sensorimotor, or sensorimotor visceral loss. Typically, sciatica affects only one side of the body. The nerve may be "pinched" on the inside or outside of the spinal canal as it passes into the leg.

Predisposing Factors
A. Inflexibility.
B. Obesity.
C. Trauma.
D. Bony osteophytes.
E. Herniated or slipped disc.
F. Piriformis syndrome.
G. Spinal stenosis.
H. Spondylolisthesis.
I. Pregnancy.

Common Findings
A. Pain around the buttocks area may occur suddenly or develop gradually.
B. Pain often associated with numbness traveling down the lateral or posterior leg.
C. Numbness.
D. Paraesthesia.

Other Signs and Symptoms
A. Difficulty walking with affected leg.
B. Positive straight leg raises.
C. Decreased sensation.

Subjective Data
A. Elicit information on onset of symptoms, duration, and what makes pain better or worse.
B. Inquire about previous episodes of pain or trauma.
C. Have the client point to the area of pain, numbness, or tingling.
D. Are the symptoms unilateral or bilateral?
E. Question the client about loss of bowel or bladder control or other deficits and/or changes.
F. Does the client notice leg weakness or difficulty walking?
G. Has the client been treated for cancer or other medical conditions?
H. Inquire about recent fever, weight loss, or night pain.

Physical Examination
A. Check pulse and blood pressure.
B. Inspect gait and movement of back and extremities.
C. Palpate and percuss spinous processes for tenderness.
D. Examine flexion and extension of spine. Assess sensation, deep tendon reflexes (DTRs), muscle strength, and motor weakness of lower extremities.
E. Examine neurologic function of back and lower extremity:
   1. Straight leg-raising sign is positive.
   2. Dorsiflexion of ankle is positive.
   3. Check for loss of sensation in radicular pattern. Light touch, pinprick, and two-point discrimination are not present.
   4. Look for decrease or loss of DTRs.
   5. Check muscle strength of lower extremities.
   6. Check motor weakness.
   7. Check for cauda equina syndrome, indicated by urinary retention, radicular symptoms, and saddle anesthesia.

Cauda equina syndrome is a surgical emergency, characterized by bowel and bladder dysfunction; saddle anaesthesia at the anus, perineum, or genitals; and widespread or progressive loss of strength in the legs or gait disturbances.

Diagnostic Tests
A. Radiology is warranted when red flags for fracture, cancer, or infection are present using Canadian C-Spine rules. www.ohri.ca/emerg/cdr/docs/cdr_cspine_poster.pdf.
B. CT scan or MRI, when cauda equina, tumour, infection, or fracture is suspected; MRI is test of choice for clients with prior back surgery.

Differential Diagnoses
A. Lumbosacral strain.
B. Herniated disc.
C. Bony osteophytes, spinal stenosis.
D. Compression fracture.
E. Neoplasm of spine.
F. Pelvic mass.
G. Epidural process causing progressive sensory, sensorimotor, or sensorimotor visceral loss.
H. Meralgia paraesthetica.

Plan

A. General interventions: Care for these clients should evolve over a three-step process. (See the following.)
B. Client teaching:
  1. *Step 1 (two to four days):*
     a. Bed rest for severe radiculopathy only.
     b. Limit walking and standing to 30 to 40 minutes each day. Alternate walking and lying as tolerated.
  2. *Step 2 (seven–14 days):*
     a. Reevaluate neurologic and back examination; advise the client to "let pain be your guide" when resuming normal daily activities.
     b. Have the client perform gentle stretching exercises.
     c. Encourage walking on flat surfaces.
     d. Educate the client regarding proper care of the back, with regard to exercises, posture, and so forth.
     e. Provide client with handouts on back exercises/stretches.
     f. Physiotherapy may be implemented at this time if no significant improvement is noted.
  3. *Step 3 (two to three weeks):*
     a. Reevaluate the client, noting degree of improvement with examination.
     b. Continue muscle toning and reconditioning exercises.
     c. If improvement is noted, gradually increase physical activities.
     d. Reinforce healthy care of the back.
     e. Continue physiotherapy until the client can perform exercises without assistance or until released by the physiotherapist.
C. Pharmacological therapy:
  1. Nonsteroidal anti-inflammatory drugs (NSAIDs) as needed: naproxen. Use caution with when recommending NSAIDS for elderly clients.
  2. Acetaminophen may also be used as needed, especially if the client is not able to tolerate ibuprofen.
  3. For more severe pain not relieved by NSAIDs, consider acetaminophen with codeine for short duration. Narcotics should not be used for more than two weeks.
  4. Muscle relaxants: Cyclobenzaprine. Muscle relaxants, which should not be used for longer than two weeks, place clients at risk for drowsiness. Warn the client not to mix medications with alcohol because it may potentiate the medication.

Follow-Up

A. Initial follow-up is needed in one to two weeks. See the "Plan" section for a stepwise approach.

Consultation/Referral

A. If cauda equina syndrome is suspected, prompt referral to a specialist is necessary.
B. If pain is severe enough that narcotics are needed for more than two weeks, consult with a specialist.
C. If bilateral sciatica is associated with vertebral collapse, osteoporosis, neoplasia, and/or vascular disease, consult with a specialist.

Individual Considerations

A. Pregnancy:
  1. Sciatica pain is common due to physiological changes of the pelvis as pregnancy progresses to term.
  2. Avoid use of NSAIDs.
  3. Physiotherapy may be used, as indicated. To avoid precipitous delivery, transcutaneous electrical nerve stimulations (TENS) may be used on a limb. Avoid use of TENS on lower back or abdomen.
  4. Noncontrast MRI may be considered.
B. Adults: For adults older than 50 years presenting with no prior history of backache, consider a differential diagnosis of neoplasm. Most common metastasis is secondary to primary site of breast or prostate, or to multiple myeloma. Pain is most prominent in the recumbent position and rarely radiates into buttock or leg.
C. Geriatrics:
  1. Bilateral sciatica is associated with vertebral collapse, osteoporosis, neoplasia, and/or vascular disease. Refer the client to a specialist immediately.
  2. Use caution when prescribing medications for pain to the elderly due to the risk for drowsiness and potential falls.

Bibliography

Beaudet, N., Courteau, J., Sarret, P., & Vanesse, A. (2013). Prevalence of claims-based recurrent low back pain in a Canadian population: A secondary analysis of an administrative database. *BMC Musculoskeletal Disorders, 14*(151), 1–8. Open access article. doi:10.1186/1471-2474-14-151

Bickley, L. S., & Szilaygi, P. G. (2017). *Bates' guide to physical examination and history taking* (12th ed.). Philadelphia, PA: Lippincott Williams & Wilkins.

Blahd, W., O'Brien, B., Thompson, E. G., Husney, A., Romito, K., Keller, B. K., & Koval, K. J. (2017). Sciatica. *Healthlink BC.* Retrieved from https://www.healthlinkbc.ca/health-topics/tp22229spec

Bussieres, A., Taylor, J., & Peterson, C. (2008). Diagnostic imaging practice guidelines for musculoskeletal findings in adults: An evidence-based approach. Part 3: Spinal Disorders. *Journal of Manipulative and Physiological Therapeutics, 31*(1), 33–88. doi:10.1016/j.jmpt.2007.11.003

Dains, J. E., Baumann, L. C., & Scheibel, P. (2015). *Advanced health assessment and clinical diagnosis in primary care* (5th ed.). Toronto, ON, Canada: Mosby.

Gray, J. (Ed.). (2011). *Therapeutic choices* (6th ed.). Ottawa, ON, Canada: Canadian Pharmacists Association.

Lewis, R. A., Williams, N. H., Sutton, A. J., Burton, K., Din, N. U., Matar, H. E., . . . Wilkinson, C. (2015). Comparative clinical effectiveness of management strategies for sciatica: Systematic review and network meta-analyses. *The Spine Journal: Official Journal of the North American Spine Society, 15*(6), 1461–1477. doi:10.1016/j.spinee.2013.08.049

Poquet, N., & Lin, C. W. (2016). Management strategies for sciatica (PEDro synthesis). *British Journal of Sports Medicine, 50*(4), 253–254. doi:10.1136/bjsports-2015-095268

Savage, N. J., Fritz, J. M., & Thackeray, A. (2014). The relationship between history and physical examination findings and the outcome of electrodiagnostic testing in patients with sciatica referred to physical therapy. *Journal of Orthopaedic & Sports Physical Therapy, 44*(7), 508–517. doi:10.2519/jospt.2014.5002

Schopflocher, D., Taenzer, P., & Joyey, R. (2011). The prevalence of chronic pain in Canada. *Pain Research Management, 16*(6), 445–450. Retrieved from https://www.hindawi.com/journals/prm/

Steffens, D., Hancock, M. J., Pereira, L. S., Kent, P. M., Latimer, J., & Maher, C. G. (2016). Do MRI findings identify patients with low back pain or sciatica who respond better to particular interventions? A systematic review. *European Spine Journal: Official Publication of the European Spine Society, the European Spinal Deformity Society, and the European Section of the Cervical Spine Research Society, 25*(4), 1170–1187. doi:10.1007/s00586-015-4195-4

Sprains: Ankle and Knee

Julie Adkins, Wanda Emberley-Burke, and Valda Duke

Definition

Sprains are ligament stretching or partial tears from forceful stress on the joint. Sprains are categorized as the following:
A. Grade 1: Microscopic tears without ligament tearing or joint instability.

B. Grade 2: Partial tearing of involved ligaments and laxity of joint with moderate function loss.
C. Grade 3: Ligament tearing with severe function loss and joint instability.

Incidence/Prevalence
A. *Ankle* sprains are among the most common injuries seen in primary care. It is estimated that there are 1 million ankle injuries per year in North America, of which 85% are sprains.
B. *Knee* injuries are among the 10 most common causes of occupational injury and worker compensation claims.

Pathogenesis
A. Sudden stress to a supporting ligament causes ligament stretching or tearing. Sprains are usually the result of jumping, falling, or rotating a joint.
B. Ankle sprains are most often inversion sprains with symptoms on the lateral side of the joint.
C. Eversion injuries affect the medial side.
D. Knee sprains most often involve the patellofemoral joint.

Predisposing Factors
A. Previous injury to ankle or knee.
B. Athletic activities.
C. Patellofemoral instability.
D. Gait and falls.

Common Findings
A. "I twisted my ankle (or knee)."
B. "I stepped off of a step and came down on the side of my foot."
C. Swelling, pain, weakness of ankle or knee from a previous injury.

Other Signs and Symptoms
A. First degree: Minimal pain; mild to moderate pain with stress, little swelling; minimal tenderness with palpation; little functional loss; unimpaired weight bearing or walking; internal microdamage with full continuity.
B. Second degree: Moderate pain with range of motion (ROM); swelling; marked tenderness on palpation; moderate loss of function; difficulty with weight bearing or walking; mechanical dissociation with partial loss of continuity.
C. Third degree: Severe pain, especially with passive inversion; severe swelling, marked tenderness; marked decrease in ROM; intolerant of weight bearing or walking; joint instability; discoloration of skin; complete rupture of a ligament.

Subjective Data
A. Inquire about history of trauma.
B. Have the client describe the injury: time, place, activity, predisposing factors, and time the symptoms developed.
C. Determine whether the symptoms are acute or chronic.
D. Inquire about the type and location of the pain.
E. Have the client describe the pain and what conditions aggravate or relieve the pain.
F. Ask whether there are symptoms of popping, clicking, locking, recurrent swelling, or giving way of the joint.
G. Ask whether there is pain or other symptoms elsewhere, such as low back, hip, or leg.
H. Explore history of any previous ankle or knee injury.
I. Determine whether the current injury was evaluated and treated previously.
J. Have the client describe ability to bear weight on the extremity and to tolerate ROM.
K. Review the client's medical history for arthritis, gout, cancer, autoimmune disorders, or metabolic disease.

Physical Examination
A. Check temperature, pulse, respirations, and blood pressure.
B. Inspect:
   1. Observe ambulation. Note overall appearance and facial grimaces during examination.
   2. Inspect injured area for swelling, discoloration, and deformity. Compare injured side to uninjured side.
C. Palpate:
   1. Palpate the injured site for tenderness.
   2. Palpate the joints above and below the injured site.
   3. Perform ROM (active and passive) and resisted ROM to evaluate strength.
   4. Check for catching or locking of the knee on extension.
   5. Assess neurovascular status of the knee or ankle and distal extremity.
   6. *Ankle*: Palpate for tender sulcus in anterolateral aspect on inversion of the ankle. Assess for pain aggravated by forced ankle inversion. Perform isometric test of plantar flexion and eversion. Perform anterior drawer test, talar tilt test.
   7. *Knee*: Palpate for tenderness on the medial and lateral joint line. Perform McMurray's test to detect a torn meniscus (*see the Section II: Procedure: Evaluation of Sprains*). Symptoms of sprained knees include the following:
      a. Meniscus tear: Locking of knee with flexion and giving way of knee.
      b. Collateral ligament tear or strain: Pain at lateral or medial sides.
      c. Anterior cruciate tear: Popping sound at injury site and immediate swelling.
      d. Posterior cruciate tear or strain: Pain in interior knee.
      e. Patellofemoral syndrome: Popping or snapping, pain under patella with motion, and pain on stairs or hills.
      f. Tendinitis: Pain over patellar tendon.
      g. Prepatellar bursitis: Swelling over patella with inability to kneel due to swelling.
      h. Nonspecific effusion: Effusion worse with exercise.

Diagnostic Tests
A. Radiology of extremity, if fracture is suspected. Following the Ottawa ankle and knee rules.
www.ohri.ca/emerg/cdr/docs/cdr_knee_card.pdf
B. MRI, if mechanical symptoms and effusion persist.
C. Bone scans, CT scans, MRI, or referral to a specialist are usually reserved for those clients who have failed to respond after six to 12 weeks of therapy.

Differential Diagnoses
A. Ankle sprain:
   1. Fracture.
   2. Acute dislocation.
   3. Infection.
   4. Ligament strain.

5. Tendinitis or tenosynovitis.
6. Nonspecific foot or ankle pain.

B. Knee sprain:
1. Fracture.
2. Dislocation.
3. Septic arthritis.
4. Infected prepatellar bursitis.
5. Inflammation.
6. Tumour.
7. Meniscus tear.
8. Collateral ligament tear.
9. Anterior cruciate tear.
10. Posterior cruciate tear.
11. Collateral ligament strain.
12. Cruciate ligament strain.
13. Patellofemoral syndrome, or chondromalacia.
14. Effusion, nonspecific.
15. Patellar tendinitis.
16. Prepatellar bursitis.
17. Nonspecific knee pain.

Plan

A. General interventions:
1. Reinforce the degree of injury and the need to take care of the extremity to prevent further damage.
2. Generally follow RICE (rest, ice, compression, and elevation) for Grade 1 and 2 (see section "Definition").
3. Prescribe an exercise program to prevent stiffness, restore function, improve ROM, and restore normal flexibility and strength.
4. A mild ankle sprain may require three to six weeks of rehabilitation, a moderate sprain may require two to three months of rehabilitation, and a severe sprain may require eight to 12 months of therapy to return to full activity.

B. Client teaching.

C. Pharmacological therapy:
1. First-line treatment:
   a. NSAIDs to reduce pain and inflammation.
   b. Consider one of the following: ASA, ibuprofen, indomethacin. Do not use these medications in the long term.
   c. If there is increased risk for bleeding, acetaminophen with codeine may be used for pain.
2. Injectable medication:
   a. Methylprednisolone acetate may be used if symptoms continue to be present six to eight weeks after injury.
   b. Repeat injection in four to six weeks if symptoms have not been reduced by 50%.

Follow-Up

A. Schedule initial follow-up in two weeks to evaluate current therapy or sooner if problems arise.
B. Follow-up appointments should be scheduled according to treatment/therapy.

Consultation/Referral

A. Refer the client to a specialist if a fracture is suspected.
B. Refer to physiotherapist as needed.
C. Refer the client to an orthopedic surgeon if therapy is unproductive and symptoms have not begun to regress within six weeks.

Individual Considerations

A. Pediatrics: In prepubertal or peripubertal clients, knee ligaments usually do not tear. Instead, the growth plate may open up on one side. In this age group, order appropriate radiology to check for fracture of the growth plate.

Bibliography

Bettin, C. C., Richardson, D. R., & Donley, B. G. (2015) Ligamentous injuries of the ankle: Sprained Ankle. In: M. Doral & J. Karlsson J. (Eds.), *Sports Injuries* (pp. 1753–1761). Berlin, Heidelberg: Springer.

Bickley, L. S., & Szilaygi, P. G. (2017). *Bates' guide to physical examination and history taking* (12th ed.). Philadelphia, PA: Lippincott Williams & Wilkins.

Canadian Orthopaedic Foundation. *Strains and sprains*. Retrieved from https://whenithurtstomove.org/about-orthopaedics/conditions-and-ailments/strains-and-sprains/

Carter, D., & Amblum-Almer, J. (2015). Analgesia for people with acute ankle sprain. *Emergency Nurse: The Journal of the RCN Accident & Emergency Nursing Association, 23*(1), 24–31. doi:10.7748/en.23.1.24.e1417

Dains, J. E., Baumann, L. C., & Scheibel, P. (2015). *Advanced health assessment and clinical diagnosis in primary care* (5th ed.). Toronto, ON, Canada: Mosby.

Gray, J. (Ed.). (2011). *Therapeutic choices* (6th ed.). Ottawa, ON, Canada: Canadian Pharmacists Association.

Janssen, K. W., van der Zwaard, B. C., Finch, C. F., van Mechelen, W., & Verhagen, E. A. (2016). Interventions preventing ankle sprains; previous injury and high-risk sport participation as predictors of compliance. *Journal of Science and Medicine in Sport/Sports Medicine Australia, 19*(6), 465–469. doi:10.1016/j.jsams.2015.06.005

Keating, J. F. (2014). Acute knee ligament injuries and knee dislocations. In G. Bentley (Ed.), *European surgical orthopedics and traumatology: The EFORT textbook* (2014th ed., pp. 2949–2971). Berlin, Germany: Springer Publishing Company.

Mau, H., & Baker, R. T. (2014). A modified mobilization-with-movement to treat a lateral ankle sprain. *International Journal of Sports Physical Therapy, 9*(4), 540–548. Retrieved from https://spts.org/member-benefits-detail/enjoy-member-benefits/journals/ijspt/ijspt-archives

McNerney, J. (2015). Treatment of lateral ankle instability. *Podiatry Management, 34*(7), 135–146. Retrieved from https://www.podiatrym.com/

Mitchell, H., Rothenberg, M. D., & Graf, B. (2016). Evaluation of acute knee injuries. *Postgraduate Medicine, 93*(3), 75–86.

Ottawa Hospital Research Institute. (1994/2013). *Ottawa ankle rules for ankle injury radiography*. Retrieved from http://www.ohri.ca/emerg/cdr/docs/cdr_ankle_card.pdf

Ottawa Hospital Research Institute. (1996/2019). *Ottawa knee rules for knee injury radiography*. Retrieved from http://www.ohri.ca/emerg/cdr/docs/cdr_knee_card.pdf

Stiell, I. G., Greenberg, G. H., Wells, G. A., McDowell, I., Cwinn, A. A., Smith, N. A., . . . Sivilotti, M. L. (1996). Prospective validation of a decision rule for the use of radiography in acute knee injuries. *JAMA, 275*, 611–615.

Stiell, I. G., McKnight, R. D., Greenberg, G. H., McDowell, I., Nair, R. C., Wells, G. A., . . . Worthington, J. R. (1994). Implementation of the Ottawa Ankle Rules. *JAMA, 271*, 827–832.

van Ochten, J. M., van Middelkoop, M., Meuffels, D., & Bierma-Zeinstra, S. M. (2014). Chronic complaints after ankle sprains: A systematic review on effectiveness of treatments. *Journal of Orthopaedic & Sports Physical Therapy, 44*(11), 862–871, C1. doi:10.2519/jospt.2014.5221

19 Neurologic Guidelines

Alzheimer's Disease

Jill C. Cash, Julie Adkins, and Donna Clare

Definition
Alzheimer's disease is a progressive, degenerative process of the brain, resulting in loss of global cognitive function, and eventually physical impairment and death. The cause of Alzheimer's disease is not yet known, and there is no cure. The onset is insidious; in the early stages it is difficult to distinguish from normal age-related changes. Early detection is associated with better quality of life for both clients and caregivers.

Incidence/Prevalence
More than 500,000 Canadians are living with dementia, with 25,000 new diagnoses being made each year. Of those over 65 years of age, 65% are women. It is projected that there will be almost one million Canadians living with dementia by 2030. The frequency of dementia increases with age: around 2% in people aged 65 to 70 years, rising to 30% to 40% in those over 85 years. As of 2016, 16,000 Canadians under the age of 65 have early-onset dementia. Alzheimer's disease is the seventh leading cause of death in Canada.

Pathogenesis
A. Alzheimer's disease is characterized by the development of extracellular amyloid-beta protein plaques, intracellular neurofibrillary tangles, and extensive neuronal death. These lesions predominate in the hippocampus and the cerebral cortex—areas associated with memory and higher cognitive functions. Defects in these areas lead to impairment of memory, orientation, learning, language composition, and judgment. Physical function declines in the later stages.
B. Alzheimer's disease is divided into three stages: preclinical (asymptomatic), mild cognitive impairment (not all go on to develop dementia), and dementia.

Predisposing Factors
Nonmodifiable
A. Age older than 50 years.
B. Positive family history.
C. Genetic factors: Down syndrome, the APOE-4 gene.

Modifiable
A. History of head trauma.
B. Diabetes and obesity.
C. Hypertension.
D. Depression.
E. Smoking (increases the risk by 45%–79%).
F. Sleep disorders (insomnia, sleep apnoea).

Common Findings
A. Problems with memory, problem-solving, and getting lost. These problems are noticed by the client, family members, and friends.

Other Signs and Symptoms
A. Impaired insight.
B. Severely impaired short-term memory.
C. Inability to follow a conversation or directions.
D. Visuospatial difficulty: trouble judging distance or colours.
E. Mood changes: depression, apathy, anxiety, agitation, delusions.
F. Disoriented to date, time, or season.
G. Unable to do familiar tasks, like follow a recipe
H. Confabulation.
I. Lack of problem-solving abilities: cannot retrace steps to find an object.
J. Poor judgment and poor decisions: gives money away, falling for scams.
K. Self-neglect (poor hygiene).
L. Social isolation and withdrawal.

Subjective Data
A. Determine the onset, course, and duration of symptoms.
B. Discuss the client's sleep–wake cycle.
C. Note any recent illnesses and new medications.
D. Review the client's history of drug and alcohol use.
E. Inquire as to driving history: accidents, getting lost, and losing parked car.
F. Inquire about incontinence and falls.
G. Review past medical history of head trauma, hypertension, cerebrovascular accident (CVA), cancer, metabolic problems, neurologic disease, infections, gastric surgery (vitamin B12 deficiency), and emotional or psychiatric problems.
H. Weight gain or weight loss is common (forgetting to eat; forgetting that they have eaten).

Physical Examination
A. Vital signs and weight.
B. Inspect overall appearance, effect, hygiene, grooming, and nutritional indicators.
C. Auscultate heart and lungs.

D. Neurologic examination:
  1. Perform a complete neurologic examination.
  2. Administer a standardized screening tool for dementia:
    a. Mini-Mental State Exam (MMSE).
    b. Montreal Cognitive Assessment (MOCA).
    c. Mini-Cog (can be used as an initial quick screening tool): mini-cog.com.
    d. Clock draw test can be used as a screening tool and as a test of executive function: www.strokengine.ca/en/assess/cdt.
  3. Administer a standardized screening tool for depression and/or depression in the context of dementia. Various tools are available through www2.gov.bc.ca/assets/gov/health/practitioner-pro/.../cogimp-appendix-d.pdf.

Diagnostic Tests
A. Complete blood count (CBC).
B. Electrolytes.
C. Thyroid function studies (thyroid-stimulating hormone [TSH]).
D. Vitamin B12 levels.
E. Calcium, magnesium, albumin.
F. Drug screen, HIV, and rapid plasma reagin (RPR; syphilis) if indicated.
G. Liver function tests.
H. MRI of brain (or CT, if MRI unavailable) only in the following circumstances, as per the Recommendations from Canadian Consensus Conference on the Diagnosis and Treatment of Dementia:[a]
  - Less than 60 years of age.
  - Rapid (one or two months) unexplained decline in cognition or function.
  - Short duration (less than two years) of dementia.
  - Recent and significant head trauma.
  - Unexplained neurological symptoms (e.g., new onset of severe headaches or seizures).
  - History of cancer (e.g., types of cancers that metastasize to the brain; cancers in sites that metastasize to the brain).
  - Use of anticoagulants; history of bleeding disorder.
  - History of urinary incontinence/gait disorder early in the course of dementia (as may be found in normal pressure hydrocephalus).
  - Any new localizing sign (e.g., hemiparesis or a Babinski reflex).
  - Gait disturbance.

Differential Diagnosis
A. Delirium.
B. Other dementias.
C. Chronic traumatic encephalopathy.
D. CVA.
E. Brain tumour.
F. Normal pressure hydrocephalus.
G. Liver failure.
H. Alcoholism.
I. Uncontrolled co-morbidity.
J. Drug interactions.

---

[a]Adapted from Gauthier, S., Patterson, C., Chertkow, H., Gordon, M., Herrmann, N., Rockwood, K., . . . Soucy, J. P. (2012). Recommendations of the 4th Canadian consensus conference on the diagnosis and treatment of dementia (CCCDTD4). *Canadian Geriatrics Journal, 15*(4), 120–126. doi:10.5770/cgj.15.49

K. Electrolyte imbalance.
L. Thyroid dysfunction.
M. Vitamin deficiency.
N. Subdural haematoma.

Plan
A. General interventions:
  1. Identify stage of dementia:
    a. Stage 1: No impairment—No evidence of symptoms.
    b. Stage 2: Very mild decline—No symptoms of dementia, has memory lapses.
    c. Stage 3: Mild decline—Difficulty in memory and concentration.
    d. Stage 4: Moderate decline—Impairment with complex tasks, trouble solving math problems, forgetting personal history.
    e. Stage 5: Moderately severe decline—Unable to remember phone number, address, confusion on the day of the week, difficulty with decisions on dressing self properly, and so forth.
    f. Stage 6: Severe decline—Difficulty with personal history, difficulty with naming family members and spouse, difficulty with dressing self, behaviour changes, may wander and get lost.
    g. Stage 7: Very severe decline—Unable to communicate appropriately with others, requires assistance with activities of daily living (ADL), abnormal reflexes, difficulty swallowing.
  There are tools available to help assess the degree of function/dysfunction:
    a. Functional Autonomy Measurement System (SMAF): msssa4.msss.gouv.qc.ca/intra/formres.nsf/ed119278eeccfe0f85256f390065cc54/566f17adf942101885256ed800456db9/$FILE/AS-755A%20(03-05).pdf
    b. Global Deterioration Scale (GDS): www2.gov.bc.ca/assets/gov/health/practitioner-pro/bc-guidelines/cogimp-global-deterioration-scale.pdf.
  2. Provide supportive measures for client and family. With sensitivity, explain to family and the client findings of the examination and possible treatment options.
  3. Treatment may include treating coexisting conditions, like depression, thyroid disease, hypertension, and vitamin deficiencies (Vitamin B12, folate and D).
  4. Discuss therapy options such as musical therapy, occupational therapy, and mind-stimulating activities. Cognitive stimulation has been shown to slow down the degenerative process.
  5. Environment: Ensure that the client has a safe environment; measures may need to be taken for environmental safety such as locks on doors, alarms on doors, relinquishing driving privileges, and so on.
  6. Exercise: Daily exercise should be encouraged.
B. Client Teaching:
  1. Educational sessions should be offered to clients, family, and the community about preventive measures for developing Alzheimer's disease.
  2. Client and family support is available through the Alzheimer Society of Canada and local provincial branches: www.alzheimer.ca or 1-800-616-8816.
  3. Legal documents (e.g., *Advanced Directives, Goals of Care, Power of Attorney*) should be completed while the affected person is still able to make decisions.
  4. If executive function is in decline, driving privileges may be rescinded.

C. Pharmacological Treatment:
1. Cholinesterase inhibitors:
   a. Rivastigmine.
   b. Donepezil.
   c. Galantamine.
2. *N*-methyl-D-aspartate (NMDA) receptor antagonist:
   a. Memantine.
3. Assess the client for secondary behaviours of dementia. Psychosis, delusions, hallucinations, anxiety, depression, and insomnia may occur and should be treated accordingly. Cognitive and behavioural interventions should be initiated in assisting the client in controlling these behaviours. The benefits and risks must be weighed, and pharmacological treatment may be necessary for those clients exhibiting extreme, aggressive behaviours with irritability and/or insomnia. Risperidone has been approved by Health Canada for short-term management of behavioural symptoms in dementia. Periodically, reduce the dosage, or trial the client off the drug, to reassess the need for antipsychotics. Note that some antipsychotics prolong the QT interval. Antipsychotic use in this population is associated with early mortality.
4. Treatment of depression should be guided by the most troublesome symptom. Selective serotonin uptake inhibitors (SSRIs) work well for most clients, but some SSRIs may potentiate the side effects of certain drugs, including cholinesterase inhibitors, warfarin, and lithium, and they may prolong the QT interval. Monitor for weight loss, decrease in seizure threshold, and tremors. Tricyclic antidepressants are not recommended. Mirtazapine is helpful for insomnia and poor appetite. Keep fall risk in mind.

Follow-Up

A. Follow-up is variable, depending on client status and needs of the client and family. Follow-up is recommended every three months to follow progression of disease. If medications are being introduced, monitor the client monthly for the first three to six months.

Consultation/Referral

A. Consider home care, social worker, and occupational and/or physical therapy.
B. Refer to a geriatric assessment service or geriatrician as required.
C. Adults:
1. Lifestyle and dietary changes should be encouraged in adults to prevent risks of developing Alzheimer's disease: Exercising, eating a healthy diet, maintaining a healthy weight, and remaining socially active and engaged. Vitamin D, B12, and folate supplements are recommended by some sources. Vitamin E, Omega 3s, and antioxidants have not been shown to be helpful.
2. Identify and treat sleep apnoea and other sleep disorders early.
3. Treat psychiatric conditions.
4. Avoid smoking. Moderate alcohol intake is beneficial.

D. Geriatrics:
1. Alzheimer's disease is primarily seen in this population.
2. Long-term prognosis: Average client lives 7 to 10 years after early symptoms appear, but those affected may live for 20 years or more.
3. Control co-morbidities.

Bibliography

Alzheimer Society of Canada. (2017). *Alzheimer's disease: The importance of early diagnosis*. Retrieved from http://alzheimer.ca/sites/default/files/files/national/core-lit-brochures/importance_early_diagnosis_e.pdf

Alzheimer's Association. (2018). *10 early signs and symptoms of Alzheimer's*. Retrieved from https://www.alz.org/alzheimers-dementia/10_signs

Annear, M. J., Eccleston, C. E., McInerney, F. J., Elliott, K. E., Toye, C. M., Tranter, B. K., . . . Robinson, A. L. (2016). A new standard in dementia knowledge measurement: Comparative validation of the dementia knowledge assessment scale and the Alzheimer's disease knowledge scale. *Journal of the American Geriatrics Society, 64*(6), 1329–1334. doi:10.1111/jgs.14142

Canadian Geriatrics Society. (2017). *Choosing wisely: Geriatrics*. Retrieved from https://choosingwiselycanada.org/geriatrics/

Guidelines & Protocols Advisory Committee. (2016). *BC guidelines: Cognitive impairment—recognition, diagnosis and management in primary care*. Retrieved from https://www2.gov.bc.ca/gov/content/health/practitioner-professional-resources/bc-guidelines/cognitive-impairment

Halloran, L. (2013). Cognitive impairment: Pearls for practice. *Journal for Nurse Practitioners, 9*(4), 254–255. doi:10.1016/j.nurpra.2013.01.011

Herrmann, N., Harimoto, T., Balshaw, R., & Lanctôt, K. L. (2015). Risk factors for progression of Alzheimer disease in a Canadian population: The Canadian outcomes study in dementia (COSID). *Canadian Journal of Psychiatry. Revue Canadienne de Psychiatrie, 60*(4), 189–199. doi:10.1177/070674371506000406

Mace, N., & Rabins, P. (2012). *The 36-hour day: A family guide to caring for people who have Alzheimer's disease, related dementias and memory loss* (5th ed.). Baltimore, MD: John Hopkins University Press. Retrieved from www.press.jhu.edu

Mendiola-Precoma, J., Berumen, L. C., Padilla, K., & Garcia-Alcocer, G. (2016). Therapies for prevention and treatment of Alzheimer's disease. *Bio Med Research International, 2016*, 1–17. doi:10.1155/2016/2589276

Plosker, G. L. (2015). Memantine extended release (28 mg once daily): A review of its use in Alzheimer's disease. *Drugs, 75*(8), 887–897. doi:10.1007/s40265-015-0400-3

Public Health Agency of Canada. (2017). *Dementia in Canada, including Alzheimer's: Highlights from the Canadian Chronic Disease Surveillance System*. Ottawa, ON, Canada: Ministry of Health. Retrieved from https://www.canada.ca/content/dam/phac-aspc/documents/services/publications/diseases-conditions/dementia-highlights-canadian-chronic-disease-surveillance/dementia-highlights-canadian-chronic-disease-surveillance.pdf

Quebec Ministry of Health and Social Services. (1983). *Functional Autonomy Measurement System (SMAF) form*. Retrieved from http://msssa4.msss.gouv.qc.ca/intra/formres.nsf/ed119278eeccfe0f85256f390065cc54/566f17adf942101885256ed800456db9/$FILE/AS-755A%20(03-05).pdf

Scheltens, N. M., Galindo-Garre, F., Pijnenburg, Y. A., van der Vlies, E. A., Smits, L. L., Koene, T., . . . van der Flier, W. M. (2016). The identification of cognitive subtypes in Alzheimer's disease dementia using latent class analysis. *Journal of Neurology, Neurosurgery, and Psychiatry, 87*(3), 235–243. doi:10.1136/jnnp-2014-309582

Statistics Canada. (2018). Table 13-10-0394-01 *Leading causes of death, total population, by age group*. Retrieved from https://www150.statcan.gc.ca/n1/pub/82-625-x/2014001/article/11896-eng.htm

Bell's Palsy

Jill C. Cash, Julie Adkins, and Donna Clare

Definition

Bell's palsy, also known as idiopathic peripheral facial palsy, is characterized by an acute onset of unilateral facial paralysis. The affected facial nerves originate in the brainstem run through long, narrow foramen through the temporal bone, exiting behind the ears. The facial nerves enervate the facial muscles including those used for eye blinking, tearing, and lid closure, all facial expressions, the stapedius muscle in middle ear, and taste sensations from the anterior two-thirds of the tongue. Usually, only one side of the face is affected.

Pathogenesis

A. Bell's palsy is an acute neuritis of the seventh cranial nerve (facial nerve). The aetiology can be viral, autoimmune, or idiopathic. Often, a triggering event or stressor induces activation of a latent virus, most likely herpes simplex virus, present within the geniculate ganglion of the facial nerve. Viral activation results in reexpression of dormant viral particles and leading to neural inflammation, then entrapment of the nerve, with subsequent ischaemia, and degeneration.
B. The degree of paralysis and synkinesis (involuntary muscle contractions with each facial expression) is closely associated with rate and degree of recovery. Those who are only mildly or moderately affected are more likely to recover completely than those more severely affected. Facial grading scales are available to aid in prognosis (sunnybrook.ca/uploads/FacialGradingSystem.pdf). Residual effects may include synkinesis and gustatory lacrimation, and corneal ulceration, keratitis, and vision loss.

Incidence/Prevalence

A. Bell's palsy is estimated to occur at rates of 20 to 30 per 100,000, with a lifetime incidence of 1 in 60. It accounts for approximately 75% of all cases of facial paralysis. Approximately 5% of those affected will experience a recurrence. Both genders are affected, as well as all ages; the majority of cases occur between the ages of 15 and 60 years.

Predisposing Factors

A. Diabetes.
B. Pregnancy.
C. Recent infection.
D. Positive family history.
E. Hypertension.
F. Hypothyroidism.

Common Findings

A. Acute onset of unilateral facial weakness with inability to close one eye.
B. Sagging of one eyelid.
C. Ipsilateral retroauricular pain with or preceding paralysis.
D. Mouth drawn to affected side.

Other Signs and Symptoms

A. Loss of nasolabial fold.
B. Hyperacusis or hypersensitivity to sound.
C. Dysgeusia, or perversion of taste, in the anterior two-thirds of the tongue.
D. Facial paraesthesia.
E. Drooling.
F. Decreased tearing.

Subjective Data

A. Elicit onset, duration, and course of symptoms.
B. Have the client describe all neurologic symptoms present.
C. Note associated symptoms such as disruption of taste and disturbances in visual function or hearing.
D. Note predisposing factors such as trauma, infection, or pregnancy.
E. Review the client's family history for presence of Bell's palsy.
F. Review the client's medical history; especially note cerebrovascular or cardiac risk factors, as well as for the presence of autoimmune diseases. A focused history should include contraindications to use of steroids.

Physical Examination

A. Check temperature, pulse, respiration, and blood pressure.
B. Inspect:
  1. Note facial appearance.
  2. Observe symmetry of eyes. Check corneal reflex (decreased).
  3. Assess the skin for lesions. Assess in and behind ears for zosteriform lesions.
  4. Ears: Complete ear examination to rule out infection.
  5. Mouth and nose.
C. Palpate:
  1. Palpate skull for evidence of temporal bone fracture.
D. Auscultate:
  1. Heart.
  2. Lungs.
E. Neurologic examination:
  1. Perform a complete neurologic examination; test all cranial nerves.
  2. Assess paralysis of all the muscles supplied by one facial nerve. Paralysis may be of varying degrees and need not be complete.

Subjective decreased sensation may be present in the trigeminal distribution.

Diagnostic Tests

A. Lyme titre (only if tick exposure suspected: see www.canada.ca/en/public-health/services/diseases/lyme-disease/risk-lyme-disease.html): Positive in clients with secondary facial weakness from Lyme disease.
B. CT scan or MRI is indicated if the paralysis is progressing or not improving as expected; facial nerve tumours are rare, but should be ruled out.

Differential Diagnoses

A. Parotid gland tumour.
B. Stroke.
C. Lyme disease.
D. Neoplasms.
E. Ramsay Hunt syndrome, herpes zoster oticus.
F. Acoustic neuroma.
G. Sarcoidosis.
H. Temporal bone fracture.
I. Sjögren's syndrome.
J. Carcinomatous meningitis.

Plan

A. General interventions:
  1. The condition is usually short term (three to four weeks) and may be managed with oral steroids and antivirals, and acetaminophen as needed for discomfort.
  2. Physical therapy may be beneficial for muscle weakness and strengthening muscles after the acute stage.
  3. Ensure the client gets reassurance and emotional support.

Recovery may take three to six months or longer and is complete in approximately 80% of the cases.

B. Client teaching:
  1. *Refer to Client Teaching Guide: Bell's Palsy*. Provide eye protection by means of the following:
      a. Apply methylcellulose drops as needed and as ocular lubricant at bedtime.
      b. Tape eye closed, especially at night.
      c. Wear dark glasses when outdoors to minimize exposure.
  2. Application of heat/cold packs may be useful for pain as needed.
C. Pharmacological treatment:
  1. Prednisone.

  Recent studies suggest that a brief course of prednisone conveys modest benefits with minimal risks.

  2. Acyclovir may be added to a regimen of corticosteroids. Consider acyclovir for clients without renal insufficiency and with no other contraindications to therapy. Acyclovir alone has not been shown to be of benefit and is discouraged as monotherapy for Bell's palsy.
  3. Analgesics, such as acetaminophen, when necessary for ear pain.

Follow-Up
A. For clients with severe symptoms, follow up in three to four days, then again in two weeks.
B. If symptoms worsen or do not resolve within four weeks, have the client return to the clinic.

Consultation/Referral
A. Consult a neurologist for the following:
  1. Failure to resolve after four to six weeks. Only 5% to 8% of clients report distressing residual signs and symptoms, including contracture of facial muscles at rest and synergistic mass innervation because of defective nerve regeneration, manifested as either crocodile tears secondary to abnormal secretory fibres intended for the salivary glands or ipsilateral eyelid shutting.
  2. Other cranial nerve involvement or other abnormalities on neurologic examination.
  3. Recurrence of facial palsy: About 5% to 7% of clients experience recurrence of symptoms. Known causes of recurrent palsy include sarcoidosis, diabetes, leukaemia, and infectious mononucleosis.
  4. Bilateral facial palsies.
B. Consult an ophthalmologist for persistent ocular pain or development of a corneal abrasion or ulceration.
C. Consult an otolaryngologist if decompression is considered.

Individual Considerations
A. Pregnancy: The incidence of Bell's palsy is increased in pregnancy, with the highest incidence in the third trimester or immediately postpartum. May treat with prednisone during pregnancy.

Bibliography
de Almeida, J. R., Guyatt, G. H., Sud, S., Dorion, J., Hill, M. D., & White, C. (2014). Management of bell palsy: Clinical practice guideline. *Canadian Medical Association Journal*, 186(12), 917–922. doi:10.1503/cmaj.131801

National Institute of Neurological Disorders and Stroke. (2016). *Bell's palsy fact sheet*. Retrieved from http://www.ninds.nih.gov/Disorders/Client-Caregiver-Education/Fact-Sheets/Bells-Palsy-Fact-Sheet

Carpal Tunnel Syndrome (CTS)

Jill C. Cash, Julie Adkins, and Donna Clare

Definition
A. Carpal tunnel syndrome (CTS) is a nerve entrapment condition of the median nerve of the wrist.

Incidence/Prevalence
A. CTS occurs in approximately 1% of the general population. It is primarily seen in 30- to 60-year-old adults. Women and older people are more likely to develop the condition.

Pathogenesis
A. CTS occurs from compression of the median nerve in the carpal canal. Compression occurs because of swelling of the flexor tenosynovium; the pressure blocks the nerve fibres, which produces numbness and discomfort in the digits/hands. Repetitive flexion and extension of the wrists create increased pressure in the carpal canal.
B. Potential causes of CTS include blunt trauma or structural changes; tumours; systemic diseases, such as rheumatoid disorders, diabetes mellitus, thyroid disorders, endocrine diseases, and so forth; mechanical overuse syndrome; and infectious diseases, such as tuberculosis (TB) and leprosy. Consider multifactorial causes of CTS. Heredity is likely an important factor, as the carpal tunnel may be smaller in some people or anatomic differences change the amount of space of the nerve; therefore, this trait can run in families.

Predisposing Factors
A. Women.
B. Hobbies or jobs that require repetitive wrist or hand movement and the use of vibratory tools.
C. Pregnancy.
D. Heredity.

Common Findings
A. Pain.
B. Tingling/numbness/burning, primarily in the thumb and index, middle, and ring fingers; sensations in the wrists, hands, and fingers that radiates up into the forearm.
C. Dropping things because of weakness and numbness or loss of proprioception.
D. Nighttime symptoms that are worse than daytime symptoms.

Other Signs and Symptoms
A. Paraesthesia in wrists, hands, and fingers.
B. Localized pain of radial three digits of the hand.
C. Weakness with grasp.
D. Decreased dexterity.
E. Night pain in wrists or waking with numbness of fingers.
F. Referred pain to elbow and/or shoulder.
G. Long-term pressure in the carpus can produce ischqemic changes and may lead to axonal death, muscular atrophy, and pain. Long-term nerve compression may produce irreversible changes.

Subjective Data
A. Determine the onset, duration, and course of presenting symptoms.

B. Note the progression of symptoms since the initial occurrence.
C. Assess whether the symptoms increase with hand or wrist activity and decrease with the joint at rest.
D. Identify what factors precipitate symptoms, what makes symptoms worse, and what alleviates symptoms.
E. Inquire whether the client awakens at night with numbness and tingling sensations.
F. Have the client describe the pain, and note if radiation is present. Are symptoms bilateral?
G. Note the client's occupation, hobby, and/or daily routines that require hand or wrist use.
H. Identify what treatment and/or relief measures have been used, and note results.

Physical Examination
A. Inspect:
  1. The hands for deformities. Note wasting or atrophy.
B. Palpate:
  1. Perform sensory motor evaluation of the hand and arm.
  2. Perform Tinel's test: Tap over transverse carpal ligament; result is positive if tingling in fingers is noted.
  3. Perform Phalen's test: Have client place elbows on flat surface and hold forearms in vertical position, then flex wrists; result is positive if pain, numbness, or tingling is noted within the next 60 seconds.

Diagnostic Tests
A. Electromyogram (EMG).
B. Nerve conduction velocity studies.
C. If an underlying systemic illness or condition exists, consider the following:
  1. Erythrocyte sedimentation rate (ESR).
  2. Blood glucose.
  3. Thyroid profile.
  4. Inflammatory disease studies.

Differential Diagnoses
A. Peripheral neuropathy.
B. Cervical spondylosis and cervical disc herniation.
C. Brachial plexus lesion.
D. Trauma.
E. Thenar atrophy and neuropathy.
F. Osteoarthritis.
G. Neurologic disorders: Polyneuritis, multiple sclerosis (MS), tumours, and so on.

Plan
A. General interventions:
  1. Help the client identify causative agents, eliminate activity if possible, decrease repetitive use, or use alternative methods to accomplish the same task.
  2. Advise resting arms and wrists as much as possible.
  3. Encourage daily stretching exercises.
  4. Give instructions on applying wrist splints, especially at bedtime, while sleeping.
B. Client teaching:
  1. Assist the client to learn how to splint their wrists.
  2. Demonstrate stretching exercises. Invite the client to do a return demonstration of stretching exercises.
  3. Stress the importance of rest. Emphasize the importance of minimizing/eliminating the causative activity.
C. Pharmacological treatment:
  1. Nonsteroidal anti-inflammatory drugs (NSAIDs) as needed for up to two weeks:
    a. Ibuprofen.
    b. Naproxen.
  2. Consider corticosteroid injections in carpal canal.

Follow-Up
A. Depending on treatment, consider follow-up in one month to evaluate status.

Consultation/Referral
A. Refer the client to a surgeon for severe symptoms that could require carpal tunnel release.
B. Consider occupational therapy consult.

Individual Considerations
A. Pregnancy: CTS is the most frequent complaint during pregnancy. About 15% of the cases will progress and continue several months postpartum.

Bibliography
Faust, K., & Jennings, C. (2016). *Carpal tunnel syndrome*. Retrieved from www.orthoinfo.aaos.org/topic.cfm?topic=A00005

Dementia

Jill C. Cash, Julie Adkins, and Donna Clare

Definition
A. Neurocognitive disorders are characterized by deficits in cognitive function, with a significant decline from a previous level of function. Decline may be evident in one or more areas of function, including attention, language, memory, visuospatial skills, or executive function (e.g., complex tasks such as organizing, sequencing, judgment, and reasoning).
B. Neurocognitive disorders include Alzheimer's disease, vascular dementia, Lewy body dementia, and other dementias (frontotemporal dementia, Parkinson's dementia, HIV dementia, neurosyphilis, and Korsakoff's dementia).
C. Clinical features that differentiate these disorders:
  1. Alzheimer's disease.
    a. Gradual onset and a course of progressive decline.
    b. Memory, language, and visuospatial deficits.
    c. Depressive symptoms, which may precede diagnosis.
    d. Delusions, hallucinations, agitation, and apathy.
  2. Vascular dementia:
    a. Abrupt onset and a stepwise course of progression.
    b. Aphasia.
  3. Lewy body dementia:
    a. Visual hallucinations and delusions.
    b. Extrapyramidal symptoms (muscle rigidity, Parkinsonism).
    c. Fluctuating mental status.
    d. Increased sensitivity to antipsychotic medications.
  4. Frontotemporal dementia:
    a. Change in personality.
    b. Hyperorality.
    c. Impairment in executive function, with relatively well-retained visuospatial skills.
    d. Loss of social awareness.
D. The diagnosis of dementia must be differentiated from delirium, a disturbance in cognition that develops over

a short period and is characterized by an alteration in attention that fluctuates in severity during the course of the day. Delirium may be the consequence of an acute medication condition, hospitalization, or medication/substance induced. Delirium typically may last weeks to months, with gradual improvement in cognition.

Incidence/Prevalence

A. The Public Health Agency of Canada reported that as of 2014, there were more than 400,000 Canadians with dementia. There is an annual increase of 76,000 dementia clients: However, the incidence per 1000 is falling. Dementia risk increases with age, and women are more likely to be affected than men, especially after age 80.

Pathogenesis

A. The most common cause of dementia is Alzheimer's disease, accounting for 60% to 80% of cases, with the other cases due to mixed causes, such as multi-infarct, or vascular dementia (being the second most common cause.) A number of other diseases alter cerebral metabolism resulting in dementia such as Huntington's disease (HD) and Parkinson's disease (PD). A variety of diseases that can produce or mimic dementia may be arrested or reversed. These are classified as pseudodementia, such as hypothyroidism or depression. Dementia is caused by damage to brain cells.

Predisposing Factors

A. Definite risks:
  1. Advanced age.
  2. Atrial fibrillation.
  3. Depression.
  4. Family history.
  5. Down syndrome.
B. Possible risks:
  1. Delirium.
  2. Head trauma (e.g., sports, accidents, boxing).
  3. Heavy smoking.
  4. Chronic poor sleep (e.g., sleep apnoea, insomnia).

Common Findings

Interview the client, family members, and/or friends/caretakers who spend quality time with the client to assess for social, neurologic, and cognitive changes experienced by the client:
A. Memory impairment.
B. Change in behaviour and inability to perform normal activities of self-care.

Other Signs and Symptoms

A. Disoriented to date and/or place.
B. Naming difficulties (anomia).
C. Impaired recent recall.
D. Decreased insight.
E. Impaired judgments.
F. Social withdrawal.
G. Problems managing finances, inability to pay bills and manage finances, spending money in unusual ways.
H. Getting lost in familiar environments.
I. Lack of safety awareness: leaving the stove on, taking medications incorrectly, increased vulnerability to strangers.

Impairment of remote memory carries a graver prognosis than the loss of recent memory alone.

Subjective Data

A. Elicit the onset and duration of symptoms; commonly, this information comes from family members.
B. Question the family members and/or caregivers regarding personality changes in the client, or any changes in personal hygiene.
C. Review the client's history for sexually transmitted infections.
D. Is there a loss of interest in things the client used to find important?
E. Review medications, specifically those medications with anticholinergic side effects, including over-the-counter (OTC) products such as diphenhydramine.
F. Evaluate the client's history for any recent major life events such as the death of a spouse, a move to a new living environment, or loss of purpose following retirement.

Physical Examination

A. Evaluate blood pressure, pulse, respiration, and weight.
B. Inspect:
  1. Observe general appearance; note grooming, interest in conversation, and apathy.
  2. Note the presence of slurred speech and slowed body movements.
  3. Inspect the nail beds and mucous membranes for anaemia.
C. Auscultate:
  1. Heart.
  2. Lungs.
  3. Abdomen.
D. Palpate:
  1. Thyroid.
E. Neurologic examination:
  1. Perform a complete neurologic examination, including cranial nerves, gait, motor function, and cerebellar function.
  2. Note facial asymmetry, distal weakness, and any focal neurologic findings.
  3. Complete a mental status examination with instrument of choice. See the section "Diagnostic Tests."
  4. Assess functional status. May use a functional assessment tool such as Physical Self-Maintenance Scale, Instrumental Activities of Daily Living Scale, or Reisberg Functional Assessment Staging (FAST) scale. Available at geriatrics.uthscsa.edu/tools/FAST.pdf.
  5. Complete depression screening with instrument of choice:
      a. Geriatric Depression Scale (GDS). Available at consultgeri.org/try-this/general-assessment/issue-4.pdf.
      b. Client Heath Questionnaire (PHQ)-9. Available at www.phqscreeners.com.
      c. Beck Depression Inventory. Available at www.bmc.org/Documents/Beck-Depression-Inventory-BDI.pdf.

Diagnostic Tests

A. Mini-Mental State Examination (MMSE). Available at www.uml.edu/docs/Mini%20Mental%20State%20Exam_tcm18-169319.pdf.
B. Pfeiffer's Short, Portable, Mental Status Questionnaire or other mental examination of choice. Pfeiffer's mental status questionnaire is available at geriatrics.stanford.edu/culturemed/overview/assessment/assessment_toolkit/spmsq.html.

C. The clock draw test (CDT) may also be administered and used as a screening tool. The CDT is available at www.rehabmeasures.org.
D. Rule out possible reversible causes of dementia; not all are required, so use discretion:
   1. Thyroid function tests, to rule out either hypothyroidism or hyperthyroidism.
   2. Complete blood count (CBC).
   3. Vitamin B12 level: Anaemia or B12 deficiency.
   4. Serum chemistry profile: Hyponatraemia, hypomagnesia.
   5. Toxicology screen or serum drug screen: Toxicity or intoxication.
   6. Rapid plasma reagin (RPR), fluorescent treponemal antibody absorption (FTA-ABS), or microhaemagglutination assay for antibody to *Treponema pallidum* (MHA-TP; cerebrospinal fluid [CSF]) to confirm syphilis, if indicated.
   7. HIV-1 antibody titre, if indicated: AIDS–dementia complex.
   8. Liver function tests: Liver disease.
   9. CT scan or MRI: Vascular dementia, tumour, chronic subdural haematoma (SDH), normal pressure hydrocephalus, and AIDS–dementia complex.
   10. EKG: Creutzfeldt–Jakob disease, if indicated.
   11. Neuropsychological evaluation.

The history is the key to the diagnosis of dementia. The physical examination may be normal. Dementia is not a normal part of aging; normal aging intelligence scores decrease by only about 10% by age 80 years. A thorough search for a potentially reversible cause is required.

Differential Diagnoses
A. Completely reversible dementia, rarely.
B. Depression and adverse reactions to medications are the most common reversible causes of dementia.
Use the DEMENTIA mnemonic:
D: Drugs or depression.
E: Emotional upset.
M: Metabolic, for example, vitamin B12 deficiency or hypothyroidism.
E: Ear or eye impairment or sensory impairment.
N: Normal pressure hydrocephalus.
T: Tumours or masses, for example, SDH.
I: Infection or sepsis.
A: Anaemia.
C. Alzheimer's disease.
D. Dementia with Lewy bodies.
E. PD with dementia.
F. Vascular dementia.
G. Frontotemporal dementia.

Plan
A. General interventions:
   1. The goal is to treat identifiable abnormalities.
   2. Supportive care for the family and client should be arranged.
   3. Caring for clients with dementia can be overwhelming. Caregivers need support when caring for these clients as well.
   4. Encourage healthy behaviours, including regular exercise, healthy diet, and stress management.
   5. Maintain brain function through involvement in stimulating social activities.
   6. Consider driving evaluation for safety if the client is still driving.
   7. Recommend the use of a safe-return bracelet.
   8. Evaluate the home for safety features.
   9. Arrange for supportive care for the family and client.
   10. Information regarding support groups for caregivers and family is helpful.
B. Client/family teaching:
   1. *Refer to Client Teaching Guide: Dementia.* Discuss the diagnosis, disease process, and progression with the client and family.
   2. Discuss advance directives and planning for future care needs.
   3. Encourage client and family caregivers to become involved in dementia support groups.
   4. Avoid medications such as anticholinergic medications, including diphenhydramine, hydroxyzine, tricyclic antidepressants (TCAs), and oxybutynin.
   5. Recommended book for the family: *The 36-Hour Day: A Family Guide to Caring for People Who Have Alzheimer's Disease, Related Dementias and Memory Loss* (Mace & Rabins, 2017).
   6. Refer clients and families to the Alzheimer's Society of Canada for more information and resources on coping with dementia and caregiver stress.
C. Pharmacological therapy:
   1. There are not any medications that have been found to decrease the rate of decline in cognitive behaviour. However, studies have shown that clients can be treated with medications for agitation, hallucinations, and depression and to improve mental alertness. Studies indicate that clients with a diagnosis of mild to moderate Alzheimer's disease, vascular dementia, Lewy body dementia, and Parkinson's dementia may trial and benefit from a cholinesterase inhibitor:
      a. Donepezil.
      b. Rivastigmine patch.
      c. Galantamine.
   2. Clients with moderate to severe Alzheimer's disease:
      a. Memantine.

Follow-Up
A. Routine follow-up in one month to evaluate client's status, response to medication, and side effects.
B. Clients and families have an ongoing need for education and support in learning to deal with the diagnosis.
C. Subsequent follow-up visits can be scheduled every three to six months.

Consultation/Referral
A. Refer the client to a neurocognitive specialist if diagnosis is unclear.
B. Refer clients and families to support groups in the community.
C. Geriatric psychiatry may be appropriate for management and treatment of behavioural and psychological symptoms of dementia.
D. Refer to home care, social services, or geriatric case management for assistance with respite care and placement options.

▶ Client Teaching Guides are available at https://connect.springerpub.com/content/reference-book/978-0-8261-9498-5

Individual Considerations
A. Paediatrics: A client who presents at a young age with dementia requires a thorough workup to evaluate the cause of the symptoms.
B. Geriatrics: Irreversible dementia or Alzheimer's disease begins in the fourth to fifth decade of life and is characterized by loss of recent memory, inability to learn new information, language problems, mood swings, and personality changes.

Resources
Alzheimer Society of Canada: https://alzheimer.ca.
Alzheimer's Association: www.alz.org.
Alzheimer's Disease Education and Referral Center: www.nia.nih.gov/alzheimers.
Alzheimer's Society of Canada: https://alzheimer.ca/en/Home.
Frontotemporal Dementia: National Institute of Neurological Disorders and Stroke: www.ninds.nih.gov.
Lewy Body Dementia Association: www.lbda.org.

Bibliography
Canadian Geriatrics Society. (2017). *Choosing wisely: Geriatrics*. Retrieved from https://choosingwiselycanada.org/geriatrics/
Delgado-Alvarado, M., Gago, B., Navalpotro-Gomez, I., Jiménez-Urbieta, H., & Rodriguez-Oroz, M. C. (2016). Biomarkers for dementia and mild cognitive impairment in parkinson's disease. *Movement Disorders*, *31*, 861–881. doi:10.1002/mds.26662
Gauthier, S., Patterson, C., Chertkow, H., Gordon, M., Herrmann, N., Rockwood, K., & Soucy, J. P. (2012). Recommendations of the 4th Canadian consensus conference on the diagnosis and treatment of dementia (CCCDTD4). *Canadian Geriatrics Journal*, *15*(4), 120–126. doi:10.5770/cgj.15.49
Guidelines & Protocols Advisory Committee. (2016). *BC guidelines: Cognitive impairment—recognition, diagnosis and management in primary care*. Retrieved from https://www2.gov.bc.ca/gov/content/health/practitioner-professional-resources/bc-guidelines/cognitive-impairment
Halloran, L. (2013). Cognitive impairment: Pearls for practice. *Journal for Nurse Practitioners*, *9*(4), 254–255. doi:10.1016/j.nurpra.2013.01.011
Reisberg, B., Ferris, S. H., de Leon, M. J., & Crook, T. (1982). The global deterioration scale for assessment of primary degenerative dementia. *American Journal of Psychiatry*, *139*(9), 1136–1139. doi:10.1176/ajp.139.9.1136

Guillain–Barré Syndrome (GBS)

Cheryl A. Glass, Julie Adkins, and Donna Clare

Definition
A. Guillain–Barré syndrome (GBS) is an acute immune-mediated polyneuropathy of the peripheral nervous system. GBS often follows an infection.
B. GBS is the most common cause of acute flaccid paralysis in healthy infants and children.
C. GBS in not contagious, and there is no known cure.
D. GBS usually presents with ascending, progressive, multifocal, symmetric muscle weakness, and paraesthesia. The first symptom of GBS is weakness or tingling sensations of the legs. Most people reach the stage of greatest weakness within the first two weeks after symptoms appear. By the third week of the illness, 90% of all clients are at their weakest.
E. GBS is considered monophasic and remits spontaneously, but may also recur in 3% of clients. About 20% to 30% of clients will have persistent disability measured by tools such as the Overall Disability Sum Score (ODSS; see Table 19.1). An electronic version of the ODSS is available online at farmacologiaclinica.info/scales/overall-disability-sum-score. This application grades the arm (range 0–5) and the leg (range 0–7) to provide an overall range score. A total score of 0 equals no disability and a total score of 12 equals maximum disability.

There are several variants of GBS:
1. Miller Fisher syndrome (MFS) often follows an infection, especially *Campylobacter jejuni* gastroenteritis.
2. Acute inflammatory demyelinating polyradiculoneuropathy (AIDP): Approximately two-thirds occur after an infection, including *C. jejuni*, cytomegalovirus (CMV), *Mycoplasma pneumonia*, or influenza virus.
3. Acute motor axonal neuropathy (AMAN).
4. Acute sensorimotor axonal neuropathy (AMSAN).
5. Acute panautonomic neuropathy (rare).
6. Bickerstaff's brainstem encephalitis (BBE).

Incidence/Prevalence
A. The incidence of GBS is 1/100,000 adults.
B. GBS occurs in all age groups. GBS is more common in older adults, with people older than 50 years at the greatest risk.
C. The incidence of GBS in children is 0.6 to 2.4 cases per 100,000.
D. Eighty percent to ninety percent become nonambulatory during the illness.
E. Relapses are not uncommon in adults who have been treated with intravenous immunoglobulin (IVIG) and plasma exchange.
F. Approximately 30% have a residual weakness after 3 years.
G. GBS severe enough to require mechanical ventilation is associated with both incomplete recovery and up to 20% mortality.
H. Approximately 5% of clients with GBS die from medical complications such as sepsis, pulmonary emboli, and cardiac arrest related to dysautonomia.
I. GBS is reported throughout the world.

Pathogenesis
A. GBS is believed to be an immune-mediated response linked to an antecedent infection wherein a patchy demyelination of the motor component of multiple peripheral nerves occurs. This causes a failure of neuromuscular transmission and leads to abrupt, distal weakness and symmetrical onset of paraesthesia. The sensory disturbance is quickly followed by a rapid progressive limb weakness and sometimes paralysis. Most clients are able to identify a specific date of onset of sensory and motor symptoms.

Predisposing Factors
A. Illness:
   1. Up to two-thirds of clients with GBS have experienced a viral upper respiratory infection (URI) or gastroenteritis 10 to 14 days before onset.
   2. *C. jejuni* gastroenteritis.
   3. CMV (CMV is the second most common reported infection preceding GBS).
   4. Epstein–Barr virus (EBV).
   5. *Mycoplasma pneumonia*.
   6. HIV.
   7. *Haemophilus influenzae*.
   8. Enteroviruses.
   9. Hepatitis A and B.
   10. Herpes simplex.
   11. *Chlamydophila* (formerly *Chlamydia*) pneumonia.
   12. Zika virus.
B. Trauma.
C. Surgery.
D. Parturition.

TABLE 19.1 Overall Disability Sum Score (ODSS) for Guillian–Barré Syndrome

Area of Body	Activities	Functional Ability Scale for Each Activity	Disability Scale Grade
Arm disability	A. Dressing upper part of body (excludes buttons/zippers). B. Washing and brushing hair. C. Turning a key in a lock. D. Using a knife and fork (use of spoon applies if never used a fork/knife). E. Doing/undoing buttons and zippers.	Not affected; affected, but does not prevent activity; prevents activity	0 = Normal function for all activities 1 = Minor S/S in one or both arms, but does not affect the activity 2 = Moderate S/S in one or both arms affecting, but not preventing, any activity 3 = Severe S/S in one or both arms preventing at least one, but not all, activities 4 = Severe S/S in both arms preventing all functions; purposeful movements still possible 5 = Severe S/S in both arms preventing all purposeful movements

Leg disability	A. Do you have any problems walking?
	B. Do you walk with a walking aid?
	C. How do you get around for 25 feet (10 m)?
	  1. Without aid.
	  2. With one stick or crutch or holding someone's arm.
	  3. With two sticks or crutches or one stick and a crutch and holding someone's arm.
	  4. With a wheelchair.
	D. If you use a wheelchair, can you stand and walk a few steps with help?
	E. If you are restricted to bed most of the time, are you able to make some purposeful movements?
		No; yes; does not apply	0 = Walking is not affected
			1 = Walking is affected, but does not look abnormal
			2 = Walks independently, but gait looks abnormal
			3 = Usually uses unilateral support (stick, crutch, one arm) to walk 25 feet (10 m)
			4 = Usually uses bilateral support (stick, crutch, two arms) to walk 25 feet (10 m)
			5 = Usually uses a wheelchair to travel 25 feet (10 m)
			6 = Restricted to wheelchair, unable to stand and walk a few steps with help, but able to make some purposeful leg movements
			7 = Restricted to wheelchair or bed most of the day, preventing all purposeful movements of the legs (e.g., unable to reposition legs in bed)

S/S, signs/symptoms.
Source: Adapted from Merkies, I. S., Schmitz, P. L., van der Meché, F. G., Samihn, J. P., & van Doorn, P. A. (INCAT Group). (2016). *Overall disability sum score: Overall disability scale online calculator.* Retrieved from http://farmacologiaclinica.info/scales/overall-disability-sum-score/

E. Immunization:
  1. In 1976, there was a small increase in GBS following the flu vaccine formulated to protect against swine flu.
  2. Rabies vaccine is prepared from infected brain tissue.
F. There is no genetic factor for GBS.

Common Findings
A. The classic clinical features:
  1. Progressive, fairly symmetric muscle weakness:
    a. Difficulty walking.
    b. Nearly complete paralysis, including:
      i. All extremities, generally starts in the proximal legs.
      ii. Facial muscles/oropharyngeal weakness.
      iii. Respiratory muscles.
      iv. Bulbar (ocular) muscles.
  2. Accompanying absent or depressed deep tendon reflexes (DTRs).
B. Acute weakness in hands, dropping things, trouble picking up small objects or buttoning buttons, inability to feel textures.
C. Acute onset of persistent tingling or pins and needles "crawling-skin" sensation in feet, possibly in hands, inability to feel pain.
D. Prominent severe lower back pain.

Other Signs and Symptoms
A. Sinus tachycardia or other arrhythmias.
B. Bilateral generally symmetric muscle weakness not improved by rest.
C. Urinary retention.
D. Ileus-gastric motility disorders.
E. Severe residual fatigue that may persist for years.
F. Loss of sweating.
G. Facial or pharyngeal weakness.

Subjective Data
A. Ask the client about any dyspnaea. If there is shortness of breath (SOB), assess the need to go immediately by ambulance to a hospital.
B. Elicit information regarding the onset and duration of symptoms.
C. Question the client regarding change or progression of symptoms.
D. Ascertain whether the client has had recent URI, flu, gastroenteritis, other infections, recent trauma, or surgery: Determine whether there was an associated fever.
E. Look for paraesthesia preceding weakness by approximately 24 to 48 hours.
F. Look for recent exposure to environmental hazards: lead, toxins (botulism), pesticides, volatile solvents, or ticks.

Physical Examination

A. Check temperature, pulse, respiration, and blood pressure (persistent hypotension, hypertension alternating with hypotension, or orthostatic hypotension). Hypertension is seen in about one-third of clients with GBS and can be labile or followed by hypotension.
B. Inspect:
  1. Observe overall appearance.
  2. Look for gait disturbance.
  3. Assess for difficulty with breathing or respiratory distress.
C. Auscultate:
  1. Note heart rate and rhythm. Tachycardia is common; bradycardia and other arrhythmias may be noted.
  2. Auscultate the lung fields.
  3. Abdomen assessment for bowel sounds/dysfunction. Gastrointestinal motility disorders occur in 15% of severely affected GBS clients.
D. Palpate:
  1. Palpate the extremities.
  2. Note muscle tone and normal muscle bulk.
  3. Assess DTRs, muscle strength, areflexia (lack of reflexes), or hyporeflexia (diminished).
  4. Look for symmetric weakness. Incidence of weakness in the ankle and knee is greater than in biceps and triceps.
  5. Palpate the abdomen: Assess urinary retention.
E. Neurologic examination:
  1. Perform complete neurologic examination: Generally, no sensory deficits to touch or pinprick are noted. Decreased proprioception or vibration may be seen. In approximately 50% of clients, GBS may progress rapidly, sometimes within hours, to severe respiratory muscle weakness and respiratory failure. The knee-jerk reflex is usually lost.

Diagnostic Tests

Prompt treatment mandates that the clinician make the diagnosis of GBS solely on history and examination. Testing done in the inpatient setting includes the following:
A. Lumbar puncture (LP).
  1. The LP primarily rules out other infectious diseases.
  2. Most GBS clients have elevated cerebrospinal fluid (CSF) protein levels with normal CSF cell counts.
B. Needle electromyogram (EMG).
C. Nerve conduction studies used to confirm the presence, pattern, and severity of neuropathy.
D. Antibody testing.
E. Serum blood testing: Electrolytes, liver function tests, creatine phosphokinase (CPK), and erythrocyte sedimentation rate (ESR).

Differential Diagnoses

A. Myasthenia gravis (MG).
B. Poliomyelitis.
C. Acute intermittent porphyria.
D. West Nile encephalomyelitis.
E. Tick paralysis: Lyme neuroborreliosis.
F. Diphtheria.
G. HIV.
H. Cervical myelopathy.
I. Sarcoidosis.
J. Poisoning:
  1. Heavy metal poisoning (arsenic, lead, or thallium).
  2. Hexacarbon abuse (glue-sniffing neuropathy).
  3. Organophosphate poisoning.
  4. Botulism.
K. Zika virus.

Plan

A. General interventions:
  1. Early diagnosis is crucial to appropriate management. A possible diagnosis of GBS requires *immediate* hospitalization at a facility with ICU capabilities and consultation with a neurologist who has experience managing GBS. The most critical part of treatment consists of keeping the client's body functioning during recovery.
B. Client teaching:
  1. Talk to the client and family about GBS; discuss the characteristics of the disease.
  2. Acknowledge to the client and family that there is no cure for GBS; however, there are several treatments and therapies that may lessen the symptoms and speed up recovery time.
  3. Recovery period may take several weeks or months. Reinforce the critical nature of the syndrome, which may include hospitalization in the ICU for paralysis and severe complications.
  4. Along with physical impairments/weakness, the client may also experience emotional problems from the sudden onset of the syndrome, requiring dependence on family and friends for physical and emotional support.
  5. Offer resources to the client and family. For example, the GBS/CIDP Foundation of Canada: www.gbscidp.ca/.
C. Hospital medical management:
  1. Plasmapheresis (plasma exchange).
  2. IVIG administration.
  3. Steroids have not been shown to be helpful and may be detrimental.
  4. Because of the associated autonomic instability, hypertension should be treated with short-acting intravenous agents.
  5. The presence of at least four of the six predictors indicate the need for support/mechanical ventilation:
     a. Onset of symptoms less than seven days.
     b. Inability to cough.
     c. Inability to stand.
     d. Inability to lift the elbows.
     e. Inability to lift the head.
     f. An increase in liver enzymes.
  6. Heparin and support/pressure stockings are used for nonambulatory clients because of the risk of deep vein thrombosis (DVT) and pulmonary embolus.
D. Pharmacological treatment:
  1. Pain therapy:
     a. Gabapentin.
     b. Carbamazepine.
     c. Narcotics may be necessary.
     d. Tricyclic antidepressants (TCAs).
  2. Immunizations:
     a. Immunizations are not recommended during the acute phase and up to approximately 1 year after the onset of GBS.
     b. Influenza, tetanus, and typhoid immunizations have been most commonly associated with relapse of GBS symptoms.

Follow-Up

A. Clients generally follow up with a neurologist once they have been discharged from the hospital or rehabilitation facility.
B. Full recovery can take up to 3 years with severe cases and even 30% of clients at this point may have residual weakness

and 3% of clients experience recurrence. Severe fatigue is a sequel of GBS in two-thirds of adults.

C. The most critical part of treatment consists of keeping the client's body functioning during recovery of the nervous system. Physical rehabilitation with a multidisciplinary team including occupational, speech, and physical therapists focuses on proper limb positioning, posture, orthotics, exercise, and strengthening swallowing muscles:
   1. Foot and wrist drop are not uncommon and may require orthotics.
   2. Joint contracture requires active and passive range of motion (ROM).

D. Psychological counseling may be required to help with adaptation.

Consultation/Referral

A. If GBS is suspected, send client to the nearest emergency department (ED).

Individual Considerations

A. Paediatrics:
   1. GBS is the most common cause of acute flaccid paralysis in healthy infants and children.
   2. The Pediatric Evaluation of Disability Inventory Computer Adaptive Test (PEDI-CAT) is designed for the assessment of children from birth to 20 years of age for physical and behavioural conditions in daily activities, mobility, and social/cognitive domains.

B. Geriatrics:
   1. Age >55 years is a poor prognostic factor.

Resources

Canadian Immunization Guide: Part 2 Vaccine Safety: https://www.canada.ca/en/public-health/services/canadian-immunization-guide.html.
GBS/CIDP Foundation International: www.gbs-cidp.org

Bibliography

American Academy of Neurology. (n.d.). *Guillain-Barré syndrome*. Retrieved from http://clients.aan.com/disorders/indexcfm?event=view&disorder_id=935

Cruse, R. P. (2013, February 1). Overview of Guillain-Barré syndrome in children. *UpToDate*. Retrieved from www.uptodate.com/contents/overview-of-guillain-barre-syndrome-in-children?topicKey=PEDS%2F6235

MD Guidelines. (n.d.). *Guillain–Barré syndrome*. Retrieved from www.mdguidelines.com/guillain-barre-syndrome

Merkies, I. S., Schmitz, P. L., van der Meché, F. G., Samihn, J. P., van Doorn, P. A., & INCAT Group. (2016). *Overall disability sum score: Overall disability scale online calculator*. Retrieved from http://farmacologiaclinica.info/scales/overall-disability-sum-score/

National Institute of Health. (2016). *Guillain-Barré syndrome fact sheet*. Retrieved from www.ninds.nih.gov/Disorders/Client-Caregiver-Education/Fact-Sheets/Guillain-Barré-Syndrome-Fact-Sheet

Vriesendorp, F. J. (2013). Treatment and prognosis of Guillain-Barré syndrome in adults. *UpToDate*. Retrieved from http://www.uptodate.com/contents/treatment-and-prognosis-of-guillain-barre-syndrome-inadults?topicKey=NEURO%2F5172

Živković, S. (2015). Intravenous immunoglobulin in the treatment of neurologic disorders. *Acta Neurologica Scandinavica*, *133*(5), 84–96. doi:10.1111/ane.12444

Headache

Cheryl A. Glass, Julie Adkins, and Donna Clare

Definition

A. Headache is a discomfort of the head that is produced from inflammation and/or tightness of the arteries, nerves, and/or muscles of the cranium. Primary headaches are a major cause for missed school and work, loss of productivity at work (presenteeism), and disability in children and adults.

B. There are multiple types of headaches: Tension-type headaches (TTHs), and trigeminal autonomic cephalalgias, including cluster headaches, chronic daily headaches, and new daily persistent headaches (NDPH; see Table 19.2). Migraines are discussed separately in this chapter under the section "Migraine Headache." Posttraumatic headaches occur within 7 days after head trauma. Tension headaches are the most frequent type, occurring as part of the postconcussive syndrome.

C. NDPHs have many similarities to TTHs and migraines. Other types of headaches, including posttraumatic headache, low cerebrospinal fluid (CSF) volume headache, raised CSF pressure headache, and headaches attributed to infection should be ruled out. NDPH is unique in that the headache is daily and unremitting from or almost from the moment of onset, typically in individuals without a prior headache history. There are two subtypes:
   1. Self-limiting, which typically resolves without therapy within several months.
   2. Refractory, which is resistant to aggressive treatment programs.

Incidence/Prevalence

Headaches are very common, and their incidence depends on age, gender, and type:

A. TTHs are the most common primary headaches, affecting 31% to 74% of the population. Up to 15% of children and teens have experienced tension headaches, compared with 4% for migraines.

B. Headaches occur in 90% of school-aged children.

C. Cluster headaches have been reported in children as young as age three years. The prevalence of cluster headaches is in <1% of the population, with men affected more than women.

D. Chronic daily headaches are more common in females than in males.

E. Medication overuse headaches (MOHs) are reported in 20% to 36% of adolescents with daily headaches.

Pathogenesis

A. Because there are different types of headaches, the origin of each type differs. Many people have a combination of the different types of headaches. Headache causes range from systemic illness such as infections, medical disorders such as tumours or haemorrhage, medications, drug use, and/or stress. Tension headaches are headaches that occur because of contracted muscles of the scalp and neck. Cluster headaches have an uncertain aetiology; however, they appear to be caused by extracerebral vasodilation.

B. Review environmental/seasonal factors. Headaches may be cyclic in the spring and summer months with allergic rhinitis and in the fall and winter for carbon monoxide poisoning from gas heaters.

C. Medications commonly associated with headaches include the following:
   1. Nitroglycerine.
   2. Nifedipine.
   3. Dipyridamole.
   4. Selective serotonin reuptake inhibitor (SSRI).

Predisposing Factors

A. Tension, stress.
B. Cervical, or back, disorders.
C. Medications (e.g., nitroglycerin, sildenafil).

International Headache Society Classification of Headaches

NDPH[a]	TTH[b]	Cluster Headache	MOH[c]
Headache that is daily and unremitting from the moment of onset or very rapidly builds up to continuous and unremitting pain. The pain is typically bilateral, pressing, or tightening in quality and of mild to moderate intensity. There may be photophobia, phonophobia, or mild nausea.	Episodic headache lasting minutes to days. Pain is mild to moderate, typically bilateral, pressing, or tightening quality. Pain does not worsen with activity.	Episodic or chronic attacks separated by pain-free periods lasting a month or longer. Pain almost always recurs on the same side during a cluster period. May be provoked by alcohol, histamine, or nitroglycerine.	Variable headache that often has a peculiar pattern with characteristics shifting, even within the same day, from migraine-like to TTH.
Diagnostic Criteria	**Diagnostic Criteria**	**Diagnostic Criteria**	**Diagnostic Criteria**
A. Headache that fulfills criteria B–D within three days of onset.	**A.** At least 10 episodes, less than one day per month on average and fulfills B–D criteria.	**A.** At least five attacks that fulfill B–D criteria.	**A.** Present on 15 days per month, which fulfills B–D criteria.
B. Headache is present daily and is unremitting for greater than three months.	**B.** Headache lasts 30 minutes to days.	**B.** Severe or very severe unilateral orbital, supraorbital, and/or temporal pain lasting 15–180 minutes if untreated.	**B.** Regular overuse for three months of one or more drugs that can be taken for acute and/or symptomatic treatment of headaches.
C. At least two of the following pain characteristics exist: 1. Bilateral location. 2. Pressing/tightening (nonpulsating) quality. 3. Mild to moderate intensity. 4. Not aggravated by routine physical activity such as walking or climbing.	**C.** At least two of the following characteristics exists: 1. Bilateral location. 2. Pressure/tightening, nonpulsating quality. 3. Mild to moderate quality. 4. No increase with routine physical activity such as walking or climbing stairs.	**C.** Accompanied by at least one of the following: 1. Ipsilateral conjunctival infection and/or lacrimation. 2. Ipsilateral nasal congestion and/or rhinorrhea. 3. Ipsilateral eyelid oedema. 4. Ipsilateral forehead and facial sweating. 5. Ipsilateral miosis and/or ptosis. 6. Restlessness or agitation (usually unable to lie down and characteristically pace the floor).	**C.** Developed or markedly worsened during medication overuse.
D. Both of the following: 1. No more than one of photophobia, phonophobia, or mild nausea. 2. Neither moderate or severe nausea nor vomiting.	**D.** Both of the following: 1. No nausea or vomiting. 2. No more than one photophobia or phonophobia.	**D.** Attacks have a frequency from one every other day to eight per day.	**D.** Headache resolves or reverts to its previous pattern within two months after discontinuing the overused medication. Examples of medications include ergotamine, triptans, analgesics, opioids, and combination analgesics.
E. Not attributed to another disorder	**E.** Not attributed to another disorder	**E.** Not attributed to another disorder	

[a] The client must clearly recall and unambiguously describe the daily headache as unremitting at the moment of onset and build to continuous/unremitting pain.
[b] Previously called common muscle contraction, stress, ordinary, or psychogenic headache.
[c] Previously called rebound, drug-induced, or medication misuse headache.
MOH, medication overuse headache; NDPH, new daily persistent headaches; TTH, tension-type headache.
Source: Adapted from the International Headache Society ICHD-II. (2018). *International classification of headache disorders* (3rd ed.). Retrieved from https://www.ichd-3.org/; International Headache Society ICHD-II. (n.d.). *Migraine.* Retrieved from https://www.ichd-3.org/1-migraine.

D. Bruxism.
E. Sleep disorders (e.g., snoring, insomnia).
F. Foods/caffeine/alcohol.
G. Hormonal changes.
H. Family history of headaches.
I. Sexual activity.
J. Cough.
K. Exertion/exercise.
L. Viral/infectious aetiologies.
M. Poor-fitting dentures.
N. Faulty/inefficient gas heating.
O. Trigeminal neuralgia.
P. Valsalva maneuvers.
Q. Head trauma.

Common Findings
A. Depending on the type of headache, other symptoms may coexist, such as lacrimation, nasal congestion, restlessness, and visual changes.
B. Pain and location depend on the type of headache.
C. Characteristics of the headache depend on the type of headache.

Other Signs and Symptoms
A. Crying.
B. Behavioural problems.
C. Neurological signs (e.g., hemiparesis, numbness, facial droop).

Subjective Data
A. Use the following acronym for subjective information: PQRST:
   P: Provocation, or worsening, of factors stimulating headaches.
   Q: Quality of pain, severity of pain.
   R: Region of headache.
   S: Strength of pain; evaluate pain on a scale of 1 to 10.
   T: Time, including onset, frequency, and duration of headaches.
B. Assess whether the client frequently has migraine headaches. Is this the first or worst headache ever experienced by the client?
C. If recurrent headaches exist, note the frequency and patterns of similar headaches.
D. Note whether the client has ever identified potential triggers of recurring headaches such as dietary issues, stressors, and odours (e.g., perfumes, cigarette smoke).
E. Identify the location of pain, along with radiation if present.
F. Describe the type of pain: throbbing, constant, or burning.
G. Assess the presence of associated symptoms: nausea or vomiting, photophobia, noise sensitivity, or the presence of halos around lights.
H. Determine whether the client experiences any neurologic symptoms and/or prodromal symptoms before a headache.
I. Review the methods used in the past to abort and/or prevent headaches and the results.
J. Inquire about past diagnostic evaluations for headaches.
K. Note a family history of headaches.
L. List current medications, including over-the-counter (OTC) medications and herbals.
M. Review the client's medical history for head trauma, allergies, presence of a ventriculoperitoneal (VP) shunt, or other neurologic diagnoses.
N. Is the client in the second or third trimester of pregnancy?
O. Does the client present with a fever or have a recent history of infection?
P. Rule out gas exposure.

Physical Examination
Physical examination may be normal unless client presents with a headache:
A. Check blood pressure, pulse, and respiration (temperature if meningeal signs are present).
B. Inspect:
   1. Observe overall appearance for the presence of discomfort, photosensitivity (use of sunglasses indoors), and level of consciousness (LOC).
   2. Examine the eyes; perform funduscopic examination.
   3. Inspect the ears, nose, and throat.
C. Auscultate:
   1. Listen for bruit at neck, eyes, and head for clinical signs of arteriovenous (AV) malformation.
D. Palpate:
   1. Palpate the head, eyes, ears, temporomandibular joint (TMJ), sinus cavities, and temporal and neck arteries.
   2. Palpate cervical vertebrae, cervical muscles, and shoulder regions. Identify potential trigger areas: Occipital nerves lead halfway between the middle of the neck at the back of the neck and lateral to this area. When palpating this trigger area, pain may be reproduced with palpation.
   3. Examine the spine and neck muscles.
   4. Assess cervical range of motion (ROM).
E. Perform neurologic examination:
   1. Cranial nerves.
   2. Extraocular movements (EOM).
   3. Pupil response.
   4. Getting up from a seated position without any support.
   5. Walking on tiptoes and heels.
   6. Tandem gait.
   7. Romberg test.
   8. Symmetry on motor, sensory, deep tendon reflexes (DTRs), and coordination tests.
   9. Assess neck flexion for nuchal rigidity.

Diagnostic Tests
Tests are selected based on history and physical examination:
A. Sinus films to rule out sinusitis or a lesion.
B. Sleep studies for obstructive sleep apnoea.
C. CT scan or MRI: Needed if headache is severe; no results are achieved with drug therapy.
D. People, especially children, with any positive neurologic signs of an intracranial process should have neuroimaging.
E. Lab tests are rarely needed for headaches, unless an infectious process is suspected.

Differential Diagnoses
A. Headache:
   1. Tension.
   2. Cluster.
   3. MOH.
   4. Migraine.
   5. Combination headache.
   6. NDPH.
B. Sinusitis:
C. Meningitis: Meningism, acute headache with fever, lethargy, nausea or vomiting, irritability, photophobia, and systemic infection.
D. Space-occupying lesion: Subacute and progressive pain; new onset for adults older than 40 years.

E. Temporal arteritis: New-onset progressive headache for adults older than 50 years, with presenting symptoms of temporal artery swelling, pain, pulselessness, visual changes, mental sluggishness, systemic symptoms (fever, anorexia, malaise), and erythrocyte sedimentation rate (ESR) >50 mm/hr.
F. Carotid dissection: Sudden headache with neck pain, radiating to the face, ear, or eye; onset related to neck movement or trauma; Horner's syndrome; tinnitus; ipsilateral tongue weakness; cervical bruit or tenderness; diplopia; and syncope.
G. TMJ syndrome: Jaw claudication, clicking, and locking sensation, ill-fitting dentures, bruxism.
H. Carbon monoxide poisoning.
I. Trigeminal neuralgia.
J. Pregnancy-induced hypertension (PIH).
K. Medication-induced headache: Review side effects of current medications (individual and/or combination of drugs).
L. Musculoskeletal condition: arthritis, atlas/axis subluxation.

Plan
A. General interventions:
  1. Encourage the client to restrict associated triggers such as caffeine, alcohol, chocolate, and odours. Some foods or food additives may be triggers for some (e.g., monosodium glutamate).
  2. Encourage daily exercise.
  3. Have the client begin a stress management routine, including yoga, meditation, and massage.
  4. Tell the client to take medications as prescribed: control and abortive medications.
  5. Advise that cluster headaches can be exacerbated by alcohol.
  6. Use ice/heat for muscular tension.
  7. Individual and/or family psychotherapy should be considered.
  8. Complementary and alternative medicine (CAM):
     a. Nutraceutical options for prevention of migraines:
        i. Magnesium citrate.
        ii. Riboflavin.
        iii. Coenzyme Q10.
     b. Herbal preparations:
        i. Feverfew.
        ii. Butternut root.
     c. Acupuncture.
     d. Oxygen/hyperbaric oxygen therapy.
     e. Transcutaneous electrical nerve (TEN) stimulation unit.
     f. Gentle chiropractic manipulation.
     g. Physiotherapy.
     h. Continuous positive airway pressure (CPAP) for sleep apnoea.
     i. Biofeedback.
     j. Relaxation training.
     k. Sleep may abort a migraine.
     l. Ergonomic evaluation.
     m. Dental appliance to reduce bruxism.
B. Client teaching:
  1. Encourage the client to keep a diary of headaches and associated factors to try to pinpoint headache triggers.
  2. Talk to clients who have menstrual headaches about possibly avoiding precipitating factors, such as alcohol, tyramine, or phenylethylamine foods; missed meals; and sleeping late.
  3. Discuss sleep hygiene guidelines (see the section "Sleep Disorders" in Chapter 22, Psychiatric Guidelines). Encourage a minimum of 7 hours of sleep per night.
  4. For muscular headaches that are nonmenstrual, biofeedback, breathing exercises, and visualization are helpful. Prevention must be stressed. Encourage lifestyle changes and daily exercise.
  5. When clients overuse various analgesics for headaches, paroxysmal migraines can convert into chronic daily headaches. Caution clients regarding this effect.
  6. MOHs occur with the highest incidence with opioids, butalbital-containing combinations, and ASA/acetaminophen/caffeine combinations as well as triptans and acetaminophen. Withdrawal of the overused medication is the first-line treatment for MOHs.
C. Pharmacological treatment: Therapy should be started at the lowest dosage and titrated up as tolerated, avoiding overuse. For some conditions, both preventative and abortive drugs may be used:
  1. Nonsteroidal anti-inflammatory drugs (NSAIDs):
     a. ASA.
     b. Ibuprofen.
  2. Combination medications:
     a. Acetaminophen, butalbital, and caffeine with or without codeine.
     b. ASA, butalbital, and caffeine.
     c. Acetaminophen, ASA, and caffeine.
  3. Cluster or vascular headaches:
     a. Verapamil is the first-line therapy for cluster headache prevention.
     b. Intranasal zolmitriptan or sumatriptan may be used as an abortive medication.
     c. Oxygen 100% therapy has been effective for relieving cluster headache episodes.
  4. Menstrual headaches:
     a. Estrogen supplements or continuous cycling is used to decrease headaches.
     b. Naproxen.
     c. Ibuprofen.
     d. Fluoxetine is also used for clients with premenstrual syndrome with luteal phase defect.
  5. Medications may be used for preventive treatment. Medications used include ergot derivatives, anticonvulsants, antidepressants, tricyclic antidepressants (TCAs), muscle relaxers, and antihistamines.
  6. Pharmacological treatment for chronic daily and NDPHs combine therapies that are used for tension-type and migraine headaches.

Follow-Up
A. See the client in 2 weeks to evaluate how therapies have worked.
B. Evaluate the client's "headache log" to assist him or her in identifying headache triggers, if present.

Consultation/Referral
A. If medications do not help with headaches, refer the client to a neurologist.

Individual Considerations
A. Pregnancy:
  1. PIH often presents with a headache.
B. Paediatrics:
  1. Antihistamines are useful as a preventive agent, as are biofeedback and relaxation techniques.

2. Avoid using ASA-containing products because of the potential of Reye's syndrome. Differentiating the causative factor is essential for this population.
   3. Medication therapy is dependent on the child's age.
C. Adults:
   1. Clients who are premenopausal may see improvement when their estrogen levels are constant, instead of being cyclic.
   2. Tension headaches may actually be migraines. Migraines may develop into tension headaches. Treat as for migraine.
D. Geriatrics:
   1. Headaches decrease with age. Serious causes of headaches increase with age. Such causes include the following:
      a. Temporal arteritis.
      b. Trigeminal neuralgia.
      c. Sleep apnoea.
      d. Postherpetic neuralgia.
      e. Cervical spondylosis.
      f. Subarachnoid haemorrhage (SAH).
      g. Intracerebral haemorrhage.
      h. Intracranial neoplasm.
      i. Postconcussive syndrome.
   2. Hypnic headache occurs only in the elderly.
   3. Consider imaging studies in the elderly with unusual presentations of headaches.
   4. Consider chronic subdural haematomas (SDH) with clients who have frequent falls who complain of headaches; perform CT scan or MRI for evaluation.
   5. Elderly clients may not exhibit any symptoms other than a headache.
   6. When medicating the elderly for headaches, start dosages low and increase as tolerated.
      a. Naproxen and hydroxyzine are commonly used oral rescue therapies for older adults with migraine or tension headaches.
      b. Oral agents for the prevention of hypnic headaches include caffeine and lithium.
      c. Consider renal function before prescribing NSAIDs.
   7. Consider all contraindications when prescribing medications; many elderly clients have cardiovascular disease, which is contraindicated with ergot derivatives.

Bibliography

American Family Physician. (2016). *Headache*. Retrieved from http://www.aafp.org/afp/topicModules/viewTopicModule.htm?topicModuleId=10

Becker, W. (2013). Headache currents—Clinical review. Cluster headache: Conventional pharmacological management. *Headaches, 53*(7), 1191–1196. doi:10.1111/head.12145

Becker, W., Findaly, T., Moga, C., Scott, N. A., Harstall, C., & Taenzer, P. (2015). Clinical review. Guideline for primary care: Management of headache in adults. *Canadian Family Physician, 61*(8), 670–679. Retrieved from https://headachesociety.ca/wp-content/uploads/2017/12/Becker-Can-Fam-Physician-2015.pdf

Cruccu, G., Finnerup, N. B., Jensen, T. S., Scholz, J., Sindou, M., Svensson, P., . . . Nurmikko, T. (2016). Trigeminal neuralgia: New classification and diagnostic grading for practice and research. *Neurology, 87*(2), 220–228. doi:10.1212/WNL.0000000000002840

El-Chammas, K., Keyes, J., Thompson, N., Vijayakumar, J., Becher, D., & Jackson, J. L. (2013). Pharmacologic treatment of pediatric headaches: A meta-analysis. *Journal of the American Medical Association Pediatrics, 167*(3), 250–258. doi:10.1001/jamapediatrics.2013.508

Family Doctor. (n.d.). *Headaches in elderly people*. Retrieved from www.familydoctor.co.uk/node/530

Frishberg, B., Rosenberg, J., Matchar, D., McCrory, D., Pietrzak, M., Rozen, R., . . . Silberstein, S. (n.d.). *Evidence-based guidelines in the primary care setting: Neuroimaging in clients with nonacute headache*. Retrieved from www.aan.com/professionals/practice/pdfs/gl0088.pdf

Illinois Neurological Institute. (2013). *Headaches and sleep*. Retrieved from www.ini.org/services/sleep-disorders/conditions-treated/headaches-and-sleep.html

International Headache Society ICHD-II. (2018). *International classification of headache disorders* (3rd ed.). London: International Headache Society. Retrieved from https://www.ichd-3.org/

International Headache Society ICHD-II. (n.d.-a). *Cluster headache*. Retrieved from https://www.ichd-3.org/3-trigeminal-autonomic-cephalalgias/3-1-cluster-headache

International Headache Society ICHD-II. (n.d.-b). *New daily-persistent headache (NDPH)*. Retrieved from https://www.ichd-3.org/other-primary-headache-disorders/4-10-new-daily-persistent-headache-ndph

International Headache Society ICHD-II. (n.d.-c). *Tension-type headache (alternative criteria)*. Retrieved from https://www.ichd-3.org/appendix/a2-tension-type-headache-alternative-criteria

Lopez, J. I. (2013, January 28). Pediatric headache treatment & management. *Medscape*. Retrieved from http://emedicine.medscape.com/article/2110861-treatment

Oomens, M. A., & Forouzanfar, T. (2015). Pharmaceutical management of trigeminal neuralgia in the elderly. *Drugs & Aging, 32*(9), 717–726. doi:10.1007/s40266-015-0293-6

Zakrzewska, J. M. (2015). Trigeminal neuralgia: Unilateral episodic facial pain. *Journal of Pain & Palliative Care Pharmacotherapy, 29*(2), 182–184. doi:10.3109/15360288.2015.1037523

Zakrzewska, J. M., & Linskey, M. E. (2016). Trigeminal neuralgia. *American Family Physician, 94*(2), 133–135. Retrieved from https://www.aafp.org/journals/afp/explore/past.html

Živković, S. (2015). Intravenous immunoglobulin in the treatment of neurologic disorders. *Acta Neurologica Scandinavica, 133*(5), 84–96. doi:10.1111/ane.12444

Migraine Headache

Cheryl A. Glass, Julie Adkins, and Donna Clare

Definition

A. Migraine headaches are a common medical complaint responsible for a significant disability and loss of quality of life. The economic impact involves loss of workdays, school, social interaction, and loss of productivity while at work (presenteeism). There are three types of migraines described by the International Headache Society (IHS) by type and diagnostic criteria (see Table 19.3).

B. Migraine headaches have been associated with increased risk of cerebral ischaemia and an increased risk of cardiac ischaemia.

Incidence/Prevalence

Headaches are one of the most common medical complaints. The exact incidence of migraines is unknown, as clients self-treat, are underdiagnosed, and are commonly misdiagnosed. About 10% to 16% is the overall estimated incidence of migraines in North America and Europe; however, several subsets of migraine headaches are noted in the literature. In 2010/2011, an estimated 2.7 million Canadians reported that they had been diagnosed with migraine headaches; this is likely an underestimation. Females are more likely to report migraines than males. Migraines are heterogeneous in frequency, duration, and disability. Although there are differences between provinces/territories, national rates of migraine headaches are as follows:

A. 0 to 11 years: <1% of Canadian children aged birth to 11 years have migraines.

B. 12 to 29 years: Migraines occur in 8.1% of the population in this age category. Migraines may be abdominal in school-aged children.

C. 30 to 49 years: This age cohort has the highest occurrence of migraine headaches in Canada at 12.1%.

D. 50 to 64 years: Adults in this age group have a 9.9% occurrence of migraines.

TABLE 19 International Headache Society Classification of Migraines

Migraine Without Aura	Migraine With Aura (Six Subtypes)	Chronic Migraine[a]
Recurrent headache attack lasting 4–72 hours meeting the diagnostic criteria.	Recurrent disorder manifesting reversible focal neurologic symptoms that usually develop gradually over 5–20 minutes and last for <60 minutes. Typical aura consists of visual and/or sensory and/or speech symptoms.	Chronic migraine that meets the criteria for migraine without aura that occurs with a frequency of at least 15 headache days per month for longer than three months' duration
Diagnostic Criteria	**Diagnostic Criteria**	**Diagnostic Criteria**

A. At least two attacks that fulfill criteria B–D.
B. Headache attacks last 4–72 hours (untreated or unsuccessfully treated).
C. Has at least two of the following:
  1. Unilateral location.
  2. Pulsating quality.
  3. Moderate or severe intensity.
  4. Aggravated by or causing avoidance of routine physical activity.
D. During headache at least one of the following:
  1. Nausea and/or vomiting.
  2. Photophobia and phonophobia.
E. Not attributed to another disorder.
	A. At least two attacks that fulfill criteria B–D.
	B. Aura consists of at least one of the following, but no motor weakness:
	  1. Fully reversible visual symptoms, including positive features (e.g., flickering lights, spots, or lines) and/or negative features (e.g., loss of vision).
	  2. Fully reversible sensory symptoms, including positive features (e.g., pins and needles) and/or negative features (e.g., numbness).
	  3. Fully reversible dysphasic speech disturbance.
	C. At least two of the following:
	  1. Homonymous visual symptoms (e.g., additional loss or blurring of central vision) and/or unilateral sensory symptoms.
	  2. At least one aura symptom develops gradually over five minutes or longer and/or different aura symptoms occur in succession over five minutes or longer in duration.
	  3. Each symptom lasts 5 minutes or longer and is 60 minutes or less in duration.
	D. Headache fulfilling criteria B–C: Migraine without aura begins during the aura or follows the aura within 60 minutes.
	E. Not attributed to another disorder.
		A. Headache, in the absence of MOH, on 15 days per month or greater, for at least three months.
		B. Occurring in a client who has had at least five attacks fulfilling criteria for migraine without aura.
		C. On eight days per month or greater, for at least three months headache fulfills C1 and/or C2 criteria noted as follows:
		C1. Has at least two of the following:
		  1. Unilateral location.
		  2. Pulsating quality.
		  3. Moderate or severe pain intensity.
		  4. Aggravation by or causing avoidance of routine physical activity *and* at least one of the following:
		    a. Nausea and/or vomiting.
		    b. Photophobia and phonophobia C2; treated and relieved by triptan(s) or ergot before the expected development of C1 symptoms.
		D. No medication overuse and not attributed to another causative disorder.

[a]A proposed alternative criteria is defined as a chronic headache for at least 4 migraine days and at least 15 total headache days, with at least 50% of headache days meeting criteria for migraine.
MOH, medication overuse headache.
Source: Adapted from the International Headache Society ICHD-II. (2018). *International classification of headache disorders* (3rd ed.). Retrieved from https://www.ichd-3.org/; International Headache Society ICHD-II. (n.d.). *Migraine.* Retrieved from https://www.ichd-3.org/1-migraine.

E. 65 years and older: 5.1% of older adults report migraine headaches.

Pathogenesis

Migraines have broad sensory processing dysfunction, with a prominent perception of pain in the dense somatosensory innervation of intracranial vessels. Current pathophysiologic concepts of migraine and migraine aura include a possible dysfunction of neuromodulatory structures in the brainstem and cortical spreading depression (CSD). An anti-CGRP drug, erenumab, has been approved in Canada as a preventative of episodic and chronic migraine in adults, and a migraine vaccine is under development. Different receptors, including cannabinoid receptors in the brain, are currently being investigated for migraine therapeutics.

Predisposing Factors
A. Family history of migraines.
B. Chronic use of over-the-counter (OTC) analgesics (rebound).
C. Posthead trauma.
D. Food, fasting, odour, light, sound, sleep, weather changes, hormonal changes, and stress triggers.
E. Menstruation.
F. Obesity.
G. Daily habitual snoring is a modest risk factor.
H. Estrogen use.

Common Findings
A. Unilateral headache (bilateral in children).
B. Frontotemporal area (occipital in children).
C. Photophobia, or sensitivity to light (young children may cover their eyes).
D. Phonophobia, or sensitivity to sound (young children may cover their ears).
E. Osmophobia, or hypersensitivity/aversion to smells/odours.

F. Nausea with/without vomiting.
G. Prodrome phase: fatigue, reduced concentration, agitation, craving, fatigue, irritability, depression, frequent yawning, or hyperexcitability hours to days before the onset of aura and headache.
H. Aura: Precedes onset of headache by 20 to 30 minutes. Can involve any of the sensory systems; scotoma are the most common.

Other Signs and Symptoms
A. Muscle tension and neck pain.
B. Cutaneous allodynia (pain from stimulus to normal skin or scalp).
C. Sinus congestion.
D. Prodrome phase can last 25 hours accompanied by fatigue and a "hangover" headache.
E. Abdominal pain (children).

Subjective Data
A. Use the following acronym for subjective information: PQRST:
   P: Provocation, or worsening of factors stimulating headaches.
   Q: Quality of pain, severity of pain.
   R: Region of headache.
   S: Strength of pain, evaluate pain on a scale of 1 to 10.
   T: Time, including onset, frequency, and duration of headaches.
B. Assess whether the client frequently has migraine headaches. Is this the first or worst headache ever experienced by the client? A "worst headache in my life" should be assessed via an ED. New onset of migraine after the age of 50 is suspicious for alternative aetiology.
C. If recurrent headaches exist, note frequency and patterns of similar headaches. Have client complete a headache diary. Headache diary templates are available online (e.g., Canadian Headache Society, Migraine Canada: migrainecanada.org/diaries/; local health region: www.albertahealthservices.ca/assets/programs/ps-1008788-champ-headache-diary.pdf).
D. Note whether the client has ever identified potential triggers of recurring headaches such as dietary issues, stressors, and odours (e.g., perfumes and cigarette smoke).
E. Identify the location of the pain, along with radiation if present.
F. Describe the type of pain: throbbing, constant, or burning.
G. Assess the presence of associated symptoms: nausea or vomiting, photophobia, and noise sensitivity.
H. Determine whether the client experiences any neurologic symptoms and/or prodromal symptoms before headache. Some clients with migraines experience transient hemiplegia or localized peripheral numbness.
I. Review the methods used in the past to abort and/or prevent headaches and the results.
J. Inquire about past diagnostic evaluations for headaches.
K. Note a family history of headaches.
L. List current medications, including OTC medications and herbal products.
M. Review the client's medical history for head trauma, infection, allergies, presence of a ventriculoperitoneal (VP) shunt, or other neurologic diagnoses.

Physical Examination
Physical examination may be normal:
A. Check blood pressure, pulse, and respiration (temperature if meningeal signs are present).
B. Inspect:
   1. Observe overall appearance for the presence of discomfort, photosensitivity (use of sunglasses indoors), and level of consciousness (LOC).
   2. Examine the eyes; perform funduscopic examination.
   3. Inspect the ears, nose, and throat.
   4. Assess for signs of physical trauma.
C. Auscultate:
   1. Listen for bruit at neck, eyes, and head for clinical signs of arteriovenous (AV) malformation.
D. Palpate:
   1. Palpate the head, eyes, ears, temporomandibular joint (TMJ), sinus cavities, temporal, and neck arteries.
   2. Palpate cervical vertebrae, cervical muscles, and shoulder regions. Identify potential trigger areas: Occipital nerves leave halfway between the middle of the neck at the back of the neck and lateral to this area. When palpating this trigger area, pain may be reproduced with palpation.
   3. Examine the spine and neck muscles.
   4. Assess the cervical range of motion (ROM).
E. Perform neurologic examination:
   1. Extraocular movements (EOM).
   2. Pupil response.
   3. Getting up from a seated position without any support.
   4. Walking on tiptoes and heels.
   5. Tandem gait.
   6. Romberg test.
   7. Symmetry on motor, sensory, deep tendon reflexes (DTRs), and coordination tests.

Diagnostic Tests
A. Neuroimaging, CT, and MRI are based on the history and physical examination:
   1. Adults and children with stable headaches, a normal examination, and absence of seizures do not require neuroimaging.
   2. Neuroimaging should be considered for children with headaches with abnormal neurologic examination and/or seizures.
   3. Neuroimaging should be considered for children with severe headaches, change in headaches, or associated neurologic dysfunction.
   4. An emergent noncontrast CT should be obtained when the client complains of "the worst headache ever" or when focal neurologic findings, nuchal rigidity, or altered mental status exist.
   5. The presence of personality changes, depression, and a migraine may indicate a temporal lobe tumour.
   6. The presence of orbital bruit requires neuroimaging.
   7. Neuroimaging is recommended for adults with onset of headache after the age of 50 years.
   8. Onset of headache with exertion, cough, or sexual activity should be considered for neuroimaging.
B. A lumbar puncture may be indicated in children with altered mental status or focal findings.
C. Sinus films to rule out sinusitis or a lesion, if indicated.
D. Laboratory tests are not required for most clients with typical symptoms and a negative physical examination:
   1. Drug screen may be indicated.
   2. Complete metabolic panel (CMP).
   3. Complete blood count (CBC).
   4. Thyroid-stimulating hormone (TSH).
   5. C-reactive protein (CRP).

Differential Diagnoses

A. Other types of headaches:
1. Medication overuse headaches (MOH).
2. Common headache.
3. Cluster headache.
4. Combination headache.
5. Chronic daily headache.
6. Tension headache.
7. Hypnic headaches (geriatrics).

B. Sinusitis.
C. Space-occupying lesion: Subacute and progressive pain, new onset for adults older than 40 years.
D. Temporal arteritis: New-onset progressive headache for adults older than 50 years.
E. Carotid dissection: Sudden headache with neck pain radiating to the face, ear, or eye.
F. TMJ syndrome.
G. Meningitis.
H. Brain abscess.
I. Encephalitis.
J. Idiopathic intracranial hypertension.

Plan

A. General interventions: There are four main approaches to migraine therapy:
1. Nonpharmacological interventions:
   a. Adjust habits to maintain a routine pattern of sleeping. This is especially important to maintain on weekends and vacations.
   b. Do not skip breakfast. Eat regular meals as well as healthy snacks.
   c. Avoid food triggers identified by the client's migraine diary.
   d. Encourage drinking no more than two caffeinated beverages a day.
   e. Hydration is important.
   f. Encourage at least 30 minutes of exercise three to seven days a week.
   g. Cold compresses.
2. Behavioural interventions:
   a. Use relaxation techniques such as yoga, deep breathing, meditation, and guided imagery.
   b. Biofeedback is an adjunct to relaxation training.
   c. Cognitive behavioural therapy.
   d. Psychiatric therapy.
3. Complementary and alternative interventions:
   a. Acupuncture.
   b. Nutraceuticals, including magnesium citrate, coenzyme Q10, and butternut root extract.
   c. Vitamins: Riboflavin (B_2).
   d. Medicinal cannabis.
   e. Physical therapy.
   f. Hypnosis.
   g. Transcutaneous electrical nerve stimulation (TENS), chiropractic manipulation, and occlusal adjustment are also noted in the literature.
   h. Onabotulinumtoxin A has been tested extensively and has been found to be ineffective in episodic migraines, but has been approved for chronic headaches.
4. Pharmacological interventions: Clients should be counseled to take medications as prescribed. When clients overuse various analgesics for headaches, paroxysmal migraines can convert into chronic daily headaches.

B. Client teaching:
1. Encourage the client to keep a headache diary. The diary may help the client identify triggers for the migraine headaches:
   a. Common food triggers are aspartame, saccharin, red wine, alcohol, chocolate, aged cheese, oranges, tomatoes, avocado, nuts, onions, tyramine, phenylethylamine, monosodium glutamate (MSG), and nitrates and nitrites found in hot dogs, luncheon meat, and sausage.
   b. Examples of odour triggers include tobacco smoke, perfumes, and strong odours.
   c. Examples of visual triggers include strobe lights, bright lights/sunlight, fluorescent lights, and glare.
   d. Other triggers are missing meals, medication side effects, barometric weather changes, too much/too little sleep, and high altitude.
2. There is an increased stroke risk in women who have migraine headaches with auras and who smoke. It is reasonable to recommend and support strategies for smoking cessation.

C. Pharmacological treatment (see Table 19.4). The choice of drug therapy prophylactic agents depends on the client's comorbid conditions such as cardiac, respiratory, psychiatric, sleep, and gastrointestinal disorders:
1. Many drugs commonly used for migraines are not approved for migraine therapy, including amitriptyline, nortriptyline, and selective serotonin reuptake inhibitors (SSRIs).
2. Antiepileptic medications, including valproic acid and topiramate, are approved for migraine prophylaxis. Topiramate should not be prescribed or discontinued for a history of kidney stones.
3. Beta-blockers are approved for migraine prophylaxis; however, they must be used with caution for clients with co-morbidities such as asthma, depression, diabetes, and thyroid disease.
4. There are currently several triptans and one triptan/nonsteroidal anti-inflammatory drug (NSAID) combination. Triptans are widely used for menstrual migraines. Triptans should be used cautiously in clients with cardiovascular co-morbidities, and some are not approved for children. Triptans should not be given within 24 hours of an ergot.
5. Dihydroergotamine mesylate is not to be used for clients during pregnancy or with heart disease, or ischaemic or vasospastic circulatory disease. Use ergot derivatives selectively. These medications are not to be used on a long-term basis or more than three times per week. There is an associated risk of strokes when using these medications because of the vasoconstrictive mechanisms of the medications.
6. Ergots and triptans should not be given within 14 days of a monoamine oxidase (MAO) inhibitor.
7. Anti-emetics are prescribed as needed for nausea/vomiting associated with migraines.
8. Multiple drugs are used off-label for migraines.
9. A two-month trial of prophylaxis is required before efficacy can be evaluated. Fifty percent fewer headaches is considered effective.

Follow-Up

A. See the client in two weeks to evaluate how therapies have worked.
B. Evaluate the client's headache diary to assist in identifying headache triggers or patterns. Use the information

TABLE 19.4 Medications for Migraines

Medication	Class	Acute vs. Prophylaxis
Sumatriptan	Triptan	Acute treatment
Sumatriptan	Triptan	Acute treatment and cluster headaches
Sumatriptan iontophoretic system	Triptan	Acute treatment migraine with and without aura
Rizatriptan	Triptan	Acute treatment
Zolmitriptan	Triptan	Acute treatment
Naratriptan	Triptan	Acute treatment
Almotriptan	Triptan	Acute treatment
Eletriptan	Triptan	Acute treatment
Frovatriptan	Triptan	Acute treatment
Sumatriptan with naproxen sodium	Triptan + NSAID	Acute treatment
Dihydroergotamine mesylate	Ergot derivative	Acute treatment
Ergotamine tartrate + caffeine	Ergot derivative	Acute treatment migraines and cluster headaches
Propranolol	Beta-blocker	Migraine prophylaxis
Timolol	Beta-blocker	Migraine prophylaxis
Topiramate	Antiseizure	Migraine prophylaxis
Valproic acid	Antiseizure	
Amitriptyline	Antidepressant	Migraine prophylaxis
Nortriptyline	Antidepressant	Migraine prophylaxis
Fluoxetine	SSRI	Migraine prophylaxis

NSAID, nonsteroidal anti-inflammatory drug; SSRI, selective serotonin reuptake inhibitor.

documented in the diary as a tool for reevaluating the need for other tests and consultations.
C. Monitor liver enzymes and CBC periodically with antiseizure medication prophylaxis.

Consultation/Referral
A. If medications do not help with headaches, refer the client to a neurologist/paediatric neurologist or headache clinic.
B. Send the client to the ED for any neurologic, life-threatening signs.

Individual Considerations
A. Pregnancy: Many medications are contraindicated in pregnancy.
B. Paediatrics:
  1. Avoid using ASA-containing products because of the potential of Reye's syndrome.
  2. Differentiating the causative factor is essential for this population.
  3. Adolescents may see improvement when their estrogen levels are constant instead of cyclic.
  4. The choice of medication management is age dependent. Antiepileptics, antidepressants, antihistamines, calcium channel blockers, and NSAIDs are prescribed for children.
C. Geriatrics:
  1. Headaches decrease after the age of 50 years. Headache onset after age 50 years is associated with epilepsy, essential tremor, ischaemic stroke, mood disorders, asthma, and patent foramen ovale.
  2. Consider imaging studies for elderly clients who present with unusual headaches.
  3. Consider chronic subdural haematomas (SDH) with clients who have had falls; perform CT scan or MRI for evaluation. Elderly clients may not exhibit any symptoms other than a headache.
  4. Consider all contraindications when prescribing medications; many elderly clients have cardiovascular disease, which is contraindicated with ergot derivatives.

Bibliography
Chawla, J. (2013, March 28). Migraine headache. *Medscape*. Retrieved from http://emedicine.medscape.com/article/1142556
International Headache Society ICHD-II. (n.d.). *Migraine*. Retrieved from https://www.ichd-3.org/1-migraine
Loder, E., Burch, R., & Rizzoli, P. (2012). The 2012 AHS/AAN guidelines for prevention of episodic migraine: A summary and comparison with other recent clinical practice guidelines. *Headache*, 52(6), 930–945. doi:10.1111/j.1526-4610.2012.02185.x
Pringsheim, T., Davenport, W., Mackie, G., Worthington, I., Aubé, M., Christie, S. N., & Canadian Headache Society Prophylactic Guidelines Development Group. (2012). Canadian Headache Society guideline for migraine prophylaxis. *Canadian Journal of Neurological Sciences*, 39(2), S1–S61. Retrieved from https://headachesociety.ca/wp-content/uploads/2017/12/Pringsheim-prophyl-guideline-CJNS-2012.pdf
Ramadan, N., Silberstein, S., Frietag, F., Gilbert, T., & Frishberg, B. (2016). *Evidence-based guidelines for migraine headaches in the primary care: Pharmacological management for prevention of migraine*. Retrieved from http://www.neurologiaszakvizsga.usn.hu/pdfs/71.pdf
Ramage-Morin, P. L., & Gilmour, H. (2014, June). Prevalence of migraine in the Canadian household population. *Health Reports*, 25(6), 10–16. Statistics Canada, Catalogue no. 82-003-X, Health Matters. Retrieved from https://www150.statcan.gc.ca/n1/pub/82-003-x/2014006/article/14033-eng.htm

Mild Traumatic Brain Injury (Concussion)

Kimberly D. Waltrip and Donna Clare

Definition
A. Mild traumatic brain injury (MTBI), also known as concussion, refers to an acute neurophysiological event resulting

from direct impact to the head, or indirect forces transmitted of the brain, such as sudden acceleration, deceleration, or rotational mechanical forces of the head, neck, or body. Brain function is affected, including an initial loss of consciousness or decreased level of consciousness (LOC), memory loss around the time of the event, altered mental status, and sometimes impairment of motor strength, balance, vision, sensation, and speech.

B. The severity of the injury does not always correlate with the degree of symptoms. Most MTBI clients do not experience decreased LOC. MTBI-related deficits are often mild without overt symptoms.

C. MTBI is on the low end of the brain injury spectrum: Head injuries with associated brain damage range from mild to severe.

D. Multiple MTBIs can result in chronic traumatic encephalopathy (CTE). CTE is an irreversible degenerative brain disorder that appears years after the injuries have occurred and significantly impairs brain function, resulting in a dementia-like syndrome and premature death.

E. A closed head injury (CHI) may result in an MTBI but may also include damage to the scalp, skull, neck, meninges, and blood vessels. Damage to these tissues must be considered with any head injury. Intracranial haemorrhage (ICH) must be ruled out.

Incidence/Prevalence

A. MTBI is common. In the province of Ontario alone, there are approximately 500 cases per 100,000 persons per year. Concussions commonly occur from falls, occupational injuries, assault, natural disasters, military blasts, motor vehicle accidents, and from sport and recreation injuries.

Pathogenesis

A. Head-injured clients can potentially sustain two different types of injuries: *primary* injury and *secondary* injury:
   1. A primary injury is the direct result of a head injury, occurring at the time of the initial traumatic impact or force. This type of injury is purely mechanical and may be *focal* (contusion or laceration, bone fragmentation) or *diffuse*, as in concussion or diffuse axonal injury (DAI). These injuries do not require surgical intervention.
   2. Secondary injury is caused by a flow-metabolism mismatch, and is therefore a complication of primary brain injury. Secondary injury includes any subsequent ischaemic and hypoxic changes in the brain, cerebral oedema, ICH, and the effects of prolonged increased intracranial pressure (ICP), hydrocephalus, and infection. Secondary injury presents with delayed onset of signs and symptoms, occurring anytime from seconds to minutes, hours, or days.
     Therefore, it is important to identify MTBI early on, and then follow the client for at least two hours, after which the client may be monitored by another responsible adult for up to 48 hours.

B. There are no consistent structural changes associated with MTBI. Even in the case of persistent symptoms, beyond the usual three-month period of resolution, dysfunction cannot be attributed to a consistent pattern of structural change. Functional changes in the absence of detectable structural change is thought to reflect disruption at the neuronal level. Research is ongoing.

Predisposing Factors

A. Motor vehicle accidents (MVAs).
B. Assaults.
C. Sports- and recreation-related trauma.
D. Male gender.
E. Ages of increased incidence:
   1. 0 to 4 years.
   2. 15 to 19 years.
   3. 65 years and older.
F. Military occupation (e.g., exposure to blasts).
G. Falls.

Common Findings

A. Headaches that are often constant, generalized in nature; may report frontal headache pain; symptoms may persist for days or weeks.
B. Brief amnestic epoch surrounding the initial injury.
C. Faintness.
D. Nausea/vomiting.
E. Changes in vision, often slight blurring.
F. Drowsiness.
G. Loss of consciousness.
H. Confusion.

Other Signs and Symptoms

Other presenting symptoms and complaints are identified in four categories as follows: *Physical, emotional, cognitive,* and *sleep-cycle disturbances.*

A. Physical:
   1. Reported or observed injury to the head.
   2. Dizziness.
   3. Fatigue.
   4. Impaired balance.
   5. Photophobia.
   6. Sensitivity to noise.
   7. Numbness/tingling.
   8. Seizures, delayed onset after initial injury.
B. Emotional:
   1. Irritability.
   2. Nervousness.
   3. Depression.
   4. Labile mood.
C. Cognitive:
   1. Difficulty concentrating.
   2. Impaired memory:
      a. Short-term memory loss.
      b. Repetition.
   3. Confusion.
   4. Slow responses/difficulty processing information.
   5. Changes in reaction time.
   6. Changes in speech.
   7. Disorientation.
   8. Fatigue.
D. Sleep-cycle disturbance:
   1. Feeling "drowsy."
   2. Difficulty falling asleep.
   3. Sleeping more or less than usual.

Subjective Data

A. Obtain a description of injury from the client or witness of the traumatic event, if possible. Identify the cause of the head injury, how it occurred (direct or indirect impact), and what type of force was exerted. Significant head injury may result from impact injuries, especially a pedestrian struck by a vehicle, ejection of an occupant from a vehicle, and a fall from 3 feet or more or more than five stairs. These clients should be assessed in an emergency facility.

B. Ask about the event, if it was observed by others, and its duration (e.g., an assault). Confirm the client's LOC at the

time of injury and afterward. Inquire about amnesia (retrograde and anterograde), which might predict increased severity of the injury. Being unable to recall events about 30 minutes *before* the injury warrants a CT scan.
C. Review initial and current symptoms. Include the description, location, severity, and onset of symptoms. It is important to note what has occurred since the initial injury. It is not uncommon for clients to report symptoms that recur or worsen on exertion.
D. Obtain the client's medical history, especially details of any previous head injuries. Learning disabilities (e.g., attention deficit hyperactivity disorder [ADHD]), developmental disorders, depression, anxiety, sleep disorders, and mood disorders should be documented because these can affect recovery.
E. Review current medications; certain medications like warfarin can be predisposing factors for complications.
F. Document any recreational drug and/or alcohol history.
G. Ask family members/significant others whether they have noticed any related signs or symptoms, behavioural changes, or evidence of seizure activity.

Physical Examination
A. Check pulse, respiration, and blood pressure.
B. Inspect:
   1. Observe overall appearance. Note LOC.
   2. Inspect the skin and head for obvious injury. Periorbital ecchymosis (raccoon's eyes), postauricular/mastoid ecchymosis (Battle's sign), or evidence of a cerebrospinal fluid (CSF) leak (otorrhoea, rhinorrhoea) can indicate a basal skull fracture. Any sign of a basal skull fracture warrants cranial imaging with CT.
   3. Examine the eyes for the presence of papilloedema (optic disc swelling caused by increased intracranial pressure [ICP]), proptosis, and periorbital oedema.
   4. Examine the ears (haemotympanum or possible laceration to the external canal), nose, and throat.
   5. Examine for facial fractures.
   6. Examine for any trauma (e.g., vertebral malalignment, abnormal curvature) to the cervical spine; if necessary, place the client on spine precautions (immobilize the head and neck) and refer to orthopaedics or neurosurgery for further evaluation.
C. Auscultate:
   1. Over the globes of the eyes if warranted (bruit may indicate traumatic carotid-cavernous fistula).
   2. Carotid arteries bilaterally if warranted (bruit may indicate carotid dissection).
   3. The heart and lungs, if cardiovascular aetiology is suspected.
   4. The abdomen, if other incidental injuries are suspected (e.g., from a contact sport or MVA).
D. Palpate:
   1. Palpate for instability of the facial bones, including the zygomatic arch—may detect a palpable step-off with orbital rim fractures.
   2. If appropriate, palpate the abdomen and the entire posterior spine to rule out any other incidental injuries.
E. Neurologic examination:
   1. Assess mental status and memory. Determine whether the client is awake, alert, cooperative, and oriented to *person, place, time,* and *situation*. Temporary impaired memory is one of the most common deficits after a head injury.
   2. Assess cranial nerve function:
     a. Ophthalmoscopic/visual examination (cranial nerve II).
     b. Pupillary response (cranial nerve III).
     c. Extraocular eye movements (EOMs; cranial nerves III, IV, and VI).
     d. Facial sensation and muscles of mastication (cranial nerve V).
     e. Facial expression and taste (cranial nerve VII).
   3. Perform a motor examination on all four extremities.
   4. Perform a sensory examination on all four extremities.
The Acute Concussion Evaluation (ACE) tool for use in an setting can be found in the Guidelines for Concussion/Mild Traumatic Brain Injury and Persistent Symptoms (2013) at onf.org/system/attachments/190/original/ONF_mTBI_Guidelines_2nd_Edition_MODULE_1.pdf.

Diagnostic Tests
A. A plain film of the skull is no longer recommended for any minor traumatic injury. If the client has a suspected skull fracture or clinical indications for imaging, a CT scan is preferred. This type of imaging will usually reveal any linear or basilar skull fractures.
B. CT scan is indicated for clients with the following (order and perform within one hour)[b]:
   1. Decreasing consciousness during or after the injury (e.g., Glasgow Coma Scale <13).
   2. Glasgow Coma Scale <15 at two hours postinjury.
   3. Potential, penetrating, or depressed skull fractures.
   4. Vomiting greater than or equal to two episodes.
   5. Age <16 years or ≥65 years.
   6. Any signs of basal skull fracture or neurological deficit.
   7. Posttraumatic amnesia (PTA), including amnesia before the impact.
   8. Dangerous mechanism of injury.
   9. Use clinical judgment regarding certain co-morbidities and conditions (e.g., client is taking warfarin or has a coagulopathy).

Differential Diagnoses
A. Contusion.
B. ICH.
C. Shearing injury.
D. Skull fracture.
E. Subarachnoid haemorrhage (SAH), traumatic.
F. Subdural haematomas (SDH).
G. Epidural haematoma (EDH).
H. Vascular occlusion or dissection.
I. Diffuse axonal injury (DAI).

Plan
A. General interventions:
   1. Initial observation for at least four hours, then discharge home if the following are noted after MTBI:
     ■ Awake, alert, oriented (AAO) × 4 (date, place, person, situation), demonstrating improvement after concussion.
     ■ No risk factors warranting a head CT or negative head CT results when risk factors are present.
     ■ No signs/symptoms or conditions indicating the need for prolonged hospital observation or admission.
   2. Direct admission to the hospital for decreased LOC, seizure activity, focal deficits, penetrating or depressed skull fracture, vomiting, serious facial injuries, and positive head CT findings.

---

[b]Adapted from Stiell, I. G., Wells, G. A., Vandemheen, K., Clement, C., Lesiuk, H., Laupacis, A., . . . Worthington, J. (2001). Canadian CT head rule for clients with minor head injury. *Lancet, 357,* 1391–1396.

3. Hospitalization may be required if the client has an injured middle meningeal artery or if venous sinus or fractures posteriorly in the skull are suspected. Posterior fossa haematomas may present suddenly (will see a wide pulse pressure).
   4. Consider possible secondary injuries, including cerebral oedema, cerebral infarction, cerebral haemorrhage, hydrocephalus, and infection.
   5. The client should not be impaired by alcohol or other drugs when leaving the health-care area, which can affect neurologic function and potentially mask evolving deficits.
   6. Hospital admission should be considered for clients without home observation/supervision.
   7. Discuss suspected abuse with the client in a private setting.
B. Client teaching:
   1. *Refer to Client Teaching Guide: Head Injury: Mild Concussion*. Discuss safety and accident prevention, including the following:
      a. Use safety helmets.
      b. Use safety belts.
      c. Do not drive or operate machinery under the influence of alcohol or other substances.
      d. Use age-appropriate car seats and booster seats for children.
      e. Remove scatter rugs and other objects that increase risk for falls.
      f. Use nonslip mats in the shower/bathtub.
      g. Install grab bars in the shower/bathtub.
      h. Use safety gates at the bottom and top of the stairs in homes with small children.
      i. Keep stairs, floors, and hallways clean and clear from clutter.
      j. Install handrails in stairways.
      k. Wear adequate, correct protective gear specific to athletic games and work.
      l. Use helmets for biking, in addition to other sports.
C. Pharmacological treatment therapy:
   1. Analgesics: Acetaminophen.
   2. Tricyclic antidepressants (TCAs) or triptans may be used for posttraumatic migraines.
   3. Short-term use of opioids may be required for some clients.

Follow-Up

A. Clients with injuries mild enough to be discharged may be observed. Clients with normal examinations in the outpatient setting generally do not require routine follow-up.
B. Assessment of driving ability in older adults should be done after MTBI from MVAs.
C. Postconcussion symptoms may continue for some period of time (usually around three months, but possibly years in certain cases). The use of the Rivermead Post-Concussion Symptoms Questionnaire may be helpful for serial evaluation. The Rivermead tool is available at www.maa.nsw.gov.au/media/publications/for-professionals/Rivermead-Post-Concussion-Symptoms-QuestionnaireMAA218.pdf.

Consultation/Referral

a. Refer all clients to the ED for the following:
   1. Focal neurologic deficit(s).
   2. Decreasing LOC.
   3. Persistent headaches, nausea, and vomiting.
   4. Seizures, any other evidence of skull fractures.
   5. Neuropsychological dysfunction.
b. Refer to a neurologist for evaluation of postconcussive syndrome with continued complaints (e.g., irritability, fatigue, headaches, difficulty concentrating, dizziness, and memory problems). Further evaluation, including MRI and EEG testing, may be needed.
c. Refer to a psychologist specifically trained to perform neuropsychological testing, as indicated for clients with mild head injury. The assessment tools used will evaluate brain function in the areas of attention/concentration, initiation/planning, motor/sensory skills, visual perception, learning and memory, language, speed of processing information/reaction time, and complex problem-solving.
d. Refer to a psychiatrist for evaluation and treatment of any associated disorders emerging within a month or longer after MTBI, or upon noting increased signs/symptoms (anxiety, depression, posttraumatic stress disorder [PTSD] secondary to assault or combat).

Individual Considerations

All clients with moderate or severe head trauma should have a CT scan of the head and neck.
A. Paediatrics:
   1. Children are at risk for traumatic brain injury (TBI) caused by falls (3 feet or higher or twice their own height), bicycle and MVA accidents, sports injuries, and nonaccidental trauma.
   2. Children under 2 years who have a large boggy haematoma on the head should be imaged with a skull x-ray or CT scan. Children under 2 years of age should be evaluated through ED.
   3. Skull x-rays are indicated if there is a suspicion of nonaccidental trauma.
   4. Seizures may occur in children within the first 24 hours postinjury.
   5. Teens are at increased risk for TBI caused by sports, MVAs, and at-risk behaviours.
B. Geriatrics:
   1. The primary risk factor for a head injury in older adults is a fall(s).
   2. MVAs are the second highest risk factor for adults above age 65 years, because of vision problems, slower reaction times/reflexes, and alcohol and medication use.
   3. Medications, such as ASA and anticoagulants, increase the complications of a head injury.

Resources

Adult Concussion Guidelines: Concussions Ontario: http://concussionsontario.org/resources/adult-concussion-guidelines/
After a Concussion Guidelines for Return to Play/Sport Strategy: http://www.parachutecanada.org/downloads/resources/return-to-play-guidelines.pdf
Canadian Paediatric Society, Sport-related concussion: Evaluation and management: https://www.cps.ca/en/documents/position/sport-related-concussion-evaluation-management
Concussion guide for parents and caregivers: http://www.parachutecanada.org/downloads/resources/Concussion-Parents-Caregivers.pdf
Ontario Neurotrauma Foundation: Pediatric Concussion Guidelines: http://onf.org/documents/guidelines-diagnosing-and-managing-pediatric-concussion

Bibliography

Farrell, C. A. (2013/2018). Management of the paediatric client with acute head trauma. *Paediatric Child Health, 18*(5), 253–258. Retrieved from https://www.cps.ca/en/documents/position/paediatric-client-with-acute-head-trauma

▶ Client Teaching Guides are available at https://connect.springerpub.com/content/reference-book/978-0-8261-9498-5

Levin, H. S., & Diaz-Arrastia, R. R. (2015). Diagnosis, prognosis, and clinical management of mild traumatic brain injury. *Lancet Neurology, 14*(5), 506–517. doi:10.1016/S1474-4422(15)00002-2

Marshall, S., Bayley, M., McCullagh, S., Velikonja, D., Berrigan, L., Ouchterlony, D., . . . Weegar, K. (2015). Updated clinical practice guidelines for concussion/mild traumatic brain injury and persistent symptoms. *Brain Injury, 29*(6), 688–700. doi:10.3109/02699052.2015.1004755

McCrory, P., Meeuwisse, W. H., Echemendia, R. J., Iverson, G. L., Dvořák, J., & Kutcher, J. S. (2013). What is the lowest threshold to make a diagnosis of concussion? *British Journal of Sports Medicine, 47*(5), 268–271. doi:10.1136/bjsports-2013-092247

Purcell, L. K. (2014). Sport-related concussion: Evaluation and management. *Pediatric Child Health, 19*(3), 153–158. Retrieved from https://www.cps.ca/en/documents/position/sport-related-concussion-evaluation-management

Rose, S. C., Weber, K. D., Collen, J. B., & Heyer, G. L. (2015). The diagnosis and management of concussion in children and adolescents. *Pediatric Neurology, 53*(2), 108–118. doi:10.1016/j.pediatrneurol.2015.04.003

Stiell, I. G., Wells, G. A., Vandemheen, K., Clement, C., Lesiuk, H., Laupacis, A., & Worthington, J. (2001). Canadian CT head rule for clients with minor head injury. *Lancet, 357,* 1391–1396.

Sweeney, T. E., Salles, A., Harris, O. A., Spain, D. A., & Staudenmayer, K. L. (2015). Prediction of neurosurgical intervention after mild traumatic brain injury using the national trauma data bank. *World Journal of Emergency Surgery, 10,* 23. doi:10.1186/s13017-015-0017-6

Wells, E. M., Goodkin, H. P., & Griesbach, G. S. (2016). Challenges in determining the role of rest and exercise in the management of mild traumatic brain injury. *Journal of Child Neurology, 31*(1), 86–92. doi:10.1177/0883073815570152

Multiple Sclerosis (MS)

Kimberly D. Waltrip and Donna Clare

Definition

Multiple sclerosis (MS) is an autoimmune degenerative disease that damages neuronal axons and ultimately replaces myelin with scar tissue. The process of inflammatory demyelination varies in progression, with recurrent relapse and remission of symptoms over time. The most common symptoms include visual disturbances, spastic paraparesis, and bladder dysfunction. The course of MS is typically intermittent with periodic exacerbations occurring in various areas of the central nervous system (CNS). MS can also present more acutely regarding the severity, progression, and variety of symptoms. Early diagnosis is difficult, but crucial to treatment. An attack or exacerbation of MS lasts at least 24 hours, without associated fever or any infectious process. Complete recovery after the first attack is common, often presenting as a *clinically isolated syndrome (CIS),* but typically converting to MS within five years. Subsequent progression with exacerbations leads to permanently damaged nerve fibres with diminished function over time.

The loss of myelin leads to neurologic deficits involving vision, speech, gait, writing, memory, and/or the swallowing or cough reflexes. Clients typically use the ED when they experience relapse; 80% present with exacerbations of previous MS-related deficits. Diagnosis is supported when at least one reported exacerbation correlates with MS-related findings obtained from the neurological examination, MRI, or visual evoked potential (VEP) studies when any visual disturbances have been noted.

MS is classified as relapsing–remitting or progressive, and further described as *active* versus *not active, with* or *without progression.* Progressive MS is further differentiated with the following two subtypes:

A. *Relapsing–remitting (RR)* affects approximately 85% of MS clients; exacerbations of symptoms and periodic remission occur.
B. *Primary progressive (PP)* is a less common form of MS, accounting for around 10% of MS cases; primary progressive multiple sclerosis (PPMS) progresses slowly without periods of relapse or remission.
C. *Secondary progressive (SP)* is not unusual for clients with relapsing–remitting multiple sclerosis (RRMS) to progress to secondary progressive multiple sclerosis (SPMS) over time. Progression of the disease process continues with or without periods of remission. Symptoms do not necessarily decrease or stabilize in terms of severity.

Incidence/Prevalence

A. MS affects approximately 1 in every 500 Canadians; this is one of the highest rates of MS in the world. It is most commonly diagnosed in young adulthood but ranges from age 15 to 40. Occasionally, it can be found in the very young and in older adults.

Pathogenesis

The cause of MS is unknown. A suspected combination of genetic predisposition and a trigger (e.g., viral infections, environmental factors, metabolic issues) may create an autoimmune disorder that facilitates the degenerative disease process. Autoimmune attacks the myelin sheaths of the CNS (brain, spinal cord) and initiate an inflammatory response followed by eventual plaque formation and scarring, the hallmark characteristics of MS. There is a loss of saltatory conduction. Axonal death occurs during this acute inflammatory response, which explains any permanent disability. The associated inflammation and oedema around an MS lesion, along with myelin and axonal loss, contribute to the associated neurologic deficit. A limited amount of remyelination and the eventual resolution of inflammation will allow a certain amount of recovery with remission. Over time, multiple plaques will continue to develop in diffuse areas of the CNS. With each attack, there is a lesser degree of recovery with subsequent decrease in function.

Predisposing Factors
A. Family history of MS.
B. Female gender (two times more likely than men to develop MS).
C. Age 20 to 50 years (onset can vary from age 10 years to 59 years).
D. Caucasian race (Northern European ancestry).
E. Environment (living in temperate zones, e.g., Canada, northern United States, Europe):
   1. A northern latitude is associated with prevalence, but no direct link has been established at this time. It is suspected that distance from the equator causes a vitamin D deficiency secondary to a lack of direct sunlight, contributing to the development of MS.
F. Previous viral infection (e.g., Epstein–Barr virus [EBV], varicella zoster) *may* increase susceptibility.
G. Smoking.

Common Findings
A. Sensory loss (e.g., paraesthesia) is often reported early in the course of the disease.
B. Visual disturbances (diplopia on lateral gaze occurs in 33% of clients, blurred vision, loss of vision, eye pain).
C. Urinary incontinence, frequency, hesitancy, or urgency (more than 90% of MS clients report bladder dysfunction).
D. Fatigue (in up to 90% of MS clients).

E. Weakness in one or more extremities.
F. Gait disturbance (50% will require assistance with ambulation within 15 years of the onset of MS).

Other Signs and Symptoms
A. Babinski response.
B. Spasticity (usually in the lower extremities).
C. Depression (occurs in nearly 50% of MS clients; also affects memory, attention, and concentration).
D. Hyperreflexia.
E. Loss of proprioception.
F. Impotence (males).
G. Impaired cognition: Subjective difficulties with attention span, concentration, short-term memory, planning, and judgment; dementia is reported in 3% of clients with late-stage MS.
H. Dysarthria.
I. Reduced libido (both genders).
J. Constipation.
K. Pain.
L. Trigeminal neuralgia (rare).
M. Dysphagia (may also have recurrent respiratory infections secondary to aspiration).

Subjective Data
A. Establish location and onset of symptoms. Is this the first time the client has experienced the symptom in question? Was the onset acute or insidious?
B. Ask the client to describe the quality and severity of the symptom, and how it has evolved over time, including duration. Is there an *RR* pattern? Is there progression regarding severity of the symptom?
C. Ask the client if there are any factors that aggravate or alleviate the symptom. Does hot weather/environment (e.g., hot tubs, saunas, and overexertion) aggravate the condition? Does rest help? Did the symptom resolve on its own?
D. Establish if there have been any known viral or bacterial infections before any reported symptoms.
E. Evaluate visual complaints, including the presence of scotoma, decreased colour perception, diplopia, decreased acuity, or painful extraocular eye movements (EOMs). Is visual deterioration induced by exercise, a hot meal, or a hot bath (known as the Uhthoff phenomenon)?

Physical Examination
A. Check temperature, blood pressure, pulse, and respiration.
B. Inspect:
  1. Conduct a complete eye examination (Snellen eye chart, test cranial nerves II, III, IV, and VI):
    a. 50% of MS clients present with retrobulbar involvement, yet funduscopy results are negative for any related pathology.
    b. Anterior involvement causes papillitis; look for the presence of macular star.
    c. Assess pupillary response bilaterally; look for pendular nystagmus or sinusoidal involuntary oscillations of one or both eyes, and/or loss of smooth eye pursuit.
  2. Conduct a neurologic and musculoskeletal examination:
    a. Sensory: Test for perception of sharp versus dull stimulus, heat versus cold stimulus, local pain perception, proprioception; use the tuning fork to evaluate sense of vibration.
    b. Motor strength: Test all extremities and assess for any increased tone (spasticity), clonus, and/or tremors.
    c. Heel-to-toe tandem gait testing (assess for ataxia, any cerebellar involvement); Romberg test.
    d. Finger-to-nose testing, heel-to-shin testing (rule out dystaxia).
    e. Check deep tendon reflexes (DTRs); assess for Babinski response, hyperreflexia.
    f. Assess mental status (orientation to person, place, time, and situation); also test short-term memory and ability to plan (impaired planning is another cognitive issue secondary to MS).
    g. Assess for pain: Location, onset, duration, timing/setting, aggravating factors, alleviating factors, and any other associated data.
    h. Assess for depression, especially with progression of MS-related symptoms.

Diagnostic Tests
A. There is no specific confirmatory test for MS. Rule out any competing differentials.
B. MRI is the designated radiologic test to support clinical diagnosis of MS. An MRI of the head will reveal any associated plaques of MS. However, MRI cannot determine whether the identified lesions are specific to MS when other diseases may have similar findings:
  1. Transverse myelitis (TM) lesions identified with MRI may convert to MS over time.
C. Cerebrospinal fluid (CSF) analysis: Characteristics specific to MS include the presence of oligoclonal bands (in 85%–90% of MS clients), elevated immunoglobulin G (IgG; >12%), and elevated white blood cells (WBCs; >5%).
D. Evoked response tests (ERTs) or evoked potential (EP) studies: Several different types of tests/studies evaluate brain function and the peripheral nervous system (PNS) using EEG with nerve conduction/velocity (NCV):
  1. Brain auditory evoked response (BAER) studies can detect subtle changes in brainstem function.
  2. Visual evoked potential (VEP) studies focus on visual interpretation and perception, evaluating optical responses to strobe light and/or frequent pattern reversal (typically checkerboard patterns).
  3. Somatosensory evoked potential (SSEP) studies evaluate nerve conduction from the extremities via the spinal cord to the brain.
E. Complete blood count (CBC) with differential, antinuclear antibody (ANA), rheumatoid factor, C-reactive protein (CRP), thyroid-stimulating hormone (TSH), B12, antiphospholipid antibodies; and vitamin D, Lyme titre, and rapid plasma reagin (RPR) if indicated.
F. Serum glucose levels will rule out hypoglycaemia and chronic hyperglycaemia as potential causes of neurologic findings.

Differential Diagnoses
A. CNS lymphoma.
B. CNS infection.
C. Acute disseminated encephalomyelitis (ADEM).
D. Tumour: brainstem, cerebellar, or spinal cord.
E. Amyotrophic lateral sclerosis (ALS).
F. Systemic lupus erythematosus (SLE).
G. Syringomyelia.
H. Progressive multifocal leukoencephalopathy (PML).

I. Sarcoidosis.
J. Sjögren's syndrome.
K. Acute transverse myelitis (TM).
L. Myasthenia gravis (MG).
M. Guillain–Barré syndrome (GBS).
N. Cerebrovascular accident (CVA) or transient ischaemic attack (TIA).
O. Diabetes mellitus.
P. Spinal cord compression (stenosis, ruptured disc).
Q. Behcet's disease.
R. Neuromyelitis optica (NMO).
S. Lyme disease.
T. Tertiary syphilis, HIV, tuberculosis.

Clients with co-morbidities at the time of diagnosis (e.g., depression, cardiovascular disease, smoking, or diabetes) can expect faster progression of the disease. Controlling co-morbidities is essential in MS management.
MS, multiple sclerosis.

Plan

A. Client teaching:
 1. Discuss heat sensitivity and how it can aggravate symptoms: Individuals with MS must avoid hot tubs, saunas, prolonged exposure to hot/humid conditions, and choose appropriate clothing for the season:
    a. Approximately 60% of individuals with MS experience heat sensitivity, facilitating a *pseudoexacerbation* in which symptoms may worsen, but do not necessarily indicate additional axon/myelin degeneration.
 2. For visual disturbances, offer advice on resting the eyes at various times during the day may be helpful; for double vision, an eyepatch may be used temporarily.
 3. Discuss the importance of exercise and its effect on MS-related fatigue and spasticity; overactivity/overwork is another issue to address at this time. Rest periods are needed during exacerbations of MS. For health maintenance, 30 minutes of daily exercise is recommended.
 4. Engage in teaching Kegel exercises and timed voiding (habit training) to improve bladder function; also advise individuals with MS to avoid alcohol and caffeinated beverages.
 5. Discuss increasing daily water intake, dietary fibre intake, and physical activity for increased bowel motility.
 6. Discuss signs and symptoms of infection, especially urinary tract infections (UTIs) and how infection can trigger exacerbations.
 7. Engage in teaching regarding self-intermittent catheterization (SIC) when necessary for urinary retention.
 8. Discuss the purpose and availability of local MS support groups.
 9. Discuss counseling for adaptive coping techniques, improving family dynamics/relationships with significant others, adjusting to physical disability, and addressing anticipatory grief issues.
 10. Familiarize client and family on all medications, including side effects and any follow-up for pertinent laboratory tests or other testing.
 11. Suggest strategies for short-term memory and planning ability: Individuals with MS can benefit from writing things down, making lists, drawing pictures, and allocating more time for planning.

B. Pharmacological therapy is prescribed specifically for the type of MS and for the specific symptoms experienced. Medications may include any combination of the following:
 1. Disease-modifying drugs suppress the immune system to slow progression of MS, decreasing the frequency and severity of exacerbations, and reducing MS-related plaques):
    a. Injectable medications (recommended for first-line therapy for RRMS):
       i. Interferon beta-1a: An immunomodulator.
       ii. Glatiramer acetate: An immunomodulator.
       iii. Peginterferon beta-1a: A more tolerable form of interferon.
    b. Oral medications:
       i. Teriflunomide: An immune modulatory with anti-inflammatory properties. Recommended for first-line therapy.
       ii. Dimethyl fumarate: An anti-inflammatory that provides some neuronal protection. Recommended for first-line therapy.
       iii. Fingolimod: An immunomodulator that reduces lymphocytic infiltration into the brain and spinal cord. Recommended for second-line therapy.
    c. Intravenous (IV) infusions:
       i. Alemtuzumab: A selective immunomodulator. Recommended for second-line therapy.
       ii. Mitoxantrone: An antineoplastic, immune modulating drug. Recommended for second-line therapy.
       iii. Rituximab: Monoclonal antibody therapy. Off-label use for RRMS when second-line medications have been ineffective.
       iv. Natalizumab: Monoclonal antibody therapy. Recommended for second-line therapy.
 2. Short-term steroid use (e.g., methylprednisolone or prednisone for three to five days) may shorten a period of exacerbation. Long-term use is not recommended. IV steroids may be prescribed initially, then converted to oral steroids (e.g., prednisone, dexamethasone) and tapered off over time:
    a. Repository corticotropin injection (ACTH) is an option when individuals cannot tolerate the side effects of high-dose corticosteroids, do not respond to corticosteroid therapy, have no available IV infusion services, or when individuals have difficult/inadequate peripheral IV access.
 3. Dalfampridine is a Food and Drug Administration (FDA)–approved drug that has been shown to improve ambulation and possibly decrease fatigue in the MS population. Dalfampridine is a potassium channel blocker that targets channels located on the outside of nerve fibres, subsequently improving nerve conduction when myelin sheaths are damaged.
 4. Meclizine may be prescribed for dizziness or vertigo.
 5. Various medications (antiepileptics and antidepressants) may be considered for the treatment of neuropathic or spasticity-related pain:
    a. Phenytoin.
    b. Amitriptyline.
    c. Clonazepam.
    d. Gabapentin.
    e. Nortriptyline.
    f. Carbamazepine.
    g. Nabiximols is a cannabinoid-like drug used for MS pain and is approved for use by Health Canada.

6. MS-related spasticity may be treated with the following drugs:
   a. Baclofen.
   b. Tizanidine.
   c. Clonazepam, diazepam (watch for sedation, dependence).
   d. Dantrolene sodium (use only when other drugs are ineffective, as it can cause liver damage).
   e. Botulinum toxin injections.
   f. Intrathecal (IT) pump placement is another option for continuous IT administration of baclofen or clonidine for spasticity.
   g. Cannabis is being used off-label for control of both pain and spasticity.
7. Stool softeners, bulk-forming agents, and/or laxatives may be prescribed for complaints of constipation, depending on the severity of symptoms.
8. Tamsulosin or terazosin can be used to improve urinary flow.
9. Oxybutynin chloride, imipramine hydrochloride, and tolterodine are several examples of medications commonly used to treat bladder spasms.
10. Options for treatment of depression include the following:
    a. Selective serotonin-norepinephrine reuptake inhibitors (SSNRIs): duloxetine hydrochloride, velafaxine.
    b. Selective serotonin reuptake inhibitors (SSRIs): fluoxetine, sertraline, paroxetine.
    Individuals with protracted, painful, and/or progressive medical conditions are at risk for suicide.
11. Modafinil, amantadine hydrochloride, or fluoxetine can be used to treat fatigue symptoms.
12. Stem cell transplantation for RRMS is emerging in the literature. Clinical trials present encouraging results that indicate reversal of symptoms while offering a way to "reset" the immune system. Stem cell transplantation shows promise as a future treatment option for RRMS.
13. Optimize vitamin D intake: 4000 units daily, orally. Vitamin D has a role to play in the remyelination of nerves.

There is insufficient evidence to recommend nutritional supplements (other than Vitamin D), acupuncture, dental mercury amalgam removal, or bee sting therapy as adjuncts or treatments for MS.
MS, multiple sclerosis.

Follow-Up

A. A neurologist who specializes in MS management should coordinate and prescribe therapies for this client population. Nurse practitioner comanagement with a primary care physician for follow-up depends on the individual's clinical presentation, diagnosis, and therapies.

Consultation/Referral

A. Neurology referral for diagnosis; followed by a referral to an MS clinic for treatment and management.
B. Ophthalmology for visual disturbances, optic neuritis.
C. Urology for genitourinary (GU) disturbances (impotence in males, UTIs, and other urinary symptoms of hesitancy, frequency, incontinence, and urgency).
D. Occupational therapy (OT) will address any barriers or problems with performing activities of daily living (ADLs), deficits in fine motor skills (coordination, strength in the upper extremities), and prescribe any necessary adaptive equipment.
E. Speech therapy (ST) will address any issues with language, cognition, or swallowing (including any evaluations necessary for feeding tube placement and for specific dietary recommendations).
F. Physiotherapy will address gait disturbances, motor weakness, spasticity, and range of motion (ROM), and prescribe any necessary adaptive equipment for impaired physical mobility.
G. Psychiatry referral and consultation for pharmacological management of depression and/or dementia may be necessary in specific cases; also consider referrals to a psychologist or counsellor for any behavioural therapy or counseling needs.
H. Social work (SW) referrals may be necessary for assistance with insurance issues, locating community resources, applying for disability, arranging home care, obtaining placement in a skilled nursing facility, and for counseling (individual and family).

Individual Considerations

A. Pregnancy:
   1. Symptoms of MS may stabilize or remit during pregnancy, but 20% to 40% of MS clients experience relapse within 3 months postpartum.
   2. No evidence suggests that pregnancy affects the long-term course of MS. There is no acceleration in the rate of disability or disease progression over time.
   3. Neither epidural anaesthesia nor breastfeeding have an adverse effect on the rate of relapse or progression of disability with MS.
   4. There are no accepted guidelines for recommending for or against pregnancy in females with MS. MS history and current neurologic deficits should be considered independently per client.
   5. Pregnancy may affect the treatment regimen; some of the medications used to treat MS are known teratogens. For instance, glucocorticoids may cause neonatal adrenal suppression and maternal glucose intolerance.
      a. Intravenous immunoglobulin (IVIG) is an alternative to consider during pregnancy or while breastfeeding, after weighing the risks and benefits carefully before administration. The adverse effects are few, but may present complications that can be severe (e.g., aseptic meningitis, thromboembolism).
B. Paediatrics:
   1. MS is rarely diagnosed in children younger than 16 years.
   2. Children with MS generally have a similar clinical presentation to adults. Most diagnoses of paediatric MS are classified as RRMS.
C. Geriatrics:
   1. The occurrence of MS is rare in individuals older than 60 years of age.
   2. Spinal infarcts are seen more often in older individuals when evaluating specific inflammatory lesions.

Resources

Multiple Sclerosis Society of Canada: www.mssociety.ca
The Canadian Agency for Drugs and Technologies in Health (CADTH): www.cadth.ca

Bibliography

Gilmour, H., Ramage-Morin, P. L., & Wong, S. L. (2018, January). Multiple sclerosis: Prevalence and impact. *Health Reports*,

29(1), 3–8. Statistics Canada, Catalogue no. 82-003-X, Health Matters. Retrieved from https://www150.statcan.gc.ca/n1/pub/82-003-x/2018001/article/54902-eng.pdf

Gullo, H. L., Hatton, A. L., Bennett, S., Fleming, J., & Shum, D. H. K. (2016). Habitual and low-intensity physical activity in people with multiple sclerosis. *Brain Impairment*, *17*(1), 77–86. doi:10.1017/BrImp.2016.9

McCarthy, C., & Thorpe, J. (2016). Some recent advances in multiple sclerosis. *Journal of Neurology*, *263*(9), 1880–1886. doi:10.1007/s00415-016-8124-1

Multiple Sclerosis Society of Canada. (2018). *What is MS?* Retrieved from https://mssociety.ca/about-ms/what-is-ms

Roy, S., Benedict, R. H., Drake, A. S., & Weinstock-Guttman, B. (2016). Impact of pharmacotherapy on cognitive dysfunction in clients with multiple sclerosis. *CNS Drugs*, *30*(3), 209–225. doi:10.1007/s40263-016-0319-6

Torkildsen, O., Myhr, K.-M., & Bø, L. (2016). Disease-modifying treatments for multiple sclerosis: A review of approved medications. *European Journal of Neurology*, *23*(Suppl. 1), 18–27. doi:10.1111/ene.12883

Myasthenia Gravis (MG)

Jill C. Cash, Julie Adkins, and Donna Clare

Definition

A. Myasthenia gravis (MG) is a chronic autoimmune neuromuscular disorder that affects the neuromuscular junction and is characterized by fatigability and weakness of voluntary muscles. The hallmark of MG is muscle weakness that increases during periods of activity and improves after periods of rest. Function is usually highest in the morning with increasing weakness as the day progresses.

Incidence/Prevalence

The prevalence is 0.5 to 11.5 cases per one million people. There are two peaks in MG incidence that are age and gender related—one is women in their 20s and 30s, and the other is men in their 60s and 70s—but MG can occur at any age. Cases of neonatal MG are temporary and usually disappear within two to three months after birth. MG in juveniles is uncommon.

Pathogenesis

MG is believed to be an antibody-mediated autoimmune attack that destroys variable numbers of acetylcholine receptors (AChR) at the postsynaptic junction. The decrease in AChRs results in weakness with repeated activities and recovery after rest. MG is often associated with thymic hyperplasia or tumours; the thymus plays an unclear role in the autoimmune process of MG. The thymus is large in infants, grows until puberty, and then gets smaller with age. In MG, the thymus gland remains large and abnormal.

Predisposing Factors

A. No predisposing factors have been identified.
B. Not inherited or contagious. Occasionally, the disease may occur in more than one family member.

Common Findings

A. Classic triad: Ptosis, diplopia, and dysphagia:
    1. Fluctuating symptoms such as droopy eyelid(s).
    2. Blurry or double vision.
    3. Sense of choking.
B. Difficulty chewing.
C. Slurring of speech.
D. Easy fatigability.
E. Symptoms are more pronounced with fatigue or in the evening.

Other Signs and Symptoms

A. Selected voluntary muscles that fatigue with activity.
B. Motor function that improves with rest, but then decreases with use.
C. Signs of impending MG crisis:
    1. Sudden onset of inspiratory distress.
    2. Difficulty swallowing.
    3. Visual difficulty.
    4. Tachycardia.
    5. Rapid onset of weakness.

Subjective Data

A. Establish onset of symptoms and possible progression.
B. Ask the client what makes the symptoms better or worse: Does rest help?
C. Ask whether the client feels better in the morning, or in the afternoon, or in the evening.
D. Look for difficulties with chewing or swallowing.
E. Investigate medications the client is currently taking or has recently taken such as antibiotics.

Physical Examination

Both the presentation and course of MG are highly variable; therefore MG can be very difficult to diagnose.
MG, myasthenia gravis.

A. Check temperature, pulse, respiration, and blood pressure.
B. Inspect:
    1. Observe overall appearance.
    2. Perform complete eye examination. Subtleties of eye movement dysfunction are often key in differentiating MG from other disorders.
C. Palpate:
    1. Assess deep tendon reflexes (DTRs); note normal to increased reflexes.
D. Neurologic examination:
    1. Perform complete neurologic examination.
    2. Test the following:
        a. Muscle strength: Weakness is increased with repetition or sustained activity; arm raise cannot be sustained.
        b. Eyes:
            i. Upward or lateral gaze cannot be maintained for longer than 30 seconds.
            ii. Ptosis occurs with repetitive lid closure.
            iii. Ice pack test—Fill a plastic bag or glove with ice and place over closed eyelid for two minutes. Remove ice and evaluate the degree of ptosis. Noted to be very sensitive with prominent ptosis.
        c. Voice: Voice quality or speech changes when counting out loud to 100.

Normal coordination, normal sensory perception, and normal pupillary response are noted in MG.
MG, myasthenia gravis.

Diagnostic Tests

A. Antibody titre for acetylcholine receptor (AChR-Ab) positive in 90% of clients with MG. May also perform an anti-muscle-specific receptor tyrosine kinase (MuSK) antibody

titre. Approximately 6% to 12% of clients will have negative antibody titres for both titres.
B. Cholinesterase-inhibiting drug test: Improvement in strength following injection of edrophonium.
C. Repetitive muscle stimulation test: Decremental response.
D. Single-fibre electromyography (EMG) and/or repetitive nerve stimulation (RNS) studies are diagnostic studies performed for diagnosis.

Initial diagnostic tests may be equivocal with some negative test results, but this does not absolutely rule out MG.
MG, myasthenia gravis.

Differential Diagnoses
A. Incomplete extraocular nerve palsy.
B. Polymyositis.
C. Brainstem transient ischaemic attack (TIA).
D. Amyotrophic lateral sclerosis (ALS).
E. Brainstem vascular accident: "Dizziness" is a symptom rarely seen with MG but often associated with brainstem ischaemia.
F. Guillain–Barré syndrome (GBS).
G. Brainstem tumour.
H. Hyperthyroidism or hypothyroidism.
I. Cholinergic crisis: Although it is useful to distinguish myasthenic crisis (weakness from MG exacerbation) from cholinergic crisis (weakness from too much medication), both can rapidly lead to respiratory failure. Transportation to an ED for evaluation should not be delayed by attempts to differentiate the two.
J. Eaton–Lambert myasthenic syndrome: Often associated with bronchogenic carcinoma but may precede detection of the carcinoma by as many as two years.

Plan
A. General interventions:
  1. MG is primarily managed by a neurologist, given the difficulty in diagnosing it, the variable course of the disease, and the highly individualized medication regimen required.
  2. The course of MG fluctuates most during the first three to five years after diagnosis.
  3. Autoimmune disorders, such as thyroid disease, rheumatoid arthritis, and systemic lupus erythematosus (SLE), should also be screened for inpatients diagnosed with MG.
B. Client teaching:
  1. *Refer to Client Teaching Guide: Mysthenia Gravis.* Clients should have a Medic Alert tag. Clients should carry a list of their medications and dosing schedules in case of an emergency.
C. Medical and surgical management:
  1. Thymectomy is an early consideration; an MRI of the chest is obtained once the diagnosis is made to assess for thymic enlargement. Some clients develop thymomas, which can become malignant.

Thymectomy lessens the severity of MG, but rarely results in complete elimination of the need for medication.
MG, myasthenia gravis.

  2. Plasmapheresis, or plasma exchange to remove antibodies, is used emergently for the management of myasthenic crisis. Opinion is mixed regarding its use in the long-term management of myasthenia.
  3. A myasthenic crisis occurs when the muscles that control breathing are weakened to the point of requiring ventilation. This usually is triggered by an infection, fever, or adverse reaction to a medication.
D. Pharmacological treatment:
  1. Many medications can cause worsening of myasthenic symptoms, so changes and additions of any medication require consultation with the client's neurologist. Cholinesterase-inhibiting medications:
     a. Pyridostigmine sustained release (SR).
     b. Neostigmine methylsulphate.
  2. Steroids may be used when inpatient and then tapered on an outpatient basis, tapering every three days.
  3. Effectiveness of medication regimen is gauged by changes in ptosis, diplopia, dysphagia, chewing ability, and muscle fatigue.
  4. Care should be used with medications that may worsen symptoms of weakness.

Follow-Up
A. Clients with MG require lifelong management by a neurologist, given the variable course both of the disease and of the client's response to treatment.
B. The client is initially followed every one to two months, then every three to four months.

Consultation/Referral
A. If MG is suspected, consider neurologic referral.

Individual Considerations
A. Pregnancy:
  1. MG is considered high risk for both the woman and the fetus.
     a. Pregnancy requires management by the client's neurologist and a perinatologist.
  2. MG frequently manifests for the first time during pregnancy. Refer to an obstetrician.
B. Paediatrics:
  1. MG is associated with prematurity, and the infant may have transient neonatal myasthenia. The neonate will need a neonatology consult.
  2. Myasthenia is less severe and commonly remits spontaneously in children, so thymectomy is not recommended.
C. Adults:
  1. Oral contraceptives may worsen myasthenic symptoms.

Bibliography
Alkhawajah, N. M., & Oger, J. (2015). Treatment of myasthenia gravis in the aged. *Drugs & Aging, 32*(9), 689–697. doi:10.1007/s40266-015-0297-2
Kalita, J., Kohat, A. K., & Misra, U. K. (2014). Predictors of outcome of myasthenic crisis. *Neurological Sciences, 35*(7), 1109–1114. doi:10.1007/s10072-014-1659-y
Liew, W. K., & Kang, P. B. (2013). Update on juvenile myasthenia gravis. *Current Opinion in Pediatrics, 25*(6), 694–700. doi:10.1097/MOP.0b013e328365ad16

▶ Client Teaching Guides are available at https://connect.springerpub.com/content/reference-book/978-0-8261-9498-5

Parkinson's Disease (PD)

Jill C. Cash, Julie Adkins, and Donna Clare

Definition
A. Parkinson's disease (PD) is an idiopathic, progressive, chronic neurologic syndrome characterized by a combination of akinesia or bradykinesia, or reduction of spontaneous activity and movement; rigidity, or increase in spontaneous muscle tone and involuntary movements; tremor; and postural instability.

Incidence/Prevalence
A. There are approximately 67,000 Canadians living with PD. The mean age of onset is 55 to 60 years. The risk increases with age. There is no gender difference in prevalence. PD is seen most frequently in people of European ancestry.

Pathogenesis
For reasons that are unclear, degenerative changes occur in the basal ganglia and deplete the dopaminergic neurons in the substantia nigra, resulting in dopamine reduction in the striatum. This interrupts neuronal circuits and produces akinesia and rigidity. The pathophysiology of tremor is less clear, but thalamic involvement is implicated. Symptoms are caused by loss of neurons that produce dopamine. Certain nerve cells (neurons) in the brain break down or die.

Predisposing Factors
A. Antecedent encephalitis.
B. Arteriosclerosis.
C. History of head trauma.
D. Toxins, pesticide exposure.
E. Drugs, particularly phenothiazines.
F. Familial neurodegenerative diseases in which Parkinsonism is a prominent feature.
G. Presence of Lewy bodies.

Common Findings
Cardinal symptoms:
A. Resting tremor: May be intermittent, but progresses over time. "Pill-rolling" tremor of the hands is common and may be unilateral or bilateral.
B. Rigidity: Joints are more rigid. Increased resistance to passive movement. Appears unilaterally and then progresses to the opposite side. Usually asymmetrical. Appears as decreased movement in arm swing when ambulating, stooped posture, cogwheel rigidity—resistance with tremor.
C. Bradykinesia, or slow voluntary movement, especially with daily activities such as cutting food, dressing self, and so forth. When walking, shorter steps are taken, shuffle-step, feeling of unsteadiness with walking. Postural instability.

Other Signs and Symptoms
A. Micrographia (handwriting that decreases in size when writing out name).
B. Voice changes: Fading, softness, hoarseness, and mumbling.
C. Saliva escaping mouth, especially at night.
D. Dysphagia.
E. Neuropsychiatric changes: Cognitive impairment/dementia/memory loss, sleep disturbance, fatigue, anxiety, depression, pain, and sensory changes.
F. Oily, greasy skin.
G. Excessive perspiration.
H. Constipation.
I. Urinary hesitancy or frequency.
J. Visual loss: Impaired vision, reflex, upward gaze, and convergence.
K. Impaired posture and balance.

Subjective Data
A. Elicit information regarding onset of symptoms. Note changes in progression of symptoms.
B. Talk with the client and family to establish if there have been behavioural changes, problems with activities such as eating or getting out of chairs, or personality changes.
C. Determine whether other family members have had similar symptoms.
D. Ascertain the client's medical history, including current medications, both prescription and over the counter (OTC).
E. Particularly in clients younger than 55 years, investigate substance abuse and exposure to herbicides or pesticides.

Physical Examination
A. Check temperature, pulse, respiration, blood pressure, and weight; note orthostatic hypotension.
B. Inspect:
  1. Observe overall appearance.
  2. Note asymmetric tremor at rest.
  3. Note subtle facial masking, decreased frequency and amplitude of eye blinks.
  4. Note posture and gait disturbances: Festination, or shuffling, increasingly tiny steps; usually walking with arms down to side; difficulty turning; freezing, or inability to continue to move.
C. Palpate:
  1. Palpate extremities, noting increased tone in resting muscles.
D. Neurologic examination:
  1. Perform complete neurologic examination. Assess all cranial nerves. Assess deep tendon reflexes (DTRs).
  2. Assess rapid alternating movements. Note difficulty with rapid alternating movements such as tapping fingers or turning palm alternately up and down.
  3. Check for cogwheel phenomenon, which is a stepwise rigidity of movement with passive range of motion (ROM), rather than anticipated smooth movement through ROM. Best tested in wrists.
  4. Perform mental state examination.
  5. Assess the progression of the disease state with the scale of choice. Scales commonly used include the following:
     a. Unified Parkinson's Disease Rating Scale: www.mdvu.org/library/ratingscales/pd.
     b. International Parkinson and Movement Disorder Society: This site hosts a list of rating scales and questionnaires: www.movementdisorders.org.
     c. Hoehn and Yahr Scale: neurosurgery.mgh.harvard.edu/Functional/pdstages.htm.
     d. Scales for Outcomes in Parkinson's Disease—Psychiatric Complications (nonmotor evaluation) and Nonmotor Symptom Screening Questionnaire: www.neurology.org/cgi/content/abstract/61/9/1222.

Diagnostic Tests
A. There is no definitive diagnostic test for PD. Consider serum blood tests or other testing to rule out competing differentials.

B. Urinalysis to rule out urinary tract infection (UTI) with any urinary symptoms.
C. Speech therapy evaluation of dysarthria and dysphagia to assess aspiration risk.
D. Brain CT scan or MRI to exclude mass lesion, multiple infarcts, or normal pressure hydrocephalus.
E. Diagnostic imaging of cervical spine may be indicated if there is increased gait disturbance after a fall.

Differential Diagnoses
A. Essential tremor.
B. Multi-infarct dementia.
C. Alzheimer's disease.
D. Brain tumour.
E. Progressive supranuclear palsy.
F. Normal pressure hydrocephalus.
G. Shy–Drager syndrome.
H. Hypothyroidism.
I. Hereditary disease such as Huntington's chorea or Wilson's disease.
J. Medication effect.

Plan
A. General interventions:
  1. Encourage regular exercise to maintain or improve flexibility.
  2. The client should follow a diet that is high in fibre and calcium, with adequate fluid intake, to limit complications caused by constipation and osteoporosis. In some clients, protein intake may need to be timed to limit interactions with medications such as levodopa.
  3. Emphasize the importance of the nonmotor symptoms being addressed and adequately treated. Encourage the family to notify the provider if these symptoms are not being controlled. Anxiety, depression, fatigue, mood changes, and behavioural issues need to be assessed, addressed, and controlled for quality of life for the client and family. Geriatric psychiatry may be consulted as needed.
  4. Home safety evaluations are recommended because the symptoms of PD place clients at high risk of falls and accidental injury.
  5. Surgery, such as pallidotomy or thalamotomy, is an option for severe PD in which tremor is poorly controlled with medications.
▶ **B.** *Refer to Client Teaching Guide: Parkinson's Disease Management.* Pharmacological treatment:
  1. Polypharmacy is the hallmark rather than the exception with PD. Always comanage with a neurologist.
  2. Lower doses of several medications, rather than high doses of a single agent, aid in maximizing function while minimizing side effects.
  3. Drug dosages are always tapered, not stopped abruptly.
  4. First-line drug:
    a. Levodopa, combined with a decarboxylase inhibitor, is the mainstay of treatment. A levodopa and carbidopa combination drug is most often used:
      i. The dose and dosing frequency are very individualized.
      ii. Clients are often on a combination of sustained release and short-acting preparations.
      iii. See literature for individual dosing.
      iv. Long-term use is often associated with adverse effects, requiring careful medication dosage. Dyskinesias are the most common complication of levodopa therapy.
  5. Second-line therapy: Dopamine agonists are generally given in conjunction with levodopa; these allow use of lower doses of levodopa that can delay or reduce levodopa-associated problems. Examples include pramipexole and ropinirole.
  6. Ergot derivatives include the following:
    a. Bromocriptine and pergolide are the two dopamine agonists most often used:
      i. Bromocriptine mesylate.
      ii. Pergolide mesylate.
    b. Nonergot drugs are preferred because of fewer side effects:
      i. Pramipexole.
      ii. Ropinirole.
  7. Neuroprotective agents: Selegiline, a monoamine oxidase-B (MAO-B) inhibitor, may have neuroprotective effects and slow progression of symptoms.
    a. Often an initial treatment, a drug is usually continued throughout the course of the disease.
    b. Amantadine is used as short-term monotherapy in clients younger than 60 years with mild to moderate PD in which akinesia and rigidity are more prominent than tremor:
      i. Its effects tend to wane, and it should be tapered once other antiparkinsonian drugs are started.
      ii. Adjust the dose gradually.
      iii. Caution should be used with these medications because of the interactions with other medications and foods that can precipitate high blood pressure to dangerous levels. Advise to avoid foods high in tyramine such as some cheeses, tofu, yeast extracts, and so forth.
  8. Anticholinergics: These are useful for treating resting tremor, but not akinesia or impaired postural reflexes.
    a. The centrally acting drug trihexyphenidyl hydrochloride is the most common anticholinergic used:
      i. Dosage should always be tapered, never stopped abruptly.
      ii. Use is not recommended in clients older than 60 years or with dementia.
    b. Benztropine mesylate may also be used in PD.
  9. Sleep disorders are common in PD and respond well to tricyclic antidepressants (TCAs), benzodiazepines, diphenhydramine, or low-dose chloral hydrate.
  10. Excessive daytime sleepiness should first be evaluated as a symptom of depression before it is attributed to medications or effects of PD.

As PD progresses, clients often develop clear "on" and "off" times of medication effectiveness and functional ability; therefore, medication schedules are very carefully customized to maximize "on" times.

Follow-Up
A. PD requires lifelong management by a neurologist.
B. Frequency of appointments depends on severity of disease and response to medication. Depression and neuropsychiatric side effects of medications are often seen in clients

▶ Client Teaching Guides are available at https://connect.springerpub.com/content/reference-book/978-0-8261-9498-5

with PD; therefore, any office visit should involve screening for these. Inquire particularly about memory loss, vivid dreams or nightmares, hallucinations, symptoms of depression or anxiety, and occurrence of panic attacks. Discuss findings with the client's neurologist, as medication adjustments could be required.

Consultation/Referral
A. Managing PD requires referral to a neurologist to initiate and adjust medications.
B. If a PD client requires the addition of medication for other conditions, consult the client's neurologist to evaluate for possible serious adverse effects.
C. Involvement with a support group can be helpful for the client and family. Information about PD and local support groups can be obtained from Parkinson Canada at www.parkinson.ca.

Individual Considerations
A. Paediatrics:
  1. When PD is seen in this age group, it is usually secondary to another condition or treatment.
B. Geriatrics:
  1. It is most commonly seen in this population.

Bibliography
Besser, L. M., Litvan, I., Monsell, S. E., Mock, C., Weintraub, S., Zhou, X. H., . . . Kukull, W. (2016). Mild cognitive impairment in Parkinson's disease versus Alzheimer's disease. *Parkinsonism & Related Disorders, 27*, 54–60. doi:10.1016/j.parkreldis.2016.04.007

Kang, M. Y., & Ellis-Hill, C. (2015). How do people live life successfully with Parkinson's disease? *Journal of Clinical Nursing, 24*(15–16), 2314–2322. doi:10.1111/jocn.12819

Khoo, T. K., Yarnall, A. J., Duncan, G. W., Coleman, S., O'Brien, J. T., Brooks, D. J., . . . Burn, D. J. (2013). The spectrum of nonmotor symptoms in early Parkinson disease. *Neurology, 80*(3), 276–281. doi:10.1212/WNL.0b013e31827deb74

Mayo Clinic. (2016). *Parkinson's disease*. Retrieved from www.mayoclinic.org

Wong, S. L., Gilmour, H., & Ramage-Morin, P. L. (2014, November). Parkinson's disease: Prevalence, diagnosis, and impact. *Health Reports, 25*(11), 10–14. Statistics Canada, Catalogue no. 82-003-X. Retrieved from https://www150.statcan.gc.ca/n1/pub/82-003-x/2014011/article/14112-eng.htm

Restless Legs Syndrome (RLS)

Julie Adkins and Donna Clare

Definition
Restless legs syndrome (RLS) is a neurologic disorder usually involving throbbing, pulling, creeping, or other unpleasant sensations of the legs with sometimes an overwhelming urge to move them. Symptoms occur usually at night when in a relaxing, resting position, but can increase in severity throughout the night. Moving the legs usually relieves the discomfort, but only momentarily, causing disorders of sleep. Left untreated, RLS can cause exhaustion and fatigue, which is often associated with daytime concentration, memory, and can cause depression.

Incidence/Prevalence
About 5% to 10% of Canadians may have RLS. Moderate to severe symptoms affect 2% to 3% of adults. Children can also have RLS; almost one million school-age children are affected and one-third have moderate to severe symptoms. RLS occurs in both men and women, but the incidence is about twice as high in women. It may begin at any age. Symptoms seem to become more frequent and last longer with age.

Pathogenesis
A. RLS is classified as a movement disorder as people are required to move their legs in order to get any relief. More than 80% of people with RLS also may experience a condition, periodic limb movement of sleep (PLMS), which involves leg twitching or jerking movements during sleep occurring every 15 to 40 seconds. Although many clients with RLS develop PLMS, most people with PLMS do not have RLS or any other cause of PLMS. Periodic limb movement disorder (PLMD) may be a variant of RLS and responds to similar treatments but occurs only during sleep. The cause of RLS is unknown; however, it may have a genetic component. Evidence indicates that low levels of iron in the brain may be responsible for RLS.
B. Considerable evidence suggests that RLS is a dysfunction in the brain's basal ganglia that uses the neurotransmitter dopamine. Disruption of this pathway frequently results in involuntary movements.
C. Alcohol and sleep deprivation may aggravate or trigger RLS symptoms.

Predisposing Factors
A. Alcohol use.
B. Sleep deprivation.
C. Chronic diseases such as kidney failure, diabetes, anaemia, and peripheral neuropathy.
D. Certain medications such as antiemetic, antipsychotic drugs, antidepressants, and some cold and allergy medications.
E. Pregnancy, especially during the third trimester.
F. Family history of RLS.
G. Withdrawal from selective serotonin reuptake inhibitors (SSRIs).

Common Findings
A. Uncomfortable sensations in the legs with an irresistible urge to move the limb. Sensations may occur on only one side of the body, but most often affect both sides.
B. Need to keep legs in motion such as pacing the floor, moving legs while sitting, and tossing and turning in bed.
C. A classic feature of RLS is that the symptoms are worse at night with a distinct symptom-free period in the early morning. RLS is absent while asleep.

Other Signs and Symptoms
A. May vary day to day, in severity and frequency, and from person to person.
B. Triggering factors may include long car trips; sitting for long periods of time, such as at a movie theater or long-distance flights; immobilization of a cast; or relaxation exercises.
C. Worsening of symptoms occurs with sleep deprivation.
D. In severe cases, interruption and impairment of daytime function occur.
E. Some people are affected in the upper limbs as well.

Subjective Data
A. Ask the client to describe the sensations (urge to move legs) that he or she is complaining of. Do sensations occur in one leg or both legs?
B. What makes symptoms worse? What makes symptoms better?

C. What does the client do to make the sensations better?
D. Do symptoms occur during rest or activity? Is there a particular activity that usually makes the symptoms worse or better? Do they improve with movement?
E. How often are symptoms present? Do the symptoms occur during the daytime or night-time? Daily, nightly, several times a day, once a week, and so forth?
F. Does the client have other medical or behavioural conditions that can be attributed to the symptoms that occur?
G. Are symptoms triggered by rest, relaxation, or sleep?
H. Determine sleep patterns and disturbances.
I. Review current medications being taken and discuss chronic conditions.
J. Inquire regarding the amount of alcohol ingested each day.
K. Inquire regarding the use of tobacco.
L. If pregnant, are symptoms new during the pregnancy or has she always had the symptoms?

Physical Examination
A. Check blood pressure, pulse, respirations, and weight.
B. Inspect:
  1. Overall appearance and hygiene.
C. Auscultate:
  1. Heart.
  2. Lungs.
D. Neurologic examination:
  1. Perform full neurologic examination.

Diagnostic Tests
A. Laboratory tests may be performed to rule out other conditions, which include the following:
  1. Iron studies: Serum ferritin level.
  2. Complete blood count (CBC).
  3. Vitamin B_{12} and folic acid.
  4. Complete metabolic panel (CMP).
  5. Haemoglobin A1c.
  6. Thyroid studies.
B. Sleep study.

Differential Diagnoses
A. RLS: There is no specific test for RLS. The basic criteria for diagnosing the disorder are the following:
  1. Symptoms are worse at night and are absent or negligible in the morning.
  2. A strong and often overwhelming need or urge to move the affected limb(s), often associated with paraesthesias or dysaesthesias.
  3. Sensory symptoms that are triggered by rest, relaxation, or sleep.
  4. Sensory symptoms that are relieved with movement, in which the relief persists as long as the movement continues.
  5. None of the previously noted symptoms are caused by another medical condition.
B. Sleep apnoea.
C. Alcoholism.
D. Specific vitamin deficiencies.
E. Pregnancy (third trimester).
F. Parkinson's disease (PD).

Plan
A. General interventions:
  1. Activities that worsen symptoms should be discontinued.
  2. Medications can be prescribed and are effective for many clients.
  3. Some chronic conditions may contribute to RLS, such as diabetes or peripheral neuropathy, or vitamin deficiency, and should be evaluated.
B. Client teaching:
  1. Advise client to discontinue activities that worsen symptoms.
  2. Lifestyle changes may be suggested such as discontinuing the use of alcohol, tobacco, and caffeine.
  3. Bedtime rituals should be encouraged. Regular sleep patterns should be encouraged. Avoid exercise at least one to two hours before bedtime. Encourage relaxation techniques before going to bed.
  4. The use of relieving techniques, such as massage or cold compresses, is encouraged.
C. Pharmacological treatment:
  1. Dopaminergic agents are recommended first-line treatment for frequent or nightly symptoms. However, caution should be used. Long-term use can lead to worsening symptoms. This is reversible with withdrawal of the medication.
      a. Health Canada–approved nonergotamine dopamine agonists for moderate to severe RLS include the following:
          i. Ropinirole.
          ii. Pramipexole.
          iii. Rotigotine transdermal patch.
      b. Levodopa formulation.
          i. Levodopa/carbidopa or levodopa/benserazid.
  2. Pregabalin.
  3. Analgesics, such as acetaminophen, nonsteroidal anti-inflammatory drugs (NSAIDs), and opioids, may be used as needed for pain.
  4. Benzodiazepines, such as clonazepam at bedtime, may be used as needed.
  5. Anticonvulsants, such as gabapentin at bedtime.
  6. Vitamin deficiencies should be treated with appropriate vitamins as diagnosed.

Follow-Up
A. Follow up in one to two weeks to evaluate effect(s) of medications.
B. Evaluate severity or minimization of symptoms.
C. Reassure clients that a diagnosis of RLS does not indicate the onset of another neurologic disorder such as PD.

Consultation/Referral
A. Consider referral to a neurologist if symptoms are not improving with treatment.

Individual Considerations
A. Pregnancy:
  1. Symptoms are usually worse in the third trimester.
B. Paediatrics:
  1. Diagnosing RLS can be difficult in children because of the child's difficulty describing symptoms such as where it hurts, when and how often it occurs, and how long symptoms last.
  2. Paediatric RLS can sometimes be misdiagnosed as "growing pains" or attention deficit disorder.
C. Geriatrics:
  1. Symptoms progress with age. Other chronic diseases are also usually present; it can be difficult to pinpoint the diagnosis of RLS because of other chronic problems.

Bibliography

Cuellar, N. G., & Dorn, J. M. (2015). Peripheral diabetic neuropathy or restless legs syndrome in persons with type 2 diabetes mellitus: Differentiating diagnosis in practice. *Journal of the American Association of Nurse Practitioners, 27*(12), 671–675. doi:10.1002/2327-6924.12311

Heim, B., Djamshidian, A., Heidbreder, A., Stefani, A., Zamarian, L., Pertl, M. T., . . . Högl, B. (2016). Augmentation and impulsive behaviours in restless legs syndrome: Coexistence or association? *Neurology, 87*(1), 36–40. doi:10.1212/WNL.0000000000002803

Hoogwout, S. J., Paananen, M. V., Smith, A. J., Beales, D. J., O'Sullivan, P. B., Straker, L. M., . . . Champion, D. (2015). Musculoskeletal pain is associated with restless legs syndrome in young adults. *BioMed Central Musculoskeletal Disorders, 16*, 294. doi:10.1186/s12891-015-0765-1

Klingelhoefer, L., Bhattacharya, K., & Reichmann, H. (2016). Restless legs syndrome. *Clinical Medicine (London, England), 16*(4), 379–382. doi:10.7861/clinmedicine.16-4-379

Lee, C. S., Kim, T., Lee, S., Jeon, H. J., Bang, Y. R., & Yoon, I. Y. (2016). Symptom severity of restless legs syndrome predicts its clinical course. *American Journal of Medicine, 129*(4), 438–445. doi:10.1016/j.amjmed.2015.12.020

National Institute of Neurological Disorders and Stroke. (2015). *Restless legs syndrome fact sheet.* Retrieved from http://www.ninds.nih.gov/Disorders/Client-Caregiver-Education/Fact-Sheets/Restless-Legs-Syndrome-Fact-Sheet

Rizek, P., & Kumar, N. (2017). Restless legs syndrome. *Canadian Medical Association Journal, 13*(189), E245. doi:10.1503/cmaj.160527

Suzuki, K., Miyamoto, M., Miyamoto, T., & Hirata, K. (2015). Restless legs syndrome and leg motor restlessness in Parkinson's disease. *Parkinson's Disease, 2015*, 490938. doi:10.1155/2015/490938

Seizures

Cheryl A. Glass, Julie Adkins, and Donna Clare

Definition

Accurate classification of seizures is dependent on observations of witnessed seizures; full medical history, including co-morbidities; and clinical findings. Epilepsy is not diagnosed until the client has more than one seizure secondary to an underlying condition in the brain. The clinical signs and symptoms depend on the location of the epileptic discharges. Status epilepticus is a continuous state of seizure and is usually defined as 30 minutes of uninterrupted seizure activity.

A. Infantile spasms begin at 3 months to 2 years of age. They are characterized by clusters of quick, sudden movements, including the head falling forward, arm flexion, and knees drawn up to the chest.

B. Partial (focal) seizures generally only involve one portion of the brain. They are the most common type of seizure and may be accompanied by visual or auditory hallucinations:

    1. Simple partial seizures (SPSs) are not associated with altered consciousness or loss of consciousness.

    2. Common SPS includes jerking of a limb and may be preceded by an aura, including epigastric discomfort, fear, or unpleasant smells.

    3. Complex partial seizure (CPS) is notable for impaired consciousness. Confusion, fatigue, and headaches may follow a CPS.

    4. An SPS may last a few seconds and develop into a CPS with symptoms that include staring, repetitive motor behaviours, clouded consciousness, and automatisms (swallowing, chewing, or lip smacking).

C. Generalized seizures are notable for EEG changes as both hemispheres of the brain are involved. Almost all generalized seizures involve loss/impaired consciousness. There are four subtypes of generalized seizures:

    1. Tonic–clonic, also known as grand mal seizures, generally last one to two minutes and are notable for falls, cries, rigidity (tonicity), jerking (clonicity), with possible cyanosis, and urinary incontinence. They may be preceded by a prodome of unease or irritability (hours or days). A grand mal seizure is followed by a postictal phase.

    2. Absent seizures, also called petit mal seizures, last 2 to 15 seconds and are notable for beginning and ending abruptly. Symptoms noted include staring, eye flutters or eye rolling, and automatisms. First aid is not required.

    3. Myoclonic seizures are characterized by rapid, brief contraction of muscles (sudden jerks or clumsiness), usually on both sides of the body, arm, or sudden jerk of a foot during sleep. First aid is generally not required. A single spasm upon transition to sleep is considered normal.

    4. Atonic seizures, also called drop seizures, are characterized by abrupt loss of muscle tone, loss of posture, or sudden collapse. These seizures tend to be resistant to medication. Protective headgear may be needed. Generally first aid is not required unless an injury occurs.

D. Lennox–Gastaut syndrome (LGS) is a rare form of epilepsy consisting of multiple seizure types. It includes cognitive impairment and drop seizures. LGS clients may require antiseizure medications, steroids or immune globulin, vagus nerve stimulation, surgical resection, and ketogenic diet.

E. Eclampsia can occur anytime in pregnancy, from the second trimester to the puerperium. It is notable for the occurrence of one or more generalized convulsions and/or coma in women with preeclampsia (in the absence of other neurologic conditions):

    1. Eclampsia is self-limited, and delivery is the treatment.

    2. The tonic–clonic seizure generally lasts 60 to 75 seconds.

    3. Fetal bradycardia lasts three to five minutes, but does not necessitate an emergent cesarean section delivery. Compensatory fetal tachycardia and transient fetal heart rate decelerations occur. Delivery should be considered for the lack of improvement in 10 to 15 minutes after maternal/fetal resuscitative interventions.

    4. Seizures caused by eclampsia generally resolve within a few hours to days postpartum. HELLP (haemolysis, elevated liver enzymes, low platelets) syndrome develops in approximately 10% to 20% of women with preeclampsia/eclampsia.

F. Idiopathic seizures, gelastic seizures, dacystic seizures, post-trauma, and nonepileptic seizures are other types noted in the literature. Pseudoseizures are common in mental illness presentations.

Incidence/Prevalence

A. Epilepsy affects 0.6% of Canadians, with over 15,000 new diagnoses every year. New cases of epilepsy commonly occur in young children (99%) and the elderly (1%). Half of childhood epilepsy cases resolve completely.

B. Stroke is the leading cause of new-onset epilepsy in adults over age 65 years.

C. Eclampsia.

    1. Mild preeclampsia: 0.5%.

    2. Severe preeclampsia: From 2% to 3%.

    3. Forty-eight hours postpartum: Up to 33%.

D. Photosensitivity (flickering lights) seizures are more common in children and adolescents.

Pathogenesis

Epilepsy is a functional disorder of the brain in which neurons signal abnormally. The exact cause of epilepsy and eclampsia is unknown. Seizure activity can occur in all areas of the brain, including the temporal and frontal lobes, which may elicit specific patterns of behaviour, emotion, or sensory disorders, before or during the seizure. Occasionally, orthostatic syncope may result in a brief seizure.

Predisposing Factors

A. Tumour.
B. Alcohol/drugs.
C. Cerebral infarction/stroke.
D. Hypoglycaemia.
E. Alzheimer's disease.
F. Posttrauma (head injury).
G. Surgery.
H. Pregnancy (eclampsia).
I. Febrile illness.
J. Photosensitivity.
K. Risk factors for recurrent seizures:
   1. Identifiable brain disease.
   2. Developmental disorders.
   3. Abnormal neurologic examination/EEG.
   4. Seizures: Onset after age 10 years.
   5. Multiple types of seizures.
   6. Family history/genetics.
   7. Poor response to antiepileptic drugs (AEDs)/combination therapy at time of withdrawal.
   8. Chronic alcoholism.
L. Eclampsia risk factors:
   1. Nulliparous.
   2. Pregnancy-induced hypertension (PIH).
   3. Teens to lower 20s and again older than 35 years.
   4. Other conditions to be ruled out:
      a. Stroke.
      b. Hypertensive disease.
      c. Space-occupying lesion.
      d. Metabolic disorders (e.g., hypoglycaemia, uraemia, water intoxication).
      e. Meningitis or encephalitis.
      f. Drug use (e.g., methamphetamines, cocaine).
      g. Idiopathic epilepsy.
      h. Thrombotic thrombocytopenia purpura (TTP).
M. Breath-holding in children.

Common Findings

A. Aura: Epigastric discomfort, fear, or unpleasant smells; can involve any sensory system.
B. Automatisms (e.g., swallowing, chewing, fumbling, picking clothes, or lip smacking).
C. Stiffening, then jerking of limbs.
D. Staring with/without repetitive motor behaviours.
E. Eclampsia:
   1. Headache: Severe or persistent frontal or occipital.
   2. Blurred vision.
   3. Photophobia.
   4. Right upper quadrant pain/epigastric pain.
   5. Altered mental status.
   6. Nausea and vomiting.
   7. Hyperreflexia.

Other Signs and Symptoms

A. Lack of memory of seizure.
B. Impaired consciousness.
C. Postictal:
   1. Confusion.
   2. Amnesia.
   3. Fatigue.
   4. Headaches.
   5. Loss of urine or bowel control.

Subjective Data

A. Obtain a history from the client or a person who witnesses the seizure:
   1. Have the witness describe the duration, part of the body affected, and qualities of the seizure.
   2. Does the client have a recollection of the seizure?
   3. How long did it take to feel better after the seizure?
B. Evaluate whether the client has ever had seizures, and ask whether this was an isolated event:
   1. Were there any warning symptoms before the seizure?
   2. What kind of warning was noted?
C. Did the client have a fever or an active/recent infection?
D. Do a thorough review of the client's medical history, including head injury, pregnancy, diabetes, and cancer.
E. Ask whether there is a family history of seizures.
F. Take a full medication history, including over-the-counter (OTC) and herbal products.
   1. Is the client on an AED?
   2. Has the client missed any doses?
   3. When was the last blood level checked to evaluate therapeutic dosing?
G. Review alcohol intake. Alcohol interferes with the efficacy of AEDs.

Physical Examination

A. Check blood pressure, pulse, respiration, and temperature (if indicated to rule out infection).
B. Inspect:
   1. Assess level of consciousness (LOC), orientation.
   2. Perform general overall examination for secondary injuries from fall or striking objects.
C. Auscultate:
   1. Lungs for possible aspiration.
D. Palpation (if applicable for any injuries):
   1. Elevate neck for nuchal rigidity.
E. Neurologic examination:
   1. Cranial nerves testing:
      a. Wrinkle forehead/raise eyebrows.
      b. Smile and show teeth.
      c. Stick out the tongue/lateral tongue movement.
      d. Ocular movements.
      e. Visual field.
      f. Finger-to-nose test.
   2. Motor strength:
      a. Shrug shoulders.
      b. Test muscle strength: Grasp hands and squeeze.
      c. Check reflexes of biceps, triceps, patellar, brachioradial, and Achilles.
   3. Sensory testing: Pinprick.
   4. Gait and posture.

Diagnostic Tests

A. Diagnosis is confirmed by the client's history, witness accounts, neurologic examination, blood work, and clinical testing such as EEG. Psychogenic seizures are notable for the absence of injury, daytime occurrence, unusual seizure movements (e.g., shaking of the head), and always being witnessed.
B. EEG.

C. Neuroimaging MRI.
D. Blood glucose.
E. Drug/alcohol screen.
F. Serum level of anticonvulsant.
G. Lumbar puncture if indicated for signs of infection/meningitis.
H. Complete blood count (CBC), electrolytes, calcium, magnesium, liver function tests, creatinine, urea, and C-reactive protein.

Differential Diagnoses
A. Brain tumour.
B. Central nervous system (CNS) infection.
C. Drug/alcohol use.
D. Stroke/transient ischaemic attack (TIA).
E. Hypoglycaemia.
F. Trauma.
G. Migraine.
H. Ménière's disease.
I. Syncope:
  1. Cardiac arrhythmic syncope.
  2. Reflex.
  3. Orthostatic.
J. Psychogenic.
K. Breath-holding (children).

Plan
A. General interventions:
  1. Emergency transport may be required. Seizures longer than 5 to 10 minutes require emergent care. If the client has a persistent headache after a rest period, unconsciousness with failure to respond, unequal pupil size or excessively dilated pupils, or weakness of the limbs, immediate medical attention is essential.
  2. Obtain a consultation with a neurologist for a thorough evaluation if at least two seizures occur.
  3. Driving restrictions are similar across provinces/territories in Canada. Clients and health-care providers should access their provincial/territorial ministry of transportation for guidelines. Guidelines are specific as to the seizure-free interval required to resume driving, or when medication doses are lowered or in the case of noncompliance or several missed doses:
    a. A person with epilepsy has the risk of motor vehicle accident (MVA) while driving. It is considered similar or slightly higher than in clients with other medical conditions (diabetes, cardiovascular disease) and compares with the risk of MVA with persons with sleep apnoea, alcoholism, dementia, and cellular phone use.
B. Client teaching:
  1. Keeping a seizure diary is extremely helpful in identifying seizure trends, maintaining drug compliance, monitoring side effects, and evaluating the need for changing the course of therapy. The frequency or time of day that seizures occur is used in the adjustment of AED dosage and timing of administration.
  2. Seizure triggers:
    a. Most common cause is missed AED and/or sudden discontinuation of meds.
    b. Sleep deprivation.
    c. Alcohol/drug intake.
    d. Stress.
    e. Hormone fluctuations.
    f. Pregnancy.
    g. Photosensitivity/strobe or flashing light/intense lights.
    h. TV and video games (flicker frequency).
    i. Contrasting visual patterns (e.g., grids, checkerboard, and stripes).
    j. Computer monitors.
    k. Visual fire alarms.
    l. Sunlight shimmering off water/through trees/through window blinds.
  3. Review the importance of medication adherence:
    a. Give oral and written dosing instructions.
    b. Refill the prescription before running out.
    c. Take the medication on a schedule (set a watch alarm, use a pill container, mark off the calendar). Taking an extra pill when a seizure aura occurs will not stop the seizure, as it is not absorbed fast enough.
    d. New prescription interaction profiles should be evaluated before starting new drugs.
    e. Clients should not use supplements, herbals, or over-the-counter (OTC) medications without checking with their health-care provider.
  4. Alcohol lowers the seizure threshold. Excessive alcohol use (greater than three drinks daily) increases the likelihood of seizures. Clients should have no more than one to two drinks a day.
  5. First aid for grand mal seizure:
    a. Stay calm.
    b. Time the seizure. Call 911 if the seizure lasts longer than 5 to 10 minutes.
    c. Clear the area to prevent harm from surrounding objects.
    d. Turn the person to the side and do not put anything in his or her mouth.
    e. Do not hold the person down.
    f. Place a soft object under the head to prevent head injury.
    g. Cardiopulmonary resuscitation (CPR) is not necessary unless the person stops breathing after the seizure.
    h. Stay with the person and reassure him or her.
    i. Help get the person home; call family or friends.
    j. Immediate transport to the ED is necessary for known conditions such as the following:
      i. Diabetes/hypoglycaemia.
      ii. Heat exhaustion.
      iii. Pregnancy.
      iv. Infection/high fever.
      v. Poisoning.
      vi. Head injury.
  6. First aid for petit mal seizures:
    a. Stay calm.
    b. Guide the client away from any dangers.
    c. Block access to hazards.
    d. Do not restrain the person.
    e. Stay with the person until full awareness returns.
C. Pharmacological treatment:
  1. There is controversy concerning whether to start AED therapy for the first seizure. AEDs are generally started after a second seizure. At least two seizures are required for a diagnosis of epilepsy.
  2. The prescription of AEDs should be individually weighed with a risk-versus-benefit decision that includes factors such as age; gender; family planning/desire for pregnancy; current driver; type/recurrence of seizure; abnormal EEG; concurrent medications used for other co-morbid conditions; history of depression, anxiety, suicidal ideation, and hepatic and renal disease; cost; client preference and lifestyle issues; and side-effect profile of medications (see Table 19.5).

TABLE: Antiepileptic Medications

Generic	Seizure Type	First-Line Treatment
Ethosuximide	Absence seizures	Adjunctive treatment
Lacosamide	Partial seizures	Adjunctive treatment
Zonisamide	Partial seizures	Adjunctive treatment
Rufinamide	LGS	Adjunctive treatment
Divalproex sodium	Absence seizures	First-line treatment
	Complex partial seizure	
Phenytoin	Tonic–clonic seizures	First-line treatment
	Psychomotor and neurosurgical-induced seizures	
Felbamate	Partial seizures LGS	Not first line in partial seizures and used as an adjunctive for LGS
Tiagabine	Partial seizures	Adjunctive treatment
Levetiracetam	Partial onset seizures	Adjunctive treatment for all types of seizures
	Myoclonic seizures	
	Generalized tonic–clonic seizures	
Clonazepam	Absence seizures LGS	First-line treatment
	Myoclonic seizures	
Lamotrigine	Partial seizures LGS	First-line treatment for LGS
Pregabalin	Partial onset seizure	Adjunctive treatment
Primidone	Focal and psychomotor seizures; tonic–clonic seizures	Not first-line treatment
Gabapentin	Partial seizures	Adjunctive treatment
Carbamazepine	Partial or mixed seizures	First-line treatment
	Generalized tonic–clonic seizures	
Topiramate	Partial onset seizures	First-line treatment and adjunctive for LGS
	Generalized tonic–clonic seizures LGS	
Oxcarbazepine	Partial seizures	Monotherapy or adjunct treatment
Valproate	LGS	First-line treatment in LGS
Magnesium sulphate	Eclamptic tonic–clonic seizure	First-line treatment

LGS, Lennox–Gastaut syndrome.

3. A neurological consultation should be obtained for full evaluation and prescription of AED with a neurologist or primary health-care providers managing subsequent follow-up.
4. A single-agent AED is started and titrated slowly to the lowest dose that is the most effective in seizure control with the least number of side effects:
   a. Ideally, the client should be maintained on one AED; however, combination therapy may be required or the first agent discontinued.
   b. When a second AED is required, the second additional medication is started by titration, a therapeutic level is achieved, and the first AED is subsequently tapered off. During this period of time there is an increase in side effects.
   c. Switching to a generic formulation has been noted to increase seizure activity.
   d. Rectal diazepam gel may be prescribed for use at home for clients with a history of prolonged seizures.
5. Stevens–Johnson syndrome (SJS) and toxic epidermal necrolysis (TEN) can occur up to four months after the institution of AEDs, including carbamazepine, oxcarbazepine, phenytoin, and lamotrigine.
6. Women of childbearing age should be routinely prescribed folate supplements. The folic acid supplements should be taken one to three months before conception when the client is on valproate or carbamazepine.

Follow-Up

A. Follow-up by primary health-care providers is dependent on the frequency of seizures, toxicity profile of AED, and other co-morbid conditions.
B. Subsequent visits include the following evaluations:
   1. Drug compliance.
   2. Seizure log/diary: a seizure diary is available through www.canadianepilepsyaliance.org.
   3. Drug levels, blood counts, and hepatic and renal function.
   4. Premenstrual serum levels when there is an increase in seizure activity the week before menstruation.
   5. Yearly drug levels are required for clients on a stable dose with no seizures.

C. There is an increased risk of suicide associated with several AEDs. Mood evaluation of the client one week after institution of therapy is prudent. Instructions should be given to notify the office concerning depression or suicidality:
   1. Perform serial depression/suicide screening.
   2. Psychiatric co-morbid conditions should be treated promptly.
D. Bone loss is noted with long-term therapy with AEDs; therefore, a dual-energy x-ray absorptiometry (DEXA) scan is warranted at intervals:
   1. Vitamin D and calcium may be prescribed with AEDs.
E. Clients taking AEDs need regular dental/oral care.
F. Address the legislative requirements around driving privileges in the client's province.
G. Consider a sleep study to evaluate for obstructive sleep apnoea.

Consultation/Referral

A. A neurology consultation is necessary for the evaluation and medication initiation. Ketogenic diets are usually reserved for exceptional cases when medications are insufficient for control; these clients require the expertise of a dietician to ensure healthy nutrient content and to recommend supplements.
B. A neurosurgical consultation is necessary to evaluate a vagus nerve stimulator (VNS) or surgical options:
   1. The VNS has been approved for intractable epilepsy refractory to medications.
C. Refer to an obstetrician for preconception consultation as well as for prenatal care.

Individual Considerations

A. Women:
   1. Preconception counseling and a planned pregnancy are imperative:
      a. Discuss the teratogenicity of AEDs:
         i. Attempt to decrease to monotherapy.
         ii. Taper doses of AEDs to the lowest possible dose.
         iii. If there is an absence of seizures for two to five years, consider a complete withdrawal of AEDs.
         iv. First-trimester use of one AED has been noted to have a two- to five-fold increase in major fetal anomalies such as neural tube defects, cleft lip and palate, and cardiac anomalies.
      b. Increase folic acid to 4 mg daily to help prevent neural tube defects.
      c. Stress the need for regular prenatal care.
      d. Offer maternal alpha-fetoprotein screening test.
      e. A fetal echocardiogram may be considered to diagnose cardiac defects.
      f. All care providers, including nurses, paediatricians, and anaesthesiologists, should be aware that the client has epilepsy on admission.
      g. Chronic hypertension develops in up to 78% of women with preeclampsia/eclampsia.
   2. Oral contraceptives are less effective on AEDs. The failure rate is 0.7 to 3.1 per 100 women. Women taking enzyme-inducing AEDs should use a backup method or alternative birth control like an intrauterine device (IUD). Enzyme-inducting AEDs include the following:
      a. Phenytoin.
      b. Phenobarbital.
      c. Carbamazepine.
      d. Ethosuximide.
      e. Felbamate.
      f. Topiramate.
      g. Oxcarbazepine.
   3. Estrogen and progesterone act on the temporal lobe where partial seizures often begin. Seizure patterns may change during menopause.
B. Paediatrics: A ketogenic diet may be prescribed under the care of a specialist.
C. Geriatrics:
   1. Seizures are likely to begin from 60 to 80 years of age.
   2. Management may be more difficult dependent on co-morbidities and the use of other medications.
   3. Older clients have an increase of falls and loss of independence.
   4. After stroke and dementia, epilepsy is the most common serious neurologic disorder in the elderly.
   5. Focus on cardiovascular and neurologic systems in the clinical physical evaluation in the elderly.
   6. Commonly prescribed AEDs include the following:
      a. Phenytoin:
         i. Most commonly prescribed AED in the elderly.
         ii. Use caution, as phenytoin interacts with digoxin and warfarin.
         iii. Causes sedation.
      b. Sodium valproate:
         i. Ataxia and tremor are not uncommon.
         ii. Can cause reversible extrapyramidal symptoms.
      c. Carbamazepine:
         i. Hyponatraemia can occur, especially with coadministration of a diuretic.
         ii. Increases warfarin metabolism.
      d. Lamotrigine:
         i. Requires a slow titration in the elderly.
      e. Levetiracetam:
         i. Mood and behavioural problems may occur.
      f. Ginkgo biloba is the most commonly used herbal for seizures in the elderly.

Resources

Canadian Epilepsy Alliance: www.canadianepilepsyalliance.org
Epilepsy Canada: www.epilepsy.ca

Bibliography

Cavazos, J. E. (2013, March 11). Epilepsy and seizures. *Medscape*. Retrieved from http://emedicine.medscape.com/article/1184846-overview

Cramer, J. A. (2010). *Seizure severity questionnaire v2.2 (baseline and follow-up versions)*. Retrieved from https://www.epilepsy.com/sites/files/atoms/files/SSQ%20BL%2BFU%20for%20academia%20use.pdf

Epilepsy Foundation. (n.d.-a). *Driver and the law*. Retrieved from http://www.epilepsy.com/search/site/driving?f[0]=bundle%3Adriving_laws

Epilepsy Foundation. (n.d.-b). *Febrile convulsions (3 months to 5 years)*. Retrieved from http://www.epilepsy.com/information/professionals/about-epilepsy-seizures/idiopathic-epileptic-seizures-and-syndromes-1

Epilepsy Foundation. (n.d.-c). *First aid for seizures*. Retrieved from http://www.epilepsy.com/learn/treating-seizures-and-epilepsy/first-aid/first-aid-resources

Epilepsy Foundation. (n.d.-d). *Injuries from seizures*. Retrieved from http://www.epilepsy.com/get-help/staying-safe/types-injuries

Epilepsy Foundation. (n.d.-e). *Photosensitivity and epilepsy*. Retrieved from http://www.epilepsy.com/learn/triggers-seizures/photosensitivity-and-seizures

Epilepsy Foundation. (n.d.-f). *Seizure provoking triggers*. Retrieved from http://www.epilepsy.com/learn/triggers-seizures

Epilepsy Foundation. (n.d.-g). *Seizures*. Retrieved from http://www.epilepsy.com/learn/types-seizures

Epilepsy Foundation. (n.d.-h). *Suicide risk*. Retrieved from http://www.epilepsy.com/article/2014/3/antiepileptic-drugs-and-suicidality

Epilepsy Foundation. (n.d.-i). *Treatment*. Retrieved from http://www.epilepsy.com/learn/treating-seizures-and-epilepsy

Seizure, Febrile (Child)

Cheryl A. Glass, Julie Adkins, and Donna Clare

Definition
Febrile seizures are the most common seizure of early childhood. The average age of onset is 18 to 22 months. Febrile seizures are of short duration, usually less than 5 minutes, and are generalized tonic–clonic convulsions; 4% to 16% have focal features. The seizures are associated with fever in the absence of central nervous system (CNS) infection, acute electrolyte imbalance, or any other defined cause for a seizure. Seizures lasting longer than 15 minutes require immediate medical attention. The majority of children with febrile seizures do not develop epilepsy.

There are three types of febrile seizures:

A. Simple seizures are brief (<15 minutes), generalized (without a focal component), and occur once during a 24-hour period. More than 90% of febrile seizures are simple.
B. Complex febrile seizures have at least one of the following features: Duration lasting longer than 15 minutes, multiple seizures in 24 hours, and focal features.
C. Symptomatic febrile seizure is noted with children with preexisting neurologic abnormality or acute illness.

Incidence/Prevalence
A. About 3% to 5% of children up to the age of 6 years develop seizures with a febrile illness. Approximately 35% of children have recurrent febrile seizures during subsequent illnesses within one year. It is estimated that 24% of children have a family history of febrile seizures, and 4% have a family history of epilepsy.
B. The risk of febrile seizures has been noted to increase slightly after the administration of measles, mumps, and rubella (MMR) and the measles, mumps, rubella, varicella (MMRV) vaccines. Studies show the risk is increased approximately 5 to 12 days after the first MMR is given.
C. Risk of febrile seizure has also been noted to increase the first 24 hours after receiving the inactivated influenza vaccine (IIV) at the same time as the pneumococcal 13-valent conjugate (PCV13) vaccine or the diphtheria, tetanus, acellular pertussis (DTaP) vaccine. It was not shown to occur when vaccines are given separately on different days. There has been an increased risk of seizure when giving the PCV13 alone.

Pathogenesis
A. Fever is characterized by a cytokine-mediated rise in core temperature as well as immunologic, neurologic, endocrinologic, and physiological changes. A febrile seizure is an abnormal electrical discharge of neurons in the cerebral cortex, causing tonic–clonic muscular contractions, induced by fever in children.
B. Febrile seizures have been identified from a combination of genetic and environmental factors. They are to an autosomal dominant inheritance, and a few other genes and chromosomal loci have been identified.

Predisposing Factors
A. Fever:
  1. Temperature of at least above 38.5°C. Most seizures occur with fever >39°C.
  2. More likely to occur with the maximal rate of temperature rise.
  3. May occur early or late in the course of the febrile illness.
  4. May occur before fever is apparent.
B. Family history of febrile seizures.
C. Family history of seizures.
D. Age:
  1. It occurs between six months and six years.
  2. Median age of onset is 18 months.
  3. Fifty percent of children have febrile seizures between 12 and 30 months.
E. Recent childhood immunizations.
F. Other neurologic abnormalities.
G. Viral infections.
H. Bacterial infections.

Common Findings
A. Fever.
B. Generalized tonic–clonic seizure lasting less than 5 minutes.
C. Staring and loss of muscle tone.
D. Staring and muscle stiffness/rigidity.

Other Signs and Symptoms
A. An altered state of consciousness after the seizure.
B. Vomiting.
C. Decreased feeding.

Subjective Data
A. Ascertain whether the child had a fever at the time of the seizure.
B. Ask the caregiver to describe how the child appeared before the seizure: lethargic, normal, or irritable.
C. Review what happened during the seizure: jerky movements of one extremity, blinking, and general convulsions with loss of consciousness.
D. After the seizure, determine whether the child was sleepy, confused, or normal.
E. Review what other symptoms, such as vomiting or diarrhoea, the child has and what treatment(s) have been given before presentation.
F. Note if this has ever happened before. If so, was it the same?
G. Assess the client's medical history and developmental course.
H. Elicit information about any family history of any type of seizures.
I. Is anyone else in the family or day care ill?

Physical Examination
A. Check temperature, pulse, respirations, blood pressure, and pulse oximetry.
B. Inspect:
  1. Observe overall appearance. Observe for seizure activity and level of consciousness (LOC): Unable to arouse? If able to arouse, is the client having trouble staying awake?
  2. Presence of difficulty breathing, grunting, and retractions.
  3. Presence and quality of crying: weak, high-pitched, or continuous crying.
  4. Inspect the head for the presence of bulging fontanelle (if applicable).
  5. Evaluate the eyes for the presence of petechiae; are they sunken?

6. Ears: Evaluate the tympanic membrane.
   7. Nasal examination for signs of sinusitis and nasal flaring.
   8. Oral examination for dry mucous membranes, erythema, and enlarged tonsils.
   9. Dermal assessment for cyanosis and pallor; check skin tone and turgor; evaluate for the presence of a rash.
   10. Nails: Check for prolonged capillary refill. A capillary refill of three seconds or greater is an intermediate risk for serious illness such as meningococcal disease.
   11. Check for nuchal rigidity/stiffness.
C. Auscultate:
   1. Heart.
   2. All lung fields for crackles and decreased breath sounds.
   3. All quadrants of the abdomen.
D. Palpate:
   1. Fontanelle (if applicable for age).
   2. Evaluate lymphadenopathy.
   3. Palpate the abdomen for masses, tenderness, and rebound.
E. Neurologic examination: Perform a complete neurologic examination, assessing all cranial nerves. Be alert for signs and symptoms of CNS infection: Stiff neck, lethargy, and confusion are highly indicative of CNS infection. The neurologic examination should be normal. Any abnormal neurologic findings are inconsistent with febrile seizures.

Diagnostic Tests
A. Pulse oximetry.
B. Complete blood count (CBC).
C. Blood chemistries are not indicated with febrile seizures unless electrolyte imbalance or other specific indications exist. Seizures that continue for more than five minutes should have electrolytes and glucose evaluated.
D. Urinalysis.
E. EEG is not indicated for febrile seizures; however, if neurologic signs are present or seizures are recurrent, an EEG and neurologic workup should be done.
F. Lumbar puncture is indicated if there are positive neurologic signs, especially in children 12 to 18 months and infants younger than 12 months who present after their first febrile seizure.
G. Consider chest x-ray for respiratory problems.
H. Consider stool cultures if indicated for diarrhoea.
I. CT and MRI imaging are not required for children with simple febrile seizures.

Differential Diagnoses
A. Rigours from fever.
B. Metabolic imbalances: hypoglycaemia, hyponatraemia, and hypomagnesaemia.
C. Syncope.
D. CNS infection: encephalitis, meningitis, and abscess.
E. Epilepsy.
F. Brain tumour.

Plan
A. General interventions:
   1. Tepid sponge baths have not been shown to be effective in the prevention of febrile seizures and are not recommended for the treatment of fever.
   2. Children with fevers should not be undressed or overwrapped.
   3. Support the client with positioning to prevent aspiration and trauma; maintain airway and administer oxygen. Do not try to pry the jaws open to place an object between the teeth.
B. Client teaching:
   1. *Refer to Client Teaching Guide: Febrile Seizures (Child).* Advise family that neurologic sequelae, intellectual impairment, and behavioural disorders are rare following febrile seizures.
   2. Advise parents that, if a child has a seizure, to lay the child on his or her side and do not try to restrict the child's movements or convulsions. Nothing should be placed in the mouth.
   3. Recommend timing the seizure to see how long the seizure lasts. Seizures that last five minutes or longer need immediate attention, and the child should be taken to the ED by calling 911.
   4. Never leave a child alone during a seizure.
   5. Acknowledge the parent's experience, including fear and helplessness.
C. Pharmacological treatment:
   1. Antipyretic agents do not prevent febrile seizures and are not used for prophylaxis. Ibuprofen or acetaminophen, using age and weight-appropriate doses every 4 hours, may be given for temperature elevation of 37.5°C.
   2. Antibiotics are not indicated for a fever without an apparent source.
   3. Neither continuous nor intermittent anticonvulsant therapy is recommended for children with one or more simple febrile seizures.

Follow-Up
A. See the client for repeat seizures and as needed.
B. Seizures lasting longer than 15 minutes require immediate medical attention.

Consultation/Referral
A. Consult a neurologist for uncontrolled or repeated seizures. When no fever is present, it may signal the onset of epilepsy and should be referred. Children who have experienced prolonged febrile seizures are more likely to develop a particular type of epilepsy (temporal lobe epilepsy [TLE]).
B. When meningitis cannot be eliminated by history and physical examination, the child should be admitted to the hospital.
C. If seizures are continuous, this is a medical emergency. The client should be sent to the hospital immediately by ambulance, and a neurologist should be consulted.

Individual Considerations
A. Paediatrics:
   1. The majority of seizures occur in children between the ages of 12 and 18 months, but can occur at any age.
   2. Approximately 30% to 35% of children who have had one febrile seizure are at risk of having another seizure.

Bibliography
Duffy, J., Weintraub, E., Hambidge, S. J., Jackson, L. A., Kharbanda, E. O., Klein, N. P., . . . DeStefano, F. (2016). Febrile seizure risk after vaccination in children 6 to 23 months. *Pediatrics*, *138*(1), 1–12. doi:10.1542/peds.2016-0320
El-Radhi, A. S. (2015). Management of seizures in children. *British Journal of Nursing*, *24*(3), 152–155. doi:10.12968/bjon.2015.24.3.152

▶ Client Teaching Guides are available at https://connect.springerpub.com/content/reference-book/978-0-8261-9498-5

Jeong, J. H., Lee, J. H., Kim, K., Jo, Y. H., Rhee, J. E., Kwak, Y. H., . . . Noh, H. (2014). Rate of and risk factors for early recurrence in clients with febrile seizures. *Pediatric Emergency Care*, *30*(8), 540–545. doi:10.1097/PEC.0000000000000191

National Institute of Neurological Disorders and Stroke. (2016). *Febrile seizures fact sheet*. Retrieved from www.ninds.nih.gov/disorders/febrile_seizures

Patel, N., Ram, D., Swiderska, N., Mewasingh, L. D., Newton, R. W., & Offringa, M. (2015). Febrile seizures. *British Medical Journal (Clinical Research Ed.)*, *351*, h4240. doi:10.1136/bmj.h4240

Patterson, J. L., Carapetian, S. A., Hageman, J. R., & Kelley, K. R. (2013). Febrile seizures. *Pediatric Annals*, *42*(12), 249–254. doi:10.3928/00904481-20131122-09

Transient Ischaemic Attack (TIA)

Cheryl A. Glass, Julie Adkins, and Donna Clare

Definition
A. Transient ischaemic attacks (TIAs) are brief focal brain deficits, spinal cord issues, or retinal ischaemia (without acute infarction) caused by vascular occlusion. Symptoms generally last less than an hour; however, they may have permanent sequelae. TIAs are considered as part of the stroke continuum: TIA, mild stroke, moderate stroke, and severe stroke. Approximately 15% of diagnosed strokes are preceded by TIAs. TIAs can be difficult to diagnose, as symptoms are transient. TIAs are considered a medical emergency.
B. TIAs present a unique opportunity to reduce the risk of stroke in individuals.

Incidence/Prevalence
A. The risk of stroke after a TIA is approximately 10% at two days, and up to 17% (17 out of 100 people) will have a stroke in the next 90 days.
B. Strokes occur at an earlier age in men and at a higher rate; however, over a lifetime, women have more strokes than men each year, because they live longer.
C. Fifteen percent of strokes are preceded by a TIA.
D. TIAs are a sign of atherosclerosis; coronary artery disease should be investigated in anyone presenting with TIA.

Pathogenesis
A. The pathogenesis is a neurologic event secondary to a temporary reduction of blood flow to the brain from a partially occluded vessel or related to an acute thromboembolic event.

Predisposing Factors
A. Hypertension is the greatest risk factor:
   1. Systolic blood pressure >140 mmHg.
   2. Diastolic blood pressure >90 mmHg.
B. Atherosclerosis.
C. African American.
D. Age older than 40 years.
E. Hypotensive episodes.
F. Oral contraceptives.
G. Atrial fibrillation.
H. Smoking.
I. Familial hyperlipidaemia.
J. Diabetes mellitus.
K. Valvular heart disease.
L. Infective endocarditis.
M. Migraine with aura.
N. Medications alter bleeding time and interact with warfarin:
   1. Feverfew.
   2. Garlic.
   3. Ginkgo biloba.
   4. Ginger.
   5. Ginseng.

Common Findings
Signs and symptoms depend on the affected vessel and surrounding brain tissue.
A. Acute onset of focal neurologic deficit:
   1. Limb weakness or numbness.
   2. Facial weakness.
   3. Speech difficulty to aphasia.
   4. Visual loss/blurring.
   5. Ataxia.
B. Acute change in level of consciousness (LOC) or confusion.
C. Posterior circulation TIAs may have a headache as one of the prodromal symptoms that precedes a stroke by days or weeks.
D. Basilar artery occlusion TIAs have vertigo, nausea, and headaches that may occur as early as two weeks or more before the onset of stroke.

Other Signs and Symptoms
A. Dysarthria.
B. Dysphagia.
C. Near syncope.
D. Hemiparesis.
E. Temporary monocular blindness.
F. Behaviour changes.
G. Vertigo.
H. Dizziness.
I. Diplopia.

Subjective Data
A. Ask detailed questions about symptoms before, during, and after the spell:
   1. Review the exact timing of onset of symptoms.
   2. How intense were the symptoms?
   3. What was the duration and the presence of any fluctuation of symptoms?
   4. Has there been a pattern that is becoming more frequent or escalating in symptoms?
B. Interview the client, family members, witnesses, and emergency personnel for their description of behaviour, speech, gait, memory, and movement.
C. Focus on precipitating factors and state of consciousness after the acute event.
D. Question the client about risk factors such as hypertension, smoking, cardiac disease, and heredity.
E. Review all medications, including anticoagulants, over-the-counter (OTC), herbals, and illicit drug use such as cocaine.
F. Review the medical history:
   1. Recent surgeries, specifically carotid or cardiac surgeries.
   2. Seizures.
   3. Central nervous system (CNS) infection.
   4. Illicit drug use.
   5. Presence of any metabolic disorders.
   6. Recent trauma (blunt or torsion injury to the neck).
   7. Atrial fibrillation.
   8. Heavy cannabis use or synthetic cannabis use.

Physical Examination
A. Check temperature, pulse, respiration, and blood pressure, including orthostatic blood pressure and pulse and pulse oximetry.

B. General observation:
  1. Observe overall appearance, LOC, ability to interact, language, difficulty swallowing, tremors, spasticity, as well as memory skills.
  2. Observe the client walking (cerebellar and motor systems).
C. Inspect:
  1. Dermal examination:
    a. Overall hydration status.
    b. Look for postcarotid endarterectomy scars, presence of a pacemaker, implantable cardioverter defibrillator, or other cardiac surgical scars.
  2. Check pupil size and reactivity to light.
  3. Perform a funduscopic examination to evaluate optic disc margins, retinal plaques, and pigmentation.
D. Auscultate:
  1. Heart for rate, rhythm, murmurs, or rubs.
  2. Lungs: Note respiratory rate and pattern.
  3. Carotid arteries for the presence of bruit.
E. Palpate extremities for irregular pulses and peripheral oedema.
F. Neurologic examination:
  1. Cranial nerve testing:
    a. Wrinkle forehead/raise eyebrows.
    b. Smile and show teeth.
    c. Stick out the tongue/lateral tongue movement.
    d. Ocular movements.
    e. Visual field.
  2. Motor strength:
    a. Shrug shoulders.
    b. Test muscle strength: Grasp hands and squeeze.
    c. Check reflexes of biceps, triceps, patellar, brachioradial, and Achilles.
  3. Sensory testing: Pinprick.
  4. Gait and posture (cerebellar system evaluation):
    a. Ocular movements.
    b. Gait.
    c. Finger-to-nose test.
    d. Heel-to-knee test.

Diagnostic Tests

A. Pulse oximetry and blood pressure.
B. Laboratory tests:
  1. Emergent labs:
    a. Glucose.
    b. Serum chemistry profile, including creatinine.
    c. Coagulation and hypercoagulablity testing.
    d. Complete blood count (CBC).
  2. Urgent labs:
    a. C-reactive protein.
    b. Cardiac enzymes.
    c. Lipid profile.
  3. Other laboratory tests based on history:
    a. Urine drug screen.
    b. Blood alcohol level and gamma-glutamyl transferase (GGT).
    c. Antiphospholipid antibodies.
    d. Rapid plasma reagin (RPR) for syphilis.
C. MRI or CT scan within 24 hours of symptom onset to rule out differentials like tumour or haemorrhage.
D. Carotid Doppler ultrasonography identifies clients with urgent surgical needs.
E. Cardiac imaging to evaluate cardioembolic sources (e.g., persistent foramen ovale or atrial septal defect).
F. EKG to evaluate for dysrhythmias (such as atrial fibrillation).
G. Lumbar puncture to rule out infection, demyelinating disease, and subarachnoid haemorrhage (SAH).
H. EEG as indicated for seizure activity.
I. Consider cardiac multiple-day Holter monitor for suspected intermittent atrial fibrillation.

Differential Diagnoses

A. Ischaemia stroke.
B. SAH/subdural haematoma (SDH).
C. Migraine.
D. Hypoglycaemia/hyperglycaemia.
E. Epilepsy—postictal period.
F. Malignant hypertension.
G. Brain tumour.
H. Bell's palsy.
I. Multiple sclerosis (MS).
J. Syncope.
K. Drug induced.
L. Concussion.
M. Vertigo.

Plan

A. General interventions:
  1. Carefully assess the client to timely diagnose TIA.
  2. Perform a full workup to determine the underlying disease process.
  3. Prevent stroke by modification of risk factors.
B. *Refer to Client Teaching Guide: Transient Ischaemic Attack.* ◀ Medical and surgical management.
  1. Treat TIAs with antiplatelet drugs as soon as intracranial bleeding is ruled out.
  2. Consider carotid endarterectomy.
  3. Hypertension and dyslipidaemia control.
  4. Glucose control.
  5. Smoking cessation.
  6. Eliminate or reduce alcohol consumption.
  7. Start exercise plan for losing weight. Recommend starting with about 30 minutes of exercise three times per week as tolerated.
C. Pharmacological treatment: The mainstay of treatment for TIA is pharmacological management with antithrombotic agents:
  1. Antiplatelet therapy:
    a. ASA.
    b. Dipyridamole may be given as an adjunct with warfarin therapy.
    c. ASA + dipyridamole extended release.
    d. Clopidogrel. ASA is not routinely recommended with clopidogrel because of the risk of haemorrhage. No dosage adjustment is necessary with clopidogrel for elderly clients or clients with renal disease.
    e. Ticlopidine is a second-line antiplatelet therapy for clients who cannot tolerate or do not respond to ASA therapy. In some circumstances, it can be an alternative to clopidogrel.
    f. Warfarin. Titrate for a goal international normalized ratio (INR) of 2.0 to 3.0.
    g. Direct oral anticoagulants (DOACs) like dabigatran and apixaban can also be used and are recommended for stroke prevention.
  2. Antihypertensive therapy as indicated to maintain blood pressure below 140/90 mmHg with an angiotensin

converting enzyme (ACE) inhibitor or an angiotensin receptor blocker alone or in combination with a diuretic.
3. Initiate a daily statin to a goal of low-density lipoprotein-cholesterol (LDL-C) <100 mg/dL.

Follow-Up
A. Rapid transfer is essential for a client with positive symptoms for risk stratification.
B. Clients with a suspected TIA who are not admitted to the hospital should have rapid access (within 12 hours) for an urgent assessment and evaluation with CT or MRI brain scan, EKG, and carotid Doppler testing.
C. Clients accessing outpatient services should know they should return to the clinic or ED immediately, if symptoms recur.
D. Specific follow-up depends on a etiology, severity, frequency, and duration of TIAs.
E. Follow-up laboratory testing as indicated (e.g., CBC, cholesterol, INR).
F. Monitor the client for occult bleeding if started on antiplatelet, antithrombic medications.

Consultation/Referral
A. TIA should be viewed as a medical emergency because these clients have salvageable neurologic function; consult with a specialist.
B. Cardiology and neurology consultations should be obtained when cardioembolic TIAs are treated with anticoagulation therapy.
C. Ophthalmologic consultation is indicated to assess the nature of transient visual symptoms.
D. Vascular surgeon consultation is necessary for clients with significant stenosis or occlusion. Clients with symptomatic carotid artery stenosis should have a surgical evaluation immediately.

Individual Considerations
A. Children: TIA aetiologies in children include the following:
   1. Congenital heart disease with cerebral thromboembolism.
   2. Drug abuse (e.g., cocaine).
   3. Clotting disorders.
   4. CNS infection.
   5. Marfan disease.
   6. Tumour.
   7. Idiopathic.
B. Adults:
   1. TIAs that occur in the younger adult population should be evaluated for embolism.
   2. Anticoagulation is not recommended for women younger than 65 years of age with atrial fibrillation who are otherwise at low risk for stroke. Antiplatelet therapy is recommended for this population.
C. Geriatrics:
   1. TIAs are most commonly seen in this population.
   2. Screen for atrial fibrillation in women, especially older than 75 years of age.

Resources
Client information on stroke prevention: *Taking Charge* http://www.strokebestpractices.ca
Heart and Stroke Foundation of Canada (2013): www.heartandstroke.com
Heart and Stroke Foundation *Stroke Assessment & Prevention Pocket Guide* http://www.strokebestpractices.ca

Bibliography
Hargroves, D., & Ward, L. (2015). Anticoagulants for stroke prevention in clients with atrial fibrillation. *British Journal of Neuroscience Nursing*, *11*(Suppl. 2), 31–37. doi:10.12968/bjnn.2015.11.Sup2.31
Jauch, E. (2016, March). Acute management of stroke. *Medscape*. Retrieved from http://emedicine.medscape.com/article/1159752-overview#a8
Nanda, A. (2016). Transient ischemic attack. *Medscape*. Retrieved from http://emedicine.medscape.comarticle/1910519-overview
National Institute of Neurological Disorders and Stroke. (2013). *NINDS transient ischemic attack information page*. Retrieved from www.ninds.nih.gov/disorders/tia/tia.htm?css=print
National Stroke Association. (n.d.). *National Stroke Association guidelines for the management of TIA*. Retrieved from www.stroke.org/site/Docserver/TIA_Guidelines_070506_sm.pdf?docID=2361
Nentwich, L. M. (2013, March 4). Transient ischemic attack. *Medscape*. Retrieved from http://emedicine.medscape.com/article/1910519-overview
Oikarinen, A., Engblom, J., Kääriäinen, M., & Kyngäs, H. (2015). Risk factor-related lifestyle habits of hospital-admitted stroke clients—An exploratory study. *Journal of Clinical Nursing*, *24*(15–16), 2219–2230. doi:10.1111/jocn.12787
Silver, B. (2015). Stroke prevention. *Medscape*. Retrieved from http://emedicine.medscape.com/article/323662-overview
Wein, T., Lindsay, M. P., Côté, R., Foley, N., Berlingieri, J., Bhogal, S., & Gladstone, D. J. (2017). Prevention of stroke. In *International Journal of Stroke* (6th ed.). Retrieved from http://www.strokebestpractices.ca/prevention-of-stroke/

Vertigo

Jill C. Cash, Julie Adkins, and Donna Clare

Definition
A. Vertigo is the illusion of self or environmental movement, typically rotating, spinning, tilting, and even a sensation that one is going to fall down. Older clients have an increased risk of falls and depression secondary to vertigo.
B. Vertigo is often classified as either central or peripheral in origin.

Incidence/Prevalence
A. Approximately 5% to 10% of the general population experience dizziness, vertigo, and imbalance. It reaches 40% in clients older than 40 years and decreases to 25% in clients older than 65 years.
B. It is estimated that approximately 0.5% of the population consults their primary health-care provider each year regarding vertigo.
C. All genders, as well as all age groups, are affected.
D. Benign paroxysmal positional vertigo (BPPV) is the most common cause of vertigo, excluding central nervous system (CNS) lesions:
   1. The prevalence of BPPV is 2.4%.
   2. BPPV rarely occurs in people younger than 35 years unless there is a history of head trauma.
   3. BPPV recurs in approximately one-third of clients after one year and in about 50% in all clients treated after five years.

Pathogenesis
A. Distinguishing between peripheral and central vertigo is critical because the evaluation, treatment, and progress vary significantly. Central vertigo suggests brainstem dysfunction affecting the vestibular nuclei or their connections. This may be secondary to a structural lesion such as neoplasm or ischaemia.
B. Vertigo, because of vascular insufficiency, is rarely isolated, and other symptoms of brainstem involvement are usually seen such as diplopia, dysphagia, motor weakness, or

disruption in sensation. Neoplasms are usually slow growing, and the vestibular dysfunction is often insidious. Other considerations for causes of central vertigo include multiple sclerosis (MS), seizures, and migraines.

C. Vertigo of peripheral origin is more common and may be caused by dysfunction of the inner ear or vestibular nerve. BPPV is the most commonly diagnosed peripheral vestibular disorder. The cause of BPPV is unknown. The most common explanation is free otoconia within the semicircular canals that are dislodged by trauma, infection, or degeneration. The debris relocates when the head is repositioned and provokes vertigo. Causes of labyrinthine dysfunction include infection, trauma, ischaemia, or toxins such as drugs or alcohol.

D. Ménière's disease causes vertigo, hearing loss, and ringing of the ears. The exact cause is unknown, but a hypothesis is a buildup of fluid in the inner ear.

E. Viral infections may lead up to vestibular neuritis (labyrinthitis). The vertigo experienced with vestibular neuritis is sudden and severe and may last days.

F. Other possible causes of vertigo are psychogenic, cardiovascular, metabolic, head trauma, and migraines.

G. Medications that cause dizziness:
 1. Anticonvulsants.
 2. Antidepressants.
 3. Antipsychotics.
 4. Anxiolytics/sedatives.
 5. Antihypertensives.
 6. Nitrates.
 7. Diuretics.
 8. Insulin/oral hypoglycemic agents.

Predisposing Factors
A. Head or body movement:
 1. Rolling over in bed.
 2. Getting out of bed.
 3. Bending down from the waist.
 4. Looking up.
B. Fear or anxiety.
C. Stress.
D. Recent infection, usually upper respiratory in cases of vestibular neuronitis.
E. Family history, especially in cases of vertiginous migraine.
F. Head trauma.
G. Migraines.
H. Idiopathic with no cause identified.
I. Hypoglycaemia.
J. Alcohol intoxication.
K. Medication side effects.
L. Cerebellar or brainstem stroke.
M. Tumours.
N. MS.
O. Dehydration.

Common Findings
A. Dizziness with or without change in body positioning.
B. Nausea/vomiting.
C. Tinnitus.
D. Aural fullness.
E. Hearing loss.

Other Signs and Symptoms
A. Central origin, including vascular insufficiencies, strokes, neoplasms, migraine, MS, and seizures:
 1. Double vision.
 2. Dysarthria.
 3. Dysphagia.
 4. Paraesthesias.
 5. Changes in motor or sensory examination.
 6. Mild to moderate vertigo.
 7. Multiple episodes of vertigo lasting seconds to minutes in duration with vascular insufficiency and seizures.
 8. Constant complaints of vertigo with neoplasms or strokes.
 9. Multiple episodes of vertigo lasting hours with migraines.
 10. Single episodes of vertigo with MS.
 11. Dix–Hallpike test: Habituation common with delayed nystagmus.
B. Peripheral origin, including BPPV, Ménière's disease, labyrinthitis, vestibular dysfunction, vestibular neuritis, and acoustic neuroma:
 1. No associated signs of brainstem dysfunction.
 2. Vertigo, usually described as severe.
 3. Multiple episodes of vertigo lasting hours with Ménière's disease.
 4. Single or multiple episodes of vertigo with labyrinthitis.
 5. Vestibular dysfunction, described as constant vertigo.
 6. Severe nausea or vomiting.
 7. Hearing loss or tinnitus; aural fullness may be present, as well as a roaring sound.
 8. Triad of vertigo, tinnitus, and hearing loss is suggestive of Ménière's disease.
 9. Dix–Hallpike test: No habituation: Nystagmus occurs immediately.

Subjective Data
A. Elicit onset, frequency, duration, and course of presenting symptoms:
 1. Is this recurrent or new?
    a. Acute vertigo is seen with trauma, stroke, meningitis, otitis media, mastoiditis, drug use, vestibular neuronitis, MS, and labyrinthitis.
    b. Recurrent vertigo is seen in migraines, BPPV, motion sickness, seizures, and Ménière's disease.
B. Elicit from the client a verbal description of the sensation(s) experienced.
C. Note triggering and alleviating factors.
D. Query the client regarding associated symptoms such as hearing loss, tinnitus, nausea, difficulty with gait, aural fullness, or other neurologic manifestations such as nystagmus.
E. Review the client's past medical history, including recent infections, trauma, risk factors for cardiovascular disease such as smoking, diabetes, and hyperlipidaemia.
F. Review over-the-counter (OTC) medications, herbal products, and medication use: aminoglycoside, antibiotics, diuretics, antihypertensives, and antidepressants.
G. Has the client had any previous treatments for vertigo such as an Epley procedure?
H. Has the client had any previous testing, such as the following:
 1. Audiometric testing.
 2. Electronystagmography (ENG)/videonystagmography (VNG) to evaluate balance.
 3. Rotational/balance platform test.
 4. CT or MRI.
 5. Computerized dynamic posturography (CDP) to evaluate postural stability/motor control.

Physical Examination
A. Check temperature (if indicated), pulse, respirations, and blood pressure; note orthostatic hypotension.

B. Inspect:
1. Observe overall appearance.

Generalized muscle weakness may be observed.

2. Note gait. Difficulty with tandem gait. Note global weakness.
3. Inspect the eyes. Assess for nystagmus; a few beats of nystagmus on extreme lateral gaze may be normal.
4. Ear examination. Rule out otitis media.
5. Evaluate for aphasia that may indicate a stroke.
C. Palpate extremities. Note pulses and oedema.
D. Neurologic examination:
1. Perform complete neurologic examination.
2. Perform Rinne and Weber's test.
3. Assess cranial nerves:
   a. Brainstem involvement is frequently seen with detailed neurologic examination. Signs of cerebellar dysfunction include difficulty with finger-to-nose testing, rapid alternating supination or pronation of hands, and gait disturbance.
4. Perform Romberg test: The client stands with feet together and closes his or her eyes. A positive result is when the client sways. This may be seen with vestibular disease and acoustic neuroma.
5. The Dix–Hallpike test (also called the Nylen–Bárány's maneuver test) is a provocative positional test. Perform the Dix–Hallpike: While the client is seated on the middle third of the examination table, turn the client's head 45 degrees toward the affected side (problem ear). While holding the head in that position, assist the client to the reclining position past the supine position. BPPV has a distinctive nystagmus in which there is involuntary eye movement (predominantly in a rotating fashion) starting slowly, progressing to a fast phase, and then entering a resetting phase. The nystagmus generally lasts <20 seconds and reverses itself upon the client sitting upright.

The Dix–Hallpike maneuver is considered the gold standard for diagnosing benign paroxysmal positional vertigo (BPPV). However, a negative test does not rule out BPPV if the client is asymptomatic on the date of the test. If a positive response is observed on the initial side, no further testing is required.

6. Test for nuchal rigidity if fever is present.
E. Auscultate:
1. Heart, neck, and carotid arteries. Auscultation may reveal cardiovascular abnormalities such as a carotid bruit.
2. Lungs—deep inspirations may cause dizziness.
3. Abdomen.

Diagnostic Tests
A. Laboratory testing:
1. Thyroid function studies: To rule out hypothyroidism.
2. Rapid plasma reagin (RPR): To rule out secondary or early tertiary syphilis, which can have symptoms similar to Ménière's disease.
3. Complete blood count (CBC): To rule out infection or severe anaemia.
4. Electrolytes: To rule out hyponatraemia, hypokalaemia, and dehydration.
5. Urine drug screen (if indicated).
6. Cardiac panel (if indicated).
7. Urinalysis to rule out a urinary tract infection (UTI) in the elderly.
B. CT scan for head trauma.
C. MRI with and without contrast to assess for mass, especially if a central origin is suspected.
D. Caloric test: Definitive procedure for identifying vestibular pathology.
E. Electronystagmography: Most useful in chronic peripheral disorders to determine the degree and progression of vestibular deficit.
F. Audiogram: Test for possible hearing loss.
G. Rotating chair test: Interprets the slow component velocity of the nystagmus response with bilateral canals stimulated.
H. Lumbar puncture if meningitis is suspected.

Differential Diagnoses
A. Vascular insufficiencies.
B. Stroke.
C. Neoplasms.
D. Migraine.
E. MS.
F. Seizures.
G. BPPV.
H. Ménière's disease.
I. Labyrinthitis.
J. Vestibular dysfunction.
K. Vestibular neuritis.
L. Acoustic neuroma.
M. Syncope.
N. Multiple sensory defects.
O. Parkinson's disease (PD).
P. Adverse reaction to medications.

Plan
A. General interventions: Treatment of vertigo depends on the underlying pathology and duration of the symptoms:
1. Acute vertigo: Maintain the client on bed rest, with the reassurance that most clients with acute vertigo recover spontaneously over a period of several weeks to months.
2. Chronic vertigo: Refer the client for physical therapy with emphasis on vestibular rehabilitation:
   a. Cawthorne Cooksey physical exercise regimen encourages eye, head, and body movements to facilitate recalibration of the vestibulo-ocular and vestibulo-spinal reflexes.
   b. Encourage ambulation when tolerated to induce central compensatory mechanism.
3. Ménière's disease: The client needs bed rest in the acute phase and nutritional therapy with restrictions of sodium, caffeine, alcohol, and tobacco.
4. BPPV:
   a. The client needs bed rest for acute symptoms. Keep head of bed up to allow canaliths to settle.
   b. Canalith repositioning procedures (CRP) provide immediate resolution of vertigo in 85% to 95% of clients. Epley procedure: The CRP is safe, simple, inexpensive, quick, and easy to perform. It is likely to be unsuccessful in clients with bilateral positional nystagmus, and it is not recommended for clients with acute vertigo, many of whom may have vestibular neuronitis. See Section II: Procedure, "Canalith Repositioning (Epley) Procedure for Vertigo." Potential referral to a physiotherapist or chiropractor trained in CRP, or a vertigo clinic, or a neurovestibular program.

Contraindications to performing the Epley procedure are the following:
  i. Recent neck fracture or neck instability.
  ii. A history of unstable carotid disease.
  iii. Recent retinal detachment.
  iv. Any physical condition that prevents the client from lying down quickly or rolling over required for the procedure.
  c. Instead, meclizine may be used for 1 to 2 weeks, and then the client is reassessed. Stop meclizine on the day the client returns; it may suppress the positional nystagmus.
  d. For clients with severe positional vertigo during the Dix–Hallpike maneuver, premedicate with a prochlorperazine suppository 1 hour before performance of the CRP.
  e. If the Dix–Hallpike is positive on the left, use a left-sided CRP. Conversely, if it is positive on the right, use a right-sided CRP. If the client has bilateral disease, refer him or her to an otolaryngologist or treat the more symptomatic side first. The condition may be bilateral.
  f. After the Epley procedures, different types of recommendations are made to prevent the otoconia from returning to their posterior semicircular canal, including the following:
    i. Wear a cervical collar for 2 nights after the maneuver.
    ii. Stay upright for 24 hours after the procedure or have the head elevated 30 degrees for 1 to 2 nights after the procedure.
    iii. Avoid sleeping with the affected ear down.
    iv. Counsel to avoid abrupt head changes for 1 week after the procedure.
    v. Avoid exercise, such as yoga and sit-ups, which would make similar motions.
    vi. Avoid looking up, such as looking at items on the top shelves at the grocery.
    vii. Symptoms may reoccur after tilting backward in dental chairs.
    viii. Symptoms may reoccur after turning in the hairdresser's chair and/or tilting backward for a shampoo.
B. Client teaching: Encourage compliance with bed rest and exercises.
C. Pharmacological treatment:
In Canada, American guidelines regarding pharmacological treatment are followed. The American Academy of Otolaryngology—Head and Neck Surgery does not recommend the use of vestibular suppressant medications to control BPPV. The American Academy of Neurology also reports that there is no evidence to support the routine use of vestibular suppressant therapy as the treatment for BPPV:
  1. Acute vertigo:
    a. Metoclopramide.
    b. Ondansetron.
    c. Dimenhydrinate.
    d. Promethazine.
    e. Dimenhydrinate.
    f. Diphenhydramine.
    g. Vestibular sedative:
      i. Cinnarizine.
      ii. Meclizine.
      iii. Diazepam.
  2. Chronic vertigo:
    a. Cinnarizine.
    b. Clonazepam.
    c. Carbamazepine.
  3. Ménière's disease:
    a. Diuretics such as hydrochlorothiazide and triamterene together will help with vertigo, but may not reduce hearing loss.
    b. Tricyclic antidepressants (TCAs) may be used in resistant cases.
  4. Antivirals are not useful for treatment of vestibular neuritis.
  5. Steroids have been used in the treatment of vestibular neuritis.
  6. Vestibular migraines respond to antimigraine medications.
D. Surgery:
  1. Pneumatic equalization tubes.
  2. BPPV surgery: canal partitioning or canal plugging.
  3. Vestibular nerve section (vestibular neurectomy) is a treatment for intractable violent episodes of BPPV.
  4. Labyrinthectomy to remove the semicircular canals, utricle, and saccule, the balance organs. This procedure is considered only when a person has already lost all hearing function in the affected ear.
  5. Chemical labyrinthectomy: Gentamicin infusion destroys the vestibular hair cells.

Follow-Up
A. Canadian practitioners refer to the American Academy of Otolaryngology—Head and Neck Surgery Foundation that recommends managing clients with BPPV as follows:
  1. CRP/Epley procedure should be offered unless there is a risk for impaired mobility or balance or the client is at increased risk of falls.
  2. Clients should be reevaluated in one month after an Epley procedure/CRP in order to confirm that the procedure resolved the symptoms of vertigo.
  3. The recurrence rate after an Epley procedure is 30% to 50%.
B. Follow up as needed according to the origin of the diagnosis and the client's needs.
C. If indicated, transfer to the ER/call 911 for cardiovascular and cerebrovascular symptoms for treatment of stroke or cardiac events.

Consultation/Referral
A. Refer to a specialist if the client does not experience improvement in two to four weeks. If symptoms worsen, consider referring to an ear, nose, and throat specialist.
B. Refer to an otolaryngologist for testing, including the following:
  1. Audiometric testing.
  2. ENG to evaluate balance.
  3. Rotational/balance platform test.

Individual Considerations
A. Paediatrics:
  1. The most common causes of dizziness in children are otitis media, migraine headaches, and BPPV.
  2. Concussion: Nausea, vertigo, and nystagmus are classic symptoms of a concussion.
  3. Drug overdoses and other poisons cause vertigo and nystagmus.
B. Geriatrics:
  1. Many of the medications, individually and especially in combination, used for vestibular suppression are on the

American Geriatrics Society Beers Criteria list of potentially inappropriate medications for older adults.

Resources
American Speech–Language-Hearing Association (ASHA): www.asha.org
Vestibular Disorders Association: www.vestibular.org

Bibliography
American Academy of Neurology Professional Association Model Policy. (n.d.). *Canalith repositioning procedure performed for patients with BPPV*. Retrieved from https://www.aan.com/policy-and-guidelines/quality/quality-measures2/quality-measures/other/canalith-repositioning-procedure-performed-for-patients-with-bppv/

American Academy of Otolaryngology—Head and Neck Surgery. (2016). *Mènière's disease*. Retrieved from www.entnet.org/Healthinformation/menieresDisease.cfm

Bhattacharyya, N., Baugh, R. F., Orvidas, L., Barrs, D., Bronston, L. J., Cass, S., . . . Fuller, D. C. (2017). Clinical practice guideline: Benign paroxysmal positional vertigo. *Otolaryngology—Head and Neck Surgery, 156*(3), S1–S47. doi:10.1177/0194599816689667

Furman, J. M. (2013). Client information: Dizziness and vertigo (beyond the basics). *UpToDate*. Retrieved from http://www.uptodate.com/contents/dizziness-and-vertigo-beyond-the-basics?view=print

Lo, A. X., & Harada, C. N. (2013). Geriatric dizziness: Evolving diagnostic and therapeutic approaches for the emergency department. *Clinics in Geriatric Medicine, 29*(1), 181–204. doi:10.1016/j.cger.2012.10.004

Vestibular Disorder Association. (n.d.-a). *Benign paroxysmal positional vertigo (BPPV)*. Retrieved from http://vestibular.org/understanding-vestibular-disorders/types-vestibular-disorders/benign-paroxysmal-positional-vertigo

Vestibular Disorder Association. (n.d.-b). *Mènière's disease*. Retrieved from http://vestibular.org/menieres-disease

Vestibular Disorder Association. (n.d.-c). *Surgical procedures for vestibular dysfunction*. Retrieved from http://vestibular.org/understanding-vestibular-disorders/treatment/vestibular-surgery

Vestibular Disorder Association. (n.d.-d). *Vestibular neuritis and labyrinthitis*. Retrieved from http://vestibular.org/labyrinthitis-and-vestibular-neuritis

20 Endocrine Guidelines

Addison's Disease

Jill C. Cash, Melissa A. Hall, and Kelly Power-Kean

Definition
A. Primary adrenal insufficiency resulting in glucocorticoid and mineralocorticoid insufficiency.

Incidence/Prevalence
A. Approximately 40 to 60 cases per million people; idiopathic autoimmune disease is more common in women and children. There is no racial predilection.

Pathogenesis
A. Autoimmune dysfunction of the adrenals accounts for up to 80% of cases; 10% to 20% of cases are attributed to tuberculosis (TB). At least 90% of the adrenal gland is destroyed, resulting in chronic cortisol deficiency, reduced aldosterone, and decreased adrenal androgens. As a result, volume and sodium depletions occur with potassium excess. The risk of death in clients with Addison's disease is two-fold that of the general population due to higher rates of cardiovascular disease, cancer, and infectious disease.

Predisposing Factors
A. Other autoimmune disorders:
  1. Diabetes mellitus (DM) type 1.
  2. Pernicious anaemia.
  3. Thyroid disorders.
B. Disseminated TB.
C. Gonadal failure.
D. Hypoparathyroidism.
E. Vitiligo.
F. Alopaecia areata.
G. Chronic active hepatitis.
H. Metastatic disease (especially lung and breast cancer).
I. AIDS.
J. Certain medications (e.g., ketoconazole, anticoagulants).
K. Fungal disease.
L. Bleeding diathesis (e.g., disseminated intravascular coagulation [DIC]).
M. Sepsis.
N. Metabolic stress.
O. Trauma.
P. Bilateral nephrectomy.
Q. Pituitary tumours.

Common Findings
A. Weakness.
B. Fatigue.
C. Anorexia.
D. Nausea.
E. Diarrhoea.
F. Abdominal pain.
G. Weight loss.
H. Hyperpigmentation.
I. Hypoglycaemia (more often in children).
J. Low libido.
K. Salt craving.

Other Signs and Symptoms
A. Proximal muscle weakness.
B. Failure to gain weight (children).
C. Muscle and joint pain.
D. Reduced axillary/pubic hair in women.
E. Amenorrhoea.
F. Hypotension.
G. Anaemia with the following:
  1. Lymphocytosis.
  2. Eosinophilia.
  3. Neutropaenia.
  4. Hyponatraemia.
  5. Hyperkalaemia.
  6. Hypoglycaemia.
  7. Hypercalcaemia.
H. Positive antiadrenal antibodies.
I. Low plasma cortisol or failure to rise after corticotropin (adrenocorticotropic hormone [ACTH]) administration.
J. ECG changes: decreased voltage, prolonged PR and QT intervals, and general slowed rhythm.

Missed or delayed diagnosis can lead to acute adrenal crisis, a medical emergency evidenced by sudden low back, abdominal, or leg pain; severe vomiting or diarrhoea; hypotension; and loss of consciousness.

Subjective Data
A. Determine extent of fatigue.
B. Elicit degree and location of weakness.
C. Question the client regarding appetite, nausea, or diarrhoea.
D. Evaluate food intake.
E. Determine the amount of weight loss or weight gain (children).
F. Discuss hypopigmentation or hyperpigmentation and whether it occurs on unexposed areas as well as exposed areas of the skin.
G. Note presence of abdominal, muscle, and joint pain.
H. Assess for light-headedness and/or fainting and when it occurs.

I. Inquire about the client's history of cancer or fungal infections.
J. Note last date of TB evaluation (purified protein derivative [PPD]) and results.
K. Determine HIV status or risk.
L. For women, discuss axillary and pubic hair distribution and note menstrual patterns.
M. Inquire about libido.
N. Inquire regarding cold intolerance.
O. Ask about recent illness and treatments.
P. Determine client's occupation in order to assess safety risk if weakness or dizziness present.

Physical Examination
A. Check pulse, respirations, and blood pressure (BP); pulse and BP while seated and standing; and weight.
B. Inspect:
   1. Observe overall appearance.
   2. Note hair distribution and skin pigmentation, especially sun-exposed surfaces.
C. Auscultate heart, lungs, and abdomen.
D. Palpate abdomen.
E. Musculoskeletal: Perform complete musculoskeletal examination.

Diagnostic Tests
A. Serum chemistry, electrolytes, urea, creatinine, glomerular filtration rate (GFR).
B. Complete blood count (CBC).
C. PPD.
D. Rapid ACTH test: Rapid ACTH stimulation test excludes or establishes adrenal insufficiency but does not differentiate between primary and secondary adrenal insufficiencies; with abnormal results (plasma cortisol <18–20 mcg/dL), proceed to plasma ACTH levels.
E. Plasma ACTH level.
F. Serum creatinine kinase (CK) levels.

Plasma ACTH level differentiates among primary (adrenal) and secondary (pituitary) or tertiary (hypothalamus) aetiologies (high plasma ACTH with primary insufficiency whereas normal or low with secondary insufficiency). The clinician can use ACTH–corticotropin-releasing hormone (CRH) to distinguish between pituitary and hypothalamic aetiologies.

G. Antiadrenal antibodies: A negative adrenal antibody test is observed in only 30% to 50% of persons with idiopathic Addison's disease and does not rule out adrenal insufficiency of autoimmune aetiology.
H. CT scan of adrenals.

Differential Diagnoses
A. Secondary adrenal insufficiency (usually after exogenous glucocorticoid therapy).
B. Hypothalamic/pituitary lesions.
C. Diabetic coma.
D. Salt-losing nephritis.
E. Acute infections.
F. Occult cancer.
G. Anorexia nervosa.
H. Hemochromatosis.
I. Acute poisoning.
J. Myasthenia gravis.
K. Pigmentation due to racial/ethnic variations.
L. Premature primary ovarian failure.
M. Testicular failure.
N. Pernicious anaemia.
O. Cancer.
P. Iatrogenic Cushing's syndrome.

Plan
A. General interventions:
   1. If primary adrenal insufficiency is established and the cause is not apparent, order adrenal CT scan to look for metastatic disease, sarcoidosis, and TB.
B. Client teaching:
   1. *Refer to Client Teaching Guide: Addison's Disease.* ◄
   2. Educate the client regarding adrenal crisis and encourage treatment before symptoms begin.
   3. Encourage the client to avoid contacts that predispose him or her to infections.
C. Pharmacological therapy:
   1. For adults, once-daily flurocortisone and hydrocortisone (first-line treatment) or cortisone acetate in two to three daily doses. The highest dose should be given in the morning when rising, the second dose in early afternoon (two hours after lunch in two-dose regimen) or at lunch, and the smallest dose in the afternoon not later than four to six hours before bedtime (in a three-dose regimen). Prednisone may be given as an alternative to hydrocortisone.
   2. Increase hydrocortisone dose or add prednisone if ill; if accompanied by diarrhoea, excessive sweating, or fever, the client should double the routine dose.
   3. Simultaneously decrease fludrocortisone about 50% to avoid salt retention and elevated BP.
   4. If serum aldosterone is undetectable, mineralocorticoid replacement is likely necessary in addition to glucocorticoid.
   5. Abrupt discontinuation of exogenous glucocorticoid administration after a course as short as three weeks may induce temporary secondary adrenal insufficiency, leading to decreased cortisol but normal or near-normal aldosterone production. This may occur up to 12 months after discontinuation of glucocorticoid therapy.
   6. Paediatrics:
      a. Hydrocortisone.
      b. Fludrocortisone acetate can be used in place of hydrocortisone, but caution should be used related to the variable 11 B-hydroxysteroid dehydrongenase type 1 activity in children and it is uncertain if the hydrocortisone dose equivalency used for the adult client applies to children.

Follow-Up
A. Plasma renin activity: When <10 ng/mL, this is a probable indication of adequate fludrocortisone dose.
B. Monitoring glucocorticoid replacement should be completed by using clinical assessment of body weight, postural BP, energy levels, and manifestations of glucocorticoid excess. Hormonal monitoring of glucocorticoid replacement is discouraged and dosage should be adjusted based on clinical response only.
C. Monitoring of mineralocorticoid replacement should be based primarily on clinical assessment, including salt craving, postural hypotension or ooedema, and serum electrolytes.
D. Consider annual TSH /T4 and hemoglobin A1C to rule out concomitate autoimmune disease.

▶ Client Teaching Guides are available at https://connect.springerpub.com/content/reference-book/978-0-8261-9498-5

Consultation/Referral
A. If Addison's disease is suspected, consult with an endocrinologist.
B. Consider Addison's disease in any client with hypotension and hyperkalaemia.
C. Clients should be seen annually by an endocrinologist or health-care provider with endocrine expertise. Infants should be seen every three to four months.

Individual Considerations
A. Pregnancy:
  1. Due to changes in plasma cortisol, diagnosis is based on lack of rise in plasma cortisol concentration after ACTH administration.
  2. Pregnant clients should be monitored for manifestations of over- or underreplacement with at least one assessment per trimester.
  3. An increased hydrocortisone dose should be implemented, especially in the third trimester, based on the individual's clinical course.
  4. If nausea and vomiting are problems, intramuscular glucocorticoid may be necessary.
  5. During labour an increased glucocorticoid dose, similar to surgery or stress dosing, should be implemented.
B. Paediatrics:
  1. Leading causes of Addison's disease are hereditary enzymatic defects, resulting in congenital adrenal hyperplasia (CAH), as well as idiopathic causes.
  2. Although rare in paediatrics, common presentations include malaise, nausea, vomiting, and weight loss. Poor vascular tone, hyperpigmentation, hyponatraemia, hyperkalaemia, and ketonaemia are classic findings.
  3. Medications should be adjusted with the child's growth.
C. Geriatrics:
  1. Urinary excretion rate of cortisol decreases by about 25%; serum level and response to ACTH stimulation are unchanged.

Safety Consideration: Clients receiving long-term replacement should carry a medication card as well as wear a medical alert bracelet or necklace. Parenteral therapy is required if clients are unable to take required replacement medication orally.

Bibliography
American Geriatric Society. (2014). GNRS: A core curriculum in advanced practice geriatric nursing. In Flaherty, E., & Resnick, B. (Eds.), *GNRS geriatric nursing review syllabus: A core curriculum in advanced practice geriatric nursing* (4th ed., pp. 506–529). New York, NY: American Geriatrics Society.

Arlt, W. (2015). Disorders of the adrenal cortex. In D. L. Kasper, A. S. Fauci, S. L. Hauser, D. L. Longo, & J. L. Jameson (Eds.), *Harrison's principles of internal medicine* (19th ed.). New York, NY: McGraw-Hill.

Bornstein, S. R., Allolio, B., Arlt, W., Barthel, A., Don-Wauchope, A., Hammer, G. D., & Torpy, D. J. (2016). Diagnosis and treatment of primary adrenal insufficiency: An endocrine society clinical practice guideline. *Journal of Clinical Endocrinology and Metabolism, 101*(2), 364–389. doi:10.1210/jc.2015-1710

Donohoue, P. A. (2016, March). Treatment of adrenal insufficiency in children. *UpToDate.* Retrieved from http://www.uptodate.com

El-Hussein, M. T., Power-Kean, K., Zettel, S., Huether, S. E., McCance, K. L., Brashers, V. L., & Rote, N. S. (2018). *Understanding pathophysiology.* Milton, ON: Elsevier.

Lee, A. (Ed.). (2016). *NPPR: Nurse practitioners' prescribing reference.* New York, NY: Haymarket Media.

Medical Council of Canada. (2018). *Clinical laboratory tests: Normal values.* Retrieved from https://mcc.ca/objectives/normal-values/?cn-reloaded=1

Nieman, L. K. (2014a, December). Diagnosis of adrenal insufficiency in adults. *UpToDate.* Retrieved from http://www.uptodate.com

Nieman, L. K. (2014b, December). Treatment of adrenal insufficiency in adults. *UpToDate.* Retrieved from http://www.uptodate.com

Prescriber's Letter. (2015). Appropriate medication use in older adults: 2015 updated. *Beer's Criteria, 22*(12), 311218. Retrieved from http://prescribersletter.therapeuticresearch.com

Stewart, P. M., & Newell-Price, J. D. (2016). The adrenal cortex. In S. Melmed, K. S. Polonsky, P. R. Larsen, & H. M. Kronenberg (Eds.), *Williams textbook of endocrinology* (13th ed., pp. 490–556). Philadelphia, PA: Elsevier.

Cushing's Syndrome

Jill C. Cash, Melissa A. Hall, and Kelly Power-Kean

Definition
A. Cushing's syndrome is a cluster of symptoms, signs, and biochemical abnormalities arising from glucocorticoid overproduction. Iatrogenically induced Cushing's syndrome is the most common cause.

Incidence/Prevalence
A. The prevalence in Canada of Cushing's syndrome is 5.5 clients per 100,000; it is five times more frequent in women.

Pathogenesis
The cause is exogenous (chronic glucocorticoid or adrenocorticotropic hormone [ACTH] administration) or endogenous (increased ACTH secretion). The endogenous type is due to either excessive pituitary or ectopic ACTH secretion (ACTH dependent), resulting in signs of androgen excess or autonomous cortisol overproduction (ACTH independent [of ACTH regulation]), as well as depressed ACTH production and absent signs of androgen excess. The aetiology of spontaneous Cushing's (adults) comprises the following:
A. 70% to 80% pituitary ACTH hypersecretion (90% pituitary adenoma, 10% pituitary hyperplasia).
B. 10% to 15% autonomous adrenal tumour (adenoma or carcinoma).
C. 5% to 15% ectopic ACTH secretion (nonpituitary neoplasm, usually lung).
D. <1% bilateral nodular hyperplasia without ACTH.
E. Among children younger than 12 years, the cause is usually iatrogenic. Cortisol excess precipitates generalized protein catabolism, reduced intestinal calcium reabsorption, elevated hepatic gluconeogenesis and glycogenosis, impaired collagen production leading to atrophy of connective and fatty tissues, impaired immune and inflammatory responses, and accelerated atherosclerosis.

Predisposing Factors
A. Exogenous glucocorticoid administration.
B. Excessive alcohol intake.
C. Pituitary adenoma.
D. Thoracic tumours.
E. Adrenal neoplasms.
F. Tumours of the pancreas.
G. Thyroid and thymus disease.
H. Pheochromocytoma.

Common Findings
A. Excessive coarse hair on face, chest, and back.
B. Rapid weight gain.
C. Easy bruising.

D. Muscle weakness.
E. Oligo- or amenorrhoea.
F. Impotence.
G. Depression.
H. Poorly controlled diabetes.
I. Irregular menses.

Other Signs and Symptoms
A. Cervicodorsal and supraclavicular fat pad.
B. Hirsutism in women.
C. Acne and/or folliculitis.
D. Increased intraocular pressure.
E. Purple striae.
F. Increased blood pressure (BP).
G. Polydipsia/polyuria, increased serum glucose, and glycosuria.
H. Osteopaenia/osteoporosis.
I. Mood lability/changes.
J. Growth deceleration (children).
K. Delayed skeletal maturation (children).
L. Spontaneous hypokalaemia.
M. Erythrocytosis.

Subjective Data
A. Ask whether the client has taken exogenous glucocorticoids.
B. Determine whether the onset of complaints was acute or subacute.
C. Assess for bruising and determine whether bruising was precipitated by trauma.
D. Assess for muscle weakness and, if present, whether it is proximal weakness.
E. Review the client's menstrual history, including characteristics of menstrual periods.
F. Identify the client's family history of similar problems.
G. Question the client regarding any vision impairment.
H. Rule out the presence of abdominal pain.
I. Review the client's history of neoplasms and location.
J. Identify the current pattern of sexual function.
K. Question the client regarding mood swings or recent treatment for psychiatric disorder.
L. Identify the pattern of weight gain and effectiveness of weight-loss interventions, if implemented.
M. Assess for the presence of leg or arm pain.
N. Review the client's history of fractures, especially if postmenopausal.
O. Determine the amount of alcohol consumed.

Physical Examination
A. Check pulse, height, and weight.
B. Inspect:
   1. Inspect the skin, noting hair distribution, lesions, bruising, and striae.
   2. Observe the face and note shape.
   3. Observe the neck.

Note that a "moon-shaped" face and fat pads in posterior neck ("buffalo hump") are characteristics of clients with Cushing's syndrome.

   4. Complete a funduscopic examination. Be alert for cataracts, glaucoma, and/or signs of benign intracranial hypertension.

C. Auscultate:
   1. Auscultate the heart and lungs.
   2. Hypercoagulable state should be considered with risk for pulmonary embolism.
D. Musculoskeletal:
   1. Complete musculoskeletal examination. Be alert for septic necrosis of femoral and/or humeral head.
   2. Assess for kyphosis or back pain associated with osteoporosis and long-term cortisol excess.
E. Peripheral vascular: Assess for deep vein thrombosis due to the hypercoagulable state.

Diagnostic Tests
A. Serum electrolytes.
B. Complete blood count (CBC) and glucose.
C. 24-hour urine-free cortisol (at least two measurements).
D. Late-night salivary cortisol (at least two measurements).
E. Late-night serum cortisol (typically inpatient study).
F. Overnight dexamethasone suppression test.
G. Bone density studies.

The overnight dexamethasone suppression test has a false-positive rate of 20% to 30%; false positives can occur with obesity, stress, depression, alcoholism, pregnancy, or medications that increase the hepatic metabolism of cortisol and dexamethasone (e.g., antiseizure drugs, estrogen, and rifampin). The false-negative rate is <3%. Use the low-dose dexamethasone test as an alternative. The 24-hour urinary-free cortisol is the most sensitive and specific test and is the best choice for screening.

If any of the earlier initial lab screenings are positive, the client should be referred to endocrinology for additional evaluation.

Differential Diagnoses
A. Iatrogenically induced Cushing's syndrome.
B. Depression.
C. Severe obesity.
D. Chronic stress.
E. Familial cortisol resistance.
F. Medication induced (e.g., phenytoin, phenobarbital, primidone).
G. Pituitary adenoma.
H. Adrenal and other neoplasms.
I. Alcoholism.
J. Nephrolithiasis.
K. Psychosis.

Plan
A. General interventions:
   1. Taper glucocorticoid dose as appropriate for the underlying disease.
   2. Begin alcohol detoxification if applicable.
   3. Consider hormone replacement therapy for postmenopausal women.
B. Client teaching: *Refer to Client Teaching Guide: Cushing's Syndrome.*
C. Medical/surgical management: If noniatrogenic aetiology, surgery is the treatment of choice followed by irradiation and/or chemotherapy.
D. Pharmacological therapy:
   1. Calcium and vitamin D.

2. Mitotane for control of adrenocortical carcinoma progression.
3. Metyrapone inhibits adrenal steroid biosynthesis.
4. Ketoconazole (most useful for blocking adrenal steroidogenesis) and suramin inhibit adrenal steroid biosynthesis. Ketoconazole is associated with hepatic failure and drug–drug interactions, resulting in fatal ventricular arrhythmias. An endocrinologist should be consulted before the use of oral ketoconazole. Avoid use in pregnancy.
5. Hydrocortisone may be given in physiological doses to avoid adrenal insufficiency.

Most persons on a daily steroid program for more than two to four weeks have some degree of hypothalamic–pituitary–adrenal axis suppression.

6. Mifepristone is given for ectopic ACTH production or adrenal carcinoma. Mifepristone is an abortifacient.

Follow-Up
A. At the provider's discretion, one to two weeks after tests are complete, follow up to discuss results and possible therapy.

Consultation/Referral
A. If Cushing's syndrome is suspected, consult with an endocrinologist regarding treatment and therapy.

Individual Considerations
A. Pregnancy: Urinary-free cortisol increases in the third trimester, but women still have normal 17-hydroxycorticosteroids and normal diurnal variability of serum cortisol. Dexamethasone testing is not recommended in the initial screening for Cushing's syndrome during pregnancy.
B. Paediatrics: It is possible to differentiate between exogenous obesity and Cushing's syndrome by the child's growth rate; exogenous obesity is characterized by normal or slightly increased growth rate.

Resource
National Adrenal Diseases Foundation: www.nadf.us/links-resources/international-adrenal-disease-groups-resources

Bibliography
Centers for Disease Control and Prevention, NCHS National Center for Health Statistics. (n.d.). *Clinical growth charts*. Retrieved from https://www.cdc.gov/growthcharts

El-Hussein, M. T., Power-Kean, K., Zettel, S., Huether, S. E., McCance, K. L., Brashers, V. L., & Rote, N. S. (2018). *Understanding pathophysiology*. Milton, ON: Elsevier.

James, P. A., Oparil, S., Carter, B. L., Cushman, W. C., Dennison-Himmelfarb, C., Handler, J., & Ortiz, E. (2013, December 18). 2014 Evidence-based guidelines for the management of high blood pressure in adults report from the panel members appointed to the Eighth joint national committee (JNC 8). *Journal of the American Medical Association, 311*(5), 507–520. doi:10.1001/jama.2013.284427

Lee, A. (Ed.). (2016). *NPPR: Nurse practitioners' prescribing reference*. New York, NY: Haymarket Media.

Medical Council of Canada. (2018). *Clinical laboratory tests: Normal values*. Retrieved from https://mcc.ca/objectives/normal-values/?cn-reloaded=1

Nieman, L. K. (2014, May). Causes and pathophysiology of cushing's syndrome. *UpToDate*. Retrieved from http://www.uptodate.com

Nieman, L. K. (2015a, June). Establishing the diagnosis of cushing's. *UpToDate*. Retrieved from http://www.uptodate.com

Nieman, L. K. (2015b, July). Epidemiology and clinical manifestations of cushing's syndrome. *UpToDate*. Retrieved from http://www.uptodate.com

Nieman, L. K., Biller, B. M. K., Findling, J. W., Murad, M. H., Newell-Price, J., Savage, M. O., & Tabarin, A. (2015). Treatment of cushing's syndrome: An endocrine society clinical practice guideline. *Journal of Clinical Endocrinology and Metabolism, 100*(8), 2807–2831. doi:10.1210/jc.2015-1818

Skelton, J. A. (2016, November). Management of childhood obesity in the primary care setting. *UpToDate*. Retrieved from http://www.uptodate.com

Stewart, P. M., & Newell-Price, J. D. (2016). The adrenal cortex. In S. Melmed, K. S. Polonsky, P. R. Larsen, & H. M. Kronenberg (Eds.), *Williams textbook of endocrinology* (13th ed., pp. 490–556). Philadelphia, PA: Elsevier.

Uum, S. V., Hurry, M., Petrella, R., Koch, C., Dranitsaris, G., & Lacroix, A. (2014). Management of clients with cushing's disease: A Canadian cost of illness analysis. *Journl of Population Therapeutics and Clinical Pharmacology, 21*(3), 508–517.

Diabetes Mellitus

Jill C. Cash, Melissa A. Hall, and Kelly Power-Kean

Definition
Diabetes is a group of diseases characterized by high levels of blood glucose with a defect in insulin secretion or action caused by a chronic disorder of carbohydrate, fat, and protein metabolism. There are four categories of diabetes: type 1, type 2, gestational, and other specific types including genetic-defined forms and those related to other diseases or medication use.
A. Type 1 diabetes, formerly referred to as insulin-dependent diabetes mellitus (IDDM) or juvenile-onset diabetes, is an endocrine condition in which there is complete destruction of pancreatic beta cells or a complete absence of insulin.
B. Type 2 diabetes, formerly referred to as noninsulin-dependent diabetes mellitus (NIDDM) or adult-onset diabetes, describes a condition in which individuals have an impairment in insulin production and/or insulin resistance.
C. Gestational diabetes is diagnosed during pregnancy. It usually disappears when the pregnancy is completed. It will increase the woman's risk of developing type 2 diabetes later in life.
D. Diabetes resulting from other specific causes is due to genetic defects and/or diseases of the pancreas, such as cystic fibrosis or other endocrinopathies. Other causes of this type of diabetes can be medication/chemical-induced diabetes from therapies used when treating HIV/AIDS, in clients who receive treatments after organ transplantation, and other chronic diseases.
E. People with diabetes are more prone to have unhealthy low-density lipoprotein cholesterol (LDL-C) and therefore are at increased risk for atherosclerotic cardiovascular disease (ASCVD). The incidence of cardiovascular disease (CVD) is two to four times higher in adults with diabetes. The risk of stroke is two to four times higher because 60% to 65% of the clients have hypertension.

Incidence/Prevalence
A. It is estimated that 3.4 million Canadians have diabetes, 9.3% of the population. It is also estimated that 5.7 million Canadians over the age of 20 years have prediabetes, 22.1% of the population. Approximately one million Canadians have diabetes but have not been diagnosed. It is estimated that by the year 2025, five million, or 12.1% of the population, will have diabetes. Type 1 diabetes accounts for approximately 9% to 10% of diagnosed cases. Some populations are at a greater risk of type 2 diabetes, such as those of South Asian, Asian, African, Hispanic, and Indigenous descent; and those

who are overweight, older, or have low income. Diabetes rates are 3.5% higher in Indigenous populations.

Pathogenesis

A. Type 1 diabetes is an inherited defect causing an alteration in immunologic integrity, placing the beta cell at risk for inflammatory damage. The mechanism of damage is autoimmune. Environmental factors that may influence the aetiology of diabetes include viral illnesses: mumps, coxsackievirus, cytomegalovirus, and hepatitis. Other factors that may influence the disease include diets high in dairy products, emotional and physical stress, and/or environmental toxins.
B. Type 2 diabetes involves impaired insulin secretion, insulin resistance, and/or an abnormally elevated glucose production by the liver. Genetics and obesity are major risk factors.
C. The severity of carbohydrate intolerance in gestational diabetes is unknown. Women identified as high risk of undiagnosed type 2 diabetes should have early screening at <20 weeks' gestation with a hemoglobin A1C. All women without known preexisting diabetes should have screening done during the second and 28th weeks of gestation.
D. Genetic defects and medications/chemicals are thought to affect the beta-cell function and alter insulin function. Hemoglobin A1C levels may not be interpreted correctly in clients with blood disorders such as anaemia/hemoglobinopathies. See www.ngsp.org/interf.asp for a complete list of laboratory methods recommended to be used to measure hemoglobin A1C values for clients with hemoglobin variants (sickle cell trait, HbC, HbS, HbE, HbD trait, or elevated HbF).

The Diabetes Canada (formally the Canadian Diabetes Association) has published comprehensive clinical practice guidelines for the prevention and management of diabetes in Canada. A free copy of this document may be obtained at guidelines.diabetes.ca/cpg

Predisposing Factors

A. Body mass index (BMI) ≥ 27 kg/m^2.
B. Physical inactivity.
C. First-degree relative with type 1 or type 2 diabetes
D. Hemoglobin A1C $\geq 5.7\%$, impaired glucose tolerance (IGT) or impaired fasting glucose (IFG) on previous testing.
E. Indigenous, Hispanic, Asian, and African American.
F. Hypertension with systolic pressure >140 mmHg and diastolic pressure >90 mmHg.
G. High-density lipoprotein (HDL) level of 1.0 mmol/L or less and/or triglyceride level of ≥ 1.7 mmol/L.
H. History of giving birth to babies larger than nine pounds or gestational diabetes.
I. History of IGT or fasting glucose.
J. Acanthosis nigricans or severe obesity.
K. Polycystic ovarian syndrome (PCOS).
L. History of CVD.
M. History of gestational diabetes.
N. Diabetes Canada recommends screening for type 2 diabetes using a fasting plasma glucose and/or A1C every three years in individuals ≥ 40 years of age or in individuals at high risk on a risk calculator (Canadian Diabetes Risk [CANRISK] www.healthycanadians.gc.ca/diseases-conditions-maladies-affections/disease-maladie/diabetes-diabete/canrisk/index-eng.php). It is advised to screen earlier and more frequently (every six to 12 months) for those with additional risk factors for diabetes or those at very high risk, using the diabetes risk calculator.

Common Findings

A. Classic triad of symptoms:
  1. Polyuria.
  2. Polydipsia.
  3. Polyphagia.
B. Weight loss.
C. Lack of energy.
D. Recurrent infections (urinary tract, vaginal, skin breakdown that is slow to heal).
E. Asymptomatic.

Other Signs and Symptoms

A. Weakness.
B. Fatigue.
C. Nausea and vomiting.
D. Abdominal pain.
E. Anorexia.
F. Sexual dysfunction, including impotence or dyspareunia.
G. Itching.
H. Visual disturbances.
I. Signs and symptoms related to nephropathy, neuropathy, and/or retinopathy.

Subjective Data

A. Obtain a detailed history regarding onset, duration, and course of presenting symptoms.
B. Question the client regarding all characteristic signs and symptoms of diabetes.
C. Determine the client's nutritional status, 24-hour recall, weight history, and eating patterns.
D. Review the family history of diabetes or other endocrine disorders.
E. Note predisposing factors to diabetes.
F. Review the client's social history, including smoking, alcohol, and exercise.

Physical Examination

A. Check pulse, respirations, blood pressure (BP), weight, and waist circumference.
B. Inspect:
  1. Observe overall appearance.
  2. Perform oral examination. Diabetic clients are prone to thrush, gingivitis, plaque, and infections. A dental examination should be done every six months.
  3. Complete funduscopic examination. Proliferative diabetic retinopathy is the most common eye disease in Canada. Clients with diabetes are 25 times more at risk for blindness and have four to six times the increased risk for cataracts and twice the increased risk for glaucoma.
  4. Inspect the skin, including feet, with monofilament testing, hands, fingers, and skin folds for erythema and insulin injection sites.
C. Auscultate the heart, lungs, and carotid arteries.
D. Percuss the chest, abdomen, and deep tendon reflexes.
E. Palpate:
  1. The neck (thyroid).
  2. The abdomen.
  3. The extremities for oedema and assess peripheral pulses.

Diagnostic Tests

A. Serum glycosylated hemoglobin A1C of 6.5% or higher.
B. Fasting plasma glucose: ≥ 7 mmol/L. All clients should have a baseline fasting blood sugar (fasting for at least eight hours) performed at 40 years of age, then repeated every

three years. The baseline should be performed earlier if any predisposing factors exist.
C. Random plasma glucose: ≥11.1 mmol/L with symptoms of diabetes.
D. Oral glucose tolerance test (OGTT): After a 75-g glucose load, a two-hour plasma glucose ≥11.1 mmol/L; IGT is a fasting plasma glucose between 7.8 and 11.0 mmol/L.

According to the Diabetes Control and Complications Trial, a hemoglobin A1C of 7.2% or below decreases the risk of retinopathy, neuropathy, and nephropathy by 50% to 70%.

Differential Diagnoses
A. Benign pancreatic insufficiency.
B. Pheochromocytoma.
C. Cushing's syndrome.
D. History of corticosteroid use.
E. Stress hyperglycaemia.
F. Acromegaly.
G. Hemochromatosis.
H. Somogyi phenomenon: Early-morning hyperglycaemia due to very early morning (2:00–3:00 a. m.) hypoglycaemia.

Plan
A. General interventions:
  1. Establish, review, and evaluate individual goals with the client on a routine basis.
  2. Center goals around normal metabolic control and the prevention and delay of complications while maintaining a flexible, normal, high-quality life.
  3. After a new diagnosis is made and treatment has begun, be alert for an initial remission or a honeymoon phase with decreased insulin needs and better control that may last three to six months.
  4. Include the following in the treatment plan:
   a. Exercise plan:
     i. Develop a consistent, individualized exercise plan with the client to improve insulin sensitivity, blood sugars, weight reduction, and reduction of cardiovascular complications. At least 150 minutes per week of aerobic exercise and at least two sessions per week of resistance exercise are recommended, though smaller amounts of activity still provide some health benefits.
     ii. Evaluation by a health-care provider, including a complete physical examination, should precede any exercise program. A resting EKG should be performed, and an exercise EKG stress test should be considered, for individuals with typical or atypical chest discomfort, unexplained dyspnoea, peripheral arterial disease, carotid bruits or history of angina, myocardial infarction (MI), stroke, or transient ischaemic attacks who wish to undertake exercise more intense than brisk walking.
     iii. Generally, the goals for physical activity are to reduce LDL-C and non-HDL-C and to lower the BP. The exercise should be of moderate to vigorous intensity.
     iv. In individuals with type 2 diabetes, exercise should be completed with caution if the fasting blood sugar is >16.7 mmol/L. The individual should ensure good hydration, be feeling well, and monitor for signs and symptoms of dehydration during the exercise regimen. In the individual with type 1 diabetes, if the fasting blood sugar is >16.7 mmol/L and the person does not feel well, urine or blood ketones should be tested. If ketone levels are elevated in the blood (≥1.5 mmol/L) or in the urine (2 + or ≥4 mmol/L), it is suggested that vigorous exercise be postponed until insulin is given (with carbohydrate, if necessary) and ketones are no longer elevated. If ketones are negative or "trace" and the person feels well, it is not necessary to defer exercise due to hyperglycaemia.
     v. Because exercise can lower the blood sugar concentration, special precautions such as medication adjustment and meal planning should be done before and after exercise if the client is taking insulin or a glucose-lowering medication.
   b. Self-monitoring blood glucose (SMBG): The process of monitoring the client's blood gives valuable information to the client on a daily basis and assists the provider in identifying trends:
     i. Several different metres are available with a variety of options. A certified diabetes educator or a pharmacist can show examples of different types before the client purchases one.
     ii. Frequency of testing depends on the type of medication the client is taking and the client's compliance and motivation.
     iii. Additional testing should be done at times of changes in medication, meal plans, and/or exercise, and during illness or stress.
     iv. An automatic blood glucose suspend feature for continuous blood glucose monitoring is recommended for clients with hypoglycaemia unawareness or frequent nocturnal hypoglycaemia.
   c. Psychosocial support: It is important from the beginning of treatment to give the client a sense of control:
     i. Consistent involvement of family members will influence compliance.
     ii. Assess and discuss psychosocial issues at each visit, including depression.
B. Client teaching:
  1. *Refer to Client Teaching Guide: Diabetes.* ◀
  2. Topics in the educational plan include the pathophysiology of diabetes, procedures for SMBG and medication therapies, recognition and treatment of hypoglycaemia, and instructions for special situations such as illness and traveling.
  3. Include preventive care, instructions for family members, and the importance of a MedicAlert tag (available at www.medicalert.ca/).
  4. Smoking cessation and avoidance of all tobacco products should be advised to all clients. Counselling regarding smoking/tobacco cessation methods and classes should be offered.
C. Dietary/physical activity management:
  1. Nutritional plan: The client should meet with a dietitian who has experience with diabetes nutritional therapy.

▶ Client Teaching Guides are available at https://connect.springerpub.com/content/reference-book/978-0-8261-9498-5

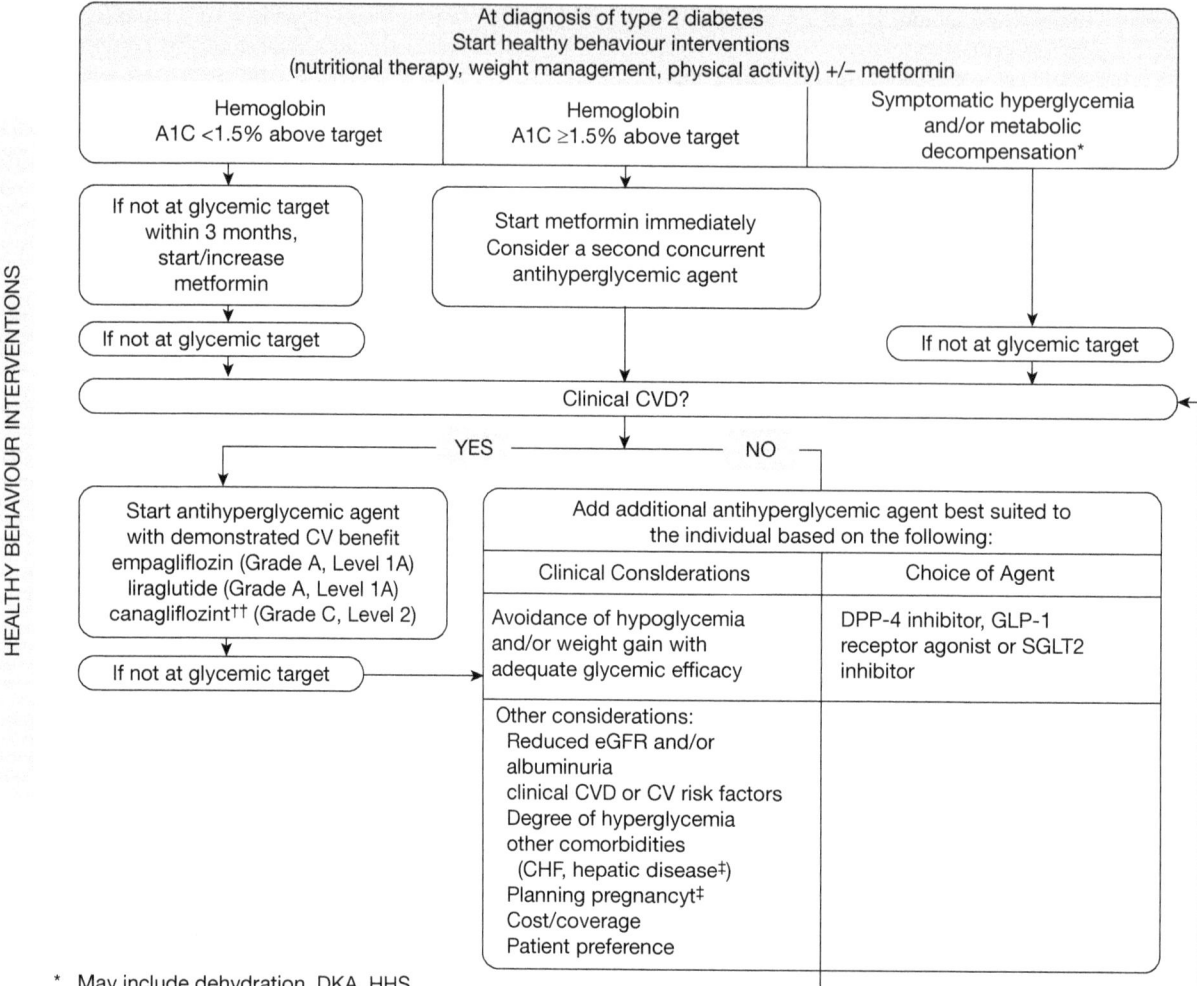

FIGURE 20.1 Management of hyperglycemia in type 2 diabetes.
Source: http://guidelines.diabetes.ca/cpg

2. Eating patterns and ideal percentage of calories from protein, carbohydrates, and fat should be individualized for each client and determined along with a dietitian.
3. Involve the family to improve compliance with the individualized meal plan.
4. Overweight/obese clients are encouraged to set a goal of healthy eating strategies to enhance weight loss. Along with dietary management, exercise programs should be encouraged as soon as the primary care provider has approved that the client is safe to perform physical exercise on a routine basis. It is recommended to perform at least 150 min/wk of aerobic exercise and at least two sessions per week of resistance exercise are recommended. Resistance training is recommended for all clients with type 2 diabetes at least two days a week after authorized by the primary care provider.

D. Pharmacological therapy:
1. Type 1 diabetes depends on exogenous insulin for treatment.
2. Type 2 diabetes is dependent on the severity of disease at the diagnosis. If the hemoglobin A1C is <1.5% above the person's individualized target, antihyperglycaemic pharmacotherapy should be added if glycaemic targets are not achieved within three months of initiating healthy behaviour interventions. In people with type 2 diabetes with hemoglobin A1C >1.5% above target, antihyperglycaemic agents should be initiated together with healthy behaviour interventions, and consideration should be given to initiating combination therapy with two agents:

   a. Monotherapy for type 2 diabetes: Metformin is the preferred oral medication for type 2 diabetes. If using monotherapy at the maximum dose and goal is not achieved within three to six months, a second oral medication should be added. Insulin may eventually be required for clients who are not controlled on oral agents:
      i. Insulin should be considered initially for clients presenting with metabolic decompensation and/or symptomatic hyperglycaemia (i.e., marked hyperglycaemia, ketosis, or unintentional weight loss) regardless of hemoglobin A1C level.
      ii. Recommended therapies:
      iii. Complicated, uncontrolled clients on previously mentioned therapy require insulin.
   b. Criteria for initiation of insulin therapy:
      i. Clients presenting with metabolic decompensation and/or symptomatic hyperglycaemia (i.e., marked hyperglycaemia, ketosis, or unintentional weight loss) regardless of hemoglobin A1C level

Table: Types of Insulin

Insulin Type (Trade Name)	Onset	Peak	Duration
Bolus (preprandial or mealtime) insulins			
Rapid-acting insulin analogues (clear)			
Insulin aspart (NovoRaipd®)	9–20 minutes	1–1.5 hour	3–5 hours
Insulin glulisine (Apidra®)	10–15 minutes	1–1.5 hour	3.5–5 hours
Insulin lispro (Humalog®) U-100 U-200	10–15 minutes	1–2 hours	3–4.75 hours
Faster-acting insulin aspart (Fiasp®)	4 minutes	0.5–1.5 hour	3–5 hours
Short-acting insulins (clear)			
Insulin regular (Humulin®-R, Novolin® ge Toronto)	30 minutes	2–3 hours	6.5 hours
Insulin regular (Entuzity® [U-500])	15 minutes	4–8 hours	17–24 hours
Basal insulins			
Intermediate-acting insulins (cloudy)			
Insulin neutral protamine Hagedorn	1–3 hours	5–8 hours	Up to 18 hours
(Humulin®-N, Novolin® ge NPH)			
Long-acting insulins (clear)			
Insulin detemir (Levemir®)	90 minutes	Not applicable	U-100 glardine 24 hours
Insulin glargine U-100 (Lantus®)			detemir 16–24 hours
Insulin glargine U-300 (Toujeo®)			U-300 glargine >30 hours
Insulin glargine biosimilar (Basaglar®)			degludec 42 hours
Degludec U-100, U-200 (Tresiba®)			

(*continued*)

Table 20.1 Types of Insulin (continued)

Insulin Type (Trade Name)	Onset	Peak	Duration
Premixed insulins			
Premixed regular insulin–NPH (cloudy)			
Humulin® 30/70	A single vial or cartridge contains a fixed ratio of insulin		
Novolin® ge 30/70, 40/60, 50/50			
Premixed insulin analogues (cloudy)			
Biphasic insulin aspart (NovoMix® 30)	(Percentage of rapid-acting or short-acting insulin to percentage of intermediate-acting insulin)		
Insulin lispro/lispro protamine			
(Humalog® Mix25 and Mix50)			

Data represent estimations derived from pooled data analysis using various experimental conditions. There is significant inter- and intraindividual variation in pharmacokinetics and pharmacodynamics depending on a variety of clinical factors, including dose.
Physicians should refer to the most current edition of Compendium of Pharmaceuticals and Specialties (Canadian Pharmacists Association; Ottawa, Ontario, Canada) and products monographs for detailed information.

NPH, neutral protamine Hagedorn.
Source: http://guidelines.diabetes.ca/cpg

Although clients with type 2 diabetes do not depend on exogenous insulin, many will require supplemental insulin during times of stress, illness, injury, pregnancy, or routinely along with oral medication (see Tables 20.1 and 20.2).

    c. Additional medications that may need to be considered:
      i. Angiotensin-converting enzyme (ACE) inhibitors are the first-line antihypertensive drugs to retard renal dysfunction associated with diabetes.
      ii. ACE inhibitors or angiotensin II receptor blockers (ARBs) are recommended for clients with clinical CVD, age ≥ 55 years with an additional cardiovascular (CV) risk factor or end-organ damage (albuminuria, retinopathy, left ventricular hypertrophy), or microvascular complications.
      iii. Statin therapy should be used to reduce CV risk in adults with type 1 or type 2 diabetes with any of the following features:
3. Clinical CVD.
4. Age >40 years.
5. Age <40 years and one of the following:
    a. Diabetes duration >15 years and age >30 years.
    b. Microvascular complications.
    c. Warrants therapy based on the presence of other CV risk factors:
For those not at LDL-C goal while taking statins, a combination of statin therapy with a second-line agent may be used to achieve the goal. The agent used should be chosen based on the amount of decrease in the LDL-C in order to reach target. Ezetimibe should be considered first. In individuals with diabetes and concomitant clinical CVD, ezetimibe or evolocumab may be used to reduce major adverse cardiac events and should also be considered for those who have concomitant familial hypercholesterolaemia.
      i. ASA therapy is recommended for clients with type 1 or type 2 diabetes that have established CVD. ASA should not be used routinely for the primary prevention of CVD events in people with diabetes. For clients who have a history of CVD with an allergy to ASA, clopidogrel 75 mg/d should be used. ASA may be used in the presence of additional CV risk factors.
    d. Some medications adversely affect diabetes:
      i. Nicotinic acids affect glycaemic control by increasing the insulin resistance.
      ii. Beta-blockers increase the risk of hypoglycaemia episodes in clients taking oral hypoglycaemia agents.
      iii. Thiazide diuretics increase insulin resistance.

Follow-Up

A. Determine follow-up appointments by the type of diabetes, age, client compliance, any treatment changes, and presence of any complications related to diabetes or other health problems.
B. A glycosylated hemoglobin determination can assist the provider in measuring the control and should be measured at least every three months when glycaemic targets are not being met and when antihyperglycaemic therapy is being adjusted.

Diabetes Medication/Class

Drug	Brand Name	Drug Class
Acarbose	Precose	Alpha-glucosidase inhibitor
Pioglitazone + metformin	ActoPlus Met	Thiazolidinedione plus biguanide
Glimepiride	Amaryl	Sulphonylurea
Rosiglitazone + metformin	Avandamet	Thiazolidinedione plus biguanide
Rosiglitazone + glimepiride	Avandaryl	Thiazolidinedione plus sulphonylurea
Exenatide	Byetta	Incretin mimetic
Exenatide ext. release	Bydureon	GLP-1 receptor agonist
Glyburide	DiaBeta	Sulphonylurea (second generation)
Pioglitazone + glimepiride	Duetact	Thiazolidinedione plus sulphonylurea
Glucagon	N/A	Antihypoglycaemic
Metformin ext. release	Glucophage	Biguanide
Glipizide ext. release	Glucotrol	Sulphonylurea (second generation)
Glyburide + metformin	Glucovance	Sulphonylurea plus biguanide
Glyburide micronized	Glynase Pres Tab	Sulphonylurea (second generation)
Miglitol	Glyset	Alpha-glucosidase inhibitor
Sitagliptin + metformin	Janumet	Dipeptidyl peptidase-4 inhibitor plus biguanide
Sitagliptin	Januvia	Dipeptidyl peptidase-4 inhibitor
Linagliptin	Tradjenta	Dipeptidyl peptidase-4 inhibitor
Liraglutide	Victoza	GLP-1 receptor agonist
Metformin + glipizide	Metaglip	Biguanide plus sulphonylurea
Glyburide	Micronase	Sulphonylurea (second generation)
Miglitol	Glyset	Alpha-glucosidase inhibitor
Nateglinide	Starlix	Insulin secretagogue
Insulin isophane suspension NPH	Novolin	Intermediate-acting insulin
Saxagliptin	Onglyza	Dipeptidyl peptidase-4 inhibitor
Pioglitazone	Actos	Thiazolidinedione
Repaglinide + metformin	Prandimet	Meglitinide analog plus biguanide meglitinide
Pramlintide	Symlin	Amylin analog/amylinomimetic
Repaglinide	Prandin	Meglitinide analog
Rosiglitazone	Avandia	Thiazolidinedione
Dapagliflozin	Farxiga	SGLT2 Inh SGLT2 Inh with DPP-4 Inh
Empagliflozin + linagliptin	Glyxambi	SGCT2 Inh + DDP-4 Inh
Canagliflozin + metformin	Invokamet	SGLT2 Inh + biguanide
Canagliflozin	Invokana	SGCT2 Inh
Empagliflozin	Jardiance	SGCT2 Inh
Alogliptin + metformin	Kazano	DDP-4 Inh + biguanide
Saxagliptin + metformin	Kombiglyze XR	DDP-4 inhibitor + biguanide
Empagliflozin + linagliptin	Synjardy	SGCT2 Inh + biguanide
Albiglutide	Tanzeum	GLP-1
Dulaglutide	Trulicity	GLP-1
Dapagliflozin	Xigduo XR Afrezza	SGLT2 Inh + biguanide Insulin for oral inhalation

DPP-4 Inh, dipeptidyl peptidase-4 inhibitor; GLP-1, glucagon-like peptide-1; N/A, not available; NPH, neutral protamine Hagedorn; SGLT2 Inh, sodium-glucose co-transporter 2 inhibitor.

TABLE 20.3 Screening for Retinopathy

When to initiate screening:
- Type 1 diabetes: five years after diagnosis in all individuals ≥15 years.
- Type 2 diabetes: children, adolescents, and adults at diagnosis.

Screening methods:
- Seven-standard field, stereoscopic-colour fundus photography with interpretation by a trained reader (gold standard).
- Direct ophthalmoscopy or indirect slit-lamp fundoscopy through dilated pupil.
- Digital fundus photography.
- If retinopathy is present:
  - Diagnose retinopathy severity and establish appropriate monitoring intervals (one year or less).
  - Treat sight-threatening retinopathy with laser, pharmacological, or surgical therapy.
  - Review glycaemic, BP, and lipid control, and adjust therapy to reach targets as per guidelines.[a]
  - Screen for other diabetes complications.
- If retinopathy is not present:
  - Type 1 diabetes: rescreen annually.
  - Type 2 diabetes: rescreen every one to two years.
  - Review glycaemic, BP, and lipid control, and adjust therapy to reach targets as per guidelines.[a]
  - Screen for other diabetes complications.

[a] See Targets for Glycaemic Control chapter, p. S42; Hypertension chapter, p. S186; Dyslipidaemia chapter, p. S178.
BP, blood pressure.
Source: Chart from http://guidelines.diabetes.ca/cpg.

C. The Canadian Diabetes management goals:
1. Fasting plasma glucose (FPG) or preprandial glucose 4 to 7 mmol/L.
2. A glucose level of 5.0 to 10.0 mmol/L two hours after meals.
3. Hemoglobin A1C <7% for most adults with type 1 or type 2 diabetes, or 7.1% to 8.5% in functionally dependent, 7.1% to 8.5% in recurrent hypoglycaemia and/or hypoglycaemia unawareness, limited life expectancy or the frail elderly, and/or with dementia. A target of <6.5% may be recommended for adults with type 2 diabetes to reduce the risk of chronic kidney disease (CKD) and retinopathy if at low risk of hypoglycaemia.
4. Diabetes Canada recommends those with diabetes should be treated to attain a systolic BP of <130 mmHg and a diastolic blood pressure of <80 mmHg.
5. Other lipid related goals are to achieve LDL-C consistently <2.0 mmol/L, apo B <0.8 g/L and non-HDL-C <2.6 mmol/L. For individuals with diabetes with fasting serum triglycerides (TG) >10.0 mmol/L, a fibrate should be used to reduce the risk of pancreatitis. If lipid-lowering treatment is not initiated, a lipid profile should be repeated every one to three years based on CV risk. Repeat testing should be performed three to six months after treatment for dyslipidaemia is initiated to verify lipid targets are being met.

D. In relation to diabetic retinopathy, the performance of a dilated funduscopic examination by an ophthalmologist, to screen for retinopathy, varies according to the individuals age and type of diabetes (see Table 20.3).

Other suggested screening, as appropriate, include an ECG every three to five years (age >40 years, duration of diabetes >15 years + age >30 years, end-organ damage, greater than one CV risk), regular monofilament foot examination (annually or every visit if diabetic foot complications exist), annual flu vaccination and other adult vaccines (pneumococcal once and repeat once if >65 years), thyroid studies, serum creatinine, urea, glomerular filtration rate (GFR), lipid panel, urinalysis, and urine for albuminuria (annual). Additional tests may be needed if complications develop.

Consultation/Referral

It is recommended that diabetes care should be managed by an interprofessional team who have training in diabetes and have the ability to provide ongoing self-management education and support. Care should be organized around the person living with diabetes and their supports. The person with diabetes should be an active participant in his or her own care.

A. Refer to endocrinology if the client experiences the following:
1. Diabetic ketoacidosis.
2. Paediatric clients with hyperglycaemia/new onset diabetes (type 1 or type 2).
3. Severe or frequent hypoglycaemia that is unresponsive to conventional pharmacological therapy.
4. Hyperosmolar hyperglycaemic nonketotic syndrome.
5. Pregnancy.
6. Symptoms from an acute complication related to retinopathy.
7. Nephropathy develops 35% to 45% of the time in type 1 and 20% of the time in type 2 diabetes; it is the leading disease requiring kidney dialysis.
8. Neuropathy: 60% to 70% of clients experience impaired sensation or pain in feet/hands, carpal tunnel syndrome; over half of all amputations of lower extremities are related to diabetes. All clients should be screened for neuropathy at the diagnosis of type 2 diabetes and at five years after the diagnosis of type 1 diabetes, and then annually. Early diagnosis is imperative to prevent nerve damage from occurring. Tight control of the blood glucose levels can slow down the progression of nerve damage but cannot reverse neuronal loss. The pain experienced with neuropathy can be treated with oral medications. Pregabalin and duloxetine are both approved by Health Canada for neuropathic pain. Other medications that may be used include opioids such as tramadol and morphine, along with venlafaxine, amitriptyline, gabapentin, or valproate.
9. Persistent uncontrolled diabetes.

Individual Considerations

A. Pregnancy/preconceptual:
  1. All women with preexisting diabetes and considering pregnancy should receive preconception care to optimize glycaemic control, assess for complications, review medications (switch to insulin or an oral agent with safe pregnancy rating), and begin folic acid supplementation:
     a. Fetal anomalies increase proportionally to uncontrolled diabetes.
     b. Hemoglobin A1C goal before conception is ≤7% (optimally ≤6.5% if possible) and ≤6.5% (ideally ≤6.1% if possible) during pregnancy.
     c. Gestational diabetes screening criteria remain controversial; however, guidelines identify a "preferred" and an "alternate" screening approach. The preferred approach is an initial 50-g glucose challenge test, followed, if abnormal, with a 75-g oral glucose tolerance test. A diagnosis of gestational diabetes is made if one plasma glucose value is abnormal (i.e., fasting ≥5.3 mmol/L, 1 hour ≥10.6 mmol/L, 2 hours ≥9.0 mmol/L). The alternate approach is a one-step approach of a 75-g oral glucose tolerance test. A diagnosis of gestational diabetes mellitus (GDM) is made if one plasma glucose value is abnormal (i.e., fasting ≥5.1 mmol/L, 1 hour ≥10.0 mmol/L, 2hours ≥8.5 mmol/L).
     d. Care by an interprofessional diabetes health-care team, preferably including a diabetes nurse educator, dietitian, obstetrician, and endocrinologist/internist with expertise in diabetes, prior to conception and during pregnancy, has been shown to minimize maternal and fetal risks in women with preexisting diabetes.
  2. Hypertensive medications may need to be changed if considering pregnancy because ACE inhibitors, beta-blockers, and diuretics are contraindicated during pregnancy.
  3. Increased monitoring of blood glucose is necessary during pregnancy. The use of the continuous glucose monitor during pregnancy should be considered in order to improve glycaemic control and neonatal outcomes.

B. Paediatrics: Screening for type 2 diabetes takes place every two years using a combination of a hemoglobin A1C and an FPG or random plasma glucose in children and adolescents with any of the following conditions:
  1. At least three risk factors in nonpubertal children beginning at 8 years of age or at least two risk factors in pubertal children. Risk factors include obesity (BMI ≥95th percentile for age and gender), member of a high-risk ethnic group (e.g., African, Arab, Asian, Hispanic, Indigenous, or South Asian descent), first-degree relative with type 2 diabetes and/or exposure to hyperglycaemia in utero, signs or symptoms of insulin resistance (including acanthosis nigricans, hypertension, dyslipidaemia, non-alcoholic fatty liver disease [NAFLD; ALT >3X upper limit of normal or fatty liver on ultrasound]).
  2. PCOS.
  3. IFG and/or IGT.
  4. Use of atypical antipsychotic medications.
  5. Children are encouraged to perform ≥60 minutes of physical activity on a daily basis.
  6. Children with type 2 diabetes should be screened for neuropathy, retinopathy, dyslipidaemia, CKD, and comorbid conditions associated with insulin resistance, including NAFLD, obstructive sleep apnoea (OSA), and PCOS in pubertal females, at diagnosis and annually thereafter.
  7. Children with type 2 diabetes should be screened for hypertension, depression, and disordered eating beginning at diagnosis of diabetes and at every diabetes-related clinical encounter thereafter (at least biannually).
  8. Children diagnosed with type 1 diabetes symptoms of classic or atypical celiac disease should be screened for celiac disease by ordering laboratory studies that include immunoglobulin A (IgA) antitissue transglutaminase or antiendomysial antibodies. If positive, the child should be treated with a gluten-free diet to improve symptoms.

  These children should also be screened for thyroid disease by ordering a thyroid-stimulating hormone (TSH) level test and thyroid peroxidase antibodies. If normal, screen every two years.

C. Elderly:
  1. Risk for hypoglycaemia should be reviewed in clients using insulin or oral agents that can cause hypoglycaemia. Medical alert bracelets and emergency care for hypoglycaemic episodes should be reviewed during each follow-up.
  2. Treatment goals for older diabetic clients should be individualized with goals equal to those of younger clients based on life expectancy.

D. Indigenous populations:
  1. Indigenous populations are among the highest-risk populations for diabetes and related complications in Canada. Screening for diabetes should be carried out earlier and more frequently for this population.
  2. Particular attention is needed for Indigenous females of childbearing age, as the high incidence of hyperglycaemia in pregnancy and maternal obesity increases the risk of childhood obesity and diabetes in future generations. As a result, early diagnosis diabetes in pregnancy is important.
  3. Prevention strategies are essential and should be implemented after considering appropriate social, cultural, and health service resources of the community.

Bibliography

American Diabetes Association. (2016). Standards of medical care in diabetes—2016. *Diabetes Care*, 39(Suppl. 1): S1–S112. Retrieved from http://care.diabetesjournals.org/content/suppl/2015/12/21/39.Supplement_1.DC2/2016-Standards-of-Care.pdf

Atkinson, M. A. (2016). Type 1 diabetes mellitus. In S. Melmed, K. S. Polonsky, P. R. Larsen, & H. M. Kronenberg (Eds.), *Williams textbook of endocrinology* (13th ed., pp. 1451–1483). Philadelphia, PA: Elsevier.

BMI Calculator. (n.d.). *BMI calculator*. Retrieved from http://www.bmi-calculator.net

Bulun, S. E. (2016). Physiology and pathology of the female reproductive axis. In S. Melmed, K. S. Polonsky, P. R. Larsen, & H. M. Kronenberg (Eds.), *Williams textbook of endocrinology* (13th ed., pp. 590–663). Philadelphia, PA: Elsevier Saunders.

The Canadian Task Force on the Periodic Health Examination. (2017). *Periodic preventive health visits: A more appropriate approach to delivering preventive services*. Retrieved from https://canadiantaskforce.ca/guidelines/periodic-preventive-health-visits/

Centers for Disease Control and Prevention. (2011). *Adult BMI calculator: English version*. Retrieved from https://www.cdc.gov/healthyweight/assessing/bmi/adult_bmi/english_bmi_calculator/bmi_calculator.html

Centers for Disease Control and Prevention. (2015, December). *Diagnosed diabetes*. Retrieved from https://www.cdc.gov/diabetes/statistics/prevalence_national.htm

Centers for Disease Control and Prevention. (n.d.). *BMI percentile calculator for child and teen: English version*. Retrieved from https://nccd.cdc.gov/dnpabmi/calculator.aspx

Centers for Disease Control and Prevention, NCHS National Center for Health Statistics. (n.d.). *Clinical growth charts*. Retrieved from https://www.cdc.gov/growthcharts

Coustan, D. R. (2016, March). Diabetes mellitus in pregnancy: Screening and diagnosis. *UpToDate*. Retrieved from http://www.uptodate.com

Diabetes Canada. (2018a). Diabetes Canada clinical practice guidelines. *Canadian Journal of Diabetes*, *42*(Suppl. 1), S1–S325. doi:10.1016/j.jcjd.2017.10.051

Diabetes Canada. (2018b). *Eye damage (Diabeteic retinopathy)*. Retrieved from https://www.diabetes.ca/diabetes-and-you/complications/eye-damage-diabetic-retinopathy

The Diabetic Children's Foundation. (2018). *Statistics on type 1 diabetes*. Retrieved from https://www.diabetes-children.ca/en/type-1-diabetes/t1d-t2d/

Eckel, R. H., Jakicie, J. M., Ard, J. D., Hubbard, V. S., de Jesus, J. M., Lee, I-Min., . . . Yanovski, S. Z. (2013). AHA/ACC guideline on lifestyle management to reduce cardiovascular risk: A report of the American college of cardiology/American heart association task force on practice guidelines. *Circulation*, *129*(25 Suppl. 2), S76–S99. doi:10.1161/01.cir.0000437740.48606.d1

El-Hussein, M. T., Power-Kean, K., Zettel, S., Huether, S. E., McCance, K. L., Brashers, V. L., & Rote, N. S. (2018). *Understanding pathophysiology*. Milton, ON: Elsevier.

Genest, J., McPherson, R., Frohlich, J., Anderson, T., Campbell, N., Carpentier, A., & Ur, E. (2009). Canadian cardiovascular society/canadian guidelines for the diagnosis and treatment of dyslipidemia and prevention of cardiovascular disease in the adult-2009 recommendations. *Canadian Journal of Cardiology*, *25*(10), 567–579.

Goff, D. C., Lloyd-Jones, D. M., Bennett, G., Coady, S., D'Agostino, R. B., Sr., Gibbons, R., . . . Wilson, P. W. F. (2013, November 12). 2013 ACC/AHA guideline on the assessment of cardiovascular risk: A report of the American college of cardiology/American heart association task force on practice guidelines. *Circulation*, *129*, S49–S73. doi:10.1161/01.cir.0000437741.48606.98

James, P. A., Oparil, S., Carter, B. L., Cushman, W. C., Dennison-Himmelfarb, C., Handler, J., & Ortiz, E. (2013, December 18). 2014 Evidence-based guidelines for the management of high blood pressure in adults report from the panel members appointed to the Eighth joint national committee (JNC 8). *Journal of the American Medical Association*, *311*(5), 507–520. doi:10.1001/jama.2013.284427

Laffel, L., & Svoren, B. (2015, March). Epidemiology, presentation, and diagnosis of type 2 diabetes mellitus in children and adolescents. *UpToDate*. Retrieved from http://www.uptodate.com

Lee, A. (Ed.). (2016). *NPPR: Nurse practitioners' prescribing reference*. New York, NY: Haymarket Media.

Levitsky, L. L., & Misra, M. (2016, March). Epidemiology, presentation, and diagnosis of type 1 diabetes mellitus in children and adolescents. *UpToDate*. Retrieved from http://www.uptodate.com

McCulloch, D. K., & Munshi, M. (2015, November). Treatment of type 2 diabetes mellitus in the older client. *UpToDate*. Retrieved from http://www.uptodate.com

McCulloch, D. K., & Robertson, R. P. (2014, September). Pathogenesis of type 2 diabetes mellitus. *UpToDate*. Retrieved from http://www.uptodate.com

Medical Council of Canada. (2018). *Clinical laboratory tests: Normal values*. Retrieved from https://mcc.ca/objectives/normal-values/?cn-reloaded=1

National Institutes of Health. (2015). *Third report of the national cholesterol education program (NCEP) expert panel on detection, evaluation, and treatment of high blood cholesterol in adults (ATP III): final report*. Bethesda, MD: Author. Retrieved from https://www.nhlbi.nih.gov/sites/www.nhlbi.nih.gov/files/Circulation-2002-ATP-III-Final-Report-PDF-3143.pdf

Polonsky, K. S., & Burant, C. F. (2016). Type 2 diabetes mellitus. In S. Melmed, K. S. Polonsky, P. R. Larsen, & H. M. Kronenberg (Eds.), *Williams textbook of endocrinology* (13th ed., pp. 1386–1450). Philadelphia, PA: Elsevier Saunders.

Powers, A. C. (2015). Diabetes mellitus: Diagnosis, classification, and pathophysiology. In D. L. Kasper, A. S. Fauci, S. L. Hauser, D. L. Longo, & J. Jameson (Eds.), *Harrison's principles of internal medicine* (19th ed., pp. 2399–2424). New York, NY: McGraw-Hill.

Skelton, J. A. (2016, November). Management of childhood obesity in the primary care setting. *UpToDate*. Retrieved from http://www.uptodate.com

Stone, N. J., Robinson, J., Lichtenstein, A. H., Bairey Merz, C. N., Lloyd-Jones, D. M., & Blum, C. B. (2013, November 7). 2013 ACC/AHA guidelines on the treatment of blood cholesterol to reduce atherosclerotic cardiovascular risk in adults: A report of the American college of cardiology/American heart association task force on practice guidelines. *Journal of the American College of Cardiology*, *63*(25), S0735–S1097. Retrieved from https://circ.ahajournals.org/content/early/2013/11/11/01.cir.0000437738.63853.7a.full.pdf

U.S. Department of Health and Human Services. (2015a, March). *Screening for abnormal blood glucose and type 2 diabetes mellitus: U. S. Preventive services task force recommendation statement*. Retrieved from http://www.guideline.gov/content.aspx?id=49928#Section420

U.S. Department of Health and Human Services. (2015b, March). *2014 National diabetes statistics report*. Centers for Disease Control and Prevention. Retrieved from http://www.cdc.gov/diabetes/data/statistics/2014statisticsreport.html

U.S. Department of Health and Human Services. (2015c, May). *2015 recommendations for physical activity*. Retrieved from https://www.nhlbi.nih.gov/health/health-topics/topics/phys/recommend

Galactorrhoea

Jill C. Cash, Melissa A. Hall, and Kelly Power-Kean

Definition

A. The production of a milky discharge excreted from the nipple, occurring beyond the six-month period of pregnancy and/or breastfeeding cessation.

Incidence/Prevalence

A. It is estimated that 1% to 50% of reproductive women will experience galactorrhoea at some time in their life.

Pathogenesis

A. The pathogenesis depends on the aetiology. Physiologic galactorrhoea is caused by pregnancy. The anterior pituitary gland secretes prolactin, which stimulates milk production. Milk production is normal for six months after pregnancy and/or after breastfeeding has ceased. The majority of cases are from a benign aetiology. Malignancy is responsible for 5% to 15% of cases.

Predisposing Factors

A. Reproductive women (15–50 years old).
B. Medications: oral contraception, first- and second-generation antipsychotics, tricyclic antidepressants, selective serotonin reuptake inhibitor (SSRI) antidepressants, antiemetics, opioid analgesics, and antihypertensives.

Common Findings

A. Milky discharge from the nipple.

Subjective Data

A. Note the onset, duration, and course of presenting symptoms.
B. Ask whether the client has been pregnant and/or breastfed within the past six months. If so, how long did she nurse?
C. Review her menstrual history and pattern.
D. Ask her to describe the discharge, noting colour, consistency, and/or presence of blood.
E. Determine the mechanism of production of discharge: spontaneous or with manual expression.
F. Assess for any palpable mass in the breast.
G. Review current medications, including use of oral contraceptives.
H. Note any previous experience with galactorrhoea. Discuss testing performed and treatment, if any.
I. Identify any family history of breast cancer or other tumours.

Physical Examination

A. Check pulse, respirations, and blood pressure (BP).
B. Inspect:
    1. Inspect the breast and nipples for symmetry.
    2. Assess the discharge.
    3. Inspect the skin; note dimpling, retraction, and irregularities.

4. Eyes: complete funduscopic examination.
5. Perform visual field testing.

C. Palpate:
1. Palpate the breasts for masses and fibrocystic changes.
2. Squeeze the nipple to induce discharge.
3. Palpate the axillary lymph nodes.
4. Palpate the neck, thyroid, and lymph nodes.

Diagnostic Tests
A. Prolactin level: normal level is 4 to 30 μg/L.
B. Thyroid-stimulating hormone (TSH).

Many cases of galactorrhoea are considered idiopathic. Usually endocrine studies will be normal.

C. Beta human chorionic gonadotropin (beta hCG).
D. Hemoccult of breast discharge.
E. Breast discharge for pathology.
F. Periareolar ultrasound (all ages).
G. CT/MRI of sella turcica if pituitary mass is suspected.
H. Mammogram in women older than 30 years if tumour is suspected.
I. Breast sonography.
J. Ductography/ductoscopy.
K. Breast MRI.
L. Skin-punch biopsy for abnormal skin presentations.

Differential Diagnoses
A. Fibrocystic disease.
B. Mastitis.
C. Breast tumour.
D. Medication induction.
E. Breast cancer: bloody nipple discharge; painless, firm fixed mass.
F. Pituitary adenoma: Can produce permanent visual field loss and headaches.
G. Hypothalamic disorders.
H. Chiari-Frommel: Galactorrhoea occurring after six months postpartum.
I. Pregnancy.

Plan
A. General interventions:
1. Treat underlying cause of nipple discharge.
2. If induced by medications, consider stopping medications if the side effect outweighs benefits.
3. If benign cause, no treatment is necessary with medication. Monitor symptoms. If symptoms progress, reevaluate.

B. Client teaching: Teach self-examination of the breast.
C. Pharmacological therapy: No pharmacological therapy is advised with the exception of tapering or discontinuing medications that are causing the discharge. This is recommended only after cautious consideration of why the medication is being used (antipsychotics).

Follow-Up
A. Monitor prolactin level every six to 12 months.
B. Recommend yearly vision evaluation.
C. Order MRI of brain at one year, then every two to five years if symptoms persist.

Consultation/Referral
A. Consult an oncologist regardless of normal imaging results if breast tumour is suspected with bloody discharge or palpable mass noted.

Individual Considerations
A. Pregnancy:
1. Galactorrhoea during pregnancy is a normal physiologic response.
2. If galactorrhoea persists after pregnancy/lactation has ceased for six months, a full workup evaluation is required.

B. Adults: Men: Galactorrhoea is rare in men; however, it can occur with prolactinoma.

Bibliography
Bulun, S. E. (2016). Physiology and pathology of the female reproductive axis. In S. Melmed, K. S. Polonsky, P. R. Larsen, & H. M. Kronenberg (Eds.), *Williams textbook of endocrinology* (13th ed., pp. 590–663). Philadelphia, PA: Elsevier Saunders.
Golshan, M., & Iglehart, D. (2013, June). Nipple discharge. *UpToDate*. Retrieved from http://www.uptodate.com
Lee, A. (Ed.). (2016). *NPPR: Nurse practitioners' prescribing reference*. New York, NY: Haymarket Media.
Medical Council of Canada. (2018). *Clinical laboratory tests: Normal values*. Retrieved from https://mcc.ca/objectives/normal-values/?cn-reloaded=1
Toward Optimized Practice. (2014a). *Laboratory endocrine testing: Galactorrhea a summary of the clinical practice guideline*. Retrieved from http://www.topalbertadoctors.org/download/334/galactorrhea_summary.pdf?_20180914052444
Toward Optimized Practice. (2014b). *Laboratory endocrine testing: Galactorrhea clnical practice guideline*. Retrieved from http://www.topalbertadoctors.org/download/333/galactorrea_guideline.pdf?_20181119154145

Gynaecomastia

Jill C. Cash, Melissa A. Hall, and Kelly Power-Kean

Definition
A. Gynaecomastia is an enlargement of the breast tissue in males.

Incidence/Prevalence
A. Common in newborns; approximately 40% to 69% of adolescent boys will experience breast enlargement. It is also seen in men (between the ages of 50 and 80 years) with excessive weight gain.

Pathogenesis
A. Male breast duct proliferation occurs due to a hormonal imbalance of estrogen. Pathologic conditions, such as pituitary tumours, systemic disorders, kidney disease, thyroid disorders, and liver disease, can cause symptoms to occur. Medications can also induce symptoms. These medications include antiandrogens, antidepressants, cimetidine, ranitidine, omeprazole, chemotherapeutic agents, amiodarone, diltiazem, nifedipine, digoxin, methyldopa, reserpine, hormones, and sedatives.

Predisposing Factors
A. Newborns.
B. Puberty.
C. Age (men older than 65 years).
D. Family history.

E. Klinefelter's syndrome.
F. Malnutrition with severe weight loss.
G. Peutz–Jeghers syndrome.
H. Obesity in males.

Common Findings
A. Enlargement of breast tissue with or without discomfort.

Other Signs and Symptoms
A. Asymptomatic.
B. Type I: nodule present under areolar tissue area.
C. Type II: nodule palpable under and beyond areolar area.
D. Type III: breast enlargement without contour separation of tissue.

Subjective Data
A. Identify when breast development first appeared.
B. Determine whether enlargement is unilateral or bilateral.
C. Review the progression of enlargement.
D. Note any pain, discharge, or masses that are palpable.
E. List current medications, drugs, and alcohol and substance abuse.
F. Review the client's medical history.
G. Note the client's family history of gynaecomastia or breast malignancy.
H. Explore nutritional intake.
I. Discuss the client's level of physical activity (sports, hobbies, etc.).
J. Note the use of herbal products.

Physical Examination
A. Inspect breasts bilaterally and surrounding nodes for enlargement or skin changes.
B. Palpate breast tissue systematically and surrounding nodes. Gynaecomastia can usually be appreciated once the glandular tissue reaches 0.5 cm or larger.
C. Palpate testes for masses or atrophic changes.
D. Check body mass index (BMI).

Diagnostic Tests
A. Prolactin level.
B. Thyroid-stimulating hormone (TSH).
C. Human chorionic gonadotropin (hCG).
D. Serum luteinizing hormone (LH).
E. Testosterone level.
F. Estradiol level.
G. Mammography for suspicious breast masses in adult males.

Differential Diagnoses
A. Obesity: fatty breast enlargement without glandular involvement.
B. Breast cancer: fixed, firm nodule in tissue with dimpling and/or breast discharge.
C. Neurofibroma.
D. Lipoma.

Plan
A. General interventions: Identify any pathologic condition. If none is identified, reassure the client that normal resolution will occur over time.
B. Client teaching: Reinforce weight reduction if weight gain is a factor in the condition.
C. Pharmacological therapy:
 1. Antiestrogens (tamoxifen).
 2. Androgens (testosterone replacement).
 3. Aromatase inhibitors (anastrozole).

Follow-Up
A. Follow-up is dependent on aetiology and/or client needs.
B. Follow up pubertal boys every four to six months for evaluation of development or regression.

Consultation/Referral
Refer to an endocrinologist if the male client:
A. Is noted to have breast enlargement for longer than two years.
B. Is a pubertal boy without genital development.

Individual Consideration
A. Newborns: Commonly seen in newborns due to maternal estrogen. This breast enlargement spontaneously regresses over time.

Bibliography
Bhasin, S., & Jameson, J. L. (2015). Disorders of the testes and male reproductive system. In S. Melmed, K. S. Polonsky, P. R. Larsen, & H. M. Kronenberg (Eds.), *Williams textbook of endocrinology* (13th ed., pp. 785–832). Philadelphia, PA: Elsevier.
BMI Calculator. (n.d.). *BMI calculator*. Retrieved from http://www.bmi-calculator.net
Braunstein, G. D. (2014, June). Causes, evaluation, and management of gyenocomastia. *UpToDate*. Retrieved from http://www.uptodate.com
Braunstein, G. D. (2015, October). Epidemiology, pathophysiology, and causes of gynecomastia. *UpToDate*. Retrieved from http://www.uptodate.com
Centers for Disease Control and Prevention. (2011). *Adult BMI calculator: English version*. Retrieved from https://www.cdc.gov/healthyweight/assessing/bmi/adult_bmi/english_bmi_calculator/bmi_calculator.html
Centers for Disease Control and Prevention. (n.d.). *BMI percentile calculator for child and teen: English version*. Retrieved from https://nccd.cdc.gov/dnpabmi/calculator.aspx
El-Hussein, M. T., Power-Kean, K., Zettel, S., Huether, S. E., McCance, K. L., Brashers, V. L., & Rote, N. S. (2018). *Understanding pathophysiology*. Milton, ON: Elsevier.
Lee, A. (Ed.). (2016). *NPPR: Nurse practitioners' prescribing reference*. New York, NY: Haymarket Media.
Medical Council of Canada. (2018). *Clinical laboratory tests: Normal values*. Retrieved from https://mcc.ca/objectives/normal-values/?cn-reloaded=1

Hirsutism

Jill C. Cash, Melissa A. Hall, and Kelly Power-Kean

Definition
A. An excessive production of an androgenic hormone causes the development of male features in females, particularly hair distribution.

Incidence/Prevalence
A. Approximately 5% of women develop hirsutism after puberty.

Pathogenesis
A. The pathogenesis depends on the aetiology: Excessive amounts of androgenic hormones from the ovary, adrenal gland, and/or a hormonal imbalance. The two major adrenal gland conditions responsible for hirsutism or virilism are congenital adrenal hyperplasia (CAH) and Cushing's syndrome.

Predisposing Factors
A. Females who have a family history of endocrine disorders.

B. Usually occurs in the second to third decade of life.
C. Southern European ancestry.
D. Polycystic ovary syndrome.
E. CAH.
F. Ovarian tumours.
G. Adrenal tumours.
H. Cushing's syndrome.
I. Hyperthecosis.
J. Severe insulin-resistance syndrome.
K. Medications.
L. Obesity.
M. Medications containing androgens, including oral contraceptives.

Common Findings
A. An excessive amount of hair production on the face (upper lip and chin), chest, areola, linea alba, lower back, buttock, and inner thigh.

Other Signs and Symptoms
A. Irregular periods.
B. Infertility.
C. Acne.
D. Virilization (temporal hair recession, large muscle mass, deep voice, decreased breast size, clitoromegaly).

Subjective Data
A. Note the age of onset, duration, and distribution pattern of the excessive hair growth.
B. Review any previous experiences with similar symptoms. What were the diagnosis, treatment, and results?
C. Note the client's menstrual history. Note amenorrhoea and galactorrhoea. Has the client ever had a history of infertility?

Physical Examination
A. Check pulse, respirations, and blood pressure (BP), body mass index (BMI; >30 kg/m^2), central obesity pattern.
B. Inspect:
  1. Look for excessive hair growth on face, breasts, abdomen, back, and shoulders.
  2. Assess for signs of virilization.
  3. Confirm expected development of secondary sexual characteristics.
  4. Assess for acne.
  5. Assess for striae acanthosis nigricans, or skin tags.
C. Palpate: Perform a pelvic examination to assess for enlarged ovaries or masses.

Diagnostic Tests
No laboratory investigation is required for mild hirsutism:
A. Total testosterone.
B. Free serum testosterone thyroid-stimulating hormone (TSH), luteinizing hormone (LH), follicle-stimulating hormone (FSH), estradiol, and progesterone in clients presenting with menstrual disorders.
C. Dehydroepiandrosterone sulfate (DHEA-S).
D. Androstenedione (drawn after 10 a.m.).
E. CT of ovaries/adrenal glands if abnormally elevated blood tests.

Differential Diagnoses
A. Hirsutism: can be secondary to primary diagnosis (idiopathic, hypothyroidism, infertility, obesity, ovarian disease, hyperprolactinaemia).
B. Hypothyroidism: elevated TSH.
C. Ovarian tumour: testosterone level >200 ng/dL.
D. Adrenal tumour: DHEA >800 mcg/dL.
E. Excessive steroid use: the client medicates self with excessive steroids.
F. Cushing's syndrome: centripetal obesity and muscle wasting.

Plan
A. General interventions:
  1. Medications are not recommended for mild cases. Hair removal by other mechanisms is recommended as the client desires (plucking, waxing, bleaching, etc.).
  2. Moderate to severe cases require treatment with medications. Drug therapy may stop excessive hair growth. Current hair growth will not spontaneously resolve. Hair removal may also be desired until the drug shows an effect.
  3. If acne is severe, institute appropriate therapy (see section "Acne Vulgaris" in Chapter 4, Dermatology Guidelines).
B. Client teaching:
  1. If obese, reinforce weight loss management. Consider nutritional consult.
  2. Educate the client that it may take three to six months on medication to see results.
C. Pharmacological therapy:
  1. Use combined oral contraceptives daily if no contraindication; any brand is effective.
  2. Use high-estrogen pills to increase steroid-binding globulins if no contraindication.
  3. Use high-progesterone pills to influence the clearance of testosterone.
  4. Antiandrogens:
      a. Spironolactone.
      b. Cyproterone acetate.
      c. Finasteride.
      d. Flutamide.
  5. Gonadotropin-releasing hormone (GnRH) agonists.
  6. Topical therapy: Topical cream to be applied twice daily to reduce growth of unwanted facial hair. Results should be noted after four to six weeks of use.

Ovarian and/or adrenal tumour must be ruled out before medication therapy is instituted.

Follow-Up
A. Follow-up depends on the treatment. If medication is used, follow up in three months to evaluate effectiveness.

Consultation/Referral
A. Consult an endocrinologist if Cushing's syndrome is suspected.
B. Refer clients who have virilization and elevated testosterone levels to an endocrinologist.

Individual Considerations
A. Pregnancy:
  1. If conception occurs, discontinue medications, which may be teratogenic to the fetus.
  2. If anovulation is diagnosed, fertility measures are needed if pregnancy is desired.
B. Geriatric:
  1. Hirsutism may be seen in women after menopause.

2. Hirsutism that occurs in the middle to late years in life should be closely monitored for adrenal hyperplasia and adrenal and/or ovarian tumours.

Bibliography

Barbieri, R. L. (2013, August). Treatment of hirsutism. *UpToDate*. Retrieved from http://www.uptodate.com

Barbieri, R. L., & Ehrmann, D. A. (2015a, January). Evaluation of premenopausal women with hirsutism. *UpToDate*. Retrieved from http://www.uptodate.com

Barbieri, R. L., & Ehrmann, D. A. (2015b, August). Pathogenesis and causes of hirsutism. *UpToDate*. Retrieved from http://www.uptodate.com

Bhasin, S., & Jameson, J. L. (2015). Disorders of the testes and male reproductive system. In S. Melmed, K. S. Polonsky, P. R. Larsen, & H. M. Kronenberg (Eds.), *Williams textbook of endocrinology* (13th ed., pp. 785–832). Philadelphia, PA: Elsevier.

BMI Calculator. (n.d.). *BMI calculator*. Retrieved from http://www.bmi-calculator.net

Bulun, S. E. (2016). Physiology and pathology of the female reproductive axis. In S. Melmed, K. S. Polonsky, P. R. Larsen, & H. M. Kronenberg (Eds.), *Williams textbook of endocrinology* (13th ed., pp. 590–663). Philadelphia, PA: Elsevier Saunders.

Centers for Disease Control and Prevention. (2011). *Adult BMI calculator: English version*. Retrieved from https://www.cdc.gov/healthyweight/assessing/bmi/adult_bmi/english_bmi_calculator/bmi_calculator.html

Centers for Disease Control and Prevention. (n.d.). *BMI percentile calculator for child and teen: English version*. Retrieved from https://nccd.cdc.gov/dnpabmi/calculator.aspx

Ehrmann, D. A. (2015). Hirsutism. In D. L. Kasper, A. S. Fauci, S. L. Hauser, D. L. Longo, & J. L. Jameson (Eds.), *Harrison's principles of internal medicine* (19th ed.). New York, NY: McGraw-Hill.

Lee, A. (Ed.). (2016). *NPPR: Nurse practitioners' prescribing reference*. New York, NY: Haymarket Media.

Medical Council of Canada. (2018). *Clinical laboratory tests: Normal values*. Retrieved from https://mcc.ca/objectives/normal-values/?cn-reloaded=1

Stewart, P. M., & Newell-Price, J. D. (2016). The adrenal cortex. In S. Melmed, K. S. Polonsky, P. R. Larsen, & H. M. Kronenberg (Eds.), *Williams textbook of endocrinology* (13th ed., pp. 490–556). Philadelphia, PA: Elsevier.

Toward Optimized Practice. (2014). *Laboratory endocrine testing: Gonadal disorders: Hirsutism clincal practice guideline*. Retrieved from http://www.topalbertadoctors.org/download/336/hirsutism_guideline.pdf?_20180529191140

Hypogonadism

Jill C. Cash, Melissa A. Hall, and Kelly Power-Kean

Definition
A. Hypogonadism in men is failure of the testes to produce physiological levels of testosterone and a normal number of spermatozoa.

Incidence/Prevalence
A. An estimated 38.7% of men older than 45 years of age have below-normal values of serum testosterone.

Pathogenesis
A. Hypogonadism in men can be the result of testicular dysfunction or nondevelopment (primary hypogonadism) or dysfunction of the pituitary or hypothalamus (secondary hypogonadism). The two clinical manifestations of impaired spermatogenesis are infertility and decreased testicular size. There are several possible clinical manifestations of testosterone deficiency, which are determined by its time of onset during reproductive development:
   1. In utero first or second trimesters: incomplete virilization of external genitalia, incomplete development of Wolffian ducts to form male internal genitalia.
   2. Third trimester in utero: micropenis.
   3. Prepuberty: incomplete pubertal maturation, eunuchoid body habitus, poor muscle development, reduced peak bone mass.
   4. Postpuberty: decreased energy, mood, and libido; decrease in sexual hair, haematocrit, muscle mass and strength, and bone mineral density.

Predisposing Factors
A. Hypogonadism associated with Klinefelter's syndrome.
B. Chemotherapy.
C. Radiation therapy.
D. Excessive alcohol consumption.
E. Painful testicular swelling.
F. Anosmia associated with Kallmann's syndrome.
G. Use of medications that cause hypogonadism: ketoconazole or extended-release opiates.

Common Findings
A. Decreased vigour and libido.
B. Depression.
C. Adolescent and young adult males: failure to begin or complete puberty.

Other Signs and Symptoms
A. Fatigue.
B. Difficulty concentrating.
C. Hot flashes.
D. No change in deepening of the voice.

Subjective Data
A. To client or parent: history of known chromosomal abnormalities in family or client.
B. History of cryptorchidism.
C. History of muscular weakness.
D. History of varicocele unresolved within six months of birth.
E. Known infections affecting the scrotum and testes.
F. Therapeutic radiation to area.
G. History of chemotherapy.
H. History of long-term ketoconazole, glucocorticoid, or long-acting opiate use.
I. Known testicular trauma.
J. Known torsion.
K. History of autoimmune disorder.
L. Alcohol consumption (amount, duration, and frequency).
M. Chronic illnesses, including cirrhosis, chronic renal failure, or HIV.
N. Decreased spontaneous erections.

Physical Examination
A. Inspect:
   1. Testes for appropriate size.
   2. Upper and lower body musculatures.
   3. Full/dense male-pattern beard.
   4. Expected Tanner development for age.
   5. Testes should be bilaterally descended.
   6. Rule out eunuchoid appearance.
   7. Gynaecomastia.
   8. Clinical findings of hypogonadism are more obvious after puberty and takes years to develop.
   9. Inspect penis for hypospadias.
   10. Long-term alcohol abuse: palmar erythema, rhinophyma, telangiestasia, hand tremour.

B. Palpate:
 1. The scrotum and testes for masses.
 2. The breasts for masses (both male and female).

Diagnostic Tests

A. Total serum testosterone (between 7 and 11 a.m., or within three hours after waking). Borderline low or low-normal testosterone (repeat for confirmation).
B. If total testosterone is low, complete a comprehensive laboratory evaluation including follicle-stimulating hormone (FSH), luteinizing hormone (LH), prolactin, SHBG, cFT or cBAT, thyroid-stimulating hormone (TSH), ferritin (or % iron saturation), complete blood count (CBC), and prostate-specific antigen (PSA).
C. Avoid lab tests during acute illness.

Differential Diagnoses

A. Moderate obesity.
B. Nephrotic syndrome.
C. Hypothyroidism.
D. Use of glucocorticoids, progestins, and androgenic steroids.
E. Acromegaly.
F. Diabetes mellitus.
G. Hepatic cirrhosis.
H. Hypopituitarism.
I. Malnutrition.
J. Klinefelter's syndrome.
K. Depression.
L. Psychological sexual dysfunction.

Plan

A. General interventions:
 1. Testosterone replacement's effect on reducing adverse health outcomes in the general population is unknown.
 2. Testosterone levels vary significantly with circadian rhythms, illness, and medications.
 3. Measurement of bone mineral density is recommended to assess fracture risk.
 4. LH and FSH concentrations can help distinguish between primary and secondary hypogonadism.
 5. Differentials for secondary hypogonadism should evaluate for pituitary neoplasia, hyperprolactinaemia, hemochromatosis, obstructive sleep apnoea (OSA), and genetic disorders.
 6. Testosterone replacement should be initiated only after a baseline PSA and digital prostate examination. PSA levels should be followed routinely.
B. Client teaching:
 1. Both men and women with hypogonadism can lead normal lives with hormone replacement therapy.
 2. Hormone replacement should continue throughout life.
 3. Potential side effects of testosterone replacement therapy should be discussed before therapy, including gynaecomastia, worsening benign prostatic hyperplasia (BPH), sleep apnoea, peripheral oedema, potential increased risk for myocardial infarction (MI), and cerebrovascular accident (CVA).
 4. Reduced sperm production and fertility is a potential side effect of testosterone replacement.
 5. Clients using topically absorbed testosterone gel or creams can transfer testosterone to female partners or children by direct skin-to-skin contact.
C. Pharmacological therapy:
 1. Injectable testosterone.
 2. 1% testosterone gel.
 3. Transdermal testosterone patch.
 4. Buccal testosterone.
 5. Axillary transdermal testosterone solution 2%.

Follow-Up

A. Clients receiving hormone replacement should be reevaluated every six months or more frequently, including screening for prostate cancer as recommended.
B. Testosterone replacement is contraindicated in metastatic prostate cancer and breast cancer. Routine screening should be performed.

Consultation/Referral

A. Endocrinology referral is recommended for males not responsive to the replacement therapy.
B. Clients with primary hypogonadism should be referred to an endocrinologist for initial workup and management.

Individual Considerations

A. Geriatrics: Current recommendations are *not* in favour of testosterone therapy for all older males. Providers should cautiously consider the benefits compared to the risks for older males. The benefits of testosterone replacement are unproven, and the long-term risks are unknown.
B. HIV clients: Short-term testosterone replacement should be considered for HIV men with low testosterone, weight loss, and muscular wasting.

Bibliography

American Geriatric Society. (2014). GNRS: A core curriculum in advanced practice geriatric nursing. In E. Flaherty & B. Resnick, (Eds.), *GNRS geriatric nursing review syllabus: A core curriculum in advanced practice geriatric nursing* (4th ed., pp. 506–529). New York, NY: American Geriatrics Society.

Bhasin, S., & Jameson, J. L. (2015). Disorders of the testes and male reproductive system. In S. Melmed, K. S. Polonsky, P. R. Larsen, & H. M. Kronenberg (Eds.), *Williams textbook of endocrinology* (13th ed., pp. 785–832). Philadelphia, PA: Elsevier.

Lee, A. (Ed.). (2016). *NPPR: Nurse practitioners' prescribing reference.* New York, NY: Haymarket Media.

Medical Council of Canada. (2018). *Clinical laboratory tests: Normal values.* Retrieved from https://mcc.ca/objectives/normal-values/?cn-reloaded=1

Morales, A., Bebb, R. A., Manjoo, P., Assimakopoulos, P., Axler, J., Collier, C., & Lee, J. C. (2015). Diagnosis and management of testosterone deficiency syndrome in men: Clinical practice guideline. *CMAJ*. doi:10.1503/cmaj.150033. Retrieved from http://www.cmaj.ca/content/cmaj/early/2015/10/26/cmaj.150033.full.pdf.

Prescriber's Letter. (2015). Appropriate medication use in older adults: 2015 updated. *Beer's Criteria, 22*(12), 311218. Retrieved from http://prescribersletter.therapeuticresearch.com

Snyder, P. J. (2015, January). Clinical features and diagnosis of male hypogonadism. *UpToDate.* Retrieved from http://www.uptodate.com

Metabolic Syndrome/Insulin Resistance Syndrome

Jill C. Cash, Melissa A. Hall, and Kelly Power-Kean

Definition

A. Metabolic syndrome is an association of several complex disorders: obesity, insulin-resistant type 2 diabetes, hypertension, and hyperlipidaemia. This coexistence of conditions leads to atherosclerotic cardiovascular (CV) disease. Metabolic syndrome is considered a proinflammatory and prothrombotic state. Elevated triglycerides and low high-density lipoprotein (HDL) cholesterol are strong predictors of vascular events. Triglycerides and the waist circumference are considered the strongest predictors for the development of metabolic syndrome.

The inclusion of type 2 diabetes in the definition of metabolic syndrome is debated. Currently, there is no consensus on definition for metabolic syndrome in children. A harmonized definition of the metabolic syndrome was established in 2009 (see Table 20.4) to assist in diagnosis.

Complications associated with metabolic syndrome include fatty liver disease, cirrhosis, chronic kidney disease, polycystic ovarian syndrome (PCOS), obstructive sleep apnea (OSA), and gout.

Metabolic syndrome is noted in the literature under other names, including insulin resistance syndrome and obesity dyslipidaemia syndrome. Previously, the term "Syndrome X" was used; however, Syndrome X is noted to have normal coronary arteries and the occurrence of angina.

Incidence/Prevalence

A. Age-dependent increase in incidence; overall incidence is estimated at 19.1% of the population. With the increase in childhood obesity, metabolic syndrome is being increasingly diagnosed in children. The Canadian prevalence of metabolic syndrome in children is 2.1%.
B. Asians living in the United States and Mexican Americans have the highest age-adjusted prevalence. Among African Americans and Mexican Americans, the prevalence is higher in women than in men. There are limited Canadian data available regarding the prevalence of metabolic syndrome in the Indigenous population. Considering the increasing prevalence of type 2 diabetes in Indigenous communities across North America, this raises concerns about metabolic syndrome in these populations.
C. Ethnic background:
   1. Indigenous peoples are at the greatest risk (60% females and 45% males).
   2. Mexican Americans have the highest prevalence (31.9%).
   3. Black and Hispanic females are 1.5 times more likely than non-Hispanic White females.

Pathogenesis

A. The exact aetiology is unknown; however, abdominal obesity has been associated with insulin resistance. Vascular endothelial dysfunction occurs secondary to insulin resistance, hyperglycaemia, hyperinsulinaemia, and adipokines. Along with high blood pressure (BP) and abnormal lipids, vascular inflammation places the individual at high risk of a CV insult.

Predisposing Factors

A. Genetic predisposition.
B. Weight gain, especially central/abdominal obesity.
C. Females, especially postmenopausal.
D. Childhood obesity.
E. Smoking.
F. High-carbohydrate diet, especially soft drink consumption.
G. Lack of exercise:
   1. Sedentary lifestyle.
   2. Television or other electronic device use more than two hours per day.
H. Insulin resistance.

Common Findings

A. Complaints are all related to the individual coexisting comorbid symptoms.

Other Signs and Symptoms

A. All are related to the individual coexisting comorbid symptoms.

TABLE 20.4 Harmonized Definition of the Metabolic Syndrome: At Least Three Measures to Make the Diagnosis of Metabolic Syndrome

Measure	Categorical Thresholds	
	Men	Women
Elevated waist circumference (cm; population and country specific cut points):		
• Canada; United States	≥102 cm	≥88 cm
• Europids; Middle Eastern; Sub-Saharan African; Mediterranean	≥94 cm	≥80 cm
• Asians; Japanese; South and Central Americans	≥90 cm	≥80 cm
Elevated TG (mmol/L; drug treatment for elevated TG is an alternate indicator[a])	≥1.7 mmol/L	
Reduced HDL-C (mmol/L; drug treatment for reduced HDL-C is an alternate indicator[a])	<1.0	<1.3
Elevated BP (mmHg; antihypertensive drug treatment in a person with a history of hypertension is an alternate indicator)	Systolic ≥130 and/or diastolic ≥85	
Elevated FPG (mmol/L; drug treatment of elevated glucose is an alternate indicator)	≥5.6	

[a]The most commonly used drugs for elevated TG and reduced HDL-C are fibrates and nicotinic acid. A person taking one of these drugs can be presumed to have high TG and reduced HDL-C. High-dose omega-3 fatty acids presumes high TG.
BP, blood pressure; FPG, fasting plasma glucose; HDL-C, high-density lipoprotein cholesterol; TG, triglycerides.
Source: Adapted from: Alberti, K. G., Eckel, R., Grundy, S., Zimmet, P. Z., Cleeman, J. I., Donato, K. A., . . . International Association for the Study of Obesity. (2009). Harmonizing the metabolic syndrome. Circulation, 120(16), 1640–1645. doi:10.1161/CIRCULATIONAHA.109.192644.

Subjective Data

A. Review the client's medical history related to comorbid conditions, including obesity, hypertension, and any abnormal laboratory testing (lipids, triglycerides, and glucose tolerance tests [GTTs]).
B. Review the client's family history.
C. Review all prescription medications, over-the-counter (OTC) drugs, and herbals.
D. Review the client's current level of exercise.
E. Review the client's usual diet (24-hour recall), noting high fat and high glucose consumption, including fast food and processed food consumption.
F. Review the client's reproductive history.

Physical Examination

A. Check height, weight, waist circumference, BP, pulse, and respirations.
B. Calculate the body mass index (BMI) and waist-to-hip measurement. Several websites have BMI, body fat, and waist-to-hip ratio calculators. Document on a growth chart BMI results for visual teaching support for client and parent.
C. Make general observations for acanthosis nigricans and skin tags (insulin resistance).
D. A full physical examination is guided by the client's medical history and presenting signs and symptoms.

Diagnostic Tests

A. Fasting plasma glucose (FPG).
B. Fasting lipid panel.
C. Triglycerides.
D. Consider thyroid function.
E. Consider C-reactive protein (CRP; optional).

Differential Diagnoses

A. Metabolic syndrome:
  1. Obesity.
  2. Hypertension.
  3. Hyperlipidaemia.
  4. High FPG.
B. Cushing's syndrome.

Plan

A. General interventions: Aggressive lifestyle modification focusing on increased physical activity and weight reduction is a cornerstone for treatment.
B. Client teaching: A team approach to managing metabolic syndrome draws upon the expertise of physicians, nurses, dietitians, and kinesiologists, and makes efficient use of each professional's time:
  1. Dietary recommendations include low-fat, low-cholesterol, and/or dietary approaches to stop hypertension (DASH). Decrease simple sugar consumption, as well as saturated and trans fats and cholesterol (see Appendix B). The Mediterranean diet has also shown to be quite effective in the prevention of metabolic syndrome and has been shown to prevent major cardiovascular events in high-risk clients. The Mediterranean diet suggests including foods that are high in monounsaturated fat (mainly from olive oil), high in complex carbohydrates from legumes and grains, high in fiber (mainly from vegetables and fruit) and high in fish; limiting foods with refined carbohydrates, processed foods/fast foods, red meat, and animal fat.
  2. Exercise recommendations include a minimum of 30 minutes a day of walking at a brisk pace or other activity at a moderate intensity. Start by using a pedometer, walking at breaks, or performing household work.
  3. Weight loss of 5% to 10% or more should be encouraged (gradual weight loss of 1–2 kg/mo). Even small losses are associated with health benefits.
  4. BP control strategies include DASH, smoking cessation, and alcohol in moderation.
  5. Counsel on smoking cessation.
  6. Abdominoplasties do not lower the risk for coronary artery disease (CAD) or insulin sensitivity.
C. Pharmacological therapy:
  1. Currently, the treatment for metabolic syndrome is to treat each individual component/diagnosis for the individual.
  2. Insulin-resistant clients usually are not treated by insulin.
  3. Statins are the most common classification used for elevated lipids.
  4. Low-dose ASA may be prescribed related to the client's risk of CV disease, with an increased risk of the client having a prothrombotic state.
  5. Oral hypoglycaemic agents used to treat type 2 diabetes are not currently recommended for the prevention of metabolic syndrome.
  6. Hypertension should be controlled with appropriate antihypertensives.

Follow-Up

A. Follow-up involves assessing clients for metabolic syndrome at a minimum of three-year intervals for anyone with one or more risk traits. Follow-up testing includes the following:
  1. BMI calculation.
  2. Waist-to-hip calculation.
  3. Fasting lipid profile.
  4. Fasting glucose or other diabetic screening methods (hemoglobin A1C, GGT).
  5. BP.

Consultation/Referral

A. Refer to an obstetrician/gynaecologist for consultation and management for infertility/pregnancy.
B. Refer to a specialist for any comorbid condition as needed.

Individual Considerations

A. Individual considerations for pregnancy, paediatrics, and geriatrics are specific to their comorbid condition.

Bibliography

Alberti, K. G., Eckel, R., Grundy, S., Zimmet, P. Z., Cleeman, J. I., Donato, K. A., . . . International Association for the Study of Obesity. (2009). Harmonizing the metabolic syndrome. *Circulation, 120*(16), 1640–1645. doi:10.1161/CIRCULATIONAHA.109.192644

American Geriatric Society. (2014). GNRS: A core curriculum in advanced practice geriatric nursing. In E. Flaherty & B. Resnick (Eds.), *GNRS geriatric nursing review syllabus: A core curriculum in advanced practice geriatric nursing* (4th ed., pp. 506–529). New York, NY: American Geriatrics Society.

American Heart Association, World Heart Federation, International Atherosclerosis Society, and International Association for the Study of Obesity. (2009). Harmonizing the metabolic syndrome: a joint interim statement of the international diabetes federation task force on epidemiology and prevention; National heart, Lung, and blood institute; American heart association; World heart federation; International atherosclerosis society; and international association for the study of obesity. *Circulation, 120*, 1640–1645.

BMI Calculator. (n.d.-a). *BMI calculator*. Retrieved from http://www.bmi-calculator.net

BMI Calculator. (n.d.-b). *Waist to hip ratio calculator*. Retrieved from http://www.bmi-calculator.net/waist-to-hip-ratio-calculator

Bray, G. A. (2015a, January). Obesity in adults: Overview and management. *UpToDate*. Retrieved from http://www.uptodate.com

Bray, G. A. (2015b, October). Client information: Weight loss treatments, beyond the basics. *UpToDate*. Retrieved from http://www.uptodate.com

Bray, G. A. (2016a, February). Obesity in adults: Prevalence, screening, and evaluation. *UpToDate*. Retrieved from http://www.uptodate.com

Bray, G. A. (2016b, March). Obesity in adults: Drug therapy. *UpToDate*. Retrieved from http://www.uptodate.com

Bray, G. A. (2016c, March). Obesity in adults: Health hazards. *UpToDate*. Retrieved from http://www.uptodate.com

Bulun, S. E. (2016). Physiology and pathology of the female reproductive axis. In S. Melmed, K. S. Polonsky, P. R. Larsen, & H. M. Kronenberg (Eds.), *Williams textbook of endocrinology* (13th ed., pp. 590–663). Philadelphia, PA: Elsevier Saunders.

The Canadian Task Force on the Periodic Health Examination. (2017). *Periodic preventive health visits: A more appropriate approach to delivering preventive services*. Retrieved from https://canadiantaskforce.ca/guidelines/periodic-preventive-health-visits/

Centers for Disease Control and Prevention. (2011). *Adult BMI calculator: English version*. Retrieved from https://www.cdc.gov/healthyweight/assessing/bmi/adult_bmi/english_bmi_calculator/bmi_calculator.html

Centers for Disease Control and Prevention. (n. d.). *BMI percentile calculator for child and teen: English version*. Retrieved from https://nccd.cdc.gov/dnpabmi/calculator.aspx

Eckel, R. H. (2015). The metabolic syndrome. In D. L. Kasper, A. S. Fauci, S. L. Hauser, D. L. Longo, & J. L. Jameson (Eds.), *Harrison's principles of internal medicine* (19th ed., pp. 2449–2454). New York, NY: McGraw-Hill.

Eckel, R. H., Jakicie, J. M., Ard, J. D., Hubbard, V. S., de Jesus, J. M., Lee, I-Min., . . . Yanovski, S. Z. (2013). AHA/ACC guideline on lifestyle management to reduce cardiovascular risk: A report of the American college of cardiology/American heart association task force on practice guidelines. *Circulation*, 129(25 Suppl. 2), S76–S99. doi:10.1161/01.cir.0000437740.48606.d1

Ervin, B. (2009). Prevalence of metabolic syndrome among adults 20 years of age and older by sex, age, race, ethnicity, and body mass index United States 2003–2006. *National Health Statistics Reports*. No. 13. Retrieved from http://www.cdc.gov/nchs/data/nhsr/nhsr013.pdf

Genest, J., McPherson, R., Frohlich, J., Anderson, T., Campbell, N., Carpentier, A., & Ur, E. (2009). Canadian cardiovascular society/canadian guidelines for the diagnosis and treatment of dyslipidemia and prevention of cardiovascular disease in the adult-2009 recommendations. *Canadian Journal of Cardiology*, 25(10), 567–579.

Goff, D. C., Lloyd-Jones, D. M., Bennett, G., Coady, S., D'Agostino, R. B., Sr., Gibbons, R., . . . Wilson, P. W. F. (2013, November 12). 2013 ACC/AHA guideline on the assessment of cardiovascular risk: A report of the American college of cardiology/American heart association task force on practice guidelines. *Circulation*, 129, S49–S73. doi:10.1161/01.cir.0000437741.48606.98

International Diabetes Foundation. (2009). *The IDF consensus worldwide definition of metabolic sydrome*. Retrieved from https://www.idf.org/e-library/consensus-statements/60-idfconsensus-worldwide-definitionof-the-metabolic-syndrome

James, P. A., Oparil, S., Carter, B. L., Cushman, W. C., Dennison-Himmelfarb, C., Handler, J., & Ortiz, E. (2013, December 18). 2014 Evidence-based guidelines for the management of high blood pressure in adults report from the panel members appointed to the Eighth joint national committee (JNC 8). *Journal of the American Medical Association*, 311(5), 507–520. doi:10.1001/jama.2013.284427

Klish, W. J. (2014, October). Clinical evaluation of the obese child and adolescent. *UpToDate*. Retrieved from http://www.uptodate.com

Klish, W. J. (2015, November). Comorbidities and complications of obesity in children and adolescents. *UpToDate*. Retrieved from http://www.uptodate.com

Klish, W. J. (2016, March). Definition; epidemiology; and etiology of obesity in children and adolescents. *UpToDate*. Retrieved from http://www.uptodate.com

Lee, A. (Ed.). (2016). *NPPR: Nurse practitioners' prescribing reference*. New York, NY: Haymarket Media.

MacPherson, M., de Groh, M., Loukine, L., Prud'homme, D., & Dubois, L. (2016). Prevalence of metabolic syndrome and its risk factors in Canadian children and adolescents: Canadian health measures survey cycle 1 (2007–2009) and Cycle 2 (2009–2011). *Health Promotion and Chronic Disease Prevention in Canada*, 36(2), 32–40.

Mantzoros, C. (2015, July). Insulin resistance: Definition and clinical spectrum. *UpToDate*. Retrieved from http://www.uptodate.com

Medical Council of Canada. (2018). *Clinical laboratory tests: Normal values*. Retrieved from https://mcc.ca/objectives/normal-values/?cn-reloaded=1

Metabolic Syndrom Canada. (2018). *About metabolic syndrome*. Retrieved from https://www.metabolicsyndromecanada.ca/about-metabolic-syndrome

Meigs, J. B. (2015, March). The metabolic syndrome (insulin resistance syndrome or syndrome X). *UpToDate*. Retrieved from http://www.uptodate.com

National Institutes of Health. (2015). *Third report of the national cholesterol education program (NCEP) expert panel on detection, evaluation, and treatment of high blood cholesterol in adults (ATP III): final report*. Bethesda, MD: Author. Retrieved from https://www.nhlbi.nih.gov/sites/www.nhlbi.nih.gov/files/Circulation-2002-ATP-III-Final-Report-PDF-3143.pdf

Prescriber's Letter. (2015). Appropriate medication use in older adults: 2015 updated. *Beer's Criteria*, 22(12), 311218. Retrieved from http://prescribersletter.therapeuticresearch.com

Skelton, J. A. (2016, November). Management of childhood obesity in the primary care setting. *UpToDate*. Retrieved from http://www.uptodate.com

Stone, N. J., Robinson, J., Lichtenstein, A. H., Bairey Merz, C. N., Lloyd-Jones, D. M., & Blum, C. B. (2013, November 7). 2013 ACC/AHA guidelines on the treatment of blood cholesterol to reduce atherosclerotic cardiovascular risk in adults: A report of the American college of cardiology/American heart association task force on practice guidelines. *Journal of the American College of Cardiology*, 63(25), S0735–S1097. Retrieved from https://circ.ahajournals.org/content/early/2013/11/11/01.cir.0000437738.63853.7a.full.pdf

U.S. Department of Health and Human Services. (2015, May). *2015 recommendations for physical activity*. Retrieved from https://www.nhlbi.nih.gov/health/health-topics/topics/phys/recommend

Polycystic Ovarian Syndrome (PCOS)

Jill C. Cash, Melissa A. Hall, and Kelly Power-Kean

Definition

Polycystic ovarian syndrome (PCOS) is characterized by ovulatory dysfunction and hyperandrogenism. PCOS was previously called Stein–Leventhal syndrome. PCOS is a risk factor for metabolic syndrome, infertility, glucose intolerance, and type 2 diabetes mellitus (DM). PCOS itself is not considered a disease; instead, it is a syndrome of coexisting conditions (see Table 20.5).

The following are the Androgen Excess Society diagnostic criteria for PCOS:
A. Hyperandrogenism.
B. Ovarian dysfunction.
C. Exclusion of other androgen excess or related disorders.

Although obesity is one of the hallmarks of PCOS, lean women may also have insulin resistance/PCOS. The diagnosis of PCOS is based on medical history, physical examination, and laboratory tests. Aggressive lifestyle modification is the mainstay of all adolescents and women with PCOS.

Incidence/Prevalence

A. The incidence of PCOS is 6.5% up to 12% in the literature. It is the most common cause of infertility. It is also the most common worldwide endocrinopathy in women, with 5 to 7 million women in the Canada experiencing its effects.

Pathogenesis

A. The exact aetiology is unknown; however, PCOS is noted to have insulin resistance and abnormal pituitary function, as well as abnormal steroidogenesis.

TABLE: PCOS-Associated Symptoms

Cutaneous Signs	Hirsutism
Menstrual irregularity Obesity Polycystic ovaries	Severe acne Alopaecia Oligomenorrhoea Amenorrhoea Dysfunctional uterine bleeding >88 cm waist circumference for women and adolescents ≥16 years ≥90th percentile for ages 10 to <16 years Noted on pelvic ultrasound

PCOS, polycystic ovarian syndrome.

Predisposing Factors
A. Obesity.
B. Genetic predisposition, including Mexican American women.
C. Metabolic syndrome.
D. Women with oligo-ovulatory infertility.
E. Type 1, type 2, or gestational diabetes.
F. History of premature adrenarche.
G. First-degree relatives with PCOS.
H. Antiepileptic medications.

Common Findings
A. Hirsutism.
B. Menstrual problems.
C. Obesity.
D. Infertility.

Other Signs and Symptoms
A. Acne.
B. Alopaecia (male pattern).
C. Hyperhidrosis.
D. Acanthosis nigricans.
E. Seborrhoea.

Subjective Data
A. Review the client's menstruation history:
   1. Premature puberty (younger than 8 years).
   2. Primary amenorrhoea: lack of menses by age 15 years.
   3. Oligomenorrhoea: missing four periods per year.
   4. Dysfunctional uterine bleeding (DUB): bleeding at irregular intervals, heavy cycles, periods longer than seven days.
B. Review the client's history of weight gain, increased waist circumference, and obesity.
C. Review the client's history of any skin/hair changes.
D. Review the family history for the presence of diabetes, metabolic syndrome, and infertility.

Physical Examination
A. Check height, weight, waist circumference, blood pressure (BP), pulse, and respirations.
B. Calculate the body mass index (BMI) and waist-to-hip measurement. Several websites have BMI, body fat, and waist-to-hip ratio calculators.
C. Inspect:
   1. Skin:
      a. Evaluate hirsutism (upper lip, chin, nape of the neck, periareolar, abdomen—linea alba).
      b. Pigmentation patterns for acanthosis nigricans (neck, axilla).
   2. Observe fat distribution.
D. Perform pelvic examination to evaluate enlarged ovaries and pelvic masses.

Diagnostic Tests
A. Fasting glucose.
B. Oral glucose tolerance test (OGTT) if fasting glucose is elevated.
C. Thyroid function tests (thyroid-stimulating hormone [TSH], free T_4).
D. Random serum cortisol only if suspicion of Cushing's syndrome.
E. Serum luteinizing hormone (LH) and prolactin to rule out hypothalamic and pituitary diseases.
F. Ultrasound to rule out ovarian pathology (as indicated: Not required for definitive diagnosis).
G. Insulin-like growth factor (IGF-I).
H. Dehydroepiandrosterone-sulphate (DHEA-S) to rule out adrenal hyperandrogenism.
I. Free testosterone level.
J. Lipid profile.
K. Serum follicle-stimulating hormone (FSH) to rule out primary ovarian failure.
L. Pregnancy test.

Differential Diagnoses
A. Adrenal disorders:
   1. Congenital adrenal hyperplasia (CAH).
   2. Cushing's syndrome.
   3. Cortisol resistance.
B. Hyperprolactinaemia.
C. Acromegaly.
D. Insulin resistance (types 1 and 2 diabetes).
E. Thyroid dysfunction.
F. Virilizing tumours.
G. Drug-induced:
   1. Anabolic steroids.
   2. Valproic acid.

Plan
A. General interventions: Aggressive lifestyle modification focusing on increased physical activity and weight reduction is a cornerstone for treatment.
B. Client education:
   1. Exercise recommendations include a minimum of 30 minutes a day of walking at a brisk pace or other activity at a moderate intensity. Start by using a pedometer, walking at breaks, or performing household work.
   2. Weight loss of 5% to 10% or more. Gradual weight loss of 1 to 2 kg/mo is recommended. Even small amounts of weight loss are associated with health benefits.

TABLE 20.6 Androgen Excess Society Screening and Treatment Requirements for IGT

All clients with PCOS, regardless of BMI, should be screened for IGT using a two-hour OGTT.
Clients with a normal glucose test should be rescreened at least once every two years or earlier if additional risk factors are identified.
Clients with IGT should be screened annually for the development of type 2 DM.
Adolescents with PCOS should be screened for IGT using a two-hour OGTT every two years. If IGT develops, the treatment with metformin should be considered.
The mainstay of treatment with PCOS and IGT is intensive lifestyle modification (diet, exercise, and weight loss).
Insulin-sensitizing agents should be considered for clients with PCOS and IGT.

BMI, body mass index; DM, diabetes mellitus; IGT, impaired glucose tolerance; OGTT, oral glucose tolerance test; PCOS, polycystic ovarian syndrome.
Source: Adapted from Salley, K. E. S., Wickham, E. P., Cheang, K. I., Essah, P. A., Karjane, N. W., & Nestler, J. E. (2007). Position statement: Glucose intolerance in polycystic ovary syndrome—A position statement of the Androgen Excess Society. *Journal of Clinical Endocrinology & Metabolism, 92*(12), 4546–4556. Retrieved from http://press.endocrine.org/doi/pdf/10.1210/jc.2007-1549.

3. Weight loss may cause a resumption of ovulation and the ability to get pregnant.
4. High-fiber, low-fat diet and reduction of refined sugar.
5. Hair removal can be achieved with shaving, waxing, or use of depilatories. Electrolysis and laser treatment are more expensive therapies for hirsutism.

C. Pharmacological therapy:
  1. Oral contraceptive pills (OCPs) are the most commonly used treatment for endometrial prevention and hirsutism:
    a. Due to sodium and water retention, weight reduction while on OCPs is more difficult.
    b. OCPs that contain 30 to 35 mcg of ethinyl estradiol and progestins, such as norethindrone, norgestimate, desogestrel, or drospirenone, are prescribed for PCOS.
  2. Metformin is used to manage oligomenorrhoea, cause weight loss, lower insulin levels, and induce ovulation for women with PCOS:
    a. Titrate slowly because of the gastrointestinal side effects (diarrhoea).
    b. Check a metabolic panel before and every three to six months to evaluate for lactic acidosis.
    c. Metformin is contraindicated in clients with renal impairment; assess renal function before instituting metformin and monitor regularly.
    d. Metformin must be stopped before any procedure with radiographic dye.
  3. Medroxyprogesterone acetate is used for a withdrawal bleed, or micronized progesterone. This withdrawal bleeding is advised to protect the endometrium.
  4. Spironolactone is used after a four- to six-month oral contraceptive trial as antiandrogen therapy:
    a. Spironolactone is also a good alternative when OCPs are contraindicated. However, spironolactone can be used in combination with OCPs.
    b. Alternative methods of birth control should be used when spironolactone is used alone secondary to potential congenital defects such as abnormal development of the male fetus' external genitalia.
    c. Monitor potassium level during spironolactone therapy.
  5. Eflornithine topical may be prescribed to prevent facial hair regrowth.
  6. Clomiphene citrate is used to induce ovulation. Weight loss should be attempted before starting ovulation induction treatment.

Follow-Up
A. Glucose tolerance needs to be evaluated regularly for type 2 diabetes in women with PCOS (see Table 20.6).

Consultation/Referral
A. Refer to an obstetrician/gynaecologist or a reproductive endocrinologist for consultation and management of the following:
  1. Infertility/pregnancy.
  2. Menstrual bleeding that is not controlled despite OCPs.
B. An endocrinologist may be an appropriate consultation.
C. Consider a nutritional consultation for weight-loss recommendations.

Bibliography

Androgen Excess and Polycystic Ovarian Syndrome Society. (2016). *Polycystic ovarian syndrome*. Retrieved from http://ae-society.org/sub/resources.php

Azziz, R. (2015, August). Epidemiology and pathogenesis of polycystic ovarian syndrome in adults. *UpToDate*. Retrieved from http://www.uptodate.com

Barbieri, R. L., & Ehrmann, D. A. (2015, March). Treatment of polycystic ovary syndrome in adults. *UpToDate*. Retrieved from http://www.uptodate.com

BMI Calculator. (n.d.-a). *BMI calculator*. Retrieved from http://www.bmi-calculator.net

BMI Calculator. (n.d.-b). *Waist to hip ratio calculator*. Retrieved from http://www.bmi-calculator.net/waist-to-hip-ratio-calculator

Centers for Disease Control and Prevention. (2011). *Adult BMI calculator: English version*. Retrieved from https://www.cdc.gov/healthyweight/assessing/bmi/adult_bmi/english_bmi_calculator/bmi_calculator.html

Centers for Disease Control and Prevention. (n.d.). *BMI percentile calculator for child and teen: English version*. Retrieved from https://nccd.cdc.gov/dnpabmi/calculator.aspx

El-Hussein, M. T., Power-Kean, K., Zettel, S., Huether, S. E., McCance, K. L., Brashers, V. L., & Rote, N. S. (2018). *Understanding pathophysiology*. Milton, ON: Elsevier.

Hall, J. E. (2015). Menstrual disorders and pelvic pain. In D. L. Kasper, A. S. Fauci, S. L. Hauser, D. L. Longo, & J. L. Jameson (Eds.), *Harrison's principles of internal medicine* (19th ed.). New York, NY: McGraw-Hill.

Lee, A. (Ed.) (2016). *NPPR: Nurse practitioners' prescribing reference*. New York, NY: Haymarket Media.

Lujan, M. E., Chizen, D. R., & Pierson, R. A. (2008). Diagnostic criteria for polycystic ovary syndrome: Pitfalls and controversies. *Journal of Obstetrics and Gynaecology Canada, 30*(8), 671–679. doi:10.1016/S1701-2163(16)32915-2

Medical Council of Canada. (2018). *Clinical laboratory tests: Normal values*. Retrieved from https://mcc.ca/objectives/normal-values/?cn-reloaded=1

Rosenfield, R. L. (2014a, October). Treatment of polycystic ovary syndrome in adolescents. *UpToDate*. Retrieved from http://www.uptodate.com

Rosenfield, R. L. (2014b, October). Definition, clinical features, and differential diagnosis of polycystic ovary syndrome in adolescents. *UpToDate*. Retrieved from http://www.uptodate.com

Salley, K. E. S., Wickham, E. P., Cheang, K. I., Essah, P. A., Karjane, N. W., & Nestler, J. E. (2007). Position statement: Glucose intolerance in polycystic ovary syndrome—A position statement of the Androgen excess society. *Journal of Clinical Endocrinology & Metabolism, 92*(12), 4546–4556. Retrieved from http://press.endocrine.org/doi/pdf/10.1210/jc.2007-1549

Stewart, P. M., & Newell-Price, J. D. (2016). The adrenal cortex. In S. Melmed, K. S. Polonsky, P. R. Larsen, & H. M. Kronenberg (Eds.), *Williams textbook of endocrinology* (13th ed., pp. 490–556). Philadelphia, PA: Elsevier.

Wjjeyaratne, C. N., Udayangani, S. A. D., & Balen, A. H. (2013). Ethnic-specific polyovarian syndrome. Epidemiology, significance, and implications. *Expert Review in Endocrinology and Metabolism, 8*(1), 71–79.

Thyroid Disease: Hyperthyroidism

Jill C. Cash, Melissa A. Hall, and Kelly Power-Kean

Definition
A. Hyperthyroidism is a condition in which thyroid hormone exerts greater than normal responses. Hyperthyroidism may be subclinical and may not be easily recognized or exhibit overt symptoms. The most common hyperthyroid conditions are Graves' disease and toxic multinodular goiter. The The Canadian Task Force on the Periodic Health Examination does not recommend screening for thyroid dysfunction in asymptomatic adults who are not pregnant.

Incidence/Prevalence
A. Overall prevalence of Graves' disease is 1% of the Canadian population. Graves' disease is the underlying cause for 50% to 80% of cases of hyperthyroidism.
B. Female gender:
  1. 5:1 ratio higher in women than men.
  2. Older women: 4% to 5% incidence.
  3. Graves' disease is more common in younger women.
  4. Toxic nodular goiter is more common in older women.
C. Children:
  1. Graves' disease in children 0.02% (1:5000).
  2. Most often occurs in 11- to 15-year-olds.
D. Elderly: Toxic multinodular goiter (Plummer disease) occurs in 15% to 20% of clients with thyrotoxicosis.
E. Symptomatology incidence:
  1. Ophthalmopathy is more common in smokers.
  2. Atrial fibrillation 10% to 25% incidence and is more common in the elderly.
  3. Autoimmune thyroid diseases have a peak incidence in people aged 20 to 40 years.

Pathogenesis
A. Hyperthyroidism is one form of thyrotoxicosis, in which an excess of hormone is excreted by the thyroid gland. The diseases that can cause hyperthyroidism include Graves' disease, toxic multinodular goiter, thyroid cancer, and increased secretion of the thyroid-stimulating hormone (TSH). Thyrotoxicosis not related to hyperthyroidism may be subacute thyroiditis, ectopic thyroid tissue, and ingestion of excessive thyroid hormone. Postpartum thyroiditis can precipitate a short-term mild hyperthyroidism, which has an onset at two to six months postpartum. Severe thyrotoxicosis of any cause is called thyrotoxic crisis or storm.

In Graves' disease, the normal feedback mechanisms that regulate hormone secretion are taken over by some abnormal thyroid-stimulating mechanism. Thyroid autoantibodies of the immunoglobulin G (IgG) class are present in more than 95% of clients with Graves' disease. The hyperfunctioning of the thyroid gland causes suppression of TSH and thyrotropin-releasing hormone (TRH). There are profound increases in iodine uptake and thyroid gland metabolism, which are believed to be the causes of the gland enlargement. The resulting increase in the level of circulating thyroid hormone is responsible for the thyrotoxic symptoms.

In the condition called toxic multinodular goiter, the thyroid gland enlarges in response to some bodily needs such as puberty; pregnancy; iodine deficiency; and immunologic, viral, and genetic disorders. As TSH levels rise, the gland enlarges; when the condition demanding increased thyroid hormone resolves, TSH levels usually return to normal and the gland slowly assumes its original size.

Predisposing Factors
A. Graves' disease:
  1. Women in the second through fifth decades of life.
  2. Familial autoimmune thyroid disease.
  3. Concomitant disorders believed to be autoimmune.
  4. Increased in clients diagnosed with trisomy 21.
  5. Higher incidence in persons who smoke.
B. Toxic multinodular goiter:
  1. Older people.
  2. Recent exposure to iodine-containing medications (amiodarone and radiocontrast dye).
  3. Long-standing simple goiter.
  4. Conditions such as puberty, pregnancy, iodine deficiency, and immunologic, viral, or genetic disorders.

Common Findings
A. Graves' disease:
  1. Prominence/protrusion of the eye (exophthalmos).
  2. Prominent "stare."
  3. Visual changes:
    a. Diplopia.
    b. Photophobia.
    c. Eye irritation: gritty feeling or pain.
B. Weight loss with no change in diet or an increase in appetite.
C. Anorexia (may be prominent in the elderly).
D. Weakness and fatigue.
E. Tachycardia.
F. Decreased tolerance of heat.
G. Thinning scalp hair.
H. Fingernail separation from the nail bed.
I. Smooth, thin skin.
J. Heart palpitations (atrial fibrillation).
K. Bowel symptoms:
  1. Increase in frequency and loose bowel movements (not diarrhoea).
  2. Constipation (more frequent in the elderly).
L. Swelling of feet and ankles.

Other Signs and Symptoms
A. Goiter: **Approximately 50% of clients will not have an enlargement of the thyroid gland.** Elderly clients are less likely to have a goiter.
B. Periorbital oedema.
C. Flushing, warm skin.
D. Fine hand tremors.
E. Dyspnoea (especially elderly).
F. Exertional fatigue/exercise intolerance.
G. Insomnia.
H. Irritability.
I. Nervousness.
J. Mood swings.

K. Inability to concentrate.
L. Depression and apathy (elderly).
M. Hyperactivity (children).
N. Decreased menses.
O. Impotence and decreased libido in men.
P. Gynaecomastia.
Q. Galactorrhoea (TSH-mediated hyperthyroidism).
R. Atrial dysrhythmias (atrial fibrillation), left ventricular dilation (common in elderly).
S. Urinary frequency and nocturia (enuresis is common in children).
T. A combination of these noted symptoms should lead to the assessment of hyperthyroidism.

Subjective Data
A. Identify when symptoms began, duration, and any change or progression.
B. Identify whether the client has noticed enlargement of the thyroid gland, difficulty swallowing, or change in voice.
C. Assess for change in weight over the past three months, past six months, and last year. Ask the client whether his or her appetite has changed.
D. Explore the client's family history of thyroid problems.
E. Obtain the client's medical history of associated diseases (especially those of autoimmune pathogenesis: pernicious anaemia, type 1 diabetes mellitus [DM], myasthenia gravis, receptor agonist [RA], ulcerative colitis).
F. Review the client's medication history including amiodarone, interferon alpha, levothyroxine (overdose), expectorants, and health food supplements containing seaweed.
G. Ask the client to identify any changes in bowel habits, loose (nondiarrhoea) stools, frequency of bowel movements, or constipation.
H. Ask about moods; changes in concentration; feelings of restlessness, nervousness, anxiety; and change in sleep habits.
I. Assess for any cardiac symptoms, such as palpitations, chest pain, shortness of breath, and decreased tolerance for activities previously done.
J. Ask whether the client has noticed any swelling or puffiness anywhere.
K. Determine whether the client has experienced changes in vision and/or eye irritation.
L. Assess for hand tremors, increase in the moistness and coolness of the skin, flushing, and blushing.
M. Ask the client to identify any menstrual changes or whether the client has had a recent pregnancy, or is in the postpartum period.
N. Review for a recent history of a viral infection.
O. Review recent trauma to the neck (significant trauma can cause thyrotoxicosis).

Physical Examination
A. Check temperature, if indicated, pulse (tachycardia), respirations (dyspnoea), blood pressure (BP; systolic hypertension), and weight. Children: Plot height/weight on growth curve. (Accelerated growth is noted.)
B. Inspect:
  1. Observe overall appearance: Does the client have any difficulty with breathing, including dyspnoea, or difficulty swallowing from tracheal obstruction secondary to a large goiter?
  2. Note eyelid retraction, lid lag, and exophthalmos. The clinician may see periorbital oedema and an elevated upper eyelid, which leads to decreased blinking and a staring quality in Graves' disease.
  3. Note tremors that are best demonstrated from outstretched hands.
  4. Inspect the skin for temperature and texture.
  5. Inspect the fingernails for the following:
    a. Onycholysis, also known as Plummer's nails (loosening of the nails from the nail beds).
    b. Softening of the nails.
  6. Inspect scalp hair.
  7. Assess Tanner stage in preadolescence/adolescence. Puberty may be delayed.
C. Auscultate:
  1. The thyroid for bruits.
  2. The heart and pulse rate. Clients with subclinical hyperthyroidism frequently present with atrial fibrillation.
  3. The carotid arteries for bruits.
  4. Bowel sounds.
D. Palpate:
  1. Palpate the neck and thyroid for nodules, thrills, and enlargement. Depending on the aetiology of the hyperthyroidism, the thyroid may range from normal to massive (Graves' disease or toxic multinodular goiter). Palpation of the thyroid can induce the gland to release increased hormone; be alert for signs and symptoms of thyroid storm.
  2. If the thyroid is tender and painful to palpation, granulomatous thyroiditis may be the aetiology of hyperthyroidism.
  3. Palpate the heart for thrills.
  4. Palpate extremities for oedema. Pretibial myxoedema is noted in Graves' disease.
E. Neurologic examination:
  1. Assess deep tendon reflexes (DTRs).
  2. Tests for lid lag:
    a. Have the client follow your finger as it moves up and down.
    b. Have the client look down and observe if sclera can be seen above the iris.
  3. Have the client stick out the tongue to observe for presence of tremours.

Diagnostic Tests
A. TSH, free thyroxine (T4), triiodothyronine (T3; see Table 20.7).
B. Radioactive iodine (131I) uptake (RAIU) if needed. If the client has ophthalmopathy, clinical symptoms of hyperthyroidism, and a diffusely enlarged thyroid gland, the RAIU test is not necessary to confirm Graves' disease. Pregnancy and breastfeeding are absolute contraindications to radionuclide imaging.
C. Consider additional laboratory testing:
  1. Complete blood count (CBC; may have normochromic, normocytic anaemia).
  2. Serum ferritin (may be high).
D. If T4 and T3 are high, but TSH is normal or high, an MRI of the pituitary should be ordered to look for a pituitary mass.
E. An echocardiogram should be considered whether an irregular heart rate and signs of heart failure are noted on examination.

Differential Diagnoses
A. Hyperthyroidism:
  1. Graves' disease.
  2. T3-toxicosis.

Test Results in Hyperthyroidism

Disorder	TSH	Free T4	T3	RAIU and Thyroid Scan
Overt hyperthyroidism	L	H	H	H
Graves' disease	L	H	H	H
Multinodular goiter	L	H	–	H
T3 thyrotoxicosis (may be caused by antithyroid drug therapy)	L	N or H	H	N or H

H, high; L, low; N, normal, RAIU, radioactive iodine uptake; TSH, thyroid-stimulating hormone.

3. T4-toxicosis.
4. Thyroid adenoma.
5. Drug-induced hyperthyroidism, that is, iodine-rich amiodarone.
6. Subclinical hyperthyroidism.
7. TSH-induced hyperthyroidism (TSH-secreting pituitary adenoma).
8. Hyperthyroidism during pregnancy.
9. Hashitoxicosis (combination of Hashimoto and thyrotoxicosis), rare autoimmune thyroid disease.

B. Cardiovascular disease such as coronary artery disease (CAD) and heart failure.
C. Gastrointestinal disorders such as irritable bowel syndrome (IBS), ulcerative colitis, and Crohn's disease.
D. Cancer: Testicular germ cell tumours.
E. Neurologic disorder.
F. Hydatidiform mole (molar pregnancy).
G. Psychological disorder.

Plan

A. General interventions:
 1. Carefully assess for complications of hyperthyroidism—cardiac, ophthalmologic, gastrointestinal, musculoskeletal, and psychological—and address each area identified.
 2. Clients with tachycardia, palpitations, tremours, anxiety, and eyelid lag can be treated with a beta-adrenergic antagonist for some relief from those symptoms until they become euthyroid.
 3. For infiltrative dermopathy over the lower extremities, the use of occlusive wraps on the affected side is recommended.
 4. Only 5% of clients with Graves' disease develop severe ophthalmopathy. An initial ophthalmologic examination is recommended as baseline, with follow-up determined by the ophthalmologist.
B. Client teaching:
 1. Clients taking propylthiouracil (PTU) or methimazole (MMI) should be instructed to immediately report any side effects, including rash, hives, fever, jaundice, abdominal pain, and clay-coloured stools.
 2. Less than 1% of clients develop agranulocytosis, but all clients should be instructed to call the provider immediately if a fever, sore throat, or joint ache develops due to their susceptibility to serious infection.
 3. Clients receiving radioactive iodine (RAI) should be informed that they most likely need to take lifelong hormone replacement after the RAI treatment is completed.
 4. Teach safety measures to guard against the possibility of fractures due to bone density loss secondary to hyperthyroidism.
 5. Inform clients that an episode of serious depression may follow successful treatment of hyperthyroidism.
 6. No special diet is required; however, clients should be told to avoid herbal supplements and sushi that contains seaweed.
C. Medical/surgical management:
 1. RAI is a common first-line therapy for adults. It is administered in capsule form or in water:
  a. One dose is usually sufficient; however, a second dose may be given if necessary.
  b. Permanent hypothyroidism requiring lifelong hormone replacement is the only notable complication.
 2. A thyroidectomy is seldom used except in limited client conditions:
  a. Pregnancy if women are noncompliant or cannot tolerate thionamides because of allergies or agranulocytosis.
  b. Severe hyperthyroidism in children.
  c. Clients who refuse RAI therapy.
  d. Refractory amiodarone-induced hyperthyroidism.
  e. Clients with unstable cardiac conditions that require quick normalization of thyroid function.
D. Pharmacological therapy:
 1. Antithyroid drugs: The first-line treatment depends on clinician experience, the severity of the disease, and client preference. Provide titration of antithyroid drug dose every four weeks until thyroid function normalizes and to ensure the client does not become hypothyroid. Graves' disease may go into remission after treatment for 12 to 18 months and drug therapy can be discontinued:
  a. PTU:
   i. Not a first-line agent in paediatrics.
   ii. Except in thyroid storm, PTU is considered a second-line drug therapy. It is reserved for use in clients who are allergic to or intolerant of MMI and in women who are in the first trimester of pregnancy or planning pregnancy.
  b. MMI:
   i. MMI is more potent than PTU and has a longer duration of action.
   ii. MMI is not recommended for use in the first trimester of pregnancy.
 2. RAI therapy is one of the most common treatments in adults. It is administered orally as a single dose. RAI is contraindicated in pregnancy and lactation.
 3. Beta-blockers, such as propranolol (Inderal), are also used for hyperthyroidism.
 4. Atrial fibrillation treatment is directed toward restoring an euthyroid state. Other therapies include the following:
  a. Beta-blockers (unless contraindicated, including chronic obstructive pulmonary disease [COPD] and asthma).
  b. Calcium channel blockers if unable to use beta-blocker.
  c. Oral anticoagulation (keeping the international normalized ratio [INR] between 2 and 3).
  d. Antiarrhythmic drugs and cardioversion may be unsuccessful until euthyroid.

Follow-Up
A. Depending on the experience of the clinician, a specialist, such as an endocrinologist, best performs treatment and therapy, including RAI and antithyroid medication.
B. Clients receiving PTU or MMI should be seen in the office every four to six weeks for evaluation and have blood drawn for serum TSH and free T4 measurements until euthyroid state is achieved and maintained.
C. Clients are usually maintained on these drugs for one to two years, with office visits every three months. The drug is then gradually withdrawn and 25% to 90% of clients experience permanent remission.
D. Clients with RAI therapy should be seen in the office to monitor thyroid levels. It is anticipated that most of them will require lifelong hormone replacement medication following treatment.
E. Due to the increased risk of bone loss, perform dual-energy x-ray absorptiometry (DEXA) scans to evaluate for osteopaenia/osteoporosis.
F. Consider testing for impaired glucose tolerance (IGT) in untreated clients.

Consultation/Referral
A. Ophthalmology consultation is recommended for clients with ophthalmologic involvement.
B. If surgery is the choice of treatment, refer the client to an endocrinologist and a surgeon.
C. An experienced obstetrician or perinatologist should follow pregnant women.

Individual Considerations
A. Pregnancy:
   1. Pregnant clients with mild hyperthyroidism may be followed with treatment.
   2. If an antithyroid drug is necessary, PTU is the first-line treatment in the first trimester. MMI has been associated with congenital anomalies such as tracheoesophageal fistula and choanal atresia. After the first trimester, mothers may be switched to MMI.
   3. Monitor thyroid function every four to six weeks during pregnancy.
   4. RAI therapy is contraindicated during pregnancy and breastfeeding.
   5. Thyrotoxicosis may improve during pregnancy; however, symptoms may relapse during the postpartum period.
   6. Hyperthyroidism in the third trimester may increase the risk of low birth weight.
   7. Prolonged high-dose iodine therapy can cause fetal goiter.
   8. Ultrasounds should be performed to evaluate fetal hyperthyroidism such as goiter, poor growth, cardiac failure, and hydrops fetalis.
B. Paediatrics:
   1. Low thyroid function at birth is present in approximately half of the neonates whose mother received PTU or MMI during pregnancy.
   2. Graves' disease can occur in prepubescent girls. Symptoms can be vague and include hyperactivity or slowness and fatigue.
   3. Carefully assess for goiter in children who present with a variety of symptoms otherwise unexplained.
   4. PTU should not be used in paediatrics unless there is allergy to or intolerance of MMI and other options are not available.
C. Adults: Sympathetic activation (anxiety, hyperactivity, etc.) is seen in adult years more commonly than in the elderly population.
D. Geriatrics:
   1. Older clients exhibit only three clinical signs (tachycardia, fatigue, and weight loss), whereas younger clients may exhibit as many as 12 symptoms.
   2. Rare signs in this population include atrial fibrillation, hyperactive reflexes, increased sweating, heat intolerance, tremours, nervousness, polydipsia, and increased appetite. Goiter is much less common.
   3. Elderly women with hyperthyroidism are at increased risk for accelerated bone loss.

Bibliography
American Geriatric Society. (2014). GNRS: A core curriculum in advanced practice geriatric nursing. In E. Flaherty & B. Resnick (Eds.), *GNRS geriatric nursing review syllabus: A core curriculum in advanced practice geriatric nursing* (4th ed., pp. 506–529). New York, NY: American Geriatrics Society.
Centers for Disease Control and Prevention, NCHS National Center for Health Statistics. (n.d.). *Clinical growth charts*. Retrieved from https://www.cdc.gov/growthcharts
El-Hussein, M. T., Power-Kean, K., Zettel, S., Huether, S. E., McCance, K. L., Brashers, V. L., & Rote, N. S. (2018). *Understanding pathophysiology*. Milton, ON: Elsevier.
Jameson, J. L., Mandel, S. J., & Weetman, A. P. (2015). Disorders of the thyroid gland. In D. L. Kasper, A. S. Fauci, S. L. Hauser, D. L. Longo, & J. L. Jameson (Eds.), *Harrison's principles of internal medicine* (19th ed.). New York, NY: McGraw-Hill.
Lee, A. (Ed.). (2016). *NPPR: Nurse practitioners' prescribing reference*. New York, NY: Haymarket Media.
LaFranchi, S. (2015, April). Clinical manifestations and diagnosis of hyperthyroidism in children and adolescents. *UpToDate*. Retrieved from http://www.uptodate.com
Medical Council of Canada. (2018). *Clinical laboratory tests: Normal values*. Retrieved from https://mcc.ca/objectives/normal-values/?cn-reloaded=1
National Guideline Clearinghouse. (2015, May). *Screening for thyroid dysfunction: U. S. Preventative services task force recommendation statement*. Retrieved from http://www.guideline.gov/content.aspx?id=49227&search=thyroid+screening
Prescriber's Letter. (2015). Appropriate medication use in older adults: 2015 updated. *Beer's Criteria*, 22(12), 311218. Retrieved from http://prescribersletter.therapeuticresearch.com
Ross, D. S. (2015, February). Hypothyroidism during pregnancy: Clinical manifestations, diagnosis, and treatment of hyperthyroidism during pregnancy. *UpToDate*. Retrieved from http://www.uptodate.com
Rubin, D. I. (2015, April). Neurologic manifestations of hyperthyroidism and graves disease. *UpToDate*. Retrieved from http://www.uptodate.com

Thyroid Disease: Hypothyroidism

Jill C. Cash, Melissa A. Hall, and Kelly Power-Kean

Definition
A. Hypothyroidism is a condition in which the body does not produce enough thyroid hormone. In general, hypothyroidism is considered permanent, requiring lifelong therapy to restore a euthyroid state. The most common physical finding is a goiter. The most common worldwide cause of hypothyroidism is iodine deficiency, whereas the most common cause in the United States is Hashimoto thyroiditis, an autoimmune thyroid disease.

Incidence/Prevalence
A. Hypothyroidism occurs in 2% of the Canadian population.
B. It occurs in women more than men (five to eight times higher).

C. The incidence is higher in Whites (5.1%) and Mexican Americans (5.1%) than in African Americans (1.7%).
D. It may present in up to 15% of people older than 65 years.
E. In adolescents, approximately 6% have acquired hypothyroidism.
F. Approximately 10% of clients with type 1 diabetes will develop chronic thyroiditis.
G. After pregnancy, up to 10% of women develop lymphocytic thyroiditis in the postpartum period (up to 10 months postpartum).
H. Approximately one in every 3,000 to 4,000 newborns in Canada have congenital hypothyroidism (cretinism).

Pathogenesis

Hypothyroidism is caused by an insufficient production of thyroid hormones by the thyroid gland, either by a primary or a secondary cause.

A. Primary causes include decreased hormone production caused by autoimmune thyroiditis, endemic iodine deficiency, congenital defects, or decreased thyroid activity after treatment for hyperthyroidism.

The most common cause of primary hypothyroidism is chronic autoimmune thyroiditis, called Hashimoto's thyroiditis. In this disease, circulating thyroid antibodies and the infiltration of lymphocytes destroy thyroid tissue. Autoimmune thyroiditis may also be a result of an inherited immune defect.
B. Secondary causes are much less common, but may include insufficient stimulation from the pituitary or hypothalamus and peripheral resistance to thyroid hormones.

Acute thyroidism is a rare cause of hypothyroidism in which the cause is an acute bacterial infection. Subacute thyroiditis, a nonbacterial inflammation of the thyroid, is often preceded by a viral infection. Both of these conditions cause inflammation of the thyroid gland by lymphocytic and leukocytic infiltration into the thyroid tissue, resulting in hypothyroidism.

Predisposing Factors

A. Iodine deficiency.
B. Women older than 40 years at highest risk.
C. Presence of other autoimmune disorders (diagnosed and previously undiagnosed).
D. Recent acute bacterial or viral infection.
E. Treatment with radioactive iodine (RAI) for thyroid gland problems.
F. Surgical removal of thyroid gland.
G. Exposure to external radiation.
H. Evidence of pituitary or hypothalamic disease.
I. Postpartum period.
J. Type 1 (autoimmune) diabetes mellitus (DM).
K. Chromosomal disorders:
   1. Down syndrome.
   2. Turner's syndrome.
   3. Klinefelter's syndrome.
L. Celiac disease.
M. Drug-induced:
   1. Amiodarone.
   2. Interferon alpha.
   3. Thalidomide.
   4. Lithium.
   5. Stavudine.
   6. Dopamine.

Common Findings

A. Weight gain/obesity.
B. Fatigue/sluggishness.
C. Cold intolerance.
D. Constipation.
E. Dry and flaky skin.
F. Coarseness or loss of hair, inability of hair to hold a curl, hair loss at eyebrows, and reduced growth of hair.
G. Reduced growth of nails.
H. Hoarseness.
I. Memory or mental impairment, difficulty concentrating, and slowed speech or thinking.
J. Periorbital oedema and facial puffiness.
K. Irregular or heavy menses and infertility.
L. Muscle aching and stiffness.
M. Children:
   1. Short stature.
   2. Delayed skeletal maturation.
   3. Overweight.
   4. Delayed puberty.
   5. Some adolescents have sexual precocity:
      a. Girls: Breast development.
      b. Boys: Macro-orchidism.

Other Signs and Symptoms

A. Asymptomatic if subclinical hypothyroidism and have no overt symptoms.
B. Delayed reflexes.
C. Elevated blood pressure (BP).
D. Hyperlipidaemia.
E. Jaundice.
F. Painful subacute thyroiditis:
   1. Sudden neck pain with sore throat, radiating to jaw and ears, and pain shifting to sides of the neck.
   2. Late stage: Myxoedema, thick scaly skin, muscle weakness/joint pain, enlarged tongue, hearing loss, bradycardia, cardiac hypertrophy, pleural effusion, and ascites.
G. Pituitary or hypothalamic failure:
   1. Loss of axillary and pubic hair.
   2. Cessation of menses.
   3. Postural hypotension.
H. Exercise intolerance:
I. Carpal tunnel syndrome is a common occurrence.
J. Depression.
K. Ataxia.
L. Decreased concentration/memory impairment.

Subjective Data

A. Note history of recent illness and/or pregnancy.
B. Evaluate the client's medical/surgical history for any treatment of hyperthyroid, including radioactive treatment or thyroidectomy.
C. Review dietary and weight history, how much weight has been gained, and over what period of time.
D. Review any changes in health status or symptoms associated with other body systems (thyroid symptoms usually involve multiple body systems).
E. Review any history of obstructive sleep apnea (OSA).
F. Assess for pain or swelling of the neck or difficulty swallowing.
G. Inquire as to the client's history of supervoltage x-ray therapy to the neck for nonthyroid cancer or for polio.
H. Identify family history:
   1. Does the client have a first-degree relative with thyroid disease?

2. Is there a family history of any endocrine problems, including thyroid, type 1 DM, and/or receptor agonist (RA)?
I. Review the client's medication history for current medication, over-the-counter (OTC) medications, vitamins, or herbal supplements.
J. Review the client's menstrual history or history of infertility.
K. Inquire about constipation (new onset or worsening).

Physical Examination
A. Check pulse (bradycardia), respirations, BP (decreased systolic BP and increased diastolic BP), and weight. Plot the height/weight on a growth curve for children.
B. General observation:
   1. Gait problems, such as ataxia or rigidity, and spasticity of the trunk and proximal extremities.
   2. Quality of the client's voice (hoarseness).
   3. Signs of depression, decreased concentration, or memory impairment.
C. Inspection:
   1. Inspect the skin (dry/flaky) for presence of jaundice.
   2. Inspect the hair (coarse, thin, brittle) and decrease in pubic/axillary hair pattern.
   3. Perform oral examination for evaluation of macroglossia (enlarged tongue).
   4. Inspect the face/eye for periorbital puffiness/oedema.
   5. Inspect the neck for the presence of a goiter and surgical scar.
   6. Child: Assess Tanner stage of puberty.
D. Auscultate:
   1. The thyroid and carotids.
   2. The heart.
   3. The lungs.
   4. The abdomen for bowel sounds in each quadrant (hypoactive).
E. Palpate:
   1. The neck, thyroid gland, and lymph nodes.
   2. The abdomen for presence of abdominal distension, ascites, masses in left lower quadrant, and haepatomegaly.
   3. Palpate/evaluate extremities for oedema.
F. Musculoskeletal examination: Perform a detailed musculoskeletal examination.
G. Neurologic examination:
   1. Check visual fields (restricted with hypothyroidism).
   2. Test hearing:
      a. Whisper words and have the client repeat.
      b. Use a ticking watch.
      c. Use a tuning fork:
         i. Weber test: Place vibrating fork on top midline of head (sound hearing equally in both ears).
         ii. Rinne test: Place vibrating tuning fork on mastoid, begin counting, and ask the client to tell you when he or she no longer hears; then quickly reposition 1/2 to 1 inch from the ear and ask the client when he or she no longer hears (hearing should be twice as long as bone conduction).
   3. Check for loss or reduction of deep tendon reflexes (DTRs).
   4. Evaluate proximal muscle weakness/strength.
   5. Test for abnormal tandem gait: Have the client walk across the room in a heel–toe, heel–toe fashion.
   6. Check for sensory loss:
      a. Evaluate the first three fingers and one half of the fourth finger on testing loss of sensation from carpal tunnel syndrome.
      b. Evaluate sensory loss of the feet/legs (generally symmetrical in a "stocking-glove" distribution).

Diagnostic Tests
A. Thyroid-stimulating hormone (TSH).
B. When a high TSH is noted, repeat the test and add a free T4.
C. T3 resin uptake.
D. Thyroid antibodies (see Table 20.8).
E. TSH assay (if TSH assay is elevated, it indicates hypothyroidism).
F. Thyroid scan.
G. Complete blood count (CBC; anaemia).
H. Lipid profile.
I. Ultrasound of the neck and thyroid to detect nodules (not a first-line test).

Differential Diagnoses
A. Hypothyroidism:
   1. Hashimoto's thyroiditis.
   2. Subclinical hypothyroidism.
   3. Hypothyroidism secondary to treatment/intervention for hyperthyroidism.
   4. De Quervain thyroiditis.
   5. If TSH and free T4 are both low, consider hypothyroidism secondary to pituitary or hypothalamic failure.
B. Obesity: Clients with elevated total cholesterol levels or triglyceride levels are often misdiagnosed by assuming that these symptoms are caused by obesity and high-fat diets.
C. Depression.
D. Ischaemic heart disease.
E. Nephrotic syndrome.
F. Cirrhosis.
G. Side effects/adverse effects of medications.
H. Constipation.
I. Sleep apnea/sleep disorder.
J. Fibromyalgia.
K. Infectious mononucleosis.

Plan
A. General interventions:
   1. The Canadian Task Force on the Periodic Health Examination does not recommend screening for thyroid dysfunction in asymptomatic adults who are not pregnant.
   2. Clients with underactive thyroids require lifelong treatment with levothyroxine.
   3. In clients with subacute thyroiditis, relatively large doses of nonsteroidal anti-inflammatory drugs (NSAIDs) or prednisone may be prescribed.
   4. For clients with enlarged thyroid glands, surgery may be recommended if the gland begins obstructing the airway.
   5. The treatment of clients with malignant thyroid nodules depends on the type of cancer.
B. Client teaching:
   1. Teach the client about the nature and course of the disease, as well as the signs and symptoms. Frequently, clients are relieved that their perceived symptoms are real and that there is treatment. This may also improve client compliance.
   2. Teach the client to report any of the following side effects of the drug:
      a. Tachycardia.
      b. Palpitations.
      c. Chest pain.

Test Results in Hypothyroidism

Disorder	TSH	Free T4	T3	RAIU and Thyroid Scan	Peroxidase Antibodies
Hypothyroid	H	L	Sometimes L	N or L	n/a
Hashimoto's disease	H or variable	N or L	Not helpful	Variable	Positive
Subacute hypothyroidism	L	H	H or variable	L or absent	Usually thyroiditis
Silent lymphocytic thyroiditis (usually postpartum)	L when toxic; H when hypothyroid	n/a	L when toxic	Positive	

H, high; L, low; N, normal; RAIU, radioactive iodine uptake; TSH, thyroid-stimulating hormone.

3. Emphasize the need for lifelong treatment with levothyroxine and the dangers of noncompliance.
4. **Thyroid replacement should be taken on an empty stomach.**
5. The beneficial effects of thyroid replacement occur in about three days to one week; the client may not feel the clinical effects for several months.
6. When switching brands or using a generic, the serum TSH should be checked in six weeks.

C. Pharmacological therapy:
1. **Clients requiring therapy with levothyroxine should be treated with the same brand/generic consistently because potency varies between brand and generics.**
   a. Levothyroxine.
   b. Desiccated thyroid.
2. The medication should be titrated to the lowest dosage needed to maintain euthyroidism and a nonelevated serum TSH and a normal or slightly elevated T4.
3. Elderly clients and those with cardiovascular disease (CVD) should be started on very low doses. Close monitoring for the development of cardiac complications such as angina, arrhythmias, and myocardial infarction needs to be undertaken.
4. Thyroid hormones should be taken on an empty stomach in the mornings to avoid insomnia.
5. Other drugs can reduce the effectiveness/affect the absorption of thyroid hormone:
   a. Cholesterol-reducing drugs.
   b. Cholestyramine, which interferes with absorption in the gut.
   c. Calcium carbonate.
   d. Aluminum hydroxide.
   e. Sucralfate.
   f. If taking one of these drugs and levothyroxine, they should be taken four to six hours apart.
6. Dietary fibre can interfere with levothyroxine absorption. Coffee reduces the absorption of levothyroxine.
7. Pharmacological treatment of the client with subclinical hypothyroidism is controversial. If goiter is present, treatment may be considered.

Follow-Up
A. Clients who are not treated with medication should be seen every six to 12 months for reevaluation.
B. When medication is instituted, monitor laboratory values and client well-being in the office every four to six weeks.
C. After the dosage is stabilized, the client with an elevated serum TSH level should be seen every six to 12 months.
   1. Undetectable TSH levels are indicative of overmedication.
   2. High TSH levels are indicative of insufficient medication or client noncompliance.
D. After the TSH is normalized, regular annual follow-up visits are required.
E. Order dual-energy x-ray absorptiometry (DEXA) scan as indicated to screen for bone loss/osteopaenia/osteoporosis.

Consultation/Referral
A. Consultation with an endocrinologist is recommended for the following:
   1. Children/teens younger than 18 years.
   2. Clients unresponsive to therapy.
   3. Pregnant clients.
   4. Presence of goiter, nodule, or other structural changes in the thyroid.
   5. Compression symptoms of dysphagia.
   6. Any client with myxoedema, significant cardiac disease, or involvement or hypothyroidism secondary to pituitary or hypothalamic failure should be referred to an endocrinologist for continued care.
   7. If fine-needle aspiration biopsy is required.

Individual Considerations
A. Pregnancy:
   1. Monitor TSH levels monthly during the first trimester.
   2. Small increases in medication dosage may be required.
   3. Some women develop postpartum thyroiditis and hypothyroidism after taking hyperthyroid medication during pregnancy or immediately thereafter.
   4. Postpartum: Monitor TSH level at six weeks' postpartum examination.
   5. A common cause of congenital hypothyroidism is maternal and infant iodine deficiency.
   6. Monitor the TSH to avoid overtreatment in postpartum women because excess thyroid hormone levels increase the risk of osteoporosis.
   7. Hypothyroidism in pregnancy is associated with preeclampsia, anaemia, postpartum hemorrhage, cardiac ventricular dysfunction, spontaneous abortion, low birth weight, impaired cognitive development, and fetal mortality.

B. Geriatrics: Some elderly clients who are actually hyperthyroid exhibit symptoms of hypothyroidism.

Bibliography

Alberta Health Services. (2018). *Congenital hypothyroidism (CH)*. Retrieved from https://www.albertahealthservices.ca/assets/info/hp/nms/if-hp-nms-ch.pdf

American Geriatric Society. (2014). GNRS: A core curriculum in advanced practice geriatric nursing. In E. Flaherty & B. Resnick (Eds.), *GNRS geriatric nursing review syllabus: A core curriculum in advanced practice geriatric nursing* (4th ed., pp. 506–529). New York, NY: American Geriatrics Society.

Centers for Disease Control and Prevention, NCHS National Center for Health Statistics. (n.d.). *Clinical growth charts*. Retrieved from https://www.cdc.gov/growthcharts

El-Hussein, M. T., Power-Kean, K., Zettel, S., Huether, S. E., McCance, K. L., Brashers, V. L., & Rote, N. S. (2018). *Understanding pathophysiology*. Milton, ON: Elsevier.

Jameson, J. L., Mandel, S. J., & Weetman, A. P. (2015). Disorders of the thyroid gland. In D. L. Kasper, A. S. Fauci, S. L. Hauser, D. L. Longo, & J. L. Jameson (Eds.), *Harrison's principles of internal medicine* (19th ed.). New York, NY: McGraw-Hill.

LaFranchi, S. (2015, November). Clinical features and detection of congenital hypothyroidism. *UpToDate*. Retrieved from http://www.uptodate.com

Medical Council of Canada. (2018). *Clinical laboratory tests: Normal values*. Retrieved from https://mcc.ca/objectives/normal-values/?cn-reloaded=1

National Guideline Clearinghouse. (2015, May). *Screening for thyroid dysfunction: U. S. Preventative services task force recommendation statement*. Retrieved from http://www.guideline.gov/content.aspx?id=49227&search=thyroid+screening

Lee, A. (Ed.). (2016). *NPPR: Nurse practitioners' prescribing reference*. New York, NY: Haymarket Media.

Prescriber's Letter. (2015). Appropriate medication use in older adults: 2015 updated. *Beer's Criteria*, 22(12), 311218. Retrieved from http://prescribersletter.therapeuticresearch.com

Ross, D. S. (2015, December). Diagnosis and screening for hypothyroidism in non-pregnant adults. *UpToDate*. Retrieved from http://www.uptodate.com

Ross, D. S. (2016, February). Treatment of hypothyroidism. *UpToDate*. Retrieved from http://www.uptodate.com

Thyrotoxicosis/Thyroid Storm

Jill C. Cash, Melissa A. Hall, and Kelly Power-Kean

Definition

A. Severe thyrotoxicosis of any cause is called thyrotoxic crisis or storm.

Incidence/Prevalence

A. It is rare; the incidence varies, depending on the cause of the thyrotoxicosis.

Pathogenesis

A. Thyrotoxic crisis or storm usually develops in clients either undiagnosed as being hyperthyroid or those who are known to be severely hyperthyroid, are being treated insufficiently, and are subjected to excessive stress from other causes. Oversecretion of T3 and T4 is followed by a release of epinephrine. Metabolism is dramatically increased. The adrenal glands produce excessive corticosteroids, which is a response to stress.

Predisposing Factors

A. Severe, uncontrolled hyperthyroidism.
B. Noncompliance with antihyperthyroid medication.
C. Inadequate preparation for thyroid surgery.

Common Findings

A. Sudden onset of the following:
  1. Hyperthermia.
  2. Tachycardia (usually atrial tachydysrhythmias).
  3. High-output cardiac failure.
  4. Altered sensorium (usually agitation, restlessness, delirium).
  5. Nausea, vomiting, and diarrhoea.

Other Signs and Symptoms

A. Symptoms of a thyrotoxic crisis or storm are similar to those of hyperthyroidism, but they are more sudden, severe, and extreme. Other common symptoms include:
  1. persistent
  2. sweating
  3. shaking
  4. unconsciousness

Subjective Data

A. Elicit information regarding the onset, duration, and nature of symptoms.
B. Determine the presence of cardiac symptoms.
C. Take a complete drug history, including whether or not the client has been taking antithyroid medication as prescribed.
D. Rule out any excessive acute stressors such as infection, pulmonary or cardiac problems, dialysis, plasmapheresis, and/or emotional stressors.

Physical Examination

A. Check temperature, pulse, respirations, and blood pressure (BP).
B. Inspect the skin.
C. Auscultate the heart and lungs.
D. Palpate the neck carefully for thyroid nodules and enlargement.

Diagnostic Tests

A. Serum T3 and free T4.
B. Thyroid-stimulating hormone (TSH).

Differential Diagnoses

A. Thyroid storm.
B. Thyrotoxic crisis.

Plan

A. General interventions:
  1. Closely monitor temperature, pulse, respirations, and BP.
  2. Assess the need to hospitalize the client for supportive therapy: intravenous (IV) fluids, medication treatment, antipyretics, and/or oxygen.

B. Client teaching: See "Client Teaching" in the "Hyperthyroidism" section.
C. Pharmacological therapy: See "Pharmacological therapy" in the "Hyperthyroidism" section.

Follow-Up

A. Following resolution of the crisis, see the client in the office every three to four weeks for evaluation and monitoring of serum TSH and free T4 levels.
B. See "Follow-Up" in the "Hyperthyroidism" section.

Consultation/Referral
A. Consider hospitalization.

Individual Considerations
A. Pregnancy: See "Individual Considerations" in the "Hyperthyroidism" section.

Bibliography
Jameson, J. L., Mandel, S. J., & Weetman, A. P. (2015). Disorders of the thyroid gland. In D. L. Kasper, A. S. Fauci, S. L. Hauser, D. L. Longo, & J. L. Jameson (Eds.), *Harrison's principles of internal medicine* (19th ed.). New York, NY: McGraw-Hill.

Lee, A. (Ed.). (2016). *NPPR: Nurse practitioners' prescribing reference*. New York, NY: Haymarket Media.

Medical Council of Canada. (2018). *Clinical laboratory tests: Normal values*. Retrieved from https://mcc.ca/objectives/normal-values/?cn-reloaded=1

National Guideline Clearinghouse. (2015, May). *Screening for thyroid dysfunction: U. S. Preventative services task force recommendation statement*. Retrieved from http://www.guideline. gov/content.aspx?id=49227&search=thyroid+screening

Ross, D. S. (2015, February). Thyroid storm. *UpToDate*. Retrieved from http://www.uptodate.com

Stewart, P. M., & Newell-Price, J. D. (2016). The adrenal cortex. In S. Melmed, K. S. Polonsky, P. R. Larsen, & H. M. Kronenberg (Eds.), *Williams textbook of endocrinology* (13th ed., pp. 490–556). Philadelphia, PA: Elsevier.

21 Rheumatological Guidelines

Ankylosing Spondylitis (AS)

Jill C. Cash and Kelly Power-Kean

Definition
A. Ankylosing spondylitis (AS) is a chronic, inflammatory joint disease that causes chronic joint pain/swelling, which primarily affects the spine and sacroiliac (SI) joints; however, larger peripheral joints can also be affected.

Incidence/Prevalence
A. It is estimated that AS occurs in approximately 1% of the Canadian population.
B. The prevalence of AS is estimated to be 0.9% and affects between 150,000 and 300,000 people in Canada.

Pathogenesis
A. Inflammation occurs at the entheses (insertion site of the ligaments and tendons of the bone) throughout the body. Primary sites of involvement include the lower back, SI joint, and lower extremities. Inflammatory cells invade the joint and erode the bone and fibrocartilage of the joints. The body responds by trying to repair the area, by which fibrous scar tissue is formed. The structure is replaced by the ossified scar tissue, which causes fusion of the joint; as a result, flexibility of the joint is lost. The eroded joint tries to repair itself by osteoblast formation in building new bone tissue. This results in the production of new enthesis that deposits itself on top of the existing enthesis. Calcification of the spinal ligaments also occurs and the appearance of the vertebral bodies looks more "square" and distinct. This is referred to as a "bamboo spine."

Predisposing Factors
A. Gender (men > women, 3:1 ratio).
B. Race (White more prevalent, occurring more in the northern European countries).
C. Age: Onset of symptoms usually occurs during the early 20s. However, diagnosis usually is made several years after the onset of symptoms, more into the late 20- to 30-year range. AS rarely occurs after the age of 50.
D. Family history of AS.
E. Thought to have a genetic predisposition: Serum human leukocyte antigen (HLA)-B27 positive. Approximately 90% of clients with AS have a positive HLA-B27. However, only 5% of clients with a positive HLA-B27 develop any type of spondyloarthropathy.

Common Findings
A. Gradual onset of low back pain with initial onset of symptoms occurring in the early 20s.
B. SI joint pain.
C. Joint pain occurring for more than three months, with morning stiffness.
D. Low back pain/joint pain that improves with activity, worsens with rest.
E. Dactylitis (sausage digits of the fingers/toes).
F. Enthesitis (inflammation/pain at insertion site of the tendon or ligament to the bone).

Other Signs and Symptoms
A. Peripheral joint pain and swelling.
B. Decreased range of motion (ROM) in joints/back/neck.
C. Extra-articular features such as anterior uveitis or iritis.
D. Fatigue.
E. Weight loss.
F. Shortness of breath (SOB).
G. Psoriasis.

Subjective Data
A. Ask the client when back pain/joint pain began. Have symptoms been present for several months/years? At what age did pain initially begin?
B. Is pain intermittent or constant?
C. Does pain improve or worsen with activity? Inflammatory back pain improves with activity and worsens with rest.
D. Does client have complaints of other joint pain?
E. Has the client noted any weight gain/loss, fatigue, or fever?
F. Any history of psoriasis or other skin rashes?
G. Any gastrointestinal (GI) changes or chronic problems such as Crohn's disease, ulcerative colitis, or diarrhoea?
H. Any pulmonary problems such as SOB, difficulty breathing, or SOB with activity?
I. Any cardiac changes or problems?
J. Any history of amyloidosis?

Physical Examination
A. Check vital signs, blood pressure (BP), pulse, respirations, and temperature as indicated.
B. Inspect:
  1. Assess the cervical spine. Ask the client to stand straight and assess the degree of cervical change. Ask the client to perform flexion, extension, and lateral flexion, and rotate the head.

2. Inspect the thoracic and lumbar spine. Note degree of chest expansion of thoracic spine. Assess lumbar spine, noting the ROM with flexion/extension. Have the client bend to the right and left side and note any difference in flexion.
3. Assess gait. If abnormal gait, assess for hip pain/involvement.
4. Inspect hands/feet for sausage digits.
5. Inspect joints in hands/wrists/feet/knees for tender, swollen joints.
C. Auscultate heart and lungs.
D. Palpate:
1. Examine the SI joints by palpating the SI joint while lying supine and while lying on the side. Have the client flex one knee while lying supine, and externally rotate the hip. Assess for pain at the SI joint area while pressure is applied on the knee.
2. Assess for pain at the entheses site. Assess Achilles tendon and plantar fascia areas where the tendon attaches to the calcaneus.

Diagnostic Tests

A. Serum blood work:
1. HLA-B27 commonly positive.
2. C-reactive protein (CRP) or erythrocyte sedimentation rate (ESR).
3. Complete blood count (CBC).
4. Comprehensive metabolic panel (CMP).
5. Alkaline phosphatase.
6. Additional testing may also be appropriate depending upon the differential diagnosis generated from the presenting features and other abnormalities identified.
B. Radiographic studies for client with chronic back pain (greater than three months) and onset before age 45:
1. Anteroposterior (AP) plain radiograph of the pelvis (SI joint assessment).
2. Clients who are negative for AS by plain radiography of the pelvis, the presence or history of each of 11 features of AS should be ascertained. A client with at least four of the 11 features can usually be diagnosed with nonradiographic axial spondyloarthritis. These clients should have positive imaging and/or positive test for HLA-B27; the absence of both of these two findings makes AS less likely. Radiographs of the spine are generally not required for the diagnosis of AS, but AP and lateral views should be performed in clients diagnosed with an AS for assessment of the severity of disease and disease progression. The 11 features characteristic of AS are the following:
- Inflammatory back pain.
- Heel pain (enthesitis).
- Dactylitis.
- Uveitis.
- Positive family history for AS.
- Inflammatory bowel disease.
- Alternating buttock pain.
- Psoriasis.
- Asymmetric arthritis.
- Positive response to nonsteroidal anti-inflammatory drugs (NSAIDs).
- Elevated acute-phase reactants (ESR or CRP).

3. MRI of the SI joints in clients suspected of AS but with nondiagnostic plain radiographs is usually indicated in clients without evidence of sacroiliitis on plain radiographs in whom AS is suspected based upon other symptoms and findings characteristic of AS, to help establish the diagnosis of nonradiographic axial spondyloarthritis. A positive MRI finding alone is not sufficient to make the diagnosis of AS in the absence of other features of AS. An MRI should only be ordered if there is a reasonable degree of suspicion of AS.
4. Consider bone mineral density screening: High incidence of osteoporosis noted in clients diagnosed with AS.

Differential Diagnoses

A. Acute or chronic mechanical nonspecific back pain and inflammatory back pain without spondyloarthropathy (SpA).
B. Fibromyalgia and myalgia.
C. Diffuse idiopathic skeletal hyperostosis.
D. Vertebral compression fracture.
E. Sacroiliac joint infection.

Plan

A. General interventions:
1. Treatment for AS includes nonpharmacological and pharmacological interventions.
2. Osteoporosis screening and treatment are recommended for these clients.
3. Systemic steroids are not routinely prescribed; however, for severe symptoms of pain and swelling, joint injection may be considered.
B. Client teaching:
1. Encourage a healthy, active lifestyle. Activity improves symptoms. Regular exercises are recommended as tolerated. Physical therapy and/or structured exercises recommended most days of the week.
2. Medications prescribed should be used on a routine basis.
3. Fall prevention should be reviewed with the client. The home should be modified to prevent falls. Suggestions include installing grab-bars in the bathroom tub/shower, removing loose rugs in the house, and keeping walkways in the home clear and clutter free.
4. Seat belts should always be worn properly.
5. For persons with severe spinal involvement, contact sports and high-impact exercises/sports should be avoided.
C. Pharmacological therapy:
1. NSAIDs are the first-line therapy for pain/symptoms produced from AS. The American College of Rheumatology/Spondylitis Association of America/Spondyloarthritis Research and Treatment Network (ACR/SAA/SPARTAN) conditionally recommend continuous treatment with NSAIDs over an on-demand approach in clients with active AS. There is no preferred NSAID, with choice based on consideration of the client's past history of NSAID use, risk factors for adverse effects, and comorbidities. Adults with stable AS are conditionally recommended to use an on-demand approach to NSAID usage.
   a. Ibuprofen.
   b. Naproxen.
   c. Celecoxib.
   d. Indomethacin.
   e. Meloxicam.
   f. Diclofenac.
2. Tumour necrosis factor alpha antagonists (anti-TNF) medications may be prescribed by a rheumatologist after failed NSAID use.
D. Nonpharmacological therapy:
Clients with active AS are strongly recommended to access physical therapy. Active physical therapy

interventions (supervised exercise) are conditionally recommended over passive physical therapy interventions (massage, ultrasound, heat). Land-based physical therapy interventions are preferred over aquatic therapy interventions.

Follow-Up
A. Clients treated with NSAIDs should have routine follow-up at two weeks following initial diagnosis, or sooner if not improving with treatment.
B. Clients treated with NSAIDs should be followed every three months with close monitoring of kidney and liver function.

Consultation/Referral
A. Clients diagnosed with AS should be referred to rheumatology for evaluation and treatment.

Individual Considerations
A. Adults:
   1. Young adults, typically during the 20- to 30-year range, are diagnosed with AS. Clients commonly present to the office with complaints of low back pain and are treated for noninflammatory chronic back pain. These clients may go years without the proper diagnosis and treatment. Therefore, delayed diagnosis is not uncommon in these clients.
   2. Standard precautions should be followed for NSAIDs for clients with renal insufficiency and clients taking anticoagulants, systemic glucocorticoids, and other interacting medications.
B. Geriatrics:
   1. Not commonly diagnosed in this group of clients.

Bibliography
American College of Rheumatology. (2015). *American College of Rheumatology/Spondylitis Association of America/Spondyloarthritis Research and Treatment Network 2015 recommendations for the treatment of ankylosing spondylitis and nonradiographic axial spondyloarthritis*. Retrieved from https://www.rheumatology.org/Practice-Quality/Clinical-Support/Clinical-Practice-Guidelines/Axial-Spondyloarthritis

The Arthritis Society. (2018a). *Ankylosing spondylitis*. Retrieved from https://www.arthritis.ca/about-arthritis/arthritis-types-(a-z)/types/ankylosing-spondylitis

Di Lorenzo, A. L. (2015). HLA-B27 syndromes. *Medscape*. Retrieved from http://emedicine.medscape.com/article/1201027-overview#a1

Fujita, T., Kutsumi, H., Sanuki, T., Hayakumo, T., & Azuma, T. (2013). Adherence to the preventive strategies for nonsteroidal anti-inflammatory drug- or low-dose aspirin-induced gastrointestinal injuries. *Journal of Gastroenterology, 48*(5), 559–573. doi:10.1007/s00535-013-0771-8

Kinkade, S. (2007). Evaluation and treatment of acute low back pain. *American Family Physician, 75*(8), 1181–1188.

Rahman, P., Choquette, D., Bensen, W. G., Khraishi, M., Chow, A., Zummer, M., & Shawi, M. (2016). Biologic Treatment Registry Across Canada (BioTRAC): A multicentre, prospective, observational study of patients treated with infliximab for ankylosing spondylitis. *BMJ Open, 6*(4), e009661. doi:10.1136/bmjopen-2015-009661

Smith, W. M. (2013). Gender and spondyloarthropathy-associated uveitis. *Journal of Ophthalmology, 2013*, 928264. doi:10.1155/2013/928264

Fibromyalgia (FM)

Jill C. Cash and Kelly Power-Kean

Definition
Fibromyalgia (FM) syndrome is a clinical condition characterized by generalized aching and stiffness, associated with the finding of numerous tender points in characteristic locations.

A. The most current guidelines for diagnosis are presented by the Canadian Rheumatology Association ([CRA] 2012). The criteria for diagnosis include characteristic symptoms of pain at specific trigger point locations that are displayed by the client for the last three months when there is no other reason or explanation for the associated pain.
B. Trigger point locations are found primarily in the back, neck, jaw, shoulders, chest, abdomen, arms, hips, and legs.
C. Somatic symptoms are also assessed for and present with FM. Somatic complaints may include cognitive problems, sleeping difficulties, fatigue, headaches, mood disorders, and other associated symptoms. These criteria can be found at the CRA website, www.rheum.ca/.

Areas palpated are considered positive if the client verbalized the area as being "painful" when palpated.

Incidence/Prevalence
A. The prevalence of fibromyalgia in Canada is 2% to 3% of the population, with females affected six to nine times more commonly than males. Fibromyalgia is seen most commonly in middle-aged females, but can also affect all age groups. Often clients have symptoms for longer than five years before finally being diagnosed.

Pathogenesis
A. The Canadian Guidelines for the Diagnosis and Management of Fibromyalgia Syndrome in Adults (fmguidelines.ca) note that although the cause of FM is unknown, abnormalities in pain processing have been identified at various levels in the peripheral, central, and sympathetic nervous systems, as well as the hypothalamo-pituitary-adrenal (HPA) axis stress–response system. A stressful event—which could be physical (such as a viral illness), traumatic, or psychological—can lead to a vulnerable health status and may be a trigger for FM.

Predisposing Factors
A. Life stress.
B. Depression.
C. Female gender.
D. Age: Mid-30s and older.

Common Findings
A. Common complaints are multifocal pain present longer than three months; moderate to extreme fatigue; morning stiffness; nonrestorative sleep; pain worsening with stress; exposure to cold; inactivity or overactivity; sensitivity to touch, light, and sound; cognitive difficulties; and sensitivity to changes in barometric pressure.

Other Signs and Symptoms
A. Numbness.
B. Swelling.
C. Reactive hyperaemia of skin.
D. Raynaud's phenomenon.
E. Irritable bowel syndrome (IBS) and bladder symptoms.
F. Headaches.
G. Restless legs syndrome (RLS).
H. Anxiety/depression.

Subjective Data
A. Determine onset, duration, and course of complaints.
B. Does fatigue interfere with the client's daily activity?

C. Note sleep quality. Does the client feel rested after sleeping?
D. Do exacerbations of discomfort occur with stress, activity, and cold?
E. Has the client experienced stress and/or depression in the past?
F. Does the client have a family history of rheumatoid disease?
G. Has the client ever been diagnosed with chronic fatigue syndrome, Lyme disease, or thyroid disease?

Physical Examination
A. Check temperature if indicated, pulse, and blood pressure (BP).
B. Inspect:
  1. Observe overall appearance.
  2. Observe the nails, skin, mucous membranes, eyes, joints, and spine. If clubbing is noted and tender points are minimal, consider hypertrophic osteoarthropathy.
C. Palpate the muscles as outlined in the aforementioned criteria for classification of FM. Note the following when palpating for tender points:
  1. Pressure should be insufficient to produce pain in normal clients or at uninvolved sites in affected clients.
  2. Specific tender point count is no longer required for a diagnosis of FM.
  3. "Positive pain reaction" is related to the client stating that palpation causes pain. Tenderness is not to be considered as pain.
  4. Painful points must be differentiated from trigger points of myofascial syndrome, which produce referred pain on compression.
D. Auscultate heart and lungs.

Diagnostic Tests
A. Complete blood count (CBC).
B. Erythrocyte sedimentation rate.
C. Thyroid-stimulating hormone (TSH).
D. Creatine kinase.
E. C-reactive protein (CRP).

Differential Diagnoses
A. Rheumatoid arthritis (RA).
B. Polymyalgia rheumatica.
C. Ankylosing spondylitis.
D. Myositis.
E. Hypothyroidism.
F. Chronic fatigue syndrome.

Plan
A. General interventions: Routine follow-up is recommended. Multiple therapies may be beneficial for controlling symptoms. Stress importance of daily exercises and therapy to control pain. Support groups are beneficial for clients and families.
▶ B. Client teaching: *Refer to Client Teaching Guide: Fibromyalgia.* Teach the client that fibromyalgia is a recognizable syndrome that does not progress or cripple and does not warrant further testing. Clients can be assured it is not "all in their head":
  1. Exercise: Encourage the client to exercise daily, including stretching programs along with walking, low-impact cardiovascular conditioning such as cycling, and low-impact aerobics. Initially, pain may increase with the first two weeks of exercise, then it improves with a routine exercise program.
  2. Pain control: Pain may improve with exercise, hot baths, heating pads, warm weather, and stress reduction.
C. Pharmacological therapy:
The CRA recommends that health-care providers identify the most bothersome symptom(s) in order to help direct pharmacologic treatments according to a symptom-based approach. This approach may require a combination of medications:
  1. Amitriptyline.
  2. Cyclobenzaprine or other muscle relaxants.
  3. Nonsteroidal anti-inflammatory drugs (NSAIDs) such as ibuprofen. Use at the lowest dose for the shortest period of time possible.
  4. Analgesics such as acetaminophen as needed.
  5. Selective serotonin reuptake inhibitors (SSRIs) The pain-modulating effects of antidepressant medications should be explained to clients with FM in order to dispel the concept of a primarily psychological complaint. All antidepressant medications, including trichloroacetic acids (TCAs), SSRIs, and serotonin norepinephrine reuptake inhibitors (SNRIs), may be used for treatment of pain and other symptoms in clients with FM.
  6. Pregabalin.
  7. Duloxetine HCl.
  8. Milnacipran. (Withdraw gradually. Precautions with renal impairment.)
  9. Current guidelines suggest guarded use of opioids chronically in nonmalignant pain. Opioids have not been studied in randomized controlled trials and should be considered only after all other medicinal therapies have been exhausted. Tramadol, a centrally acting analgesic with atypical opioid and antidepressant-like activity, is moderately effective in treating FM pain. The use of strong opioids is discouraged.
  10. Neurontin is approved for use in the treatment of neuropathic pain but not for FM. Only pregabalin and duloxetine have Health Canada approval for management of FM symptoms.
  11. A trial of a pharmacologic cannabinoid may be considered in a client with FM, particularly in the presence of a sleep disturbance.

Follow-Up
A. Schedule regular visits in initial two to four weeks to evaluate how therapy is helping. Educate the client at each visit, and stress positive reinforcement and supervision of treatment regimen. Visits may then be scheduled every three months to monitor progress.

Consultation/Referral
A. Consult with a specialist if the client has abnormal laboratory results.
B. Refer the client specialist if depression is suspected and current medication therapy is unsuccessful.

Individual Considerations
A. Geriatrics:
  1. FM is common in the elderly and can be more painful for this population because of other coexisting conditions, such as osteoarthritis (OA).

Bibliography

Canadian Rheumatology Association. (2012). *Canadian Fibromyalgia Guidelines*. Retrieved from https://rheum.ca/resources/publications/canadian-fibromyalgia-guidelines/

Centers for Disease Control and Prevention. (2015a). *Fibromyalgia*. Retrieved from www.cdc.gov/arthritis/basics/fibromyalgia.htm

Gota, C. E., Kaouk, S., & Wilke, W. S. (2015). Fibromyalgia and obesity: The association between body mass index and disability, depression, history of abuse, medications, and comorbidities. *Journal of Clinical Rheumatology, 21*(6), 289–295. doi:10.1097/RHU.0000000000000278

Liedberg, G. M., & Björk, M. (2014). Symptoms of subordinated importance in fibromyalgia when differentiating working from non-working women. *Work: A Journal of Prevention, Assessment and Rehabilitation, 48*(2), 155–164.

Painter, J. T., & Crofford, L. J. (2013). Chronic opioid use in fibromyalgia syndrome: A clinical review. *Journal of Clinical Rheumatology, 19*(2), 72–77. doi:10.1097/RHU.0b013e3182863447

Wolfe, F., Clauw, D. J., Fitzcharles, M. A., Goldenberg, D. L., Katz, R. S., Mease, P., . . . Yunus, M. B. (2010). The American College of Rheumatology preliminary diagnostic criteria for fibromyalgia and measurement of symptom severity. *Arthritis Care & Research, 62*(5), 600–610. doi:10.1002/acr.20140

Gout

Jill C. Cash and Kelly Power-Kean

Definition
A. Gout is an acute, sudden inflammatory disease of the joint, caused by high concentrations of uric acid in the joints and bones.
B. Three stages of gout:
  1. Acute gouty arthritis: Acute attack exhibiting severe pain, redness, and swelling of a joint, which may last from days to weeks, even if left untreated.
  2. Intercritical gout: Period without flares.
  3. Chronic/tophaceous gout: The progression of gout that has been inadequately treated, resulting in urate crystal deposits (tophaceous deposits) in the joints that can cause deformity and disability of the joint.

Incidence/Prevalence
A. Gout is most common in men from ages 30 to 60 years. Women become increasingly susceptible to gout after menopause. It is estimated that gout occurs in approximately 5.2% of adult Canadian men and 2.4% of Canadian women. People aged 65 years or older are more commonly affected.

Pathogenesis
A. Primary: High levels of uric acid result from either increased production or decreased excretion rates of uric acid.
B. Secondary: Hyperuricaemia results from primary disease processes such as hypertension, renal failure, kidney disorders, and so forth. See the following section "Predisposing Factors."
C. Medications/toxins can also cause hyperuricaemia.

Predisposing Factors
A. Chronic conditions: Hyperuricaemia, chronic kidney disease, hypertension, diabetes mellitus, ischaemic cardiovascular disease, hyperlipidaemia, obesity.
B. Gender (men older than 30 years).
C. Medications that alter uric acid level (diuretics, acetylsalicylic acid, alcohol, nicotinic acid, ethambutol, pyrazinamide).
D. Dietary factors (high intake of beer and meat/fresh seafood products).

Presentation
A. Redness, swelling, warmth, and/or pain in the joint (usually one joint only)—podagra (big toe). The pain is likely to be the most severe in the first 12 to 24 hours.
B. History of having severe joint pain with inflammation in other joints, followed by pain-free episodes.

Other Signs and Symptoms
A. Tophi are seen from several years of untreated gout.
B. Fever may be present in acute stages.

Subjective Data
A. Note when initial symptoms began.
B. Review client history of gout.
C. Determine what makes the symptoms worse or better.
D. List medications/therapies used and the result of the different therapies used.

Physical Examination
A. Check temperature, pulse, respirations, and blood pressure (BP).
B. Inspect:
  1. Inspect the joints.
  2. Note the presence of tophi on other joints.
C. Palpate the joints for tenderness, pain, and increase in temperature of skin.

Diagnostic Tests
A. Joint fluid aspiration for urate crystals is the gold standard in diagnosing gout. Inspect fluid with a polarized light microscopy to identify uric acid crystals.
B. Complete blood count (CBC): White blood cell count elevated.
C. Erythrocyte sedimentation rate (ESR): Elevated in gout.
D. Serum uric acid level: Uric acid >404.46 umol/L. Serum uric acid level may be normal during acute attacks. Perform test at least two weeks after acute attack or when flare has resolved.
E. Rheumatoid factor (RF) titre.
F. x-Ray or MRI: Identify bone cysts/gout tophi.

Differential Diagnoses
A. Infectious arthritis.
B. Hyperparathyroidism.
C. Pseudogout (calcium pyrophosphate deposition disease) commonly occurs in the knee, wrist, or other joints.
D. Bursitis.
E. Cellulitis.

Plan
A. General interventions:
  1. Rest the joint area; no heavy lifting or weight-bearing activity.
  2. ASA products should not be used.
B. Client teaching:
  1. Increase fluid intake to at least eight glasses of water daily.
  2. Avoid alcohol intake and excessive meat and seafood products that trigger flares.
  3. Medication treatment and compliance of taking the prescribed medications can be very effective in preventing

the development of the chronic tophaceous gout stage. *Refer to Client Teaching Guide: Gout.*

C. Pharmacological therapy:
1. Analgaesia.
   a. Nonsteroidal anti-inflammatory drugs (NSAIDs)—most effective if started within 48 hours of presenting symptoms:
      i. Indocin.
      ii. Naproxen.
      iii. NSAIDs are contraindicated for clients with the diagnosis of renal insufficiency, heart failure, ulcer disease, NSAID allergy, and anticoagulation therapy.
   b. Colchicine medication may be stopped after the client is free from symptoms after two to three days. Colchicine may also be used to prevent attacks. Colchicine warnings: Be aware of contraindications. Caution regarding drug interactions. Intolerable side effects of colchicine include nausea, vomiting, and diarrhoea. Be cautious with use in clients with kidney/liver impairment.
   c. Corticosteroids may be used for clients who cannot tolerate oral medications. Intra-articular steroid injection of methylprednisolone acetate may be given. Oral steroids may also be prescribed for clients who cannot take NSAIDs or colchicine and who cannot tolerate intra-articular steroid injection. Prednisone is safe. Be aware of rebound effects.
2. For hypersecretion of uric acid, long-term therapy is needed to decrease uric acid production: Allopurinol is the first line of treatment. The goal is to keep the uric acid level <356 μmol/L. Febuxostat is also used to lower blood uric acid levels. Initial laboratory studies include liver enzymes before beginning Febuxostat. Common side effects include liver problems, nausea, gout flares, joint pain, and rash.
3. For reduced excretion rates of uric acid, consider probenecid. Increased consumption of fluids must be encouraged.
4. Chronic gout: If clients have three or more attacks per year, consider long-term therapy, low dose of NSAIDs, or allopurinol for two to 12 months.
5. Alternative medications for intolerance, renal insufficiency, and extensive tophi include oxypurinol, febuxostat, and uricase. Refer to rheumatology specialist.

Follow-Up

A. The client should be contacted within 24 hours for evaluation.
B. Schedule follow-up visit in one month to reevaluate status.
C. Chronic gout: Obtain yearly uric acid levels; before initiating long-term therapy, obtain baseline urea level, serum lipid profile, and CBC and periodic liver enzymes.

Consultation/Referral

A. Refer to rheumatologist for aspiration of joint fluid and other treatment options.

Individual Considerations

A. Pregnancy: Colchicine not recommended.
B. Paediatrics:
   1. Colchicine not recommended.
   2. If gout is seen in this population, consider underlying primary cause (i.e., inborn error of metabolism).
C. Geriatrics:
   1. Reformation in joint areas may be seen in clients who have a history of gout from the uric acid deposits.
   2. Complications for chronic gout include nephrolithiasis and chronic urate nephropathy.
   3. Avoid indometacin in elderly clients because of the increased risk of adverse effects with other medications when compared with other NSAIDs.
   4. NSAIDs are not recommended in the elderly with a history of heart failure, gastrointestinal (GI) ulcers/disease, and renal impairment.
   5. Individual considerations must be given in this population regarding GI, cardiac, renal, and liver disease.
   6. Glucocorticoids are generally well tolerated in this population and a safer alternative if NSAIDs or colchicine may increase the risks for the client.

Bibliography

The Arthritis Society. (2018). *Gout*. Retrieved from https://arthritis.ca/about-arthritis/arthritis-types-(a-z)/types/gout

Becker, M. A. (2016a). Clinical manifestations and diagnosis of gout. *UpToDate*. Retrieved from http://www.uptodate.com/contents/clinical-manifestations-and-diagnosis-of-gout

Becker, M. A. (2016b). Prevention of recurrent gout: Pharmacologic urate-lowering therapy and treatment of tophi. *UpToDate*. Retrieved from http://www.uptodate.com/contents/prevention-of-recurrent-gout-pharmacologic-urate-lowering-therapy-and-treatment-of-tophi

Becker, M. A. (2016c). Treatment of acute gout. *UpToDate*. Retrieved from www.uptodate.com/contents/treatment-of-acute-gout

Centers for Disease Control and Prevention. (2015). *Gout*. Retrieved from www.cdc.gov/arthritis/basics/gout.htm

Choy, G., Baria, N., Bell, A., Hatcher, L., Sequeira, D., & Gagnon, D. (2014). Current gout management practices by primary-care physicians in Canada. *Canadian Rheumatology Association Journal, 24*(4), 12–14. Retrieved from http://craj.ca/archives/2014/English/Winter/PDFs/CRAJ_Winter_2014_Choy.pdf

Fujita, T., Kutsumi, H., Sanuki, T., Hayakumo, T., & Azuma, T. (2013). Adherence to the preventive strategies for nonsteroidal anti-inflammatory drug- or low-dose aspirin-induced gastrointestinal injuries. *Journal of Gastroenterology, 48*(5), 559–573. doi:10.1007/s00535-013-0771-8

Mayo Clinic. (2013). *Gout*. Retrieved from http://www.mayoclinic.org/diseases-conditions/gout/basics/Definition/con-20019400

Neogi, T., Jansen, T. L., Dalbeth, N., Fransen, J., Schumacher, H. R., Berendsen, D., . . . Taylor, W. J. (2015). 2015 Gout classification criteria: An American College of Rheumatology/European League Against Rheumatism collaborative initiative. *Annals of the Rheumatic Diseases, 74*(10), 1789–1798. doi:10.1136/annrheumdis-2015-208237

Osteoarthritis (OA)

Jill C. Cash and Kelly Power-Kean

Definition

A. Osteoarthritis (OA), formerly known as degenerative joint disease, is a chronic noninflammatory disease that affects the movable joints. OA is characterized by destruction of the cartilage with resultant decrease in the joint spaces and bony overgrowth. OA is considered to be primary when there are no underlying conditions, and secondary to conditions such as trauma, septic arthritis, inflammatory arthritis, metabolic disorders, or congenital or acquired joint abnormalities.

Incidence/Prevalence
A. OA is the most common form of arthritis, affecting approximately five million Canadians or one in every six persons. It is estimated one in four Canadians will be affected by OA by 2035. The incidence clearly increases with age, as up to 85% of the general population older than 65 years of age have radiographic changes suggestive of OA.

Pathogenesis
A. Damage to the articular cartilage and subchondral bone may be because of local trauma and results in chondrocyte injury.
B. Chondrocytes release proteolytic enzymes that assist in repair of the cartilage.
C. In OA, the remodeling process of chondrocytes and release of enzymes is impaired and results in a loss of strength and greater trauma and destruction of the subchondral bone. The end result is joint destruction and bony overgrowth.

Predisposing Factors
A. Increasing age: Among clients older than 55 years.
B. Gender: Women are more commonly affected and exhibit greater disease severity.
C. Genetic predisposition; distal interphalangeal (DIP) joint involvement.
D. Trauma such as previous fractures, ligamentous injuries, or occupationally related repetitive stress.
E. Altered joint anatomy or instability.
F. Obesity: Mechanical injury in the knee may increase OA.
G. Secondary inflammation such as infections, inflammatory arthropathies, and metabolic disorders.

Common Findings
A. Unilateral joint pain frequently involving the joints of the hands, neck, lower back, knees, and hips.
B. Morning stiffness lasting less than one hour.

Other Signs and Symptoms
A. Unilateral joint pain involving the DIP and proximal interphalangeal (PIP) joints, first carpometacarpal joint, hips, knees, cervical and lumbar spine, and first metatarsophalangeal joint.
B. Mild OA or early disease; pain that increases with joint use and decreases with rest.
C. Severe OA, or late disease, pain that is present with rest.

Subjective Data
A. Elicit the client's age at onset of pain.
B. Has the pain gradually gotten worse over the months or years?
C. How long does the pain last in the morning? Does the pain get worse with joint use and better with rest?
D. What joints are involved?
E. Is the joint pain described as "aching"?
F. What does the client take to relieve the pain?
G. Is there any joint deformity, redness, swelling, or warmth?
H. Is there any decrease in range of motion (ROM) of the joint?
I. Is there any family history of OA?

Physical Examination
A. Check pulse and blood pressure (BP).
B. Inspect the joints for enlargement, oedema, and erythema.
C. Palpate:
   1. Palpate the joints, noting temperature, oedema, and tenderness. Joints are cool; bony enlargement may be present in the PIP (Bouchard's nodes) or DIP joints (Heberden's nodes) and other weight-bearing joints.
   2. Palpate extremities. Perform assisted and active ROM exercises. With examination, limited ROM of the joint and/or pain on palpation may be present, along with crepitus.

Diagnostic Tests
A. Erythrocyte sedimentation rate (ESR): OA does not cause an increase of the ESR.
B. Chemistry profile.
C. Complete blood count (CBC).
D. Rheumatoid factor (RF).
E. Radiography: Confirms disease severity and presence of joint narrowing.
F. CT scan or MRI: Considered with nerve impingement syndrome (spine) or spinal stenosis.

Differential Diagnoses
A. Rheumatoid arthritis (RA).
B. Gout or pseudogout.
C. Septic arthritis.
D. Bursitis or tendonitis.
E. Systemic lupus erythematosus.
F. Fracture or trauma.

Plan
A. General interventions:
   1. Confirm diagnosis.
   2. Provide the client with support and education to improve client well-being and reduce discomfort.
   3. Physical therapy and/or occupational therapy should be initiated, if indicated.
B. Client teaching:
   1. *Refer to Client Teaching Guide: Osteoarthritis.* Reinforce the importance of joint protection; avoid repetitive stress or trauma.
   2. Encourage daily exercises and strengthening.
   3. Encourage weight loss if the client is obese.
C. Pharmacological therapy:
   1. First-line agents: The goal of treatment is to preserve joint mobility. First-line agents should be used in a stepwise approach:
      a. Acetaminophen: In early disease, this may be given on an as-needed basis.
      b. Nonsteroidal anti-inflammatory drugs (NSAIDs) if acetaminophen has failed to control the pain. Use with caution. Consider renal function and risk factors for peptic ulcer disease (PUD) and cardiovascular disease:
         i. Naproxen.
         ii. Inflammatory OA: Consider naproxen. Recommend taking this medication for two to four weeks for maximum effects.
         iii. Ibuprofen may also be considered. Doses may be increased at a gradual pace for maximum benefit as tolerated. If one NSAID does not work, consider other NSAIDs:

1) Cox-2 inhibitors such as celecoxib may also be considered.
   2) Meloxicam.
   c. For high-risk clients, an H$_2$ receptor blocker may decrease gastritis and be helpful in preventing duodenal ulcers. Consider diclofenac sodium/misoprostol.
   d. Misoprostol may be considered in clients who are at high risk of gastric ulcers. It should not be used by pregnant women. It is considered high risk for foetal death and possible congenital abnormalities.
   e. Topical creams:
      i. Diclofenac gel may be applied to affected area; recommended for clients with severe pain who are not able to tolerate oral NSAIDs.
      ii. Capsaicin cream may be applied to the affected area. Capsaicin creams may cause local burning at the site of application for the first several days.
2. Second-line agents: Second-line agents, such as intra-articular corticosteroid injections, may prevent some joint erosion and decrease pain. The same joint should not be injected more than three to four times a year in three-month intervals. If the joint is injected at this frequency for more than one year, alternative options, such as surgery, should be considered. Narcotics may provide relief from more severe OA pain, but they carry a risk of dependence.
3. The use of glucosamine and chondroitin has not been established and is not recommended for clients. There do not appear to be any risks associated with using glucosamine and chondroitin. If the client does not notice any relief within the first six months of use, then recommendations are to discontinue this product.
4. Physical therapy to create an individualized exercise regimen to strengthen muscles, increase ROM, and reduce pain.
5. Lubrication injections may also be considered. Referral to the rheumatologist should be considered for this treatment.

Follow-Up
A. Follow-up is based on disease severity and therapeutic treatment. If the client is treated with first-line agents, follow up on pain control, nonpharmacological interventions, and possible side effects of medications within two to four weeks.

Consultation/Referral
A. Referral to an orthopedic surgeon may be considered for moderate to severe pain as indicated.

Individual Considerations
A. Pregnancy: NSAIDs should not be used in pregnancy unless clearly indicated. Misoprostol should be used with great caution in women of childbearing age because of its potential for foetal abnormalities and abortive properties.
B. Adults and geriatrics: Clients on chronic NSAIDs should be monitored closely for toxicity such as renal insufficiency, gastritis, and PUD. Elderly clients and those with preexisting gastrointestinal (GI) disease, diabetes, congestive heart failure, and cirrhosis should be monitored closely.
The Arthritic Alliance of Canada, together with the Centre for Effective Practice and the College of Physicians of Canada, have developed the OA Tool for primary care providers who are managing clients with new or recurrent joint pain consistent with OA in the hip, knee, or hand. This tool assists primary care providers to identify symptoms and provide evidence-based, goal-oriented nonpharmacological and pharmacological management while identifying triggers for investigations or referrals. The tool can be accessed at www.cfpc.ca/uploadedFiles/CPD/OATOOL_FINAL_Sept14_ENG.pdf.

Bibliography
The Arthritis Society. (2018). *Osteoarthritis*. Retrieved from https://www.arthritis.ca/about-arthritis/arthritis-types-(a-z)/types/osteoarthritis

Centers for Disease Control and Prevention. (2015). *Osteoarthritis (OA)*. Retrieved from www.cdc.gov/arthritis/basics/osteoarthritis.htm

Fujita, T., Kutsumi, H., Sanuki, T., Hayakumo, T., & Azuma, T. (2013). Adherence to the preventive strategies for nonsteroidal anti-inflammatory drug- or low-dose aspirin-induced gastrointestinal injuries. *Journal of Gastroenterology, 48*(5), 559–573. doi:10.1007/s00535-013-0771-8

Kalunian, K. C. (2014). Diagnosis and classification of osteoarthritis. *UpToDate*. Retrieved from http://www.uptodate.com/contents/diagnosis-and-classification-of-osteoarthritis

Kalunian, K. C. (2015a). Nonpharmacologic therapy of osteoarthritis. *UpToDate*. Retrieved from www.uptodate.com/contents/nonpharmacologic-therapy-of-osteoarthritis

Kalunian, K. C. (2015b). Treatment of osteoarthritis resistant to initial pharmacologic therapy. *UpToDate*. Retrieved from www.uptodate.com/contents/treatment-of-osteoarthritis-resistant-to-initial-pharmacologic-therapy

National Institute for Health and Care Excellence. (2014, February). *Osteoarthritis: Care and management. Clinical guideline, No, 177* (p. 36). London, England: Author.

Solomon, D. H. (2014). Overview of selective COX-2 inhibitors. *UpToDate*. Retrieved from http://www.uptodate.com/contents/overview-of-selective-cox-2-inhibitors

Osteoporosis/Kyphosis/Fracture

Jill C. Cash and Kelly Power-Kean

Definition
A. Osteoporosis is a condition of reduced bone mass resulting in bone fragility and fracture. The World Health Organization (WHO) has defined it as "spinal or hip bone mineral density (BMD) of 2.5 standard deviations or more below the mean for healthy, young women (T-score of -2.5 or below) as measured by dual-energy x-ray absorptiometry." Bone mineral density (BMD) is performed on the lumbar spine, hip, and/or forearm.
B. Clinical diagnosis of osteoporosis can also be defined as having a fragility fracture of the spine, hip, wrist, pelvis, rib, and/or humerus without evidence of a BMD.
C. Osteopaenia is defined as low bone mass of the spinal or hip BMD between 1 and 2.5 standard deviations below the mean as evidenced by the T-score (T-score between -1.0 and -2.5).
D. Kyphosis (dowager's hump) is the forward curvature of the thoracic spine. It is estimated that kyphosis occurs in approximately 20% to 40% of clients older than 60 years of age. Kyphosis may occur because of many different causes, including vertebral fractures, muscle weakness, degenerative disc disease, postural changes, and genetic/metabolic changes. Kyphosis is associated with other conditions, such as decreased pulmonary function, back pain, increased risk of fracture of the spine, limited mobility, and an increase in mortality.
E. Osteoporotic fracture occurs from a fall while standing at normal height or less, without any type of trauma and/or while performing daily activities. A vertebral compression fracture is the most common type of osteoporotic fracture.

F. Vertebral fractures: There are three primary types of vertebral fractures:
1. Biconcave deformity.
2. Wedge fracture.
3. Compression fracture.

Incidence/Prevalence
A. The Public Health Agency of Canada estimated that approximately 1.5 million Canadians aged 40 years and over (10%) are diagnosed with osteoporosis. Women are diagnosed with osteoporosis six to eight times more often than men and this is thought to be related to hormone deficiency (oestrogen). The peak incidence of fractures in men occurs 10 years later in life than for women, averaging at 70 years of age.
B. Approximately 50% to 60% of 50-year-old women sustain osteoporosis-related fractures during their remaining life. Spinal fractures occur in 25% of White women by age 65 years, causing pain, deformity, and disability. Most common fractures include 25% at distal radius (Colles' fracture), 50% in vertebrae, and 25% in the hip.
C. Approximately 33% of all women and 17% of men suffer a hip fracture before age 90 years, and 20% of those who sustain a fracture die within three months of the event.

Pathogenesis
A. Osteoporosis occurs because of bone reabsorption being greater than bone formation.

Predisposing Factors
A. Hypogonadal states, particularly menopause.
B. Small body frame, low body weight >57.6 kg).
C. Cigarette smoking.
D. Low calcium intake.
E. Lack of weight-bearing exercise.
F. Family history of hip/pelvic fracture.
G. Excessive alcohol intake.
H. Asian or White.
I. Advanced age.
J. Previous fracture.
K. Secondary causes:
1. Hyperparathyroidism.
2. Hyperthyroidism.
3. Cushing's syndrome.
4. Multiple myeloma.
5. Thyroid replacement therapy.
6. Corticosteroid therapy.
7. Renal disease.

Common Findings
A. Loss of height.
B. Kyphosis, or dowager's hump.
C. Back pain as a result of a compression fracture.

Other Signs and Symptoms
A. Cervical lordosis.
B. Fracture with little or no trauma.
C. Crush fracture of vertebra.
D. Pain.

Subjective Data
A. Explore history of the following:
1. Loss of height. Ask client to compare current height with height written on the driver's license if height unknown.
2. Low initial bone mass.
3. Early menopause, oophorectomy, postmenopause, or amenorrhoea.
4. European or Asian family origin.
5. Family history of spinal fractures and osteoporosis.
6. Sedentary lifestyle with little weight-bearing activity.
7. Endocrine disorders.
8. Review medications taken in the present and past, including over-the-counter (OTC) and herbal supplements, with attention to medications such as corticosteroids, barbiturates, heparin, and thyroid hormone.
9. Dietary review for low calcium and vitamin D intake.
10. Increased alcohol, caffeine, and protein intake.
11. Renal disease/dialysis.
B. Determine the onset, duration, location, and characteristic of back pain if present.
C. Has the client had any recent falls?

Physical Examination
A. Check pulse, blood pressure (BP), height, and weight.
B. Inspect:
1. Compare present height with previous height.
2. Observe presence of dorsal kyphosis.
3. Observe physical abnormalities that interfere with mobility.
C. Palpate the joints and over the back for pain.

Diagnostic Tests
A. Laboratory studies:
1. Women: Comprehensive metabolic panel (CMP; calcium, phosphorus, albumin, total protein, creatinine, liver enzymes, alkaline phosphatase, electrolytes), thyroid-stimulating hormone (TSH), and 25-hydroxyvitamin D level.
2. Men: CMP (calcium, phosphorus, albumin, total protein, creatinine, liver enzymes, alkaline phosphatase, electrolytes), TSH, 25-hydroxyvitamin D level, and testosterone level.
3. Complete blood count (CBC), erythrocyte sedimentation rate (ESR), and serum protein electrophoresis to rule out multiple myeloma and leukemia if concerned.
B. BMD or dual-energy x-ray absorptiometry (DEXA) scan:
1. The DEXA scan measures bone density of the lumbar spine and/or hip. Medicare will reimburse for this test to be performed every two years. If the spine is compressed or has severe scoliosis, BMD values may not be valid for the lumbar spine. Consider assessing the forearm for radial interpretation.
2. The result of this procedure is read in "T-scores" or "Z-scores." T-scores are evaluated for postmenopausal women and older men. A T-score is a number given to identify the amount of bone present when compared with other healthy adults. Z-scores are recommended for premenopausal women. A Z-score is a score given to identify the amount of bone present when compared with other people of the same age, gender, and weight.
3. The WHO Fracture Risk Assessment Tool (FRAX) was developed to determine the absolute fracture risk of breaking a bone in the next 10 years. This tool may be used with the BMD results to determine who needs to be treated with medication for prevention of fracture when treatment is unclear. FRAX should be used on women who have not previously been treated with antiresorptive therapy when T-scores are between

−1.5 and −2.5. The FRAX tool can also be used with clients who have been treated with prior antiresorptive medications if they have been off these medications for more than two years. FRAX scoring is not recommended for clients currently being prescribed antiresorptive medications.

C. Radiography: x-Ray of the lumbar and thoracic spine for suspected vertebral fracture and/or for height loss >5 cm. Consider a CT to assess for instability of a wedge fracture. An MRI is recommended to assess for the extent of a compression fracture and/or possible malignancy.

Differential Diagnoses

A. Osteoarthritis (OA).
B. Secondary causes:
   1. Thyroid disease.
   2. Glucocorticoid therapy.
   3. Malabsorption syndromes.
   4. Renal or collagen disease.
   5. Vitamin D deficiency.
   6. Metastatic cancer.
   7. Multiple myeloma.

Plan

A. General interventions: Lifestyle changes should be introduced to the client.
▶ B. Client teaching: *Refer to Client Teaching Guide: Osteoporosis:*
   1. Educate the client regarding calcium and vitamin D intake in diet:
      a. Calcium intake:
         i. Calcium supplement.
         ii. Food sources high in calcium include salmon or sardines with bones, low-fat yogurt and skim milk, green vegetables, and cheese.
      b. Vitamin D intake:
         i. Vitamin D supplement.
         ii. Food sources high in vitamin D include vitamin D–fortified milk and cereals, fish liver oils, cod liver oil, mushrooms, herring, catfish, salmon, sardines, egg yolks, cheese, and beef liver.
   2. Encourage the client to eliminate alcohol and caffeine from diet.
   3. Encourage the client to eliminate cigarette smoking.
   4. Prescribe regular moderate exercise, such as 30 minutes of walking at least three times per week. Walking 50 to 60 minutes three times per week provides optimal benefits.
   5. Fall prevention: Advise the client to avoid medications that may cause drowsiness and precipitate falls. Use extra light at night in the bathroom to help prevent falls. Remove all loose rugs and clutter from the home. Install hand rails on steps.
   6. Discuss safety issues and fall prevention with the client and family.
C. Pharmacological therapy:
   1. Calcium supplements:

   Calcium supplements may be contraindicated in clients who have a history of renal stones.

      a. Calcium carbonate.
   2. Vitamin D supplements: Clients diagnosed with vitamin D deficiency should ingest an increased dosage, according to the deficiency.
   3. Bisphosphonates: First-line therapy recommended for osteoporosis:
      a. Acts by reducing bone resorption and bone loss by preventing osteoclast activity.
      b. May be given daily, weekly, or monthly:
         i. Alendronate sodium + vitamin D tablet.
         ii. Risedronate.
         iii. Zoledronic acid: Check serum creatinine and calcium before infusion.
      c. Instruct the client to take medication with 200 ml of water one-half hour before breakfast or any medication for the day. Advise standing or sitting upright after taking medication. No food should be ingested for 30 minutes after taking the medication. Precautions should be used for clients who have upper gastrointestinal (GI) side effects.
      d. Studies support the efficacy of treatment with bisphosphonates for up to five years. After five years of treatment, reassess the treatment options. Treatment beyond five years of bisphosphonate therapy is highly individualized.
   4. Receptor activator of nuclear factor kappa B ligand (RANKL):
      a. Acts by inhibiting osteoclast formation, decreasing bone resorption, reducing bone fracture, and increasing bone density:
         i. Denosumab: Clients with chronic kidney disease and/or a risk of hypocalcaemia should have a serum calcium level checked 10 days after the administration.
   5. Selective oestrogen receptor modulator (SORM):
      a. Raloxifene.
      b. For postmenopausal women, it prevents osteoporosis, is cardio-protective, and appears to decrease oestrogen-recepted breast cancer by 65% more than eight years. Client may note side effects of increased vasomotor symptoms and increased risk of venous thromboembolism.
   6. Calcitonin:
      a. Intranasal calcitonin.
      b. Calcitonin injections.
      c. Fortical.
   7. Parathyroid hormone (PTH):
      a. Recombinant human PTH rebuilds bone density and increases strength of bone. Approved for severe osteoporosis for postmenopausal women and men with the diagnosis of osteoporosis who have failed antiresorptive therapy and are not able to tolerate bisphosphonates. See package insert for contraindications.
      b. Teriparatide: Check calcium and renal function before prescribing. Contraindicated for clients with a history of kidney stones and prior history of radiation therapy.
   8. Hormone replacement therapy (HRT).

Oestrogen therapy and oestrogen/progesterone therapy are available as tablets or transdermal patches and come in a wide variety of doses. Hormone replacement therapy (HRT) is approved for prevention of bone loss, but not approved for the treatment of osteoporosis.

▶ Client Teaching Guides are available at https://connect.springerpub.com/content/reference-book/978-0-8261-9498-5

Follow-Up
A. If the client is on calcium supplements, check urinary calcium excretion two times per year. If it is below 5.5 mmol/L, nephrocalcinosis and the risk of renal stones are decreased.
B. Bone density test is recommended every two years to evaluate effectiveness of medical plan.

Consultation/Referral
A. If fracture is suspected, consult with a specialist.

Individual Consideration
A. Geriatrics: Assessment and treatment for osteoporosis must be performed routinely to prevent the risk of fracture, which may increase the risk of morbidity and mortality rates in this population.
The 2010 Clinical Practice Guidelines for the Diagnosis and Management of Osteoporosis in Canada were developed to provide primary care providers with a quick-reference summary of the most important recommendations. A quick osteoporosis reference guide can be obtained from osteoporosis.ca/wp-content/uploads/Quick_Reference_Guide_October_2010.pdf.

Bibliography
Chang, S. F., Hong, C. M., & Yang, R. S. (2014). The performance of an online osteoporosis detection system: A sensitivity and specificity analysis. *Journal of Clinical Nursing, 23*(13–14), 1803–1809. doi:10.1111/jocn.12209

Cosman, F., de Beur, S. J., LeBoff, M. S., Lewiecki, E. M., Tanner, B., & Lindsay, R. (2014). Clinician's guide to prevention and treatment of osteoporosis. *Osteoporosis International, 25*(10), 2359–2381. Retrieved from www.Springerlink.com

Curtis, E. M., Moon, R. J., Dennison, E. M., Harvey, N. C., & Cooper, C. (2015). Recent advances in the Pathogenesis and treatment of osteoporosis. *Clinical Medicine (London, England), 15*(Suppl. 6), s92–s96. doi:10.7861/clinmedicine.15-6-s92

Farford, B., Balog, J., Jackson, K. D., & Montero, D. (2015). Osteoporosis: What about men? *Journal of Family Practice, 64*(9), 542–552.

Fontenot, H. B., & Harris, A. L. (2014). Pharmacologic management of osteoporosis. *Journal of Obstetric, Gynecologic, and Neonatal Nursing, 43*(2), 236–245; quiz E20. doi:10.1111/1552-6909.12285

Government of Canada. (2018). *Osteoporosis*. Retrieved from https://www.canada.ca/en/public-health/services/chronic-diseases/osteoporosis.html

Kado, D. M. (2014). Overview of hyperkyphosis in older persons. *UpToDate*. Retrieved from http://www.uptodate.com/contents/overview-of-hyperkyphosis-in-older-persons

Mackey, P. A., & Whitaker, M. D. (2015). Osteoporosis: A therapeutic update. *Journal for Nurse Practitioners, 11*(10), 1011–1017. doi:10.1016/j.nurpra.2015.08.010

Martin, G. M., Thornhill, T. S., & Katz, J. M. (2015). Total knee arthroplasty. *UpToDate*. Retrieved from www.uptodate.com/contents/total-knee-arthroplasty

National Osteoporosis Foundation. (n.d.-a). *Medications to prevent & treat osteoporosis*. Retrieved from https://www.nof.org/?s=osteoporosis+prevention

National Osteoporosis Foundation. (n.d.-b). *Prevention: Vitamin D*. Retrieved from https://www.nof. org/?s=osteoporosis+prevention

Rosen, H. N., & Walega, D. R. (2014). Osteoporotic thoracolumbar vertebral compression fractures: Clinical manifestations and treatment. *UpToDate*. Retrieved from http://www.uptodate.com/contents/osteoporotic-thoracolumbar-vertebral-compression-fractures-clinical-manifestations-and-treatment

Polymyalgia Rheumatica (PMR)

Jill C. Cash and Kelly Power-Kean

Definition
Polymyalgia rheumatica (PMR) is an inflammatory condition, with an insidious or abrupt onset, that causes morning muscle stiffness, pain, and decreased range of motion (ROM), primarily in the hips, shoulders, and neck.

Incidence/Prevalence
PMR occurs in all racial groups; however, it is rarely seen in the African American and Latino populations. It is commonly seen in adults older than 50 years, with an increased incidence in the 70- to 80-year-old population. Women are affected two to three times more often than men. PMR is occasionally associated with giant cell arteritis. Approximately 15% of diagnosed clients with PMR will also have giant cell arteritis. Approximately half of clients diagnosed with giant cell arteritis will be diagnosed with PMR.

Pathogenesis
The cause of PMR is unknown. Environmental and genetic factors have been shown to play a role in PMR. Studies speculate that environmental triggers, such as viruses, may cause the onset of symptoms. There are common similarities between PMR and giant cell arteritis.

Predisposing Factors
A. Age (older than 50 years).
B. Gender (women are affected two to three times more often than men).
C. Ethnicity (those of Northern European origin have a higher rate of PMR).

Common Findings
A. Early morning joint stiffness and pain, lasting for approximately 20 to 30 minutes after waking for at least two weeks.
B. Stiffness and pain commonly occur in the shoulders, hips, and neck.
C. Decreased ROM of joints.
D. Muscle pain.
E. Weakness of joints and muscles.

Other Signs and Symptoms
A. Fever.
B. Fatigue.
C. Malaise.

Potential Complications
A. Difficulty performing daily activities, such as getting up out of a chair, dressing, and bathing.
B. Decreased activity.
C. Overall decrease in general health because of limitations.

Subjective Data
A. Ask the client if there was an activity that brought about or preceded the episode of joint pain.
B. Has the client had any recent illness or injury?
C. Ask the client to describe the onset, duration, and intensity of pain, noting what particular joints are involved.
D. How long does pain and stiffness last in the morning?
E. Does the client notice a decrease in ROM? Are there activities that the client is not able to perform?
F. Ask the client to list all medications currently being taken, particularly substances not prescribed and over-the-counter (OTC) products. What medications improve pain?
G. Has the client noticed a problem with sleeping since the symptoms began?

Physical Examination
A. Vital signs: Check temperature, pulse, respirations, and blood pressure (BP).

B. Inspect:
1. Hands, wrists, elbows, shoulders, hips, and neck for erythema and synovitis.
C. Palpate:
1. Palpate joints for swelling and pain. Marked swelling is not usually seen in clients with PMR.
2. Assess ROM of the shoulders, hips, back, and neck. Perform passive ROM of the shoulders and hips.
3. Assess trigger points for tenderness, assessing for symptoms of fibromyalgia (FM).
4. Assess muscle strength of upper and lower extremities and neck.
5. Assess temporal arteries for signs of inflammation.
D. Auscultate heart and lungs.

Diagnostic Tests
A. Complete blood count (CBC)—normocytic anaemia common.
B. Erythrocyte sedimentation rate (ESR)—elevation.
C. C-reactive protein (CRP), noncardiac—elevation.
D. Rheumatoid factor (RF)—negative.
E. x-Rays or MRI of the affected joints.

Differential Diagnoses
A. Rheumatoid arthritis (RA).
B. Giant cell arteritis.
C. FM (symptoms will have been present for years).

Plan
A. General interventions:
1. Treat the client with steroid therapy to improve symptoms, starting at an adequate dose to resolve symptoms. Treatment will include slowly tapering the steroids over a period of weeks/months to keep the client symptom-free until off of steroids.
B. Client teaching:
1. *Refer to Client Teaching Guide: Polymyalgia Rheumatica.* Educate the client and family that PMR is primarily a self-limiting condition that will improve slowly over time.
2. Treatment will include several weeks/months of low-dose prednisone therapy, tapering slowly until completion of steroid therapy. Tapering slowly and patience will prevent recurrent attacks and rebound flares.
C. Pharmacological therapy:
1. Low-dose prednisone is used to treat the symptoms. Steroids should be given to relieve symptoms and then will be tapered slowly over the next six months. Gradually decreasing the steroid dose by very small increments over time has the best results, minimizing the possibility of relapse.

Follow-Up
A. A follow-up appointment is recommended two weeks after the initial appointment.
B. If symptoms are improving with the steroid therapy, a follow-up appointment is recommended every one to two months until there are not any flares of symptoms and the client has completed the steroid therapy. This treatment may take several months and even up to greater than one year.

Individual Considerations
A. Another condition to consider with the symptoms is remitting seronegative symmetrical synovitis with pitting oedema. This condition presents with hand and distal extremity swelling, noting marked pitting oedema in extremities. It is commonly seen in clients older than 50 years of age with an acute onset of swelling and pain. Symptoms respond quickly to the use of low-dose steroids. Laboratory testing for RA is negative.
B. Clients on long-term steroids should have a bone mineral density (BMD) performed to evaluate for osteoporosis.

Bibliography
Klippel, J. H. (2008). *Primer on the rheumatic diseases* (13th ed.). New York, NY: Springer Publishing Company.
Yurdakul, F. G., Bodur, H., Sivas, F., Başkan, B., Eser, F., & Yilmaz, O. (2015). Clinical features, treatment and monitoring in patients with polymyalgia rheumatica. *Archives of Rheumatology, 30*(1), 28–33. doi:10.5606/ArchRheumatol.2015.4643

Pseudogout
Jill C. Cash and Kelly Power-Kean

Definition
A. An acute inflammatory condition primarily affecting the larger joints in which crystal deposits of calcium pyrophosphate dihydrate (CPPD) occur in the connective tissues.

Incidence/Prevalence
A. Acute attacks occur more often in men than in women.
B. Women diagnosed with osteoarthritis with CPPD have a higher incidence of occurrence.
C. Approximately 50% of cases occur in clients older than the age of 84 years, 36% occur during the ages of 75 to 84 years, and 15% occur in those from 65 to 74 years old.
D. Joints affected: The knee is affected approximately 50% of the time; other joints affected include wrists, shoulders, ankles, feet, and elbows.

Pathogenesis
Pseudogout occurs from the crystal formation in the cartilage that is shed into the synovial joint. Excessive cartilage pyrophosphate production leads to calcium pyrophosphate production and CPP crystals are formed and deposited in the joint.

Predisposing Factors
A. Older adults.
B. Joint trauma.
C. Hospitalization/illness.
D. Familial chondrocalcinosis.
E. Endocrine/metabolic disorders:
1. Gout.
2. Hyperparathyroidism.
3. Hemochromatosis.
4. Hypophosphatasia.
5. Hypothyroidism.
6. Hypomagnesaemia.
7. Gitleman's syndrome.
8. Haemosiderosis.

Common Findings
A. Asymptomatic (may be visible on x-ray).
B. Acute attack of pain and swelling of affected joint, commonly a large joint.
C. Erythema.

▶ Client Teaching Guides are available at https://connect.springerpub.com/content/reference-book/978-0-8261-9498-5

D. Decreased range of motion (ROM) secondary to severe pain; inability to bear weight.

Other Signs and Symptoms
A. Fever.
B. Pain, swelling, and redness in several joints.

Subjective Data
A. Ask the client about the onset, progression, and duration of symptoms.
B. How many joints are affected?
C. Is this the first time this has occurred, or is this a chronic problem?
D. Ask the client to describe the onset of symptoms, in the order of occurrence.
E. In addition to today, has this occurred in other joints?
F. Does the client have a history of rheumatoid arthritis (RA), osteoarthritis (OA), or other types of arthritis?
G. Any previous injury to the joint?
H. What has the client used for pain or fever?

Physical Examination
A. Check vital signs, temperature as indicated.
B. Inspect:
　1. Inspect the affected joint for erythema, oedema, and synovitis.
　2. If erythema is present, note location of erythema and evaluate if erythema extends beyond joint area.
　3. While examining the joint, note facial grimaces, guarding with examination.
　4. If weight-bearing joint is affected, note if the client is able to bear weight.
C. Auscultate lungs and heart.
D. Palpate:
　1. Palpate affected joint, noting pain and swelling in the joint.
　2. Assess ROM in joint if possible.

Diagnostic Tests
A. Complete blood count (CBC).
B. Erythrocyte sedimentation rate (ESR).
C. Serum C-reactive protein (CRP).
D. Comprehensive metabolic profile (CMP).
E. Magnesium level.
F. Thyroid-stimulating hormone (TSH).
G. Iron studies (iron, total iron-binding capacity, ferritin level).
H. Joint aspiration for synovial fluid: Microscope: Synovial fluid evaluation for crystals.
I. x-Ray of joint: Results may demonstrate linear and punctate calcifications in articular hyaline or fibrocartilage, also known as chondrocalcinosis.

Differential Diagnoses
A. Pseudogout: Joint aspiration of synovial fluid recommended for diagnosis. Diagnosis made by crystals identified by polarized light microscopy or radiographic changes of CPPD crystals noted in the tissue or synovial fluid.
B. Gout.
C. Septic arthritis.
D. RA.
E. OA.

Plan
A. General interventions:
　1. Acute attacks should be treated with rest, immobilization, and education.
　2. Differentiate between acute and chronic attacks and treatment.
　3. Recurrent attacks should have long-term management.
B. Client teaching: *Refer to Client Teaching Guide: Pseudogout.*
　1. For acute attacks, encourage rest and elevation of affected joint.
　2. Encourage no weight bearing until symptoms subside. Suggest the use of crutches or cane for assistance.
　3. Warm, moist compresses may be used as needed for comfort.
　4. As symptoms improve, suggest ROM exercises for affected joint.
　5. Once symptoms have improved, weight-bearing activities may resume.
　6. Symptoms should continue to improve over the next seven to 10 days. Full recovery should be expected.
C. Pharmacological therapy:
　1. For acute attack, with one to two joints affected and no signs of infection:
　　a. Large joints (knees/shoulders): Joint aspiration and glucocorticoid steroid injection: Triamcinolone acetonoid mixed with 1% procaine. Smaller joints require less steroid.
　2. If not meeting the criteria discussed earlier, the next treatment option recommended is the use of nonsteroidal anti-inflammatory (NSAID) medications:
　　a. Naproxen.
　　b. Indomethacin (not recommended in high-risk clients with heart failure, gastrointestinal [GI] effects, or decreased renal function).
　　c. Sulindac.
　3. If NSAIDs are contraindicated, use colchicine.
　4. If injection and use of NSAIDs are contraindicated, use oral prednisone until flare begins to resolve, then taper prednisone over the next seven to 10 days.
　5. Recurrent attacks (more than three attacks in one year) should be treated with colchicine. Monitor liver and kidney function. Consult with or refer to rheumatologist.

Follow-Up
A. The client should return to the office in 48 to 72 hours after diagnosis and treatment.
B. Client follow-up in one week is recommended for continued care.
C. If symptoms are not improving or are worsening, client should return to the clinician's office or present to the ED for further evaluation and treatment.

Consultation/Referral
A. Refer all clients who appear to have a septic joint to the ED for evaluation and treatment. Refer to an orthopaedic surgeon for consult.
B. Consider referring clients with pseudogout to rheumatology for evaluation and continued care.

▶ Client Teaching Guides are available at https://connect.springerpub.com/content/reference-book/978-0-8261-9498-5

Individual Considerations
A. Adults:
  1. Most commonly seen in adults older than 60 years.
  2. Precautions should be used in treating clients with long-term NSAIDs. Active GI ulcers or history of GI disease should avoid NSAID use.
  3. Clients on blood thinner medications should avoid the use of NSAIDs.
  4. All precautions for the use of NSAIDs in adults should be considered, including chronic kidney disease.
  5. Clients diagnosed with diabetes who are prescribed oral or injection steroids should be advised that steroids may increase blood sugar and to monitor blood sugar values at home as indicated.

B. Geriatrics:
  1. Most common in the older adult.
  2. Precaution should be used with using NSAIDs in the older adult.
  3. Monitor renal function.

Bibliography
Sholter, D. E., & Russell, A. S. (2016). Synovial fluid analysis. *UpToDate*. Retrieved from www.uptodate.com/contents/synovial-fluid-analysis

Psoriatic Arthritis (PsA)
Jill C. Cash and Kelly Power-Kean

Definition
A. Psoriatic arthritis (PsA) is a systemic inflammatory condition that occurs in the joints that presents with symptoms of joint pain, stiffness, and swelling around the tendons and ligaments. Other symptoms include psoriasis and inflammatory back pain. PsA is a chronic disease; and when left untreated, it can cause irreversible joint damage.

B. Five different types of psoriatic arthritis:
  1. Symmetrical polyarthritis.
  2. Asymmetric oligoarthritis (fewer than four joints involved).
  3. Distal interphalangeal (DIP) joint involvement.
  4. Arthritis mutilans (destructive and deforming, causes resorption of the phalanges).
  5. Axial arthritis (spondyloarthritis).

C. The 2006 Classification of Psoriatic Arthritis (CASPAR) was developed to assist in diagnosing clients with PsA. The client must score at least three points from the following list:
  1. Skin psoriasis:
  Present: Two points.
  Previous history of skin changes: One point.
  Family history of psoriasis if client not affected: One point.
  2. Nail lesions (onycholysis, pitting): One point.
  3. Dactylitis (present or past): One point.
  4. Rheumatoid factor (RF) negative: One point.
  5. x-Ray evidence of new bone formation near a joint: One point.

Incidence/Prevalence
A. Approximately 10% to 30% of clients with psoriasis will develop PsA. PsA affects both men and women in equal numbers and usually appears between the ages of 20 and 50 years.
B. It is estimated that approximately 0.25% of Canadians have PsA.

Pathogenesis
A. Individuals are genetically susceptible to PsA. It is thought that the immune system is triggered by something in the environment, which may include infection and/or trauma. The immune system is stimulated, activating T-cells that produce inflammatory cytokines and mediators that attack the joints, causing inflammation, pain, and/or erosions that can potentially destroy the joint. This response occurs in the joint and causes damage to the ligament or tendon attachment area (enthesium), (bone spurs), skin, and/or nails.

Predisposing Factors
A. Gender: Men and women are affected equally.
B. Commonly seen in adults ranging from 30 to 55 years of age.
C. The client has a first-degree relative with psoriasis.
D. More common in Whites.

Common Findings
A. Pain and stiffness in joints, usually lasting longer than 30 minutes in the morning after wakening.
B. Pain and stiffness that usually improves with activity.
C. Enthesopathy (pain and inflammation at the ligament or tendon attachment site of the bone, commonly seen on the Achilles tendon, plantar fascia, or tibial tuberosity area).

Other Signs and Symptoms
A. Skin and nail psoriasis, nail pitting.
B. Uveitis.

Subjective Data
A. Does the client have a history of skin rash, plaques, and so forth? If present, ask the client when psoriasis began. What treatments have been used, including topical, light therapy, oral, and subcutaneous treatments?
B. Does the client complain of photosensitivity?
C. Ask the client to describe joint changes, such as swelling, pain, redness, and so forth. What joints are affected with pain and swelling?
D. Have any treatments used for psoriasis improved joint pain?
E. What medications or treatments are being used for the joint pain and swelling? What is the result of medications/treatments being used?
F. Does the client have a history of back pain? If so, when did symptoms begin? Ask the client to describe his or her back pain. Does pain improve or worsen with physical activity?
G. Does the client have a history of frequent infections or high fevers?
H. Any history of frequent eye infections?

Physical Examination
A. Check vital signs and temperature as indicated.
B. Inspect:
  1. Skin for plaques or rash.
  2. Nails for pitting.
  3. Joints for inflammation, synovitis, and erythema.
  4. Eyes for erythema and injection.
C. Auscultate the heart and lungs.
D. Palpate:
  1. Palpate all joints (hands, wrists, feet, elbows, ankles, knees, and shoulders) for synovitis/pain:

a. Dactylitis (swelling of the entire finger/toe that appears as a "sausage digit") occurs in approximately 50% of clients diagnosed with PsA.
   b. Enthesopathy is commonly seen in the Achilles tendon, plantar fascia, or tibial tuberosity.
2. Note range of motion (ROM) of all joints.
3. Palpate lumbar/thoracic spine.
4. Palpate sacral/iliac joint for tenderness.

Diagnostic Tests
A. Erythrocyte sedimentation rate (ESR): May be elevated or normal.
B. C-reactive protein (CRP): May be elevated or normal.
C. Complete blood count (CBC).
D. RF: Commonly negative in these clients; only 2% to 16% of clients with PsA will have a positive RF.
E. x-Rays of affected joints.

Differential Diagnoses
A. Rheumatoid arthritis (RA).
B. Ankylosing spondylitis (AS).
C. Osteoarthritis (OA).
D. Gout.
E. Reactive arthritis.

Plan
A. General interventions:
   1. Early identification is necessary to prevent irreversible joint damage.
B. Client teaching:
   1. Nonpharmacological treatment options include the following:
      a. Exercise on most days of the week. ROM exercises are encouraged for joint stiffness.
      b. Heat application for stiffness and ice to affected joint for swelling may be used.
      c. For extended joint stiffness/pain, recommend physical therapy for assessment and treatment.
C. Pharmacological therapy:
   1. First-line treatment: The European League Against Rheumatism (EULAR) recommends the use of nonsteroidal anti-inflammatory drugs (NSAIDs) for first-line treatment. Precautions should be given for all clients using NSAIDs (cardiovascular, renal, and gastrointestinal [GI] risks should be considered). NSAIDs are used for mild symptoms.
   2. Second-line treatment: Disease-modifying antirheumatic drugs (DMARDs), such as methotrexate (MTX), sulphasalazine, and leflunomide, are used. These medications should be prescribed by a rheumatology specialist.
   3. Third-line treatment: Biological tumour necrosis factor (TNF) inhibitors (adalimumab, certolizumab pegol, etanercept, golimumab, and infliximab). These medications should be prescribed by a rheumatology specialist.

Follow-Up
A. Follow-up is recommended in two weeks if prescribing NSAIDs for treatment of early disease.
B. Recommend follow-up every three months if not referred to rheumatology.

Consultation/Referral
A. Clients diagnosed with PsA who are not controlled with NSAIDs or who have evidence of joint changes should be referred to a rheumatology specialist for evaluation and treatment. NSAIDs do not prevent joint damage and prevention of irreversible joint damage is imperative.
B. Clients presenting with uveitis should be referred to an ophthalmologist for evaluation and treatment.
C. Clients diagnosed with severe joint damage should be referred to orthopaedics for evaluation and treatment options (surgery).
D. Clients diagnosed with severe skin psoriasis should be referred to dermatology for evaluation and treatment.

Individual Considerations
A. Adults:
   1. The use of oral steroids is not recommended for clients with PsA. Oral steroids have not been found to be effective; they also present a high risk of skin psoriasis flare when tapering the steroid dose.
   2. Clients diagnosed with PsA are at higher risk for cardiovascular disease and should be screened and monitored annually.
B. Geriatrics:
   1. When prescribing NSAIDs, monitor renal, cardiac, and GI systems for adverse events with use.

Bibliography
American College of Rheumatology. (2016). *Group for research and assessment of psoriasis and psoriatic arthritis 2015 treatment recommendations for psoriatic arthritis*. Retrieved from https://onlinelibrary.wiley.com/doi/full/10.1002/art.39573
The Arthritis Society. (2018). *Psoriatic arthritis*. Retrieved from https://arthritis.ca/about-arthritis/arthritis-types-(a-z)/types/psoriatic-arthritis
Dewing, K. A. (2015). Management of patients with psoriatic arthritis. *Nurse Practitioner, 40*(4), 40–46; quiz 46. doi:10.1097/01.NPR.0000461950.23292.18
Plilipose, J., & Deodhar, A. (2012). *Classification criteria for psoriatic arthritis: CASPAR*. Retrieved from http://www.rheumatologynetwork.com/psoriatic-arthritis/classification-criteria-psoriatic-arthritis-caspar

Raynaud's Phenomenon (RP)

Jill C. Cash and Kelly Power-Kean

Definition
Raynaud's phenomenon (RP) is an idiopathic disease in which an exaggerated vascular response occurs in extreme circumstances (heat, cold, and stress). It is manifested by bilateral blanching of the skin that is well demarcated, discomfort in the fingers, then by cyanosis, then erythema after warming the digits.

Cold hands and feet are very common complaints. RP involves both cutaneous colour change and cool skin temperature. Although the hands are the most common area of attacks, RP also can occur in the toes, ears, nose, face, knees, and nipples. A Raynaud attack typically begins in a single finger and spreads symmetrically; however, the thumb is often spared.

RP may be either primary or secondary. Spontaneous remission may occur with primary RP:
A. Criteria for diagnosis of primary RP:
   1. Symmetric episodic attacks.
   2. No evidence of peripheral vascular disease.
   3. No tissue gangrene, digital pitting, or tissue injury.
   4. Negative nailfold capillary examination.
   5. Negative antinuclear antibody (ANA) test.
   6. Normal erythrocyte sedimentation rate (ESR).
B. Indications of secondary RP:
   1. Age of onset older than 40 years.

2. Painful severe attacks with signs of ulceration/ischaemia.
3. Ischaemic signs/symptoms proximal to the fingers or toes.
4. Asymmetric attacks.
5. Abnormal laboratory, suggesting vascular or autoimmune disorders.

Incidence/Prevalence
A. Raynaud's phenomenon occurs in 5% to 20% of females and 4% to 14% of males in the general population.
B. Wide global variations occur.

Pathogenesis
A. Primary RP: Occurs alone, without any other disease process. Speculated theories include digital microvascular vasospasm because of increased response of alpha 2-adrenergic receptors and a high sympathetic vascular tone.
B. Secondary RP: Symptoms occur as a secondary manifestation from other diseases or products such as autoimmune disorders (connective tissue disorders, systemic sclerosis, systemic lupus erythematosus, rheumatoid arthritis [RA], vasculitis, Sjögren's syndrome, dermatomyositis, polymyositis, etc.), atherosclerotic diseases, haematologic disorders (polycythaemia, cryofibrinogenaemia, etc.), metabolic/endocrine disorders (diabetes mellitus, pheochromocytoma, myxedema), neoplastic syndromes (lymphoma, leukaemia, polycythaemia, monoclonal/type 1 cryoglobulinaemia), infections (hepatitis B, hepatitis C, mycoplasma infections), environmental exposures/neurologic changes (frostbite, vibratory injuries from use, lead exposure, vinyl chloride exposure, arsenic exposure, organic solvents [xylene, toluene, acetone, chlorinated solvents], carpal tunnel syndrome), and some medications/drugs (cyclosporines, antineoplastics, oral contraceptives, narcotics, ergot alkaloids, bromocriptine, beta-adrenergic blocking agents, and nicotine). Symptoms may be unilateral and may affect only one or two fingers. Secondary RP usually has a poorer morbidity than the primary disease.

Predisposing Factors
A. Primary RP:
  1. Female.
  2. Onset of symptoms after menarche (15–30 years).
  3. Smoking.
  4. Emotional stress.
B. Secondary RP:
  1. Onset after age 40 years.
  2. Male gender.
C. Family history: Multiple family members.
D. Frostbite.
E. Vascular trauma (distal ulnar artery).
F. Vibration-induced/occupation exposure (jackhammers, pneumatic drills, weed eaters).
G. Medication-associated RP (see Table 21.1).

Common Findings
A. Paleness of the fingertips after exposure to cold temperatures, followed by redness and discomfort after warming fingers.
B. "White attack": Sharp, demarcated colour of skin pallor.
C. "Blue attack": Cyanotic skin.
D. White or blue attack: Usually lasting 15 to 20 minutes.
E. Age of onset between 15 and 30 years.

TABLE 21.1 Drugs That Induce Raynaud's Phenomenon

• Amphetamines	• Cyclosporine
• Beta-blockers	• Ergot
• Bleomycin	• Interferon alpha
• Cisplatin	• Nicotine
• Clonidine	• Vinblastine
• Cocaine	• Vinyl chloride

Other Signs and Symptoms
A. Paresthesias and numbness.
B. Clumsiness of the aching hand/finger.
C. Loss of pulp in pads of fingers (severe cases).

Subjective Data
A. Determine the age of onset, time, duration, and course of presenting symptoms.
B. Question the client regarding location and symptoms, noting blanching, followed by erythema and pain after hands are warm.
C. Note frequency of attacks.
D. Review the presence of any other skin alterations that have occurred. Does client also note skin mottling of the arms and legs? Livedo reticularis is a lilac or violet mottling or reticular pattern that occurs during a cold response.
E. Ask the client to identify any events that precipitate occurrences and what makes symptoms worse or better:
  1. Air-conditioning.
  2. Grocery cold/freezer food sections.
  3. Cold weather.
  4. Cold water.
  5. Emotional stress.
  6. Sudden startling.
F. Identify any other symptoms that occur at the same time, such as migraine headaches.
G. Review the client's health history for underlying disorders, such as hypothyroidism and autoimmune disorders/connective tissue disease.
H. Review current or past occupation (especially those that include the use of vibratory tools).
I. Review current medications, stimulants, herbals, and over-the-counter (OTC) medications.

Physical Examination
A. Check pulse, respirations, and blood pressure (BP).
B. Inspect:
  1. Dermal examination: Note malar/petechial rash, telangiectasias, digital pallor, or erythema. Examine for any ulceration or signs of ischaemia.
  2. Inspect joints for swelling or redness and overall ischaemic changes.
  3. Examine several fingernails using a microscope or ophthalmoscope; examine capillaries at nailfold:
    a. Normal: Fine red capillaries, lined in the same direction.
    b. Abnormal: Capillaries dilated, tortuous, and irregularly spaced; avoid using the index finger for evaluation.
C. Auscultate heart and lungs.

D. Palpate:
  1. Palpate the joints for tenderness and peripheral pulses bilaterally.
E. Neurologic examination: Sensory function:
  1. Sensory discrimination (hot/cold, sharp/dull).
  2. Location of sensation (proximal/distal to previous stimuli).
  3. Vibratory sensation with tuning fork (distal to proximal joints).
  4. Graphesthesia (draw a number or letter in the palm of the hand with a blunt object, such as a pencil, applicator stick, or pen, and have the client identify the letter/number).

Diagnostic Tests
A. There is no gold standard diagnostic test.
B. History alone is accepted as diagnostic, as no office test application consistently triggers an attack. A history of at least two colour changes, pallor, and cyanosis after cold exposure is adequate for the diagnosis of RP. Ask the client to take a picture when symptoms occur and bring it into the office for evaluation.
C. The cold water challenge test is no longer recommended.
D. Tools to assess vascular response (usually not readily available):
  1. Nailfold capillaroscopy.
  2. Videomicroscopy.
  3. Thermography.
  4. Angiography.
  5. Laser Doppler.
  6. Direct measures of the skin temperature and local blood flow.
E. Laboratory tests:
  1. ANA.
  2. ESR.
  3. Thyroid profile if hypothyroidism is suspected.
  4. Other tests are used, depending on suspected aetiology; testing should be guided by results of history and physical examination:
    a. Complete blood count (CBC).
    b. Chemistry profile with renal and liver function.
    c. Urinalysis.
    d. Rheumatoid factor (RF).
    e. Complement (C3 and C4).
    f. ANA.

Differential Diagnoses
A. Scleroderma.
B. Systemic lupus erythematosus.
C. Occupational trauma.
D. Medication induced.
E. Peripheral vascular disease.
F. Neurovascular processes (diabetes, atherosclerosis, thromboangitis obliterans).

Plan
A. General interventions:
  1. If ulcerations are present, monitor for secondary infections. Consider topical/systemic antibiotics if secondary infection. Debridement may be necessary.
  2. Biofeedback and relaxation techniques are frequently used for treatment.
B. Client teaching:
  1. Stress the importance of not smoking.
  2. Keep the body warm:
    a. If in extreme temperatures, wear extra clothing (thermal underwear) to maintain temperature.
    b. Wear mittens instead of gloves to protect hands and keep them warm.
    c. Wear a hat to conserve heat.
  3. If possible, stop all medications that could be inducing symptoms. Other drugs that should be avoided include the following:
    a. Decongestants.
    b. Herbals that contain ephedra.
    c. Medications used for migraine headaches; for example, serotonin agonists such as sumatriptan, or caffeine plus ergotamine.
  4. If vibratory injury is present, stop the repetitive activity that induces symptoms. Consider alternative methods of work. If unable to totally stop the activity, decrease the time spent using the vibratory equipment.
  5. Emotional stress can be a trigger because of the vasoconstriction of the sympathetic nervous system being triggered. Counsel the client regarding controlling the stress in his or her life and treatment (nonpharmacological/pharmacological) options that may be beneficial.
C. Surgical therapy (only recommended for clients resistant to initial therapies):
  1. Temporary sympathectomy involving a local chemical block with lidocaine or bupivacaine (without epinephrine) relieves the pain.
  2. Chemical and cervical sympathectomy may be used for severe cases with digital ischaemia for temporary measures.
  3. Vascular reconstruction is an option.
D. Pharmacological therapy:
  1. Therapy may be required only during the winter months.
  2. Long-acting calcium channel blockers are used. Doses may be adjusted every four weeks or as tolerated. Monitor by side effects: Headaches, dizziness, flushing tachycardia, and oedema:
    a. Nifedipine.
    b. Amlodipine.
  3. Low-dose ASA antiplatelet therapy may be considered in secondary RP with a history of ischaemic ulcers or other thrombotic events.
  4. Vasodilators (sildenafil) and endothelin receptor antagonists (bosentan) may be useful in refractory cases with associated digital ulcers/infarcts. However, these medications are not FDA approved for this treatment.

Follow-Up
A. Follow up in one month or as needed by client symptoms.

Consultation/Referral
A. Consult a specialist if signs of ischaemia are present and/or if refractory symptoms are present.
B. Refer to a rheumatologist if there is a moderate/high suspicion of secondary RP.
C. Refer for surgical therapies.

Individual Considerations
A. Paediatrics: RP is commonly seen in children with systemic lupus erythematosus and scleroderma.
B. Adults: The onset of RP after age 40 years is commonly associated with an underlying disease.

Bibliography
The Arthritis Society. (2018). *Raynaud's phenomena*. Retrieved from https://arthritis.ca/about-arthritis/arthritis-types-(a-z)/types/raynaud-s-phenomenon

Hansen-Dispenza, H. (2015). Raynaud phenomenon treatment & management. *Medscape*. Retrieved from http://emedicine.medscape.com/article/331197-treatment

Jordan, S., Maurer, B., Toniolo, M., Michel, B., & Distler, O. (2015). Performance of the new ACR/EULAR classification criteria for systemic sclerosis in clinical practice. *Rheumatology (Oxford, England), 54*(8), 1454–1458. doi:10.1093/rheumatology/keu530

Miller, M. L., & Viegels, R. A. (2016). Clinical manifestations of dermatomyositis and polymyositis in adults. *UpToDate*. Retrieved from www.uptodate.com/contents/clinical-manifestations-of-dermatomyositis-and-polymyositis-in-adults

Quéméneur, T., Mouthon, L., Cacoub, P., Meyer, O., Michon-Pasturel, U., Vanhille, P., . . . Hachulla, E. (2013). Systemic vasculitis during the course of systemic sclerosis: Report of 12 cases and review of the literature. *Medicine, 92*(1), 1–9. doi:10.1097/MD.0b013e31827781fd

Varga, J. (2014). Diagnosis and differential diagnosis of systemic sclerosis (scleroderma) in adults. *UpToDate*. Retrieved from www.uptodate.com/contents/diagnosis-and-differential-diagnosis-of-systemic-sclerosis-scleroderma-in-adults

Varga, J., & Steen, V. (2015). Pulmonary arterial hypertension in systemic sclerosis (scleroderma): Definition, classification, risk factors, screening and prognosis. *UpToDate*. Retrieved from www.uptodate.com/contents/pulmonary-arterial-hypertension-in-systemic-sclerosis-scleroderma-definition-classification-risk-factors-screening-and-prognosis

Rheumatoid Arthritis (RA)

Jill C. Cash and Kelly Power-Kean

Definition

Rheumatoid arthritis (RA) is a chronic systemic disease that involves articular inflammation of the joints. The disease is generally insidious, and symmetrical involvement of synovial joints is a characteristic feature. Typically, the interphalangeal joints of the fingers and thumbs are noted; however, other joints involved include the elbows, shoulders, ankles, knees, and toes. If left untreated, the client is at high risk of joint deformity and disability. Treatment goals of RA include remission, preventing functional decline of the client, and halting progression of the disease.

RA is not limited to the joints; extra-articular features of RA include anaemia, pleuropericarditis, neuropathy, myopathy, splenomegaly, Sjögren's syndrome, scleritis, vasculitis, and renal disease. Most clients with extra-articular symptoms also have the classic RA joint symptoms. Clients with RA are at increased risk of development of carpal tunnel syndrome, stroke, an osteoporotic fracture, and renal disease (secondary to drug toxicity). The Canadian Rheumatology Association (CRA) developed recommendations for the pharmacological management of RA that take into consideration Canada's current health-care system. These guidelines include a summary of RA assessment and treatment algorithms.

Clients who should be screened for RA include those who have had at least one swollen joint, with the joint swelling not being caused by any other known aetiology. The CRA algorithms may be found at www.jrheum.org/content/39/8/1559.

A. Classification criteria for screening for RA:
  1. Duration of symptoms for more than six weeks.
  2. Joint swelling involvement (synovitis).
  3. Serology: Rheumatoid factor (RF) and/or anti-citrullinated protein antibody (ACPA).
  4. Acute-phase reactants: C-reactive protein (CRP) and erythrocyte sedimentation rate (ESR).

B. Four stages of RA:
  1. Stage 1: No symptoms or signs; normal activity; RF and/or CCP antibody is present.
  2. Stage 2: Morning stiffness, warmth at joint, normal activities of daily living (ADL), minimal limitation in joint use; increased T-cells, B-cells, antibody production, and synovial cells are observed.
  3. Stage 3: Morning stiffness, warmth at joint, and extra-articular manifestations; marked limitation in ADL. Increased T-cells, B-cells, antibody production, and synovial cells are observed.
  4. Stage 4: Same as Stage 3 plus proliferating synovial membrane involved, causing injury to the bone, tendons, and cartilage. Client is now incapacitated or confined to a wheelchair.

Incidence/Prevalence

A. It is estimated that one out of every 100 adult Canadians has RA. RA occurs two to three times more often in women compared with men.

Pathogenesis

A. The cause is unknown. Articular inflammation results in joint destruction. Antibody formation in the joint area results in inflammation and pain in the joint area.

Predisposing Factors

A. Family history, including 15% prevalence in monozygotic twins.
B. Female gender.
C. Risk increases with age, commonly developing between 40 and 60 years of age.
D. Recent systemic illness or trauma. Infection may trigger RA in those who have a have genetic predisposition to RA.
E. Numerous studies have shown that cigarette smoking is a strong environmental risk for the development and increased severity of RA.

Common Findings

A. Joint pain.
B. Morning stiffness in joints for at least one hour that has been present for more than six weeks.
C. Swelling and warmth in at least three joints or more for at least six weeks. Common joints affected include the wrists and hands, the metacarpal phalangeal (MCP) joints, and the proximal interphalangeal (PIP) joints.

Other Signs and Symptoms

A. Fatigue.
B. Malaise.
C. Subcutaneous nodules.
D. Joint deformities:
  1. PIP joints: Boutonniere deformities.
  2. Fingers: Swan-neck contractures, ulnar deviation.
  3. Wrists: Loss of extension.
  4. Hips: Loss of internal rotation, followed by flexion contractures.
  5. Knees: Suprapatellar pouch distension.
  6. Elbows: Decreased extension, olecranon bursitis.
  7. Shoulders: Limited range of motion (ROM) movement.
  8. Cervical spine: Subluxation rare.
  9. Temporomandibular joint: Pain with biting.
E. Depression.
F. Low-grade fever.
G. Weight loss.
H. Myalgia.
I. Anaemia.
J. Carpal tunnel syndrome.

Subjective Data
A. Review when joint pain began and identify the joints involved. Is pain and stiffness worse in the morning? How long does it last? Is it symmetrical?
B. Elicit the client's description of pain and a description of how the pain interferes with ADL (walking, climbing stairs, using the toilet, getting up from a chair, opening a jar).
C. Review the family history of RA.
D. Has the client ever had any type of injury to the specific joint area? Rule out recent injuries.
E. Identify what makes the pain worse and alleviating factors. In clients with RA, activity typically alleviates symptoms, which is indicative of inflammation.
F. Review list of medications, including herbal and over-the-counter (OTC) medications. What therapies have specifically been used, and what were the results?
G. Review the client's history for recent infections.
H. Does the client use any assistive devices, including cane, crutches, walker, wheelchair/power mobility device, kitchen devices/grips, and so forth?

Physical Examination
A. Check temperature, if indicated, pulse, respirations, blood pressure (BP), and weight.
B. General observation:
  1. Observe the client getting up and down in the chair.
  2. Observe the client walking (may have a tendency to bear weight on heels and hyperextend toes secondary to tenderness to the metatarsophalangeal joints).
  3. Observe the client handling objects in his or her hands.
  4. Observe for signs of depression.
C. Inspect:
  1. Inspect all joints, noting deformities, erythema, and temperature. (Heat and redness are not prominent features of RA.)
  2. Evaluate for pitting oedema in the hand (may have a "boxing glove" appearance).
  3. Inspect for subcutaneous rheumatoid nodules (elbow is the most common site).
  4. Evaluate skin for ulcerative lesions (secondary from venous stasis and neutrophilic infiltration), skin atrophy and ecchymoses from glucocorticoids, and petechiae (side effect from medications causing thrombocytopaenia).
  5. Eye examination:
    a. Episcleritis: Acute redness and pain without discharge.
    b. Scleritis: Deep ocular pain with dark red discolouration.
D. Auscultate.
  1. Heart.
  2. Lungs (at risk of infectious complications from immunosuppression and pulmonary toxicity from methotrexate [MTX] if currently being treated with medications).
E. Percuss:
  1. Perform a patellar tap to evaluate synovial thickening/effusion of the knee.
F. Palpate:
  1. Palpate the lymph nodes.
  2. Perform oral examination to palpate the salivary glands (may have lymphocytic infiltration).
  3. Palpate all joints to evaluate for tenderness with pressure, pain with movement of the joint, and "bogginess" of the joint (synovial thickening).
  4. Palpate the popliteal fossa for evidence of a popliteal (Baker's) cyst.
  5. Examine abdomen for splenomegaly.
G. Musculoskeletal examination:
  1. Assess grip (a reduced grip is a useful parameter in evaluating disease activity and progression). Is the client able to close fingers to make a fist?
  2. Assess the strength of the extremities.
  3. Assess the ROM (active and passive) and flexion.

Diagnostic Tests
A. Complete blood count (CBC) and platelets.
B. ESR.
C. CRP.
D. RF, quantitative.
E. CCP antibody.
F. Uric acid level.
G. Synovial fluid (optional).
H. Plain film radiography of the hands, wrists, and feet as a baseline and to monitor disease progression.

Differential Diagnoses
A. Osteoarthritis (OA).
B. Crystalline arthritis (gout and pseudogout).
C. Polyarthritis.
D. Reactive arthritis.
E. Acute viral/infectious process:
  1. Lyme disease.
  2. Hepatitis B.
  3. Hepatitis C.
  4. Parvovirus B19.
F. Sjögren's syndrome: Keratoconjunctivitis sicca, splenomegaly, and lymphadaenopathy.
G. Sarcoidosis.
H. Polymyositis.

Plan
A. General interventions:
  1. Focus on exercise and joint mobility to maintain functional abilities.
  2. Encourage smoking cessation, especially among females on glucocorticoids because of the risk of increased bone loss/fracture.
B. Client teaching:
  1. Once diagnosed, it is recommended that treatment with medications begin to prevent joint damage. First-line medications include disease-modifying antirheumatic drugs (DMARDs). Depending on what medication is used, educate the client regarding benefits, risks, side effects, and precautions for medications. If MTX is used, educate the client that alcohol should be avoided to prevent hepatotoxicity.
  2. Stress the importance of returning for laboratory follow-up while on DMARDs.
  3. Discuss vaccinations, especially pneumonia and influenza vaccines. Emphasize the importance of keeping all vaccinations up to date. Most treatment medications suppress the immune system and increase the risk of infections.
C. Pharmacological therapy:
  1. Early disease:
    a. Daily nonsteroidal anti-inflammatory drugs (NSAIDs) and pain-relieving medications:
      i. Ibuprofen.
      ii. Naproxen.

iii. Celecoxib.
iv. Acetaminophen.

b. Comorbid conditions, such as a history of heart failure, renal disease, and peptic ulcers, should be considered before starting NSAID therapy.

c. Be aware of other medications the client is prescribed by other providers and consider possible drug-to-drug interactions. Examples include NSAIDs, antacids, anticoagulants, oral hypoglycaemic agents, antihypertensive/diuretics, lithium, MTX, and diphenylhydantoin.

d. DMARDs are recommended by CRA as soon as possible following the diagnosis of active RA. The benefits, risks, and side effects of all medications should be explained to the client before beginning therapy. Recommended blood work monitoring should also be followed according to the CRA guidelines and medication recommendations. The CRA algorithm for pharmacological management of RA can be obtained from www.jrheum.org/content/39/8/1559.figures-only:

i. MTX is increased as tolerated to control symptoms. MTX should not be given to clients who desire to become or who are pregnant or clients with liver disease.
ii. Sulphasalazine.
iii. Hydroxychloroquine. Before starting clients on hydroxychloroquine, the client must be counseled regarding the possible risks of the medication, including retinal damage that can lead to blindness. A baseline eye examination must be performed, followed by eye examination every six months to monitor for retinal changes.

2. Moderate to severe RA disease:

a. Oral glucocorticoids may be added for active joint inflammation. Prednisone may be used up to six months, but shorter courses are recommended because of the consequence of long-term steroid use. Steroids should be tapered over a period of a few months and then completely discontinued if possible.

b. Intra-articular long-acting glucocorticoid injections are used for the reduction of synovitis in inflamed joints.

c. If the response to DMARD is not adequate, biological agents, tumour necrosis factor (TNF) alpha inhibitors, and other classes of drugs may be instituted. Because of the associated side effects, rheumatology consult is recommended for treatment with these medications:

i. Examples of TNF inhibitors.
   1) Infliximab.
   2) Adalimumab.
   3) Etanercept.
   4) Golimumab.
   5) Certolizumab pegol.
ii. Janus kinase inhibitor:
   1) Tofacitinib citrate.
iii. Interleukin-6 (IL-6) inhibitor:
   1) Tocilizumab.
iv. T-cell depletion:
   1) Abatacept.
v. B-cell depleting therapy:
   1) Rituximab.

d. Clients may also use combination therapy. Examples of this include using MTX plus a TNF inhibitor or sulfasalazine.

e. Clients receiving treatment with pharmacological agents should be evaluated at routine intervals, every one to three months, regarding their functional status to identify whether treatment therapies are improving the symptoms. There are several functional forms that are available for use. The Stanford Health Assessment Questionnaire (HAQ) is a well-known questionnaire that is recommended for use. When treatment goals have been attained, disease activity should be monitored every six to 12 months.

f. Drug monitoring, by performing serum blood work, is also recommended at routine intervals when prescribing pharmacological agents to avoid adverse effects of the medications being prescribed.

Follow-Up

A. Follow-up will be guided by medication therapy. Disease activity and response to therapy should be reassessed every one to three months.

B. Follow laboratory values with certain medications, including MTX with liver function testing, albumin, CBC with differential, platelets, and urinalysis monthly.

C. Assume all clients with RA are at risk of osteoporosis. Dual-energy x-ray absorptiometry (DEXA) scan is used to evaluate bone loss secondary to glucocorticoid-induced osteopaenia. Initiate bisphosphonate therapy as indicated for signs of bone loss. Use a low threshold for starting in post-menopausal women with RA.

D. Anti-TNF agents are contraindicated in clients with an active infection and those who are at high risk of reactivation of tuberculosis (TB). A TB skin test is required before administration. Clients with a positive skin test should be treated with prophylactic anti-TB therapy one month before therapy with anti-TNF agents.

E. Clients should receive a baseline ophthalmologic examination before starting antimalarial drugs, such as plaquenil, and then follow-up examinations every six to 12 months while on therapy.

Consultation/Referral

A. Refer all clients with early inflammatory arthritis to a rheumatologist if RA is the suspected. Early intervention may prevent bone destruction of the joints and improve the long-term outcome for the client.

B. Clients with a history of chronic swelling and pain of the joints should be referred to a rheumatologist.

C. Refer all clients to the rheumatologist, orthopaedist, or ED if a septic joint is suspected.

Individual Considerations

A. Pregnancy:

1. RA activity improves substantially in pregnancy:
   a. Approximately 70% to 80% of clients will have symptoms improve during pregnancy.
   b. Approximately 90% of women will have a flare in the postpartum period. Flares usually occur within the first three months postpartum.

2. Leflunomide, etanercept, adalimumab, and infliximab are contraindicated in pregnancy and while breastfeeding.

3. Pregnancy should be avoided with the use of MTX and leflunomide. Women need to have one normal menstrual cycle following discontinuation of MTX before attempting pregnancy. Men should wait at least three months after discontinuing MTX before attempting to conceive.

4. Therapy during pregnancy should be coordinated with the perinatologist and the rheumatologist.
B. Paediatrics:
   1. In children, consider juvenile-onset RA.
   2. If suspected, consider referral to a paediatric rheumatologist for evaluation and diagnosis.
C. Geriatrics:
   1. Use NSAIDs with caution. Consider the client's age, weight, and chronic conditions when prescribing NSAIDs. NSAIDs are not recommended in clients with renal conditions.

Bibliography

Aletaha, D., Neogi, T., Silman, A. J., Funovits, J., Felson, D. T., Bingham, C. O., . . . Hawker, G. (2010). 2010 rheumatoid arthritis classification criteria: An American College of Rheumatology/European League Against Rheumatism collaborative initiative. *Arthritis and Rheumatism, 62*(9), 2569–2581. doi:10.1002/art.27584

The Arthritis Society. (2018). *Rheumatoid arthritis*. Retrieved from https://arthritis.ca/about-arthritis/arthritis-types-(a-z)/types/rheumatoid-arthritis

Behnam, B., Moghimi, J., Ghorbani, R., & Ghahremanfard, F. (2013). The frequency and major determinants of depression in patients with rheumatoid arthritis. *Turkish Journal of Rheumatology (Turkish League Against Rheumatism/Turkive Romatizma Arastima VeSavas Dernegi), 28*(1), 32–37. doi:10.5606/tjr.2013.2599

Bombardier, C., Hazlewood, G. S., Akhavan, P., Schieir, O., Dooley, A., Haraoui, B., . . . Bykerk, V. (2012). Canadian Rheumatology Association recommendations for the pharmacological management of rheumatoid arthritis with traditional and biologic disease-modifying antirheumatic drugs: Part II safety. *The Journal of Rheumatology, 39*(8), 1583–1602. doi:10.3899/jrheum.120165

Bykerk, V. P., Akhavan, P., Hazlewood, G. S., Schieir, O., Dooley, A., Haraoui, B., . . . Bombardier, C. (2012). Canadian Rheumatology Association recommendations for pharmacological management of rheumatoid arthritis with traditional and biologic disease-modifying antirheumatic drugs. *The Journal of Rheumatology, 39*(8), 1559–1582. doi:10.3899/jrheum.110207

Cakir, T., Evcik, F. D., Subasi, V., Gokce, I. Y., & Kayuncu, V. (2014). The effectiveness of aquatic exercises in the treatment of rheumatic arthritis. *Turkish Journal of Osteoporosis/Turk Osteoporoz Dergisi, 20*(1), 10–15.

Carter, S. C., Patty-Resk, C., Ruffing, V., & Hicks, D. (2015). *Core curriculum for rheumatology nursing* (1st ed.). Greenville, SC: Rheumatology Nurses Society.

Fujita, T., Kutsumi, H., Sanuki, T., Hayakumo, T., & Azuma, T. (2013). Adherence to the preventive strategies for nonsteroidal anti-inflammatory drug- or low-dose aspirin-induced gastrointestinal injuries. *Journal of Gastroenterology, 48*(5), 559–573. doi:10.1007/s00535-013-0771-8

Ikdahl, E., Rollefstad, S., Olsen, I. C., Kvien, T. K., Hansen, I. J., Soldal, D. M., . . . Semb, A. G. (2015). EULAR task force recommendations on annual cardiovascular risk assessment for patients with rheumatoid arthritis: An audit of the success of implementation in a rheumatology outpatient clinic. *BioMed Research International, 2015*, 515280. doi:10.1155/2015/515280

Klippel, J. H. (2008). *Primer on the rheumatic diseases* (13th ed.). New York, NY: Springer Publishing Company.

Marcus, D. M. (2015). *Herbal remedies, supplements & acupuncture for arthritis*. Retrieved from www.rheumatology.org/i-am-a/patient-caregiver/treatments/herbal-remedies-supplements-acupuncture-for-arthritis

Moerman, R. V., Bootsma, H., Kroese, F. G., & Vissink, A. (2013). Sjögren's syndrome in older patients: Aetiology, diagnosis and management. *Drugs & Aging, 30*(3), 137–153. doi:10.1007/s40266-013-0050-7

Palmer, D., & ElMiedany, Y. (2014). Rheumatoid arthritis: Recommendations for treat to target. *British Journal of Nursing (Mark Allen Publishing), 23*(6), 310–315. doi:10.12968/bjon.2014.23.6.310

Raza, K., Klareskog, L., & Holers, V. M. (2016). Predicting and preventing the development of rheumatoid arthritis. *Rheumatology (Oxford, England), 55*(1), 1–3. doi:10.1093/rheumatology/kev261

Schur, P. H., & Moreland, L. W. (2016). General principles of management of rheumatoid arthritis in adults. *UpToDate*. Retrieved from http://www.uptodate.com/contents/general-principles-of-management-of-rheumatoid-arthritis-in-adults

Sholter, D. E., & Russell, A. S. (2016). Synovial fluid analysis. *UpToDate*. Retrieved from www.uptodate.com/contents/synovial-fluid-analysis

Singh, J. A., Saag, K. G., Bridges, S. L., Akl, E. A., Bannuru, R. R., Sullivan, M. C., . . . McAlindon, T. (2016). 2015 American College of Rheumatology Guideline for the treatment of rheumatoid arthritis. *Arthritis & Rheumatology (Hoboken, NJ), 68*(1), 1–26. doi:10.1002/art.39480

Systemic Lupus Erythematosus (SLE)

Jill C. Cash and Kelly Power-Kean

Definition

Systemic lupus erythematosus (SLE) is a chronic, inflammatory autoimmune disorder. It may affect multiple organ systems. The body's immune system forms antibodies that attack healthy tissues and organs. The clinical course is marked by spontaneous remission and relapses. Severity varies from a mild episodic disorder to a rapidly fulminating fatal disease. The three types of lupus are as follows:

A. Discoid lupus erythematosus (DLE) affects the skin, causing a rash, lesions, or both.
B. SLE attacks body organs and systems, such as joints, kidneys, brain, heart, and lungs. SLE is usually more severe than DLE and can be life-threatening.
C. Drug-induced lupus symptoms usually disappear when medication is discontinued.

Incidence/Prevalence

A. The incidence of SLE in relation to gender, ancestry, and familial history has been repeatedly documented. About 90% of clients with SLE are women; it affects mainly young women after menarche and before menopause. The majority of clients who develop SLE during childhood or after age 50 years are also women. SLE affects about one in every 2,000 Canadians. The disorder is concordant in 25% to 75% of identical twins. The risk of developing the disease if a mother has SLE is 1:40 for a daughter and 1:250 for a son. Positive antinuclear antibody (ANA) is seen in asymptomatic family members, and the prevalence of other rheumatic diseases is increased among close relatives of clients. There is a high frequency of specific genes in SLE. SLE is much less common in the very young and the very old. Ten percent of DLE clients go on to develop SLE.

Pathogenesis

A. The exact cause of SLE is unknown, but clinical manifestations of SLE are secondary to the trapping of antigen–antibody complexes in capillaries of visceral structures, or to autoantibody-mediated destruction of host cells such as thrombocytopaenia.

Predisposing Factors

A. Female gender.
B. African Canadian, Asian, Hispanic ancestry.
C. Childbearing age.
D. Positive family history of SLE.
E. Drug use:
   1. Procainamide.
   2. Hydralazine.
   3. Isoniazid.

Common Findings

A. Joint pain: Joint symptoms occur in 90% of clients.
B. Fever.
C. Loss of appetite.
D. Fatigue.
E. Weight loss.
F. Oral or nasal ulcers.
G. Hair loss.
H. Photosensitive skin rash and skin lesions over areas exposed to sunlight.
I. Relapsing polychondritis.

Other Signs and Symptoms

A. DLE:
 1. Rash: Erythematosus, round, scaling papules 5 to 10 mm in diameter, appearing as "butterfly" shape across bridge of nose.
 2. Rash, commonly on the trunk, extremities, scalp, external ear, and neck.
 3. Photosensitivity.
B. SLE: The Systemic Lupus Erythematosus International Collaborating Clinics (SLICC) revised and validated the 1997 American College of Rheumatology (ACR) SLE classification criteria for SLE. The SLICC specify that classification requires (a) fulfillment of at least four criteria, with at least one clinical criterion AND one immunologic criterion, OR (b) lupus nephritis as the sole clinical criterion in the presence of ANA or anti-double stranded DNA (anti-dsDNA) antibodies. The revised criteria for diagnosis can be found at cmijournal.files.wordpress.com/2015/10/slicc-criteria-article.pdf:
 1. Other signs and symptoms:
  a. Weight loss.
  b. Fatigue.
  c. Acute abdominal pain.
  d. Alopaecia.
  e. Tendon involvement.
  f. Urinalysis: Active urine sediment (blood or protein without urinary tract infections [UTIs]).
  g. Fever and malaise.
  h. Lymphadaenopathy.
 2. Other complications:
  a. Hashimoto's thyroiditis.
  b. Haemolytic anaemia.
  c. Thrombocytopeania purpura.
  d. Arterial and venous thrombosis in the presence of antiphospholipid antibodies.
  e. Recurrent pleurisy.
  f. Pleural effusion, pneumonitis.
  g. Pulmonary embolism.
  h. Pericarditis, endocarditis, myocarditis.
  i. Hypertension.
  j. Splenomegaly.
  k. Recurrent miscarriages in the presence of antiphospholipid antibodies.
  l. Relapsing polychondritis.
C. Central nervous system (CNS) problems:
 1. Chronic headaches (migraine).
 2. Seizures or epilepsy.
 3. Personality changes, chronic brain syndrome.
D. Decreased haemoglobin (Hgb), white blood cells (WBC), and platelets.

Subjective Data

A. Determine systemic features and onset, course, and duration of symptoms (see the section "Other Signs and Symptoms").
B. Obtain medication history (see the section "Predisposing Factors").
C. Determine family history of rheumatoid diseases or other autoimmune disorders.
D. Review the client's recent history for possible allergen exposure.

Physical Examination

A. Check temperature, pulse, respirations, and blood pressure (BP).
B. Inspect:
 1. Observe general overall appearance and generalized movement of extremities.
 2. Conduct dermal examination for colour, petechiae, rashes, lesions, and hair loss.
 3. Conduct funduscopic examination; note photosensitivity.

Funduscopic examination: Cotton–wool exudates are the most common eye lesion.

 4. Examine mouth and nose for oral lesions/ulcers.
 5. Observe for pericardial lifts and heaves.
 6. Inspect joints for subluxation of the metacarpal phalangeal joints and swan-neck deformities of the hands.
C. Palpate:
 1. The back for tactile fremitus; palpate the heart for lifts, heaves, and thrills.
 2. The neck for thyroid enlargement.
 3. The neck, axilla, and groin for lymphadaenopathy.
 4. The abdomen for organomegaly, masses, and tenderness; palpate suprapubic area for suprapubic tenderness and assess back for costovertebral angle (CVA) tenderness.
D. Percuss:
 1. The chest, anterior and posterior lung fields, for consolidation.
 2. The abdomen for splenomegaly.
E. Auscultate heart, lungs, and abdomen.
F. Musculoskeletal examination:
 1. Examine for bone or joint swelling, tenderness, and increased warmth.
 2. Check lower extremities for evidence of phlebitis, asymmetrical swelling, calf tenderness, and palpable cord.
G. Neurologic examination: Complete neurologic examination with mental status examination.

Diagnostic Tests

A. Complete blood count (CBC) with differential.
B. Platelets.
C. ANA: Indirect immunofluorescence assay (IFA) positive. In clients with SLE, the ANA will typically be positive with a high titre ANA. Note pattern associated with positive ANA. A negative ANA by the IFA method dramatically decreases the risk of misdiagnosing SLE.
D. Complement levels (decreased C3 and C4).
E. Rheumatoid factor (RF) can be positive in clients with SLE.
F. Thyroid profile.
G. Anti-DNA antibodies, seen in approximately 30% of clients with renal disease.
H. Antiphospholipid antibodies: Lupus anticoagulant immunoglobulin A (IgA), immunoglobulin G (IgG), and immunoglobulin M (IgM) anticardiolipin antibodies; IgA, IgG, and IgM anti-beta-2-glycoprotein.
I. Erythrocyte sedimentation rate (ESR).
J. Urinalysis (check for haematuria, proteinuria, and cellular casts) and urine culture.
K. Collection of 24-hour urine for protein and creatinine clearance.
L. Skin biopsy.
M. Follow-up Coombs' test: Positive.
N. Microhemagglutination assay for *Treponema pallidum* (MHA-TP) antibodies to confirm reactive syphilis for

positive rapid plasma reagin (RPR): False-positive serologic test for syphilis needs follow-up.
O. Chest x-ray film may show changes.
P. x-Ray of joints for nondestructive arthritis.

Differential Diagnoses
A. DLE.
B. Undifferentiated connective tissue disease.
C. Drug-induced lupus.
D. Rheumatoid arthritis (RA): Lupus can resemble RA, especially early in the course of SLE. Unlike RA, the arthritis is nonerosive: There is no joint destruction.
E. Vasculitis.
F. Scleroderma.
G. Chronic active hepatitis.
H. Acute drug reactions.
I. Polyarteritis.
J. Infection.
K. Influenza.
L. Rosacea.
M. Neoplasm.

Plan
A. General interventions: After diagnosis, refer the client to a rheumatologist and comanage.
B. Pharmacological therapy:
   1. Nonsteroidal anti-inflammatory drugs (NSAIDs) for arthritis symptoms.
   2. Prednisone for the control of thrombocytopaenic purpura, haemolytic anaemia, myocarditis, pericarditis, convulsions, and nephritis.
   3. Always give the lowest dose that controls the condition.
   4. Corticosteroids can usually be tapered to low doses.
   5. Antimalarial drug, hydroxychloroquine sulfate, every day may help treat lupus rashes and joint symptoms that do not respond to NSAIDs. *Consult with a rheumatology specialist.*
   6. Alternative drug therapy: Immunosuppressive agents, such as cyclophosphamide, chlorambucil, and azathioprine, are used in cases resistant to corticosteroids. The exact role of immunosuppressive agents is controversial.

Follow-Up
A. Very close follow-up by a specialist is needed when immunosuppressants are employed.
B. If fever is present on examination, explore cause of fever to rule out infection. Monitor the client for infections, especially with opportunistic organisms.
C. Preventive heart care is important because of the presence of premature atherosclerosis seen in these clients.
D. Up-to-date immunizations.
E. Osteoporosis screening.

Infections are the leading cause of death secondary to the depression of WBCs, followed by active SLE, chiefly because of renal or CNS disease.

Consultation/Referral
A. After diagnosis, refer the client to a rheumatologist.
B. Referral to a specialist for a biopsy of the skin or kidney may be necessary to confirm the diagnosis.

Individual Considerations
A. Pregnancy:
   1. Infertility: 25% of clients have a problem getting pregnant.
   2. Clients with SLE experience frequent miscarriages and stillbirths.
   3. Clients are considered high risk when consultation and management with a perinatologist are needed.
   4. Approximately 33% of clients have an antibody (anticardiolipin) that is associated with early failure of the placenta.
   5. Approximately 10% have a related antibody (lupus anticoagulant) that allows early pregnancy, but compromises foetal growth as the placenta fails.
   6. It is estimated that 25% of the remaining pregnancies deliver prematurely.
   7. Family planning:
      a. Barrier methods or intrauterine devices (IUDs) are best and safest.
      b. Oral contraceptives may exacerbate lupus. Avoid use of oestrogen birth control pills with active SLE. Consider alternate methods of birth control.
   8. Exacerbations of lupus are sometimes caused by pregnancy.
B. Paediatrics:
   1. Prematurity is the greatest danger of lupus's effects on the baby.
   2. There are no known congenital abnormalities related to lupus.
   3. Three percent of all lupus clients have a baby with neonatal lupus. This is a syndrome, not SLE, and it is transient.
C. Geriatrics: Males are affected more than females.

Bibliography
The Arthritis Society. (2018). *Systemic lupus erythematosus*. Retrieved from https://arthritis.ca/about-arthritis/arthritis-types-(a-z)/types/systemic-lupus-erythematosus

Bartels, C. (2015). Systemic lupus erythematosus. *Medscape*. Retrieved from www.emedicine.medscape.com/article/332244-overview

Centers for Disease Control and Prevention. (2015). *Systemic lupus erythematous (SLE or lupus): Prevalence and incidence*. Retrieved from www.cdc.gov/arthritis/basics/lupus.htm

Chasset, F., Francès, C., Barete, S., Amoura, Z., & Arnaud, L. (2015). Influence of smoking on the efficacy of antimalarials in cutaneous lupus: A meta-analysis of the literature. *Journal of the American Academy of Dermatology, 72*(4), 634–639. doi:10.1016/j.jaad.2014.12.025

Fonseca, R., Bernardes, M., Terroso, G., de Sousa, M., & Figueiredo-Braga, M. (2014). Silent burdens in disease: Fatigue and depression in SLE. *Autoimmune Diseases, 2014*, 790724. doi:10.1155/2014/790724

Jordan, S., Maurer, B., Toniolo, M., Michel, B., & Distler, O. (2015). Performance of the new ACR/EULAR classification criteria for systemic sclerosis in clinical practice. *Rheumatology (Oxford, England), 54*(8), 1454–1458. doi:10.1093/rheumatology/keu530

Keeling, S. O., Alabdurubalnabi, Z., Avina-Zubieta, A., Barr, S., Bergeron, L., Bernatsky, S., . . . Santesso, N. (2018). Canadian Rheumatology Association recommendations for the assessment and monitoring of systemic lupus erythematosus. *Journal of Rheumatology, 45*(10), 1426–1439. doi:10.3899/jrheum.171459

Kim, S. J., & McMahon, M. (2013). Diagnosis and treatment of systemic lupus erythematosus. *Journal of Clinical Outcomes Management, 20*(2), 85–95.

Lalani, S., Pope, J., de Leon, F., & Peschken, C. (2010). Clinical features and prognosis of late-onset systemic lupus erythematosus: Results from the 1000 faces of lupus study. *Journal of Rheumatology, 37*(1), 38–44. doi:10.3899/jrheum.080957

Moerman, R. V., Bootsma, H., Kroese, F. G., & Vissink, A. (2013). Sjögren's syndrome in older patients: Aetiology, diagnosis and management. *Drugs & Aging, 30*(3), 137–153. doi:10.1007/s40266-013-0050-7

Montes, R. A., Mocarzel, L. O., Lanzieri, P. G., Lopes, L. M., Carvalho, A., & Almeida, J. R. (2016). Smoking and its association with morbidity in systemic lupus erythematosus evaluated by the Systemic Lupus International Collaborating Clinics/American College of Rheumatology damage index: Preliminary data and systematic review. *Arthritis & Rheumatology (Hoboken, NJ.), 68*(2), 441–448. doi:10.1002/art.39427

Petri, M., Orbai, A. M., Alarcón, G. S., Gordon, C., Merrill, J. T., Fortin, P. R., & Magder, L. S. (2012). Derivation and validation of the Systemic Lupus International Collaborating Clinics classification criteria for systemic lupus erythematosus. *Arthritis and Rheumatism, 64*(8), 2677–2686. doi:10.1002/art.34473

Sam Lim, S., Rana Bayakly, A., Helmick, C. G., Gordon, C., Easley, K. A., & Drenkard, C. (2014). The incidence and prevalence of systemic lupus erythematosus, 2002–2004: The Georgia Lupus Registry. *Arthritis & Rheumatology, 66*(2), 357–368. doi:10.1002/art.38239

Shur, P. H., & Wallace, D. J. (2014). Diagnosis and differential diagnosis of systemic lupus erythematosus in adults. *UpToDate*. Retrieved from www.uptodate.com/contents/diagnosis-and-differential-diagnosis-of-systemic-lupus-erythematous-in-adults

Tunnicliffe, D. J., Singh-Grewal, D., Kim, S., Craig, J. C., & Tong, A. (2015). Diagnosis, monitoring, and treatment of systemic lupus erythematosus: A systematic review of clinical practice guidelines. *Arthritis Care & Research, 67*(10), 1440–1452. doi:10.1002/acr.22591

Varga, J. (2014). Diagnosis and differential diagnosis of systemic sclerosis (scleroderma) in adults. *UpToDate*. Retrieved from www.uptodate.com/contents/diagnosis-and-differential-diagnosis-of-systemic-sclerosis-scleroderma-in-adults

Varga, J., & Steen, V. (2015). Pulmonary arterial hypertension in systemic sclerosis (scleroderma): Definition, classification, risk factors, screening and prognosis. *UpToDate*. Retrieved from www.uptodate.com/contents/pulmonary-arterial-hypertension-in-systemic-sclerosis-scleroderma-definition-classification-risk-factors-screening-and-prognosis

Temporal Arteritis/Giant Cell Arteritis (GCA)

Jill C. Cash and Kelly Power-Kean

Definition
A. Temporal arteritis, also known as giant cell arteritis (GCA), is a vascular illness that can affect the entire body; however, it primarily affects the blood vessels. There is inflammation of the arteries that begins in the aortic arch and branches out to the cranial arteries.

Incidence/Prevalence
A. GCA occurs in approximately one in 500 individuals older than 50 years. GCA rarely occurs in individuals younger than 50 years and is more commonly seen during later years (older than 70 years). It can also be seen in clients diagnosed with polymyalgia rheumatica (PMR). Approximately 50% of clients diagnosed with GCA will also have PMR.

Pathogenesis
A. The cause of GCA is unknown. The immune system attacks the body and causes inflammation of the medium and large arteries, which causes thickening of the arterial walls and narrowing of the lumen. When these changes occur, the result is a decrease in the blood flow, which can potentially cause an occlusion in the artery, leading to ischaemia. Arteries commonly involved include the temporal artery, medium and large vessels, and the vessels of the eyes. Blindness is the major acute morbidity with GCA.

Predisposing Factors
A. Age (older than 50 years).
B. Ethnicity (Scandinavian descent).
C. Gender (women > men).

Common Findings
A. Abrupt onset of headaches.
B. Visual impairment.
C. Joint pain (PMR).

Other Signs and Symptoms
A. Fever.
B. Anaemia.
C. Jaw or arm claudication.
D. Fatigue.
E. Weight loss.

Potential Complications
A. Visual loss, blindness.
B. Joint pain.

Subjective Data
A. Have the client describe the presenting complaints. What makes it better or worse?
B. Ask the client when presenting symptoms began. Discuss the course of new-onset symptoms. Note systemic symptoms such as fever, weight loss, fatigue, headache, vision changes, jaw/arm pain.
C. Ask the client to describe pain, for example, crushing, stabbing, or burning.
D. Have client rate pain on a scale of 1 to 10, with 1 being the least painful.
E. What has the client taken to relieve the pain or symptoms?
F. Has the client noted any visual disturbance or changes? Is vision change constant or does it occur when headache is present? What makes the headache worse? What makes the headache better?

Physical Examination
A. Vital signs: Check temperature, pulse, respirations, and blood pressure (BP; take BP in both arms and note discrepancies).
B. Inspect:
  1. Inspect overall general appearance. Clients with GCA usually appear chronically ill.
  2. Perform funduscopic examination, looking for a pale disc and blurred margins of the disc. Assess pupils equal and reactive to light and accommodation (PERLA), extraocular muscles (EOMs), and visual acuity.
C. Palpate:
  1. Palpate pulses (carotid, brachial, radial, pedal, and femoral pulses).
  2. Perform range of motion (ROM) of all joints (shoulders, neck, hips, and extremities), noting limitations because of pain and/or swelling.
  3. Assess joints for swelling and pain. (Note symptoms of PMR.)
D. Auscultate:
  1. Heart for murmurs.
  2. Carotid, brachial, and femoral arteries for bruits.
  3. Abdomen noting any bruits.

Diagnostic Tests
A. Serum laboratory studies (erythrocyte sedimentation rate [ESR], complete blood count [CBC], C-reactive protein [CRP], and comprehensive metabolic profile [CMP]).
B. Temporal artery biopsy. Any client suspicious of having temporal arteritis should have a temporal artery biopsy performed. This is the gold standard for diagnosing GCA. Recommended sample size of the artery for biopsy should be ≥4 cm. False-negative biopsy results may be up to 20%.

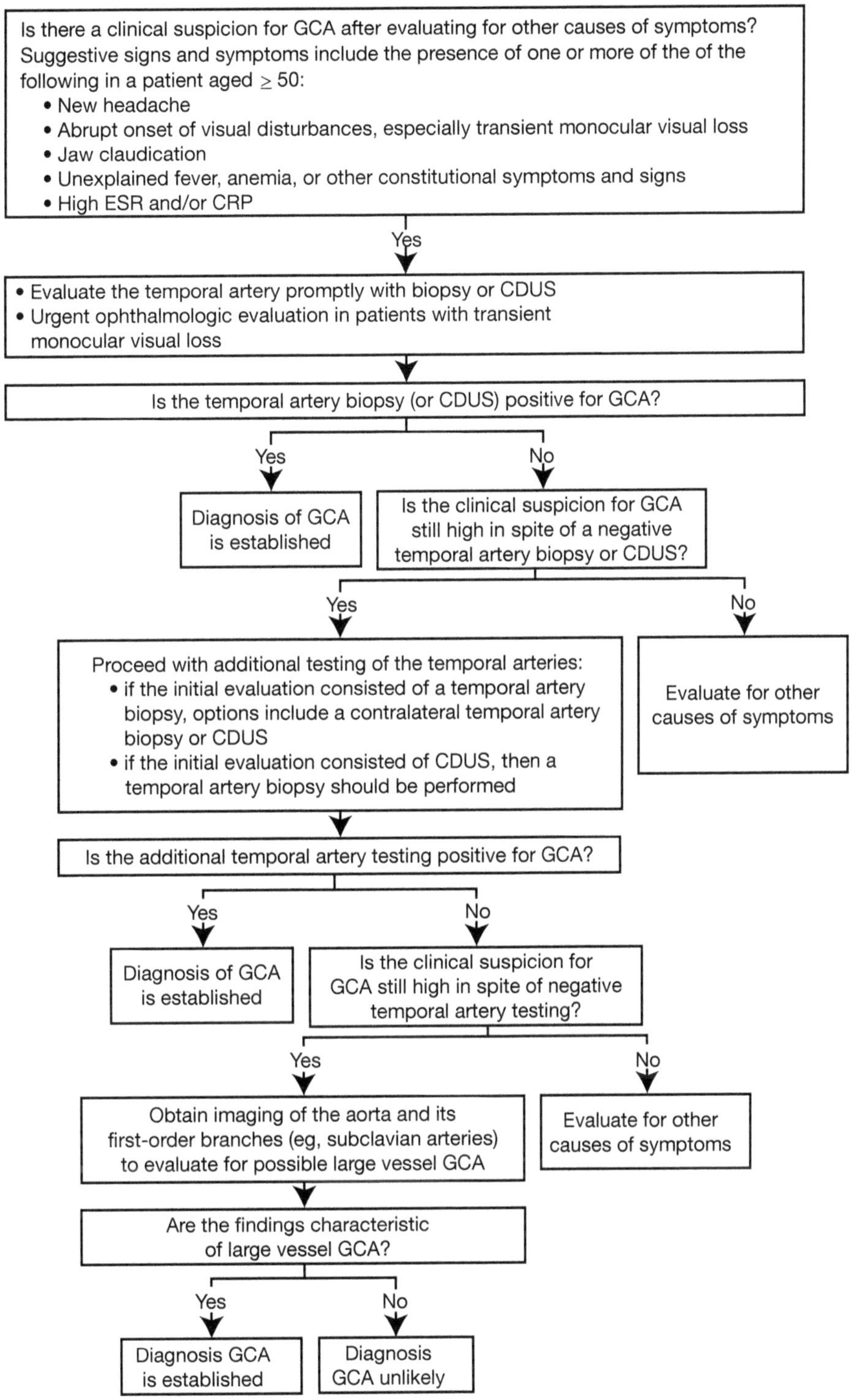

```
Is there a clinical suspicion for GCA after evaluating for other causes of symptoms?
Suggestive signs and symptoms include the presence of one or more of the of the
following in a patient aged ≥ 50:
  • New headache
  • Abrupt onset of visual disturbances, especially transient monocular visual loss
  • Jaw claudication
  • Unexplained fever, anemia, or other constitutional symptoms and signs
  • High ESR and/or CRP
                            │ Yes
                            ▼
  • Evaluate the temporal artery promptly with biopsy or CDUS
  • Urgent ophthalmologic evaluation in patients with transient
    monocular visual loss
                            │
                            ▼
          Is the temporal artery biopsy (or CDUS) positive for GCA?
           │ Yes                              │ No
           ▼                                  ▼
    Diagnosis of GCA              Is the clinical suspicion for GCA
     is established               still high in spite of a negative
                                  temporal artery biopsy or CDUS?
                                   │ Yes                │ No
                                   ▼                    ▼
     Proceed with additional testing of the temporal arteries:
       • if the initial evaluation consisted of a temporal artery
         biopsy, options include a contralateral temporal artery    Evaluate for other
         biopsy or CDUS                                             causes of symptoms
       • if the initial evaluation consisted of CDUS, then a
         temporal artery biopsy should be performed
                            │
                            ▼
        Is the additional temporal artery testing positive for GCA?
           │ Yes                              │ No
           ▼                                  ▼
    Diagnosis of GCA              Is the clinical suspicion for
     is established               GCA still high in spite of negative
                                  temporal artery testing?
                                   │ Yes                │ No
                                   ▼                    ▼
     Obtain imaging of the aorta and its
     first-order branches (eg, subclavian arteries)    Evaluate for other
     to evaluate for possible large vessel GCA         causes of symptoms
                            │
                            ▼
              Are the findings characteristic
                  of large vessel GCA?
              │ Yes               │ No
              ▼                   ▼
       Diagnosis GCA         Diagnosis
       is established        GCA unlikely
```

FIGURE 21.1 Approach to the diagnosis of giant cell arteritis.
Source: © 2019 UpToDate, Inc. and/or its affiliates. All Rights Reserved. Reproduced with permission.

Differential Diagnoses
A. Vasculitis.
B. PMR.

Plan
A. General interventions:
  1. Educate the client and family regarding the disease process of GCA.
B. Client teaching:
  1. Educate the client and family that common symptoms of GCA include headaches, vision change, and jaw/arm joint pain.
  2. Teach the client that GCA causes inflammation of the blood vessels in the head and neck, but not the blood vessels in the brain.
  3. Advise the client that PMR may also occur in some clients, in which joint pain may be present.
  4. Medications commonly used for GCA are steroids. Steroids will improve the inflammation, which in return will improve pain. The steroids are commonly used for the duration of treatment and will be tapered down over several months. Steroids are the only medication that has proven to prevent blindness. Any side effects or problems should be reported to the primary provider.
  5. A baby ASA is commonly used daily.

6. Any vision changes should be immediately reported to the primary provider. Vision loss/blindness is one of the greatest risks of GCA.
C. Pharmacological therapy:
 1. If GCA is suspected, consult with collaborating specialist and begin steroids immediately. Do not wait for biopsy results. Steroids are used to suppress the manifestations of symptoms and decrease the risk of blindness. Steroids will eventually be tapered when symptoms begin to improve, commonly after one month or so.
 2. ASA.

Follow-Up
A. Follow up with rheumatologist/surgeon as recommended.

Consultation/Referral
A. Consultation with the collaborating specialist or surgeon should be obtained regarding any client with the suspicion of having temporal arteritis.
B. Refer all clients to a rheumatologist within one week of diagnosis to manage the client with GCA.
C. All clients suspicious of having temporal arteritis should be referred to a general surgeon for a temporal artery biopsy within two to three days after beginning steroids.
D. Refer the client to the ophthalmologist for evaluation and treatment.

Individual Considerations
A. Paediatrics:
 1. Vasculitis is rare in children. It is estimated to occur in 12 to 50 per 100,000 children younger than 17 years.
B. Geriatrics:
 1. Most commonly seen in older clients. Symptoms may occur after the age of 50 years; however, GCA is most commonly seen in clients older than 70 years.

Bibliography
Docken, W. P. (2018a). Diagnosis of giant cell arteritis. *UpToDate*. Retrieved from https://www.uptodate.com/contents/diagnosis-of-giant-cell-arteritis?topicRef=8240&source=see_link
Docken, W. P. (2018b). Treatment of giant cell arteritis. *UpToDate*. Retrieved from https://www.uptodate.com/contents/treatment-of-giant-cell-arteritis
Hunder, G. G. (2014). Clinical manifestations of giant cell (temporal) arteritis. *UpToDate*. Retrieved from http://www.uptodate.com/contents/clinical-manifestations-of-giant-cell-temporal-arteritis
Seetharaman, M. (2015). Giant cell arteritis (temporal arteritis) workup. *Medscape*. Retrieved from http://emedicine.medscape.com/article/332483-workup

Vitamin D Deficiency

Jill C. Cash and Kelly Power-Kean

Definition
A. Vitamin D deficiency is defined as having a serum 25-hydroxyvitamin D (25[OH]D) level <30 nmol/L. As per the recommendations of the Institute of Medicine (IOM), vitamin D deficiency is classified as follows: deficient <25 nmol/L, insufficient 25–75 nmol/L, optimal 75–225 nmol/L, potential adverse effects >225 nmol/L, and potentially toxic >500 nmol/L. Individuals classified as deficient, or who have blood levels below 25 nmol/L, are also included in this cutoff level.

Incidence/Prevalence
A. Vitamin D deficiency is seen in all ages. It is highest in the elderly, institutionalized, and/or hospitalized clients. It is found to be more common in women than in men (83% vs. 48%), the difference most likely being less skin exposure to the sun. There is a higher incidence in the winter months, again because of less sun exposure during the winter months. It is estimated that approximately 32% of Canadians are below the deficient level. In addition, Vitamin D deficiency in mothers and their infants continues to be problematic in Canada, with Indigenous women appearing to have a higher prevalence.

Pathogenesis
A. The best source of vitamin D is direct sunlight exposure to the skin. It is also absorbed by ingesting foods that are rich in vitamin D. The liver is responsible for breaking vitamin D down. The liver hydroxylates the vitamin D to storage form, 25[OH]D, which then breaks down into the bioactive form in the kidney, 1,25-dihydroxyvitamin D (1,25[OH]2D). The 1,25(OH)2D is regulated by the parathyroid hormone and causes calcium absorption to occur in the intestine, which in return affects bone metabolism and muscle function. When any part of this cascade is interrupted, the cascade is broken and vitamin D deficiency occurs.

Predisposing Factors
A. Race (darker skin population).
B. Age: Elderly population highest risk.
C. Long-term institutionalized individuals (nursing home).
D. Obese individuals.
E. Decreased sun exposure (individuals who spend very little time outdoors in the sun). Geography is also a factor to consider. In locations in the northern hemisphere, including Canada, there are fewer ultraviolet B (UVB) photons reaching the Earth, thus predisposing the population to vitamin D absorption deficits.
F. People with serious nervous or digestive disorders (chronic kidney disease and malabsorption problems).
G. Medications: Drugs, such as phenytoin, phenobarbital, and rifampin, induce hepatic p450 enzymes and accelerate catabolism of vitamin D.

Common Findings
A. Complaints vary from none to severe.
B. Chronic muscle aches/pain/fatigue/weakness.
C. Joint pain and bone pain.

Other Signs and Symptoms
A. Fracture of bone.
B. Frequent falls and muscle weakness.
C. The most severe form of vitamin D deficiency can cause nutritional rickets.

Subjective Data
A. With clients presenting with complaints, assess onset, duration, and course of complaints.
B. Assess daily nutritional habits. Does the client get enough calcium and vitamin D in current diet?
C. Does the client live in the home or an institution? Is the client allowed to spend time outdoors in sunlight? What time of the season/year is it? Is 20 to 30 minutes in the sun without sunscreen reasonable?

D. Is the client currently taking any vitamin supplements? If so, review vitamin and ingredients in that particular vitamin.
E. Review the client history and determine if the client has a chronic condition, malabsorption condition, chronic kidney condition, or medications interfering with absorption. If there is no current diagnosis of a gastrointestinal (GI) problem, inquire regarding food intolerances, stool patterns, constipation, and diarrhea history.
F. Does the client currently take a vitamin D and/or calcium supplement?
G. Has the client had a recent vitamin D level drawn?
H. Inquire regarding the client's fatigue level.
I. Assess for muscle weakness and frequent falls, especially if a pattern of more falls in the winter months is noticed.
J. Has the client been diagnosed with osteoporosis? If so, the client needs to be screened for vitamin D deficiency.

Physical Examination
A. Check pulse and blood pressure (BP).
B. Inspect:
  1. Observe the client walk in the room and assess for stability.
  2. Observe the skin colour and overall appearance and type of skin texture.
  3. Note any deformities in the spine:
    a. Kyphosis.
    b. Bowing of the legs.
    c. Waddling of gait.
C. Palpate:
  1. Joints or areas of complained tenderness that the client presented with.
  2. The abdomen if intestinal absorption problems are suspected and workup is needed.
D. Auscultate the heart and lungs.

Diagnostic Tests
A. Serum 25(OH)D if deficiency is suspected or would affect the person's response to therapy.
B. Parathyroid hormone.
C. Calcium level.

Differential Diagnoses
A. Rickets.
B. Cystic fibrosis.
C. Malabsorption syndrome.
D. Chronic kidney disease.

Plan
A. General interventions:
  1. Educate the client regarding the importance of calcium and vitamin D for the body.
  2. Vitamin D levels should be monitored if deficiency is diagnosed. Vitamin D levels should be above 75 nmol/L.
B. Client teaching:
  1. Educate the client about vitamin D deficiency and the importance of getting vitamin D into the diet on a daily basis.
  2. Suggest eating foods that are higher in vitamin D in the diet. These foods include fish oil, cod liver, salmon, and foods fortified with vitamin D such as milk and cereals.
  3. Discuss how inadequate sun exposure can increase the risk of vitamin D deficiency. Recommend 20 to 30 minutes of sunlight during summer months without use of sunscreen, if this is not contraindicated to other chronic conditions.
  4. Foods higher in calcium should also be included in the diet on a daily basis.
  5. Health Canada recommends the daily consumption of vitamin D for both males and females: children and adults.
  6. Because of the high incidence of vitamin D deficiency and insufficiency found in Indigenous Peoples of Canada, special attention should be focused on this population.
C. Pharmacological therapy:
  1. Vitamin D:
    a. Cholecalciferol (vitamin D3) is preferred to ergocalciferol (vitamin D2) for supplementation when available.
  2. Calcium levels should be maintained.
D. For malabsorption problems, refer to a GI specialist for workup.

Follow-Up
A. Follow-up should be performed according to recommendations based on laboratory results. Initial laboratory results should be repeated in eight weeks with initial treatment. As soon as vitamin D levels are stable, repeat lab work routinely to confirm that levels remain within normal range. If levels continue to fall, refer to a specialist.

Consultation/Referral
A. Consult with or refer the client to a gastroenterologist for those who consistently have low vitamin D levels or if malabsorption problems are diagnosed.

Individual Considerations
A. Pregnancy: No contraindications for treatment during pregnancy. The same prescribing dose is safe for pregnancy and breastfeeding clients.
B. Paediatrics:
  1. The Canadian Paediatric Association recommends infants fed exclusively by breast milk should have vitamin D supplementation.
  2. Up to 1 year of age: Vitamin D2 or D3 (see CPA recommendations).
  3. Ages 1 to 18 years: Vitamin D2 (see CPA recommendations).
C. Geriatrics:
  1. Vitamin deficiencies are commonly seen in this population.
  2. All clients diagnosed with osteoporosis should be assessed for vitamin D deficiency.
  3. Clients with a serum 25(OH)D level of <10 are at risk for developing osteomalacia.

Bibliography
Angeline, M. E., Gee, A. O., Shindle, M., Warren, R. F., & Rodeo, S. A. (2013). The effects of vitamin D deficiency in athletes. *American Journal of Sports Medicine, 41*(2), 461–464. doi:10.1177/0363546513475787

Canadian Pediatric Association. (2007). Vitamin D supplementation: Recommendations for Canadian mothers and infants. *Paediatr Child Health, 12*(7), 583–589. Reaffirmed 2017

Canadian Pediatric Association. (2017). *Vitamin D supplementation: Recommendations for Canadian mothers and infants.* Retrieved from https://www.cps.ca/en/documents/position/vitamin-d

Correia, L. C., Sodré, F., Garcia, G., Sabino, M., Brito, M., Kalil, F., . . . Noya-Rabelo, M. M. (2013). Relation of severe deficiency of vitamin D to cardiovascular mortality during acute coronary syndromes. *American Journal of Cardiology, 111*(3), 324–327. doi:10.1016/j.amjcard.2012.10.006

Dawson-Hughes, B. (2014). Vitamin D deficiency in adults: Definition, clinical manifestations, and treatment. *UpToDate*. Retrieved from http://www.uptodate.com/contents/vitamin-d-deficiency-in-adults-definition-clinical-manifestations-and-treatment

Hanley, D. A., Cranney, A., Glenville, J., Whiting, S. J., Leslie, W. D., Cole, D. E. C., . . . Rosen, C. (2010). Vitamin D in adult health and disease: A review and guideline statement from Osteoporosis Canada. *Canadian Medical Association Journal, 182*, E610–E618. doi:10.1503/cmaj.080663

Statistics Canada. (2013). *Health at a glance: Vitamin D levels of Canadians*. Retrieved from https://www150.statcan.gc.ca/n1/pub/82-624-x/2013001/article/11727-eng.htm

22 Psychiatric Guidelines

Generalized Anxiety Disorder (GAD)

Moya Cook, Alyson Wolz, Lynn Miller, and Luisa Barton

Definition
Generalized anxiety disorder (GAD) is a condition, exhibited by excessive worry, tension, apprehension, and uneasiness from anticipated events or activities, that is present on most days of the week for at least six months. It is the "fight or flight" response that is part of the survival instinct. Anxiety is distinguished from fear in that fear is a response to consciously recognized external danger. The source of anxiety is largely unknown or unrecognized.

Normal anxiety allows us to get in touch with developmental learning that is part of our human growth. Anxiety in its chronic form is maladaptive and is considered a psychiatric disorder. Many cases of anxiety disorder in late life are chronic, having persisted from younger years. In its pathologic form, anxiety interferes with developmental learning because it infers significant distress.

When a client presents with anxiety, it is often comorbid with other psychiatric disorders, particularly depression. Anxiety may act as a predispositional factor to early-onset depression (before age 26 years) and to increased frequency of depressive episodes. Clients also present clinically with only anxiety, in one of its many forms, such as GAD, posttraumatic stress disorder (PTSD), obsessive-compulsive disorder (OCD), adjustment disorder with anxious mood, phobic disorders, acute anxiety, or panic disorder, with or without agoraphobia.

Incidence/Prevalence
A. There is limited research on anxiety disorders in Canada; however, statistics from 2012 suggest that 2.5% of Canadians over 15 years of age report symptoms of GAD. Anxiety is present in many medical illnesses and must be distinguished to treat it appropriately. GAD and panic disorder are associated with frequent suicide attempts.

Pathogenesis
A. Some degree of familial transmission of GAD, as well as panic disorder, has been noted. Unconscious conflict is thought to be the underlying cause of anxiety, which signals the ego to be careful expressing unacceptable impulses. Behavioural anxiety is considered a conditioned response to a stimulus associated with danger.

Clinically, however, identifying specific anxiogenic stimuli is difficult. The onset of GAD is also thought to be the cumulative effect of several stressful life events. Many studies have found that phobic/anxiety symptoms predated clinical alcoholism by a number of years. t-Aminobutyric acid–benzodiazepine receptor complex, the locus coeruleus–norepinephrine system, and serotonin are three neurotransmitter systems implicated in the biological basis of anxiety. These systems are thought to mediate "normal" anxiety and pathologic anxiety.

Predisposing Factors
A. Female; onset usually at 20 to 30 years of age.
B. Single.
C. Lower socioeconomic status.
D. A childhood anxiety disorder.
E. Excessive worrying.
F. Unresolved unconscious conflict.

Common Findings
A. Inability to control worrying.
B. Motor tension.
C. Autonomic hyperactivity vigilance.
D. Sleep disturbance.

Statements concerning self-medication with alcohol to help with sleep may indicate a coexistent alcohol misuse/dependence diagnosis that must be treated concomitantly.

E. Shortness of breath.
F. Increased heart rate and respirations.
G. Feelings of apprehension.
H. Dizziness.
I. Abdominal disturbances/nausea.
J. Increased perspiration.
K. Trembling.

Other Signs and Symptoms
A. According to the *Diagnostic and Statistical Manual of Mental Disorders, Fifth Edition* (*DSM-5*), other symptoms include excessive worry out of proportion to the likelihood or impact of the feared events that occurs for a period of six months or longer, during which the person has been bothered more days than not by these concerns.
B. At least three of the following six symptoms are present:
   1. Muscle tension.
   2. Restlessness or feeling keyed up or on edge.
   3. Easy fatigability.
   4. Difficulty concentrating or "mind going blank" because of anxiety.
   5. Trouble falling or staying asleep.
   6. Irritability.

C. If depression or bipolar disorder is present, the anxiety may be in response to fear of the following:
  1. Being embarrassed in public in the presence of a social phobia.
  2. Being contaminated in the presence of OCD.
  3. Gaining weight in the presence of anorexia nervosa.
  4. Having an illness (as in hypochondriasis or somatization disorder).
D. Impaired social or occupational function. The anxiety, worry, or physical symptoms significantly interfere with the person's normal routine or usual activities or cause marked distress.

Subjective Data
A. Review the onset, course, and duration of symptoms. How often does the anxiety occur (e.g., every day, week, month)?
B. Review any history of anxiety and age of onset. If treated, how was the previous anxiety treated and what was the success of the treatment?
C. Determine whether there is a history of suicide attempts. Does the client have a current plan or vague ideas of suicide? Ask the client, "Have you ever thought of hurting yourself or others?" If there is any concern regarding suicide/homicide, immediately refer the client to a psychiatrist.
D. Review drug history for prescription, over-the-counter (OTC) medications, and recreational/illicit drug use, and the client's use of caffeine, which precipitates anxiety symptoms.
E. Review the client's history of alcohol consumption. Mild or moderate alcohol withdrawal presents primarily with anxiety symptoms. In clients who have developed tolerance to the effects of alcohol or benzodiazepines, abrupt cessation of these agents may produce heightened anxiety over baseline, as well as a risk of seizure.
F. Review the client's history for major stressors. Are these stressors new or chronic? If chronic problems, ask what made the client come in today.
G. Determine how the client has been coping with stress up until today (e.g., exercise, medication).
H. Review the client's history of other medical problems.
I. Does anyone else in the family have the same problem? How are they treated?

Physical Examination
A. Check pulse, respirations, blood pressure, and weight.
B. Inspect: Observe general appearance. Note grooming, dress, ability to communicate, body movements, nail biting, playing with hair, inability to sit still, and so on.
C. Administer mental examination of choice:
  1. *DSM-5*, Diagnostic Criteria for GAD.
  2. Beck Anxiety Scale.
D. Physical examination as indicated by somatic complaints.

Diagnostic Tests
A. Blood alcohol level, if indicated.
B. Thyroid profile.
C. Blood glucose.
D. Medication level (e.g., theophylline) if applicable.
E. Urine drug screen.
F. Additional testing related to suspected physical pathology (e.g., drug screening).

Differential Diagnoses
A. Substance/medication-induced anxiety disorder.
B. Psychiatric syndrome:
  1. Mood disorders such as depression or bipolar disorder.
  2. Psychotic disorders.
  3. Somatoform disorders (characterized by physical complaints lacking known medical basis or demonstrable physical finding in the presence of psychological factors judged to be aetiologic or important in the initiation, exacerbation, or maintenance of the disturbance).
  4. Personality disorders.
  5. Alcoholism and drug misuse/dependence.
  6. Attention deficit hyperactivity disorder (ADHD).
C. Medical conditions. Anxiety syndromes mimic many medical illnesses, including intracranial tumours, menstrual irregularities, hyperparathyroidism and hypoparathyroidism, postconcussion syndrome, psychomotor epilepsy, and Cushing's disease:
  1. Consider hypoglycemia if anxiety is chronic.
  2. Hypothyroidism.
  3. Rapid-onset anxiety could be a symptom of hyperthyroidism.

Plan
A. General interventions:
  1. Treat medical conditions as appropriate.
  2. Refer the client for cognitive behaviour therapy (CBT). Counselling is effective for learning new techniques to help with alleviating symptoms. CBT may be effective alone or may also be used as adjunct to medication treatment.
  3. Encourage the client to perform self-calming techniques at home, such as deep breathing/relaxation techniques, meditation, and exercise.
B. Client teaching.
C. Pharmacological therapy:
  1. Selective serotonin reuptake inhibitors (SSRIs) are first-line therapies after nonpharmacological therapies (e.g., CBT):
    a. Fluoxetine: *Caution:* Long half-life; alters metabolism of cytochrome P-450 2D6-cleared agents.
    b. Paroxetine.
    c. Sertraline.
    d. Escitalopram: *Caution:* Clients with severe renal impairment are at risk for QT prolongation.
    e. Citalopram: *Caution:* Risk for QT prolongation, contraindicated in clients with congenital long QT syndrome. Check dosage if prescribed to clients also taking CYP2C19 inhibitors (e.g., cimetidine, fluconazole, and omeprazole).
    f. Fluvoxamine.
  2. Serotonin norepinephrine reuptake inhibitors (SNRIs) may also be effective for some clients.
    a. Venlafaxine.
    b. Duloxetine: *Caution:* Do not use in clients with severe renal impairment, chronic liver disease, or cirrhosis.
  3. These medications can take four to six weeks to take effect.
  4. Warn clients that they should not stop these medications abruptly; they should taper off gradually.
  5. Nonbenzodiazepine anxiolytic (buspirone): Not recommended for children younger than 18 years. Therapeutic effects delayed from one to four weeks.
  6. Short-acting benzodiazepines:
    a. Alprazolam.

b. Lorazepam:
  i. Use for initial short-term stabilization while simultaneously prescribing buspirone because therapeutic effects of buspirone are delayed from one to four weeks.
  ii. Limit use to several weeks to a few months to prevent dependence.
 7. Long-acting benzodiazepines: Clonazepam.

Follow-Up
A. Follow up in one to two weeks to assess the client's status.
B. Follow up every two to four weeks after that to check the client's progress.
C. Complete a suicide risk assessment at every office visit.

Consultation/Referral
A. Refer to a psychiatric clinician for complex medication management and psychotherapy after initial assessment.
B. If the client expresses suicidal thoughts, immediately refer to the ED (inpatient therapy) or psychiatric specialist for continuing psychotherapy.

Individual Considerations
A. Pregnancy:
 1. Caution should be used in prescribing medications for anxiety during pregnancy; the benefits must be weighed against the risks.
 2. If the client becomes pregnant while taking these medications, taper the medication dose instead of ceasing abruptly.
B. Paediatrics: Children with suspected anxiety disorders should be immediately referred to a paediatrician or psychiatrist for further evaluation.
C. Geriatrics:
 1. Anxiety is often unrecognized and inadequately treated in this population because of concomitant medical illness; overlap with cognitive disorders; and comorbid depression, ageism, and cohort effects.
 2. Start with the lowest dose of medication and increase slowly.
D. Partners:
 1. If available in the community, provide resources for partners.
 2. Psychotherapy for the client and partner is often helpful.

Bibliography
American Psychiatric Association. (2013). *Diagnostic and statistical manual of mental disorders* (5th ed.). Arlington, VA: American Psychiatric Publishing.
Dziegielewski, S. (2015). *DSM-5 in action*. Hoboken, NJ: John Wiley & Sons.
Jensen, B., & Regier, L. D. (Eds.). (2017). *RxFiles drug comparison charts*. Saskatoon Health Region, SK, Canada: Author.
Mental Health Commission of Canada. (2013). *Making the case for investing in mental health in Canada*. Retrieved from https://www.mentalhealthcommission.ca/sites/default/files/2016-06/Investing_in_Mental_Health_FINAL_Version_ENG.pdf
Pelletier, L., O'Donnell, S., McCrae, L., & Grenier, J. (2017). The burden of generalized anxiety disorder in Canada. *Health Promotion & Chronic Disease Prevention in Canada, 37*(2), 54–62. Retrieved from https://www.canada.ca/en/public-health/services/reports-publications/health-promotion-chronic-disease-prevention-canada-research-policy-practice.html
Wendell, A. D. (2013). Overview and epidemiology of substance misuse in pregnancy. *Clinical Obstetrics and Gynecology, 56*(1), 91–96. doi:10.1097/GRF.0b013e31827feeb9

Attention Deficit Disorder (ADD)/Attention Deficit Hyperactivity Disorder (ADHD)

Moya Cook, Alyson Wolz, Lynn Miller, and Luisa Barton

Definition
A. Attention deficit hyperactivity disorder (ADHD) is a syndrome that consists of a cluster of behaviours that emerge early in a child's life and persist over time. Excessively high levels of motor activity and problems with attention span, concentration, and/or impulsivity characterize ADHD. Clients with ADHD often have other psychosocial disorders, such as oppositional defiant disorder (ODD), anxiety and depression, bipolar disorder, posttraumatic stress disorder (PTSD), or Tourette's syndrome.
B. The diagnostic criteria for ADHD include symptoms of inattention and hyperactivity/impulsivity. These criteria are available at www.cdc.gov/ncbddd/adhd/diagnosis.html.

Incidence/Prevalence
A. Five to nine percent of school-aged children and teens, and 3% to 5% of adults.
B. Occurs in all races and socioeconomic groups.
C. Boys are more likely than girls to have symptoms, by a ratio of two to one.
D. Not uncommon for this disorder to persist into adulthood.
E. Approximately 33% of children with learning disabilities also have ADHD.

Pathogenesis
A. Unknown, but several studies suggest a biochemical basis involving deficits in the availability of neurotransmitters to the frontal–orbital circuits of the neurobehavioural regulatory systems of the brain. ADHD may also be inherited.
B. Associated problems with ADHD include academic, social, and emotional problems.

Predisposing Factors
A. A close relative with a mood disorder, anxiety, or ADHD.
B. Brain trauma.
C. Selective therapeutic regimens, such as intrathecal chemotherapy.
D. Recent studies have suggested a possible link to maternal smoking, alcohol misuse, or other toxins during pregnancy.
E. Some perinatal influences have been theorized to be connected to ADHD, including fetal distress, prolonged labour, prematurity, and perinatal asphyxia.

Common Findings
A. Hyperactivity, impulsivity, and/or inattentiveness.
B. Poor school performance.
C. Poor peer relationships.

Other Signs and Symptoms
A. Inattentive and easily distracted when completing tasks (e.g., daydreams, does not finish work, loses things, has difficulty concentrating).
B. Impulsive: Risk taking, impatient, very emotional.
C. Hyperactivity/overactivity: Speech and motor skills overactive.
D. Difficulty with learning, poor performance in school/work.

Subjective Data
A. Determine the presenting symptoms and ascertain when symptoms first began.
B. Note duration of symptoms:
 1. Have they been present for at least six months?
 2. Ask regarding specific behaviours as listed in the diagnostic criteria.
C. Review settings in which symptoms are present (e.g., home, school, and day care).
D. Discuss the child's past medical history.
E. Discuss the child's developmental history. Did he or she meet all of the developmental milestones?
F. Review the child's family, social, and school histories.
G. Review all current medications, including any over-the-counter (OTC) medications and herbal preparations. Specifically review medication history for theophylline, prednisone, and albuterol.
H. Review the child's diet, eating habits, and sleeping habits.
I. Review the child's routines and habits. Stimulation may come from TV, video, and computer.

Physical Examination
A. Check temperature, pulse, respirations, blood pressure, weight, and height.
B. Inspect:
 1. Observe overall appearance. Note behaviour and interactions with others.
 2. Inspect the skin, eyes, ears, nose, and throat.
C. Auscultate the heart, lungs, and abdomen.
D. Palpate the neck, thyroid, chest, and abdomen.
E. Perform neurologic examination:
 1. Hearing/vision evaluation: Evaluate constant, involuntary movement of the eyes (nystagmus).
 2. Evaluate coordination difficulties/impaired motor skills.
 3. Evaluate visual-motor control problems (hand–eye coordination).
F. Assess mental health, including assessment for anxiety and depression using age-appropriate tools.
G. Complete age-appropriate developmental assessment.

Diagnostic Tests
A. Complete blood count (CBC) with differential to rule out iron-deficiency anemia.
B. Lead level.
C. Thyroid studies to rule out other organic problems.
D. Complete age-appropriate diagnostic test for ADHD, such as the Canadian ADHD Research Alliance (CADDRA) Assessment form, available at www.caddra.ca/wp-content/uploads/CADDRA-Guidelines-4th-Edition-Feb2018.pdf.
E. Refer for psychological testing (e.g., IQ, social/emotional adjustment, presence of learning disabilities).
F. EEG may be considered.
G. MRI may be considered to rule out organic diagnoses.

Differential Diagnoses
A. ODD.
B. Autism spectrum disorder.
C. Hyperthyroidism/hypothyroidism.
D. Lead poisoning.
E. Other behavioural/psychological disorders (pervasive developmental delay, mood disorders, anxiety, or personality disorder).
F. Learning disorders.
G. Seizure disorder, nonconvulsive.
H. Impaired hearing related to chronic or recurrent otitis media.
I. Adverse reactions to medications (theophylline, prednisone, or albuterol).
J. Substance use/misuse disorder (caffeine, alcohol/drugs).

Plan
A. General interventions:
 1. A multimodal and multidisciplinary approach is imperative and includes parent education regarding the nature of ADHD. Effective behavioural management, appropriate educational placement and support, and family and/or individual therapy are strongly encouraged.
 2. Use of evidence-informed assessment tools, completed by teachers, parents, health-care providers and others who have regular contact with the client, may be helpful to guide management decisions. Examples of such tools are available at www.caddra.ca/pdfs/caddraGuidelines2011_Toolkit.pdf.
 3. The primary care provider, school nurse, school psychologist, and/or parent may function as the case manager to coordinate services.
B. Client teaching: Provide ADHD resources for parents, children, teens, and adults.
C. Pharmacological therapy:
 1. Begin with short-acting stimulants. Advance dose as needed for desired result.
 2. Consider adding a long-acting agent to a short-acting agent if needed.
 3. Long-acting agent may also be used alone.
D. First-line agents: Long-acting psychostimulants recommended, but individualization of therapy should be considered:
 1. Methylphenidate.
 2. Dextroamphetamine.
 3. Amphetamine-dextroamphetamine.
 4. Lisdexamfetamine.
E. Second-line agents: May be considered if risk of substance misuse:
 1. Nonstimulants: Atomoxetine, guanfacine XR.
 2. Short- to intermediate-acting psychostimulants.
F. Third-line agents: Consider if comorbid psychiatric diagnoses or treatment-resistant cases:
 1. Bupropion.
 2. Clonadine.
 3. Impiramine.
G. Medications:
 1. Methylphenidate hydrochloride.
 2. Lisdexamfetamine dimesylate.
 3. Atomoxetine: May take a few weeks to see the full effect. Should be taken daily at the same time every day to avoid SNRI effects.
 4. Be cautious when prescribing other medications concurrently.

Follow-Up
A. At one month: Inquire about improvements in each area of life and duration of the medication's actions.
B. Medication frequency may need to be altered.
C. Consider adding a third dose if the duration of action is very short and the child needs better afternoon or evening coverage to successfully complete homework or participate in other extracurricular activities.
D. When medication schedule is stable, subsequent visits can be every three months.

Consultation/Referral
A. Consult with the psychiatrist to help coordinate the medications.
B. Consult with psychologist if indicated for additional data.
C. Refer the client for individual and/or family therapy if indicated.

Individual Considerations
A. Paediatrics:
   1. The overall goal of ADHD therapy is to build the child's sense of competence and performance.
   2. Not all behaviour issues are ADHD. The diagnosis must be carefully and cautiously established according to the diagnostic criteria of the American Psychiatric Association (APA).
   3. Individualize medications, preparations, and timing; 80% of children respond positively to stimulants.
   4. Instituting routine drug holidays should be done with caution. It is important to occasionally stop medication to compare treated and untreated states. The child's ability to concentrate and manage behaviour at all times is critical. Not instituting drug holidays may prevent a "yo–yo" behaviour experience for the client.
   5. Use caution when medicating children with a personal or family history of Tourette's syndrome. Tics may worsen in these children.
   6. When prescribing psychostimulants to children with seizure disorders who are already on anticonvulsants, closely monitor plasma levels of both medications.
   7. Treat the child, not the parents, teachers, day-care personnel, or coaches.

B. Adults: Up to half of the affected children have some symptoms of ADHD that persist into adulthood. Adults tend to outgrow the "hyperactivity" aspect; however, they may still require treatment for the ADD. Teens and adults benefit from specific coping strategies for ADD.

Resources
CADDAC website: www.caddac.ca
CADDRA 2018 Guidelines: https://www.caddra.ca/wp-content/uploads/CADDRA-Guidelines-4th-Edition_-Feb2018.pdf
PANDA (Quebec): www.associationpanda.qc.ca

Bibliography
Almagor, D., Duncan, D., & Gignac, M. (Eds.). (2018). *Canadian ADHD practice guidelines*. Retrieved from https://www.caddra.ca/wp-content/uploads/CADDRA-Guidelines-4th-Edition_-Feb2018.pdf
Canadian ADHD Resource Alliance. (2018). *Canadian ADHD Practice Guidelines* (4th ed.). Retrieved from https://www.caddra.ca/wp-content/uploads/CADDRA-Guidelines-4th-Edition_-Feb2018.pdf
Jensen, B., & Regier, L. D. (Eds.). (2017). *RxFiles drug comparison charts*. Saskatoon Health Region, SK, Canada: Author.

Bipolar Disorder

Alyson Wolz, Lynn Miller, and Luisa Barton

Definition
A. Bipolar disorder, previously called manic-depressive disorder, is characterized by changes in moods, thoughts, and behaviours. These changes may range from mania (excessive energy, euphoria, racing thoughts, decreased need for sleep, grandiosity, pressured speech, and impulsive behaviour) to depression (low energy, sadness, diminished interest and pleasure in most activities, recurrent thoughts of death, changes in sleep patterns, cognitive impairment, and difficulty carrying out daily activities).

B. There are four types of bipolar disorder:
   1. Bipolar I disorder: Individual meets the diagnostic criteria for a manic episode, which may have been preceded or followed by a hypomanic or depressive episode.
   2. Bipolar II disorder: Individual has a pattern of depressive episodes and hypomanic episodes (no mania). Often symptoms of depression and hypomania, especially agitation, irritability, and verbal impulsivity, are displayed in the same episode (mixed).
   3. Cyclothymic disorder: A chronic pattern of hypomanic and depressive symptoms that do not meet the full criteria for hypomania or depressive episodes. Symptoms occur for at least two years (one year in children and adolescents).
   4. Unspecified bipolar and related disorder: This category applies to situations in which there are symptoms that are characteristic of bipolar disorder, but do not meet the full criteria. There may be insufficient information to make a diagnosis, or underlying medical conditions or substance use contributing to the condition.

Specific criteria for bipolar disorder as published by the APA are available at the National Institute for Mental Health website: www.nimh.nih.gov/health/topics/bipolar-disorder/index.shtml.

Incidence/Prevalence
A. One percent of adults ages 18 years or older in Canada.
B. Median age of onset is 25 years, although can range from childhood to late onset (50s).
C. Occurs in all races and socioeconomic groups.
D. Men may present with symptoms of mania earlier than women. Women are more likely to present with symptoms of depression and experience more rapid cycling.

Pathogenesis
A. No specific biological markers for bipolar disorder have been identified to date; however, studies indicate a significant genetic component as well as a potential brain structure component. Individuals with a first-degree relative with bipolar disorder are seven to 10 times more likely to develop the disorder.

Predisposing Factors
A. A family history of bipolar disorder or schizophrenia.
B. Periods of high stress.
C. Drug or alcohol misuse.
D. Major life changes, such as the death of a loved one or a traumatic experience.

Common Findings
A. Frequently seek treatment for depressive episodes.
B. Poor work or school performance; unfinished tasks.
C. Mood swings, irritability, or anger episodes.
D. Social problems.
E. Sleep disturbance.

Other Signs and Symptoms
A. Mania: Symptoms last at least one week and may include inflated self-esteem, grandiosity, decreased need for sleep, talkativeness, racing thoughts, distractibility, increased goal-directed activity, and impulsive behaviour (e.g., buying sprees, sexual indiscretions, poor business decisions). Symptoms cause marked impairment in functioning and may require hospitalization.

B. Hypomania: Symptoms last at least four days. Symptoms same as mania, but are not severe enough to cause marked impairment. Person frequently displays irritability and agitation.
C. Depression: Symptoms last for at least two weeks. Depressed mood most of the day; diminished interest in pleasure; changes in weight; sleep disturbances; restlessness or low energy; fatigue; feelings of worthlessness, guilt, and burdensomeness; cognitive changes; and thoughts of death.
D. Clients in primary care settings are more likely to present for symptoms of depression, which may look like a depressive disorder. It is important to rule out bipolar disorder before initiating treatment. Screening tool for bipolar symptoms include the following:
  1. The Mood Disorder Questionnaire, available at www.integration.samhsa.gov/images/res/MDQ.pdf.
  2. The Goldberg Bipolar Screening Quiz, available at www.ementalhealth.ca/index.php?m=survey&ID=19.
  Note: During a manic episode, individuals often do not perceive that there is anything wrong, and will often refuse treatment or become angry with those who are trying to intervene.
E. Impulse control: Client may present as extremely happy and sociable. May have rapid mood changes, such as irritability or aggression when wishes are denied, especially if using substances.
F. Suicidal or homicidal thoughts or acts. Any statements made by the client, such as "Life isn't worth living, I wish I were dead, I don't deserve to be alive, I can't deal with this," should be taken seriously. Refer the client for counselling and assessment and treatment.

Subjective Data
A. Review the onset, duration, and course of presenting symptoms.
B. Review any previous history of depression, mania, or mood disorders.
C. Determine how the previous mood disorder was treated, if applicable.
D. Evaluate the client's suicide potential. Ask: "Have you ever thought of hurting yourself or others?" Does the client have a current suicide plan or vague ideas of suicide? Has the client had any previous history of suicide attempts? If so, evaluate how life-threatening they were.
E. Review the client's medical history.
F. Review the client's drug history for prescription, over-the-counter (OTC), and recreational/illicit drug use (how much, how long, how often), and review his or her history of alcohol consumption (how much, how long, and how often).
G. Assess client's compliance with prescribed medications.
H. Review the client's history for recent major life changes, such as pregnancy, death, divorce, or any loss that may be normal throughout the stages of life. The *client's perception* of the loss is what is important.
I. Review dietary intake since the symptoms have begun.
J. Establish usual weight, review weight gain/loss, and note in what time span.
K. Review the client's activities of daily living. Does the client get up and dress daily, perform daily hygiene, put on makeup?
L. Review how many hours of sleep and quality of sleep per day.
M. Review the disruption of usual activities: return to work, return to school, exercise. Has the client been engaging in activities outside the norm?
N. Assess mood patterns, rate of cycling, seasonal changes.
O. Review the occupational/home exposure to neurodegenerative products.
P. Review any exposures to infectious diseases, including Lyme disease. Does anyone else, such as family, friends, or coworkers, have similar symptoms?
Q. If female, review for symptoms of menopause (e.g., sleep disturbances, irregular menses/amenorrhoea, hot flashes, vaginal dryness, and dyspareunia).
R. Obtain collateral information about current and past symptoms and behaviours from family and friends, if possible.

Physical Examination
A. Check pulse, respirations, blood pressure, and weight.
B. Inspect:
  1. Observe overall appearance.: Note grooming, tone of voice, eye contact, conduct of client during communication, and breath (smell of alcohol).
  2. Complete neurologic examination with screening tool of choice.
  3. Complete dermal examination for signs of substance use (refer to section "Substance Use Disorders").
C. Palpate.
  1. Palpate the neck and thyroid;: note goiter, if present.
  2. Palpate the axilla and groin for lymphadenopathy (infectious aetiology).
  3. Check the joints for swelling and arthritis and range of motion (ROM; rule out musculoskeletal cause).
D. Auscultate heart, lungs, and abdomen (as applies to physical complaints).
E. Neurologic examination: Complete the Mental State Examination (MSE), including appearance, affect/mood, thought content, perception, suicide/self-destruction, homicide/aggression, judgment/insight, and cognition.

Diagnostic Tests
A. Complete blood count (CBC) with differential to rule out iron-deficiency anemia or infection.
B. Urine/serum drug screen.
C. Thyroid studies to rule out other organic problems.
D. Glucose (fasting or random) and hemoglobin A1C to rule out diabetes.
E. Erythrocyte sedimentation rate (ESR).
F. Liver and renal panel.
G. Refer for psychological assessment to confirm diagnosis, rule out other mental health disorders, assess for social/emotional adjustment, and for the presence of learning disabilities.
H. Electrocardiogram (ECG) to assess for QT prolongation.
I. Electroencephalogram (EEG) may be considered.
J. CT scan or MRI may be considered to rule out organic diagnoses.

Differential Diagnoses
A. Substance-induced mood disorder, including caffeine, alcohol/illicit drugs.
B. Head trauma.
C. Hyperthyroidism/hypothyroidism.
D. Lead poisoning.
E. Other behavioural/psychological disorders (pervasive developmental delay, oppositional defiant disorder, seasonal affective disorder, anxiety disorder, schizoaffective disorder, schizophrenia, and personality disorder).
F. Posttraumatic stress disorder.
G. Attention deficit hyperactivity disorder (ADHD)/learning disorders (in children).

H. Seizure disorder, nonconvulsive.
I. Medical conditions (menopause, neurosyphilis, multiple sclerosis, Lyme disease, diabetes).
J. Adverse reactions to medications (theophylline, prednisone, albuterol, levaquin, and antidepressant medications [may induce mania]).

Plan
A. General interventions:
   1. Keep the client safe from self-harm.
   2. Treat physical/laboratory findings. Recommend dietary change, iron supplements, and hormone replacement therapy per findings (see related chapters).
B. Client teaching:
   1. Encourage the client to take medications as prescribed. Educate the client that some medications may take time to get into the system to work; time should be allowed to see the effects of the medication. Review side effects.
   2. Encourage the client to express feelings or worsening of symptoms if this occurs before next appointment. Have the client make a client contract with you that they will not cause harm to self or others and if the client begins having these thoughts, the client will contact you or go to the nearest ED.
   3. Encourage exercise on a daily basis for 20 to 30 minutes to increase energy and enhance a feeling of well-being.
   4. Encourage the client to get at least seven to eight hours of sleep each night. If sleep is a problem, address this issue with the client.
   5. Avoid caffeine at night and/or watching TV late at night.
   6. Encourage the client to seek counselling with a professional counsellor. Refer to the appropriate resource (e.g., psychologist, psychiatrist, and group therapy). Offer local resources to the client.
   7. Advise client to participate in activities to enhance interpersonal relationships and build self-esteem. Include family and friends in recommended therapies and advise them to encourage the client to participate in activities to enhance self-esteem.
   8. Once the client is feeling better, encourage continued use of medication, activities, and resources.

Bipolar disorder is a chronic condition requiring long-term, continuous treatment. Untreated, episodes of mania and depression may become more severe and more difficult to treat over time.

C. Pharmacological therapy:
Medication choice depends on the current episode: mania/depression. This section provides information about the medications commonly used to manage bipolar disorder. Balancing combination therapy is a complex process that requires regular monitoring; therefore, primary care providers are urged to consult with psychiatrist to guide initiation of pharmacological management as well as ongoing titration or medication changes. Refer to Canadian Network for Mood and Anxiety Treatments (CANMAT) 2018 Guidelines for specific indications, levels of evidence and combination therapy recommendations; available at www.ncbi.nlm.nih.gov/pmc/articles/PMC5947163/pdf/BDI-20-97.pdf.

1. Mood stabilizers:
   a. Divalproex sodium:
      i. Anticonvulsant and prodrug of valproic acid.
      ii. Indicated for treatment of acute mania, prevention of mania, any mood episode, and depression.
      iii. Drug–drug interactions: May increase concentrations of clonazepam, diazepam, lamotrigine, and carbamazepine.
      iv. Labs: Check valproic acid level, liver function test (LFT), and CBC after one week, then at one to two months, then every six to 12 months thereafter.
      v. Side effects include dizziness, sedation, nausea, tremor, thrombocytopenia, elevated liver enzymes, polycystic ovarian syndrome, and hepatotoxicity (rare).
      vi. Monitoring: Serum drug levels during treatment initiation; monitor weight and menstrual history every three months for the first year, then annually.
   b. Carbamazepine CR:
      i. Anticonvulsant indicated for mania and mixed episodes.
      ii. Capsules may be taken whole or opened and sprinkled on food.
      iii. Do not use with monoamine oxidase inhibitors (MAOIs) or within 14 days of using an MAOI.
      iv. Side effects include dizziness, somnolence, dry mouth, constipation, aplastic anemia, agranulocytosis, rash, toxic epidermal necrolysis (TEN), and Stevens–Johnson syndrome (SJS); clients of Asian ancestry have a 10-fold greater risk of TEN/SJS.
      v. Monitoring: Serum drug levels during treatment initiation and as clinically indicated. CBC, LFT, electrolytes, urea, creatinine monthly for three months, then annually.
   c. Lithium:
      i. Indicated for mania, prevention of mood episode, mania and depression, and maintenance.
      ii. Lithium workup before initiating the medication: ECG, urea/creatinine, urinalysis, complete metabolic panel (CMP), and thyroid-stimulating hormone (TSH).
      iii. Lithium toxicity: ausea, vomiting, diarrhea, muscular weakness, lack of coordination, giddiness, and large output of dilute urine; may involve multiple organs and organ systems.
      iv. Monitoring: Serum drug levels every three to six months once stable. Electrolytes, urea, creatinine every three to six months to exclude renal impairment. TSH, calcium, and weight after six months, then annually.
   d. Lamotrigine:
      i. Anticonvulsant indicated for maintenance therapy.
      ii. Must titrate slowly due to risk of rash/SJS.
      iii. Side effects include nausea, insomnia, somnolence, rash, leg cramps, aphasia, and SJS.
2. Atypical antipsychotics: Monitor body mass index (BMI), waist circumference, HbA1c, fasting plasma glucose, and fasting lipid panel at baseline, three months, and then annually.

[*Potential side effects for all atypical antipsychotics:*]
- *Extrapyramidal and/or withdrawal symptoms in neonates with third-trimester exposure.*
- *Lower seizure threshold.*
- *Leukopenia, neutropenia, and agranulocytosis.*
- *Metabolic changes, including hyperglycemia/diabetes, dyslipidemia, and weight gain.*
- *Orthostatic hypotension.*
- *Tardive dyskinesia.*
- *Cognitive and motor impairment.*
- *Increased risk of stroke in elderly clients with dementia-related psychosis; elderly clients with a history of cerebrovascular accidents (CVAs) treated with antipsychotic medications are at an increased risk of death.*
- *Suicidal thinking.*
- *Neuroleptic malignant syndrome: High fever, stiff muscles, confusion, sweating; changes in pulse, heart rate, and elevated blood pressure.*

a. Aripiprazole:
  i. Indicated for treatment of acute mania, mixed episodes, prevention of any mood episode and mania, and maintenance.
  ii. Side effects include akathisia (restlessness), weight gain, nausea, constipation, headache, dizziness, and stuffy nose.
b. Ziprasidone:
  i. Indicated as monotherapy for mania and mixed episodes and as an adjunct to lithium or valproate for maintenance.
  ii. Side effects include QT prolongation. Do not use in clients with recent heart failure, recent heart attack, or arrhythmias. Other more common side effects include akathisia (restlessness), sleepiness, weight gain, nausea, constipation, headache, dizziness, and stuffy nose. Less common: severe cutaneous adverse reactions (SCAR), such as SJS.
c. Risperidone:
  i. Indicated as monotherapy for mania and mixed episodes, and as an adjunct to lithium or valproate for maintenance therapy.
  ii. Side effects include dizziness, drooling, nausea, tiredness, weight gain, akathisia, tremor, blurred vision, QT prolongation, increased prolactin levels. Dose adjustment recommended for clients with severe renal or hepatic impairment. Monitor prolactin levels along with other recommended labs.
d. Asenapine:
  i. Indicated as monotherapy for mania and mixed episodes, and as an adjunct to lithium or valproate for maintenance therapy.
  ii. Side effects include orthostatic hypotension, syncope, akathisia (restlessness), weight gain, nausea, constipation, headache, dizziness, and stuffy nose. Contraindicated in clients with severe hepatic impairment.
e. Quetiapine:
  i. Indicated as monotherapy for bipolar mania, mixed, and depressive episodes, and as an adjunct to lithium or valproate for maintenance therapy.
  ii. Side effects include somnolence, dry mouth, dysarthria, increased appetite, weight gain, nausea, constipation, dizziness, stuffy nose, joint pain, QT prolongation, hypotension.
f. Olanzapine:
  i. Indicated for monotherapy for mania, mixed episodes, prevention of mania and depression, and maintenance.
  ii. Side effects include postural hypotension, akathisia (restlessness), increased appetite, weight gain, somnolence, nausea, constipation, headache, dizziness, stuffy nose, and tremors.
g. Chlorpromazine:
  i. Third-line therapy for acute for mania/mixed episode.
  ii. Drug–drug interactions: Multiple drug–drug interactions, alpha blockers, anticholinergic/antispasmodic drugs. Avoid use with other medications that may cause QT prolongation or respiratory depression.
  iii. Side effects include drowsiness, postural hypotension, akathisia (restlessness), dystonia, tremor, weight gain, nausea, constipation, headache, dizziness, stuffy nose, QT prolongation.
3. Antidepressants;
  a. Use of traditional antidepressants to treat bipolar depression is controversial.
  b. Using antidepressants alone to treat bipolar depression is not recommended due to the potential to cause hypomania, mania, and rapid cycling.
  c. According to the CANMAT guidelines, antidepressants may be used in combination with another medication, typically a mood stabilizer, when there is a history of a positive response to antidepressants or if the client relapses into a depression after an antidepressant is discontinued.
  d. Do not prescribe an antidepressant during manic or mixed episodes.

Other Therapies
Electroconvulsive therapy (ECT):
A. Evidence is limited; however, ECT has been shown to be an effective short-term treatment for severe manic or depressive episodes, especially when suicidal or psychotic symptoms are present or when medication intervention is ineffective or not well tolerated.
B. ECT is among the safest treatments for severe mood disorders and is effective in up to 75% of clients.

Follow-Up
A. Initially, monitor clients closely to assess for response to treatment, need for medication dose adjustment, side effects, and changes in level of functioning.
B. Monitor for emergence of suicidal thoughts, psychosis, mania, or depression.
C. As appropriate, order lab work to monitor serum blood levels of medications and assess for potential side effects, such as metabolic changes, elevated liver enzymes, decreased kidney functioning, cardiac changes, and blood dyscrasias.
D. After initial stabilization, follow-up appointments should be made every one to three months.
E. Client teaching related to importance of self-care and medication compliance.

Consultation/Referral

A. If the client is experiencing suicidal/homicidal ideations, refer immediately to the nearest ED to be evaluated by a mental health professional for possible emergency admission.
B. Consult with the psychiatric provider to help coordinate care.
C. Refer the client for individual and/or family therapy if indicated.

Individual Considerations

A. Pregnancy:
  1. Some of the medications used to treat bipolar disorder can potentially lower the effectiveness of hormone contraception. Women should be counselled on the use of additional methods of pregnancy prevention.
  2. Medications such as mood stabilizers cause an increased risk of birth defects in the first trimester. Women of childbearing age should be counselled on planned pregnancy to allow for medication adjustment and initiation of supportive therapy/close monitoring.
  3. Stopping bipolar medications during pregnancy puts a woman at high risk of relapse during the pregnancy and developing postpartum depression. Some bipolar medications pass through the breast milk. Risk versus benefits of medication use during pregnancy and breastfeeding should be discussed with the client and significant other, if appropriate. Refer to a psychiatric specialist for consultation.
B. Paediatrics: Bipolar disorder in children/adolescents is difficult to diagnose and does not present with the same clinical picture as adults. Children and adolescents with suspected bipolar disorder should be referred to a paediatric mental health specialist.
C. Partners/family: Provide educational materials and information on local support resources to partners and family members. The Centre for Addictions and Mental Health (CAMH) has a resource to support family members that can be found at www.camh.ca/en/your-care/planning-your-care/for-families.
D. Geriatrics:
  1. Dementia and delirium are common in the elderly. Rule out underlying medical conditions and possible medication-induced mood/cognitive changes.
  2. Caution should be used in the treatment of bipolar mania/mixed symptoms in geriatrics. Atypical antipsychotic medications increase the risk of stroke and death in elderly clients with a history of cerebrovascular accident (CVA) and dementia-related psychosis.

Bibliography

Crum, R. M., Anthony, J. C., Bassett, S. S., & Folstein, M. F. (1993). Population-based norms for the Mini-Mental State Examination by age and educational level. *Journal of the American Medical Association*, 269(18), 2386–2391. doi:10.1001/jama.1993.03500180078038
Hampton, T. (2015). *Epidemiology and pathogenesis of bipolar disorders*. Retrieved from http://www.medpagetoday.com/resource-center/bipolar-resource-center/epidemiology_pathogenesis/a/44242
Jensen, B., & Regier, L. D. (Eds.). (2017). *RxFiles drug comparison charts*. Saskatoon Health Region, SK, Canada: Author.
Mental Health Commission of Canada. (2013). *Making the case for investing in mental health in Canada*. Retrieved from https://www.mentalhealthcommission.ca/sites/default/files/2016-06/Investing_in_Mental_Health_FINAL_Version_ENG.pdf
Yatham, L. N., Kennedy, S. H., Parikh, S. V., Schaffer, A., Bond, D. J., Frey, B. N., & Berk, M. (2018). Canadian Network for Mood and Anxiety Treatments (CANMAT) and International Society for Bipolar Disorders (ISBD) 2018 guidelines for the management of clients with bipolar disorder. *Bipolar Disorders*, 20(2), 97–170. doi:10.1111/bdi.12609

Depression

Moya Cook, Alyson Wolz, Lynn Miller, and Luisa Barton

Definition

Depression is a mental health disorder that interferes with a person's daily life. Depression may be mild or severe, depending on signs and symptoms expressed, as well as the length of time symptoms are present. Depression affects multiple body systems and may impact one emotionally, cognitively, and physically, as well as one's behaviour. Symptoms of depression may include difficulty sleeping, depressed mood, inability to function at work, change in appetite, and inability to enjoy activities that bring one pleasure. There are many forms of depression, and treatment varies depending on the specific diagnosis. Types of depression include (a) major depression, single episode or recurrent (mild, moderate, or severe with or without psychotic features); (b) persistent depressive disorder (dysthymia); (c) premenstrual dysphoric disorder; (d) postpartum depression; (e) seasonal affective disorder (SAD); and (f) bipolar disorder. Depression is frequently a concomitant diagnosis with other physical or mental disorders.

Incidence/Prevalence

A. One in eight adults in Canada experiences depression at some point during their lifetime. Depression can occur at any age, but was highest in 15- to 24-year-olds in recent Statistics Canada data. Women have a two-fold higher rate of depression than men. Estimated rates of major depression in the elderly are 3% to 5% for those living in the community, with a higher risk for those with a chronic disease, acting as the primary caregiver for a spouse or family member, and living in a long-term care facility.
B. Only 10% to 25% of people with depressive disorders seek treatment. There is a high mortality from suicide if untreated (see section "Suicide," which follows).
C. No single causal factor has been identified. Depressive syndromes are so varied in course and symptomatology that a single cause is unlikely. Several factors appear to contribute, including genetics, neurochemical abnormalities (reductions in adrenergic or serotonergic neurotransmission), electrolyte disturbances, and neuroendocrine abnormalities such as hypothalamic, pituitary, adrenal cortical, thyroid, and gonadal functions. Depression is frequently a concomitant diagnosis with other physical or mental disorders. Personality and psychodynamic factors of depression include low self-esteem, self-criticism, and interpersonal loss. A childhood history of emotional, physical, and/or sexual misuse can also contribute to adult-onset depression.

Predisposing Factors

A. Age (between 25 and 32 years and the elderly).
B. Lack of social support/living alone.
C. A history of early parental loss.
D. Female gender:
  1. Most common in childbearing years, from ages 25 to 45.
  2. Premenstrual.
  3. Perimenopausal.
  4. Postpartum.
E. Family history of depression.
F. Frequent exposure to stressful events.
G. Nutritional disorders:
  1. Vitamin B12 deficiency.
  2. Pellagra (niacin deficiency).

H. Personality characteristics that include absence of resilience, flexibility, and optimism in response to stress.
I. Anger not dealt with and turned in on the self.
J. Negative interpretation of one's life experiences.
K. Poor physical health.
L. Postsurgical diagnosis of cancer.
M. Chronic pain.
N. Chronic medical problems, such as hypothyroidism and hyperthyroidism, Cushing's syndrome, hypercalcaemia, hyponatraemia, diabetes mellitus, lupus erythematosus, fibromyalgia, rheumatoid disease, and chronic fatigue syndrome.
O. Neurologic disorders, such as stroke, subdural haematoma, multiple sclerosis, brain tumour, Parkinson's disease, epilepsy, dementias, and Huntington's disease.
P. Alcoholism/drug misuse or dependence/withdrawal.
Q. Infectious aetiology, such as mononucleosis and other viral infections, syphilis, HIV, and Lyme disease.
R. Side effect of prescription drugs, such as methyldopa, antiarrhythmic, benzodiazepines, barbiturates/central nervous system (CNS) depressants, beta-blockers, cholinergic drugs, corticosteroids, digoxin, H_2-blockers, and reserpine.

Common Findings
A. Lack of interest in pleasurable activities.
B. Digestive problems.
C. Chronic aches and pains that are not otherwise explained.

Other Signs and Symptoms
A. Vegetative:
   1. Changes (increased or decreased) in sleep, appetite, and weight.
   2. Changes in appearance: poor grooming and hygiene.
   3. Poor eye contact, staring downward, flat affect.
   4. Loss of energy.
   5. Decreased interest in sex.
   6. Psychomotor retardation or agitation.
B. Cognitive:
   1. Sense of guilt, worthlessness, low self-esteem.
   2. Problems with attention span, concentration or memory; frustration tolerance,;negative distortions; mild paranoia; and psychosis.
C. Impulse control: Suicidal or homicidal thoughts or acts. Any statements made by the client, such as "Life isn't worth living, I wish I were dead, I don't deserve to be alive, I can't deal with this," should be taken seriously. Refer the client for counselling and assessment and treatment.
D. Behavioural:
   1. Depressed mood, anxiety, and irritability.
   2. Isolation, decreased motivation, fatigability, and anhedonia (unable to derive gratification from pleasurable activities).
E. Physical symptoms:
   1. Digestion problems, nausea, constipation, diarrhea (less common), and dry mouth.
   2. Fatigue, but difficulty sleeping.
   3. Physical pain, chronic aches and pains that cannot be explained.
   4. Recurrent headaches, backaches, or stomach aches that have no cause.
   5. Migrating pain that disappears when depression lifts.
   6. Increased muscle tension.

Subjective Data
A. Review the onset, duration, and course of presenting symptoms.
B. Review any previous history of depression (such as postpartum depression).
C. Determine how the previous depression was treated.
D. Evaluate the client's suicide potential. Ask: "Have you ever thought of hurting yourself or others?" Does the client have a current suicide plan or vague ideas of suicide? Has the client had any previous history of suicide attempts? If so, evaluate how life threatening they were.
E. Review the client's medical history (see section "Predisposing Factors").
F. Review the client's drug history for prescription, over-the-counter (OTC) medications, and recreational/illicit drug use (how much, how long, and how often), and review his or her history of alcohol consumption (how much, how long, how often).
G. Review the client's history for recent major life changes, such as pregnancy, death, divorce, or any loss that may be normal throughout the stages of life. The *client's perception* of the loss is what is important.
H. Review dietary intake since the symptoms have begun.
I. Establish usual weight, review weight gain/loss, and note in what time span.
J. Review the client's activities of daily living. Does the client get up and dress daily, perform daily hygiene, put on makeup?
K. Review how many hours of sleep and quality of sleep per day.
L. Review the disruption of usual activities: return to work, return to school, exercise.
M. Review the amount of crying per day, for what length of time (days and weeks).
N. Assess whether the depression is cyclic/seasonal (starts in the fall, ends in the spring).
O. Review occupational/home exposure to lead and lead-based products.
P. Review any exposures to infectious diseases, including Lyme disease (refer Chapter 16, Infectious Disease Guidelines for specific questions). Does anyone else, such as family, friends, or coworkers, have similar symptoms?
Q. If female, review for symptoms of menopause (sleep disturbances, irregular menses/amenorrhoea, hot flushes, vaginal dryness, and dyspareunia).
R. Collateral information from family or friends may be helpful.

Physical Examination
A. Check pulse, respirations, blood pressure, and weight.
B. Inspect:
   1. Observe overall appearance; note grooming, tone of voice, conduct of client during communication, and breath (smell of alcohol).
   2. Complete neurologic examination and Mini-Mental State Examination (MMSE), available for download at www.uml.edu/docs/Mini%20Mental%20State%20Exam_tcm18-169319.pdf.
   3. Complete dermal examination for signs of substance use (refer to section "Substance Use Disorders" in Chapter 2).
C. Palpate:
   1. Palpate the neck and thyroid; note the goiter.
   2. Palpate the axilla and groin for lymphadenopathy (infectious aetiology).
   3. Check the joints for swelling and arthritis and range of motion (ROM); rule out musculoskeletal cause.
D. Auscultate heart, lungs, and abdomen (as applies to physical complaints).

Diagnostic Tests
Diagnostic tests are indicated to rule out organic causes of symptoms, but should not delay initiation of treatment. Diagnostic tests should be selected based on history and physical examination findings; therefore, this list represents options to consider.
A. Complete blood count (CBC) with differential.
B. Electrolytes, serum calcium, and phosphorus.
C. Thyroid profile.
D. Liver profile.
E. Vitamin D25 hydroxy.
F. Vitamin B12/folate.
G. Lead level.
H. Follicle-stimulating hormone/luteinizing hormone (FSH/LH).
I. Viral cultures.
J. Blood alcohol.
K. Urine drug screen.
L. Monospot.
M. CT and MRI scans if indicated to rule out organic cause for symptoms.
N. Dexamethasone suppression test.
O. Perform mental state examination with depression rating scale of choice:
   1. Beck Depression Inventory Scale: beckinstitute.org/get-informed/tools-and-resources/professionals/client-assessment-tools/.
   2. Geriatric Depression Scale (GDS), short version: www.dementia-assessment.com.au/depression/geriatric_depression_scale_short.pdf.
   3. The SIG-E-CAPS tool: www.unmc.edu/media/intmed/geriatrics/reynolds/pearlcards/depression/sigecaps.htm. SIG-E-CAPS stands for: **S**leep changes, loss of **I**nterest, feelings of **G**uilt or worthlessness, lack/loss of **E**nergy, changes in **C**ognition / **C**oncentration, **A**ppetite changes, **P**sychomotor changes, thoughts of **S**uicide or death.
   4. Client-administered tests such as Patient Health Questionnaire (PHQ-9).

Differential Diagnoses
A. Mood disorder due to another medical condition.
B. Adjustment disorder with depressed mood.
C. Chronic untreated anxiety disorders such as generalized anxiety disorder (GAD), posttraumatic stress disorder (PTSD), or obsessive-compulsive disorder (OCD).
D. Personality disorders.
E. Schizoaffective disorder.
F. SAD.
G. Alcoholism and drug misuse/dependence.
H. Early dementia.
I. Endocrine aetiologies (see the section "Predisposing Factors").
J. Infectious aetiologies (see the section "Predisposing Factors").
K. Menopause.
L. Side effect of medication (see the section "Predisposing Factors").
M. Cancer: 50% of clients with tumours (particularly of the brain and lung) and carcinoma of the pancreas develop symptoms of depression before the diagnosis of tumour is made.
N. Heavy metal poisoning.
O. Nutritional deficit (see section "Predisposing Factors").

Plan
A. General interventions:
   1. Attempt to keep the client safe from self-harm.
   2. Treat physical/laboratory findings.
   3. Recommend dietary change, iron supplements, hormone replacement therapy per findings.
B. Client teaching.
   1. Encourage the client to take medications as prescribed. Educate the client that some medications may take time to get into the system to work and time should be allowed to see the effects of the medication. Review side effects.
   2. Encourage the client to express feelings or worsening of symptoms if this occurs before next appointment. Have the client make a contract with you that he or she will not harm self or others and if he or she begins having these thoughts, the client will contact you or go to the nearest ED.
   3. Encourage exercise on a daily basis for 20 to 30 minutes to increase energy and enhance a feeling of well-being.
   4. Encourage the client to get at least seven to eight hours of sleep each night. If sleep is a problem, address this issue with the client.
   5. Avoid caffeine at night and/or watching TV late at night.
   6. Encourage the client to seek counselling with a professional counsellor. Refer to appropriate site (e.g., psychologist, psychiatrist, or group therapy). Offer local resources to the client.
   7. Advise client to participate in activities to enhance interpersonal relationships and build self-esteem. Include family and friends in recommended therapies and advise them to encourage the client to participate in activities to enhance self-esteem.
   8. Once the client is feeling better, encourage continued use of medication, activities, and resources for at least six months after the client has started feeling better to prevent relapse.
C. Pharmacological therapy: Table 22.1 presents dosage information listed alphabetically.
   1. First-line treatment: Selective serotonin reuptake inhibitor (SSRI) antidepressants. Caution should be used when coadministering SSRIs with drugs that have a narrow therapeutic window, such as carbamazepine, warfarin, tricyclic antidepressants (TCAs), antiarrhythmics, and some antipsychotic medications (risperidone, haloperidol, and phenothiazine), as well as other drugs, including diazepam and monoamine oxidase (MAO) inhibitors:
      a. Most antidepressant therapy takes three to four weeks for onset of action to elicit visible changes.
      b. Never prescribe more than a week's supply or a total of 2g of a TCA if there is a risk of suicide.
      c. Medication should not be changed until a trial of six to eight weeks has been given to measure the progress.
      d. Before concluding that the antidepressant is ineffective, verify that the client is taking the medication correctly.
      e. Dosing must be adjusted in older adult clients, with first-line therapy being SSRIs, which have significantly fewer side effects than the traditional TCAs. Paroxetine and sertraline have short half-lives and can be withdrawn quickly.
      f. Taper the medication off instead of abruptly withdrawing.
D. Second-line therapies include TCAs, quetiapine, and trazadone. These agents have a higher incidence of drug interactions and side effects.

TABLE 22-? Drugs Used for Depression With Mechanism of Action

Generic Name	Mechanism
Bupropion	NDRI
Citalopram	SSRI
Desvenlafaxine	SNRI
Duloxetine	SNRI
Escitalopram	SSRI
Fluoxetine	SSRI
Fluvoxamine	SSRI
Mirtazapine	a2-Adrenergic agonist; 5-HT2 antagonist
Paroxetine	SSRI
Sertraline	SSRI
Venlafaxine	SNRI

Source: Table adapted from Jensen, B., & Regier, L. D. (Eds.). (2017). RxFiles drug comparison charts. Saskatoon, SK, Canada: Saskatoon Health Region; Kennedy, S. H., Lam, R. W., McIntyre, R. S., Tourjman, S. V., Bhat, V., Blier, P., . . . CANMAT Depression Work Group. (2016). Canadian Network for Mood and Anxiety Treatments (CANMAT) 2016 Clinical guidelines for the management of adults with major depressive disorder: Section 3. Pharmacological treatments. *The Canadian Journal of Psychiatry, 61*(9) 540–560. doi:10.1177/0706743716659417. NDRI, noradrenaline and dopamine reuptake inhibitor; SNRI, serotonin norepinephrine reuptake inhibitor; SSRI, selective serotonin reuptake inhibitor.

E. Monamine oxidase inhibitors (MAOIs) are third-line agents and should only be prescribed by or after consultation with a psychiatrist.

Follow-Up

A. Follow up in one to two weeks to assess client's status, drug effectiveness, and adverse reactions.
B. Clients can become suicidal after the depression is treated and they begin to have more energy to act on the suicidal ideation. **Assess risk of suicide at every office visit.**
C. Follow up every two to four weeks afterward to check client's progress.
D. Once positive change is seen, the client can be seen monthly.
E. Refer to other applicable medical diagnoses for the follow-up recommendations.

Consultation/Referral

A. If there is any potential for suicidal/homicidal behaviour, refer client immediately to emergency care or a psychiatrist for management.
B. Consult and/or comanage with a specialist, especially if symptoms are resistant to treatment or for concerns with recurrent suicidal ideation.
C. Clients who fail to respond to antidepressants after one to two months of appropriate antidepressant therapy should have a psychiatric consultation.

Individual Considerations

A. Pregnancy:
  1. Women with a history of depression or previous postpartum depression are at a high risk of postpartum depression (recurrent). Caution should be used in prescribing antidepressants during pregnancy. Review the benefits versus risks.
  2. Refer Chapter 13, Obstetrics Guidelines, for the section "Postpartum Depression."
B. Paediatrics: Children with depression are more difficult to diagnose and do not necessarily meet adult criteria. The clinical picture can be completely different (i.e., acting-out behaviour). Children suspected to be depressed should be referred to a child psychiatrist.
C. Adolescence:
  1. Teens are at risk for suicide after recent losses from death (especially if one of their friends/family members commits suicide) or other relationship events, such as breaking up.
  2. If a teen has had a depressive episode, he or she may be at a higher risk for suicide if he or she is suddenly happy and things are "just fine." He or she may have decided on a suicide plan and may be experiencing a sense of relief because plans have been made.
D. Partners:
  1. If available in the community, provide resources for partners and support persons.
  2. Frequently, partners will take too much responsibility for the depressed client's state of mind and, over time, also become depressed. Relating to other people with depressed partners will assist them in dealing with their significant other's depression.
E. Geriatrics:
  1. Dementia masked as "pseudodepression" is common in the elderly. Check for memory impairment and disorientation, because delirium can often be mistaken for depression.
  2. Elderly clients who are depressed may experience agitation rather than retardation in psychomotor function.
  3. Look for depression in caretakers of clients with Alzheimer's disease.

Elderly clients who are suicidal may present with atypical symptoms of depression and may not express their distress directly. Three identified behaviours are impaired ability to communicate, intractable tinnitus, and feelings of helplessness.

Bibliography

Beck, A. T., Ward, C. H., Mendelson, M., Mock, J., & Erbaugh, J. (1961). An inventory for measuring depression. *Archives of General Psychiatry, 4*(6), 561–571. doi:10.1001/archpsyc.1961.01710120031004

Crum, R. M., Anthony, J. C., Bassett, S. S., & Folstein, M. F. (1993). Population-based norms for the Mini-Mental State Examination by age and educational level. *Journal of the American Medical Association, 269*(18), 2386–2391. doi:10.1001/jama.1993.03500180078038

Guidelines and Protocols Advisory Committee. (2013). *Major depressive disorder in adults: Diagnosis and management.* Retrieved from https://www2.gov.bc.ca/gov/content/health/practitioner-professional-resources/bc-guidelines/depression-in-adults#diagnosis

Jensen, B., & Regier, L. D. (Eds.). (2017). *RxFiles drug comparison charts.* Saskatoon Health Region, SK, Canada: Author.

Kennedy, S. H., Lam, R. W., McIntyre, R. S., Tourjman, S. V., Bhat, V., Blier, P., . . . CANMAT Depression Work Group. (2016). Canadian Network for Mood and Anxiety Treatments (CANMAT) 2016 Clinical guidelines for the management of adults with major depressive disorder: Section 3. Pharmacological treatments. *The Canadian Journal of Psychiatry, 61*(9), 540–560. doi:10.1177/0706743716659417

Yesavage, J. A. (1988). Geriatric depression scale. *Psychopharmacology Bulletin, 24*(4), 709–711. Retrieved from https://medworksmedia.com/product-category/psychopharmacology-bulletin/

Failure to Thrive

Moya Cook, Alyson Wolz, Lynn Miller, and Luisa Barton

Definition
Failure to thrive (FTT) is an abnormality in growth in which an individual fails to gain or maintain weight or develop as expected for the client's age. FTT is a manifestation of an underlying problem, whether the problem be mental, physical, or psychological.

A. Children: In a growing child, measuring below the third to fifth percentile on the growth curve or exhibiting a drop greater than two percentiles on the growth curve in the past several months is referred to as FTT.
B. Adults: FTT is seen in adults who have a weight <80% of the ideal average body weight for the adult.
C. Geriatrics: FTT in the geriatric population is defined as a deterioration in functional status disproportional to their disease burden. Signs are decreased appetite, weight loss of >5% of their weight, and decreased physical activity, along with dehydration, depression, and compromised immune status.

Incidence/Prevalence
A. Incidence and prevalence data for Canada is not available; however, literature suggests that the diagnosis in children is connected to low birth weight, poverty, and other social determinants of health, while in seniors it is related to living circumstances, either living along or in a long-term care facility.

Pathogenesis
A. Organic causes for FTT:
1. Gastrointestinal (reflux, celiac disease, Hirschsprung's disease, and malabsorption).
2. Cardiopulmonary (cardiac diseases, congestive heart failure).
3. Pulmonary (asthma, bronchopulmonary dysplasia, cystic fibrosis).
4. Renal (diabetes insipidus, renal insufficiency, urinary tract infections).
5. Endocrine (hypothyroidism, adrenal diseases, parathyroid disorders, thyroid disorders, pituitary disorders).
6. Neurologic (intellectual disability, cerebral haemorrhages).
7. Metabolic disorders (inborn errors of metabolism).
8. Congenital (syndromes such as fetal alcohol syndrome, chromosomal abnormalities, perinatal infections).
9. Infectious (gastrointestinal infections, tuberculosis, HIV).

B. Inorganic (or psychosocial) causes pertain to family dynamics among the parents, siblings, and the client. It is common to see both organic and inorganic problems as causative factors for FTT.
C. Geriatric population:
1. Feel fuller with less food, which may be an endorphin response that decreases the adaptive relaxation of the fundus of the stomach.
2. Increased number of cytokines, which contributes to anorexia.
3. Diminished sense of smell or taste.
4. Dysphagia.
5. Medications.
6. Depression, delirium, dementia.
7. Alcohol or substance misuse.

Predisposing Factors
A. Children: Low birth weight, prematurity.
B. Geriatrics: Dementia, comorbidities (cancer, chronic infections, malabsorption syndromes, and psychiatric disorders), limited mobility, despair.
C. Poverty.
D. Organic conditions with the major organs (noted earlier).
E. Parents with psychosocial disorders.
F. Altered family processes.

Common Findings
A. Failure to grow and gain weight.
B. Weight loss.

Clients do not always present for this problem. Many clients are diagnosed at a routine examination in the ambulatory setting.

Other Signs and Symptoms
A. No growth in height.
B. Loss of subcutaneous fat tissue.
C. Muscle atrophy.
D. Alopecia.
E. Dermatitis.
F. Marasmus.
G. Kwashiorkor.

Subjective Data
A. Obtain detailed history of the client's diet. Note the differences between foods offered and foods eaten.
B. Assess quality of nutrients offered to the client. Consider knowledge deficit of care provider if inadequate:
1. Children: If breastfeeding, note frequency, duration, milk supply, medications, or foods that would alter breast milk. If formula is used, note type, frequency, amount taken each feeding, emesis, and so on.
2. Geriatrics: Is client able to chew and swallow food offered? Are supplements being offered?

C. Inquire about financial resources and, if needed, family participation in social support services.
D. Evaluate cultural, religious, or unusual dietary beliefs/habits that may contribute to food choices and preparation.
E. For infants and children, obtain a detailed perinatal history, noting complications with mother or baby.
F. For infants and children, determine whether the formula is being prepared correctly (e.g., powder, concentrate, ready to feed).
G. Rule out any difficulty in swallowing or retaining ingested food.
H. Note regular bowel/bladder habits.
I. Note any recent illness, chronic or acute.
J. Inquire about any recent travel and locale.
K. Query regarding lead exposure.
L. Rule out family history of cystic fibrosis or lactose intolerance.
M. Note whether a short/small stature runs in the family history.
N. Geriatrics: Evaluate nutritional screening using an appropriate tool such as the Mini Nutritional Assessment™, available at www.mna-elderly.com/forms/MNA_english.pdf.

Physical Examination

A. Check temperature, pulse, respirations, blood pressure, height, and weight:
  1. Measure head circumference in children.
  2. Calculate body mass index (BMI) or determine percentile on appropriate growth chart.
B. Inspect:
  1. Observe overall appearance.
  2. Observe oral pathology, including dentition, caries and any lesions on gums or tongue; for geriatrics, check for ill-fitting dentures, dental, and gum condition.
  3. Examine throat and neck, including posterior pharynx.
  4. Note muscle tone, strength, and movement.
  5. Note social interactions among family members.
  6. Note social skills of the client.
  7. Perform developmental assessment using appropriate tool;
     a. The Rourke Baby Record can be accessed at www.rourkebabyrecord.ca/default.
     b. The Greig Health Record, for children between 6 and 17 years of age, can be accessed at www.cps.ca/en/tools-outils/greig-health-record.

Note any changes in growth curve, especially if crossing over percentiles and if height and weight are not concordant. If premature, adjust for gestational age as appropriate. Use appropriate growth charts for ethnic (e.g., Indigenous or oriental heritage), breast versus bottle-fed babies, or specific preexisting conditions (e.g., Down syndrome). World Health Organization Growth Charts for Canada can be accessed at cpeg-gcep.net/content/who-growth-charts-canada.

C. Palpate neck, specifically thyroid; abdomen, back; and extremities.
D. Percuss the abdomen
E. Auscultate the heart and lungs

Diagnostic Tests

A. Complete blood count (CBC).
B. Urinalysis and culture, if indicated.
C. Electrolytes.
D. Thyroid panel, if indicated.
E. Lead screen.
F. Sweat test, if indicated.
G. x-Rays, CT scan, or MRI as appropriate and if indicated, looking for evidence of fractures.
H. Serum albumin.
I. Mini-Mental State Exam in older adults.
J. Purified protein derivative (PPD) skin test if tuberculosis (TB) exposure suspected.
K. HIV, rapid plasma reagin (RPR).

Differential Diagnoses

A. FTT inorganic versus organic aetiology.
B. Weight loss.
C. Depression.
D. Impaired physical function.
E. Cognitive impairment.
F. Depression.
G. Malnutrition related to malabsorption (e.g., bariatric surgery).
H. Eating disorder spectrum (e.g., anorexia nervosa and bulimia).

Plan

A. General interventions:
  1. The plan is based on the cause of FTT. Children with organic aetiologies need follow-up regarding the specific problem.
  2. Severe malnutrition requires hospitalization.
  3. Geriatrics: Obtain nutritional consult to evaluate the dietary needs for protein, iron, and other nutrients.
B. Client teaching:
  1. Reinforce positive eating habits and encourage dietary meal planning.
  2. Offer nutrition counselling with dietitian.
  3. Educate the client and family about the importance of meeting the dietary requirements for protein, iron, calcium, and other nutrients to prevent weight loss, loss of muscle and bone mass, and to prevent infection and other complications that can stress the body.
C. Dietary management:
  1. Meal suggestions: Offer adequate time for meals (20–30 minutes), offer solid food before drinks/juices, and provide a pleasant environment for eating.
  2. Encourage all family members to sit down and eat at least one meal a day together. This time will also enhance family social interactions.
  3. Provide handout for high-calorie foods (e.g., peanut butter, cheese, and whole milk).
  4. Consider exercise sessions for geriatrics to stimulate appetite.
  5. Encourage clients to attend centers where meals are served as a group, or have meals delivered to the home.
  6. Encourage small frequent meals with snacks between meals and before bedtime.
D. Pharmacological therapy:
  1. High-calorie supplements are recommended for some clients (e.g., Polycose, Pediasure, and Ensure).

Weight gain with high-calorie supplements is commonly seen with clients who have psychosocial aetiology of failure to thrive.

  2. Geriatrics: Short-term aggressive caloric replacement has been shown to be effective in reversing FTT. Severe malnutrition may require hospitalization with total parental nutrition. Medications used to increase appetite:
     a. Megestrol.
     b. Antidepressants such as selective serotonin reuptake inhibitors (SSRIs), tricyclic antidepressants (TCAs), and mirtazapine have been shown to be beneficial to help stimulate appetite and increase weight.

Follow-Up

A. Two-week evaluation for weight/height measurements and to evaluate compliance with regimen at home. Routine visits recommended every two to four weeks to monitor progress.
B. Reevaluate client in one to two months. After two months, if no improvement or further loss is noted, refer to a specialist.

Consultation/Referral

A. Consult with a specialist if height/weight measurements are noted below the third percentile on a growth chart or if crosses two percentiles on chart.

B. For the majority of clients, a nutrition consultation is needed to assist the parents or food provider in providing adequate resources/calories for the client.
C. Consider social services and home care for assistance in the home.

Individual Considerations
A. Paediatrics:
   1. The prognosis for inorganic aetiologies of children in the first year of life is ominous due to the poor brain growth. These children will be at high risk for developmental delay, poor cognitive and emotional developments, and social/emotional problems.
   2. Approximately 10% of children are normally small children by genetic makeup. These children are not diagnosed with FTT. FTT is most commonly seen in children younger than 3 to 5 years.
   3. Consider keeping small children on formula past the 12-month age mark if FTT is diagnosed.
   4. Early intervention programs should be considered for children.
B. Geriatrics:
   1. FTT in the elderly may lead to a decline in physical and mental functions. Aggressive treatment should be employed to improve the nutritional status of these clients.
   2. FTT increases the risk of morbidity and mortality.
   3. FTT increases the risk of depression and social isolation in the elderly.

Bibliography
Canadian Pediatric Endocrine Group. (2018). *WHO growth charts for Canada*. Retrieved from https://cpeg-gcep.net/content/who-growth-charts-canada

Dhekney, K., Faghih, S., & Secord, E. (2013). Fever and failure to thrive in toddler. *Contemporary Pediatrics, 30*(1), 35–40.

Greig, A. A., Constantin, E., LeBlanc, C. M. A., Riverin, B., Tak, P., & Li, S. (2016). An update to the Greig Health Record: Preventive health care visits for children and adolescents aged 6 to 17 years–Technical report. *Community Paediatrics Committee*. Retrieved from https://www.cps.ca/en/documents/position/greig-health-record-technical-report

National Initiative for Children's Healthcare Quality. (2014). *Scoring instructions for NICHQ vanderbilt assessment scales*. Retrieved from http://www.aap.org/en-us/Documents/sodbp_vanderbilt_scoringinstructions.pdf

Rourke, L. (2017). *The rourke baby record*. Retrieved from http://www.rourkebabyrecord.ca/default

Grief

Moya Cook, Alyson Wolz, Lynn Miller, and Luisa Barton

Definition
A. Grief is defined as the normal, appropriate emotional response caused by a loss. This feeling of loss is a response to a particular event in one's life. It is unique to the individual experiencing it, and there is no general timetable for completing it. Grief is commonly seen following the death of a loved one, but grief also follows other losses (e.g., loss of independence, loss of affection, loss of body parts; pain, distress). Mourning is defined as the process by which grief is resolved. Mourning is individual and helps in reaching acceptance of a loss.
B. One model used to describe the process through which one resolves grief is adapted from the Kübler-Ross Grief Cycle, which was original developed to describe stages experienced through death and dying:
   1. Denial: Denial occurs when one refuses to accept the circumstance that has occurred. It is a natural defense mechanism that occurs to protect the body.
   2. Anger: Pain, tears, anxiousness, anger, and feelings of guilt may be seen.
   3. Bargaining: In this stage, the person tries to negotiate alternatives that will make him or her feel better.
   4. Depression: One begins to understand what has happened and may show feelings of sadness and fear.
   5. Acceptance: One begins to rebuild one's life and think about the past with pleasure. In this phase, one regains interest in activities and forms new relationships.
C. It is important to distinguish between the normal grief reactions, pathologic grief, and major depression. Approximately 10% to 15% of individuals experience a severe grief reaction. Often depressive symptoms are a pervasive part of the grief response, and a clear delineation of grief versus depression is not always possible.

Incidence/Prevalence
A. Grief or bereavement is an emotional response that may follow any loss that impacts an individual's life. Incidence and prevalence rates are not available.

Pathogenesis
A. Grief is an emotional response to a loss. Abnormal, pathologic grief can occur if the mourner is not encouraged to grieve losses. Normal grief resolution begins to subside at approximately six months but may sometimes take longer.

Predisposing Factors
A. Sudden, unexpected, or traumatic deaths.
B. Excessive dependency on the deceased and feelings of ambivalence.
C. Traumatic losses earlier in life.
D. Social isolation.
E. Actual or imagined responsibility for "causing" the death.
F. Avoidance of grief and denial of loss.
G. Survived a traumatic experience that killed the deceased.

Common Findings
A. Anger at deity or medical personnel for not doing more, anger at oneself for not seeing the warning signs, anger at the deceased for not taking better care of himself or herself.
B. Anger at being left alone and not making proper financial/legal preparations may also occur.
C. Sleeping all the time or inability to sleep without medication.
D. Change in eating habits with significant weight loss or gain.
E. Fatigue, lethargy, or lack of motivation.
F. Decreased concentration and memory, forgetfulness.
G. Increased irritability.
H. Unpredictable bouts of crying.
I. Fears:
   1. Of being alone or with people.
   2. Of leaving the house.
   3. Of staying in the house.

Other Signs and Symptoms
A. Normal grief:
   1. Protest, disbelief, shock, and denial.
   2. Profound sadness and survivor guilt.
   3. Multiple somatic symptoms without actual organic disease.

4. Sense of unreality and withdrawal from others.
   5. Disruption of normal patterns of conduct, with restlessness and aimlessness.
   6. Preoccupation with memories of the deceased, dreams of the deceased, hallucinations, fear of going crazy, and transient psychotic symptoms.
B. Complicated or prolonged grief:
   1. Persistence of denial with delayed or absent grief.
   2. Depression with impaired self-esteem, suicidal thoughts, and impulses with self-destructive behaviour.
   3. Actual organic disease and medical illness.
   4. Progressive social isolation.
   5. Persistent anger and hostility, leading to paranoid reactions, especially against those involved in medical care of the deceased, or suppression of any expression of anger and hostility.
   6. Continued disruption of normal patterns of conduct, often with a persistent hyperactivity unaccompanied by a sense of loss or grieving.
   7. Continued preoccupation with memories of the deceased to the point of searching for reunion (sustained depressive delusions).
   8. Conversion symptoms similar to the symptoms of the deceased.
   9. Self-blame.
   10. Prolonged grief longer than six months is commonly linked to complications and impairment for the next one to two years.

Subjective Data
A. Review onset, duration, and course of presenting symptoms. Review the client's grief symptoms.
B. Obtain an in-depth personal history, including client's relationship to the identified loss or with the deceased.

Understanding the bereaved person's history is critical to understanding the individual's loss.

C. Identify anniversary dates pertinent to the client's relationship with the deceased/loss.
D. Determine whether the client has suicidal ideation (especially with a plan). Be sure to ask, "Have you ever thought of hurting yourself or others?"
E. Assess whether the client experiences self-blame.
F. Review the client's appetite.
G. Establish usual weight, review weight gain/loss, and in what time span.
H. Review activities of daily living. Does the client get up and dress daily and perform daily hygiene?
I. Review sleep quality.
J. Review daily routines: return to work, return to school, and exercise.
K. Review amount of crying per day, for what length of time (days and weeks).
L. Review drug (prescribed and illicit) and alcohol consumption since the loss.

Statements suggesting self-medication with alcohol to facilitate sleep could indicate a coexistent alcohol misuse-dependence diagnosis.

M. Review usual medical problems and how the loss/grief has affected these problems.

Physical Examination
A. Check temperature, pulse, respirations, blood pressure, and weight.
B. Inspect:
   1. Observe overall appearance. Note grooming habits, dress, and appearance.
   2. Note social interactions among family members.
   3. Note social skills of the client.
C. Auscultate the heart and lungs.

Diagnostic Tests
A. As indicated to rule out other pathology.
B. Blood glucose.
C. Thyroid studies.
D. If depression is suspected, complete assessment using appropriate tools. See section "Depression."

Differential Diagnoses
A. Depressive disorder.
B. Posttraumatic stress disorder (PTSD).
C. Somatoform disorders (characterized by physical complaints lacking known medical basis or demonstrable physical findings in the presence of psychological factors).
D. Alcohol use disorder.
E. Substance use disorder.

Plan
A. General interventions:
   1. Evaluate the nature of the grief and any accompanying psychiatric symptoms.
   2. Treat physical/laboratory findings as indicated.
   3. Encourage the client to eat a healthy diet, exercise daily, and maintain normal sleep habits/activities.
   4. Encourage support by family and friends.
   5. Offer counselling with professional psychologist or group sessions.
   6. Assess for depression at each office visit and treat accordingly.
B. Client teaching: *Psychology Works Fact Sheet: Grief in Adults* may be a helpful resource; at cpa.ca/docs/File/Publications/FactSheets/PsychologyWorksFactSheet_GriefIn Adults.pdf.
C. Pharmacological therapy: Antidepressants should not be prescribed for acute grief, but reserved for a possible subsequent major depression. Clinical data suggest that selective serotonin reuptake inhibitors (SSRIs) may assist the client with mobilizing the energy necessary to assist him or her through the grieving process.

Resist sedation of individuals suffering from acute grief because this tends to delay and prolong the mourning process. Refer section "Depression" for Pharmacological therapy.

   1. First-line treatment: Sedative to help sleep:
      a. Sedative anxiolytic hypnotics may be prescribed for no more than two weeks at a time. Try initially for one week to establish a sleep pattern. If insomnia continues, refer the client to a specialist:
         i. Temazepam *or* Flurazepam.
         ii. Zolpidem (not to be used for more than two weeks).
         iii. Zopiclone.

2. Sedating antihistamines_Hydroxyzine hydrochloride. Avoid use in older adults.
3. Antidepressant with sedating properties:
   a. Trazodone hydrochloride.
   b. Paroxetine.
   c. Mirtazapine.

Follow-Up
A. Follow up in one week to assess the client's status and symptoms.
B. Then follow up every two weeks to assess the client's progress.
C. Assess for depression and suicide at every office visit.
D. Once positive change is seen, the client can be seen monthly.

Consultation/Referral
A. Provide immediate referral/consult for continuing psychotherapy for severe depression and/or suicidal threats.
B. Consult with a specialist for evaluation of pharmacologic agents.

Individual Considerations
A. Pregnancy:
   1. Miscarriage, stillbirth, and neonatal death should be considered a major loss and treated as a grief reaction.
   2. Grief is also seen in pregnancy termination. The woman who terminates a pregnancy (regardless of gestational age and reason for termination) may exhibit a major response to this loss.
   3. Hospitals often provide photographs, footprints, and identification bracelets and connect families with perinatal grief support groups.
   4. Use the baby's name when discussing feelings about the loss of a child.
   5. Suggest that friends and family not put away the baby clothes and bedroom furniture. The couple should do this as part of their closure process.
B. Paediatrics:
   1. Grief in children may be delayed or difficult to identify.
   2. Children who suddenly experience behavioural problems not present before the death of a significant person should be immediately referred to a child psychiatrist.
   3. Children should not be told the deceased person is "asleep" or died because they were "sick"; this may connote fears of falling asleep and becoming sick themselves.
   4. Use proper terms: heart attack, stroke, "Your baby brother had a congenital heart defect." Use the correct terms and draw pictures to help explain.
   5. Young children do not understand death is forever and may continue to ask to see the deceased.
C. Adults: Grief responses vary from among individuals. Look for behaviours outside the norm.
D. Geriatrics: Grief in the elderly should be closely assessed to rule out medical diagnoses.
E. Partners: Involvement in grief/loss psychotherapy groups is extremely helpful.

Bibliography
Chan, D., Livingston, G., Jones, L., & Sampson, E. L. (2013). Grief reactions in dementia carers: A systematic review. *International Journal of Geriatric Psychiatry, 28*(1), 1–17. doi:10.1002/gps.3795

Jensen, B., & Regier, L. D. (Eds.). (2017). *RxFiles drug comparison charts.* Saskatoon Health Region, SK, Canada: Author.

Sleep Disorders

Moya Cook, Alyson Wolz, Lynn Miller, and Luisa Barton

Definition
Insomnia disorders are categorized as situational, persistent, or recurrent.
A. In normal sleepers, transient insomnia occurs in those who have traveled to another time zone (e.g., "jet lag"), are under situational stress, or are sleeping in unfamiliar surroundings. Treatment is not required in these situations as the problem is usually self-limiting.
B. With short-term insomnia, the normal sleeper experiences difficulty sleeping that does not resolve within a few days. This can be the result of stress, such as financial difficulty and/or divorce. These clients may require short-term symptomatic relief of insomnia.
C. Long-term insomnia is persistent and disabling. Studies suggest that 40% to 50% have an associated psychiatric disorder, most commonly depression, an associated substance use disorder, or an associated medical disorder.

Incidence/Prevalence
Difficulties with sleep are among the most common client complaints and affect a large percentage of the population. Prevalence ranges from 6% to 48% depending on the severity of symptoms, which are used to define the specific diagnostic type of insomnia. Sleep disorders are implicated in decreased work efficiency, impaired industrial productivity, and increased risk of traffic accidents, and have been suggested to enhance the propensity for cardiovascular disease and increase the risk of death. Insomniacs are also at increased risk for the development of depression and anxiety disorders. Clients with obstructive sleep apnoea (OSA) syndrome have significant performance impairments on complex motor tasks.

The risk of depression increases with time if insomnia is left untreated.

Pathogenesis
Other than situational stress, jet lag, and sleeping in unfamiliar surroundings, difficulty with sleep can be related to psychiatric illness or medical problems. It is most frequently due to chronic depression and/or anxiety. Antisocial and obsessive-compulsive features are also common among these clients. Clients may self-medicate, which produces more insomnia.

Predisposing Factors
A. Alcohol use: Initially assists with sleep but produces fragmented sleep.
B. Hypnotic medications can produce tolerance, which causes sleep disruption and rebound insomnia with withdrawal from the medication.
C. Substances such as caffeine, nicotine cigarettes, amphetamines, steroids, methylphenidate, hallucinogens, aminophylline, ephedrine, decongestants, bronchodilators, weight loss/diet pills, thyroid preparations, monoamine oxidase (MAO) inhibitors, and anticancer agents.
D. Women with fibromyalgia syndrome.
E. Women experiencing menopausal symptoms.
F. Upper respiratory symptoms.

G. OSA disorders such as nasal obstruction, large uvula, low-lying soft palate, craniofacial abnormalities, excessive pharyngeal tissue, pharyngeal masses (tumours, cysts), macroglossia, tonsillar hypertrophy, and vocal cord paralysis.
H. Obesity.
I. Hypothyroidism.
J. Acromegaly.
K. Chronic pain.
L. Urinary frequency possibly due to prostatism, diabetes, diuretics, and infection.

Common Findings
A. Statements regarding impaired sleep pattern:
  1. Inability to fall asleep.
  2. Restlessness throughout the night.
  3. Early morning awakening with inability to fall back to sleep.
  4. Difficulty concentrating during the daytime hours.
  5. Feeling fatigued after eight hours of sleep, no energy.
  6. Partner complains of the client's snoring.

Other Signs and Symptoms
A. Excessive daytime sleepiness.
B. Tension, irritability, and agitation.
C. Heightened anxiety and aggressiveness (occasionally).
D. Reports of prolonged pauses in respiration during sleep.
E. Weight gain.
F. Frontal headaches on awakening.
G. Difficulty with short-term recall.

Subjective Data
A. Review the onset, course, and duration of problems and symptoms.
B. Take a thorough history of the sleep problem, including the 24-hour sleep–wake cycle: sleep–wake habit history, sleep hygiene history, meal and exercise times, ambient noise, and light and temperature.
C. Identify the pattern: trouble falling asleep, trouble staying asleep (frequent awakenings), and early morning awakenings.
D. Inquire about life stresses, drug and alcohol use, and marital and family problems.

Statements suggesting self-medication with alcohol to facilitate sleep could indicate a coexistent alcohol use disorder. In clients who have developed tolerance to alcohol or sleep medications, abrupt cessation of these agents may produce increased insomnia and anxiety.

E. Determine whether the insomnia is simply normal sleep. Some "insomniacs" get ample sleep (pseudo-insomnia), and the problems are psychological.
F. Review the client's smoking and caffeine intake history.
G. Review all medications, including prescribed and over-the-counter (OTC), herbal preparations, recreational drug use, and weight-loss medications.
H. Review the client's medical history: thyroid pathology, hypertension, steroid use, diabetes, and cancer.
I. If possible, interview the client's bed partner to provide information about snoring, breathing pauses, and unusual body positions or movements. Is the partner concerned/frightened about the apneic pauses?
J. Review cardiopulmonary dysfunction: orthopnoea, paroxysmal nocturnal dyspnoea, or nocturnal angina.
K. If female, establish last menses to rule out pregnancy or menopause. Are there regular menses, vaginal dryness, and/or hot flashes?
L. If male, review for signs of prostatism (greater than age 50 years, hesitancy, dribbling, nocturia, frequency, incomplete emptying, etc.).

Physical Examination
A. Check pulse, respirations, blood pressure, and weight.
B. Inspect:
  1. Observe general overall appearance; note grooming and behaviours during interview.
  2. Evaluate eyes: pupil dilation/constriction (may indicate recent prescription/nonprescription drug use).
  3. Inspect nasal mucosa for erythema, oedema, discharge, and nasal patency; look for septal deviation and polyps. Transluminate sinus (if indicated).
  4. Inspect the mouth for erythema, the teeth for uneven surfaces (grinding), and the retropharynx for abnormality.
C. Auscultate heart, lungs, and abdomen.
D. Palpate:
  1. Conduct a neurologic examination.
  2. Palpate the neck and thyroid; note goiter.
  3. Check the joints for swelling, arthritis, and range of motion (ROM) to rule out musculoskeletal cause.
  4. Rectal examination if indicated for men with prostate symptoms.
  5. Perform speculum/bimanual examination if indicated to evaluate menopausal atrophy and bladder complaints.

Diagnostic Tests
A. Complete blood count (CBC) with differential.
B. Electrolytes.
C. Thyroid-stimulating hormone (TSH) or full thyroid profile,
D. Follicle-stimulating hormone (FSH), luteinizing hormone (LH).
E. Prostate-specific antigen (PSA) for men.
F. Serum creatinine and urea.
G. Urinalysis: Check for hematuria and urine culture (if indicated).
H. Glucose tolerance test.
I. Urine drug screen.
J. Sinus x-rays.
K. Urodynamic tests if bladder issues suspected.
L. Post void residual (catheterization or ultrasound).
M. Nocturnal polysomnography or actigraphy.
N. Psychiatric evaluation, if indicated.
O. Sleep studies to rule out OSA.

Differential Diagnoses
A. Insomnia/sleep disorder:
  1. Inadequate sleep hygiene: Habitual behaviours that harm sleep, such as delaying morning awakening time or napping.
  2. Insufficient sleep syndrome: Curtailing time in bed in response to social and occupational demands over long periods of time (shift work, circadian rhythm sleep–wake disorder).
  3. Adjustment sleep disorder: Acute emotional stressors (job loss or hospitalization) resulting in difficulty falling asleep because of tension and anxiety.
  4. Psychophysiologic insomnia: Anticipatory anxiety over the prospect of another night of sleeplessness and the next day of fatigue.
  5. Narcolepsy: Persistent daytime sleepiness with brief naps accompanied by vivid dreams:

a. Cataplexy or abrupt paralysis or paresis of skeletal muscles following anger, surprise, laughter, or physical exercise.
b. Hypnagogic hallucinations (vivid and often frightening dreams that occur shortly after falling asleep or on awakening).
c. Sleep paralysis, a transient global paralysis of voluntary muscles that occurs shortly after falling asleep and lasts a few seconds or minutes.
d. Disturbed and restless sleep.
B. Alcohol use disorder.
C. Substance use disorder.
D. Major depressive disorder.
E. Acute psychosis, mania, and hypomania.
F. Medical problems such as chronic pain, anxiety, depression, hyperthyroidism, epilepsy, general paresis, diabetes, benign prostatic hypertrophy, urinary problems related to age/diuretic use, cardiopulmonary dysfunction, and menopause.

Plan
A. General interventions:
1. Identify cause of insomnia.
2. Treat physical/laboratory findings if underlying condition exists. Treat condition according to diagnosis made (e.g., hormone replacement therapy, thyroid medications, diabetes) as indicated.

B. Client teaching:
1. Have the client record a two-week log for sleep–wake habits. A sleep diary is available from HealthLink BC: www.healthlinkbc.ca/sites/default/libraries/healthwise/media/pdf/hw/form_tm4434.pdf.
2. Advise the client to avoid alcohol, caffeine, and stimulating agents during the evening hours.
3. Avoid exercising before going to bed.
4. Encourage smoking reduction/cessation. Avoid smoking in the evening hours.
5. Encourage regular sleep habit/hygiene. Recommend going to bed the same time every night and waking up the same time every day.
6. Recommend keeping the bedroom cool, quiet, and dark while sleeping.
7. Encourage relaxation exercises before going to bed.
8. If stress/anxiety contributes to sleeping disorder, recommend counselling with psychologist or counsellor to identify and deal with issues.

C. Pharmacological therapy:
1. Eliminate prescription medications (when possible) and OTC products as part of your management plan *before writing another prescription.*
2. Only after making the assumption that the insomnia cannot be adequately treated by addressing the underlying medical problem responsible for causing the insomnia should medications for sleep be prescribed.

Do not prescribe medications for sleep to clients with alcohol use disorder, substance use disorder, or depressive disorders.

3. Use short-term pharmacological therapy. Restrict duration of prescription to two weeks.
4. First-line treatment: Sedative anxiolytic hypnotics: Try initially for one week to establish a sleep pattern. If insomnia continues for more than one month, refer the client to a specialist:
   a. Zopiclone.
   b. Flurazepam.
   c. Zolpidem.
   d. Temazepam.
   e. Eszopiclone.

Anxiolytic agents, such as diazepam and alprazolam, tend to increase the duration and frequency of sleep apneas and are contraindicated for clients with possible/undiagnosed apnea spells.

5. Sedating antihistamines are not recommended for use over four months: hydroxyzine hydrochloride.
6. Antidepressants with sedating properties:
   a. Trazodone hydrochloride.
   b. Paroxetine.

Follow-Up
A. Follow up for one week to assess the client's status, and then follow up every two weeks to check the client's progress.
B. Once positive change is seen, the client can be seen monthly as needed.
C. Assess the client's potential for suicide with every office visit.
D. If coexisting medication conditions exist, refer to medical diagnosis for follow-up recommendations.

Consultation/Referral
A. Refer to a psychiatrist for medication management and psychotherapy after initial assessment if psychiatric differential diagnosis is made.
B. Refer for psychological testing.
C. If insomnia continues for more than one month, refer to a specialist if the client requires a sedative anxiolytic hypnotic for more than four weeks.

Individual Considerations
A. Pregnancy: Sleep difficulties are more prevalent in second and third trimesters of pregnancy because of the growing size of the uterus and difficulty finding comfortable sleeping positions. Treat with comfort measures.
B. Paediatrics:
1. Children normally require about 10 hours of sleep.
2. Children younger than 18 years with sleep problems should be referred to a paediatrician or paediatric psychiatrist, depending on clinical findings.

C. Adults:
1. The "right" amount of sleep results in optimal daytime alertness and a sense of mental efficiency and well-being.
2. Daytime naps often interfere with the quality of night sleep. Encourage eliminating naps during the day.
3. Nocturia and disturbed sleep are the symptoms that cause older men to seek medical help with prostatism.

D. Geriatrics:
1. With aging, it is normal for sleep time to decrease (less than seven hours), with a tendency toward sleep fragmentation and an increase in the frequency of awakenings and brief arousals. Explain this to older adults to avoid "worry over sleeplessness."
2. Always assess for depression in elderly clients.
3. Start with the lowest dose of pharmacological agents.
4. Chronic pain is a leading cause for sleep disruption in elderly persons with degenerative joint pain.
5. Review elderly clients' medications, time of dosing and dosage because of known side effects or medication toxicity.

6. Gastroesophageal reflux is commonly seen in geriatric clients at nighttime and causes them to wake up at night. Correcting the reflux with sleeping position, avoiding late-night meals and spicy food, prescribing medications (proton pump inhibitors [PPIs]), and making possible weight-loss interventions could improve sleep disturbance in these clients.

7. Clients with end-stage renal disease may have nocturnal leg movement disorders and anemia due to renal failure. Improving the anemia will improve the insomnia and will decrease the leg movements.

E. Partners: Those who find it necessary to sleep in another room because of their partner's snoring should refer the snorer to the primary care provider to rule out an OSA syndrome.

Resource
Canadian Sleep Society: https://css-scs.ca/

Bibliography
Brandt, N. J., & Piechocki, J. M. (2013). Treatment of insomnia in older adults: Re-evaluating the benefits and risks of sedative hypnotic agents. *Journal of Gerontological Nursing, 39*(4), 48–54. doi:10.3928/00989134-20130220-99

Buysse, D. J. (2013). Insomnia. *Journal of the American Medical Association, 309*(7), 706–716. doi:10.1001/jama.2013.193

Canadian Sleep Society. (2018). *Healthy sleep for healthy Canadians.* Retrieved from https://css-scs.ca/

Jensen, B., & Regier, L. D. (Eds.). (2017). *RxFiles drug comparison charts.* Saskatoon Health Region, SK, Canada: Author.

Suicide

Moya Cook, Alyson Wolz, Lynn Miller, and Luisa Barton

Definition
Suicide is defined as the intentional destruction of one's own life. It is the most critical consequence of mental illness and occurs in all diagnostic psychiatric categories, therefore knowing the risk factors for suicide and eliciting key clinical features that differentiate the truly suicidal client from the attention seeker are of utmost importance. Symptoms are often missed because they can be very subtle. Because there are important legal, social, cultural, and religious implications from suicide, the general health-care practitioner should not attempt to treat these high-risk clients. This section focuses on identifying the suicidal client for immediate referral to a psychiatrist or psychiatric inpatient facility.

Incidence/Prevalence
A. Suicide accounts for 24% of all deaths in 15- to 24-year-olds and 16% in 25- to 44-year-olds.
B. Approximately 60% of Canadians who die from suicide suffered from a depressive illness.
C. Many people who attempt suicide have seen their primary care provider within four to six weeks prior to the attempt.
D. Suicide was the ninth leading cause of death in Canada in 2009 and the second leading cause of death for those between 15 and 24 years of age.
E. Canada averages 11.5 suicides per 100,000 population annually, with men having a suicide rate three times higher than women; however, women attempt suicide three to four times more frequently.

Pathogenesis
A. Recent studies confirm that some changes in the noradrenergic system along with reduced serotonin levels are associated with suicide. Research has identified a suicidality syndrome consisting of hopelessness, ruminative thinking, social withdrawal, and lack of activity as core symptoms.
B. Familial, genetic, early life-loss experiences, and comorbid alcoholism may be causal factors. In adolescence, depression is the largest single risk factor for suicidal behaviour, although family relationship difficulties make a significant independent contribution to this.
C. Environmental stressors in the presence of psychiatric disorders may also be responsible for initiating the impulsive behaviour, leading to suicide.
D. The risk of suicidal behaviours is higher in those with mental disorders than those with mood disorders.

Predisposing Factors
A. Predisposing factors for suicide are summarized in the following acronym, which is a useful screening/diagnostic tool as well.

SAD PERSONS
S = Sex.
A = Age.
D = Depression.
P = Previous attempts.
E = Ethanol misuse.
R = Rational thinking loss.
S = Social support loss.
O = Organized plan.
N = No spouse.
S = Sickness.

Also, consider gender, race and ethnicity, medications, and other medical conditions.

Common Findings
A. Overt or indirect suicide talk or threats: "You won't be bothered by me much longer."

Any mention of dying or ending one's life must be taken seriously.

B. Depressed or anxious mood due to depression.

Every depressed client must be assessed for suicide risk.

C. Significant recent loss, such as spouse, job, or self-esteem.
D. Unexpected change in behaviour, such as making a will, intense talks with friends, and giving away possessions.
E. Unexpected change in attitude, such as sudden cheerfulness, anger, or withdrawal.
F. Atypical symptoms of depression in the elderly, such as impaired ability to communicate, intractable tinnitus, and feelings of helplessness.

Other Signs and Symptoms
Indications for hospitalization of suicidal clients:
A. Psychosis.
B. Intoxication with drugs or alcohol that cannot be evaluated and treated over a period of time in the ED.

C. No change in affect or symptoms despite the intervention of the primary health-care provider, family, and friends.
D. Command hallucinations.
E. Lack of access to, or low availability of, outpatient resources.
F. Family exhaustion.
G. Escalating number of suicide attempts.
H. Uncertainty about the risk of suicide.
I. Severe psychic anxiety, anxious ruminations, and global insomnia are acute risk factors.

Subjective Data
A. Ascertain the client's intention. Ask, Why he or she wants to die? Asking the client about suicide does not give the client any ideas about suicide.
B. Determine whether the client has thought of a suicide plan. The more specific the plan, the more likely the act. A well-worked out, realistic, and potentially lethal plan suggests great risk.
C. Rule out the presence of psychiatric or organic factors such as psychotic depression, thought disorder, or sedative self-medication.
D. Determine whether the precipitating crisis is resolving satisfactorily to the client.
E. Take an "inventory of loss." Determine the losses the client has incurred in the last several months or years.
F. Review the client's plans for the future.
G. Determine whether the client thinks he or she is going to commit suicide.
H. Evaluate whether the client has a caring family or other support systems.

Physical Examination
A. Check pulse, respirations, blood pressure, and weight.
B. Inspect:
   1. Observe overall appearance; note grooming, eye contact, posture, tone of voice, conduct of client during communication.
   2. Complete dermal examination. Check for physical evidence of suicidal behaviour, such as wrist lacerations or rope burns around the neck. Look for signs of substance use.
C. Palpate:
   1. The neck and thyroid; note any goiter.
   2. The axilla and groin for lymphadenopathy (infectious aetiology).
D. Auscultate heart, lungs, and abdomen (as applies to physical complaints).
E. Neurologic examination:
   1. Complete mental status review: Specific concern exists when client displays a flat affect when discussing thoughts or plans for suicide.
   2. Assess for thought disorder: Is the client having command hallucinations telling him or her to harm or kill him- or herself? Is the client having delusions or a strong sense of "burdensomeness," thinking that others will be better off without him or her?
   3. Is the client exhibiting obsession with taking his or her own life?

Diagnostic Tests
A. Complete blood count (CBC) with differential.
B. Electrolytes, serum calcium, and phosphorus.
C. Thyroid profile.
D. Liver profile.
E. Urea, creatinine.
F. Blood alcohol.
G. Urine drug screen.
H. EKG.
I. Rapid plasma reagin (RPR).
J. CT and MRI scans if indicated to rule out organic cause.
K. Perform the Mini-Mental State Examination to rule out dementia/delirium.
L. Perform suicide assessment using an assessment tool. Examples include SAD PERSONS, IS PATH WARM, or the Suicide Behavior Questionnaire-Revised (SBQ-R) available at www.integration.samhsa.gov/images/res/SBQ.pdf.

Differential Diagnoses
A. Mood disorder due to another medical condition.
B. Adjustment disorder with depressed mood.
C. Personality disorders.
D. Psychotic disorder.
E. Alcoholism and drug misuse/dependence.
F. Dementia/delirium.
G. Side effect of medications (e.g., antidepressants and antipsychotics).

Plan
A. General interventions:
   1. If the client is suicidal, refer immediately. Make sure there is someone with the client at all times.
   2. If the client came to the office alone, call a family member or friend to accompany the client to the hospital ED or treatment center.
   3. If you are fearful, the client will try to escape or leave unaccompanied, call an ambulance to escort the client to the hospital ED where commitment papers for involuntary hospital admission can be completed.

Documentation is critical. Make sure all statements are recorded and the decision-making process followed. Be sure to advise the hospital staff of your concerns regarding the client's suicidal status.

B. Client teaching:
   1. Educate client and family regarding pharmacological treatment. Discuss benefits/risks of medication and side effects.
   2. Encourage the client to enroll in counselling with a psychologist/therapist to discuss current problems/needs.
   3. Determine whether social services may be needed for client support.
   4. Provide local resources for counselling and social services as appropriate.
   5. If the client is not hospitalized, make sure that family or friends are aware of the client's status and that he or she has someone to talk to and monitor his or her condition until the next office appointment.
C. Pharmacological therapy:
   1. See sections on "Depression" and/or "Bipolar Disorder" in this chapter for complete pharmacological interventions for specific mood disorders.
   2. Antidepressants, such as serotonin reuptake inhibitors (SSRIs), serotonin norepinephrine reuptake inhibitors (SNRIs), and antianxiety medications, can help to reduce symptoms of depression and severe anxiety, which may help the client to feel less suicidal.
   3. Clozapine is approved for reduction of suicidal behaviour in clients with schizophrenia.

4. Quetiapine and lithium have been shown to prevent suicide in clients with bipolar depression.

Follow-Up
A. After emergency admission for suicidal ideation or threats, clients should be closely observed, especially in the first year after the serious suicide attempt.
B. With each visit, question the client regarding suicidal ideation or a plan (see section "Subjective Data" for important questions to ask).

Consultation/Referral
A. Consult with the client's psychiatrist.
B. Be sure the client continues to follow up with psychiatric counselling and medication management (see section "Depression").

Individual Considerations
A. Pregnancy: A woman with a history of depression or previous postpartum depression is at high risk for postpartum depression (recurrent; see section "Postpartum Depression" in Chapter 13, Obstetrics Guidelines).
B. Adolescents.
  1. Teens are at risk after recent losses from death (especially if a friend/family member commits suicide). Recent loss includes breaking up with a boyfriend or girlfriend.
  2. If a teen has had a depressive episode, he or she may be at a higher risk if he or she suddenly seems happy and things are "just fine." The teen may have decided on a suicide plan and is experiencing a sense of relief because he or she has made plans.
C. Geriatrics.
  1. Suicide is the eighth leading cause of death in males older than 65 years.
  2. Older persons use the usual means for suicide as well as a slower plan, including not eating, stopping prescription drugs or overmedicating, increasing alcohol intake, and refusing treatment.
  3. The elderly population is more susceptible to the adverse effects of medications.
  4. Antidepressants should be started at the lowest doses and slowly increased for the elderly. The SSRIs are considered the first line of antidepressant therapy in the elderly population (see section "Depression" in this chapter).

Resource
IS PATH WARM tool: https://www2.gnb.ca/content/gnb/en/departments/health/Suicide_Prevention/content/Warning_Signs.html
SAD PERSONS tool: http://www.capefearpsych.org/documents/SADPERSONS-suiciderisk.pdf
Suicide Behavior Questionnaire-revised (SBQ-R): www.integration.samhsa.gov/images/res/SBQ.pdf

Bibliography
Government of New Brunswick. (2018). *Suicide prevention: Warning signs*. Retrieved from https://www2.gnb.ca/content/gnb/en/departments/health/Suicide_Prevention/content/Warning_Signs.html
Jensen, B., & Regier, L. D. (Eds.). (2017). *RxFiles drug comparison charts*. Saskatoon Health Region, SK, Canada: Author.
Mamo, D. C. (2007). Managing suicidality in schizophrenia. *Canadian Journal of Psychiatry, 52*(6 Suppl. 1), 59S–70S.
Navaneelan, T. (2017). *Suicide rates: An overview*. Statistics Canada. Retrieved from https://www150.statcan.gc.ca/n1/pub/82-624-x/2012001/article/11696-eng.htm
Osman, A., Bagge, C., Guitierrez, P., Konick, L., Kooper, B., & Barrios, F. (2001). The Suicidal Behaviors Questionnaire—Revised (SBQ-R): Validation with clinical and nonclinical samples. *Assessment, 8*(4), 443–454. doi:10.1177/107319110100800409. Retrieved from http://www.integration.samhsa.gov/images/res/SBQ.pdf
Patterson, W. M., Dohn, H. H., Bird, J., & Patterson, G. A. (1983). Evaluation of suicidal clients: The SAD PERSONS scale. *Psychosomatics, 24*(4), 348–349, 343–345. doi:10.1016/S0033-3182(83)73213-5
World Health Organization. (2018, August). *Suicide fact sheet*. Retrieved from http://www.who.int/mediacentre/factsheets/fs398/en

23 Assessment Guide for Sport Participation

Kimberley Lamarche

Student athletes who plan to participate in sport activities are required by most jurisdictions to have a preparticipation sports physical examination. The primary goals of this examination include (a) to ensuring that the student is safe to participate in the specified sport; (b) to assessing growth and development, evaluating the maturation and size of the athlete; (c) to identifying any congenital or new anomalies or conditions that would pose a threat of injury with activity; (d) to assessing the preparticipation condition of the athlete that would put the athlete at risk while participating in the sport; and (e) to eliminate any unnecessary barriers that would restrict the student's participation in the identified sport.

Ideally, the examination should be performed several weeks (typically six weeks) before sport activity. In the event that any conditions need to be addressed, this time frame would allow adequate time for evaluation and resolution, if possible, of the problem before participation in the sport. There is controversy regarding the frequency of these sports examinations. However, many jurisdictions address this controversy by resorting to an annual physical examination. The annual examination would suffice for each sport in which the athlete is engaged throughout the academic year.

The physical examination may be performed by the primary care provider or by attending an arranged multistation setting. These settings are frequently arranged by schools, in which multiple providers in a specialty will perform an assessment on a particular part of the body. The evaluation includes vital signs (blood pressure, pulse, respirations, height, weight, body mass index [BMI]), vision, dental and physical examination, musculoskeletal examination, nutrition, flexibility/strength, speed/agility, and balance. A lead primary care provider will then evaluate the results from each substation and determine the clearance of the athlete. In Canada, there is no official mandate or published preparticipation screening requirements. Canadian health providers make use of guidelines widely accepted worldwide. The American Academy of Pediatrics (AAP) has developed four forms to use for completing the athlete history and physical examination.

The sports physical forms are available on the AAP website at www.aap.org.
1. Preparticipation Physical Evaluation History Form.
2. Preparticipation Physical Evaluation Physical Examination Form.
3. Preparticipation Physical Evaluation Clearance Form.
4. Preparticipation Physical Evaluation of the Athlete With Special Needs: Supplemental History Form (used with permission from American Academy of Family Physicians, American Academy of Pediatrics, American College of Sports Medicine, American Medical Society for Sports Medicine, 2010).

A thorough medical history is imperative to identify potential risk factors for the athlete. A complete review of systems should be discussed with the athlete to identify possible risks. Prior personal conditions/injuries should be reviewed and assessed, such as previous head concussions. See the section "Mild Traumatic Brain Injury" in Chapter 19, Neurologic Guidelines, for assessment and treatment guidelines. The morbidity rate increases with repetitive concussions, and new guidelines are emerging regarding assessment and clearance for these athletes with a history of concussions. The Acute Care, Adolescent Health, Community Paediatrics, and Injury Prevention Committees of the Canadian Paediatric Society have all endorsed the following sport-specific concussion management guidelines:

- Parachute: www.parachutecanada.org/injury-topics/topic/C9.
- Centers for Disease Control and Prevention (U.S.): https://www.cdc.gov/headsup/providers/tools.html, www.cdc.gov/concussion/sports/index.html.
- Sport Concussion Assessment Tool 3: links.lww.com/JSM/A30.
- Child SCAT3: links.lww.com/JSM/A31.
- Concussion Recognition Tool: links.lww.com/JSM/A32.
- Ontario Government website: www.ontario.ca/concussions.
- McMaster Children's Hospital: www.canchild.ca/en/ourresearch/mild_traumatic_brain_injury_concussion_education.asp.

Dizziness or syncope episodes should be evaluated. There are many causes for these symptoms; however, cardiac conditions can present with these symptoms and an in-depth cardiac evaluation should be performed. There are conflicting recommendations on routine cardiac screening for all athletes because of the poor sensitivity, cost-effectiveness, and high false-positive rates of electrocardiograms (ECG). Recently, Canadian scholars have proposed a significantly different approach: complete the ECG and omit the physical exam. This recommendation is based on the premise that preparticipation screening is primarily to prevent sudden cardiac death (SCD). At this time, the American Medical Society for Sports Medicine (AMSSM) has published a framework to guide decision-making for providers related to ECG screening. The Canadian Academy of Sport and Exercise Medicine has endorsed the AMSSM position statement on cardiovascular preparticipation screening. Figure 23.1 provides the rationale and considerations for ECG screening.

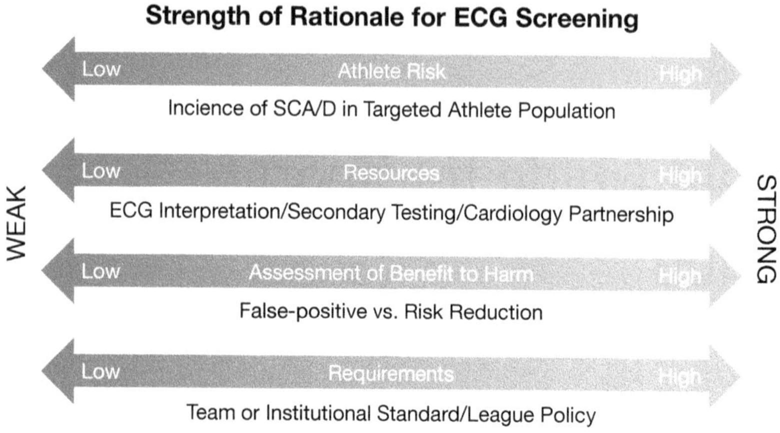

Strength of Rationale for ECG Screening

Low ← Athlete Risk → High
Incidence of SCA/D in Targeted Athlete Population

Low ← Resources → High
ECG Interpretation/Secondary Testing/Cardiology Partnership

Low ← Assessment of Benefit to Harm → High
False-positive vs. Risk Reduction

Low ← Requirements → High
Team or Institutional Standard/League Policy

WEAK ←→ STRONG

FIGURE 23.1 Major considerations and strength of rationale for ECG screening. ECG, electrocardiogram; SCA/D, sudden cardiac arrest/death.

Current work is under way to create a nationwide registry to track the factors that contribute to SCD in order to develop more accurate strategies to prevent and identify true elements specific to the Canadian population. Regardless of the choice of including an ECG or not, a thorough family history should be obtained. A family history of relevant conditions, such as exercise-related deaths or heart attacks before the age of 50 years, should be further evaluated.

Previous injuries, illnesses, fractures, or other trauma should be evaluated for complete resolution and healing. Prior history of heat illness poses a higher risk for recurrence. Prior surgery or other procedures need to be assessed to document that the athlete has been released by the surgeon and there is no risk involved with participation in the sport.

Flexibility and endurance should also be evaluated. These assessments are commonly performed by sport trainers. There are several techniques available to assess flexibility and endurance. Flexibility may be assessed by having the athlete perform range of motion of extremities and comparing the left side to the right side. A goniometer is an instrument that is useful to measure the motion of specific joints. Active and passive range of motion can be used to assess the joints. Normal degrees of range of motion of particular joints can be accessed at www.dshs.wa.gov/sites/default/files/FSA/forms/pdf/13-585a.pdf. Lower extremity range of motion can be assessed by a "sit-and-reach" test and/or with bilateral measurements using a standard goniometer. Endurance can be evaluated by having the athlete perform a timed test such as measuring the distance run in a 12-minute period.

Clearance for sport participation is determined once the history and examination are completed. There are currently two accepted classifications of participation, depending on the level of contact during participation in each sport. The athlete may be cleared for all sports without restriction or may be cleared for all sports without restriction with further evaluation or treatment for the particular condition diagnosed at the time of examination. An example of this may be an athlete with a history of well-controlled exercise-induced asthma. Clearance may be denied at the time of examination and the athlete given further recommendations. Common conditions for which the athlete may be disqualified for the clearance to participate in the sport include the following: dizziness with exercise, asthma history, musculoskeletal abnormality, heart murmur, visual impairment, elevation in blood pressure, and/or BMI outside of normal parameters.

If concerns regarding the medical history or examination are present and the athlete is unsure of clearance status, Canadian providers refer to the AAP guidelines for clearance for sports participation, which can be accessed at www.aap.org.

The time spent with the athlete during the physical examination also provides an opportunity to discuss at-risk behaviours and issues the athlete may be currently experiencing. In addition, this is an ideal time to review preventive health strategies with the athlete to help achieve optimal health and participation to the full extent of the athlete's ability. Topics to consider discussing include the following:

A. Preventive care and injury prevention: Discuss the use of proper equipment for each particular sport. Safety equipment, such as mouth guards, goggles, properly fitting head gear/helmets, and so forth, are an important aspect of the education for the athlete to prevent injury and enhance performance. Techniques of stretching, warming up, and cooling down should be encouraged before and after every practice, game, or competition. Stretching properly can prevent musculoskeletal injuries; coordination with an athletic trainer and/or physiotherapist can be beneficial as an education strategy.

B. Respiratory considerations: Use of appropriate medications for chronic conditions, such as asthma, is imperative to prevent complications. Similar to other conditions in sport, athletes with a history of asthma or exercise-induced bronchospasm should be risk stratified based on their medical history and sport requirements. Clinicians should consider the use of pulmonary function testing, standard classification of asthma tracking, and understanding of sport-related triggers. Athletes who have a previous diagnosis of asthma and present asymptomatic both at rest and during exertion can be cleared for participation. If the clinical picture is less clear, pulmonary function testing can be considered to distinguish between exercise-induced bronchospasm and undiagnosed asthma. Based on history and presentation, it is prudent to restrict athletes from participation until they are asymptomatic or stabilized to an acceptable risk level. The immediate availability of a rescue inhaler may be considered as a participation requirement for those athletes at low risk, or when returning to sport post-illness/asthma exacerbation. See Chapter 9, Respiratory Guidelines, and the section "Asthma" for assessment and treatment.

C. Substance abuse: The Canadian Centre on Substance Abuse (CCSA) has been investigating the relationship between sport and patterns of substance abuse. The group commissioned a literature review, which concluded broadly that sport participation was linked to higher alcohol use and decreased marijuana and other drug use. Clinicians should focus their efforts on education and risk screening for athletes. Using a harm reduction approach, clinicians can work with athletes to support sport as a means for substance abuse prevention. See Chapter 2, Public Health Guidelines, and the section "Substance Use Disorders" for screening questions and treatment.

D. Sport participation and mental health: Mental health challenges dominate the Canadian primary care landscape; athletes are not immune. Depression, generalized anxiety disorder, and eating disorders are common. Recognizing that athletes are at risk, there are critical times when an individual athlete typically needs additional support. Athletic progression (to the next level of sport), plateauing of performance, postinjury/illness, and pre-retirement are sensitive times when additional screening may be warranted. The Canadian Centre for Mental Health and Sport (CCMHS) tries to address these challenges, specifically that the nature of high-level sport can sometimes contribute to mental strain in elite athletes 16 years of age and older. Mental health challenges are not unique to older athletes; however, experts contend that early specialization of sport may play a role in the development of anxiety at a younger age. Whatever the age, when considering who to screen, a clinician may gain risk factor information from a general evaluation (e.g., problems with concentration, changes in appetite, loss of energy, changes in sleep pattern, and decreased interest/motivation).

Clinicians frequently use depression screenings (e.g., Patient Health Questionnaire [PHQ-9] and Beck Depression Inventory) in their primary care practice, and should make these mandatory inclusions for sport preparticipation screening. See Chapter 22, Psychiatric Guidelines, and the section "Depression" for screening questions and treatment. While conducting a screening for mental health disorders is ideal, primary health clinicians should ensure that there is also an appropriate and timely avenue for referral of athletes who screen positive. Engagement of multiple stakeholders (coaches, sport psychologists, and counsellors) will ensure that the athlete is mentally prepared to participate in or return to sport.

E. Stigma of mental illness in sport: The primary care clinician has an advocacy role to play in the reduction of stigma of mental illness in sport. Athletes may be given the message to "tough it out" and overtrain. The stigma surrounding mental illness for Canadian athletes has historically left individuals to struggle in silent suffering and isolation. The shame and stigma some athletes feel can be countered with resiliency tools, mental health resources, and self-care. Initiatives such as the Bell Let's Talk (www.letstalk.bell.ca/en/) campaign and the Student-Athlete Mental Health Initiative (SAMHI) for Canadian mental health have started to attempt to publically reverse this trend. Working with coaches, sporting regulatory bodies, and teams, clinicians can play a role in creating an environment that supports seeking help for mental health challenges and assists in effective treatment and appropriate participation. Provision of appropriate resources such as those though SAMHI found in the Huddle (www.samhi.ca/the-huddle/) ensures that the athlete is well positioned to thrive. Clinicians can advocate for the adoption of a mental health plan or charter for sport on a larger level and on an individual level by educating, advocating for, and supporting athletes in all their health and performance concerns.

F. Sport nutrition: It is the position of the Academy of Nutrition and Dietetics, Dietitians of Canada, and the American College of Sports Medicine that the performance of, and recovery from, sporting activities are enhanced by well-chosen nutrition strategies. Together, these organizations have published a joint position statementto promote optimal health and performance for athletes across a wide range of scenarios and levels of training. It is imperative to also recognize that younger athletes are at increased risk of the health effects of poor nutrition and inappropriate supplement use. Before puberty, energy requirements for both boys and girls are relatively equal; however, extra energy requirements occur with the expenditure of calories. Education from clinicians and dietitians can promote healthy development, decrease fatigue, and increase performance of prepubertal athletes. In addition to nutritional considerations, hydration is of particular concern. Assessment of hydration status and sport drink use as well as reinforcing the importance of water intake should form part of an athletic nutritional assessment. Healthy nutrition is an area of sport participation where interprofessional collaboration can greatly benefit the athlete. Community-based and specialized sport dietitians should be engaged wherever possible to participate in the nutritional plan for your athlete.

Useful resources for the clinician include the following:

- Nutrition and Athletic Performance Position Statement. https://www.dietitians.ca/Downloads/Public/noap-position-paper.aspx.
- Sport Nutrition: Coach.ca. https://www.coach.ca/sport-nutrition-s14783.
- Adult Sport Nutrition (including information for vegetarian athletes). https://www.dietitians.ca/Your-Health/Nutrition-A-Z/Sports-Nutrition-(Adult).aspx.
- Canadian Paediatric Society Practice Point: Sport Nutrition for Young Athletes. https://www.cps.ca/en/documents/position/sport-nutrition-for-young-athletes.
- Canadian Centre for Ethics in Sport: Sport Nutrition. https://cces.ca/sport-nutrition.

G. Performance-enhancing substances: The ethical use of supplements is an evolving area causing concern for health and the sporting community. In Canada, it is important to note that dietary and sport supplements are *not* classified by the Canada Food and Drugs Act. As such, they are subject to little government regulation and may contain ingredients not on the label. The use of supplements is rapidly increasing within the casual and elite sporting community. According to the Canadian Centre for Ethics in Sport, in 2012, 87% of athletes disclosed using supplements. Of that high percentage of supplement users, a few reported receiving advice on their use from a professional (4% obtained advice from a medical doctor; 0.8% were advised by a dietitian). In a 2016 Canadian study of athletes aged 11–18 years, 100% of athletes reported using dietary supplements in the preceding three months, most commonly multivitamins, sports bars, protein powders and drinks, plant extracts, and gels/gummies. Although their use is pervasive within athletic culture, medical consensus in the literature is that supplementation is generally not required. The possible exception to this would be the use of vitamin D and iron, which should be under the supervision of a prescribing clinician.

Ongoing participation at the elite level in sport may cause the athlete to require a supplement-directed "Medical Review." Clinicians need to be aware, as they may be asked to provide documents pertaining to the athlete's training plan and medications confirming that they match the information provided by the athlete. This occurs when athletes are asked to demonstrate additional information related to a banned substance being found in a doping control test. When conducting an athletic screening, specific questions about their supplement use should be incorporated. Although athletes have the ultimate responsibility for the ingestion of banned substances, clinicians can continue to counsel with the intent to minimize any potential risks of unintended doping. Their use remains controversial and athletes should be counseled appropriately.

Useful resources for the clinician include the following:

- Dietitians of Canada-Sport Supplements Get the Facts. https://www.dietitians.ca/Downloads/Factsheets/FACTSHEET-Sport-Supplements-ENG.aspx.
- Canadian Centre for Ethics in Sport – Medical Review. https://cces.ca/medicalreview.
- Facts on Sports Supplements. http://www.unlockfood.ca/en/Articles/Physical-Activity/Sports-Nutrition-Facts-on-Sports-Supplements.aspxUnlockFood.ca.

H. Female athlete triad: Female athletes have unique considerations in terms of health screening. Often described as the female athlete triad, particular attention is given to low body mass index, menstrual irregularity, and low bone mineral density. The ideal time to screen for this condition is during the preparticipation screening. Regardless of body build or sport, all female athletes should be considered at risk. Specific clinical indications can include amenorrhoea, oligomenorrhoea, disordered eating (or eating disorder present for more than six months), low energy availability, minimal trauma stress fractures, and low bone density. Clinical treatment is aimed at improving adjusting energy expenditure with energy availability, correcting nutritional deficiencies, education of stakeholders, and advocacy with stakeholders to cease risk-inducing behaviours (e.g., weight loss practices). Focus on the identification of elements contributing to the female athlete triad have been reinforced through the inclusion of screening tools. To this end, the Female Athlete Triad Coalition has developed a questionnaire used widely in collegial-level sports. Support for the mandatory and more widespread inclusion/use of this screening with female athletes has come from the American College of Obstetricians and Gynecologists, the Canadian Interuniversity Sport, and the AAP. Questions centre on worries about weight or body composition, a preoccupation with foods eaten, self-esteem, the use of diuretics or laxatives, eating in secret, menstrual patterns, and the frequency of stress fractures.

Screening tools, treatment, return-to-play guidelines, risk assessment tools, and sample treatment contracts can be accessed through the following:

- Female Athlete Triad Coalition. www.femaleathletetriad.org/important-documents/).
- Canadian Academy of Sport and Exercise Medicine Position Statement: Osteoporosis and Exercise www.casem-acmse.org/wp-content/uploads/2018/06/CASEM-Osteo-position-statement-downloaded-from-CJSM.pdf

I. Female fitness and the pelvic floor: Pelvic floor health is an often overlooked element for athletic readiness. Athletes who engage in high-impact sports involving jumping, running, and high-impact landing (e.g., track, gymnastics, basketball, and cross-country skiing), especially at the elite level, need to be screened for pelvic floor health. Downward pressure and increased intra-abdominal pressure placed on the pelvic floor of female athletes can result in pelvic floor dysfunction presenting as incontinence. Although there are specific pelvic health guidelines for postpregnancy, there are currently none for primary care providers related to sport. Providers should have an understanding of how high-level athletic performance can result in fatigue of the pelvic floor musculature. Specific screening questions related to urinary continence and bladder/bowel habits should be included in each assessment. When counselling female athletes, a frank discussion about the realities of pelvic floor dysfunction and the possible actions such as targeted physical therapy and targeted training should be included for education and prevention.

J. Return to sport/play: Identifying medical concerns during screening demonstrates how primary prevention can be applied to athletes. The principles of harm reduction and secondary prevention, however, have just as strong a role to play in having an athlete return to sport. Nonconcussive sport-specific injuries (e.g., musculoskeletal injury, fracture, and surgery) need to be evaluated by the primary care team prior to return to sport/play/school. Similar to concussion rehabilitation, athletes should be risk stratified and treatment stabilized where required. Clinicians should supervise the deliberate, progressive reentry to sport while assessing the risk of relapse. All the elements of the preparticipating screening must be reevaluated (physical and psychological objectives) and in some cases sport-specific physical capabilities confirmed. When communicating return to sport plans with stakeholders, both physical and mental health plans need to be disseminated after all data from all team members (e.g., physiotherapists, athletic trainers, surgeons, and psychologists) to enable the best chance of success, and limited risk of reinjury, for the athlete.

Bibliography

American Academy of Family Physicians, American Academy of Pediatrics, American College of Sports Medicine, American Medical Society for Sports Medicine. (2010). *Preparticipation physical evaluation* (4th ed.). Elk Grove Village, IL: American Academy of Pediatrics. Copyright © 2010 American Academy of Pediatrics. Reproduced with permission. Retrieved from https://www.aap.org/en-us/professional-resources/practice-support/Documents/Preparticipation-Physical-Exam-Form.pdf

De Souza, M. J., Nattiv, A., Joy, E., Misra, M., Williams, N. I., Mallinson, R. J., . . . Matheson, G. (2013, May). 2014 Female Athlete Triad Coalition Consensus Statement on treatment and return to play of the female athlete, triad: 1st International Conference held in San Francisco, California, May 2012 and 2nd International Conference held in Indianapolis. *British Journal of Sports Medicine, 48*(4), 289–289. doi:10.1136/bjsports-2013-093218

Dietitians of Canada, the American Dietetic Association, and the American College of Sports Medicine. (2000). Joint position statement: Nutrition and athletic performance. *Medicine & Science in Sports and Exercise, 32*(12), 2130–2145. doi:10.1097/00005768-200012000-00025

Drezner, J. A., O'Connor, F. G., Harmon, K. G., Fields, K. B., Asplund, C. A., Asif, I. M., . . . O'Roberts, W. O. (2017). AMSSM position statement on cardiovascular preparticipation screening in athletes: Current evidence, knowledge gaps, recommendations and future directions. *British Journal of Sports Medicine, 51*(3), 153–167. doi:10.1136/bjsports-2016-09678

Hergenroeder, A. C. (2016). Sports participation in children and adolescents: The preparticipation physical evaluation. *UpToDate*. Retrieved from www.uptodate.com/contents/sports-participation-in-children-and-adolescents-the-preparticipation-physical-evaluation

Lithwick, D., Fordyce, C., Morrison, B., Nazzari, H., Krikler, G., Isserow, S., . . . Taunton, J. (2016). Pre-participation screening in the young competitive athlete: International recommendations and a Canadian perspective. *British Columbia Medical Journal, 58*(3), 145–151. Retrieved from https://www.bcmj.org/

Lun, V., Erdman, K. A., Fung, T. S., & Reimer, R. A. (2012). Dietary supplementation practices in Canadian high-performance athletes. *International Journal of Sport Nutrition & Exercise Metabolism, 22*(1), 31–37. doi:10.1123/ijsnem.22.1.31

Matheson, G. O., Shultz, R., Bido, J., Mitten, M. J., Meeuwisse, W. H., & Shrier, I. (2011). Return-to-play decisions: Are they the team physician's responsibility? *Clinical Journal of Sport Medicine, 21*(1), 25–30. doi:10.1097/JSM.0b013e3182095f92

McKinney, J., Lithwick, D., Morrison, B., Nazzari, H., Luong, M., Fordyce, C., . . . Isserow, S. (2016). Detecting underlying cardiovascular disease in young competitive athletes. *Canadian Journal of Cardiology, 33*(1), 155–161. doi:10.1016/j.cjca.2016.06.007

Parnell, J. A., Wiens, K. P., & Erdman, K. A. (2016). Dietary intakes and supplement use in pre-adolescent and adolescent Canadian athletes. *Nutrients, 8*(9), 526. doi:10.3390/nu8090526

Rebullido, T. R., Chulvi-Medrano, I., Faigenbaum, A. D., & Stracciolini, A. (2019). Pelvic floor dysfunction in female athletes. *Strength & Conditioning Journal.* doi:10.1519/SSC.0000000000000440

Roberts, W. O., Löllgen, H., Matheson, G. O., Royalty, A. B., Meeuwisse, W. H., Levine, B., . . . Debruyne, A. (2014). Advancing the preparticipation physical evaluation: An ACSM and FIMS joint consensus statement. *Clinical Journal of Sport Medicine, 24*(6), 442–447. doi:10.1097/JSM.0000000000000168

Thake, J. (2015). *Surveys of sport participation and substance use among Canadian youth: An environmental scan.* Unpublished study commissioned by Canadian Centre on Substance Abuse

Trojian, T. (2016). Depression is under-recognised in the sport setting: Time for primary care sports medicine to be proactive and screen widely for depression symptoms. *British Journal of Sports Medicine, 50*(3), 137–139. doi:10.1136/bjsports-2015-095582

A Normal Laboratory Values

Normal laboratory values are presented here. However, ranges of laboratory value differ from laboratory to laboratory. They differ because of age and gender. Different values are presented; all normal values are listed under the Females column (Table A.1). Values for males are the same unless otherwise noted. Legend: $10^6 = 1{,}000{,}000$; $10^3 = 1000$.

TABLE A.1   Normal Laboratory Values

	Females	Males
Complete blood count		
RBCs	3.9–5.03×10^{12} cells/L	4.3–5.72×10^{12} cells/L
Hgb ↑ polycythaemia, dehydration, ↓ blood loss, severe anaemia, low production, or death of blood cell	120–155 g/L	135–176 g/L
Hct ↓ anaemia, massive blood loss, ↑ dehydration, or haemoconcentration with shock	0.40%–0.54%	0.37%–0.47%
MCV RBC size: normocytic, microcytic, macrocytic	80–96 fL	
MCH RBC colour: normochromic, hypochromic	27–33 pg	
MCHC	334–355 g/L or %	
Reticulocyte count: Measures the number of new RBCs produced by the bone marrow	33–137×10^9/L	
WBCs		
↑ Bacterial infections, infectious diseases (mononucleosis), ↓ stress, tissue death, leukaemia, cancer, haemorrhage	3.8–11.0×10^9/L	
Differential		
Segmented neutrophils ↑ stress, trauma, inflammatory disorders, ↓ viral infections, severe bacterial infections, aplastic anaemia	2–7×10^9/L	

(continued)

Normal Laboratory Values (continued)

	Females	Males
Band neutrophils	0–0.7 × 10^9/L	
Lymphocytes ↑ chronic bacterial infection, viral infections, ↓ leukaemia, AIDS, lupus erythematosus	1–4 × 10^9/L	
Monocytes ↑ chronic inflammatory disorders, viral infections, chronic conditions, ↓ steroid therapy	300–500 × 10^6/L	
Eosinophils ↑ allergies, parasite infections, leukaemia	0.1–1.0 × 10^9/L	
Basophils ↑ leukaemia ↓ allergic reactions, stress, hyperthyroidism	0.1 × 10^9/L	
Serum iron concentration of iron bound to transferrin	11–29 μmol/L	14–33 μmol/L
TIBC amount of iron transferrin can bind	45–82 μmol/L	
ESR	Women <50	Males <50
↑ Pregnancy, inflammatory conditions, ↓ sickle cell anaemia	<20 mm/hr women >50 <30 mm/hr	<15 mm/hr males >50 <20 mm/hr
Electrolytes		
Calcium	2.2–2.6 mmol/L	
Chloride	95–107 mmol/L	
Magnesium	0.75–0.95 mmol/L	
Phosphate	0.8–1.5 mmol/L	
Potassium	3.5–5.2 mmol/L	
Sodium	135–147 mmol/L	
Urea/Creatinine-renal function tests		
Urea >20 years old	2.5–10.7 mmol/L	0.07–0.21 mmol/L
Creatine	<99.1 μmol/L	
Uric acid	149–446 μmol/L	238–505 μmol/L
Creatinine by age and gender • 20–49 years • 50–59 years • 60–69 years • 70–79 years • >80 years	44.2–97.2 μmol/L 44.2–92.8 μmol/L 44.2–87.5 μmol/L 53–82.2 μmol/L 53–77.8 μmol/L	53–119.3 μmol/L 61.9–117.6 μmol/L 61.9–110.5 μmol/L 61.9–104.3 μmol/L 61.9–100.8 μmol/L
Thyroid studies		
TSH	0.4–4.2 mU/L	
↑ Hypothyroidism, ↓ hyperthyroidism	0.16–0.2 mU/L	
T3 ↑ pregnancy and oral contraceptive use	0.9–2.8 nmol/L (total) 2.0–7.0 pmol/L (free)	

(continued)

Normal Laboratory Values (continued)

	Females	Males
Thyroxine (T4) ↑ hyperthyroidism, ↓ hypothyroidism	71–160 nmol/L (total) 12–30 pmol/L (free)	
Aminotransferases		
ALT	6–18 U/L	7–21 U/L
AST	18–40 U/L	
Bilirubin (measures bile salt conjugation and excretion)		
Direct bilirubin	0.0–3.4 μmol/L	
Indirect bilirubin	Total bilirubin minus direct bilirubin	
Total bilirubin >20 years	1.7–22.2 μmol/L; 51.3 μmol/L indicates hepatic disease, jaundice is visible	

Glucose
 Fasting 3.6–5.6 mmol/L
 2-hour postprandial 3.6–7.8 mmol/L

Serum albumin (measures protein synthesis)
 32–50 g/L
 ↑ Dehydration, inflammatory illness, liver insufficiency, malnutrition, and cancer

Lipid profile—adults
 Fasting cholesterol: <5.2 mmol/L indicates low risk for CHD
 5.2–6.2 mmol/L: Borderline risk for CHD
 >6.2 mmol/L: High risk for CHD
 Triglycerides
 <1.6 mmol/L: Low risk for CHD
 1.7–2.25 mmol/L: Borderline risk for CHD
 >2.26 mmol/L: High risk for CHD
 >5.65 mmol/L: Very high risk for CHD
 HDL: Females >1.3 mmol/L; Males >0.1 mmol/L desirable levels higher than 1.6 mmol/L

 LDL: <2.6 mmol/L is optimal
 1.6–4.1 mmol/L: Borderline CHD
 >4.1 mmol/L: High risk for CHD
 >4.9 mmol/L: Very high risk for CHD

Lipid profile—paediatrics
 Triglycerides
 Ages 0–9 years: <0.85 mmol/L; ages 10–19 years: <1.02 mmol/L
 Ages 0–9 years: 0.85–1.12 mmol/L; ages 10–19 years: 1.02–1.46 mmol/L borderline risk for CHD
 Ages 0–9 years: >1.13 mmol/L; ages 10–19 years: >1.47 mmol/L high risk for CHD
 HDL: >1.17 mmol/L
 1.03–1.17 mmol/L: Borderline risk for CHD
 <1.03 mmol/L: High risk for CHD
 LDL: <2.85 mmol/L
 2.85–3.34 mmol/L: Borderline risk for CHD
 >3.37 mmol/L: High risk for CHD

(continued)

Normal Laboratory Values (continued)

	Females	Males
Coagulation PT : 9–12.5 seconds PTT : 20–36 seconds Fibrinogen: 1.6–4.5 g/L Bleeding time: 3–7 minutes Thrombin time: 11–15 seconds Platelets: 140–450 × 10^9/L ↓ Thrombocytopaenia, acute leukaemia/aplastic anaemia during chemotherapy, interferon, infections, and drug reactions ↑ Myeloproliferative disease, cancer, and RA **Sickle cell disease** HgbS: Normal, none present Homozygous HgbS: Sickle cell disease Heterozygous HgbS: Sickle cell trait Haemoglobin electrophoresis: Determines haemoglobin types and percentages **Hepatitis B** Hepatitis B surface antigen: Negative Positive: Acute or chronic infection, further liver function tests needed Hepatitis B surface antibody: Positive indicates immunity to infection (previous infection or hepatitis B vaccine) **Serum ALP (marks liver disease)** 40–120 U/L Pregnancy value 30–200 U/L ↑ Bile stones, biliary and pancreatic cancer, viral hepatitis, cirrhosis, Paget's disease, osteomalacia, bone metastasis **D-Dimer** <1.37 nmol/L objective evidence of increased fibrinolysis/evidence of intravascular coagulation and thrombotic disease. Routine first-line assessment of patients with a suspected VTE, which can be present as a DVT or PE **Urinalysis** Colour: Pale yellow/straw to amber Clarity: Clear Specific gravity: 1.001–1.035 pH: Normal 4.6–8.0 (acidic) Glucose: Absent Ketones: Absent Protein: Negative **Urine dipstick U/A** Nitrites: Negative (positive = bacteria, infection) Leukocytes oxidase: Negative (positive = WBCs) **Arterial blood gas values** pH: 7.35–7.45 $PaCO_2$: 35–45 mmHg (4.7–5.9 kPa) HCO_3: 22–26 mmol/L O_2 saturation: 94%–100% PaO_2: 80–100 mmHg (11–13 kPa) BE: −2 to +2 mmol/L **Venous blood gas values** pH: 7.32–7.42 $PaCO_2$: 38–52 mmHg (5.1–6.9 kPa) HCO_3: 19–25 mmol/L O_2 saturation: 40%–70% PaO_2: 28–48 mmHg (3.7–6.4 kPa) BE: 0 to +4 mmol/L		
HIV ELISA: Negative ELISA: Positive: Repeat; if second ELISA positive, perform Western blot Western blot negative: No evidence of HIV Western blot positive: Evidence of HIV **Rubella** Titre: >1:10 immune Titre: <1:7 nonimmune administer rubella vaccine		

(continued)

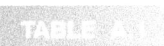

Normal Laboratory Values (*continued*)

	Females	Males		
Female hormone levels				
	FSH	LH	Progesterone	Prolactin
Follicular phases	2–25 U/L	5–30 U/L	0.2–6.0 U/L	<23 mg/L
Midcycle phase	10–90 U/L	75–150 U/L	6–30 U/L	<28 mg/L
Luteal phase	2–25 U/L	3–40 U/L	5.7–28.1 U/L	5–40 mg/L
Postmenopausal	40–350 U/L	30–200 U/L	0–0.2 U/L	<12 mg/L

ALP, alkaline phosphatase; ALT, alanine transaminase; AST, aspartate aminotransferase; BE, base excess; CHD, coronary heart disease; DVT, deep vein thrombosis; ELISA, enzyme-linked immunosorbent assay; ESR, erythrocyte sedimentation rate; FSH, follicle-stimulating hormone; Hct, haematocrit; HDL, high-density lipoprotein; Hgb, haemoglobin; HgbS, sickle cell haemoglobin; low-density lipoprotein; LH, luteinizing hormone; MCH, mean corpuscular haemoglobin; MCHC, mean corpuscular haemoglobin concentration; MCV, mean corpuscular volume; PE, pulmonary embolism; PT, prothrombin time; PTT, partial thromboplastin time; RA, rheumatoid arthritis; RBC, red blood cells; TIBC, total iron-binding capacity; TSH, thyroid-stimulating hormone; U, unit; VTE, venous thromboembolism; WBC, white blood cell.

B Diet Recommendations

Bland Diet

Cheryl A. Glass and Jill C. Cash

You have been prescribed a bland diet. This diet provides adequate nutrition along with the treatment of gastrointestinal (GI) problems such as ulcerative conditions or inflammatory problems of the stomach and intestines. It is intended to decrease irritation in the lining of the stomach and intestines.

Food Tips
Foods to Avoid

Garlic, onions, alcohol, fatty foods, fried foods, chocolate, cocoa, coffee (even decaffeinated), dried fruits, citrus fruit and juices (orange, pineapple, and grapefruit), tomato products, peppermint, whole-grain breads and cereals, prespiced foods such as processed lunch meats and ham. Avoid pepper, chili powder, and cocoa spices.

General Instructions

A. Eat at least three small meals a day.
B. Avoid alcohol and beer.
C. Avoid caffeinated drinks/colas.
D. Avoid fried, greasy foods.
E. Bake or broil your foods.
F. Trim the fat from meats before cooking.
G. Bake, broil, mash, or cream potatoes.
H. Avoid raw fruits and vegetables, such as corn on the cob, and other gas-forming vegetables such as cabbage, dried beans, and peas.
I. Avoid rich desserts.
J. Avoid bedtime snacks—they may increase acid production and cause discomfort at night.
K. Avoid eating two hours before you go to bed.
L. Ask your health-care provider if nutritional supplements are necessary.

Approved Foods by Food Group

A. Dairy products:
   1. Whole milk.
   2. Low-fat or 2% milk.
   3. Skim milk.
   4. Evaporated milk.
   5. Buttermilk.
   6. Cottage cheese.
   7. Yogurt.
   8. Cheese.
B. Meat:
   1. Beef.
   2. Veal.
   3. Fresh pork.
   4. Turkey.
   5. Chicken.
   6. Fish (canned or fresh).
   7. Liver.
   8. Egg (as a meat substitute).
C. Breads/grains:
   1. Enriched breads (plain toast).
   2. Oats.
   3. Cereal.
   4. Tortillas.
   5. English muffins.
   6. Saltine crackers.
   7. Pasta (all types).
D. Fruits/vegetables.
   1. All vegetables.
   2. All fruits and juices (except citrus).
E. Desserts.
   1. Custard.
   2. Pudding.
   3. Sherbet.
   4. Ice cream (except peppermint and chocolate).
   5. Gelatin.
   6. Angel food cake.
   7. Pound cake.
   8. Sugar cookies.
   9. Jams and jellies.
   10. Honey.
F. Drinks:
   1. Decaffeinated tea.
   2. Juices (except citrus).
   3. Caffeine-free sodas.
G. Spices:
   1. Salt.
   2. Thyme.
   3. Sage.
   4. Cinnamon.
   5. Paprika.
   6. Apple cider vinegar.
   7. Prepared mustard.
   8. Lemon and lime juices.

DASH Diet: Dietary Approaches to Stop Hypertension

Cheryl A. Glass and Jill C. Cash

The Dietary Approaches to Stop Hypertension (DASH) diet is based on a combination of different types of foods and is recommended to help control high blood pressure (BP). It is a food plan that is based on foods that are low in cholesterol and high in dietary fiber, potassium, calcium, and magnesium; it is moderately high in protein. DASH eating has a reduction in lean red meats, added sugar, and sugar-containing sodas. The DASH diet's dairy food portions make the diet high in calcium and vitamin D. Overall, Americans, especially African Americans, are deficient in vitamin D.

The DASH diet, along with weight loss and exercise, is used to control other health problems such as type 2 diabetes and heart disease. If your ethnic background is Hawaiian, American Indian, Eskimo, Hispanic, or African American, you are at higher risk for high BP. Following a DASH eating plan will also help lower the bad cholesterol, or low-density lipoprotein (LDL), which can reduce heart disease.

A major way the DASH diet helps lower BP is to limit the amount of salt (sodium). The recommendations are limiting sodium to 2300 mg a day or less. If you have high BP, you may be limited to 1500 mg or less a day. One teaspoon of salt contains 2000 mg of sodium.

Foods high in sodium make you retain extra fluid. If you notice that your hands are swelling (rings are tight) or your feet and legs swell (sock rings or shoes feel tight), you are getting too much salt. Fluid retention is bad if you have heart failure. This diet is rich in potassium, which can help you get rid of the extra sodium and decrease the fluid retention.

Sea salt, even though it may contain less sodium, is not low enough in sodium to use as a substitute for regular salt. Salt substitutes contain potassium chloride; this can cause more fluid retention. Potassium chloride salt substitutes may also interfere with your BP medications, so check with your health-care provider before using them.

Tips for Reducing Sodium

A. Slowly cut back on your salty foods and begin to use healthier products. Take the saltshaker off the table.
B. Eat fresh foods:
  1. Avoid prepackaged foods.
  2. Eat fresh vegetables instead of canned vegetables. If you use canned vegetables, choose the low-sodium option and/or rinse the vegetables.
C. Read food labels:
  1. Sodium is in almost all processed foods, including milk.
  2. Focus on the amount of sodium per food serving.
  3. Do not forget to read labels on soda and sports drink bottles.
  4. Choose your favorite food brand with low-salt or low-sodium labels on the package instead of the same product with more salt.
D. Avoid salty snacks and foods, including the following:
  1. Crackers, chips, and pretzels.
  2. Cheeses.
  3. Olives, pickles, pickled okra, and other foods.
  4. Processed foods, including jerky, hot dogs, bacon, deli meats, canned fish, and canned meats, which contain a large amount of sodium.
E. Limit using soy sauce, seasoned salts, and meat tenderizers.
F. Many seasonings, including ketchup and sauces, contain a lot of sodium. Substitute with other flavours such as fresh herbs (e.g., rosemary, thyme, oregano, cilantro, and basil). Use garlic powder, lemon and lime juice, and crushed red peppers, as well as ginger.
G. Try making your own salt-free herb blend to use on your foods. Ingredients that can add flavour without adding salt include the following:
  1. Peppers such as cayenne, black pepper, and lemon pepper.
  2. Dried herbs such as thyme.
  3. Garlic powder.
  4. Paprika.
  5. Celery seed.
H. Helpful websites for salt-free herb blend, products, and recipes are the following:
  1. Salt-free seasoning recipes:
     a. busycooks.about.com.
     b. www.tasteofhome.com/Recipes/Salt-Free-Seasoning-Mix.
  2. Websites with low-salt recipes:
     a. homecooking.about.com/library/archive/blhelp13.htm.
     b. McCormick: www.mccormick.com.
     c. Mrs. Dash: www.mrsdash.com.

Tips on Eating the DASH Way

A. Start small. Make gradual changes in your eating habits, such as eating smaller portions (see Tables B.1 and B.2).
B. Center your meal around carbohydrates such as pasta, rice, beans, or vegetables.

DASH Diet Serving Portion Sizes

Food	Portion Size	Food	Portion Size
1 baked potato	Fist	1 cup of popcorn (unbuttered)	Baseball
1 cup of flaked cereal	Baseball	1/2 cup of fresh fruit	1/2 Baseball
1 1/2 oz. cheese	4 Dice	1/2 cup of pasta, rice, or potato	1/2 Baseball
1 tbsp of margarine	1 Die	1/2 cup of ice cream	1/2 Baseball
1/4 cup of raisins	Egg	3 oz. of meat, includes fish, meat, and chicken	Deck of cards
1/4 cup almonds	Golf ball	1 pancake	CD
2 tbsp peanut butter	Ping-Pong ball	1 piece of cornbread	Bar of soap
1 cup of salad	Baseball	3 oz. of grilled or baked fish	Checkbook

Source: Adapted from the National Heart, Lung, and Blood Institute. (2013). Serving sizes and portions. Retrieved from: http://www.nhlbi.nih.gov/health/educational/wecan/eat-right/distortion.htm.

TABLE B.2 DASH Diet Daily Servings

Food Group	Daily Servings	Serving Sizes	Examples and Notes	Significance of Each Food Group to the DASH Diet Pattern
Grains and grain product	6–8	1 slice bread 1/2 cup dry cereal 1/2 cup cooked rice, pasta, or cereal	Whole-wheat bread, English muffin, pita bread, bagel, cereals, grits, oatmeal, couscous	Major sources of energy and fiber
Vegetables	4–5	1 cup raw leafy vegetables 1/2 cup cooked vegetables 6 oz. vegetable juice	Tomatoes, potatoes, carrots, peas, squash, broccoli, turnip greens, collards, kale, spinach, artichokes, beans, sweet potatoes	Rich sources of potassium, magnesium, and fiber
Fruits	4–5	6 oz. fruit juice 1 medium fruit 1/4 cup dried fruit 1/4 cup fresh, frozen, or canned fruit	Apricots, bananas, dates, grapes, oranges, orange juice, grapefruit, grapefruit juice, mangoes, melons, peaches, pineapples, prunes, raisins, strawberries, tangerines	Important sources of potassium, magnesium, and fiber
Low-fat or fat-free milk and dairy foods	2–3	1 cup milk 1 cup yogurt 1.5 oz. cheese	Skim or 1% milk, skim or low-fat buttermilk, nonfat or low-fat yogurt, part-skim mozzarella cheese, nonfat cheese	Major sources of calcium and protein
Lean meats, poultry, and fish	6 or less	1 oz. cooked meats, poultry, or fish 1 egg	Select only lean; trim away visible fat; broil, roast, or boil instead of frying; remove skin from poultry	Rich sources of protein and magnesium
Nuts, seeds, and legumes	4–5	Per week 1 1/2 oz. of nuts 1/2 oz. or 2 tbsp seeds 2 tbsp of peanut butter 1/2 cup cooled legumes	Almonds, filberts, mixed nuts, peanuts, walnuts, sunflower seeds, kidney beans, lentils	Rich sources of energy, magnesium, potassium, protein, and fiber
Sweets and added sugars	5 or less per week	1 tbsp sugar 1 tbsp jelly or jam 1/2 cup sorbet or gelatin 1 cup lemonade	Fruit-flavoured gelatin, fruit punch, hard candy, jelly, maple syrup, sugar	Sweets should be low in fat

Source: Adapted from the National Heart, Lung, and Blood Institute (NHLBI) DASH Diet Eating Plan.

C. Treat meat as only part of a whole meal instead of the main focus of the meal.
D. Use fruits or low-fat, low-calorie foods such as sugar-free gelatin for desserts and snacks.
E. Choose "whole" grains in breads and cereals.
F. Choose to eat vegetables without butter or sauce.
G. Choose lean cuts of meat. Use fresh poultry, for example, skinless turkey and chicken.
H. Choose ready-to-eat breakfast cereals that are lower in sodium.
I. Eat fruits for dessert. Use fruits that are canned in their own juice.
J. Add fruit to plain yogurt.
K. To increase eating vegetables, stir-fry with 2 oz. of chicken and use 1 1/2 cups of raw vegetables.
L. Snack on vegetables, bread sticks, graham crackers, or unbuttered/unsalted popcorn.
M. Drink water or club soda.
N. Table B.3 lists the number of servings suggested and Table B.4 offers an example of the caloric adjustment for 2000 calories a day using the DASH diet.

TABLE B.3 Total Number of Servings in 2,000 Calories per Day DASH Diet

Food Group	Servings
Grains	6–8
Vegetables	4–5
Fruits	4–5
Fat-free or low-fat milk and dairy foods	2–3
Lean meats, poultry, and fish	2 (6 oz.)
Nuts, seeds, and legumes	1 (4–5/wk)
Fats and oils	2–3
Sweets and added sugars	1 (<5/wk)

DASH, dietary approaches to stop hypertension.

TABLE 8.4 DASH Example Menu (2,000 Calories)

Food	Amount	Servings Provided
Breakfast		
Orange juice	6 oz.	1 fruit
1% low-fat milk	8 oz. (1 cup)	1 dairy
Corn flakes (with 1 tbsp sugar)	1 cup	2 grains
Banana	1 medium	1 fruit
Whole-wheat bread (with 1 tbsp jelly)	1 slice	1 grain
Soft margarine	1 tsp	1 fat
Lunch		
Chicken salad	¾ cup	1 poultry
Pita bread	½ large	1 grain
Raw vegetable medley: Carrot and celery sticks Radishes Loose-leaf lettuce	3–4 sticks each 2 2 leaves	1 vegetable
Part-skim mozzarella cheese	1.5 slice (1.5 oz.)	1 dairy
1% low-fat milk	8 oz. (1 cup)	1 dairy
Fruit cocktail in light syrup	½ cup	1 fruit
Dinner		
Herbed baked cod	3 oz.	1 fish
Scallion rice	1 cup	2 grains
Steamed broccoli	½ cup	1 vegetable
Stewed tomatoes	½ cup	1 vegetable
Spinach salad: Raw spinach Cherry tomatoes Cucumber	½ cup 2 2 slices	1 vegetable
Light Italian salad dressing	1 tbsp	½ fat
Whole-wheat dinner roll	1 small	1 grain
Soft margarine	1 tsp	1 fat
Melon balls	½ cup	1 fruit
Snacks		
Dried apricots	1 oz. (¼ cup)	1 fruit
Mini pretzels	1 oz. (¾ cup)	1 grain
Mixed nuts	1.5 oz. (½ cup)	1 nuts
Diet ginger ale	12 oz.	0

Resources

DASH Diet Calorie Adjustments for 1,200, 1,600, 2,000, and 2,400 calorie diets: http://dashdiet.org/ images/calories.pdf.

The DASH Diet Eating Plan: http://dashdiet.org/dash_diet_recipes.asp.

DASH Diet Recipes: www.mayoclinic.com/health/dash-diet-recipes/RE00089.

DASH for Health: www.dashforhealth.com/index.php.

Foods to Avoid While Taking Warfarin (Coumadin, Jantoven)

Cheryl A. Glass and Jill C. Cash

Warfarin is a medication that thins the blood to prevent blood clots. Some nutrients and foods can interfere with warfarin and make the warfarin less effective or not work as well. Therefore, it is important to closely monitor the foods that you eat daily to make sure your medication is working for you the same way every day. One nutrient that causes this problem is vitamin K. Vitamin K interferes with the warfarin and can cause problems with thinning the blood. Therefore, it is important to avoid foods and nutrients that would cause this problem. It is suggested to eat foods that contain the same amount of vitamin K every day. This will help to prevent problems with thinning your blood.

The recommended intake of vitamin K for the adult man is 120 mcg and for adult women is 90 mcg.

The following is a list of foods that have a **MODERATE to HIGH level of vitamin K and should be avoided:**

1. Broccoli (cooked).
2. Brussels sprouts.
3. Chard.
4. Collard greens.
5. Green tea.
6. Kale.
7. Mustard greens.
8. Parsley.
9. Spinach.
10. Turnip greens.

Some drinks can also interfere with warfarin and **should be avoided**. These drinks include the following:
1. Cranberry juice.
2. Alcohol.

Foods that have a **LOWER level of vitamin K** and are safer to eat in moderate portions include the following:
1. Asparagus.
2. Avocado.
3. Blackberries/blueberries.
4. Cabbage.
5. Carrots.
6. Cauliflower.
7. Cucumbers.
8. Lettuce, iceberg and romaine.
9. Peas.
10. Peppers.
11. Potatoes.
12. Prunes.
13. Squash (summer and winter).
14. Sweet potatoes.
15. Tomatoes.
16. Tuna.

Medications (prescribed and over-the-counter [OTC] medications, multivitamins, supplements, and herbal supplements) may also interfere with warfarin and should only be taken after discussing the medication, vitamin, or supplement with your health-care provider for safety.

If you have questions about certain foods or medications, you need to discuss this with your health-care provider.

Foods Rich in Vitamin K

If you are taking a blood thinner, you should be aware that certain foods are high in vitamin K.

Vitamin K can interfere with how blood thinners work.

You do not necessarily have to stop eating these foods, just be consistent and maintain your regular eating habits.

Please discuss these foods further with your health-care provider.

These vitamin K–rich foods include the following:
1. Broccoli.
2. Brussels sprouts.
3. Collard greens.
4. Endive.
5. Kale.
6. Mustard greens.
7. Parsley.
8. Swiss chard.
9. Spinach.
10. Turnip greens.

Foods that are low in vitamin K:
1. Asparagus.
2. Avocado.
3. Blackberries.
4. Blueberries.
5. Cabbage.
6. Cranberry juice.
7. Green tea.
8. Lettuce (iceberg and leafy).
9. Liver.
10. Peas.
11. Prunes.
12. Tuna.

Gluten-Free Diet

Cheryl A. Glass and Jill C. Cash

Gluten-Free Diet Tips

The symptoms from celiac disease are triggered from glutens in your diet. Three cereals that contain gluten are wheat, rye, and barley. Glutens are also present in other products, such as food additives, so it is very important to read all the ingredients on food labels (see Table B.5).

Dietary Recommendation for Celiac Disease

A. You may also be told to follow a lactose-free diet for a short time to help your symptoms.
B. Most bread sold in the grocery aisle is not allowed on a gluten-free eating plan.
C. All vegetables and fruits are gluten-free. However, frozen and canned fruits and vegetables may contain an additive with gluten.
D. Although you should not enjoy beer, wine is still on the menu when you go to dinner.
E. Specialty bakeries are able to make gluten-free cakes for special occasions. Plain hard candy, marshmallows, and other candies are usually gluten-free.
F. Caution should be taken when ordering any breaded foods such as chicken nuggets or breaded fish.
G. Deli meats may also contain gluten.
H. Gluten-free foods are often not fortified with vitamins and minerals. It is recommended to take a daily multivitamin.

Resources

Celiac Disease Foundation: www.celiac.org.
www.celiac.com.
www.chex.com/glutenfree.
www.BettyCrocker.com/glutenfree.

TABLE B.5 Examples of Foods That Are Allowed and Avoided on a Gluten-Free Diet

Allowed	Avoid
Fresh fruits and vegetables without any processing or additives	Wheat, wheat berry, wheat bran, wheat germ, wheat grass, whole-wheat berries
Meat	Flours, bread flour
Soy, soybean, tofu	Bulgur (bulgur wheat, bulgur nuts)
Brown rice	Rye
Enriched rice/instant rice/wild rice	Barley
Buckwheat	Barley malt/barley extract
Millet	Oats, oat bran, oat fiber
Sorghum	Cereals
Alfalfa	Matzo
Almond	Beer, ale, porter, stout
Canola	Farina
Chickpea	Croutons
Corn, corn flour, cornmeal	Bran
Brown rice flour	Tabbouleh
Tapioca	Soy sauce

https://celiac.org/celiac-disease/understanding-celiac-disease-2/what-is-celiac-disease/.
Gluten-free recipes: http://allrecipes.com/Recipes/Healthy-Cooking/Gluten-Free/Main.aspx.

High-Fiber Diet

Cheryl A. Glass and Jill C. Cash

Fiber is a plant cell wall component that is not broken down by the digestive system. An old term for fiber is roughage because it absorbs fluid and moves waste faster through the intestines in a bulky mass. The Food and Drug Administration (FDA) defines as high-fiber those products that contain 20% of the daily fiber value. High-fiber diets are used to help prevent constipation as well as diarrhoea. Fiber has been used to help several medical conditions such as diabetes, diverticulosis, irritable bowel syndrome (IBS), and high cholesterol, as well as weight loss. If you have a chronic health condition, check with your health-care provider about starting any new dietary change.

Fiber provides a full feeling that can help with spacing meals further apart (three to four hours). Fiber recommendations change with your age (see Table B.6).

Tips for Increasing Fiber in Your Diet

A. Read the Nutrition Facts food label for fiber content per food serving.
   1. Cereals that provide 5 g of fiber per serving give you 20% of your daily fiber.
   2. Look for "whole grain" on the label. Just because bread is brown does not mean it is whole grain.

Fiber Recommendations by Age

Group/Gender	Age (Years)	Fiber Recommendations (Grams of Fiber Each Day)
Children	1–3	19
Children	4–8	25
Boys	9–13	31
Boys	14–18	38
Girls	9–13	26
Girls	14–18	26
Men	Younger than 50	38
Women	Younger than 50	25
Men	Older than 50	30
Women	Older than 50	21

Source: Adapted from the American Heart Association. (2015). *Fiber and children's diets.* Retrieved from http://www.heart.org/HEARTORG/HealthyLiving/HealthyEating/Nutrition/Fiber-and-Childrens-Diets_UCM_305981_Article.jsp#.WGagdLnT8rM.

B. Increase fiber in your diet gradually to prevent gas. Adding too much fiber too quickly may give you abdominal pain, bloating, and constipation. Increase your fiber over several weeks so that it gives time for you to adjust.
C. As you increase fiber, it is also important to increase the amount of fluids you drink up to six to eight glasses a day, including tea, milk, fruit juices, coffee, and even soft drinks. The extra fluids that you drink along with the extra fiber makes you feel fuller, which can help control snacking.
D. Keep a food diary and review it periodically to decide on other diet adjustments that need to be made.
E. Several fiber supplements are available over the counter (OTC) to help you get your daily recommendation of fiber.

Good Food Sources of Fiber

A. Bran: Add one teaspoon of whole-grain bran to food three times a day, or take an OTC fiber supplement, such as psyllium (Metamucil), as directed.
B. Whole-grain cereals and breads: Eat oat, bran, multigrain, light, wheat, or rye breads rather than pure white bread or breads that list eggs as a major ingredient. Grains are not only a good source of fiber but also contain vitamins and minerals. Folic acid has been added to breads and cereals to help reduce neural tube defects.
C. Fresh or frozen fruits and vegetables: Citrus fruits are especially good sources of fiber. Eat raw or minimally cooked vegetables, especially squash, cabbage, lettuce and other greens, and beans. Leave the skin on fruits and vegetables; eating the whole fruit is better than drinking the juice. Whole tomatoes offer more fiber than peeling the skin off. The more colourful the fruit and vegetable (dark green, red, blue, yellow), the better; they provide a good source of antioxidants that are good for the heart and the prevention of some cancers. Apples are a good source of both fiber and water.
D. Legumes (pods): Peas and beans are a good source of fiber. Add chickpeas and kidney beans to salads for extra fiber and flavour. Add baked beans as a delicious side item to your meal.
E. Coffee is another source of fiber.
F. Nuts are an excellent source of fiber. They are considered nutrient-dense and are a good source of vitamins and folic acid. Sprinkle sunflower seeds on a salad to add flavour and fiber. The amount of nuts eaten should be limited to 1 to 2 oz. because they are also high in calories.
G. If you have diverticulosis avoid foods with seeds or indigestible material that may block the neck of a diverticulum such as nuts, corn, popcorn, cucumbers, tomatoes, figs, strawberries, and caraway seeds.

Lactose-Intolerance Diet

Cheryl A. Glass and Jill C. Cash

Lactose is the sugar present in milk. Lactose intolerance is very common; it occurs when the body is not able to appropriately digest this milk sugar content and the result is diarrhoea. You have been diagnosed as having difficulty digesting milk (lactose) products or you have problems with malabsorption. Lactose intolerance can cause gas, bloating, abdominal cramps, diarrhoea, and nausea or vomiting. You may be able to eat small portions without problems, or you may be unable to tolerate any foods containing lactose (see Table B.7).

Recommended Foods for Lactose Intolerance

Foods	Recommended	Not Recommended
Milk	Soybean milk, milk treated with lactase, nondairy creamers, whipped topping; up to 1 cup per day of buttermilk, yogurt, sweet acidophilus milk, or whole, low-fat, or skim milk	Milk products in excess of 1 cup per day, malted milk, milkshakes, hot chocolate, cocoa
Meat and protein foods	All meats; fish; poultry; eggs; peanut butter; tofu; or hard, aged, and processed cheese, if tolerated	Sandwich meat, hot dogs that contain lactose, cottage cheese, any meat prepared with milk products
Vegetables	All fresh, frozen, canned, buttered, and/or breaded vegetables	Any vegetable prepared with milk or milk products in excess of allowance (1 cup)
Fruits	All fresh, frozen, or canned fruits	Any fruits processed with lactose
Breads, cereal, and starchy food	White, wheat, rye, or other yeast breads, crackers, macaroni, spaghetti, popcorn, dry or cooked cereals	Commercial bread products (French toast, bread mixes, pancakes, biscuits), cakes/cookies containing milk or milk products

(continued)

Recommended Foods for Lactose Intolerance (*continued*)

Foods	Recommended	Not Recommended
Fats and oils	Butter/margarine, salad dressing, mayonnaise, all oils, nondairy creamers, bacon	Sour cream, salad dressings with milk products in excess of 1 cup allowance
Soups	Vegetable and meat soups, broth, and bouillon	Dried soups, creamed soups made with milk
Desserts	Plain and fruit-flavoured gelatins, sherbet, fruit pies, cakes, pudding, pastries, angel food cake, sponge cake	Ice cream, ice milk, cream pie, puddings, custards, cakes, and pastries with milk (unless count as day's allowance)
Beverages	Coffee, tea, soft drinks, fruit juices, carbonated and mineral waters	Beverages with milk over the 1 cup Allowance
Miscellaneous condiments	Catsup, mustard, soy sauce, vinegar, steak sauce, Worcestershire sauce, chili sauce	None
Seasonings	Salt, pepper, spices, herbs, and seasonings	None
Sweets	Sugar, jelly, honey, molasses, preserves, marmalade, syrups, hard candy, baker's cocoa, carob powder, artificial sweeteners	Cream or chocolate candies containing milk or milk products (unless count as day's allowance), caramels, toffee, and butterscotch

Tips for Following a Lactose-Intolerance Diet

A. Limit or omit foods that contain milk, lactose, whey, or casein.
B. Lactose-controlled diets allow up to one cup of milk per day for cooking or drinking, if you can tolerate it.
C. Read labels carefully. If you cannot tolerate any lactose, choose lactose-free foods with lactate, lactic acid, lactalbumin, whey protein, sodium caseinate, casein hydrolysates, and calcium compounds.
D. You may also choose kosher foods marked "pareve" or "parve," which do not contain lactose. Read labels carefully.
E. A low-fat diet is important if you have fat malabsorption.
F. To help with diarrhoea because of malabsorption, avoid more than one serving a day of caffeine-containing drinks.
G. Beverages with high sugar content, such as soft drinks and fruit juices, may increase diarrhoea. Juices and fruits with high amounts of fructose include apples, pears, sweet cherries, prunes, and dates.
H. "Sugarless" sorbitol-containing candies and gums may cause diarrhoea.

Low-Fat/Low-Cholesterol Diet

Cheryl A. Glass and Jill C. Cash

The connection between fat in the diet and heart attacks is cholesterol. Cholesterol is a fat-like substance produced by your liver and also found in many foods. Too much cholesterol causes heart attacks by clogging the arteries that deliver blood to your heart.

Exercising and following a low-fat/low-cholesterol diet can help control your blood cholesterol and reduce your risk of heart attack.

Tips

A. Read food labels. Use the ingredient list on labels to identify products containing saturated fat. High-fat ingredients may have many names. Remember, foods can say "no cholesterol" and still be high in saturated vegetable fat and calories.
B. Train yourself to think "low fat" in your food and cooking methods:
   1. Bake.
   2. Broil.
   3. Grill.
   4. Stir-fry.
C. Eat less fried food, fast food, and baked products.
D. Eat more fruits and vegetables.
E. Organize your shopping around low-fat foods.
F. Add flavour to foods by using herbs and spices instead of butter and sauces.
G. Choose coleslaw, sliced tomatoes, or a dill pickle instead of fries and chips.

Foods to Avoid or Limit

A. Proteins/meats:
   1. Shrimp.
   2. Fried meats, fish, or poultry.
   3. Fatty ground meat.
   4. Prime or heavily marbled meats.
   5. Bacon, sausage, high-fat deli meats, and cheeses.
   6. Liver and organ meats.
B. Breads/cereals:
   1. High-fat baked foods, such as Danish pastries, croissants, and doughnuts.
   2. Fried rice, crispy chow mein noodles.
   3. Granola bars with coconut or coconut oil.
   4. Chips, cheese, or butter crackers.
   5. High-fat cookies and cakes.
C. Fruits and vegetables:
   1. Coconut.
   2. Fried vegetables such as onion rings and breaded fried pickles, mushrooms, and okra.
   3. Cream, cheese, or butter sauces on vegetables.
D. Milk/dairy products:
   1. Whole or 2% milk.
   2. Cream, half-and-half, nondairy creamers.
   3. Ice cream, whipped cream, nondairy whipped toppings.
   4. Whole-milk yogurt, sour cream.
   5. Cheeses: Cheddar, American, Swiss cream cheese, Brie, Muenster.
E. Very high-fat foods:
   1. Butter or margarine made with partially hydrogenated oils.
   2. Lard, meat fat, and coconut or palm oils.
   3. Salad dressings made with sour cream or cheese.
   4. Chocolate.
   5. Beef tallow.

6. Hydrogenated or partially hydrogenated vegetable shortening.
7. Cream.
8. Cocoa butter.

Foods That Are Allowed
A. Proteins/meats:
  1. Fish and shellfish.
  2. Chicken and turkey cooked without the skin.
  3. Ground turkey.
  4. Eggs: limited to two yolks per week.
  5. Dried beans, lentils, tofu.
  6. Small amounts of meat and seafood.
B. Breads/cereals:
  1. Plain bread and English muffins and bagels.
  2. Plain pasta, rice.
  3. Cereals, oatmeal.
  4. Pretzels, air-popped popcorn, rice cakes, Melba toast.
  5. Low-fat baked goods: angel food cake, graham crackers, fruit cookies, and gingersnaps.
C. Fruits and vegetables:
  1. Eat several servings per day of high-nutrition, low-fat fruits and vegetables.
  2. Prepare vegetables by steaming, broiling, baking, or stir-frying.
D. Milk/dairy products:
  1. Skim or 1% milk.
  2. Low-fat milk, evaporated milk, nonfat dry milk powder.
  3. Frozen yogurt, ice milk, sherbet, sorbet.
  4. Low-fat yogurt.
  5. Low-fat cheeses: 1% cottage cheese, skim-milk ricotta, mozzarella, and American cheeses.
E. Allowed high-fat foods:
  1. Margarine made with liquid safflower, corn, or sunflower oils.
  2. Olive, canola, or peanut oils.
  3. Nut snacks in moderation (high fat and calories).
  4. Salad dressings made with saturated oils.

Nausea and Vomiting Diet Suggestions (Children and Adults)

Cheryl A. Glass and Jill C. Cash

For simple nausea and vomiting with an upset stomach, follow these steps:

Step 1: Replace Lost Fluids
A. Rest your stomach for 1 to 2 hours.
B. Infants and small children: Oral electrolyte solutions are recommended because children become dehydrated quickly.
C. Infants: Resume breast-or bottle-feeding as soon as possible.
D. Young children: Give very small sips every 10 to 20 minutes until they keep the fluid down.
E. Older children: Give sports drinks or oral electrolyte solutions.
F. Older child and adults:
  1. After vomiting stops, take sips of clear liquids at room temperature, such as flat ginger ale, flat cola, or gelatin.
  2. Suck on lollipops or Popsicles.
  3. Gradually increase the amount of liquids. If four hours pass without vomiting, progress to Step 2.

Step 2: Dry Diet
The foods in this diet do not meet all daily food requirements and should be used only for a short period before adding foods or advancing to Step 3.
A. Cheerios.
B. Crackers.
C. Corn flakes.
D. Graham crackers.
E. Crisped rice cereal.
F. Vanilla wafers.
G. Toast.
H. Dinner rolls.

Step 3: More Advanced Carbohydrates
A. Oatmeal.
B. Grits, unseasoned.
C. Rice, unseasoned.
D. Mashed potatoes.
E. Baked potato.
F. Noodles.
G. Peanut butter.
H. Pudding.

Step 4: Bland Foods With Limited Odours
After you are able to eat dry and more complex carbohydrates, a trial of bland foods may be tried. Foods with little or no odours are more easily tolerated after experiencing nausea and vomiting (see Table B.8).

BRAT Diet
You may be told to use a BRAT diet. This is a combination of foods that make up a bland diet and help with nausea and vomiting: bananas, rice, applesauce, and toast as tolerated.

Bland Foods With Limited Odours

Apple juice	Canned pears	Ice cream
Apple sauce	Chicken noodle soup	Iced tea
Baked chicken	Cottage cheese	Low-fat milk
Baked turkey	Fresh apple	Sherbet
Canned peaches	Fresh banana	½ turkey sandwich

Vitamin D and Calcium Supplementation

Cheryl A. Glass and Jill C. Cash

Sunlight exposure to the skin is also recommended for approximately 20 to 30 minutes without sunscreen. Sun exposure provides an adequate source of vitamin D. Care should be taken not to burn skin.
A. Vitamin D recommendations (Table B.9):
  1. Men and women age younger than 50: 400 to 800 IU/d
  2. Men and women 50 years and older: 800 to 1000 IU/d

Vitamin D–Enriched Foods

Food Source	Serving Size	Food International Units (IU)
Fish liver oils, cod liver oil	15 mL	1360
Mushrooms	3 oz.	2700
Fortified milk	8 oz.	100
Herring	3 oz.	1383
Catfish	3 oz.	425
Mackerel (cooked)	3.5 oz.	345
Salmon (cooked)	3.5 oz.	360
Sardines (canned in oil, drained)	1.75 oz.	250
Fortified orange juice	8 oz.	100
Fortified cereal	1 serving	100
Fortified cheese	3 oz.	100

Calcium-Rich Foods

Food Source	Serving Size	Food International Units (IU)
Yogurt	1 cup	448
Orange juice	1 cup	350
Fat-free milk	1 cup	316
Shrimp	3 oz.	275
Salmon	3 oz.	182
Instant oatmeal	1 packet	165
Tofu	½ cup	130
Broccoli	1 cup	94
Dried beans, cooked	½ cup	50
Cheddar cheese	1½ oz.	306
Turnip greens	1 cup	197
Cereal bars, snack bars (fortified)	1 bar	200

B. Calcium recommendations (Table B.10):
  1. Women 50 and younger: 1000 mg/d; women age 51 years and older: 1200 mg/d
  2. Men age younger than 70: 1000 mg/d; men 70 years and older: 1200 mg/d
C. Vitamin D assists with calcium absorption into the bones.
D. Research indicates that caffeine interferes with calcium absorption and lowers bone density. Carbonated beverages appear to be worse than coffee.
E. Vitamin D and calcium deficiency contribute to bone loss, and thus, osteoporosis.

Bibliography

American Dietetic Association Reports. (2008). Position of the American dietetic association: Nutrition guidance for healthy children ages 2 to 11 years. *Journal of the American Dietetic Association, 108*, 1038–1047.

American Heart Association. (2015). *Fiber and children's diets*. Retrieved from http:// www.heart.org/HEARTORG/HealthyLiving/HealthyEating/Nutrition/Fiber-and-Childrens-Diets_UCM_305981_Article.jsp#.WGagdLnT8rM

Banks, D. (n.d). Salt: Too much of a good thing. In *University of Illinois extension: Thrifty living*. Retrieved from http:// urbanext.illinois.edu/thrifty living/ tl-salt.html

Boyle, M., & Long, S. (2013). *Personal nutrition* (8th ed.). Belmont, CA: Wadsworth Cengage.

The DASH Diet Eating Plan. (n.d[a]). Retrieved from http:// dashdiet.org/default.asp

The DASH Diet Eating Plan. (n.d[b]). *The DASH diet and African American heart health*. Retrieved from http:// dashdiet.org/ dash _ diet_ and_ african_american.asp

The DASH Diet Eating Plan. (n.d[c]). *DASH diet FAQ*. Retrieved from http:// dashdiet.org/ dash_ diet_ faq.asp

The DASH Diet Eating Plan. (n.d[d]). *Low salt, low sodium, and the DASH diet*. Retrieved from http:// dashdiet.org/ low_ salt_ diet.asp

Dietary Fiber Guide. (n.d.). *High fiber foods*. Retrieved from http:// dietary-fiberguide.com

National Heart, Lung, and Blood Institute. (2013). *Serving sizes and portions*. Retrieved from: http:// www.nhlbi.nih.gov/ health/educational/wecan/eat-right/distortion.htm

National Heart, Lung, and Blood Institute. (2015). *In brief: Your guide to lowering your blood pressure with DASH*. Retrieved from http:// www.nhlbi.nih.gov/ files/docs/ public/ heart/ dash_brief.pdf

National Heart, Lung, and Blood Institute. (n.d[a]). *Tips for reducing sodium in your diet*. Retrieved from www.nhlbi.nih.gov/ hbp/ prevent/ sodium/tips.htm

National Heart, Lung, and Blood Institute. (n.d[b]). *Tips on how to make healthier meals*. Retrieved from www.nhlbi.nih.gov/ hbp/ prevent/h_ eating/ tips.htm

National Institute of Diabetes and Digestive and Kidney Diseases. (2015). *Lactose intolerance*. Retrieved from https:// www.niddk.nih.gov/health-information/health-topics/digestive-diseases/lactose-intolerance/Pages/facts.aspx

National Osteoporosis Foundation. (n.d.). *Calcium and vitamin D: What you need to know*. Retrieved from www.nof.org/articles/10

The University of Chicago Celiac Disease Center. (n.d.). *Is a gluten-free diet similar to a diabetic diet?* Retrieved from www.cureceliacdisease.org/?s=glutentfree+diet

Tanner's Sexual Maturity Stages

Stage	SEXUAL MATURITY STAGES IN FEMALES Breasts	SEXUAL MATURITY STAGES IN MALES Penis, Testes, and Scrotum
1	Preadolescent: Only papilla is elevated above the level of the chest wall	Preadolescent: All are the size and proportion seen in early childhood (testes 1 cm)
2	Breast budding: Breast and papilla elevated as small mound; increased diameter of areola	Slight enlargement, with alteration in colour (more reddened) and texture of scrotum (testes 2.0–3.2 cm)
3	Continued breast and areola enlargement; no contour separation	Further growth and enlargement (testes 3.3–4.0 cm)
4	Areola and papilla form secondary mound	Penis significantly enlarged in length and circumference; further development of glands; enlargement of testes and scrotum with darkening of scrotal skin (testes 4.1–4.9 cm)
5	Mature: Nipple projects; areola is part of general breast contour	Genitalia of adult size (testes 5.0 cm)
Stage	Pubic Hair	Pubic Hair
1	Preadolescent: None or vellus hair in pubis area	Preadolescent: None or vellus hair in pubis area
2	Sparse, straight, lightly pigmented along medial border of labia	Sparse, straight, lightly pigmented at base of penis
3	Darker, coarser, curlier, and in increased amount	Darker, coarser, curlier, and in increased amount
4	Abundant, but has not spread to medial surface of thighs	Abundant, but less quantity than adult type
5	Adult feminine, inverse triangle, spread to medial surface of thighs	Adult distribution, spread to medial surface of thighs

Source: Child Growth Foundation. www.childgrowthfoundation.org, with permission.

Index

AAA. *See* abdominal aortic aneurysm
AAN. *See* analgesic abuse nephropathy
abatacept, 624
abdominal aortic aneurysm (AAA), 233, 235
abdominal hernias, 286–288
abdominal pain, 231–235
abdominal trauma, 233
abdominal ultrasonography, appendicitis, 237
ABGs. *See* arterial blood gases
ablation therapy, 199
abrupt coronary artery occlusion, 189
abrupt paralysis, 651
abruptio placentae, 376, 377
    marginal abruption, 377
    moderate abruption, 377
    severe abruption, 377
absent seizures, 556
absolute contraindications, 392, 401, 417
abuse assessment screening, 54
acalculous cholecystitis, 242
ACE. *See* acute concussion evaluation
acebutolol, 199
acetazolamide, 119
acetic acid, 130
acetylcholine receptors (AChR), 550
acetylsalicylic acid (ASA), 128, 224, 456, 471, 580, 621
AChR. *See* acetylcholine receptors
AChR-Ab. *See* antibody titre for acetylcholine receptor
acne rosacea, 69–70
acne vulgaris, 70–71
acoustic neuroma, 128
acquired immune deficiency syndrome (AIDS), 499
acquired premature ejaculation, 335
ACTH. *See* adrenocorticotropic hormone
actinic keratoses, 72
Actinomyces israelii, 116
activities of daily living (ADLs), 32, 56–57
acute appendicitis, 231, 235
acute cervicitis, 397
acute cholecystitis, 231, 241
acute concussion evaluation (ACE), 115
acute diarrhoea, 258
acute epididymitis, 323, 325
acute gouty arthritis, 609
acute inflammatory demyelinating polyradiculoneuropathy (AIDP), 531
acute limb ischaemia, 223
acute myocardial infarction (MI), 189–191
acute neck pain, 515
acute obstruction, 234
acute otitis media (AOM), 125–126, 128, 131
acute pain, 59–61, 231
acute respiratory distress syndrome (ARDS), 372

acute rheumatic fever (ARF), 469–471
acute sinusitis/rhinosinusitis, 139–142
acute thyroidism, 599
acute vertigo, 567, 568
acyclovir, 83, 84, 112, 179, 434, 448, 464, 487, 527
adalimumab, 255, 619, 624
adamantane, 179
Addison's disease, 571–573
adenovirus, 110, 265
ADHD. *See* attention deficit hyperactivity disorder
adjustment sleep disorder, 650
ADLs. *See* activities of daily living
adolescents
    amenorrhoea, 390
    contraception, 402
    depression, 644
    dysmenorrhoea, 404
    herpes simplex virus-1, 82–83
    suicide, 654
adrenocorticotropic hormone (ACTH), 573
Adult Children of Alcoholics (ACOA), 48
adult risk assessment form, 27
adults
    abdominal pain, 234
    acne rosacea, 70
    acute myocardial infarction, 191
    acute sinusitis/rhinosinusitis, 142
    Alzheimer's disease, 525
    ankylosing spondylitis, 607
    appendicitis, 235, 237
    atherosclerosis, 197
    atopic dermatitis, 78
    attention deficit hyperactivity disorder, 637
    benign skin lesions, 74
    breast pain, 396–397
    candidiasis, 75
    chronic fatigue syndrome, 497
    chronic kidney disease, 319–323
    chronic obstructive pulmonary disease, 165
    constipation, 250
    contraception, 402
    cytomegalovirus, 444, 446
    dysmenorrhoea, 404
    erectile dysfunction, 328
    failure to thrive, 645
    galactorrhoea, 585
    gastroenteritis, 267
    glaucoma, acute angle-closure, 119
    gonorrhoea, 432
    grief, 649
    headache, 538
    hearing loss, 129
    heart failure, 212
    hepatitis B, 282
    hepatitis C, 285

    herpes simplex virus-1, 83
    herpes simplex virus type 2, 434
    H1N1 influenza A, 451
    human immunodeficiency virus, 502–503
    hydrocele, 332
    hyperthyroidism, 598
    influenza, 452, 454
    iron-deficiency anaemia, 509
    lower back pain, 67
    lower extremity ulcer, 101
    lymphadenopathy, 512
    meningitis, 462
    myasthenia gravis, 551
    nausea, 674
    neck and upper back disorders, 517
    obesity, 32
    obstructive sleep apnoea, 173
    oral cancer, 147
    osteoarthritis, 612
    parvovirus B19, 469
    peptic ulcer disease, 309
    periodic health examination, 21
    pernicious anaemia, 514
    premature ejaculation, 336
    pressure ulcers, 103
    preventative health care, 21
    preventive care checklist form, 21
    pseudogout, 618
    psoriasis, 93
    psoriatic arthritis, 619
    respiratory syncytial virus, 181
    rheumatic fever, 471
    roundworm, 312
    sciatica, 520
    seborrhoeic dermatitis, 96
    sleep disorders, 651
    substance use disorders, 48
    syncope, 230
    thrush, 151
    tinea corporis, 97
    transient ischaemic attacks, 565
    undescended testicles, 349
    varicella, 487–488
    varicocele, 359
    vomiting diet, 674
    Zika virus infection, 492
AED. *See* antiepileptic drugs
Aedes, 490, 492
Aerobacter aerogenes, 380
AHI. *See* apnea hypopnoea index
AIDP. *See* acute inflammatory demyelinating polyradiculoneuropathy
AIDS. *See* acquired immune deficiency syndrome
alanine transaminase (ALT), 242
albendazole, 294
albuminuria, 339
alcohol, 613, 614
alcoholism, 634, 642, 649

alemtuzumab, 548
alendronate sodium, 614
alfuzosin, 318
alkaline phosphate, 242
allergic contact dermatitis, 76–77
allergic rhinitis, 135–136
allergy testing, asthma, 153
allodynia, 334
alpha-1 antagonists, 318
alpha-reductase inhibitors, 318–319
alprazolam, 634
ALT. See alanine transaminase
aluminum hydroxide, 601
Alzheimer's disease, 523–525, 528
amantadine, 451, 553
amantadine hydrochloride, 549
Amblyomma americanum, 472
amblyopia, 107
ambulatory blood pressure monitoring (ABPM), 216
amenorrhoea, 389–390
American Medical Society for Sports Medicine (AMSSM), 655
aminoglycoside, 111, 113, 128, 132
5-aminosalicylates (5-ASA), 253, 261
amiodarone, 199, 585, 595, 596, 599
amitriptyline, 32, 82, 296, 334, 385, 405, 608
amlodipine, 621
amniocentesis, 364
amoxicillin, 70, 71, 75, 126, 141, 142, 143–145, 149, 176, 220, 261, 356, 374, 431, 458, 459, 471, 482
amoxicillin-clavulanate, 126, 357
amoxil, 130
amphetamine-dextroamphetamine, 636
ampicillin, 220, 380, 461
AMSSM. See American Medical Society for Sports Medicine
ANA. See antinuclear antibody
anabolic steroids, 593
anaemia, 181, 322, 365–366, 506, 571
analgesic abuse nephropathy (AAN), 320
analgesics, 66, 167, 338, 555
anaphylaxis, 84
anastrozole, 586
Ancylostoma ceylonicum, 292
Ancylostoma duodenale, 292, 311
androgenic hormones, 586
angiotensin II receptor blockers (ARBs), 322, 580
angiotensin-converting enzyme (ACE), 322, 580
animal bites, mammalian, 72–73
ankle brachial index (ABI), 98
ankle sprains, 521
ankylosing spondylitis (AS), 605–607
anoscopy, 274
antepartum
    anaemia, iron deficiency, 365–366
    gestational diabetes mellitus, 366–368
    preconception counselling: identifying clients at risk, 361–363
    preeclampsia, 369–370
    preterm labour, 371–372
    pyelonephritis in pregnancy, 372–374
    routine prenatal care, 363–364
    testing, 368
    vaginal bleeding, 374–378
anterior cruciate tear, 521
anteroposterior (AP), 606
anthelmintic therapy, 312
anthranilic acid derivatives, 403
anti-beta-2-glycoprotein, 626
antibiotic therapy, 124, 130, 422, 461
antibiotics, 141, 159, 167, 181, 237, 255, 259, 266

antibody titre for acetylcholine receptor (AChR-Ab), 550
anticholinergics, 114, 243, 553
anticipatory guidance, 3, 15–18
anticonvulsants, 63, 555
antidepressants, 164, 385, 640, 646, 649, 651, 653
antidiarrhoeal therapy, 266–267, 296
antiemetics, 243, 540
antiepileptic drugs (AED), 540, 557–558
antihistamines, 112, 114, 126, 142, 167, 477, 482, 487, 537
antihypertensive, 580
antimicrobial resistance rates, 142
antimicrobial therapy, 308
antimicrobials, 120
antinuclear antibody (ANA), 625, 626
antiplatelet therapy
    atrial fibrillation, 199
    transient ischaemic attacks, 563
antipyretics, 437, 456, 562
antiretroviral therapy (ART), 443, 500
antisecretory therapy, 308
antispasmodics, 245, 296, 302
antithyroid, 602
antitubercular triple therapy, 325
antiviral agents, 178, 434, 475, 568
anxiety, 633, 635
anxiolytic agents, 651
AOM. See acute otitis media
aortic regurgitation, 220, 221
aortic stenosis, 220, 221
apixaban, 199, 208
aplastic anaemia, 366
apnea hypopnoea index (AHI), 173
appendicitis, 234, 235–237
appendix, during pregnancy, 236
aqueous crystalline penicillin G, 437
ARF. See acute rheumatic fever
aripiprazole, 640
arousal disorder, 409
arrhythmias, 191–193
ART. See antiretroviral therapy
arterial blood gases (ABGs), 172
    respiratory syncytial virus, 180
arterial/ischaemic ulcer, 99
arthritis, 458, 467
arylacetic acid derivatives, 403
AS. See ankylosing spondylitis
5-ASA. See aminosalicylates
ASB. See asymptomatic bacteriuria
Ascaris lumbricoides, 311
ASCUS. See atypical squamous cells of undetermined significance
asenapine, 640
aspartate transaminase (AST), 242, 299
aspergillus, 129
AST. See aspartate transaminase
asthma, 153–157, 169
    medications for, 156–157
astrovirus, 265
asymptomatic bacteriuria (ASB), 344, 354
atenolol, 199
atherosclerosis, 194–197
atherosclerotic cardiovascular disease (ASCVD), 194, 196, 575
atomoxetine, 636
atonic seizures, 556
atopic dermatitis, 77–78
atrial fibrillation (AF), 191, 192, 197–200
atrioventricular nodal reentrant tachycardia (AVNRT), 191, 192
atrioventricular reentrant tachycardia (AVRT), 191
atrophic gastritis, 301
atrophic rhinitis, 137
atrophic vaginitis, 391–392

atropine, 253
attention deficit hyperactivity disorder (ADHD), 634, 635–637
atypical antipsychotics, 639–640
atypical squamous cells, 419
atypical squamous cells of undetermined significance (ASCUS), 419, 435
atypical squamous cells–cannot exclude HSIL (ASC-H), 435
audiogram, 133
    for vertigo, 567
augmentin, 374, 380
auscultation, 133
autoimmune disorders, 497, 571, 620
autoimmune thyroid disorders, 241
autoimmune thyroiditis, 599
avian flu, 450, 451
avulsed tooth, 143
axonal death, 546
AZA. See azathioprine
azathioprine (AZA), 251, 627
azithromycin, 79, 83, 108, 109, 111, 126, 141, 149, 220, 430, 431, 432, 433, 442, 443, 462, 471, 482

Babinski reflex, 38
baby blues, 385
Bacillus Calmette–Guérin (BCG), 334
bacitracin, 108, 111, 113
bacitracin zinc ophthalmic ointment, 113, 120
bacitracin/polymyxin B ointment, 111
bacterial and viral gastroenteritis. See gastroenteritis
bacterial vaginosis (BV), 392–394
Bacteroides, 387, 460
Bacteroides fragilis, 235
barbiturates, 63, 79
bariatric surgery, 34–41
    annual laboratory monitoring, 40
    complications, 37–38
    surgical weight loss procedures, 35
    types of, 37
    vitamin deficiencies, 36
Bartholin's cyst, 394–395
Bartonella, 442
Bartonella henselae, 441, 442
basal body temperature (BBT), 414–415
basal cell carcinoma (BCC), 73, 90
basement membrane (GBM), 320
BBT. See basal body temperature
BCC. See basal cell carcinoma
Beck Depression Inventory, 63, 529, 642
beclomethasone dipropionate, 136
behavioural therapy, 33, 42, 133, 336
Behcet's syndrome, 122
belladonna, 418
Bell's palsy, 457, 525–527
benign paroxysmal positional vertigo (BPPV), 565, 567
benign prostatic hypertrophy (BPH), 317–319, 352
benign skin lesions, 73–74
benserazid, 555
benzathine penicillin G, 437, 471
benzeneacetic acid derivatives, 403
benzodiazepines, 63, 555
benzoyl peroxide, 71
benztropine, 553
beta-blockers, 540, 597
beta-haemolytic *Streptococcus*, 379
beta-lactam, 131
beta-lactamase-resistant antibiotic, 126
betamethasone, 78, 80, 96, 378
beta-mimetic agents, 367
betaxolol, 199
Bethesda System, 419

biceps reflex tests, 516
bilateral salpingo-oophorectomy, 409
bilateral sciatica, 520
biliopancreatic diversion with duodenal switch (BPD/DS), 38
bilirubin, 242
bimanual examination
    first trimester, 375
    preterm labour, 371
biophysical profile (BPP), 368, 370
bipolar disorder, 634, 637–641
bipolar I disorder, 637
bipolar II disorder, 637
bisoprolol, 199
bisphosphonates, 614
bites, 73
bladder control diary, 353–354
bladder function, 383
bladder outlet obstruction (BOO), 317
bland diet, 667
blepharitis, 108–109
bloody discharge, 376
blues questionnaire, 386
BMD. *See* bone mineral density
BMI. *See* body mass index
BNP. *See* brain natriuretic peptide
body lice, 87
body mass index (BMI), 3, 31, 32, 591
boggy uterus, 381
bone loss, 560
bone marrow aspiration, 505
bone mineral density (BMD), 612, 613
BOO. *See* bladder outlet obstruction
Bordetella pertussis, 160
Borrelia burgdorferi, 457, 458
bosentan, 621
botulinum toxin A (BTX-A), 334
bowel function, 383
Bowen's disease, 91
BP. *See* blood pressure
BPH. *See* benign prostatic hypertrophy
BPP. *See* biophysical profile
BPPV. *See* benign paroxysmal positional vertigo
brachioradialis reflex tests, 516
bradycardia, 191, 192
bradykinesia, 552
brain natriuretic peptide (BNP), 164
BRAT diet, 674
breast abscess, 382
breast cancer, 584, 585
breast engorgement, 378–379
breast pain, 395–397
breastfeeding, 186, 241, 267, 272
British Thoracic Society, 176
bromocriptine, 553
bromocriptine mesylate, 553
bronchiolitis, 162–160
bronchitis, 160–161
bronchodilators, 159, 180
bronchoscopy, 185
    viral croup, 171
Brudzinski's sign, 447, 448, 450, 452, 458, 461, 466, 489
budesonide, 136, 253
Buerger's disease, 223
bulk-forming agents, 250
bupivacaine, 621
bupropion, 636
buspirone, 634
BV. *See* bacterial vaginosis

caesarean section, 387
caffeine, 613, 614, 621
calamine lotion, 392
calcium, 574, 614
calcium carbonate, 601
calcium deficiency, 36, 37
calcium pyrophosphate dihydrate (CPPD), 616
calcium toxicity, 36, 37
calcium-rich foods, 675
caloric test, 567
CAMH. *See* Centre for Addictions and Mental Health
campho-phenique, 83
Campylobacter species, 258
Canada Food and Drugs Act, 657
Canada's Low Risk Alcohol Drinking Guidelines, 41
Canadian Academy of Sport and Exercise Medicine, 655
Canadian Association of Gastroenterology, 239
Canadian Cancer Society, 147
Canadian Centre for Mental Health and Sport (CCMHS), 657
Canadian Centre on Substance Abuse (CCSA), 656
Canadian child welfare law, 51
Canadian National Shelter, 29
Canadian Network for Mood and Anxiety Treatments (CANMAT), 643
Canadian Paediatric Society (CPS), 456, 459
Canadian Task Force on Preventive Health Care, 31, 34
Canadian Tobacco, Alcohol and Drugs Survey (CTADS), 41
Canadian Urology Association, 333
canalith repositioning procedures (CRP), 567
cancerous skin lesions, 90–91
Candida albicans, 74, 95, 148, 150, 425
Candida krusei, 425
Candida parapsilosis, 425
Candida tropicalis, 4257
candidiasis, 74–75, 77, 116, 150
CANMAT. *See* Canadian Network for Mood and Anxiety Treatments
capsaicin cream, 612
capsule enteroscopy, 252
carbamazepine, 32, 63, 132, 463, 533, 560, 568, 639
carbidopa, 555
carbohydrates, 674
carbon monoxide poisoning, 537
carbuncle, 81
cardiac aetiology, 200
cardiopulmonary resuscitation (CPR), 190
cardioselective beta-blockers, 165
cardiovascular disease (CVD), 109, 181, 194, 319, 325, 575, 580, 601
cardiovascular guidelines
    acute myocardial infarction, 189–191
    arrhythmias, 191–193
    atherosclerosis, 194–197
    atrial fibrillation, 197–200
    chest pain, 200–204
    chronic venous insufficiency, 205–207
    deep vein thrombosis, 207–208
    heart failure, 209–212
    hyperlipidaemia, 194–197
    hypertension, 213–216
    lymphoedema, 217–218
    murmur, 218–221
    palpitations, 221–222
    peripheral arterial disease, 222–225
    superficial thrombophlebitis, 225–227
    syncope, 227–230
    varicose veins, 205–207
carisoprodol, 517
carotid dissection, 537
carotid Doppler ultrasonography, 564
carotid sinus massage, 229

carpal tunnel syndrome (CTS), 527–528
Carrion's disease, 442
cat scratch disease (CSD), 441–443
cataplexy, 651
cataracts, 109–110
cauda equina syndrome, 519, 520
CBT. *See* cognitive behaviour therapy
CCMHS. *See* Canadian Centre for Mental Health and Sport
CCSA. *See* Canadian Centre on Substance Abuse
CD. *See* Crohn's disease
cefazolin, 177, 220, 243
cefdinir, 126
cefixime, 126, 357, 432, 433
cefotaxime, 145, 461
cefoxitin, 388
cefpodoxime, 126
cefprozil, 126, 141
ceftazidim, 462
ceftriaxone, 126, 145, 149, 220, 242, 380, 422, 430, 432, 433, 458, 459, 461, 462
cefuroxime, 126, 141, 145, 458
celecoxib, 66, 606, 612, 624
celiac disease, 238–241
    histologic stages of, 238
    tests and positive results, 240
celiac sprue. *See* celiac disease
central nervous system (CNS), 465, 626
central sensitization, 61
Centre for Addictions and Mental Health (CAMH), 641
cephalexin, 81, 130, 144, 149, 356, 374, 380, 383, 471
cephalosporin therapy, 462
cephalosporins, 432, 473
certolizumab, 255
certolizumab pegol, 619, 624
cerumen impaction (earwax), 126–127
cervical cancer, 419
cervical caps, 400
cervical dysplasia, 419
cervical epithelium, 419
cervical motion tenderness (CMT), 421
cervical spine, radiology of, 516
cervical strain, 515
cervicitis, 397–398
cetirizine, 89, 136
cetirizine HCl, 78
Chadwick's sign, 375
chalazion, 110, 120
chemoprophylaxis, 461
chemotherapy, 186, 376
cherry angioma, 74
chest computed tomography for COPD, 164
chest pain, 200–204
    aetiologies, 201–202
chest radiograph (CXR)
    asthma, 153
    bronchiolitis, 159
    cholecystitis, 243
    chronic obstructive pulmonary disease, 163
    pneumonia, 176
    respiratory syncytial virus, 180
    tuberculosis, 185
    viral croup, 171
chickenpox, 83
child neglect, 49
Child Protection Services, 50, 51
Child Welfare, 50
childhood
    abuse, 49
    obesity, 31
    physical abuse, 49
    sexual abuse, 49

children
  acute sinusitis/rhinosinusitis, 141–142
  appendicitis, 235
  atherosclerosis, 197
  atopic dermatitis, 78
  failure to thrive, 645
  nausea, 674
  obstructive sleep apnoea, 173
  pyelonephritis, 342
  transient ischaemic attacks, 565
  violence, 49–52
  vomiting diet, 674
Children's Aid Society, 50
Children's Services, 50
Chlamydia, 110, 111, 112, 323, 338, 430–431
Chlamydia pneumoniae, 162, 175, 177
Chlamydia trachomatis, 148, 149, 175, 323, 324, 336, 393, 397, 430, 431
chlorambucil, 627
chloramphenicol, 473, 474
chlorpromazine, 640
cholecalciferol, 631
cholecystitis, 241–243
cholescintigraphy, 243
cholesterol, 194, 601, 672
cholesterol stones, 242
cholesterol-lowering drugs, 242
cholestyramine, 601
cholinesterase inhibitors, 525
cholinesterase-inhibiting drug test, 551
chondrocalcinosis, 617
chondrocytes, 611
chondroitin, 612
chorionic villus sampling (CVS), 364
chronic bleeding, 365
chronic cervicitis, 397
chronic daily headaches, 534
chronic diarrhoea, 258
chronic disease, 618
chronic epididymitis, 323, 324
chronic fatigue syndrome, 495–497
chronic gout, 610
chronic hypertension, 560
chronic illnesses, 29
chronic kidney disease (CKD), 582
  in adults, 319–323
  stages of, 319
chronic limb ischaemia, 223
chronic medical problems, 642
chronic meningitis, 460
chronic neck pain, 515
chronic obstructive pulmonary disease (COPD), 162–165
chronic otitis externa, 129
chronic pain, 61–64, 231, 651
chronic pulmonary disease, 452
chronic sinusitis, 139
chronic traumatic encephalopathy (CTE), 543
chronic tubulointerstitial nephritis (CTIN), 320
chronic venous insufficiency (CVI), 205–207
chronic vertigo, 567, 568
chronically homeless, 29
chronic/tophaceous gout, 609
cidofovir, 445
cimetidine, 308, 309, 334, 339, 487, 585
cinnarizine, 568
ciprofloxacin, 111, 113, 128, 255, 257, 261, 343, 356, 462
CIS. *See* clinically isolated syndrome
citalopram, 385, 418, 634
clarithromycin, 85, 126, 141, 142, 149, 220, 442, 471
clavulanate, 73, 77, 141

clavulanic acid, 126, 145, 261
clavulin, 388
clearance, for sport participation, 656
client education before exercise, 21
Client Heath Questionnaire (PHQ)-9, 529
client-administered tests, 642
clindamycin, 85, 144, 149, 220, 380, 383, 388, 394, 471, 484
clinically isolated syndrome (CIS), 546
clobetasol, 89
clobetasol propionate, 78, 80
clock draw test (CDT), 524, 530
clomiphene, 594
clonadine, 636
clonazepam, 548, 549, 555, 568, 635, 639
clonidine, 418
clopidogrel, 309, 564
closed head injury (CHI), 543
Clostridium, 387
Clostridium difficile, 258, 296
Clostridium perfringens, 380
clotrimazole, 75, 77, 97, 98, 130, 149, 426
clotrimazole troche, 151
cloxacillin, 85, 114, 116
clozapine, 32, 653
cluster headaches, 534
cluster or vascular headaches, 537
CMT. *See* cervical motion tenderness
CMV. *See* cytomegalovirus
coagulation tests
  idiopathic thrombocytopaenic purpura, 505
  secondary postpartum haemorrhage, 381
cobblestone, 135
COC. *See* combined oral contraceptive
codeine, 167, 253, 383
cognitive behaviour therapy (CBT), 634
cognitive-based therapy, 33
colchicine, 610
colic, 243–245
collateral ligament tear, 521
colonoscopy, 274, 275
  Crohn's disease, 252
Colorado tick fever, 446
colorectal cancer screening, 245–246
columnar epithelium, 419
combined oestrogen/progesterone contraceptives, 401
combined oral contraceptive (COC), 409
common cold, 166–168
common wart, 99
commonly abused drugs, 43–45
community-based care, 30
complete miscarriage, 375, 376
complex febrile seizures, 561
complex partial seizure (CPS), 556
complicated or prolonged grief, 648
compression of median nerve, 527
compressive pain, 61, 63
conductive hearing loss, 128
congenital adrenal hyperplasia (CAH), 586
congenital aganglionic megacolon, 291–292
congestive heart failure (CHF), 469
conjugate vaccines, 459
conjugated oestrogen, 392
conjunctiva, 117
conjunctivitis, 110–112
constipation, 246–250
contact dermatitis, 76–77
contraception, 398–402
contraception, emergency, 407
COPD. *See* chronic obstructive pulmonary disease
Core Back Tool, 65

cornea, 117
corneal abrasion, 112–113
corticosteroids, 157, 159, 167, 180, 240, 253, 255, 370, 372, 442, 448, 464, 612, 627
cortisone acetate, 572
cortisporin, 130
Corynebacterium diphtheriae, 148, 160
costovertebral angle (CVA), 148, 333
co-trimoxazole, 81
cough, 168–170
coumadin, 670–671
Coxiella burnetiid, 177
coxsackievirus, 110, 148
CPS. *See* Canadian Paediatric Society
CRA, 622
C-reactive protein (CRP), 498
  diverticulitis, 261
Criminal Code of Canada, 52
Crohn's disease (CD), 122, 250–256
  medications for, 254
cromolyn sodium ophthalmic, 112
CRP. *See* canalith repositioning procedures; C-reactive protein
cryotherapy, 435
cryptorchidism, 348–349
CSD. *See* cat scratch disease
CSF. *See* cerebrospinal fluid
CT. *See* computed tomography
CT urography (CTU), 330
CTADS. *See* Canadian Tobacco, Alcohol and Drugs Survey
CTE. *See* chronic traumatic encephalopathy
CTIN. *See* chronic tubulointerstitial nephritis
CTS. *See* carpal tunnel syndrome
cultural competence, 3
cultural diversity, 3–4
cultural safety, 3–4
cultural sensitivity, 3
culture, 3–4
Cushing's syndrome, 573–575, 586
CVA. *See* costovertebral angle
CVD. *See* cardiovascular disease
cyclobenzaprine, 517, 520, 608
cyclobenzaprine HCL, 66
cyclophosphamide, 627
Cyclospora cayetanensis, 256
cyclosporiasis, 256–257
cyclosporine, 242
cyclothymic disorder, 637
cyproheptadine, 32
cyproterone acetate, 587
cytomegalovirus (CMV), 336–337, 443–446

dabigatran, 199, 208, 309
dacryocystitis, 113–114, 116
dalfampridine, 548
dalteparin sodium, 208
danazol, 396, 409
darifenacin, 352
DASH diet, 667–670
debilitating disease, 130
decongestants, 137, 621
deep tendon reflexes (DTRs), 38, 60, 62, 414, 516, 547
deep tissue pressure injury (DTPI), 102
deep vein thrombosis (DVT), 38, 205, 207–208
DEET. *See* N-diethyl-m-toluamide
degenerative disorders, 65, 515
degenerative joint disease, 610
delirium, 641
dementia, 528–531, 641
  identify stage of, 524
dendritic ulcer, 116

denosumab, 614
dental abscess, 140, 144
depot medroxyprogesterone acetate (DMPA), 400
depression, 634, 638, 641–644, 647, 648, 657
  drugs used for, 644
  treatment of, 525
Dermacentor andersoni, 472
Dermacentor variabilis, 472
dermatitis, 77
dermatology guidelines
  acne rosacea, 69–70
  acne vulgaris, 70–71
  animal bites, mammalian, 72–73
  benign skin lesions, 73–74
  candidiasis, 74–75
  contact dermatitis, 76–77
  eczema or atopic dermatitis, 77–78
  erythema multiforme, 79–80
  folliculitis, 80–81
  hand, foot, and mouth syndrome, 81–82
  herpes simplex virus type 1, 82–83
  herpes zoster or shingles, 83–84
  impetigo, 84–85
  insect bites and stings, 85–86
  mammalian, 72–73
  pediculosis (lice), 86–88
  pityriasis rosea, 89–90
  precancerous or cancerous skin lesions, 90–91
  psoriasis, 91–93
  scabies, 93–94
  seborrhoeic dermatitis, 95–96
  tinea corporis (ringworm), 96–97
  tinea versicolour, 97–98
  warts, 98–99
  wound care. *See* wound care
  wounds of the skin, 103–105
  xerosis (winter itch), 105
dermatosis papulosa nigra, 74
desipramine, 296
desire disorder, 409
desloratadine, 136
desogestrel, 594
desvenlafaxine, 418
detoxification, 47
DEXA. *See* dual-energy x-ray absorptiometry
dexamethasone, 305, 378, 461, 575
dexlansoprazole, 308
dextroamphetamine, 636
dextromethorphan, 139, 167
diabetes, 362
  exercise plan, 577
  medication/class, 581
  nutritional plan, 577–578
  psychosocial support, 577
  type 1, 574, 575
  type 2, 574, 575, 578
diabetes mellitus (DM), 366, 575–583
diabetes mellitus screen (DMS), 367
diabetic foot ulcer, 99
diaper dermatitis, 77
diaphragms, 399
diarrhoea, 241, 250, 256, 258–259, 267, 271
diastasis hernia, 286
diastolic blood pressure (DBP), 213
diastolic murmurs, 220
diazepam, 370, 568
diclofenac, 113, 606
diclofenac gel, 612
diclofenac potassium, 403
dicloxacillin, 130, 383
dicyclomine, 245, 296
diet recommendations
  anti-hypertension diet, 667–670

bland diet, 667
calcium handout, 674–675
DASH diet, 667–670
gluten-free diet, 671
high-fiber diet, 671–672
lactose-intolerance diet, 672
low-fat/low-cholesterol diet, 672–674
nausea and vomiting diet suggestions, 674
vitamin D, 674–675
warfarin, foods to avoid, 670–671
dietary approaches to stop hypertension (DASH) diet, 591, 667–670
dietary fiber supplementation, 250
dietary management
  acute myocardial infarction, 190
  atherosclerosis, 195
  atrial fibrillation, 199
  cholecystitis, 243
  chronic obstructive pulmonary disease, 164
  colic, 245
  constipation, 248
  Crohn's disease, 252–253
  cyclosporiasis, 257
  diverticulitis, 261
  failure to thrive, 646
  gastroenteritis, 266
  gastro-oesophageal reflux disease, 269
  gestational diabetes mellitus, 368
  Giardia intestinalis, 272
  heart failure, 211
  hypertension, 215
  irritable bowel syndrome, 296
  malabsorption, 302
  mastitis, 383
  obstructive sleep apnoea, 174
  peptic ulcer disease, 308
  peripheral arterial disease, 224
  pneumonia, 176
  pyelonephritis in pregnancy, 374
  renal calculi, 346
  respiratory syncytial virus, 180
  shortness of breath, 183
  ulcerative colitis, 314–315
  urinary tract infections, 356
  viral croup, 172
  viral pneumonia, 178
  wound infection, 388
dietary nonadherence, 238
dietary plan, obesity, 33
digital rectal examination (DRE), 318
digoxin, 199, 471, 585
dihydroergotamine mesylate, 541
diltiazem, 199, 585
dimenhydrinate, 305, 568
dimethyl fumarate, 548
dimethyl sulfoxide (DMSO), 334
diphenhydramine, 77, 78, 83, 86, 94, 105, 112, 405, 477, 487, 568
diphenhydramine HCl, 78
diphenoxylate, 253
diphenylhydantoin, 624
diphtheria, tetanus, and pertussis (DTaP) vaccine, 267
dipyridamole, 309, 534, 564
direct inguinal hernias, 288–289
direct oral anticoagulants (DOACs), 564
discoid lupus erythematosus (DLE), 625
disease-modifying antirheumatic drugs (DMARDs), 619, 623, 624
disease-modifying drugs, 548
disopyramide, 199
disulfiram therapy, 47
diuretics, 114, 568
divalproex sodium, 639
diverticulitis, 260–262
diverticulosis, 260–262

Dix–Hallpike test, 567
dizziness, 655
DLE. *See* discoid lupus erythematosus
DM. *See* diabetes mellitus
DMARDs. *See* disease-modifying antirheumatic drugs
DMPA. *See* depot medroxyprogesterone acetate
docusate calcium, 274
docusate sodium, 274
domperidone, 305
donepezil, 525, 530
dopamine, 553, 599
dopaminergic agents, 555
dowager's hump, 612
Down's syndrome, 364
doxazosin, 32, 318
doxepin, 32
doxycycline, 70, 71, 73, 81, 108, 142, 380, 431, 432, 437, 438, 442, 443, 458, 473, 474
DRE. *See* digital rectal examination
dronedarone, 199
drop seizures. *See* atonic seizures
drospirenone, 594
drug dissolution therapy, 243
drug misuse/dependence, 634, 642
drug–drug interactions, 639
dry diet, 674
dry eyes, 114–115
dry powder inhaler (DPI), 155
DTPI. *See* deep tissue pressure injury
DTRs. *See* deep tendon reflexes
dual-energy x-ray absorptiometry (DEXA), 38, 613
duloxetine, 634
duloxetine HCl, 608
dumping syndrome, 36, 39
dutasteride, 319
dyslipidaemia, 322
dysmenorrhoea, 402–404
dyspareunia, 404–406
dyspnoea. *See* shortness of breath
dysuria, 373

ear guidelines
  acute otitis media, 125–126
  cerumen impaction (earwax), 126–127
  hearing loss, 127–129
  otitis externa, 129–131
  otitis media with effusion, 131–132
  tinnitus, 132–133
early systolic murmurs, 219
EBV. *See* Epstein–Barr virus
EC. *See* emergency contraception
eclampsia, 556, 557
ectocervix, 419
ectopic pregnancy, 237, 374, 375, 376
eczema, 77–78
eczema herpeticum, 78
eczematous otitis externa, 129
ED. *See* erectile dysfunction
edoxaban, 199, 208
effective refractory period (ERP), 192
eflornithine, 594
EFM. *See* external foetal monitor
EIA. *See* enzyme immunoassay
Eikenella, 72
ejection fraction (EF), 209
elbows, 516
elderly
  atopic dermatitis, 78
  clients, 644
  contact dermatitis, 77
  homelessness, 31
  shingles, 84

electroconvulsive therapy (ECT), 640
electroencephalography (EEG)
  attention deficit hyperactivity disorder, 636
  bipolar disorder, 638
  cholecystitis, 243
  seizures, 562
  transient ischaemic attacks, 564
electrolytes, 567
electromyography (EMG)
  carpal tunnel syndrome, 527–528
  neck and upper back disorders, 516
electronystagmography, 567
elevated liver enzymes, 262–264
  differential diagnosis with, 264
ELISA. *See* enzyme-linked immunosorbent assay
eluxadoline, 297
emergency contraception (EC), 406–407
emergent pain, 231
EMG. *See* electromyography
emotional harm, 49
empiric therapy, 308, 461
empirical treatment, 430, 432
encephalitis, 446–449
encephalopathy, 446
endocarditis, 442
endocervical cells, 420
endocervix, 419
endocrine guidelines
  Addison's disease, 571–573
  cushing's syndrome, 573–575
  diabetes mellitus, 575–583
  galactorrhoea, 584–585
  gynaecomastia, 585–586
  hirsutism, 586–588
  hypogonadism, 588–589
  metabolic syndrome/insulin, 589–591
  polycystic ovarian syndrome (PCOS), 592–594
  thyroid disease, 595–602
  thyrotoxicosis/thyroid storm, 602–603
endometrial biopsy, 415
endometriosis, 402, 408–409
endometritis, 379–380
endoscopic retrograde cholangiopancreatography (ERCP), 243
endoscopy, 269
  celiac disease, 239
enoxaparin sodium, 208
enteric cytopathic human orphan (ECHO) viruses, 110
  pharyngitis, 148
Enterobacter, 72, 342, 355, 373
Enterobius vermicularis, 309
Enterococci, 355
Enterococcus, 336, 380
enzyme immunoassay (EIA), 64, 271, 437
enzyme-linked immunosorbent assay (ELISA) test, 86, 136
EOMs. *See* extraocular movements
EP. *See* premature ejaculation
ephedra, 621
epidermidalization, 419
Epidermophyton, 96
epididymitis, 323–325, 332
epigastric hernia, 286
epiglottitis, 145
epilepsy, 556, 557
epilepsy medications, 559
epinephrine, 86, 144
epiphora, 116
episodically homeless, 29
epistaxis, 137–138
epithelial cell abnormalities, 419

Epstein–Barr virus (EBV), 146, 148, 463, 495
erectile dysfunction (ED), 318, 325–328
ergonovine maleate, 381
ergot derivatives, 553
ergotamine, 621
ergotamine tartrate, 418
ergots, 541
erupting teeth, 143
erythema, 108
erythema infectiosum (EI), 467
erythema marginatum, 148, 469
erythema multiforme, 79–80
erythrocyte sedimentation rate (ESR), 638
erythromycin, 70, 71, 77, 81, 108, 114, 116, 149, 431, 433, 438, 471, 482
erythromycin ophthalmic ointment, 108, 110, 111, 113
erythroplakia, 147
Erythrovirus, 467
Escherichia coli, 235, 242, 323, 336, 342, 373, 380, 460
escitalopram, 418, 634
esomeprazole, 308
esotropia, 120
estimated glomerular filtration rate (eGFR), 321
estradiol, 392
estradiol hemihydrate, 392
estrogen, 560
eszopiclone, 651
etanercept, 619, 624
ethacrynic acid, 128
ethinyl estradiol, 594
ethmoid sinusitis, 141
ethosuximide, 560
European League Against Rheumatism (EULAR), 619
eustachian tube dysfunction, 131
evoked response tests (ERTs), 547
excessive tears, 116
excoriated folliculitis, 80
exercise, 5, 21, 33, 64, 518
exercise-induced bronchospasm, 155
exogenous insulin, 578
exogenous platelets, 506
exostoses, 128
exotropia, 120
expectorants, 596
external foetal monitor (EFM), 377
external haemorrhoids, 273, 274
extraocular movements (EOMs), 121
eye drop application, 37
eye guidelines
  amblyopia, 107
  blepharitis, 108–109
  cataracts, 109–110
  chalazion, 110
  conjunctivitis, 110–112
  corneal abrasion, 112–113
  dacryocystitis, 113–114
  dry eyes, 114–115
  excessive tears, 116
  eye pain, 116–118
  glaucoma, acute angle-closure, 118–119
  hordeolum (stye), 119–120
  strabismus, 120–121
  subconjunctival haemorrhage, 121–122
  uveitis, 122–123
eye pain, 116–118
eyelids, 117

facial grading scales, 526
faecal immunochemical test (FIT) testing, 245
faecal impaction, 248
faecal occult blood test (FOBT), 245

failure to thrive (FTT), 244, 645–647
famciclovir, 84, 112, 434
family violence, 49
famotidine, 308
fasting plasma glucose (FPG), 576, 580
fatigue, 495, 497
febrile seizures, 561–562
febuxostat, 610
felbamate, 560
female athlete triad, 658
female condoms, 399
female fitness, and pelvic floor, 658
female sexual dysfunction, 409–411
female sterilization, 400
femoral hernias, 288–289
fesoterodine, 352
fetuses, 444
fever, 561
fevers of unknown origin (FUO), 497–499
fexofenadine, 136
FHR. *See* foetal heart rate
fiber, 671
fibromyalgia (FM), 607–608
fibrosis-4, 284
fifth disease, 467
fifth vital sign, 5
filiform wart, 99
financial exploitation, 56
finasteride, 319, 587
finger-to-nose testing, 547
fingolimod, 548
first trimester, 365, 366, 374–376
first-line drug, 553
first-line therapy, 327–328
first-line treatment, sciatica, 522
Flagyl, 380
flat wart, 99
Flavivirus, 488
flexibility, 656
fluconazole, 75, 97, 151, 426
fluocinonide ointment, 77
fluorescein, 112, 117
fluoroquinolones, 111, 113, 131
fluoxetine, 336, 418, 549, 634
flurazepam, 648, 651
flurocortisone, 572
flutamide, 587
fluticasone furoate, 136
fluticasone propionate, 136
fluvoxamine, 634
FOBT. *See* faecal occult blood test
foetal effects, 361–362
foetal fibronectin, 371, 372
foetal heart rate (FHR), 377, 378
folate deficiency, 36, 37
folic acid supplementation, 253
follicle-stimulating hormone (FSH), 415
folliculitis, 80–81
fondaparinux, 208
foscarnet, 445
fosfomycin, 356
foul odour, 381
fracture risk assessment tool (FRAX), 613
frontal sinusitis, 140
frontotemporal dementia, 528
FTT. *See* failure to thrive
full-thickness skin and tissue loss, 102
fulminant hepatitis, 275
functional incontinence, 350
funduscopic, 576
FUO. *See* fevers of unknown origin
furosemide, 128, 242
furuncle, 80

gabapentin, 32, 63, 84, 418, 533
GABHS. *See* Group A beta-haemolytic streptococcal

GAD. *See* generalized anxiety disorder
galactorrhoea, 584–585
galantamine, 525, 530
gallbladder disease, 241
ganciclovir, 445
gardnerella, 379. *See also* bacterial vaginosis
Gardnerella vaginalis, 336
garlic suppositories, 394
gastric bypass surgery, 39
gastric sleeve (GS), 35, 38
gastric varices, 304
gastroenteritis, 231, 264–267
    infectious agents causing, 265
gastroesophageal reflux, 652
gastrointestinal (GI) aetiology, 200
gastrointestinal guidelines
    abdominal pain, 231–235
    appendicitis, 235–237
    celiac disease, 238–241
    cholecystitis, 241–243
    colic, 243–245
    colorectal cancer screening, 245–246
    congenital aganglionic megacolon, 291–292
    constipation, 246–250
    Crohn's disease, 250–256
    cyclosporiasis, 256–257
    diarrhoea, 258–259
    diverticulosis and diverticulitis, 260–262
    elevated liver enzymes, 262–264
    gastroenteritis, bacterial and viral, 264–267
    gastro-oesophageal reflux disease, 268–270
    Giardia intestinalis, 271–272
    haemorrhoids, 273–275
    hepatitis A, 275–278
    hepatitis B, 278–282
    hepatitis C, 282–285
    hernias. *See* hernias
    Hirschsprung's disease, 291–292
    hookworm, 292–294
    irritable bowel syndrome, 294–297
    jaundice, 298–300
    malabsorption, 301–303
    nausea and vomiting, 303–306
    peptic ulcer disease, 306–309
    pinworm, 309–310
    roundworm, 311–312
    ulcerative colitis, 312–316
gastro-oesophageal reflux disease (GORD), 268–270
GBS. *See* Group B *Streptococcus*
GCA. *See* giant cell arteritis
GDM. *See* gestational diabetes mellitus
GDS. *See* Geriatric Depression Scale
general approach to sexually transmitted infections, 429–430
generalized anxiety disorder (GAD), 633–635
generalized lymphadenopathy, 511
genetic screening, 364
genetic testing, 239
genital candidal dermatitis, 151
genital warts, 99
genitourinary guidelines
    benign prostatic hypertrophy, 317–319
    chronic kidney disease in adults, 319–323
    cryptorchidism, 348–349
    epididymitis, 323–325
    erectile dysfunction, 325–328
    haematuria, 329–331
    hydrocele, 331–332
    interstitial cystitis, 333–335
    kidney stones, 344–347
    premature ejaculation, 335–336
    prostatitis, 336–338
    proteinuria, 339–341
    pyelonephritis, 341–344
    renal calculi, 344–347
    testicular torsion, 347–348
    undescended testicles, 348–349
    urinary incontinence, 350–354
    urinary tract infection, 354–358
    varicocele, 358–359
gentamicin, 113, 131, 380, 432, 442, 461
Geriatric Depression Scale (GDS), 529, 642
geriatrics, 115, 122, 132
    abdominal hernias, 288
    abdominal pain, 234–235
    acute myocardial infarction, 191
    acute otitis media, 126
    acute pain, 61
    acute sinusitis/rhinosinusitis, 142
    Addison's disease, 573
    Alzheimer's disease, 525
    animal bites, mammalian, 73
    ankylosing spondylitis, 607
    appendicitis, 237
    asthma, 157
    benign skin lesions, 74
    bipolar disorder, 641
    bladder outlet obstruction, 319
    breast pain, 397
    bronchitis, 161
    cancerous skin lesions, 91
    celiac disease, 241
    cerumen impaction (earwax), 127
    chest pain, 204
    cholecystitis, 243
    chronic obstructive pulmonary disease, 165
    colorectal cancer screening, 246
    common cold, 167
    constipation, 250
    cough, 170
    Crohn's disease, 256
    cytomegalovirus, 446
    deep vein thrombosis, 207
    dementia, 531
    depression, 644
    diarrhoea, 259
    encephalitis, 449
    epididymitis, 325
    epistaxis, 138
    erectile dysfunction, 328
    failure to thrive, 645, 646, 647
    fevers of unknown origin, 499
    fibromyalgia, 608
    gastroenteritis, 267
    gastro-oesophageal reflux disease, 270
    generalized anxiety disorder, 635
    grief, 649
    Guillain–Barreì syndrome, 534
    haematuria, 331
    haemorrhoids, 275
    headache, 538
    hearing loss, 129
    heart failure, 212
    hepatitis A, 278
    hepatitis B, 282
    hepatitis C, 285
    hirsutism, 587
    human papillomavirus, 436
    hypertension, 216
    hyperthyroidism, 598
    hypogonadism, 589
    hypothyroidism, 602
    idiopathic thrombocytopaenic purpura, 506
    influenza, 454
    insect bites and stings, 86
    jaundice, 300
    lymphadenopathy, 512
    malabsorption, 303
    meningitis, 462
    migraine headaches, 542
    mild traumatic brain injury, 545
    mononucleosis, 464
    multiple sclerosis, 549
    murmur, 221
    nausea (vomiting), 306
    neck and upper back disorders, 517
    obesity, 34
    osteoarthritis, 612
    osteoporosis, 615
    otitis externa, 131
    otitis media with effusion, 132
    Parkinson's disease, 554
    pelvic hernias, 290
    peptic ulcer disease, 309
    pernicious anaemia, 514
    pityriasis rosea, 90
    pneumonia, 177
    premature ejaculation, 336
    proteinuria, 341
    pseudogout, 618
    psoriatic arthritis, 619
    pyelonephritis, 344
    restless legs syndrome, 555
    Rheumatoid arthritis, 625
    scabies, 94
    sciatica, 520
    seizures, 560
    shortness of breath, 183
    sleep disorders, 651
    substance use disorders, 48
    suicide, 654
    superficial thrombophlebitis, 227
    syncope, 230
    syphilis, 438
    systemic lupus erythematosus, 627
    temporal arteritis, 630
    testicular torsion, 348
    transient ischaemic attacks, 565
    trichomoniasis, 439
    tuberculosis, 186
    urinary incontinence, 352
    urinary tract infections, 358
    vertigo, 568
    vitamin D deficiency, 631
    West Nile Virus, 490
gestational diabetes, 367, 575, 576, 583
gestational diabetes mellitus (GDM), 366–368, 583
giant cell arteritis (GCA), 628–630
    diagnosis of, 629
Giardia, 265
Giardia intestinalis, 271–272
Giardia lamblia. *See Giardia intestinalis*
giardiasis, 272
gilbert syndrome, 299
gingivitis, 148
ginkgo biloba, 560
glandular cell, 420
glatiramer acetate, 548
glaucoma, acute angle-closure, 118–119
glomerular filtration rate (GFR), 213, 321
glomerular proteinuria, 339
glomus tumours, 128
glucocorticoid gel, 150
glucocorticoid therapy, 130
glucocorticoids, 32, 456, 477, 572, 574, 610, 617
glucosamine, 612
glucose, 638
glucose tolerance test (GTT), 367, 583
gluten-free diet, 239, 671
glyburide, 368
glycerin, 128, 248
goiter, 595

Goldberg Bipolar Screening Quiz, 638
golimumab, 254, 619, 624
gonadotropin-releasing hormone (GnRH), 389, 409, 587
gonorrhea, 111, 112, 323, 430, 431–433
GORD. See gastro-oesophageal reflux disease
goserelin, 409
gout, 609–610
   stages of, 609
gram-negative bacilli, 355
grand mal seizures. See tonic–clonic seizure
granisetron, 305
Graves' disease, 595–598
gray hepatization, pneumonia, 175
grief, 647–649
griseofulvin, 97
groin hernia, 290
group A beta-haemolytic streptococcal (GABHS), 469–471, 480, 481
group A beta-haemolytic *Streptococcus*, 464
group A *Streptococci*, 455
group B *Streptococcus* (GBS), 342, 357, 371, 372, 373, 460, 462
GU. See genitourinary
guanfacine XR, 636
guiafisin, 167
Guillain–Barre syndrome (GBS), 84, 492, 531–534
gynaecomastia, 585–586
gynecologic guidelines
   amenorrhoea, 389–390
   atrophic vaginitis, 391–392
   bacterial vaginosis, 392–394
   Bartholin's cyst, 394–395
   breast pain, 395–397
   cervicitis, 397–398
   contraception, 398–402
   dysmenorrhoea, 402–404
   dyspareunia, 404–406
   emergency contraception, 406–407
   endometriosis, 408–409
   female sexual dysfunction, 409–411
   infertility, 412–415
   menopause, 415–418
   pap smear screening, 418–420
   pelvic inflammatory disease, 420–423
   premenstrual syndrome, 423–425
   vulvovaginal candidiasis, 425–427

HAART. See highly active antiretroviral therapy
haemagglutinins, 451
haematocrit (Hct), 274, 365, 366
haematocrit values for children, 507
haematuria, 329–331, 373
haemoglobin (Hgb), 321, 365, 366
haemoglobin A1C, 367
haemoglobin values for children, 507
haemolysis, elevated liver enzymes, and low platelets (HELLP) syndrome, 263
haemolytic anaemia, 366
Haemophilus influenzae, 110, 125, 140, 145, 175, 177, 451, 453, 459, 461
Haemophilus influenzae type b (Hib) vaccine, 267, 459, 460
haemorrhage, 381
haemorrhoidectomy, 274
haemorrhoids, 273–275
haemostatic deficiencies, 366
haloperidol, 32
hand, foot, and mouth syndrome, 81–82
Hashimoto's thyroiditis, 599
HD. See Hirschsprung's disease
head lice, 87
headache, 534–538
health care fraud and abuse, 56

health maintenance guidelines
   adult preventive health care, 21
   anticipatory guidance, 5, 15–18
   client education before exercise, 21
   culture, cultural safety, and cultural diversity, 3–4
   exercise, 5
   interprofessional collaborative practice, 22
   nutrition, 5, 19, 20
   paediatric well-child examination, 5
   periodic health examination, 21
   Rourke baby record, 5–14
Health Quality Ontario, 60
healthy diet, 19
hearing loss, 127–129
   types of, 127
heart failure (HF), 209–212
   New York Heart Association Functional Classification, 210
   pharmacologic treatment for, 212
   stages, 211
heavy metals, 361
heel spurs, 518
heel-to-shin testing, 547
heel-to-toe tandem gait testing, 547
Hegar's sign, 375
Helicobacter pylori, 306–309
Hemabate, 381
hemoglobin A1C, 576, 578, 582, 583
hepadnavirus, 279
heparin, 208, 613
hepatitis A, 275–278, 429
hepatitis A vaccines, 277
hepatitis B, 278–282, 429
   antigens and antibodies, 280
hepatitis B immunization, 422
hepatitis B vaccine, 267
hepatitis C, 282–285
hepatitis, serologic tests for, 264
hepatitis, viral, 264
hepatojugular reflux (HJR), 220
hepatosplenomegaly, 463
herald patch, 90
herbal remedies, 245
herbals and biotanics, 425
heredity, 527
hernias, 332
   abdominal, 286–288
   pelvic, 288–290
herpangina, 82, 148
herpes simplex encephalitis, 449
herpes simplex type 1, 78
herpes simplex virus (HSV), 113, 150, 433, 434, 444
herpes simplex virus type 1(HSV-1), 78, 82–83, 433
herpes simplex virus type 2(HSV-2), 397, 433–434
herpes virus, 495
herpes zoster, 82, 83–84, 485
herpetic keratoconjunctivitis, 111
heterophile test, 464
HF with reduced ejection fraction (HFrEF), 209
Hib vaccine, 459
high-calorie supplements, 646
high-density lipoprotein cholesterol (HDL-C), 194
high-fiber diet, 671–672
high-grade squamous intraepithelial lesions (HSILs), 419, 435
highly active antiretroviral therapy (HAART), 42, 500, 502
high-power microscope field (HPF), 329
Hirschberg's test, 121
Hirschsprung's disease (HD), 291–292
hirsutism, 586–588

histamine-2receptor antagonists, 269
HIV. See human immunodeficiency virus
H1N1 influenza A, 449–451
Hodgkin's disease, 460
Hodgkin's lymphoma, 512
homelessness, 29–31
Homelessness Partnering Strategy, 29
hookworm, 292–294
hordeolum (stye), 119–120
hormonal intrauterine device, 400
hormone disruption, 406
hormone replacement therapy (HRT), 396, 416, 417
hormones, 406
hospital medical management, Guillain–Barreì syndrome, 533
HPF. See high-power microscope field
HPV. See human papillomavirus
HSV. See herpes simplex virus
HTN. See hypertension
huffing, 48
human bocavirus (hBoV), 162
human chorionic gonadotropin (HCG) test, 232, 236
human herpesvirus 4, 463
human herpesvirus type 6(HHV-6), 474, 475
human immunodeficiency virus (HIV), 499–503
human leukocyte antigen (HLA)-B27 positive, 605, 606
human metapneumovirus (hMPV), 158–160
human papillomavirus (HPV), 397, 429, 434–436
   oral cancer, 146
human pneumovirus, 160
Hutchinson's sign, 84
hydralazine, 211, 370, 510, 625
hydrocele, 331–332
hydrocodone, 167
hydrocortisone, 78, 103, 572, 575
hydrocortisone ointment, 77
hydrogen peroxide, 127
hydroureteronephrosis, 345
hydroxychloroquine, 624
hydroxychloroquine sulfate, 627
5-hydroxytryptamine (5-HT), 294
hydroxyzine, 77, 78
hyoscyamine, 296
hyperandrogenism, 592
hyperemesis gravidarum, 303
hyperglycemia, 578
hyperkalaemia, 322
hyperlipidaemia, 194–197
hyperlipoproteinaemias, 194
hyperplasia, 317
hypertension (HTN), 213–215, 369, 370
   benign prostatic hypertrophy, 318
   chronic kidney disease, 319
hyperthyroid, 602
hyperthyroidism, 595–598, 599
hypertrophic cardiomyopathy, 220
hypnagogic hallucinations, 651
hypnic headache, 538
hypnotic medications, 649
hypoglycemia, 36, 39, 362, 368, 634
hypogonadism, 588–589
hypokalaemia, 247
hypomania, 638
hyponatraemia, 560
hypotension, 232
hypothalamic amenorrhoea, 389
hypothyroidism, 598–602
hysterectomy, 409
hysterosalpingogram (HSG), 414, 421

IADLs. *See* instrumental activities of daily living
IBS. *See* irritable bowel syndrome
ibuprofen, 66, 84, 126, 130, 161, 167, 306, 330, 376, 379, 383, 403, 451, 456, 466, 562, 606, 608, 611, 623
IC. *See* interstitial cystitis
ice therapy, 518
idiopathic peripheral facial palsy. *See* Bell's palsy
idiopathic thrombocytopaenic purpura (ITP), 504–506
idocaine, 63, 83, 104, 138, 150, 336, 405, 518, 621
IELT. *See* intravaginal ejaculation latency time
Ig. *See* immunoglobulin
IgE. *See* immunoglobulin E
IgM antibody capture enzyme-linked immunosorbent assay (MAC-ELISA), 489, 491
imipramine, 32, 296
imipramine hydrochloride, 549
imiquimod, 435
immune system, 618, 623, 625
immunizations, 21, 177, 179, 314, 322, 363, 453, 465, 533
  homelessness, 30
immunocompromised women, bacterial vaginosis, 394
immunoglobulin (Ig), 444, 477, 479, 480
immunoglobulin A (IgA), 583, 626
immunoglobulin E (IgE), 78, 85
immunoglobulin G (IgG), 279, 284, 444, 464, 468, 479, 486, 626
  idiopathic thrombocytopaenic purpura, 505
immunoglobulin M (I_gM), 443, 464, 467, 468, 479, 483, 486, 489, 626
immunomodulatory agents, 253
impetigo, 86, 84–85
impiramine, 636
impotence. *See* erectile dysfunction (ED)
impulse control, 638, 642
inactivated polio vaccine (IPV), 267
incisional hernia, 286
incomplete miscarriage, 375, 376
incontinence-associated dermatitis (IAD), 102
indirect inguinal hernias, 288–289
individual factors, 29
indocin, 610
indomethacin, 132, 378, 606, 617
induced menopause, 415
inevitable miscarriage, 375, 376
infection, 497, 516
infectious disease guidelines
  cat scratch disease, 441–443
  cytomegalovirus, 443–446
  encephalitis, 446–449
  H1N1 influenza A, 449–451
  influenza, 451–454
  Kawasaki disease, 454–457
  Lyme disease, 457–459
  meningitis, 459–462
  mononucleosis, 463–464
  mumps, 465–467
  parvovirus B19, 467–469
  rheumatic fever, 469–471
  Rocky Mountain spotted fever, 472–474
  roseola, 474–475
  rubella, 475–477
  rubeola, 477–480
  scarlet fever, 480–482
  toxoplasmosis, 482–485
  varicella, 485–488
  West Nile Virus, 488–490

Zika virus infection, 490–492
infectious diseases, 362
infertility, 409, 412–415
  pathogenesis of, 413
inflammation, 171
inflammatory bowel diseases (IBDs), 117, 123, 232, 312
inflammatory pain, 61, 63
infliximab, 93, 255, 619, 624
influenza (Flu), 451–454
influenza A virus, 449, 450, 451
influenza B virus, 450, 451, 453
influenza C virus, 450, 453
influenza vaccination, 450, 453, 456
inguinal hernias, 288
inhaled flu vaccine, 155
initial prenatal visit, 363–364
injectable medication, sciatica, 522
injectable medications, 548
injury prevention, 656
innermost mucinous layer, 114
inpatient therapy, 370
insect bites and stings, 85–86
insert intravenous, epiglottitis, 145
insomnia disorders, 649
insomnia/sleep disorder, 650
instrumental activities of daily living (IADLs), 56–57
insufficient sleep syndrome, 650
insulin, 32
  antagonism, 366
  during pregnancy, 368
  therapy, 368
  types of, 579–580
insulin-dependent diabetes mellitus (IDDM), 575
intact skin, 102
intensive behaviour therapy, 33
intercritical gout, 609
interferon alpha, 596, 599
interferon beta-1a, 548
intermittent atrial fibrillation, 197
intermittent claudication (IC), 224
internal haemorrhoids, 273, 274
International Headache Society (IHS), 538
  headaches classification, 535
  migraines classification, 539
International Prostate Symptom Score (IPSS), 317
interstitial cystitis (IC), 333–335
interstitial lung disease, 182
intertriginous dermatitis (ITD), 102
intestinal malrotation, 234
intestinal obstruction, 231, 234
intimate partner violence (IPV), 52–55, 361
intrachalazion, 110
intracranial haemorrhage (ICH), 543
intrahepatic cholestasis, 299, 300
intramuscular (IM), 366, 378, 482
intranasal zolmitriptan, 537
intraocular pressure (IOP), 118, 119
intrauterine device (IUD)
  contraception, 400
  emergency contraception, 407
  pelvic inflammatory disease, 421, 422
intravaginal ejaculation latency time (IELT), 335
intravenous immunoglobulin (IVIG), 456, 468, 471
intussusception, 234
invasive cancer, 419
IOP. *See* intraocular pressure
ipratropium bromide, 139
iprofloxacin, 130
IPV. *See* inactivated polio vaccine; intimate partner violence
iritis, 122

iron deficiency, 36
iron dextran injection, 508
iron sucrose, 508
iron toxicity, 36, 37
iron-deficiency anaemia, 241, 506–509
irritable bowel syndrome (IBS), 231, 238, 294–297
  red-flag differential diagnoses, 295
  rome IV diagnostic criteria, 296
irritant contact dermatitis, 76, 77
ischaemia, 371
isolated diastolic hypertension (IDH), 213
isolated systolic hypertension (ISH), 213
isoniazid, 325, 463, 625
isopropyl alcohol, 130
isotretinoin, 114
itraconazole, 81, 97, 130
itraconazole tablets, 97
IVIG. *See* intravenous immunoglobulin
Ixodes, 457

jantoven, 670–671
Japanese encephalitis (JE), 446, 448
jaundice, 298–300
  classification of, 298
  drugs and herbals associated with, 30299
JE. *See* Japanese encephalitis

Kawasaki disease (KD), 454–457, 482, 512
KD. *See* Kawasaki disease
keratic precipitates, 122
keratitis, 117
keratoacanthoma, 90
keratoconjunctivitis sicca, 114
Kernig's sign, 447, 448, 450, 452, 458, 461, 466, 473, 489
ketoacidosis, 367
ketoconazole, 95–98, 427, 575
ketogenic diets, 560
ketorolac, 113
ketorolac tromethamine, 112
kidney stones, 344–347
killed-virus vaccine, 478
Klebsiella pneumoniae, 342, 354, 373, 380
Klebsiella species, 323, 336
Kleihauer–Betke test, 378
knee injuries, 521
Koplik's spots, 478, 479
Kübler-Ross Grief Cycle, 647
kyphosis, 612–615

labetalol, 370
lacrimal gland, 114
lacrimal sac, 113
lactase, 245
Lactobacillus acidophilus, 394
Lactobacillus fermentum, 383
Lactobacillus reuteri, 245
Lactobacillus salivarius, 383
lactose-intolerance diet, 672
lactulose, 297
LAGB. *See* laparoscopic adjustable gastric band
lamotrigine, 559, 560, 639
lansoprazole, 308
laparoscopic adjustable gastric band (LAGB), 35
  bariatric surgery, 37–38
laparoscopy, 415
laryngoscopy, viral croup, 171
laryngotracheobronchitis. *See* viral croup
laxatives, 247, 249
LEARN model, 4
leflunomide, 619, 624
left lower quadrant (LLQ) pain, 233
left upper quadrant (LUQ) pain, 233
left ventricular ejection fraction (LVEF), 209

Legionella species, 175, 177
Lennox–Gastaut syndrome (LGS), 556
lentiviruses, 500
Leriche syndrome, 223
leucovorin calcium, 484
leukoplakia, 146
leukotrine inhibitors, 157
leuprolide acetate, 403, 409
level of consciousness (LOC), 543
levetiracetam, 560
levodopa, 132, 553, 555
levofloxacin, 142, 343, 356
levothyroxine, 596, 600, 601
Lewy body dementia, 528
lice, 86–88
lichen planus, 88–89
lidocaine, 83, 104, 138, 150, 334, 336, 405, 422
lifelong premature ejaculation, 335
linaclotide, 297
linezolid, 383
lipoprotein metabolism, 196
lisdexamfetamine, 636
lisdexamfetamine dimesylate, 636
Listeria monocytogenes, 460
lithium, 599, 639, 640, 654
liver biopsy, 284
liver chemistry tests and implications, 263
liver, disease of, 264
liver function tests (LFTs), 262
liver spots, 74
localized lympadenopathy, 511
lochia, 380, 381, 383
lone atrial fibrillation, 197
long-acting benzodiazepines, 635
long-acting psychostimulants, 636
long-term insomnia, 649
loperamide, 253, 296
loratadine, 112, 136
lorazepam, 635
low-density lipoprotein (LDL), 322, 668
low-density lipoprotein cholesterol (LDL-C), 194–196, 575, 580, 582
low-dose antidepressant therapy, 497
low-dose suppressive therapy, 338
lower back pain, 65–67
lower extremity ulcer, 99–101
lower urinary tract symptoms (LUTS), 317, 319
low-fat/low-cholesterol diet, 672–674
low-grade squamous intraepithelial lesion (LSIL), 419, 435
low-lying placenta, 376
lubiprostone, 249, 297
lumbar puncture (LP), 533, 540, 558, 562
lupus, 117, 625
luteinizing hormone (LH), 414
LUTS. *See* lower urinary tract symptoms
Lyme disease, 457–459, 526
lymph nodes, 447, 463
lymphadenitis, 442
lymphadenopathy, 500, 509–512
lymphoedema, 217–218

MAC-ELISA. *See* IgM antibody capture enzyme-linked immunosorbent assay
macrolides, 111, 126, 176, 177, 338, 357
magnesium deficiency, 37
magnesium sulphate, 370, 378
malabsorption, 301–303
malabsorptive symptoms, 272
malassezia folliculitis, 80
male condoms, 399
male lower urinary tract symptoms (MLUTS), 319
male sexual partners, 422
male sterilization, 400

malignant melanoma, 73, 90
malnutrition, 5
mammogram, breast pain, 396
mandibular repositioning appliances (MRAs), 174
mania, 637
Mantoux tuberculin skin test, 185
MAOIs. *See* monamine oxidase inhibitors
mast cell stabilizer, 112
mastalgia. *See* breast pain
mastitis, 382–383
maternal age, 361
maxillary sinusitis, 140
maxillomandibular advancement (MMA), 174
MDI. *See* metered-dose inhaler
measles–mumps–rubella (MMR) vaccine, 465, 467, 475, 476, 478, 480, 485
measles vaccine, 479, 480
measles virus, 179
measles–mumps–rubella–varicella (MMRV) vaccine, 465, 475, 476, 478, 485
mebendazole, 293, 310, 312
mechanical pain, 61, 63
meclizine, 548, 568
meconium, 371
median nerve, compression of, 527
medical adhesive–related skin injury (MARSI), 102
medical device pressure injury, 102
medical/surgical management
  Crohn's disease, 253
  diverticulitis, 261
  gastro-oesophageal reflux disease, 269
  haemorrhoids, 274
  myasthenia gravis, 551
  viral croup, 172
medication overuse headaches (MOHs), 534
medication-induced headache, 537
Mediterranean diet, 591
medroxyprogesterone acetate, 409, 594
mefenamic acid, 403
megaloblastic anaemia. *See* pernicious anaemia
megestrol, 646
meibomian gland dysfunction, 108
meibomian glands, 110
meloxicam, 606, 612
memantine, 525, 530
Ménière's disease, 128, 133, 566, 567
meningitis, 459–462, 536
meningococcal vaccines, 462
meniscus tear, 521
menopausal women, 410
menopause, 415–418
menstrual headaches, 537
menstruation, pelvic inflammatory disease, 421
mental health, and sport participation, 657
6-mercaptopurine (6-MP), 253
mesalamine, 253, 255
metabolic acidosis, 322
metabolic disturbances, 234
metabolic syndrome/insulin, 589–591
metabolism, 602
metered-dose inhaler (MDI), 155, 179
metformin, 368, 578, 594
meth mouth, 46
methicillin-resistant *Staphylococcus aureus* (MRSA), 383
methimazole (MMI), 597, 598
methocarbamol, 66
methotrexate (MTX), 255, 376, 619, 623
methylcellulose drops, 527
methyldopa, 370, 585
methylnaltrexone bromide, 250
methylphenidate, 636

methylphenidate hydrochloride, 636
methylprednisolone, 522, 610
metiamide, 308
metoclopramide, 305, 568
metoprolol, 199
metronidazole, 70, 73, 96, 261, 272, 394, 439
metronidazole gel, 394
metyrapone, 574
miconazole, 75, 77, 95, 426
microcytic anaemia, 506
micrographia, 552
microscopic haematuria, 319, 329, 356
Microsporum, 96
mifepristone, 575
migraine headaches, 538–542
migraines, medications for, 540
mild endometriosis, 409
mild intermittent, asthma, 153
mild persistent, asthma, 153
mild traumatic brain injury (MTBI), 542–545
Miller Fisher syndrome (MFS), 531
Mini-Cog, 524
Mini-Mental State Examination (MMSE), 524, 529, 642
minocycline, 70, 71, 463
minor recurrent aphthous stomatitis, 149–150
mirtazapine, 32, 649
misoprostol, 308, 309, 370, 381, 612
mitotane, 574
mitoxantrone, 548
mitral regurgitation, 219, 221
mitral stenosis, 220
mitral valve prolapse (MVP), 219, 220
mixed incontinence, 350
MMA. *See* maxillomandibular advancement
MMI. *See* methimazole
MMSE. *See* Mini-Mental State Examination
modafinil, 549
moderate infection, 130
moderate persistent, asthma, 153
Modification of Diet in Renal Disease (MDRD), 321
Modified Marsh Classification, 238
moisture-associated skin damage (MASD), 102
molluscum contagiosum, 99
mometasone furoate, 136
monamine oxidase inhibitors (MAOIs), 644
mononucleosis, 148
mononucleosis (Epstein–Barr), 463–464
montelukast, 136, 157, 160
Montreal Cognitive Assessment (MOCA), 524
Mood Disorder Questionnaire, 638
mood disorders, 634
mood stabilizers, 639
Moraxella catarrhalis, 125
morphine, 471
moxifloxacin, 111, 142
MR cholangiography, cholecystitis, 243
MRAs. *See* mandibular repositioning appliances
MS. *See* multiple sclerosis
MTBI. *See* mild traumatic brain injury
MTX. *See* methotrexate
mucocutaneous lymph node syndrome, 454
mucolytic agents, 165
mucosa, 135
mucosal erythroplasia, 146–147
mucosal membrane pressure injury, 103
Multi-Matrix System (MMX), 253
multiple sclerosis (MS), 545–549
mumps, 465–467
mumps, measles, and rubella (MMR), 323

murmur, 218–221
muscle relaxants, 520
musculoskeletal aetiology, 200
musculoskeletal guidelines
    neck and upper back disorders, 515–517
        plantar fasciitis, 517–518
        sciatica, 519–520
        sprains: ankle and knee, 520–522
myasthenia gravis (MG), 550–551
mycobacteria, 183
Mycobacterium bovis, 183
Mycobacterium tuberculosis, 160, 183, 337, 460
Mycoplasma pneumoniae, 148, 149, 162, 160, 171, 175, 177
Mycoplasma species, 323, 336, 393
myelogram, neck and upper back disorders, 516
mylase, 242
myocardial infarction (MI), 189–191, 194, 213, 234, 454
myoclonic seizures, 556
myofascial pain syndrome, 61

N-methyl-D-aspartate (NMDA) receptor antagonist, 525
NAATs. *See* Nucleic acid amplification tests
nabilone, 305
nabiximols, 548
nadolol, 199
naproxen, 66, 606, 610, 611, 617, 623
naproxen sodium, 403
narcolepsy, 650
narcotics, 370, 383, 533
nasal guidelines
    acute sinusitis/rhinosinusitis, 139–142
    allergic rhinitis, 135–136
    epistaxis, 137–138
    nonallergic rhinitis, 138–139
nasal saline, 142
nasogastric (NG), 145
nasopharyngeal, 125
natalizumab, 255, 548
National Institute for Health and Clinical Excellence (NICE), 255
National Pressure Ulcer Advisory Panel (NPUAP), 101
natural family planning (NFP), 401
natural menopause, 415
nausea (vomiting), 303–306
N-diethyl-m-toluamide (DEET), 459, 490, 492
Necator americanus, 292, 311
neck and upper back disorders, 515–517
neck pain, 515
necrotizing/malignant otitis externa, 129, 130
neglect, 56
Neisseria, 114
Neisseria gonorrhoeae, 110, 148, 323, 324, 336, 379, 395, 431, 432, 433
Neisseria meningitidis, 459, 460, 461
nematode, 309
neomycin, 111, 130
neoplasms, 497
nephrolithiasis, 344–347
nerve conduction studies, 516
neural tube defects (NTDs), 364
neuraminidases, 450
neurocognitive disorders, 528
neuroinvasive disease, 488, 489, 490
neurologic aetiology, 200
neurologic disease, 114, 442
neurologic disorders, 642
neurologic examination
    Alzheimer's disease, 524
    hyperthyroidism, 596

hypothyroidism, 600
otitis media with effusion, 131
Raynaud's phenomenon, 621
suicide, 653
tinnitus, 133
neurologic guidelines
    Alzheimer's disease, 523–525
    Bell's palsy, 525–527
    carpal tunnel syndrome, 527–528
    dementia, 528–531
    febrile seizures, 561–562
    Guillain–Barreì syndrome, 531–534
    headache, 534–538
    migraine headaches, 538–542
    mild traumatic brain injury, 542–545
    multiple sclerosis, 545–549
    myasthenia gravis, 550–551
    Parkinson's disease, 552–554
    restless legs syndrome, 554–556
    seizures, 556–560
    transient ischaemic attacks, 563–565
    vertigo, 565–569
neurontin, 608
neuropathic pain, 59, 61, 63
neuropathy, 582
neuroprotective agents, 553
new daily persistent headaches (NDPH), 534
New York Heart Association Functional Classification, 210
nicotine replacement therapy (NRT), 164
nifedipine, 274, 534, 585, 621
nipple discharge, 411, 414
nitazoxanide, 272
nitrofurantoin, 357, 374
nitroglycerin, 274, 534
nociceptive pain, 59
nociceptors, 59
nocturnal cough, 169
nocturnal penile tumescence (NPT), 327
nonallergic rhinitis, 138–139
nonbenzodiazepine anxiolytic, 634
noncardiac chest pain, 270
nonergot drugs, 553
nonhormonal intrauterine device, 400
noninsulin-dependent diabetes mellitus (NIDDM), 575
noninvasive prenatal screening, 364
nonlatex condoms, 399
nonnicotine therapy, 47
nonparalytic strabismus, 120
nonpharmacological interventions
    lymphoedema, 218
    migraine headaches, 541
    shortness of breath, 183
nonstatin drug therapy, 196
nonstress test (NST), 368, 370
nonsurgical treatment, obstructive sleep apnoea, 174
nontraumatic neck pain, 516
nontraumatic splenic rupture, 234
nontreponemal, 437
norethindrone, 594
norgestimate, 594
normal grief, 647–648
normal laboratory values, 661–665
norovirus, 265
nortriptyline, 32, 296
NRT. *See* nicotine replacement therapy
NST. *See* nonstress test
NTDs. *See* neural tube defects
nucleic acid amplification tests (NAATs), 430, 432
nutrient deficiencies, 37
nutriguides apps, 239
nutrition, 5, 362
    food servings per day, 19
    for kids, healthy diet, 19

    mineral deficiencies, 20
    vitamin, 20
    well-balanced diets, 5
nutrition therapy, 239
nutritional deficiencies, 20
Nylen–Bárány's maneuver test. *See* Dix–Hallpike test
nystatin, 75, 130, 427

OA. *See* osteoarthritis
OAB. *See* overactive bladder
OAs. *See* oral appliances
obesity, 31–34, 600. *See also* bariatric surgery
    adult, 32
    childhood, 31
obsessive-compulsive disorder, 385
obstructive sleep apnoea (OSA), 172–174, 649
obturator hernia, 286
occupational therapy (OT), 549
OCPs. *See* oral contraceptive pills
OCs. *See* oral contraceptives
oesophageal, 304
oestrogen, 242, 304, 348, 391, 417
oestrogen therapy (OT), 352, 392, 614
oestrogen-induced alteration, 242
ofloxacin, 104, 111, 113, 130, 142, 431
OGTT. *See* oral glucose tolerance test
olanzapine, 32, 640
older adults
    amenorrhoea, 390
    Bartholin's cyst, 395
    medication use in, 21
    nutrition diets, 5
    periodic health examination, 21
    violence, 55–56
olopatadine, 112
olsalazine, 255
OME. *See* otitis media with effusion
omeprazole, 270, 308, 585
ondansetron, 305, 568
onychomycosis, 97
ophthalmic drops, 120
ophthalmic ointment, 113, 120
opiate narcotic analgesics, 242
opiates, 130, 253
opioids, 63, 545, 582, 608
orabase, 150
oral antifungal agents, 426–427
oral appliances (OAs), 174
oral balsalazide, 255
oral bile acid therapy, 243
oral cancer, 146–147
oral candidiasis, 151
oral contraceptive pills (OCPs), 422, 594
oral contraceptives (OCs), 40, 71, 221, 368, 401, 551, 560, 584, 587, 627
oral decongestants, 167
oral glucose tolerance test (OGTT), 367, 577
oral hairy leukoplakia (OHL), 463
oral hormone replacement therapy, 417
oral iron replacement, 508
oral ivermectin, 87
oral medications, 548
oral oestrogen replacement therapy, 392
oral sores, 146
orchitis, 332
organisms, diarrhoea, 258
orgasm disorder, 409
orlistat, 34
oroya fever, 441
orphenadrine, 66
OSA. *See* obstructive sleep apnoea
oseltamivir, 179, 450, 451, 453, 454
osmotic laxatives, 250
osteoarthritis (OA), 610–612

osteopaenia, 612
osteoporosis, 612–615
osteoporotic fracture, 612
OTC. *See* over-the-counter
otic solution, 130
otitis externa, 127, 129–131
otitis media, 123–124
otitis media with effusion (OME), 128, 131–132
otolaryngologist, 129
otomycosis, 130
otosclerosis, 128
otoscope light, 136
outermost lipid layer, 114
ovarian dysfunction, 592
overactive bladder (OAB), 333, 350
Overall Disability Sum Score (ODSS), 531, 532
overflow incontinence, 350
overflow proteinuria, 339
oxcarbazepine, 559, 560
oxybutynin chloride, 352, 549
oxymetazoline hydrochloride, 136
oxytocin, 381

paediatric infectious diseases, 434
paediatric well-child examination, 5
Paget's disease, 129
pain, 59, 518, 520
pain disorder, 409
pain management guidelines
    acute pain, 59–61
    chronic pain, 61–64
    lower back pain, 65–67
pain therapy, 533
painful bladder syndrome (PBS), 333
palivizumab, 159, 160, 180, 181
palpable nodes, 512
palpate spine, 65
palpitations, 221–222
pancrelipase, 302
panic disorder, 385
pantoprazole, 308
Pap smear screening, 418–420
papillomavirus, 146
papule, 441
paralytic strabismus, 120, 121
Paramyxovirus, 465, 478
paromomycin, 272
parathyroid hormone (PTH), 614
parietal pain, 231
Parkinson's disease (PD), 552–554
2018PAR-Q+, 23
paromomycin, 272
paroxetine, 32, 336, 418, 634, 649, 651
paroxysmal atrial fibrillation, 191, 197
partial-thickness skin loss, 102
Partner Violence Screen (PVS), 53
parvovirus B19 (fifth disease, erythema infectiosum), 467–469
pasteurella multocida, 72
Pastia's lines, 148
patellofemoral syndrome, 521
pathogenesis of infertility, 413
Patrick's test, 66
PBS. *See* painful bladder syndrome
PCOS. *See* polycystic ovarian syndrome
PDE-5. *See* phosphodiesterase-5
Pediatric Evaluation of Disability Inventory Computer Adaptive Test (PEDI-CAT), 534
pediatrics, 107, 112, 113, 116, 119, 121
    abdominal hernias, 287–288
    abdominal pain, 234
    acute otitis media, 126
    acute sinusitis/rhinosinusitis, 142
    Addison's disease, 572
    animal bites, mammalian, 73
    appendicitis, 235, 237
    arrhythmias, 193
    asthma, 157
    attention deficit hyperactivity disorder, 637
    avulsed tooth, 144
    bipolar disorder, 641
    bronchitis, 161
    cancerous skin lesions, 91
    cat scratch disease, 443
    celiac disease, 241
    chest pain, 204
    chlamydia, 431
    cholecystitis, 243
    chronic fatigue syndrome, 497
    common cold, 167
    constipation, 249–250
    contact dermatitis, 77
    cough, 170
    Crohn's disease, 255
    cushing's syndrome, 575
    cytomegalovirus, 446
    dementia, 531
    depression, 644
    diabetes mellitus, 583
    diarrhoea, 259
    epididymitis, 325
    epiglottitis, 145
    epistaxis, 138
    erythema multiforme, 80
    failure to thrive, 647
    fevers of unknown origin, 499
    gastroenteritis, 267
    gastro-oesophageal reflux disease, 270
    generalized anxiety disorder, 635
    Giardia intestinalis, 272
    gonorrhoea, 432–433
    gout, 610
    grief, 649
    Guillain–Barre syndrome, 534
    haemorrhoids, 275
    hand, foot, and mouth syndrome, 82
    headache, 537
    hearing loss, 129
    heart failure, 212
    hepatitis A, 278
    hepatitis B, 282
    hepatitis C, 285
    herpes simplex virus-1, 83
    herpes simplex virus type 2, 434
    Hirschsprung's disease, 292
    H1N1 influenza A, 451
    homelessness, 31
    hookworm, 294
    human immunodeficiency virus, 503
    hydrocele, 332
    hyperthyroidism, 598
    idiopathic thrombocytopaenic purpura, 506
    influenza, 452, 454
    insect bites and stings, 86
    interstitial cystitis, 335
    iron-deficiency anaemia, 509
    jaundice, 300
    Kawasaki disease, 456–457
    lice, 88
    lichen planus, 89
    Lyme disease, 459
    lymphadenopathy, 512
    meningitis, 462
    migraine headaches, 542
    mild traumatic brain injury, 545
    mononucleosis, 464
    multiple sclerosis, 549
    mumps, 467
    murmur, 221
    myasthenia gravis, 551
    nausea (vomiting), 305–306
    neck and upper back disorders, 517
    obesity, 34
    oral cancer, 147
    Parkinson's disease, 554
    parvovirus B19, 469
    pelvic hernias, 290
    pelvic inflammatory disease, 423
    pernicious anaemia, 514
    pharyngitis, 149
    pinworm, 310
    pityriasis rosea, 90
    pneumonia, 177
    proteinuria, 341
    pyelonephritis, 344
    Raynaud's phenomenon, 621
    renal calculi, 347
    respiratory syncytial virus, 181
    restless legs syndrome, 555
    Rheumatoid arthritis, 625
    roseola, 475
    roundworm, 310
    rubella, 477
    rubeola, 480
    scabies, 94
    sciatica, 522
    seborrhoeic dermatitis, 95
    seizures, 560, 562
    shingles, 84
    shortness of breath, 183
    sleep disorders, 651
    stomatitis, 150
    substance use disorders, 48
    syphilis, 438
    systemic lupus erythematosus, 627
    temporal arteritis, 630
    testicular torsion, 348
    thrush, 151
    tinea corporis, 97
    toxoplasmosis, 484–485
    tuberculosis, 186
    ulcerative colitis, 316
    undescended testicles, 349
    urinary incontinence, 352
    urinary tract infections, 357–358
    varicella, 487
    varicocele, 359
    vertigo, 568
    viral croup, 172
    viral pneumonia, 179
    vitamin D deficiency, 631
    warts, 99
    West Nile Virus, 490
    Zika virus infection, 492
pediculosis, 86–88
Pediculosis capitis, 87
Pediculosis corporis, 87
peginterferon beta-1a, 548
pelvic floor health, female fitness and, 658
pelvic hernias, 288–290
pelvic inflammatory disease (PID), 420–423, 432
penicillin, 79, 176, 458, 459, 471, 473
penicillin G, 459, 461, 471
penicillin G benzathine, 482
penicillin V, 482
penicillin V potassium, 149
penile implant, 328
pentoxifylline, 224
PEP. *See* postexposure prophylaxis
peptic ulcer, 304
peptic ulcer disease (PUD), 306–309
Peptostreptococcus species, 235
percutaneous coronary intervention (PCI), 190
percutaneous nephrolithotomy, 346
perform traction tests, 66

performance-enhancing substances, 657–658
pergolide mesylate, 553
perianal disease, 256
pericarditis, 455
perimenopause, 415
perineum, 383
periodic limb movement disorder (PLMD), 554
periodic limb movement of sleep (PLMS), 554
peripheral arterial disease (PAD), 205, 222–225
peripheral vascular disease (PVD), 194, 205
peritoneal irritation, 234
peritonsillar cellulitis, 148
permanent atrial fibrillation, 191, 197
permethrin, 87–88, 94
pernicious anaemia, 512–514
persistent atrial fibrillation, 191, 197
persistent proteinuria, 339
personality disorders, 634
pertussis, 168
pesticides, 361–362
petit mal seizures. *See* absent seizures
petroleum jelly, 95, 130, 136
PHAC. *See* Public Health Agency of Canada
Phalen's test, 528
pharmacological interventions
    migraine headaches, 540
    shortness of breath, 183
pharmacological therapy
    abdominal pain, 234
    acne rosacea, 70
    acne vulgaris, 71
    acute myocardial infarction, 190
    acute otitis media, 126
    acute pain, 61
    acute sinusitis/rhinosinusitis, 141
    Addison's disease, 572
    allergic rhinitis, 136
    amenorrhoea, 390
    anaemia, iron deficiency, 366
    animal bites, mammalian, 73
    ankylosing spondylitis, 606–607
    appendicitis, 237
    arrhythmias, 193
    asthma, 155
    atherosclerosis, 195–196
    atopic dermatitis, 78
    atrial fibrillation, 199
    atrophic vaginitis, 392
    attention deficit hyperactivity disorder, 636
    avulsed tooth, 143
    bacterial vaginosis, 394
    bariatric surgery, 39–40
    Bartholin's cyst, 395
    benign skin lesions, 74
    bipolar disorder, 639
    bladder outlet obstruction, 318–319
    blepharitis, 108
    breast engorgement, 379
    breast pain, 396
    bronchiolitis, 161
    bronchitis, 161
    candidiasis, 75
    cat scratch disease, 442
    cerumen impaction (earwax), 127
    cervicitis, 398
    chalazion, 110
    children violence, 51
    chlamydia, 431
    cholecystitis, 243
    chronic fatigue syndrome, 497
    chronic kidney disease, 322
    chronic obstructive pulmonary disease, 164–165
    chronic pain, 63
    colic, 245
    colorectal cancer screening, 246
    common cold, 167
    conjunctivitis, 111
    contact dermatitis, 77
    contraception, 400–401
    corneal abrasion, 113
    cough, 170
    Crohn's disease, 253
    cushing's syndrome, 574–575
    cyclosporiasis, 257
    cytomegalovirus, 445
    dacryocystitis, 114
    deep vein thrombosis, 208
    dementia, 530
    dental abscess, 144
    depression, 643
    diabetes mellitus, 578
    diverticulitis, 261
    dry eyes, 115
    dysmenorrhoea, 403
    dyspareunia, 405
    emergency contraception, 407
    encephalitis, 448
    endometriosis, 409
    endometritis, 380
    epididymitis, 325
    epiglottitis, 145
    epistaxis, 138
    erectile dysfunction, 327–328
    erythema multiforme, 80
    excessive tears, 116
    failure to thrive, 646
    female sexual dysfunction, 411
    fevers of unknown origin, 499
    fibromyalgia, 608
    first trimester, 376
    folliculitis, 81
    galactorrhoea, 585
    gastroenteritis, 266
    gastro-oesophageal reflux disease, 269–270
    generalized anxiety disorder, 634
    gestational diabetes mellitus, 368
    Giardia intestinalis, 272
    glaucoma, acute angle-closure, 119
    gonorrhoea, 432
    gout, 610
    grief, 648
    gynaecomastia, 586
    haematuria, 331
    haemorrhoids, 274
    hand, foot, and mouth syndrome, 82
    heart failure, 211
    hepatitis A, 277
    hepatitis B, 281
    hepatitis C, 284
    herpes simplex virus-1, 83
    herpes simplex virus type 2, 434
    hirsutism, 587
    H1N1 influenza A, 450–451
    hookworm, 293
    hordeolum (stye), 120
    human immunodeficiency virus, 502
    human papillomavirus, 435
    hypertension, 214
    hyperthyroidism, 597
    hypogonadism, 589
    hypothyroidism, 601
    idiopathic thrombocytopaenic purpura, 506
    impetigo, 85
    influenza, 453
    insect bites and stings, 86
    interstitial cystitis, 334
    intimate partner violence, 55
    iron-deficiency anaemia, 508
    irritable bowel syndrome, 296–297
    Kawasaki disease, 456
    lice, 87
    lichen planus, 89
    lower back pain, 66
    lower extremity ulcer, 101
    Lyme disease, 458–459
    lymphadenopathy, 512
    malabsorption, 302
    mastitis, 383
    meningitis, 461–462
    menopause, 417–418
    metabolic syndrome/insulin, 591
    mononucleosis, 464
    multiple sclerosis, 548
    mumps, 466
    murmur, 220
    neck and upper back disorders, 517
    nonallergic rhinitis, 139
    obesity, 34
    older adults violence, 57
    oral cancer, 147
    osteoarthritis, 611–612
    osteoporosis, 614
    otitis externa, 130
    otitis media with effusion, 131–132
    parvovirus B19, 468
    pelvic inflammatory disease, 420
    peptic ulcer disease (PUD), 308
    peripheral arterial disease, 224
    pernicious anaemia, 513
    pharyngitis, 149
    pinworm, 310
    pityriasis rosea, 90
    plantar fasciitis, 518
    pneumonia, 176
    polycystic ovarian syndrome (PCOS), 594
    polymyalgia rheumatica, 616
    postpartum care, 384
    postpartum depression, 385
    preeclampsia, 370
    premature ejaculation, 336
    pressure ulcers, 103
    preterm labour, 372
    prostatitis, 338
    proteinuria, 341
    pseudogout, 617
    psoriasis, 93
    psoriatic arthritis, 619
    pyelonephritis, 343
    pyelonephritis in pregnancy, 374
    Raynaud's phenomenon, 621
    renal calculi, 346
    respiratory syncytial virus, 180–181
    Rheumatoid arthritis, 623–624
    ringworm, 97
    Rocky Mountain spotted fever, 473
    roseola, 475
    roundworm, 312
    rubella, 477
    rubeola, 479
    scabies, 94
    scarlet fever, 482
    sciatica, 520
    seborrhoeic dermatitis, 96
    second trimesters, 378
    secondary postpartum haemorrhage, 381–382
    shingles, 84
    sleep disorders, 651
    sprains: ankle and knee, 522
    stomatitis, 150
    substance use disorders, 47
    suicide, 653–654
    superficial thrombophlebitis, 227
    syncope, 229

pharmacological therapy (cont.)
  syphilis, 437–438
  systemic lupus erythematosus, 627
  temporal arteritis, 630
  third trimesters, 378
  thrush, 151
  tinea versicolour, 98
  tinnitus, 133
  toxoplasmosis, 484
  trichomoniasis, 439
  tuberculosis, 185–186
  ulcerative colitis, 315
  undescended testicles, 349
  urinary incontinence, 352
  urinary tract infections, 356–357
  uveitis, 122
  varicella, 487
  viral croup, 172
  viral pneumonia, 178–179
  vitamin D deficiency, 631
  vulvovaginal candidiasis, 426–427
  warts, 99
  West Nile Virus, 490
  wound infection, 388
  wounds of the skin, 104
  xerosis, 105
  Zika virus infection, 492
pharmacological treatment
  Alzheimer's disease, 525
  Bell's palsy, 527
  carpal tunnel syndrome, 528
  Guillain–Barreì syndrome, 533
  headache, 537
  migraine headaches, 540
  mild traumatic brain injury, 545
  myasthenia gravis, 551
  Parkinson's disease, 553
  restless legs syndrome, 555
  seizures, 558–559, 562
  transient ischaemic attacks, 564
  vertigo, 568
pharmacology, celiac disease, 240
pharyngitis, 147–149
phenazopyridine, 374
phenelzine, 32
phenobarbital, 418, 560, 630
phenothiazine, 114
phenylbutazone, 79
phenylephrine, 136, 142
phenytoin, 63, 79, 370, 463, 560, 630
phosphodiesterase-5(PDE-5), 318, 327–328
physical abuse, 49, 56
physical therapy, 526
  interstitial cystitis, 334
physiologic menopause, 415
physiological anaemia, 366
physiological saline nasal spray, 139
PID. See pelvic inflammatory disease
pigment stones, 242
pilocarpine, 119
pinworm, 309–310
pityriasis rosea, 89–90
pityrosporum, 80
Pityrosporum orbiculare, 97
Pityrosporum ovale, 95
placenta, 376
placenta previa, 376, 377
plantar fasciitis, 517–518
plantar wart, 99
plasmapheresis, 471, 533, 551
platelet count, idiopathic thrombocytopaenic purpura, 505
platelet transfusions, 506
pleural aetiology, 200
Plummer–Vinson syndrome, 146
PMDD. See premenstrual dysphoric disorder
PMR. See polymyalgia rheumatica

PMS. See premenstrual syndrome
pneumatic otoscopy, 131
pneumococcal conjugate vaccine, 267
pneumococcal vaccine, 155, 164, 322, 462, 502
pneumococcus vaccine, 459
Pneumocystis carinii pneumonia (PCP), 175
Pneumocystis jiroveci, 175
pneumonia, 175–177. See also viral pneumonia
podofilox, 435, 436
podophyllum, 435, 436
POF. See premature ovarian failure
Poiseuille's equation, 170
polycystic ovarian syndrome (PCOS), 592–594
  symptoms of, 593
polycystic ovary syndrome (PCOS), 414
polymorphous, 455
polymyalgia rheumatica (PMR), 615–616, 628
polymyxin B, 111, 130
polymyxin B sulfate, 113, 120
polysaccharide vaccine, 459, 462
Porcine circovirus (PCV), 267
postbariatric surgery, 34–41
posterior cruciate tear, 521
postexposure prophylaxis (PEP), 503
postherpetic neuralgia, shingles, 84
postmenopausal women, atrophic vaginitis, 392
postpartum
  breast engorgement, 378–379
  contraception, 368
  depression, 384–386
  endometritis, 379–380
  mastitis, 382–383
  postpartum care: six weeks postpartum examination, 383–384
  postpartum depression, 384–386
  secondary postpartum haemorrhage, 381–382
  thyroiditis, 384
  wound infection, 387–388
postpartum care: six weeks postpartum examination, 383–384
postprimary tuberculosis, 183
postpuberty, 588
posttraumatic headaches, 534
posttreatment Lyme disease syndrome (PTLDS), 457
postural hypotension, 497
postvoid residual (PVR), 334, 351
PPI. See proton pump inhibitors
pramipexole, 553, 555
prasugrel, 309
prazosin, 318
preconception counselling
  human immunodeficiency virus, 502–503
  identifying clients at risk, 361–363
preconceptional care, 361
prednisolone, 157, 253, 506, 522, 548
prednisone, 79, 89, 90, 240, 253, 505, 506, 527, 572, 610, 616, 624, 627
prednisone therapy, 505
preeclampsia, 361, 369–370
pregabalin, 63, 84, 487, 555, 608
pregnancy
  abdominal hernias, 287
  abdominal pain, 234
  acne vulgaris, 71
  Addison's disease, 573
  allergic rhinitis, 136
  animal bites, mammalian, 73
  appendicitis, 237
  asthma, 155, 157
  atopic dermatitis, 78

bacterial vaginosis, 394
bariatric surgery, 40–41
Bartholin's cyst, 395
Bell's palsy, 527
bipolar disorder, 641
breast pain, 396
candidiasis, 75
carpal tunnel syndrome, 528
celiac disease, 241
cervicitis, 398
chest pain, 204
chlamydia, 431
cholecystitis, 243
chronic obstructive pulmonary disease, 165
constipation, 249
contact dermatitis, 77
corneal abrasion, 113
cough, 170
Crohn's disease, 255
cushing's syndrome, 575
cyclosporiasis, 257
cytomegalovirus, 446
dental abscess, 144
depression, 644
diabetes mellitus, 583
dysmenorrhoea, 404
dyspareunia, 405–406
elevated liver enzymes, 263
emergency contraception, 407
endometriosis, 409
epistaxis, 138
exercise, 21
fevers of unknown origin, 499
galactorrhoea, 585
gastro-oesophageal reflux disease, 270
generalized anxiety disorder, 635
Giardia intestinalis, 272
gonorrhoea, 432
grief, 649
haematuria, 331
haemorrhoids, 275
headache, 537
heart failure, 212
hepatitis A, 278
hepatitis B, 282
hepatitis C, 285
herpes simplex virus type 2, 434
hirsutism, 587
H1N1 influenza A, 451
homelessness, 31
hookworm, 293–294
human immunodeficiency virus, 503
hypertension, 216
hypothyroidism, 601
idiopathic thrombocytopaenic purpura, 506
influenza, 451
intimate partner violence, 53, 55
iron-deficiency anaemia, 509
jaundice, 300
lice, 88
lichen planus, 89
lower back pain, 67
Lyme disease, 459
meningitis, 462
migraine headaches, 542
multiple sclerosis, 549
mumps, 466–467
murmur, 221
myasthenia gravis, 551
nausea (vomiting), 305
obesity, 34
osteoarthritis, 612
parvovirus B19, 468–469
pelvic hernias, 290
pelvic inflammatory disease, 423

peptic ulcer disease, 309
pernicious anaemia, 514
pinworm, 310
pityriasis rosea, 90
pneumonia, 177
proteinuria, 341
pyelonephritis, 343, 344
pyelonephritis in pregnancy, 373
renal calculi, 346–347
respiratory syncytial virus, 181
restless legs syndrome, 555
rheumatic fever, 471
Rheumatoid arthritis, 624
Rocky Mountain spotted fever, 474
roundworm, 312
rubella, 477
rubeola, 480
scabies, 94
sciatica, 520
shingles, 84
shortness of breath, 183
sleep disorders, 651
substance use disorders, 48
suicide, 654
superficial thrombophlebitis, 227
syphilis, 438
systemic lupus erythematosus, 627
tinea corporis, 97
toxoplasmosis, 484
trichomoniasis, 439
tuberculosis, 186
urinary incontinence, 352
urinary tract infections, 357
Varicella, 487
viral pneumonia, 179
vitamin D deficiency, 631
vulvovaginal candidiasis, 427
West Nile Virus, 490
Zika virus infection, 492
pregnancy-induced hypertension (PIH), 270, 537
premature ejaculation (EP), 335–336
premature ovarian failure (POF), 415
premature ventricular contractions (PVCs), 191, 192
premenstrual dysphoric disorder (PMDD), 423–425
premenstrual syndrome (PMS), 423–425
  medications used with, 424
prenatal vitamins, 366
prepatellar bursitis, 521
prepuberty, 588
presbycusis, 128
preseptal cellulitis, 120
pressure injury, 102–103
pressure ulcers, 101–103
preterm labour (PTL), 371–372
primary amenorrhoea, 389
primary dysmenorrhoea, 402
primary progressive multiple sclerosis, 546
primary Raynaud's phenomenon, 619, 620
probenecid, 445, 610
procainamide, 625
procaine penicillin, 437
prochlorperazine, 305, 568
proctosigmoiditis, 313
progestational steroids, 32
progesterone, 417, 560
progesterone therapy, 390, 614
progestin-only pills (POPs), 400
progestins, 589, 594
prolapse, 273
prolonged rupture, 380
promethazine, 568
prophylactic therapy, 357, 458, 473
prophylaxis, 366
  human immunodeficiency virus, 503

Propionibacterium acnes, 70
propionic acid derivatives, 403
propranolol, 32, 132, 199, 216, 597
propylthiouracil (PTU), 597, 598
prostate-specific antigen (PSA), 318, 319
prostatitis, 336–338
protein deficiency, 36, 39
protein-to-creatinine ratio (PCR), 339
proteinuria, 321, 339–341, 370
Proteus, 373
Proteus mirabilis, 342, 355, 380
Proteus species, 323
prothrombin time (PT), 239, 299, 302, 330, 375, 378, 505
proton pump inhibitors (PPI), 269–270, 308
PSA. *See* prostate-specific antigen
PsA. *See* psoriatic arthritis
pseudoephedrin, 142
pseudogout, 616–618
pseudomembrane, 148
Pseudomonas, 113, 129, 130, 235, 323, 336, 355, 373
Pseudomonas aeruginosa, 177, 380, 462
pseudostrabismus, 120
psoriasis, 91–93
psoriatic arthritis (PsA), 618–619
psychiatric disease, 247
psychiatric guidelines
  attention deficit hyperactivity disorder, 635–637
  bipolar disorder, 637–641
  depression, 641–644
  failure to thrive, 645–647
  generalized anxiety disorder, 633–635
  grief, 647–649
  sleep disorders, 649–652
  suicide, 652–654
psychiatric syndrome, 634
psychiatry referral, 549
psychogenic aetiology, 203
psychogenic seizures, 557
psychological abuse, 52, 56
psychophysiologic insomnia, 650
psychosis, 385
psychosocial distress, 247
psychotherapy, premature ejaculation, 336
psychotic disorders, 634
psyllium, 261
PTH. *See* parathyroid hormone
Pthirus pubis, 87, 88
PTL. *See* preterm labour
PTLDS. *See* posttreatment Lyme disease syndrome
PTU. *See* propylthiouracil
pubic lice, 87
Public Health Agency of Canada (PHAC), 21, 430–431, 432, 529
public health guidelines
  homelessness, 29–31
  intimate partner violence, 52–55
  obesity, 31–34
  older adults, 55–56
  postbariatric surgery, 34–41
  substance use disorders, 41–48
  violence, 49–52
PUD. *See* peptic ulcer disease
pulmonary embolism (PE), 40, 207, 225
pulmonary function tests (PFTs), 163, 165
pulmonary regurgitation, 220
pulmonic stenosis, 220
pulse oximetry, 171
purified protein derivative (PPD), 164, 185, 252
PVS. *See* Partner Violence Screen
pyelonephritis, 341–344, 354, 357, 373
  in pregnancy, 372–374
pyrantel, 312

pyrantel pamoate, 293
pyrimethamine, 484, 510

quadrivalent influenza vaccine (QIV), 450, 451
quadrivalent live attenuated influenza vaccine (QLAIV), 450, 451
quadruple therapy, 308
quality of life (QOL), 162
quetiapine, 32, 640, 654
quinidine, 128, 199, 271

RA. *See* Rheumatoid arthritis
rabeprazole, 308
rabies, 448
radioactive iodine (RAI), 596, 597
radioactive iodine uptake (RAIU), 596, 597, 601
radiofrequency ablation (RFA), 174
RAI. *See* radioactive iodine
raloxifene, 614
Ramsay Hunt syndrome, 84
random plasma glucose, 577
range of motion (ROM), 521, 615
ranitidine, 269, 308, 309, 585
rapid ACTH, 572
rapid plasma reagin (RPR), 150, 437, 530, 564, 567
rapid strep test, 148
RAS. *See* recurrent aphthous stomatitis
Raynaud's disease, 223
Raynaud's phenomenon (RP), 619–621
RBCs. *See* red blood cells
real-time reverse transcriptase-polymerase chain reaction (RT-qPCR), 266
receptor activator of nuclear factor kappa B ligand (RANKL), 614
rectal bleeding, 273
rectal prolapse, 275
rectal sparing, 252
recurrent aphthous stomatitis (RAS), 149–150
recurrent seizures, risk factors for, 557
red blood cells (RBCs), 329, 365
red hepatization, pneumonia, 175
referred pain, 231
regional lymphadenopathy, 512
regurgitation, 270
Reiter's syndrome, 122
relapsing–remitting multiple sclerosis, 546
renal calculi, 344–347
renal osteodystrophy, 322
repetitive muscle stimulation test, 551
reserpine, 585, 642
respiratory disturbance index (RDI), 173
respiratory guidelines
  acute bronchitis, 160–161
  asthma, 153–157161
  bronchiolitis, 162–160
  chronic obstructive pulmonary disease, 162–165
  common cold, 166–168
  cough, 168–170
  obstructive sleep apnoea, 172–174
  pneumonia, 175–179
  respiratory syncytial virus, 179–181
  shortness of breath, 181–183
  tuberculosis, 183–186
  viral croup, 170–172
  viral pneumonia, 177–179
respiratory syncytial virus (RSV), 162, 179–181
resting tremor, 552
restless legs syndrome (RLS), 554–556
retinopathy, 582
retinopathy screening, 582
return to sport/play, sport participation, 658

Reye's syndrome, 451, 454, 456, 487, 499, 542
rheumatic fever, 469–471
rheumatoid arthritis (RA), 622–625, 627
rheumatoid disease, 114
rheumatological guidelines
  ankylosing spondylitis, 605–607
  fibromyalgia, 607–608
  giant cell arteritis, 628–630
  gout, 609–610
  kyphosis, 612–615
  osteoarthritis, 610—612
  osteoporosis, 612–615
  polymyalgia rheumatica, 615–616
  pseudogout, 616–618
  psoriatic arthritis, 618–619
  Raynaud's phenomenon, 619–621
  Rheumatoid arthritis, 622–625
  systemic lupus erythematosus, 625–627
  temporal arteritis, 628–630
  vertebral fractures, 612–615
  vitamin D deficiency, 630–631
Rhipicephalus sanguineus, 472
RhO (D) immune globulin (RhoGAM), 376, 378
ribivarin (RBV), 285
ribonucleic acid (RNA), 499
Rickettsia rickettsii, 472
rickettsial diseases, 473
rifampin, 185, 186, 442, 461, 462, 630
right lower quadrant (RLQ) pain, 233
right upper quadrant (RUQ) pain, 233, 243
rigidity, 552
rimantadine, 179, 451
ringworm, 96–97
Rinne test, 127, 128, 131, 133, 600
risedronate, 614
risperidone, 32, 640
rituximab, 548, 624
rivaroxaban, 199, 208
rivastigmine, 525
rivastigmine patch, 530
RLS. *See* restless legs syndrome
RMSF. *See* Rocky Mountain spotted fever
RNA. *See* ribonucleic acid
Rocky Mountain spotted fever (RMSF), 472–474
ROM. *See* range of motion
Romberg test, 547, 567
ropinirole, 553, 555
rosacea, 69–70
roseola (exanthem subitum), 474–475
rotating chair test, vertigo, 567
rotavirus, 265, 267
rotavirus vaccine, 259
rotigotine transdermal patch, 555
roundworm, 309, 311–312
Rourke baby record, 5–14
routine prenatal care, 363–364
Roux-en-Y gastric bypass (RYGB), 35–38
RP. *See* Raynaud's phenomenon
RPR. *See* rapid plasma reagin
RSV. *See* respiratory syncytial virus
rubber band ligation, 274
rubella (German measles), 475–477
rubella vaccination, 384
rubeola (red measles), 477–480
Rubulavirus, 465
ruptured ectopic pregnancy, 233

sacroiliac (SI) joints, 605, 606
salbutemol, 86
salicylate, 132
saline spray, 136
Salmonella, 265, 267
sarcoidosis, 117
Sarcoptes scabiei, 93

scabies, 93–94
scarlet fever (Scarlatina), 480–482
SCC. *See* squamous cell carcinoma
SCD. *See* sudden cardiac death
sciatica, 519–520
scopolamine, 305
sebaceous hyperplasia, 74
seborrhoeic blepharitis, 95–96
seborrhoeic dermatitis, 95–96
seborrhoeic keratosis, 74
sebum, 70
secondary amenorrhoea, 389, 390
secondary dysmenorrhoea, 402
secondary engorgement, 378
secondary postpartum haemorrhage, 381–382
secondary progressive multiple sclerosis, 546
secondary Raynaud's phenomenon, 620
second-line therapy, 328, 553
secretory proteinuria, 339
sedating antihistamines, 651
sedative anxiolytic hypnotics, 648
sedatives, 245
seizure, 370, 556–560
selective oestrogen receptor modulator (SORM), 614
selective serotonin reuptake inhibitors (SSRIs), 63, 385, 525, 534, 549, 634, 643
selective serotonin-norepinephrine reuptake inhibitors (SSNRIs), 549
selenium deficiency, 37
selenium sulphide, 98
selenium toxicity, 37
self-monitoring blood glucose (SMBG), 368, 577
sensorineural hearing loss, 127
septic thrombophlebitis, 225
serologic tests for hepatitis, 264
serotonin norepinephrine reuptake inhibitors (SNRIs), 634
Serratia, 373
sertraline, 385, 634
serum blood testing, 533
serum glucose levels, 547
serum progesterone, 414
serum testosterone, 328, 587, 589
serum vitamin B12, pernicious anaemia, 513
severe persistent, asthma, 153
sexual abuse, 49, 52, 56
sexual activity, pelvic inflammatory disease, 421
sexual dysfunction, 165, 410
Sexual Health Inventory for Men (SHIM), 325
sexual intercourse, 376, 394, 404, 405, 431
sexual maturity stages, 677
sexually transmitted agents, 419
sexually transmitted diseases (STDs), 361
sexually transmitted infections (STI), 111, 317, 323, 424, 429, 434
sexually transmitted infections guidelines
  chlamydia, 430–431
  general approach to sexually transmitted infections, 429–430
  gonorrhoea, 431–433
  herpes simplex virus type 2, 433–434
  human papillomavirus, 434–436
  syphilis, 436–438
  trichomoniasis, 438–439
Shigella, 265, 267
shingles, 83–84, 485
short-acting benzodiazepines, 634
shortness of breath (SOB), 181–183, 207
short-term insomnia, 649
SI joints. *See* sacroiliac joints
SIG-E-CAPS tool, 642

sigmoidoscopy, 274
  colorectal cancer screening, 246
  Crohn's disease, 252
  gastroenteritis, 266
sildenafil, 318, 328, 621
silodosin, 318
simethicone, 245
simple partial seizures (SPSs), 556
simple seizures, 561
sinus bradycardia, 191–193
sinus tachycardia, 191–193
sinuses, 140
sinusitis, 117, 536
Sjögren's syndrome, 114, 115, 620, 623
SJS. *See* Stevens–Johnson syndrome
skeletal muscle pain, 61, 63
skin biopsy, 252
skin cancer, 90
skip lesions, 252
SLE. *See* systemic lupus erythematosus
sleep disorders, 553, 649–652
sleep paralysis, 651
sliding hernias, 288
slit-lamp examination, 119, 122
small-bowel obstruction, 304
SMBG. *See* self-monitoring blood glucose
smoking, 169, 362
SNRIs. *See* serotonin norepinephrine reuptake inhibitors
SOB. *See* shortness of breath
social work (SW) referrals, 549
Society of Obstetricians and Gynaecologists of Canada (SOGC), 361, 363
sodium bicarbonate, 270
sodium valproate, 32, 560
SOGC. *See* Society of Obstetricians and Gynaecologists of Canada
soiltransmitted helminthes, 292
solar lentigines, 74
solifenacin, 352
somatic nociceptive pain, 61
somatoform disorders, 634, 648
sotalol, 199
space-occupying lesion, 536
spasmodic croup, 170
speech therapy (ST), 549, 553
spermatocele, 332
spermicide, 399–401, 422
SPF. *See* sun protection factor
sphenoid sinusitis, 141
spiramycin, 484
spirometry, 154, 163
spironolactone, 71, 216, 587, 594
splenectomy, 506
spontaneous miscarriage, 374, 376
sport nutrition, 657
sport participation
  assessment guide for, 655–658
  clearance for, 656
  female athlete triad, 658
  female fitness, 658
  and mental health, 657
  performance-enhancing substances, 657–658
  preventive care and injury prevention, 656
  respiratory considerations, 656
  return to sport/play, 658
  sport nutrition, 657
  stigma of mental illness, 657
  substance abuse, 656
sprains: ankle and knee, 520–522
squamous cell abnormalities, 419
squamous cell carcinoma (SCC), 73, 90
squamous metaplasia, 419
SSRIs. *See* selective serotonin reuptake inhibitors
Staphylococci, 355

Staphylococcus, 72, 81, 108, 113, 129, 380, 387, 481
Staphylococcus aureus, 72, 78, 84, 103, 108, 119, 140, 175, 177, 382
Staphylococcus epidermis, 72
Staphylococcus saprophyticus, 342, 355
stapled haemorrhoidopexy, 274
statin therapy, 196, 215, 580
stavudine, 599
Stein–Leventhal syndrome, 592
stem cell transplantation, 549
sterile speculum examination
 first trimester, 375
 preterm labour, 371
sterilization, 400
steroid sprays, 136, 142
steroids, 548, 551, 568
Stevens–Johnson syndrome (SJS), 79, 559
stigma of mental illness, in sport, 657
stimulant laxatives, 249, 250, 297
STIs. *See* sexually transmitted infections
stomatitis, 82, 148, 149–150
stool softeners, 549
strabismic amblyopia, 107
strabismus, 120–121
Streptobacillus moniliformis, 72
Streptococcus, 72, 113, 129, 148, 387
Streptococcus aureus, 110
Streptococcus pneumoniae, 110, 125, 145, 175, 459, 460, 461
Streptococcus pyogenes, 84, 145, 469, 480
Streptococcus viridans, 379
stress incontinence, 350
structural factors, 29
Student-Athlete Mental Health Initiative (SAMHI), 657
subacute neck pain, 515
subacute sinusitis, 139
subacute thyroiditis, 595, 599, 600
subconjunctival haemorrhage, 121–122
subcutaneous nodules, 469
subdural haematomas (SDH), 538
subjective, objective, assessment, and plan (SOAP), 5
subjective premature ejaculation, 335
substance abuse, 41, 656
substance dependence, 41
substance use disorders, 41–48
 commonly abused drugs, 43–45
 drug addiction treatment, 42
substance withdrawal, 41
sucralfate, 150, 601
sudden cardiac death (SCD), 655
sudden infant death syndrome (SIDS), 48
suicidal or homicidal thoughts, 638
suicide, 652–654
sulfacetamide, 111
sulfamethoxazole, 431
sulfamethoxazole-trimethoprim, 261
sulfas, 132
sulfonamides, 126
sulfonylureas, 32
sulindac, 617
sulphadiazine, 471, 484
sulphasalazine, 253, 255, 619, 624
sulphonamides, 79
sumatriptan, 537, 542, 621
sun protection factor (SPF), 147
superficial thrombophlebitis, 225–227
supraventricular tachydysrhythmias (SVTs), 191
surgical weight loss procedures, 35
swollen lymph glands, 441
sydenham chorea, 469
symptomatic febrile seizure, 561
syncope, 227–230
syncope episodes, 655

syndemic, 29
syndrome X, 590
syphilis, 436–438
system factors, 29
systemic disease, 114
systemic disorders guidelines
 chronic fatigue syndrome, 495–497
 fevers of unknown origin, 497–499
 human immunodeficiency virus, 499–503
 idiopathic thrombocytopaenic purpura, 504–506
 iron-deficiency anaemia, 506–509
 lymphadenopathy, 509–512
 pernicious anaemia, 512–514
systemic exertion intolerance syndrome. *See* chronic fatigue syndrome
systemic lupus erythematosus (SLE), 625–627
Systemic Lupus Erythematosus International Collaborating Clinics (SLICC), 626
systolic blood pressure (SBP), 213
systolic murmurs, 219–220

tachycardia, 191, 192, 232, 455
tachypnoea, 176, 178
tadalafil, 319
tamoxifen, 207, 586
tamsulosin, 318, 319, 549
Tanner's sexual maturity stages, 677
Tay–Sachs disease, 361
TB. *See* tuberculosis
TCAs. *See* tricyclic antidepressants
temazepam, 648, 651
temporal arteritis, 537, 628–630
temporomandibular joint syndrome, 132
tendinitis, 521
tension headaches, 534, 538
terazosin, 318, 549
terbinafine, 97
terbutaline, 372
terbutaline sulphate, 378
terconazole, 426
terconazole vaginal antifungal cream, 426
teriflunomide, 548
teriparatide, 614
testicular torsion, 347–348
testicular tumours, 332
testosterone, 326, 327, 328, 410, 586, 588, 589
tetracycline, 70, 71, 108, 109, 144, 343, 357, 437, 438, 473, 474, 482
thalidomide, 599
theophylline, 155, 157, 165, 212
thiamine (B1) deficiency, 36
thiazide diuretics, 580
thiazolidinediones, 32
thiopurine methyltransferase (TPMT) testing, 253
third trimester, 365, 366
threatened miscarriage, 374, 376
throat and mouth guidelines
 avulsed tooth, 143
 dental abscess, 144
 epiglottitis, 145
 minor recurrent aphthous stomatitis, 149–150
 oral cancer, 146–147
 pharyngitis, 147–149
 stomatitis, 149–150
 thrush, 150–151
thromboangiitis obliterans, 223
thrombocytopaenia, 505
thrombopoietin receptor agonists, 506
thrush, 150–151
thumbprinting, 252
thymectomy, 551
thyroid disease

hyperthyroidism, 595–598
hypothyroidism, 598–602
thyroid function tests, 530
thyroid studies, 638
thyroidectomy, 597
thyroid-stimulating hormone (TSH), 222, 229, 327, 583, 595, 596, 600–601
thyrotoxicosis/thyroid storm, 602–603
thyrotropin-releasing hormone (TRH), 595
thyroxine (T4), 596
TIA. *See* transient ischaemic attacks
tick-borne diseases, 447
ticlopidine, 309, 564
timolol, 199
tincture of opium, 253
tinea capitis, 96, 97
tinea corporis, 96–97
tinea cruris, 96
tinea pedis, 96
tinea unguium, 96
tinea versicolour, 97–98
Tinel's test, 528
tinidazole, 272
tinnitus, 132–133
tissue transglutaminase (tTG), 238
TMJ syndrome, 537
TNF. *See* tumour necrosis factor
tobacco (smoking) cessation, 164
tobradex ophthalmic, 110
tobramycin, 113
tocilizumab, 624
tocolytics, 372
tolterodine, 352, 549
tongue-retaining devices (TRDs), 174
tonic–clonic seizure, 556
tonometer, 118
topical cream, 63, 274, 587, 612
topical therapy, 130
topiramate, 541, 542, 560
Torulopsis glabrata, 425
total parenteral nutrition (TPN), 253
toxic multinodular goiter, 595
toxicities, 36
Toxoplasma gondii, 482, 483, 484
toxoplasmosis, 482–485
tracheostomy, 174
tramadol, 608
tranquilizers, 55
transdermal replacement therapy, 418
transient ischaemic attacks (TIA), 563–565
transvaginal replacement therapy, 418
transverse myelitis (TM) lesions, 547
trauma, 233–234
trazodone hydrochloride, 649, 651
tremor, 552
Treponema pallidum, 323, 436, 437, 626
treponemal, 437
treponemal pallidum particle agglutination (TP-PA), 437
triamcinolone, 89, 93, 105, 150, 405, 617
triamcinolone acetonide, 77, 78, 136
triceps reflex tests, 516
trichloroacetic acid (TCA), 435
Trichomonas vaginalis, 336, 393, 397, 438
trichomoniasis, 438–439
Trichophyton, 96
Trichuris trichiura, 311
tricuspid regurgitation, 219–220
tricuspid stenosis, 220
tricuspid valve prolapse, 220
tricyclic antidepressants (TCAs), 61, 114, 525, 533, 545, 568
trifluridine, 112
trigeminal ganglia, 82
trigeminal neuralgia, 537
trigger point location, 607

triglyceride, 194
triiodothyronine (T3), 596
trimethoprim, 111, 126, 357
trimethoprim-sulfamethoxazole (TMP/SMZ), 257, 383, 442, 443, 484, 502
triple therapy, 199
triptans, 540, 545
trivalent inactivated influenza vaccines (TIV), 450, 453
trospium, 352
TSH. *See* thyroid-stimulating hormone
tuberculin skin test, tuberculosis, 185
tuberculosis (TB), 183–186, 571
tubular proteinuria, 339
tumour necrosis factor (TNF), 619, 624
tumour necrosis factor (TNF)-alpha blocker, 255
tympanic membrane, 127, 128, 133
tympanogram, 125
type 1 diabetes, 574, 575
type I hypersensitivity, 149
type IV hypersensitivity, 149

UC. *See* ulcerative colitis
UI. *See* urinary incontinence
ulcerative colitis (UC), 312–316
    medications for, 254
    stepwise management of, 315
    topical agents, 315
    treatment algorithm, 316
ulcerative proctitis, 313
ultraviolet B (UVB) light therapy, 81
umbilical hernia, 286
undescended testicles, 349
universal carrier screening, 361
unspecified bipolar and related disorder, 637
unstageable pressure injury, 102
upper respiratory infection (URI), 132, 145, 481
upper respiratory tract infection (URTI), 166
Ureaplasma, 336, 338, 397, 420
urge incontinence, 350
URI. *See* upper respiratory infection
uric acid, 609, 610
urinalysis, 330, 553
urinary incontinence (UI), 350–354
urinary tract infection (UTI), 234, 332, 341, 350, 354–358, 372, 373, 548
urolithiasis, 344, 346
urology for genitourinary, 549
uterine dehiscence, 376
uterine rupture, 376, 377
UTI. *See* urinary tract infection

uveal tract, 117
uveitis, 122–123

vaccinations, 155
vaginal antifungal creams, 426
vaginal bleeding, 374–378
    first trimester, 374–376
    second trimesters, 376–378
    third trimesters, 376–378
vaginal hormonal therapy, 392
vaginal sponge, 400
vaginismus, 404
vagus nerve stimulator (VNS), 560
valacyclovir, 83, 84, 112, 434
valproic acid, 471, 593, 639
vancomycin, 383, 461
varenalcine, 164
varenicline, substance use disorders, 47
variable premature ejaculation, 335
varicella (chickenpox and shingles), 485–488
varicella zoster, 83
varicella-zoster immune globulin, 179
varicella-zoster immune globulin (VZIG), 487
varicella-zoster virus (VZV), 443, 485
varicocele, 332, 358–359
varicose veins, 205–207
vascular congestion, pneumonia, 175
vascular dementia, 528
vascular disease, 320
vascular ulcer, 99, 100
vasomotor rhinitis, 139
venlafaxine, 418, 582, 634
venous ligation surgery, 328
venous ulcer, 99, 100
verapamil, 192, 199, 537
verruca filiformis, 99
verruca plana, 99
verruca plantaris, 99
verruca vulgaris, 99
verruga peruana, 441
vertebral fractures, 612–614
vertigo, 565–569
very-low-density lipoprotein (VLDL), 194
vestibular migraines, 568
Vincent's angina, 148
violence
    children, 49–52
    intimate partner violence, 52–55
    older adults, 55–56
viral capsid antigen (VCA), 464
viral croup, 170–172
viral culture, 433
viral pneumonia, 177–179
Virchow's triad, 207

visceral nociceptive pain, 61
visceral pain, 231
vitamin A, 479
vitamin B12, 39, 40, 253, 513, 530
    deficiency, 36, 37
vitamin D, 253, 416, 560, 574, 614, 630
    deficiency, 36, 37, 630–631
vitamin D–enriched foods, 675
vitamin K foods, 670–671
vitamins, 424, 600
    deficiencies, 36, 555
vomiting, nausea, 303–306
vulvodynia, 405
vulvovaginal candidiasis, 425–427
VZIG. *See* Varicella-zoster immune globulin
VZV. *See* Varicella-zoster virus

warfarin, 142, 193, 199, 200, 208, 221, 227, 309, 560, 670–671
warts, 98–99
Weber test, 127, 128
weight loss, 256, 269
West Nile virus (WNV), 446, 449, 488–490
Westley scoring for croup, 171
winter itch. *See* xerosis
withdrawal, contraception, 401
WNV. *See* West Nile virus
Wolff–Parkinson–White (WPW), 191
Wood's lamp, 98
wound
    bed, 100, 102
    infection, 387–388
    of skin, 103–105
wound care
    lower extremity ulcer, 99–101
    pressure ulcers, 99–103
wrists, 516

xerosis, 105
X-ray
    neck and upper back disorders, 516
    plantar fasciitis, 518
xylometazoline, 142

Yeoman Guying, 66

zanamivir, 179, 450, 451, 453, 454
Zika virus infection, 490–492
zinc deficiency, 36
ziprasidone, 640
zoledronic acid, 614
Zollinger–Ellison syndrome, 307, 309
zolpidem, 648, 651
zopiclone, 648, 651

www.ingramcontent.com/pod-product-compliance
Ingram Content Group UK Ltd.
Pitfield, Milton Keynes, MK11 3LW, UK
UKHW062230220426
53491PUK00005B/82